THIRD EDITION

DIAGNOSTIC PATHOLOGY

INFECTIOUS DISEASES

SOLOMON ▪ MILNER

LAGA ▪ CROTHERS ▪ PECORA ▪ ABEDALTHAGAFI ▪ WEISS

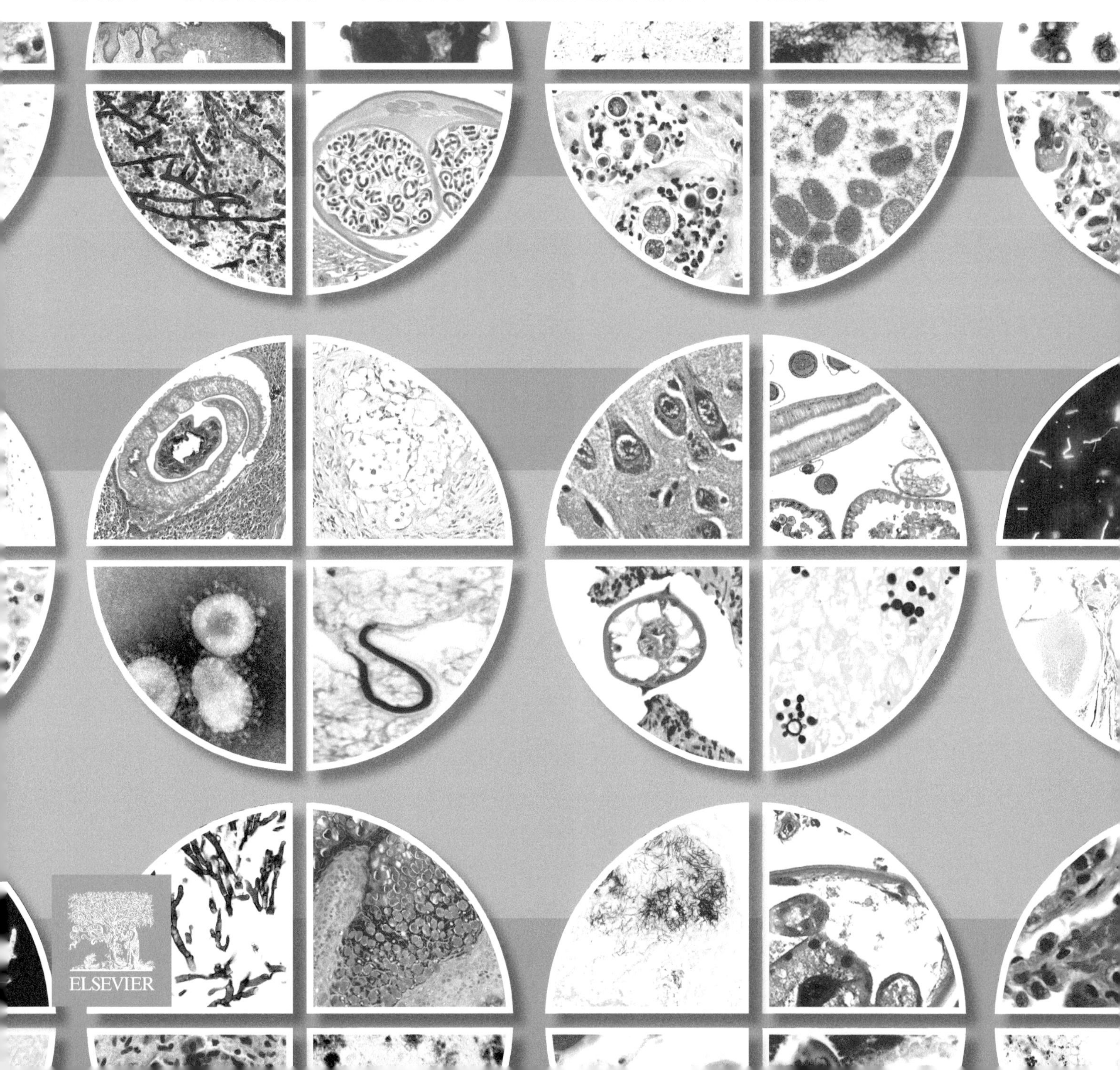

DIAGNOSTIC PATHOLOGY
INFECTIOUS DISEASES

THIRD EDITION

ISAAC H. SOLOMON, MD, PhD
Neuropathologist and Infectious Disease Pathology Consultant
Department of Pathology
Brigham and Women's Hospital
Assistant Professor of Pathology
Harvard Medical School
Boston, Massachusetts

DAN MILNER, MD, MSc(Epi), MBA
Consultant Pathologist, Executive Director, and Medical Director
Libragem Consulting, LLC
Palm Springs, California
Adjunct Professor
Department of Immunology and Infectious Diseases
Harvard T.H. Chan School of Public Health
Boston, Massachusetts

Alvaro C. Laga, MD, MMSc
Dermatopathologist and Infectious Disease Pathology Consultant
Department of Pathology
Brigham and Women's Hospital
Associate Professor of Pathology
Harvard Medical School
Boston, Massachusetts

Jessica Crothers, MD
Assistant Professor
Associate Director of Clinical Microbiology
Department of Pathology and Laboratory Medicine
Larner College of Medicine at the University of Vermont
Burlington, Vermont

Nicole Pecora, MD, PhD
Associate Director of Clinical Microbiology
Brigham and Women's Hospital
Assistant Professor of Pathology
Harvard Medical School
Boston, Massachusetts

Malak Abedalthagafi, MD, MBA
Professor
Director of Neuropathology
Department of Pathology and Laboratory Medicine
Emory University School of Medicine
Atlanta, Georgia

Zoe Freeman Weiss, MD
Assistant Professor
Division of Geographic Medicine and Infectious Diseases
Assistant Professor
Department of Pathology
Assistant Medical Director of Clinical Microbiology
Tufts Medical Center
Boston, Massachusetts

ADDITIONAL CONTRIBUTORS

Leigh Compton, MD
Brian J. Hall, MD
Lenette Lu, MD, PhD
Eleanor Russell-Goldman, MD, PhD
T. Rinda Soong, MD, PhD, MPH
Shira Winters, MD

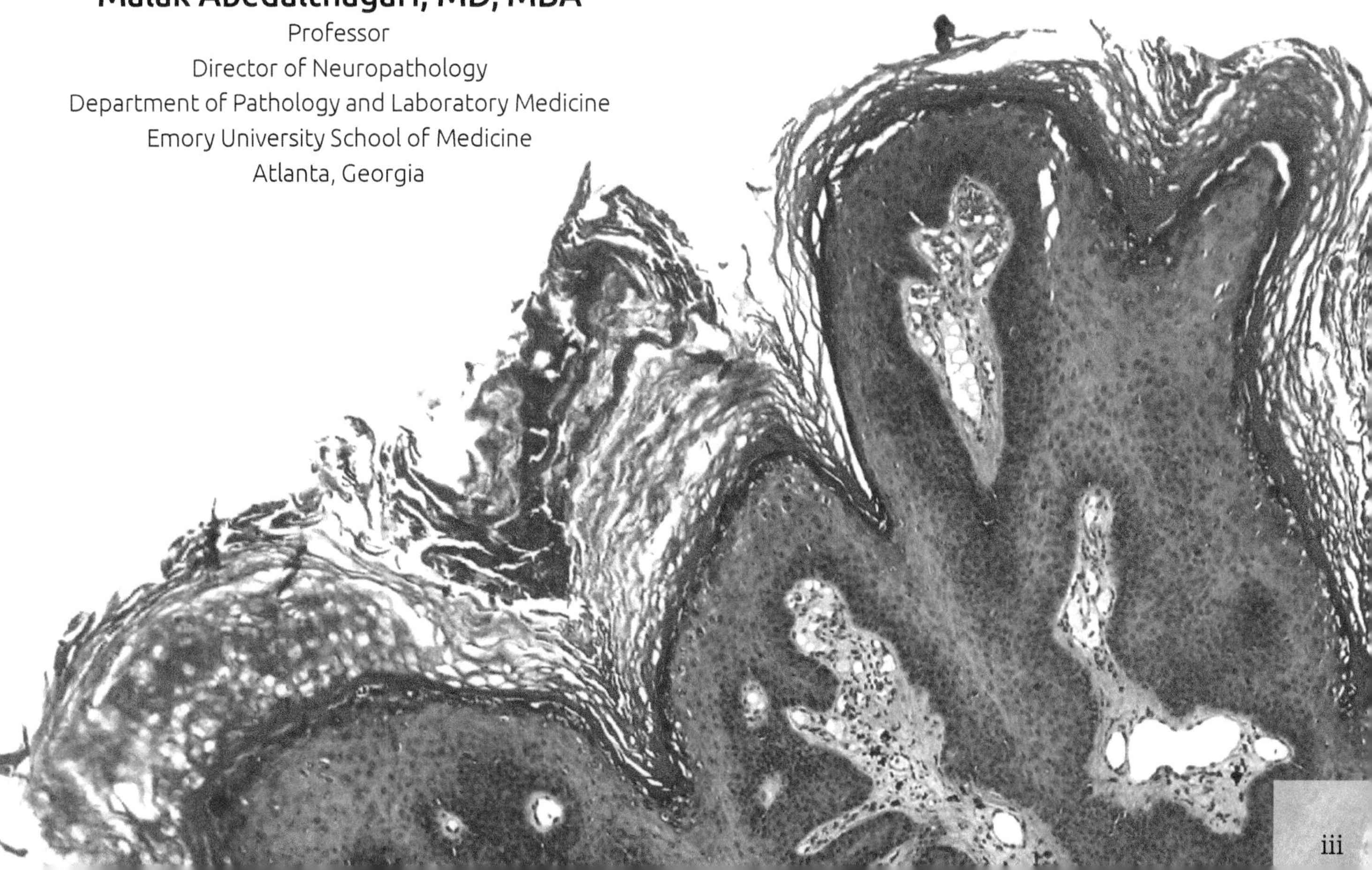

Elsevier
1600 John F. Kennedy Blvd.
Ste 1800
Philadelphia, PA 19103-2899

DIAGNOSTIC PATHOLOGY: INFECTIOUS DISEASES, THIRD EDITION ISBN: 978-0-443-12477-8

Copyright © 2024 by Elsevier. All rights reserved.

No part of this publication may be reproduced or transmitted in any form or by any means, electronic or mechanical, including photocopying, recording, or any information storage and retrieval system, without permission in writing from the publisher. Details on how to seek permission, further information about the Publisher's permissions policies and our arrangements with organizations such as the Copyright Clearance Center and the Copyright Licensing Agency, can be found at our website: www.elsevier.com/permissions.

This book and the individual contributions contained in it are protected under copyright by the Publisher (other than as may be noted herein).

Notices

Practitioners and researchers must always rely on their own experience and knowledge in evaluating and using any information, methods, compounds or experiments described herein. Because of rapid advances in the medical sciences, in particular, independent verification of diagnoses and drug dosages should be made. To the fullest extent of the law, no responsibility is assumed by Elsevier, authors, editors or contributors for any injury and/or damage to persons or property as a matter of products liability, negligence or otherwise, or from any use or operation of any methods, products, instructions, or ideas contained in the material herein.

Previous edition copyrighted 2020.

Library of Congress Control Number: 2023949823

Printed in Great Britain

Last digit is the print number: 9 8 7 6 5 4 3 2

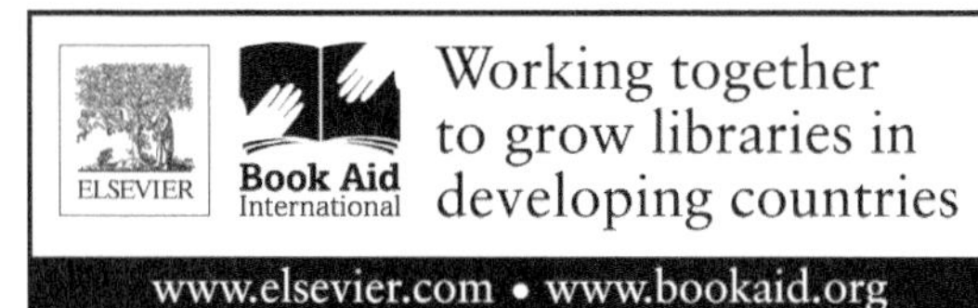

DEDICATION

To KDS, EHS, LKS, and DJS.

IHS

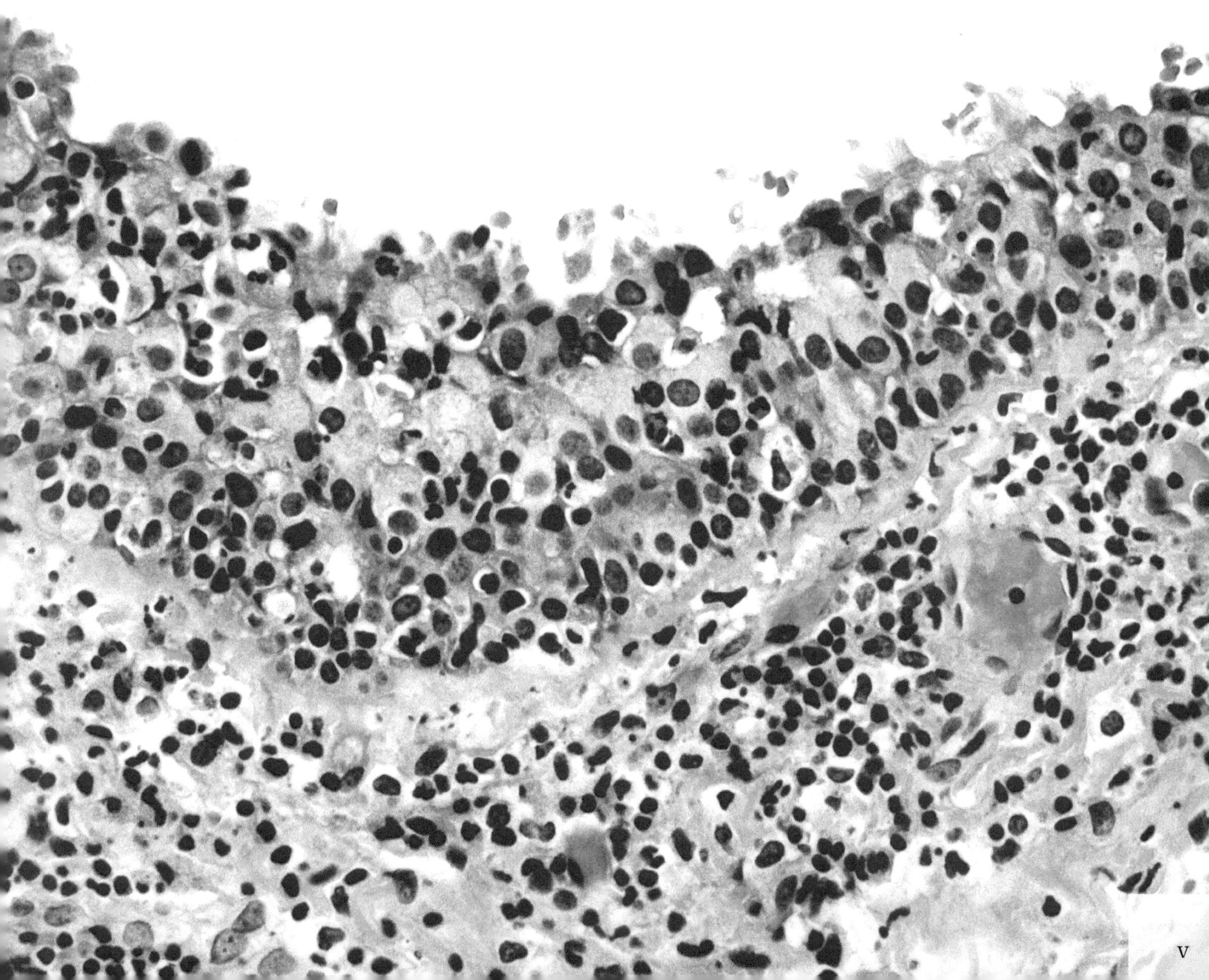

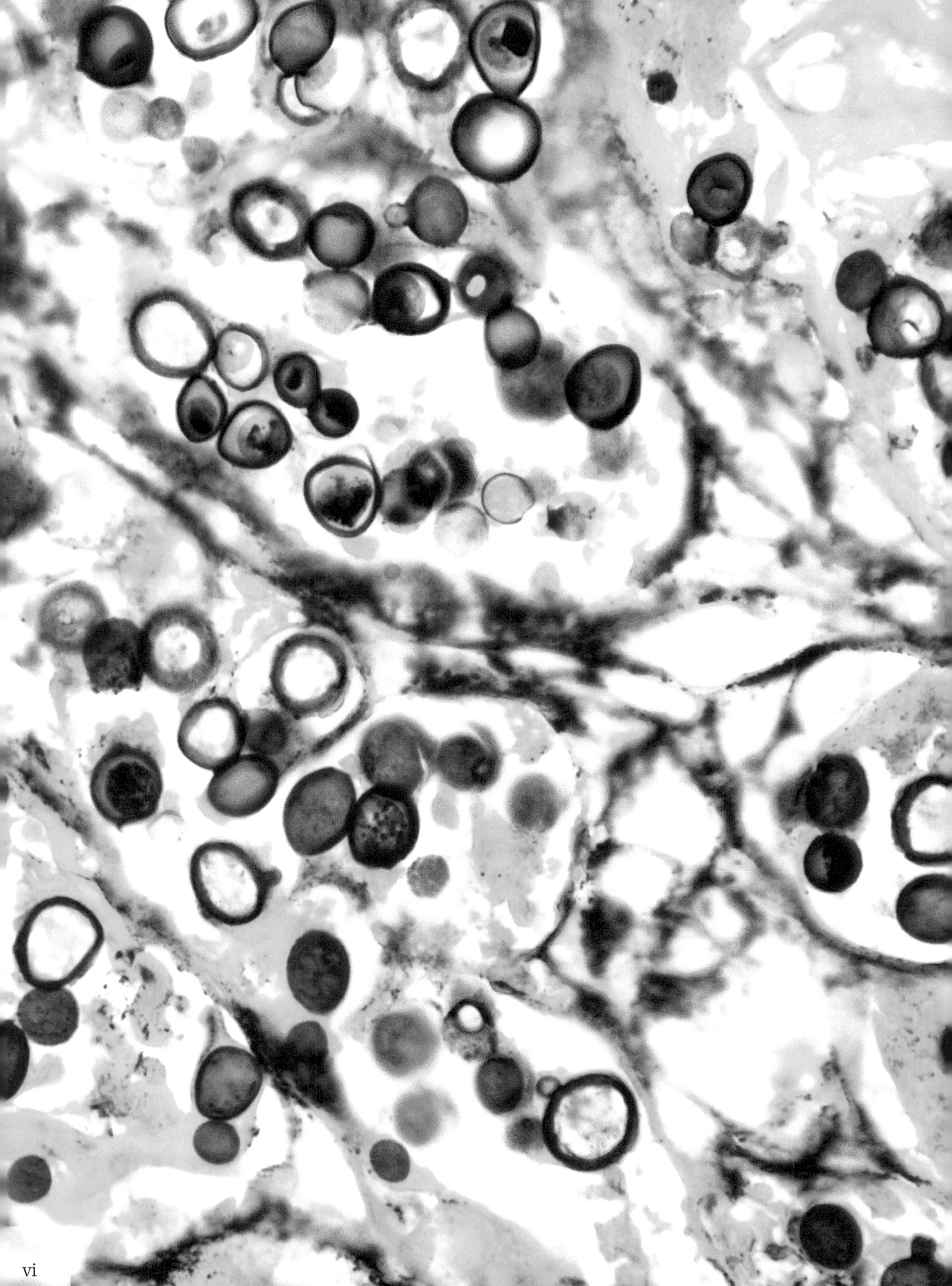

PREFACE

It would be an understatement to say that the world is a different place now than it was in 2019 when the second edition of this book was published. COVID-19 has demonstrated the need for rapid and accurate infectious disease diagnostic testing. PCR, cycle thresholds, and rapid antigen tests, all long-established terms, have now entered common vernacular. The international scientific community as a whole, albeit temporarily, came together in pursuit of a single goal: To save as many lives as possible from this highly contagious virus. Other infections, including monkeypox, now mpox, have also reemerged on a global level. At the same time, increasing use of sequencing and mass spectrometry has led to increased accuracy and precision in the identification of microorganisms, allowing for more targeted therapies.

This third edition seeks to build on the practical knowledge in the first two editions by expanding or adding new chapters on emerging or uncommon infections and illustrating more examples of common entities with less common presentations. In contrast to other textbooks organized by organ system, this book focuses on individual organisms, minimizing the potential for redundancy and allowing the reader to observe similarities across tissue types that may be outside of their particular subspecialty. This is especially helpful for infections that rarely disseminate from their primary sites of infection but are becoming more common in an era of increased iatrogenic immunosuppression. As much as possible, we have included microbiology laboratory findings (e.g., ova identified in stool preparations) for direct comparison to tissue sections to highlight both similarities and differences.

New readers of this book will find it very useful regardless of their comfort level with infectious diseases, and I believe our seasoned readers will greatly appreciate the additions we have made as well as the aspects we have kept consistent. Ancillary testing recommendations and focused differential diagnoses will help confirm a suspected infection or lead to a more likely alternative.

We wish to thank all our colleagues who contributed cases or images to this textbook, including those at Brigham and Women's Hospital and around the world. We are also appreciative of the direct and indirect contributions of the late Sherif Zaki, MD, PhD, in his role as chief of the Infectious Diseases Pathology Branch of the Centers for Disease Control and Prevention.

All my coauthors and I hope that you enjoy using this book as much as we enjoyed putting this edition together. As with the last edition, if you find something we missed or any errors (in print or online), please let us know, and we will correct them and update our material.

Isaac H. Solomon, MD, PhD
Neuropathologist and Infectious Disease Pathology Consultant
Department of Pathology
Brigham and Women's Hospital
Assistant Professor of Pathology
Harvard Medical School
Boston, Massachusetts

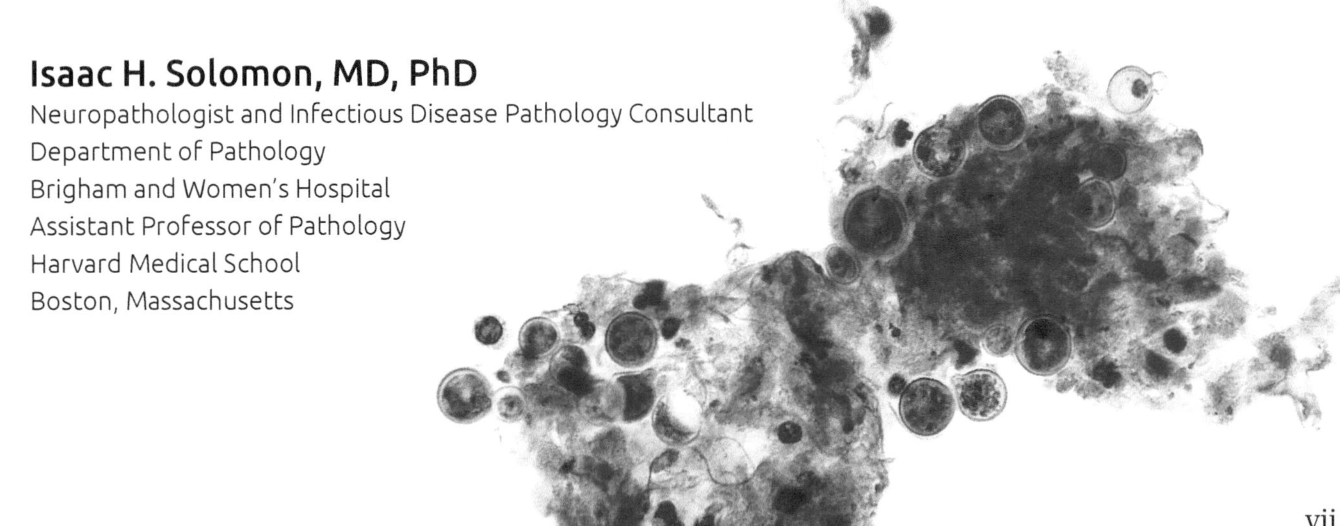

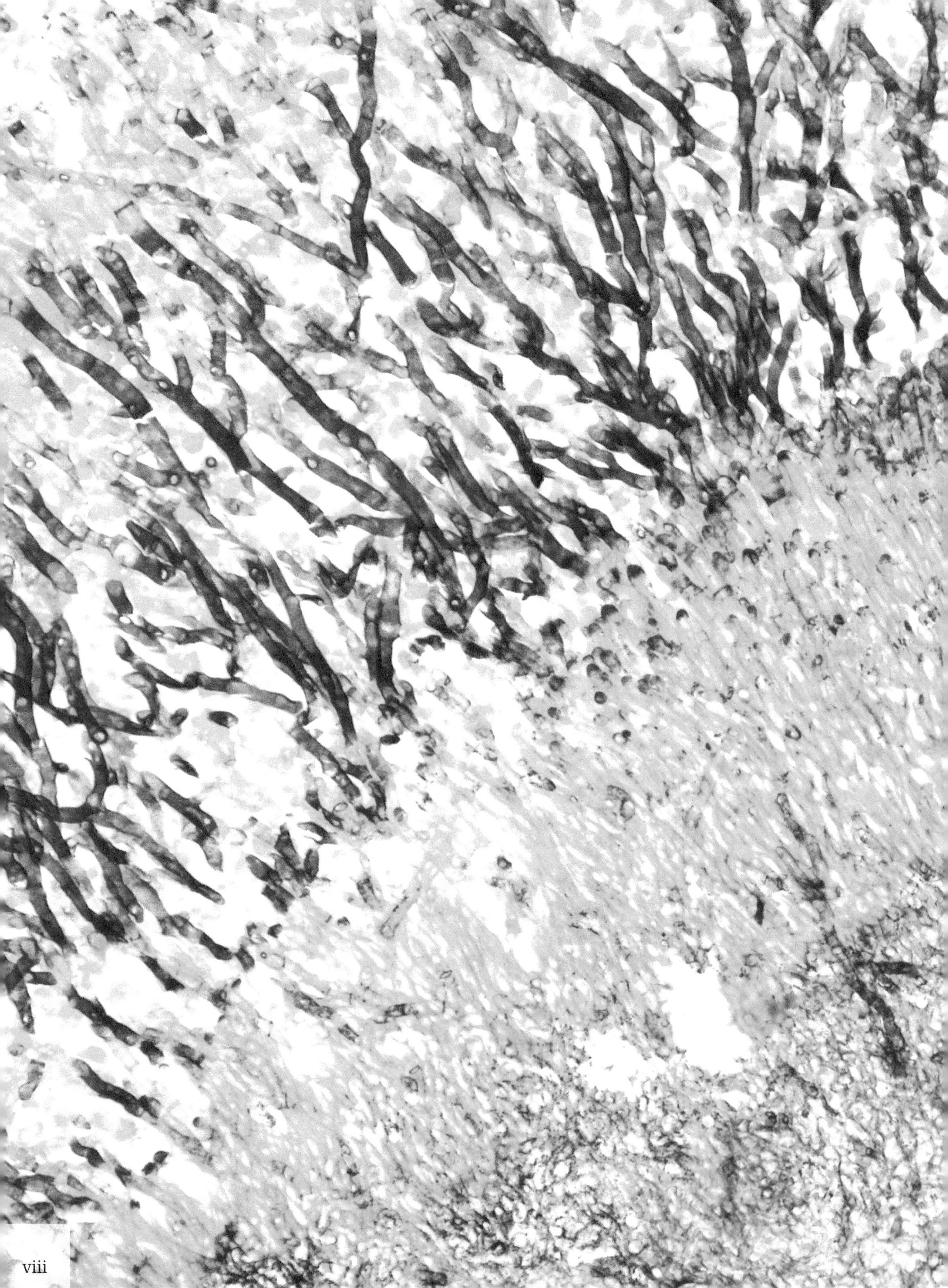

ACKNOWLEDGMENTS

LEAD EDITOR

Terry W. Ferrell, MS

LEAD ILLUSTRATOR

Lane R. Bennion, MS

TEXT EDITORS

Arthur G. Gelsinger, MA
Rebecca L. Bluth, BA
Nina Themann, BA
Megg Morin, BA
Kathryn Watkins, BA
Shannon Kelly, MA

ILLUSTRATIONS

Richard Coombs, MS
Laura C. Wissler, MA

IMAGE EDITORS

Jeffrey J. Marmorstone, BS
Lisa A. M. Steadman, BS

ART DIRECTION AND DESIGN

Cindy Lin, BFA

PRODUCTION EDITORS

Emily C. Fassett, BA
John Pecorelli, BS

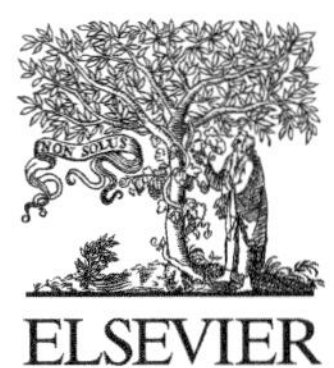

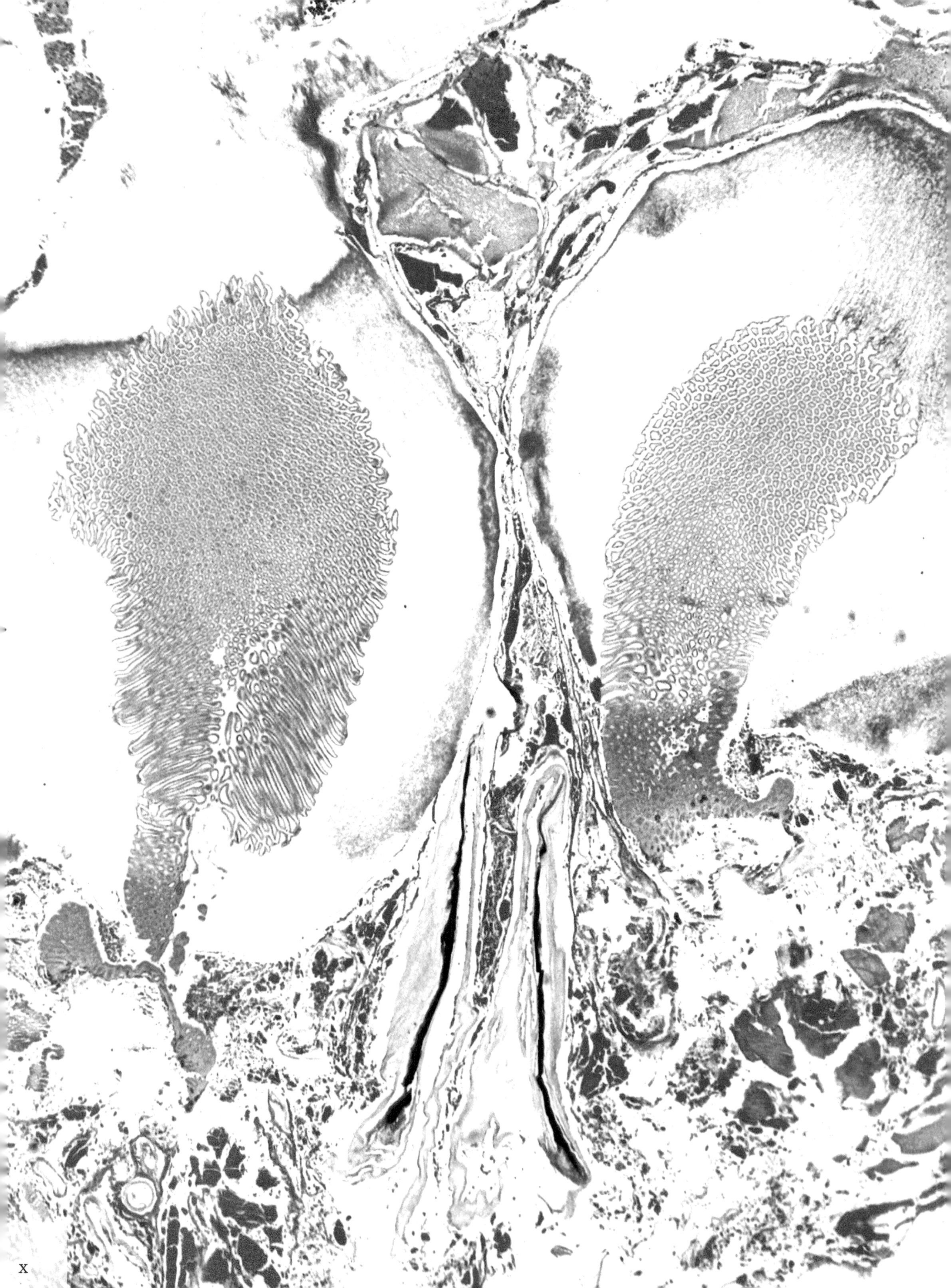
x

SECTIONS

TABLE OF CONTENTS

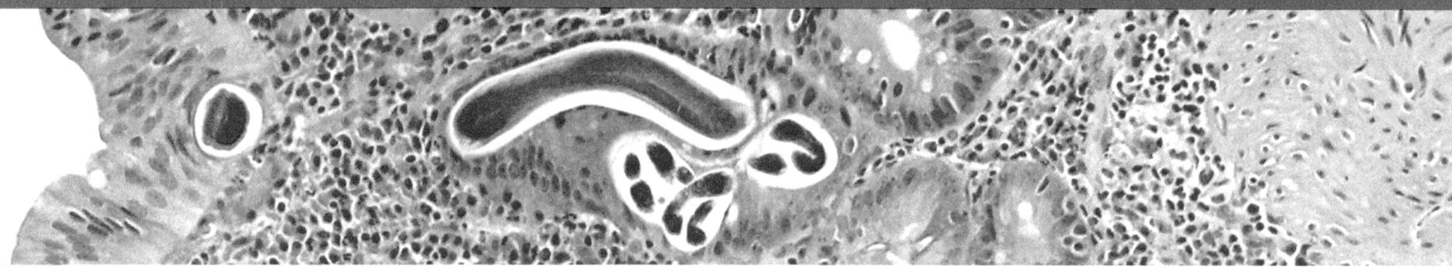

SECTION 1: OVERVIEW

SECTION 2: VIRAL INFECTIONS

DNA VIRUSES

RNA VIRUSES

TABLE OF CONTENTS

TABLE OF CONTENTS

TABLE OF CONTENTS

DEEP TISSUE PROTOZOA

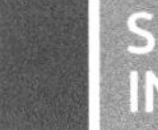

SECTION 7: HELMINTHIC PARASITIC INFECTIONS

NEMATODES

TREMATODES

CESTODES

SECTION 8: INFESTATIONS AND OTHER INVERTEBRATE-RELATED MALADIES

THIRD EDITION

DIAGNOSTIC PATHOLOGY
INFECTIOUS DISEASES

SOLOMON ▪ MILNER

LAGA ▪ CROTHERS ▪ PECORA ▪ ABEDALTHAGAFI ▪ WEISS

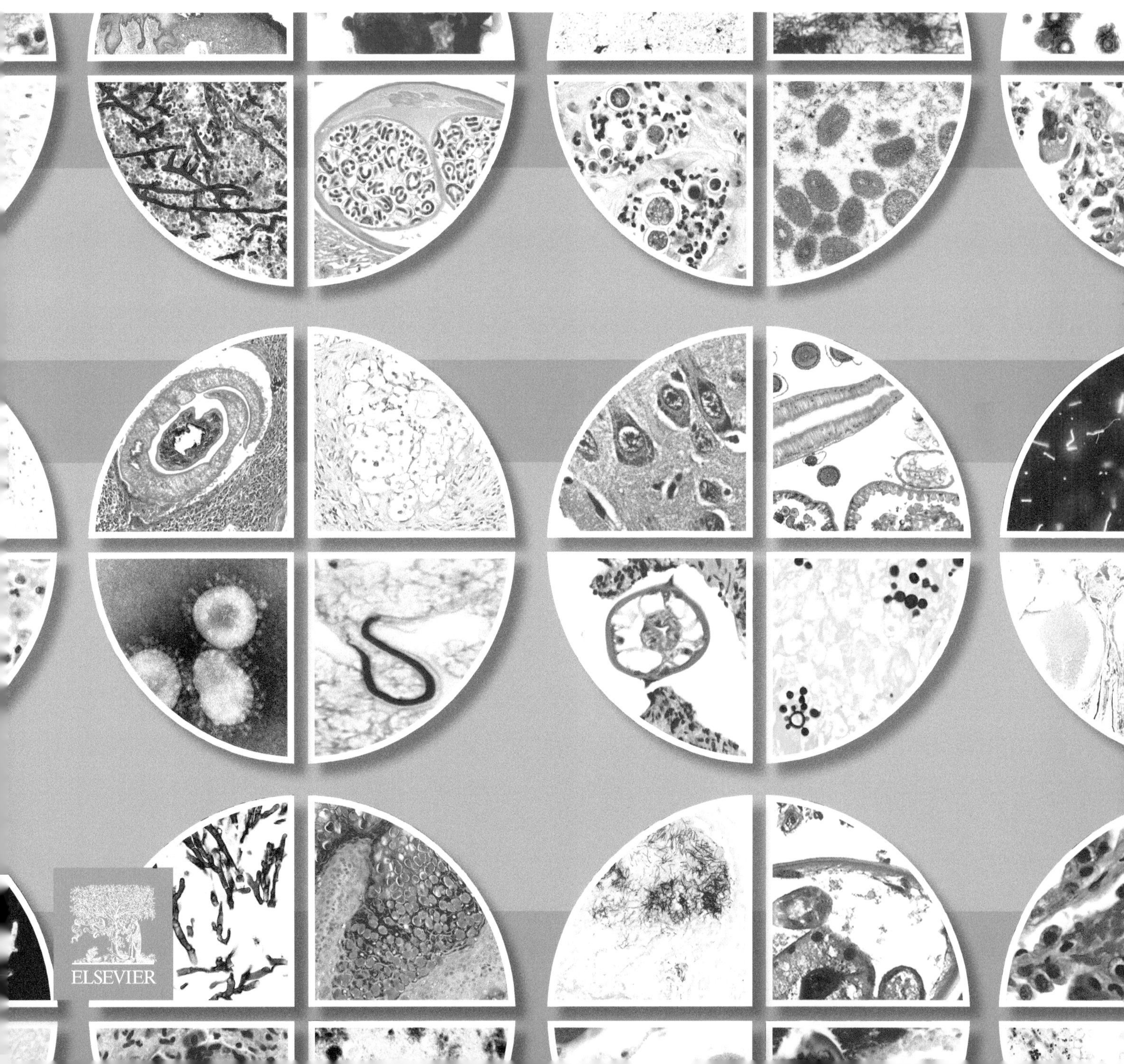

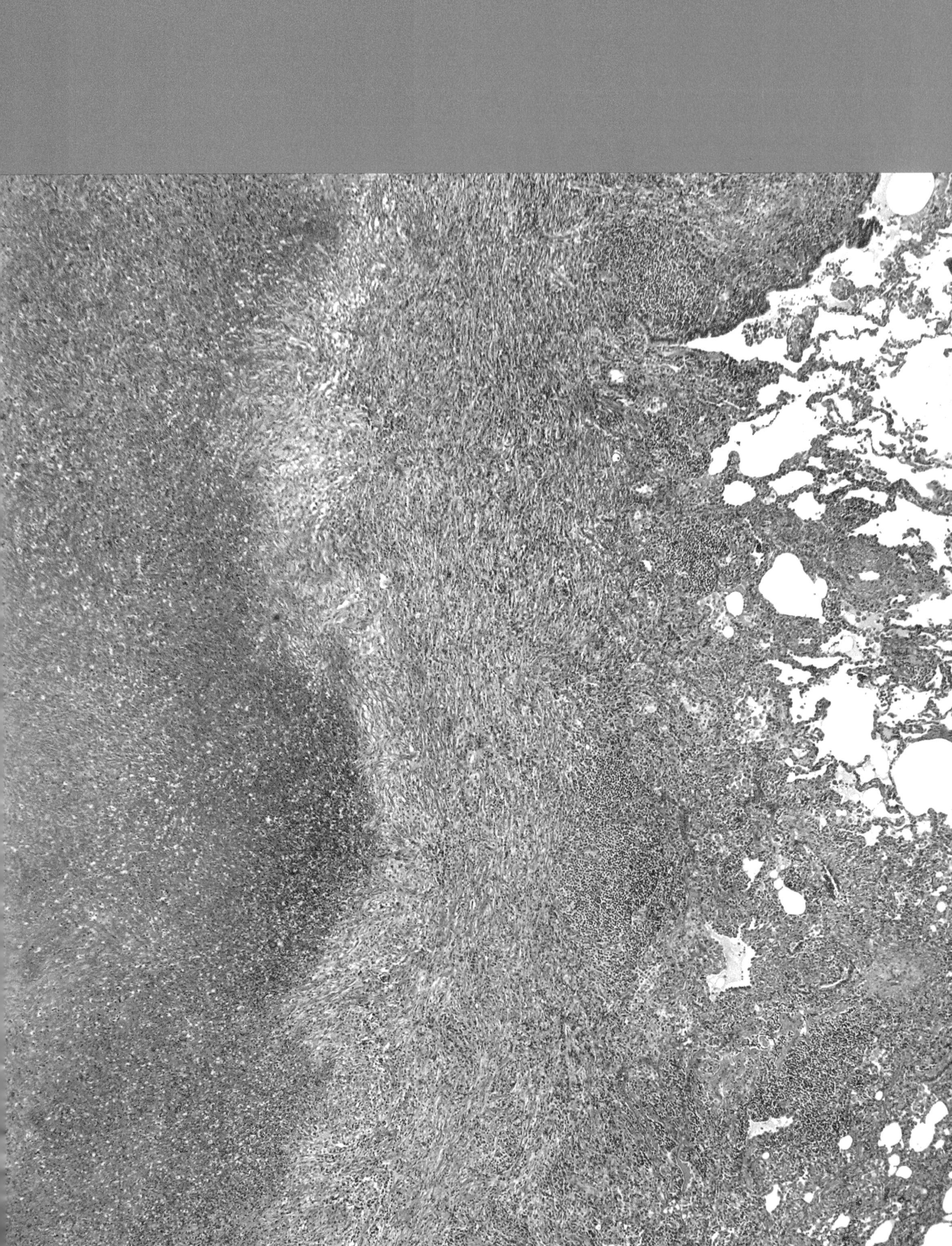

SECTION 1
Overview

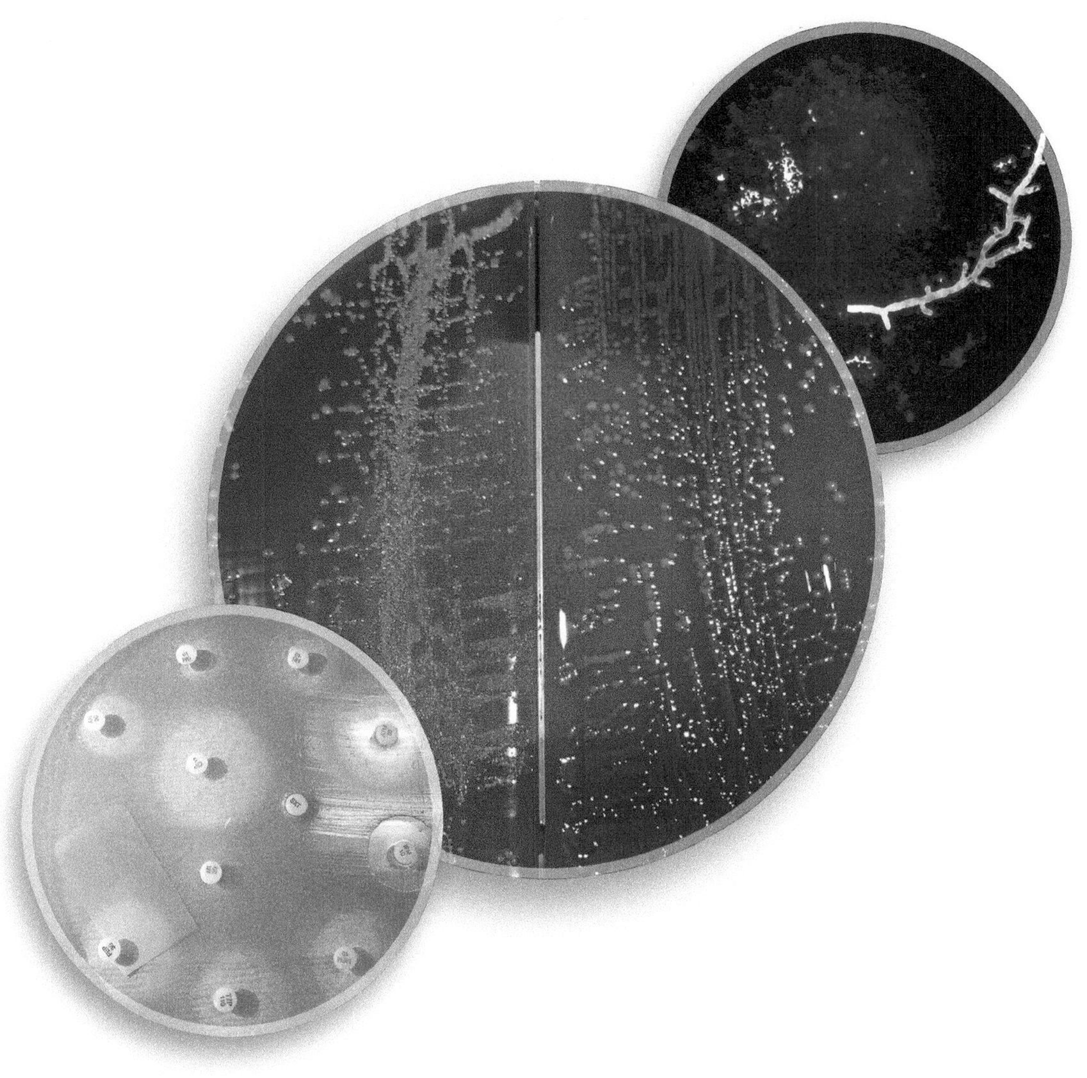

IDENTIFICATION FROM PRIMARY SPECIMENS (GENERAL TO ALL ORGANISMS)

Histopathology

- H&E-stained sections allow for visualization of most parasites and fungi, some bacteria, and viral cytopathic effects, when present
- Gram (e.g., Brown-Brenn and Lillie-Twort stains): Highlights most bacteria and some yeasts (e.g., *Candida* spp.)
- Silver: Fungal organisms, positive for many bacteria
  - Methenamine silver (e.g., GMS): Highlights fungal cell walls and many bacteria
  - Silver nitrate (e.g., Warthin-Starry, Dieterle, and Steiner): Used to highlight spirochetes and gram negatives, including *Bartonella* spp. (cat scratch), *Klebsiella* spp. (in rhinoscleroma), etc.
  - Nonspecific staining (varies with tissue type) can provide challenges in interpretation and decrease sensitivity/specificity
- PAS-D stain: Detects polysaccharides in wall of fungal organisms and bacteria, including *Tropheryma whipplei*
- Acid-fast (e.g., Ziehl-Neelsen, Kinyoun): Highlights mycobacteria, including modified AFB stains (e.g., Fite-Faraco utilizing oil to protect wall and maintain acid-fastness) for *Mycobacteria leprae* and *Nocardia* spp.
- Mucicarmine: Used to confirm *Cryptococcus* spp. (stains capsule in non-capsule-deficient strains)
- Fontana-Masson highlights melanin and melanin-like pigments: Stains *Cryptococcus* spp. but also positive in some other yeast (e.g., *Blastomyces* and *Coccidioides* spp.) as well as all dematiaceous fungi
- IHC for specific pathogens; often cross reactivity between related organisms
  - Anti-*Treponema pallidum* antibody for syphilis may also stain other spirochetes (e.g., *Borrelia* spp.)
  - Commercially available antibodies for many viruses, including HSV-1/2, VZV, CMV, HHV-8, adenovirus, polyomaviruses, SARS-CoV-2, etc.
  - Other IHC may be available at reference laboratories

Microbiology Procedures for Infectious Disease Work-Ups

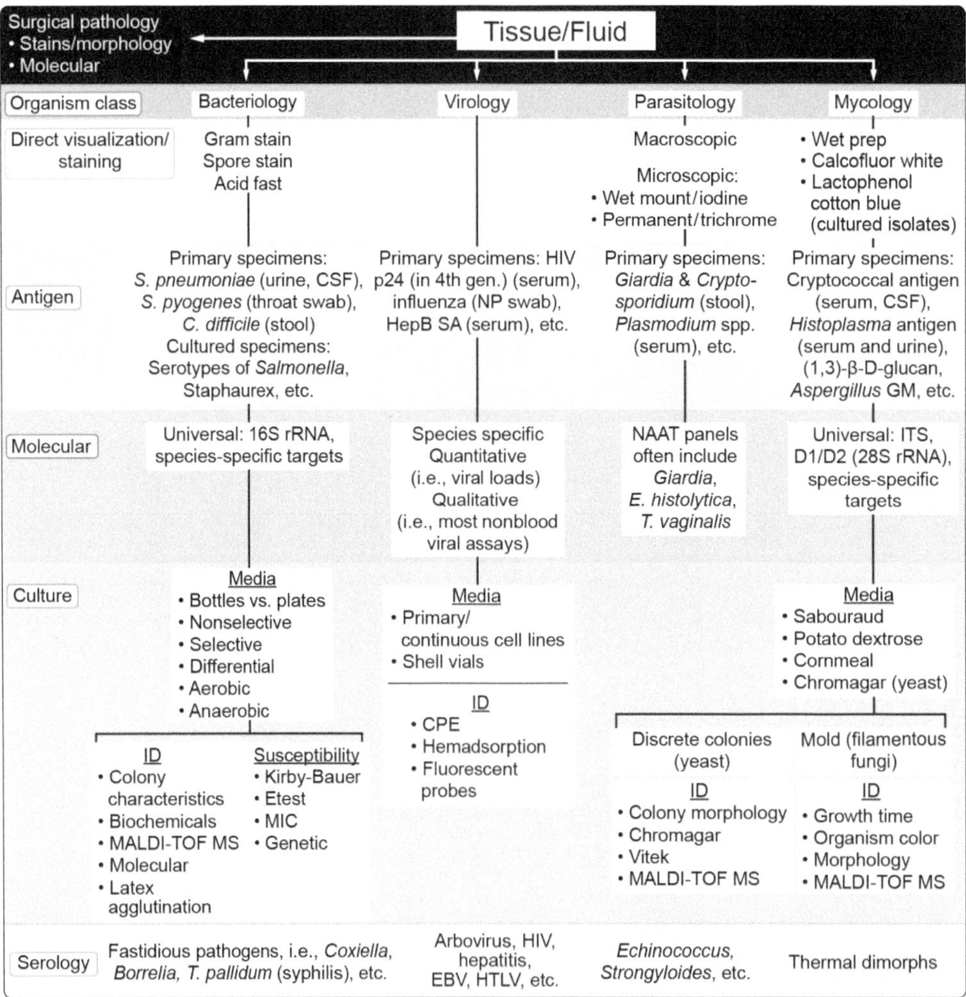

Chart shows testing in the clinical microbiology laboratory organized by technique and organism class. Common examples of different techniques are noted.

- In situ hybridization (ISH) for pathogen DNA/RNA: Excellent specificity and sensitivity
  - EBER ISH for EBV
  - HPV ISH cocktails for high- or low-risk HPV strains

Molecular Methodologies and Platforms

- Fresh or frozen primary specimens preferred; DNA cross linking in formalin-fixed paraffin-embedded (FFPE) tissue limits potential amplicon size
- Polymerase chain reaction (PCR), qualitative or quantitative
  - Relies on heat-stable polymerase to generate new amplicons after heat denaturation
  - Most widely used amplification method
  - Rapid, singleplex assays are available, e.g., Cepheid (*Mycobacterium tuberculosis* complex from sputum, enterovirus in CSF, *Clostridioides difficile* from stool, norovirus from stool, group A *Streptococcus* spp. from throat swabs, etc.)
  - Multiplexed panels are also available from variety of manufacturers and offered as "syndromic" tests, covering several bacterial, fungal, viral, and parasitic pathogens
- Isothermal methods
  - Amplification methods that do not rely on thermal cycling
  - Strand displacement amplification (SDA), e.g., BD Viper platform for chlamydia and gonorrhea testing
  - Transcription-mediated amplification (TMA), e.g., Panther platform (Hologic) for HPV and others
  - Loop-mediated isothermal amplification (LAMP), e.g., Illumigene (Meridian) for group B *Streptococcus*, *Bordetella pertussis*, *Mycoplasma*, etc.
- Sequencing methods
  - Generally reserved for cultured isolates but can be used on primary specimens
  - Ribosomal regions, such as 16S for bacteria and internal transcribed spacer (ITS) and D1/D2 region of 28S for fungi, are common targets for speciation as well as hsp65 for mycobacteria
  - Targeted next-generation sequencing (NGS) panels are available for detection of large numbers of pathogens in single assay; usually restricted to reference/commercial laboratories
  - Unbiased NGS assays can be used in select circumstances to detect any nonhuman sequences in specimen; data can be difficult to analyze/interpret and may require confirmatory testing

BACTERIOLOGY

Staining Techniques

- Gram stain: Used to determine presence or absence of bacteria and differentiate between gram-positive (purple) and gram-negative (red) organisms
  - Shape (rods, cocci), size, and arrangement (clusters, chains, pairs) are observed and aid in classification into broad categories
  - Variations include spore and capsule stains (i.e., for identification of *Bacillus anthracis*)
- Acid-fast stain
  - Fluorescent (Auramine-Rhodamine) and traditional (Kinyoun, Ziehl-Neelsen) for *Mycobacterium* spp.
  - Modified Kinyoun for partial acid-fast (e.g., *Nocardia* spp.)

Detection From Primary Specimens

- Immunoassay/antigen based
  - *Streptococcus pneumoniae* (urine and blood)
  - Group A *Streptococcus* (*Streptococcus pyogenes*) (throat swab)
  - *Helicobacter pylori* antigen (stool and biopsy)
  - *Legionella* spp. (urine)
  - *C. difficile* toxin
  - Shiga toxin
- Molecular
  - Targeted assays on primary specimens
    - *C. difficile* (stool)
    - Group A *Streptococcus* (*S. pyogenes*) (throat swab)
    - Methicillin-resistant *Staphylococcus aureus* (nares, blood)
    - *Bordetella pertussis* (respiratory)
    - *Mycoplasma pneumoniae*
    - Enteric pathogen panels (stool), e.g., BD MAX, BioFire, Verigene
    - Meningitis/encephalitis pathogen panels (CSF), e.g., BioFire
    - Respiratory/pneumonia panels (lower respiratory specimens), e.g., BioFire
    - Direct detection of bloodstream pathogens (i.e., not from positive blood bottles)
  - 16S sequencing can be used to identify occult (or partially treated) infections from primary samples when organisms cannot be grown

Culture

- Solid media
  - Variety of solid culture media are available, including aerobic and anaerobic media as well as formulations that aid in growth and differentiation of bacterial spp.
    - Rich media is ideal for growing wide variety of organisms
    - Selective media contain antibiotics or chemicals to inhibit growth of certain organisms
    - Differential media contain compounds that allow organisms to be distinguished based on visualization (typically by color change) of chemical reactions that result from biochemical differences between organisms
  - Common solid media
    - Blood agar: Rich medium; differentiates by ability to hemolyze
    - Chocolate agar: Enriched; used for *Haemophilus* spp. and *Neisseria* spp.
    - Brucella blood agar: Rich agar often used for anaerobes
    - MacConkey agar: Selective for gram-negative enteric bacteria; differentiates by ability to ferment lactose
    - Buffered charcoal yeast agar: Selective for *Legionella* and *Nocardia* spp.
    - CHROMagar: Differentiates organisms by color and, in some cases, selects by drug susceptibility (MRSA, VRE, CRE, *Candida* spp., etc.)
    - Löwenstein-Jensen agar: Selective for *Mycobacterium* spp.
- Bottle media

- Rich broth can grow many organisms
- Typically used for culture of blood and other fluids (joint, abdominal, etc.)
- If positive, broth is Gram stained and plated to solid media for further work-up
  - Several molecular panels are also available for analyzing positive blood bottles

Identification of Cultured Isolates

- Latex agglutination: Latex particles coated with antibody are mixed with bacterial specimen to detect presence of target antigen
  - Staphaurex (*S. aureus*)
  - Lancefield typing (*Streptococcus* spp.)
  - Serotyping of *Salmonella* spp.
- Biochemical testing: Assesses characteristic reactions for differentiation (commonly part of automated panels, such as VITEK 2)
  - Carbohydrate metabolism (e.g., lactose fermentation in enteric organisms)
  - Metabolic pathway end products (e.g., Voges-Proskauer and methyl red test to differentiate enteric organisms)
  - Amino acid decarboxylation (arginine, ornithine, lysine)
  - Catalase (central in differentiating *Staphylococcus* from *Streptococcus* spp.)
  - Coagulase (separates *S. aureus* positive from many other spp. of *Staphylococcus*)
  - Oxidase (differentiates organisms, such as *Pseudomonas* and *Neisseria*)
  - Urease (virulence factor used to differentiate genera, such as *Proteus* and *Klebsiella*)
  - Indole (product of tryptophan degradation used to differentiate spp., such as *Escherichia coli, Klebsiella oxytoca, Proteus vulgaris*)
  - Hydrogen sulfide production (assessed in many agars and panels to differentiate *Salmonella* positive from *Shigella* negative, among others)
  - Motility (differentiates organisms, such as *Listeria*, by their ability to move in semisolid agar)
- Matrix-assisted laser desorption/ionization time-of-flight (MALDI-TOF) mass spectrometry
  - Based on characteristic mass profile of ribosomal proteins
  - Becoming most commonly used platform for organism identification (replacing traditional biochemical approaches)
- Molecular
  - Hybridization: Detection of target sequences with complementary probes
    - Usually involves amplification of target (i.e., through growth in culture) or signal
    - Examples: AccuProbes (Hologic) for *Mycobacterium* spp., Verigene blood culture test system (Luminex)
  - PCR &/or sequencing: 16S rRNA gene (gold standard for speciation)
  - NGS is becoming more standard in clinical laboratories, particularly for epidemiologic questions and support of infection prevention initiatives

Susceptibility

- Multiple methods can be used to determine susceptibility to antimicrobials
  - Minimum inhibitory concentration (MIC)
    - Lowest concentration of antibiotic that prevents visible growth of bacteria
    - Standards exist for individual bacteria-antibiotic pairs to determine MIC at which that bacteria is considered susceptible or resistant to that antibiotic (CLSI, FDA, EUCAST)
    - Can be automated or manual
    - Novel methods emerging, e.g., single cell microscopy, microfluidics, MALDI-TOF
  - Etest
    - Reagent strip with antibiotic gradient placed on inoculated plate
    - MIC is equal to concentration of antibiotic where zone of inhibition intersects with strip
  - Kirby-Bauer disc diffusion susceptibility test
    - Zone of growth inhibition around antibiotic discs is measured to determine susceptibility
  - Molecular tests
    - Targeted nucleic acid amplification (NAAT) for resistance genes
    - Reserved for relatively common, highly predictable genes (*mecA, blaKPC*, etc.)

VIROLOGY

Detection From Primary Specimens

- Immunoassay/antigen based: Later generation HIV tests (incorporate p24 antigen)
- Molecular
  - NAAT assays are becoming preferred means of viral diagnosis
  - Both qualitative and quantitative assays are available for wide range of targets for both diagnosis and monitoring
  - Can be offered as single-pathogen assays (e.g., influenza, norovirus, HPV) or as components of large syndromic panels
  - Respiratory panels (nasopharyngeal swabs, lower respiratory specimens)
  - Meningitis/encephalitis pathogen panels (CSF), e.g., BioFire

Culture

- Traditional method utilizing variety of primary and immortalized cell preparations to assess for characteristic cytopathic effect (CPE) with viral infection
- Takes days to weeks and requires highly trained staff; gradually giving way to molecular methods
- Adenovirus: Round, grape-like clusters of cells in ~ 6 days
- CMV: Slowly progressive foci of rounded cells (fibroblasts) in ~ 8 days
- HSV: Large rounded cells and some syncytia ~ 2 days
- RSV: Syncytia in some lines (Rhesus monkey kidney and HEp-2) in ~ 6 days
- VZV: Foci of rounded, degenerating cells in ~ 6 days

MYCOLOGY

Staining Techniques

- Calcofluor white: Fluorescent stain that can be used on direct specimens or fixed tissue; binds to chitin in fungal cell wall (including *Pneumocystis* spp.)

- Lactophenol cotton blue: Standard strain for visualization of fungal morphology from cultured isolates
- India ink: Due to exclusion by capsule, can be used for *Cryptococcus* spp. in primary specimens; capsule production may be downregulated on subculture

Detection From Primary Specimens

- Immunoassay/antigen based
  - (1,3)-β-D-glucan detection for diagnosis of systemic fungal disease; negative with organisms that produce little or no antigen, such as Mucorales, *Cryptococcus*, and *Blastomyces* spp.
  - *Aspergillus* galactomannan
  - *Histoplasma* antigen (and other dimorphs), blood and urine
  - *Cryptococcus* antigen (CSF)
- Molecular
  - Generally offered as components of syndromic panels
  - Meningitis/encephalitis pathogen panels (CSF), e.g., BioFire (*Cryptococcus* spp.)
  - Direct detection of bloodstream pathogens, e.g., T2 *Candida* panel
  - *Pneumocystis* singleplex PCR assays may be available in some laboratories (on primary specimens)

Culture

- Agars include potato dextrose agar, inhibitory mold agar, and Sabouraud agar
  - Methods to visualize diagnostic reproductive structures include tape and tease preps as well as slide culture (all with lactophenol cotton blue staining)
  - Speciation has traditionally been morphologic
- CHROMagar can be used to differentiate spp. of *Candida* by colony color
- Fungemia diagnostics
  - Blood isolators (lysis centrifugation) are preferred for *Histoplasma* spp. and other thermal dimorphs
  - Standard blood culture bottles are able to support growth of *Candida* spp.

Biochemicals

- Biochemical identification is available for many yeasts (e.g., API strips, VITEK cards)

Matrix-Assisted Laser Desorption/Ionization Time of Flight

- Speciates organisms by mass spectra of ribosomal proteins
- Routine practice for many yeasts; becoming more common for filamentous fungi

Molecular

- Broad-range fungal sequencing targeting (e.g., ITS and D1/D2 28S rRNA regions) can be quick and accurate way to directly speciate many fungi; available at many reference labs and increasingly within clinical labs
- Fungal targets (*Candida* spp.) are included in several blood culture PCR panels

PARASITOLOGY

Direct Examination: Macroscopic

- Worms are occasionally submitted to clinical microbiology laboratories for morphologic identification

Direct Examination: Microscopic

- Stains include iodine, trichrome (permanent, often reserved for confirmation), and modified Kinyoun acid-fast (*Cryptosporidium*, *Cyclospora*, and *Cystoisospora* spp.)
- Stool (and other sources) are assessed by microscopy for helminth eggs and protozoa: Stool specimens must be concentrated using sedimentation or flotation methods
- Blood parasites (Giemsa-stained thick and thin smears): Can detect *Plasmodium* spp., *Trypanosoma*, microfilaria, *Babesia* spp., and *Leishmania* spp.

Detection From Primary Specimens

- Immunoassay/antigen based: Rapid, lateral flow immunoassays for common GI (e.g., *Giardia*, *Cryptosporidium* spp.) and blood parasites (e.g., *Plasmodium* spp.)
- Detection of GI parasites directly from stool is incorporated into some molecular panels (BD MAX, xTAG, BioFire, etc.)
- Molecular detection of *Trichomonas* spp. is often incorporated into PCR STD panels for use on urine, endocervical swabs, and liquid-based cytology specimens

CLINICAL IMMUNOLOGY

Serology

- Measure of patient immune response to antigen associated with pathogen
- IgM- and IgG-specific assays can provide approximate indication as to whether infection is acute or chronic/resolved
- Acute and convalescent serologies can be compared to look at relative antibody titers (standard is to look for 4x change)
- May be diagnostic test of choice for nonendemic/rare or difficult-to-culture pathogens, e.g., arboviral infections, Lyme disease, syphilis, etc.

Common Testing Modalities

- Agglutination: Inert particles coupled to reagent antigen or antibody are mixed with patient specimen; agglutination indicates presence of target
- Precipitation assay: Degree of visible precipitation of antigen-antibody complexes within gel or in solution is measured after addition of patient sample
- Enzyme immunoassay (EIA): Patient sample is added to sample well with bound reagent antibody or antigen; after addition of enzyme-conjugated antibody, substrate is added, and enzyme-substrate interaction produces quantifiable reaction
- Immunofluorescent assay: Fluorochrome-conjugated antibody is added to patient sample, typically on glass slide; fluorescent microscope is used to visualize slide and determine presence of fluorescence

SELECTED REFERENCES

1. Carroll KC et al:Manual of Clinical Microbiology. 12th ed. ASM Press, 2019
2. Miller JM et al: A guide to utilization of the microbiology laboratory for diagnosis of infectious diseases: 2018 update by the Infectious Diseases Society of America and the American Society for Microbiology. Clin Infect Dis. 67(6):e1-94, 2018
3. Buchan BW et al: Emerging technologies for the clinical microbiology laboratory. Clin Microbiol Rev. 27(4):783-822, 2014

Selective and Nonselective Media

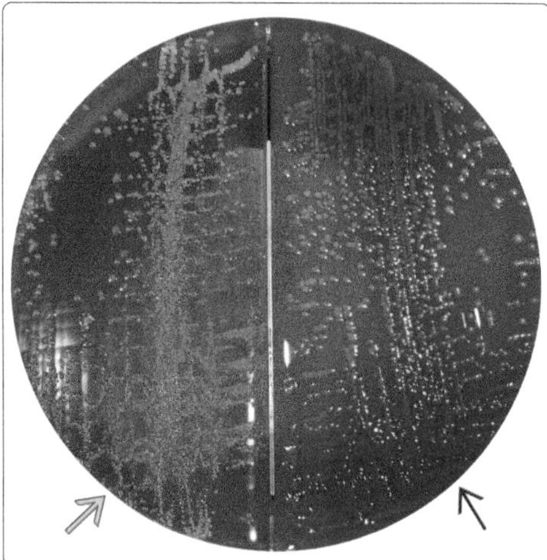

Traditional Resistance Testing

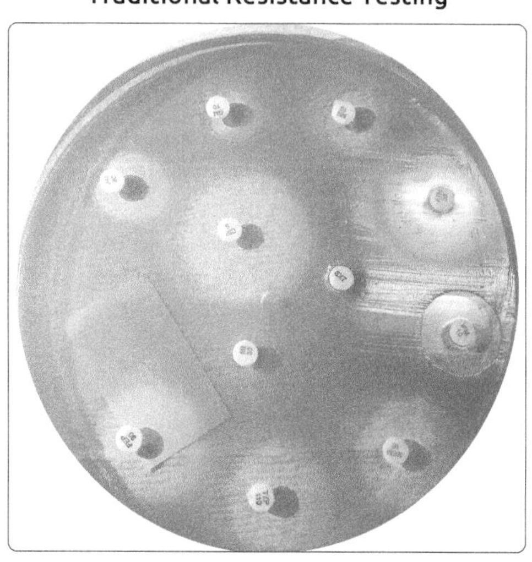

(Left) *Blood ⇒ is a rich media that differentiates by hemolysis, while MacConkey ⇒ selects for gram negatives and differentiates lactose fermenters (pink colonies). Here, a nonhemolytic, gram-negative organism that ferments lactose is shown.* **(Right)** *Kirby-Bauer disc diffusion uses drug discs on a Mueller-Hinton plate. Diameter of clearing around each disc is measured and used to determine whether the isolate is susceptible. Note the characteristic blue-green pigmentation of Pseudomonas species.*

Biochemical Identification

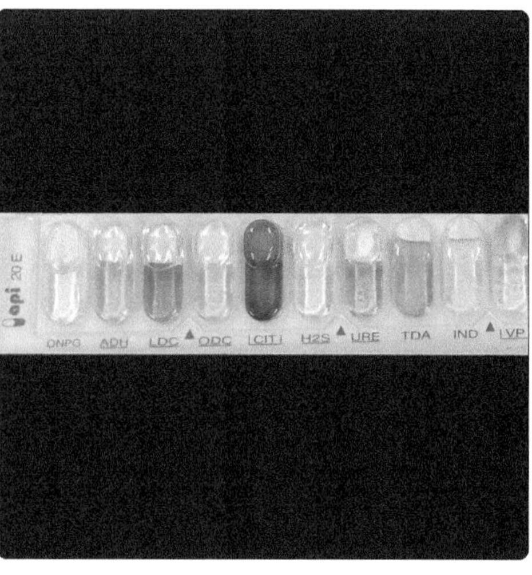

Mass Spectrometry in Microbiology

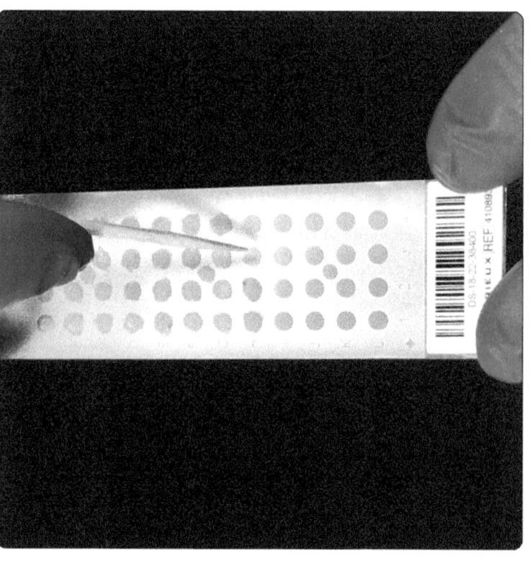

(Left) *Traditional organism identification by biochemical reactions and carbohydrate utilization (this API strip shows the biochemical patterns of Klebsiella pneumoniae) is often incorporated into larger panels on automated platforms, i.e., VITEK 2.* **(Right)** *Photograph shows the application of the organism to a spot on a MALDI slide. MALDI is supplanting many traditional (biochemical) methods of organism identification.*

Anaerobic Culture Systems

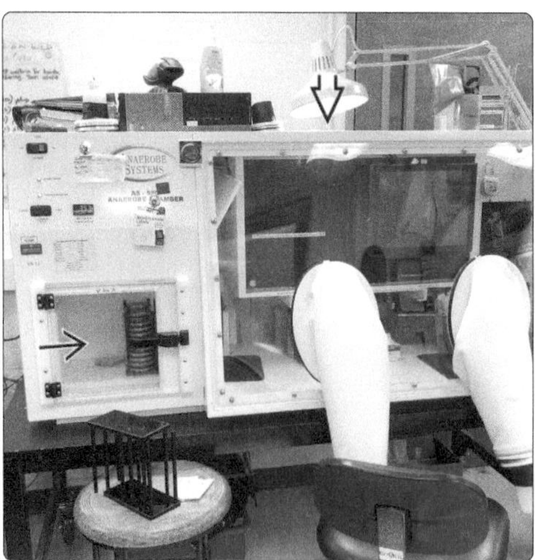

Parasitology: Morphology

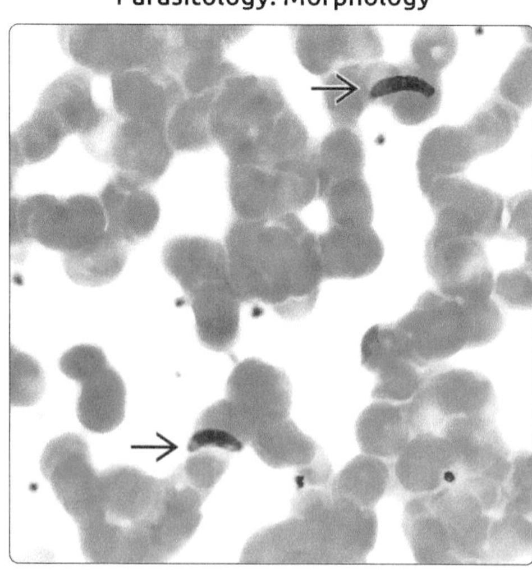

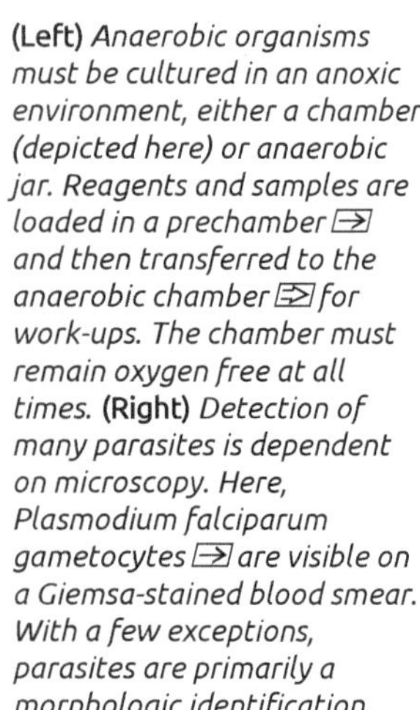

(Left) *Anaerobic organisms must be cultured in an anoxic environment, either a chamber (depicted here) or anaerobic jar. Reagents and samples are loaded in a prechamber ⇒ and then transferred to the anaerobic chamber ⇒ for work-ups. The chamber must remain oxygen free at all times.* **(Right)** *Detection of many parasites is dependent on microscopy. Here, Plasmodium falciparum gametocytes ⇒ are visible on a Giemsa-stained blood smear. With a few exceptions, parasites are primarily a morphologic identification.*

Parasitology: Gross Examination

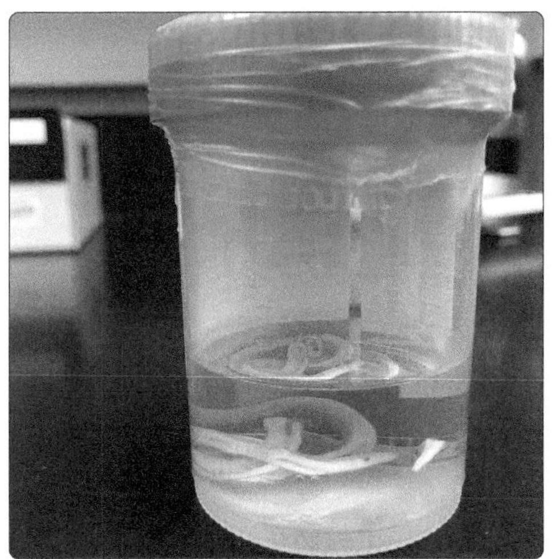

Parasitology: Stool Examination

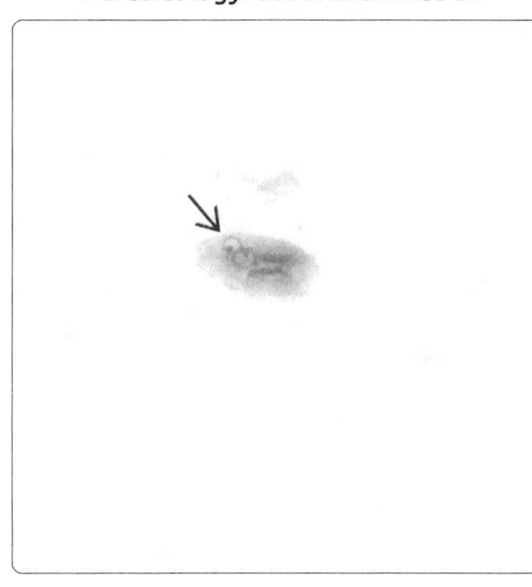

(Left) *Worms may be submitted for identification. The diagnosis of helminth infections is typically by the visualization of eggs in stool. This cup holds a preserved Ascaris worm. "Found objects" thought to be worms or other organisms are commonly received in the microbiology laboratory.* **(Right)** *Parasites are often visualized using iodine &/or a trichrome stain. A cyst form of Giardia (trichrome, 100x) is shown with 2 or 4 visible nuclei ⇒. Larvae and eggs from helminths, as well as cysts and trophozoites, are visualized.*

Fungal Culture

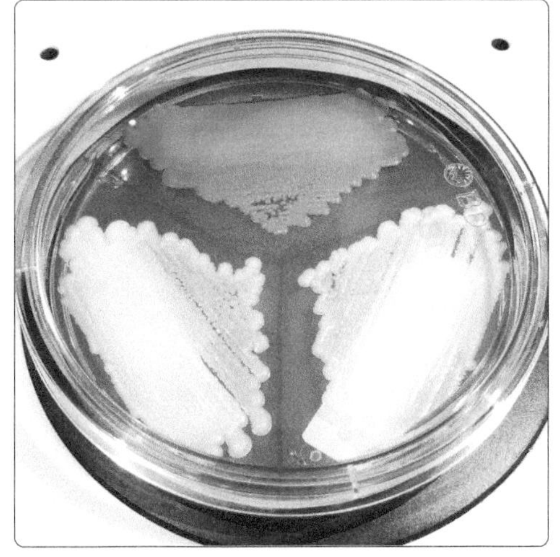

Fungal Culture

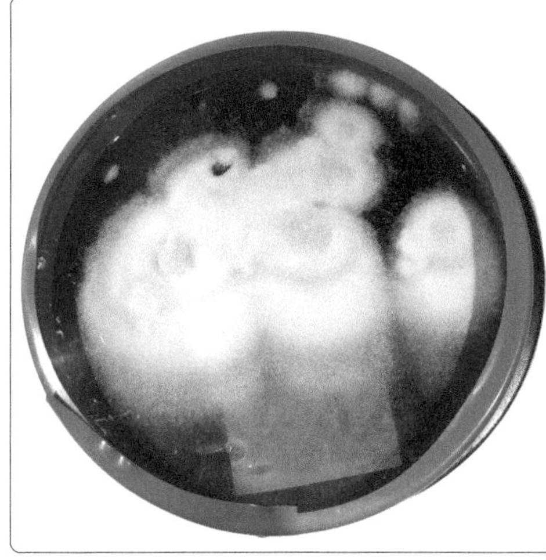

(Left) *Sabouraud and potato dextrose agars are commonly used for mycology. Yeast typically form wet, discrete colonies on agar (clockwise from top: Rhodotorula mucilaginosa, Candida guilliermondii, and Saccharomyces cerevisiae).* **(Right)** *Filamentous fungi typically form fluffy colonies on agar with distinct coloration on the back and front of the plate. Here, Trichophyton rubrum (a dermatophyte) displays a white, cottony form with some pinkish coloration; underside of the plate is a deep red.*

Fungal Morphology

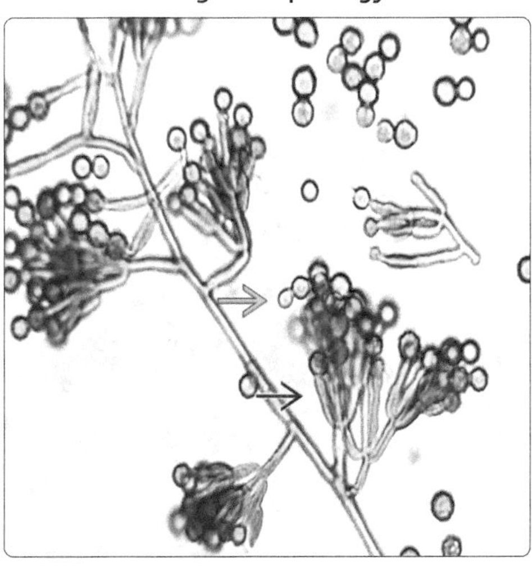

Fungal Special Stains

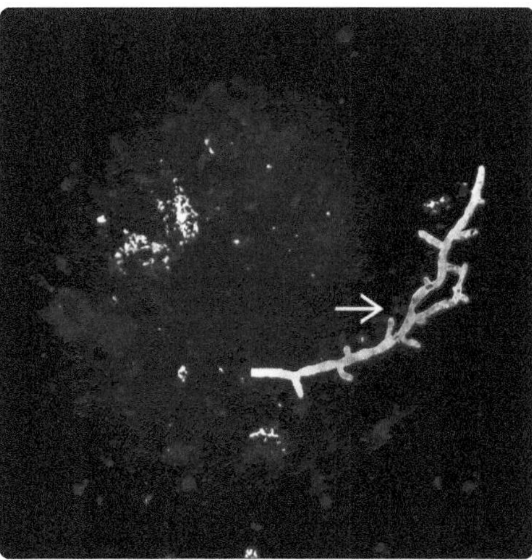

(Left) *Lactophenol cotton blue is typically used to visualize fungal structures for identification. In this image, Scopulariopsis annellides ⇒ bearing conidia ⇒ is depicted. (Courtesy C. Myers, MS.)* **(Right)** *Calcofluor white is a sensitive and common fluorescent dye used to visualize fungal elements ➡ in primary specimens. (Courtesy C. Myers, MS.)*

DIGITAL PATHOLOGY AND ARTIFICIAL INTELLIGENCE

Acid-Fast Bacilli Detection

- Artificial intelligence (AI) and machine learning algorithms are being assessed for ability to assist in detection of acid-fast bacilli (AFB) in histologic specimens from whole-slide images (WSI)
- AI-supported detection can greatly improve workflow and efficiency
- Can improve sensitivity and time to detection for *Mycobacterium tuberculosis*
- Higher sensitivity, negative predictive value, and accuracy compared with light microscopy and WSI evaluation without AI
- May have high frequency of false-positives (low specificity)

Parasite Identification

- Automated slide interpretation of blood and stool smears for parasite identification
- Avoid need for highly trained technical staff, particularly in resource-limited settings
- Clinical validation will require large image banks and databases
- Can be used to evaluate staining quality and coloration quality

Fungal Identification

- Morphologic speciation of filamentous fungi can be challenging in tissue sections
- Automated image-based species identification have potential to increase accuracy and decrease turnaround time
- Uses AI-based neural networks and classification systems
- Clinical validation requires large annotated image databases

Clinical Microbiology Laboratory

- Image analysis and AI analysis approaches are beginning to impact practice of routine microbiology
- Plate interpretation: Analysis of microbial growth on agar plates
  - Requires integration with total laboratory automation workflow
  - Rare event detection image analysis
  - AI-based screening algorithms to identify negative or mixed cultures or for use with chromogenic agars
- Score-based analyses can be used for culture and smear interpretation (Nugent score for bacterial vaginosis, primary Gram stain, urine cultures)

NUCLEIC ACID DETECTION

Multiplex Syndromic Testing

- Polymerase chain reaction (PCR)-based technology
- Amplifies and detects microorganism DNA directly from patient sample
- Particularly useful for low-volume samples (CSF)
- Multiple automated commercial platforms currently FDA approved/cleared, many with rapid (1- to 3-hour) turnaround times and on-demand testing
- Detects presence of multiple (8-22) bacterial, viral, and fungal pathogens that cause overlapping clinical signs and symptoms in single multiplex assay
- Panels developed for encephalitis/meningitis, gastrointestinal, respiratory, pneumonia, joint infections, and bloodstream infections
- Some assays include identification of antimicrobial resistance genes but do not provide complete antimicrobial susceptibility information
- Can support antimicrobial stewardship and infection prevention practices
- Detection of coinfections, DNA from nonviable organisms, or identification of unusual organisms can cause clinical confusion
- Challenges include cost, test utilization strategies, and test interpretation

Digital Pathology: AFB Detection

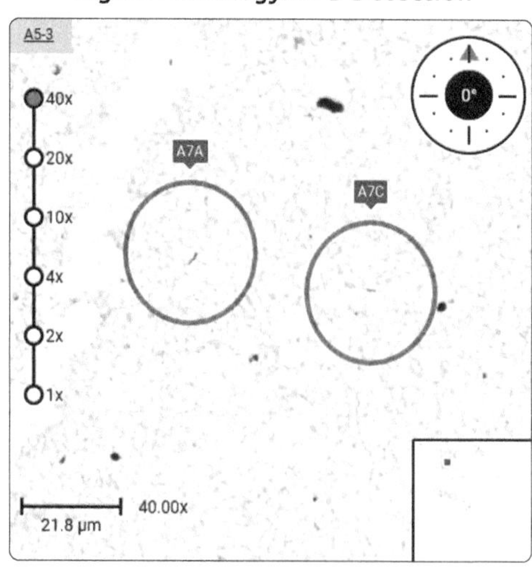

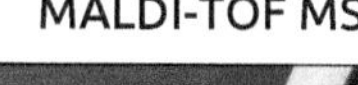

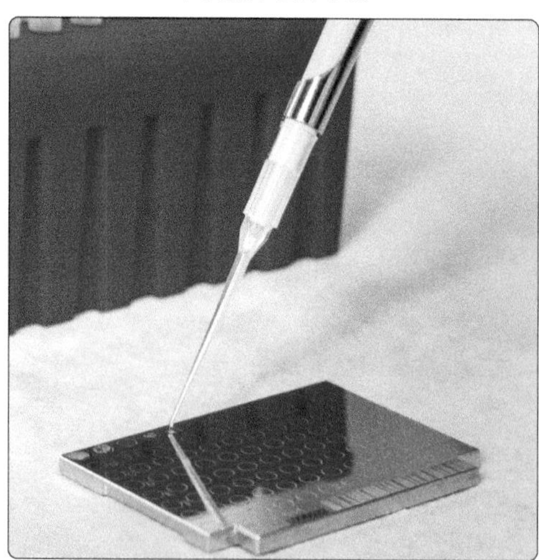

(Left) *Whole-slide scanned images of AFB-stained sections can lead to increased sensitivity and decreased pathologists' time to detection, following validation of imaging analysis algorithms to identify regions of interest (red circles) containing potential organisms.* **(Right)** *MALDI-TOF MS has an increasing number of infectious disease applications, including identification of microorganisms from culture isolates and primary specimens. (Courtesy D. Drapeau, CDC/PHIL.)*

Broad-Range Polymerase Chain Reaction With Sequencing

- Amplification and sequencing of conserved genomic regions for species-level identification
  - Bacteria: 16S ribosomal RNA (rRNA)
  - Mycobacteria: 65-kilodalton heat shock protein (hsp65)
  - Fungi: 28S rRNA, internal transcribed spacer (ITS)
  - Viruses: No broad-spectrum targets available
- Increasingly available at reference laboratories or as laboratory-developed tests
- Performed directly from patient fluid and tissue samples, including fresh, frozen, and formalin-fixed paraffin-embedded (FFPE) specimens
  - DNA recovery negatively impacted by formalin fixation (fresh or frozen tissue preferable)
  - Diagnostic yield is increased (and false-positives decreased) when organisms are observed histologically and molecular results are correlated with morphologic findings
- Species-level identification reported to be achievable in 65-91% of cases
- Can detect unculturable (leprosy, syphilis, *Tropheryma whipplei*) or difficult-to-grow organisms (*Coxiella burnetii*, HACEK bacteria)
- For some pathogens, sensitivity can be reduced compared to culture and targeted PCR-based approaches
- Detection of DNA from nonviable organisms, lack of quantitative results, detection of low-abundance organisms (contamination, colonization) can lead to difficulty in clinical interpretation
- Contamination can occur during specimen processing (collection, reagents, environment) or during sequencing (positive controls, adjacent samples)
- Additional challenges include cost and lack of antimicrobial susceptibility information

Metagenomic Next-Generation Sequencing

- Unbiased, untargeted sequencing of all RNA &/or DNA within sample
- Includes detection of bacteria, fungi, viruses, and parasites
- Must remove human DNA during bioinformatic analysis
- Offered by some commercial and reference laboratories for limited specimen types (CSF, serum)
- Detection of low-abundance or novel organisms can pose interpretive challenges
- Results may lead to escalation or deescalation of therapy; clinical management changed in 11% of cases in recent multiinstitutional study

MATRIX-ASSISTED LASER DESORPTION/IONIZATION TIME-OF-FLIGHT MASS SPECTROMETRY

Fungal Identification

- Requires different protein extraction protocol
- Bypasses need for highly experienced personnel to perform morphologic identification
- Reduces time to identification
- Can be dependent on organism growth phase

Direct Specimen Testing

- Direct testing of positive blood culture bottles, sometimes following short-term incubation, can provide more rapid organism identification than isolation-based approaches
  - Antimicrobial resistance prediction using machine learning analysis
- Mass spectrometry imaging direct from tissue has potential for rapid organism identification
  - Intraoperative frozen section evaluation
  - Potential to provide functional data (antimicrobial susceptibility)
  - Pathogens in tissue need to be inactivated prior to ionization to remove risk of infection to laboratory personnel

SELECTED REFERENCES

1. Burns BL et al: The use of machine learning for image analysis artificial intelligence in clinical microbiology. J Clin Microbiol. 61(9):e0233621, 2023
2. Rahman MA et al: Classification of fungal genera from microscopic images using artificial intelligence. J Pathol Inform. 14:100314, 2023
3. Săndulescu O et al: Syndromic testing in infectious diseases: from diagnostic stewardship to antimicrobial stewardship. Antibiotics (Basel). 12(1):6, 2022
4. Weis C et al: Direct antimicrobial resistance prediction from clinical MALDI-TOF mass spectra using machine learning. Nat Med. 28(1):164-74, 2022
5. Zaizen Y et al: Deep-learning-aided detection of mycobacteria in pathology specimens increases the sensitivity in early diagnosis of pulmonary tuberculosis compared with bacteriology tests. Diagnostics (Basel). 12(3):709, 2022
6. Zurac S et al: A new artificial intelligence-based method for identifying mycobacterium tuberculosis in Ziehl-Neelsen stain on tissue. Diagnostics (Basel). 12(6):1484, 2022
7. Basu SS et al: Bringing matrix-assisted laser desorption/ionization mass spectrometry imaging to the clinics. Clin Lab Med. 41(2):309-24, 2021
8. Carr C et al: Deciphering the low abundance microbiota of presumed aseptic hip and knee implants. PLoS One. 16(9):e0257471, 2021
9. Fida M et al: Diagnostic value of 16s ribosomal RNA gene polymerase chain reaction/sanger sequencing in clinical practice. Clin Infect Dis. 73(6):961-8, 2021
10. Hogan CA et al: Clinical impact of metagenomic next-generation sequencing of plasma cell-free DNA for the diagnosis of infectious diseases: a multicenter retrospective cohort study. Clin Infect Dis. 72(2):239-45, 2021
11. Pantanowitz L et al: Artificial intelligence-based screening for mycobacteria in whole-slide images of tissue samples. Am J Clin Pathol. 156(1):117-28, 2021
12. Egli A et al: Digital microbiology. Clin Microbiol Infect. 26(10):1324-31, 2020
13. Mathison BA et al: Detection of intestinal protozoa in trichrome-stained stool specimens by use of a deep convolutional neural network. J Clin Microbiol. 58(6):e02053-19, 2020
14. Smith KP et al: Image analysis and artificial intelligence in infectious disease diagnostics. Clin Microbiol Infect. 26(10):1318-23, 2020
15. Vetter P et al: Diagnostic challenges of central nervous system infection: extensive multiplex panels versus stepwise guided approach. Clin Microbiol Infect. 26(6):706-12, 2020
16. Zieliński B et al: Deep learning approach to describe and classify fungi microscopic images. PLoS One. 15(6):e0234806, 2020
17. Intra J et al: Genus-level identification of dermatophytes by MALDI-TOF MS after 2 days of colony growth. Lett Appl Microbiol. 67(2):136-43, 2018
18. Ramanan P et al: Syndromic panel-based testing in clinical microbiology. Clin Microbiol Rev. 31(1):e00024-17, 2018
19. Hanson KE et al: Multiplexed molecular diagnostics for respiratory, gastrointestinal, and central nervous system infections. Clin Infect Dis. 63(10):1361-7, 2016
20. Suarez S et al: [Applications of MALDI-TOF technology in clinical microbiology.] Pathol Biol (Paris). 63(1):43-52, 2015

ANATOMIC PATHOLOGY

General Considerations

- It is important to evaluate risk level of each case (clinical notes, imaging, laboratory testing results) prior to initiation of procedures (autopsy, fine-needle aspiration, frozen section evaluation)
- Pathogen exposure can occur via accidental puncture wounds from needles or other sharps, splashes into mucous membranes, inhalation, or passage of infective agent through preexistent wounds
- Universal precautions and use of standard personal protective equipment (PPE) should be routinely employed
- Barrier protection (gloves, cut-resistant gloves, gowns, eye protection, foot covers)
- Tissue fixation, decontamination of equipment and work surfaces
- Hand washing, care to not contaminate materials (paperwork) leaving procedure space
- Ongoing communication with local infection control, occupational health and safety departments to implement biosafety plan and continuing safety education
- Institutional-level biosafety measures should include engineering and administrative controls [separation of physical spaces into clean and dirty areas, basic biosafety level (BSL) risk assessment], ventilation recommendations (negative pressure, exhaustion by HEPA filters), safe exposure of contaminated waste, and access to postexposure chemoprophylaxis
- Consult with local microbiology laboratory for pathogen-specific national and state reporting requirements

Autopsy

- Consider all autopsies as potential infective source
- Clinical history/diagnoses are often incomplete or medical information insufficient to inform accurate risk level assessment

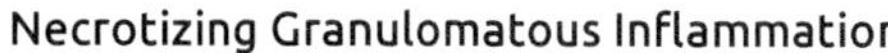

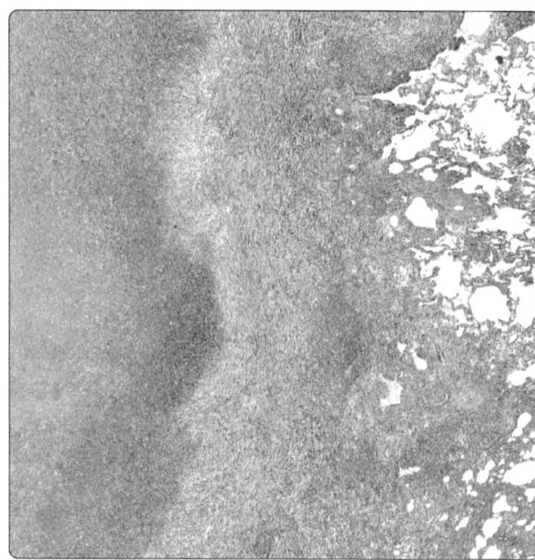

Coccidioidomycosis

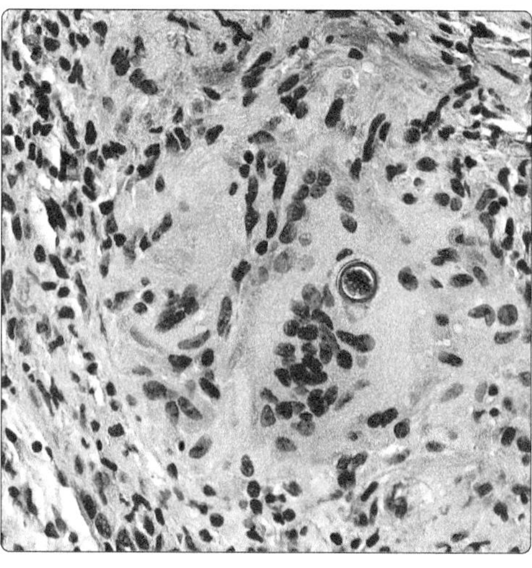

(Left) *Necrotizing granulomatous inflammation is associated with a variety of infections, including tuberculosis. Lung nodules of uncertain etiology should be treated as potentially infectious during intraoperative frozen sections and autopsy.* **(Right)** *Coccidioides species may be identified in AP specimens prior to culture identification. The microbiology laboratory should be notified to reduce risk of airborne transmission amongst laboratory personnel due to the highly infectious arthroconidia.*

Transmissible Spongiform Encephalopathy

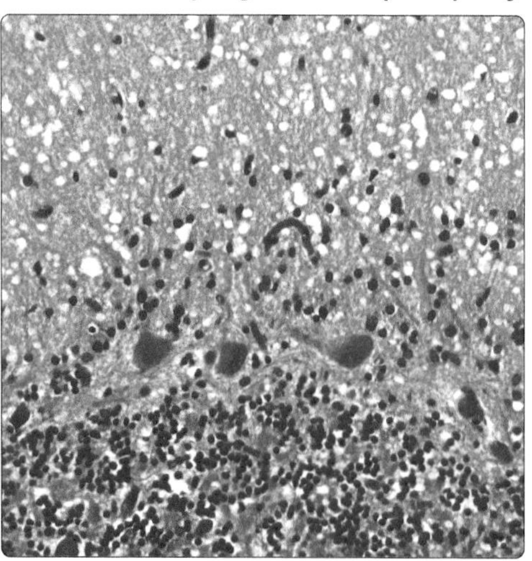

Ebola Hemorrhagic Fever

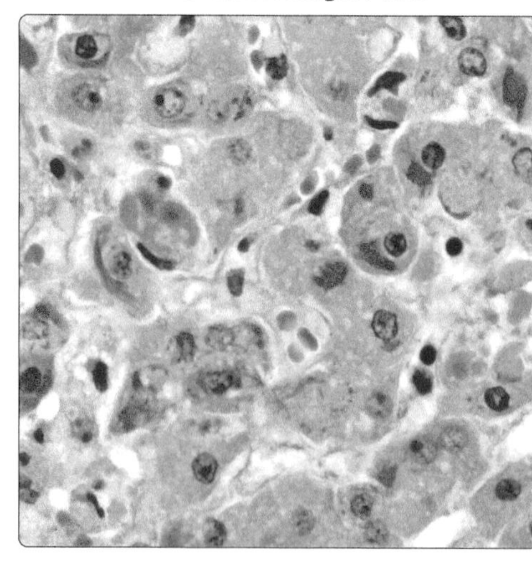

(Left) *Tissue from cases of suspected prion disease requires formic acid treatment for inactivation prior to processing and paraffin embedding. Frozen tissue should be collected for Western blotting at time of autopsy.* **(Right)** *Suspected cases of viral hemorrhagic fever requires close coordination with public health officials and timely identification of other more common pathogens (e.g., malaria). (Courtesy S. Zaki, MD, PhD.)*

- Autopsy procedures include increased exposure risks: Scalpels, needles, bones fragments, and teeth can result in percutaneous injuries; organ manipulation increases exposure to body fluids and blood; use of instruments, hoses, and saws can produce aerosols contaminating environment or allowing inhalation
- PPE should be used for all autopsies, including scrub suits, gowns, waterproof sleeves, plastic disposable aprons, caps, N95 particulate masks, eye protection (goggles or face shields), shoe covers or footwear restricted to contaminated areas, and double sets of gloves; cut-resistant and puncture-resistant hand protection (plastic or steel gloves) recommended
- Use of "isolation" room for postmortem examinations with potential for pathogens of concern: Hantavirus, hepatitis, HIV/AIDs, leprosy, multidrug-resistant bacteria (MRSA, VRE), rickettsial diseases, typhoid fever, systemic infections of unknown etiology
- Isolation rooms should limit personnel, use strictly enforced universal precautions, and include additional special safety and decontamination procedures as indicated; consider use of overhead ultraviolet lights for secondary decontamination
- Additional efforts to reduce aerosols should be included for pathogens spread by aerosol/droplet
  - Tuberculosis, meningococcal meningitis, SARS, influenza, rabies, *Yersinia pestis* (plague), legionellosis, meningococcemia, rickettsioses, coccidiomycosis, prion disease, and anthrax
  - Considerations include collecting body cavity fluids in ladle or bulb syringe instead of hose aspirator, placing plastic bags over decedent head during removal of calvarium, using saws equipped with HEPA filters, moistening bone before cutting
- Consider less hazardous sampling and testing methodologies to arrive at diagnosis: Molecular detection of viral hemorrhagic fevers using skin fragment or respiratory viruses (SARS, influenza) using nasopharyngeal swabs

Surgical Pathology

- Routine use of PPE should be used for grossing specimens (scrub suits, gowns, waterproof sleeves, plastic disposable aprons, face shields/goggles)
- It is recommended to gross specimens with concern for infective agents in biosafety cabinet, particularly when risk of spatter or aerosolization present
- Frozen section considerations include
  - Use of N95 or respiratory mask during tissue sectioning, as cryostats may produce aerosoles
  - Avoid use of freezing sprays and propellants
  - Perform regular cryostat decontamination with 70% ethyl or isopropyl alcohol
  - Obtain cultures as indicated, and alert microbiology laboratory if concern for highly infectious organism or agent of bioterrorism

Cytology

- Routine use of PPE on-site during procedures
- Fine-needle aspiration procedures and making smears can cause aerosols
- Air-dried slides are infectious; slides are generally considered to be infectious until fixed and coverslipped
- Obtain cultures as indicated and alert microbiology laboratory if concern for agent of bioterrorism

MOLECULAR LABORATORY

Nucleic Acid Detection and Sequencing

- Sample processing and inactivation should be performed in validated biosafety cabinet in BSL level 2 (BSL-2) facility with unidirectional airflow
- Extraction, reagent preparation, and amplification performed in separate rooms with unidirectional workflow

MICROBIOLOGY LABORATORY

General Considerations

- Universal precautions and PPE should be regularly employed
- Aerosolizing procedures should be performed in class II biosafety cabinet or using additional barrier precautions
- Clinical teams should alert technical staff when there is concern for infection with agent of bioterrorism
- Potential agents of bioterrorism and other highly infectious organisms should be worked with in biosafety cabinet and not on open bench top
- Culture plates with concern for growth of highly infectious organism should be taped until organism can be appropriately ruled out
- Avoid use of MALDI-TOF for definitive identification of highly infectious organisms (*Neisseria meningitidis, Brucella* spp.)

Agents of Bioterrorism

- Easily transmissible pathogens with high rate of illness in exposed individuals and low immunity in community
- Often difficult to diagnose and lack of effective therapies
- Microbiology laboratories act as sentinel laboratories and must promptly alert public health officials and refer potential agents of bioterrorism for definitive identification
- Category A: High mortality, easily grown, resistant to destruction, suited to airborne dissemination
- Category B: Highly transmissible, lower morbidity/mortality
- Category C: Emerging pathogens that could be engineered for mass dissemination with potential for significant morbidity/mortality

PATHOGENS OF SPECIAL INTEREST

Creutzfeldt-Jakob Disease, Prion Disease, Transmissible Spongiform Encephalopathies

- Disease of central nervous system in which normal prion protein (PrP) spontaneously folds into abnormal, protease-resistant isoform
- Prions are resistant to inactivation by procedures that denature nucleic acids, such as ultraviolet radiation, but are inactivated by procedures that denature or hydrolyze proteins, such as exposure to some detergents or to NaOH
- Infectious specimens include spinal fluid, brain tissue; can be spread by ingestion of prions from infected tissue or receipt of contaminated cadaver-derived tissues/hormones (growth hormone)

- Autopsy can serve vital role in confirming diagnosis and should be pursued; brain can be examined after adequate formaldehyde fixation (10-14 days) on table covered with absorbent pad and nonpermeable backing (plastic)
- Disinfect contaminated surfaces by flooding with NaOH or bleach and leaving undisturbed for at least 1 hour; use of disposable instruments recommended
- Samples for histology should be labeled [Creutzfeldt-Jakob disease (CJD) precautions] and placed in 95-100% formic acid for 1 hour, followed by fresh 10% neutral buffered formalin for at least 48 hours
- Tissue remnants, cutting debris, and contaminated formaldehyde solution should be discarded in water-tight plastic container as infective hospital waste for incineration

Mycobacterium tuberculosis

- Acid-fast bacilli capable of aerosolization; transmitted via inhalation of aerosols and droplets, traumatic inoculation, or introduction into skin through previous lesions or punctures (tuberculosis verrucosa cutis)
- Active tuberculosis often undiagnosed premortem
- Clinical tip-offs include nonspecific symptomatology, early death, positive IGRA, PPD, pulmonary lesions, presence of epidemiologic risk factors (immigration from endemic areas, history of incarceration)
- Viable organism isolated 24-48 hours after embalming
- Formalin fixation recommended prior to handling tissues; all unfixed tissues need to be manipulated in biologic safety cabinet
- Advisable to introduce 10% formalin into lungs through trachea as well as to submerse organs for 24 hours after evisceration and before dissection
- Reduce aerosolizing procedures (use hand saws in place of power equipment); restrict number of personnel involved
- Sputum, pus, tissue, and urine samples should be manipulated as little as possible to avoid splashing and aerosol formation

Middle East and Severe Acute Respiratory Syndrome Coronaviruses (MERS-CoV, SARS-CoV-1, SARS-CoV-2)

- Transmitted through inhalation of aerosol droplets or through contaminated surfaces (can persist for up to 72 hours)
- Perform autopsy in isolation room, limit aerosolizing procedures
- Primary clinical specimens can be handled in BSL-2 laboratory using standard universal precautions
- Culture isolates must be handled in BSL-3 laboratory

Hepatitis B and C

- HBV is highly transmissible (100x more transmissible by blood and aerosols than HIV); occupational risk decreased by availability of effective vaccine and postexposure prophylaxis
- HCV is more transmissible than HIV but less so than HBV; no vaccine or immunoprophylaxis currently available
- Indirect transmission possible, as virus persists on surfaces at room temperature for days
- Epidemiologic risk factors include injection drug use, hemodialysis patients, history of blood transfusions or organ transplants prior to 1992

HIV

- Occupational transmission usually occurs following accidental needle stick or scalpel injury; transmission risk related to patient's viral load, inoculated volume; postexposure prophylaxis available
- Viable virus isolated from fluids (pericardial, pleural, CSF, blood) and tissues (spleen, bone, brain) for days to weeks following storage at 6-20 °C
- Surfaces and materials should be decontaminated with 1% glutaraldehyde or 3% hydrogen peroxide
- Epidemiologic risk factors include injection drug use, men who have sex with men

BIOSAFETY LEVELS

Basic Biosafety Level 1

- Basic teaching and research laboratories, good microbiologic technique
- Open bench work, no requirement for PPE use

Basic Biosafety Level 2

- Minimum requirement for handling direct specimens, all anatomic and clinical pathology laboratories
- Good microbiologic techniques with use of PPE
- Open bench with biosafety cabinet use for potential aerosols
- Directional airflow for some laboratory activities (mycology, mycobacteriology)
- Restricted access, closed doors

Containment Biosafety Level 3

- Specialized diagnostic services and research laboratories
- Level 2 requirements plus special clothing, controlled access, directional airflow
- Biosafety cabinets &/or other primary devices for all activities

Maximum Containment Biosafety Level 4

- Highly specialized dangerous pathogen units
- Level 3 requirements plus airlock entry, shower exit, special waste disposal
- Class III biosafety cabinet or positive pressure suits in conjunction with class II biosafety cabinets, double-ended autoclave filtered air

SELECTED REFERENCES

1. CDC: Biosafety in microbiological and biomedical laboratories. Reviewed August 7, 2023. Accessed August 7, 2023. https://www.cdc.gov/labs/pdf/SF__19_308133-A_BMBL6_00-BOOK-WEB-final-3.pdf
2. Barbareschi M et al: Biosafety in surgical pathology in the era of SARS-Cov2 pandemia. a statement of the Italian Society of Surgical Pathology and Cytology. Pathologica. 112(2):59-63, 2020
3. Abdalla de Oliveira Cardoso T et al: Biosafety in autopsy room: an systematic review, Rev. Salud Publica. 21(6): 1-5, 2019
4. Andrew J et al: Autopsy biosafety. In Andrew J et al: Autopsy Pathology: A Manual and Atlas. 3rd ed. Elsevier, 2016
5. Ehdaivand S et al: Are biosafety practices in anatomical laboratories sufficient? A survey of practices and review of current guidelines. Hum Pathol. 44(6):951-8, 2013
6. Shapiro DS et al: Exposure of laboratory workers to Francisella tularensis despite a bioterrorism procedure. J Clin Microbiol. 40(6):2278-81, 2002

Microorganisms Requiring Airborne or Contact Precautions

Pathogen Category	Airborne Precautions*	Contact Precautions**
Agent of bioterrorism: Category A	Smallpox virus (variola major), *Clostridium botulinum* toxin (botulism), hemorrhagic fever viruses (Ebola, Marburg, Lassa), *Bacillus anthracis* (anthrax)^, *Yersinia pestis* (plague)^, *Francisella tularensis* (tularemia)^	
Agent of bioterrorism: Category B	*Brucella* spp. (brucellosis)^, *Coxiella burnetii* (Q fever), *Burkholderia mallei* (glanders)^, *Burkholderia pseudomallei* (melioidosis)^, *Chlamydia psittaci* (psittacosis)^, *Rickettsia prowazekii* (typhus)^, neuroinvasive arboviruses (EEE, WEE, VEE)	*Clostridium perfringens* epsilon toxin, *Salmonella* spp., *Staphylococcus* enterotoxin B, *Shigella dysenteriae, Escherichia coli* 0157:H7, *Vibrio cholerae* (cholera), multidrug-resistant organism (VRE, MRSA, CRE), *Cryptosporidium parvum*
Agent of bioterrorism: Category C	Nipah virus, hantavirus, tickborne hemorrhagic fever/encephalitis viruses, yellow fever virus	
Additional agents of special interest	*Mycobacterium tuberculosis*^, *Neisseria meningitidis*^, Creutzfeldt-Jakob disease#, MERS-CoV, SARS-CoV-1, SARS CoV-2, influenza virus, measles virus, *Coccidioides immitis*^	Hepatitis A virus, hepatitis B virus, hepatitis C virus, human immunodeficiency virus, rabies virus, *Mycobacterium leprae* (leprosy), *Rickettsia rickettsii* (Rocky Mountain spotted fever), *Candida auris*

**Avoid aerosolizing procedures, work in class II biosafety cabinet when possible, use of isolation room for postmortem examination; **PPE, including additional barrier precautions (face shield, eye protection), consider use of isolation room for postmortem examination; ^alert microbiology laboratory if cultures obtained; #label tissue cassettes and contact histology laboratory.*

Nationally Notifiable Infectious Diseases (in USA, 2023)

Bacterial/Toxin	Viral	Fungal and Parasitic
Anthrax	Arboviral diseases	*Candida auris*
Botulism	COVID-19	Coccidioidomycosis
Brucellosis	Dengue virus	Babesiosis
Campylobacteriosis	Hantavirus	Cryptosporidiosis
Chancroid	Hepatitis A	Cyclosporiasis
Chlamydia trachomatis	Hepatitis B	Giardiasis
Cholera	Hepatitis C	Malaria
Diphtheria	HIV infection	Trichinellosis
Ehrlichiosis and anaplasmosis	Influenza, pediatric mortality	
Gonorrhea	Measles	
Haemophilus influenzae	Mpox	
Hansen disease	Mumps	
Invasive pneumococcal disease	Novel influenza A virus	
Legionellosis	Poliomyelitis	
Leptospirosis	Rabies	
Listeriosis	Rubella	
Lyme disease	SARS	
Melioidosis	Smallpox	
Meningococcal disease	Varicella deaths	
Pertussis	Viral hemorrhagic fever	
Plague	Yellow fever	
Psittacosis	Zika virus	
Q fever		
Salmonella Paratyphi, *Salmonella* Typhi, salmonellosis		
Shiga toxin-producing *Escherichia coli*		
Shigellosis		
Spotted fever rickettsiosis		
Streptococcal toxic shock syndrome		
Syphilis		
Tetanus		
Tuberculosis		
Tularemia		
Vibriosis		
Carbapenemase-producing organisms		
Vancomycin-resistant *Staphylococcus aureus*		

GENERAL FEATURES

Types of Pitfalls and Artifacts

- False-positive: Presence of structures incorrectly identified as infectious organisms
  - Contamination of tissue block or slides with environmental microorganisms
  - Imitation of microorganisms by foreign material
  - Misidentification of normal human cells/tissue as microorganisms
- False-negative: True infection missed or misidentified as wrong organism
  - Special stains exhibit weak or negative signal
  - Negative or discordant molecular testing results in setting of histologically identified organisms
  - Misidentification of organisms due to orientation or miscalculation of size

Approach to Interpretation

- Always consider clinical context and correlate with concurrent cultures, serology, etc.
- Compare region of interest with all available stains when suspicious structures identified on any individual stain
- Repeat or obtain confirmatory stains with equivocal or unexpected results (and review controls)
- Rereview slides with unexpected molecular results to assess for likelihood of contamination
- Consult experts in infectious disease pathology as needed

BACTERIAL PITFALLS AND ARTIFACTS

Pigment Granules

- Distinguished from bacteria by morphology and staining characteristics; typically lack associated inflammation
- True microorganisms exhibit smooth outer contours and have homogeneous size and shape, while pigment granules are irregular with jagged and uneven contours
- **Endogenous pigments** occur widely in tissues, related to both normal physiologic (melanin, lipofuscin, bile) and pathologic (iron, copper) processes
  - Hemosiderin: Not birefringent with polarized light, stains deeply with Prussian blue (iron)

Antibiotic Treatment Effect

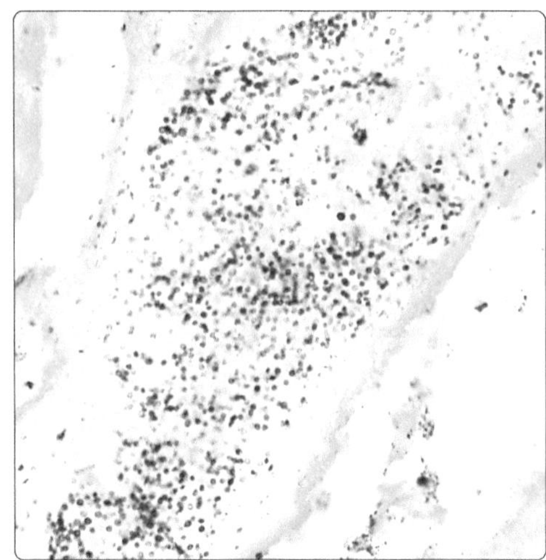

Warthin-Starry Stain: Melanocyte Dendrites Mimicking *Treponema pallidum*

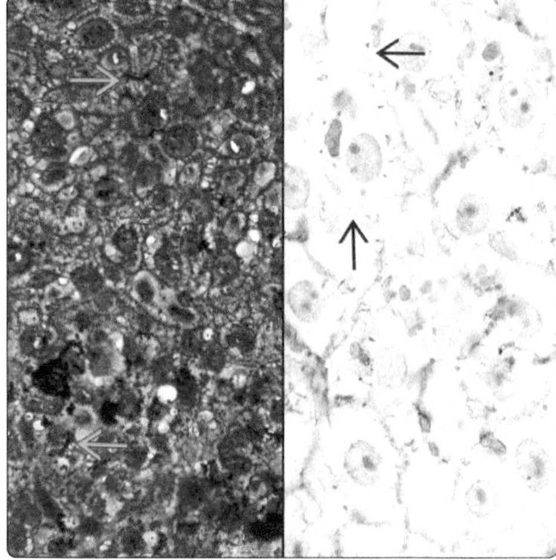

(Left) *Antibiotic treatment can cause changes in morphology and staining properties of bacteria, as in this case of gram-positive cocci with negative Gram stain (not shown) and slightly increased size, creating potential confusion with smaller yeast.* **(Right)** *Melanocyte dendrites may mimic spirochetes, given the elongated and beaded appearance ⇒, but are distinguished by the coarse nature of the reaction and intercellular localization. True treponemes are thin and delicate with spiraling corkscrew morphology ⇒.*

PAS Stain: Thin Capillaries Mimicking Fungal Hyphae

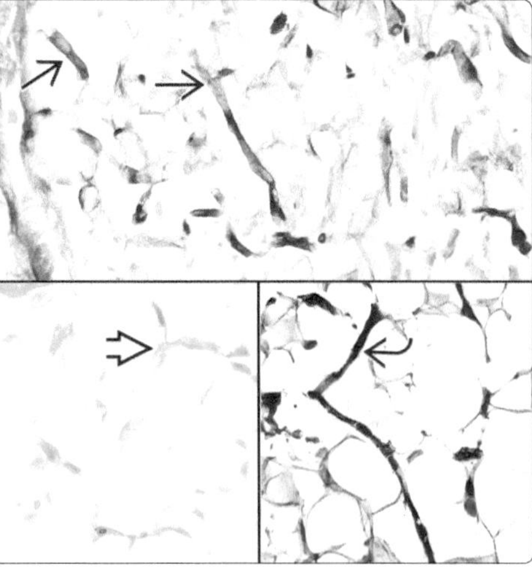

Collagen Fibers Mimicking Fungal Hyphae

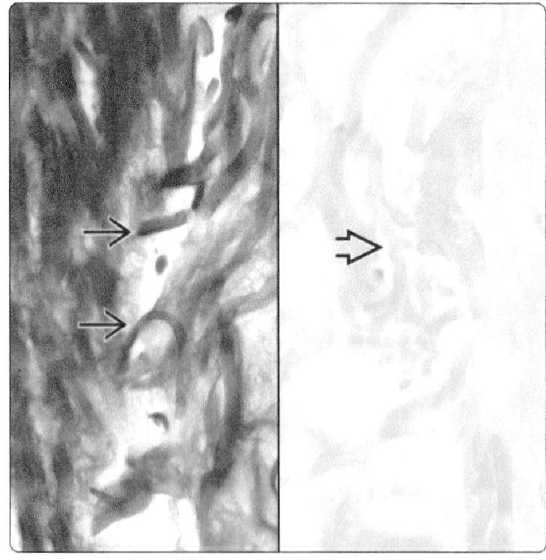

(Left) *PAS staining highlights the thin walls of capillaries simulating hyphae with apparent septation ⇒, which are negative on GMS stains ⇨ and positive with vascular markers, such as CD31 ⇨.* **(Right)** *Collagen fibers in dense connective tissue can mimic fungal hyphae ⇒ and may even appear to show branching. The wavy, uneven appearance of the fibers, the lack of associated inflammation, and negative GMS staining ⇨ can help rule out infection.*

- Melanin: Normally along basal layer of epidermis and as "protective cap" on keratinocytes but can be seen in phagocytic cells, subset of neurons (neuromelanin), and leptomeninges
  - Highlighted by stains used for microorganisms (GMS, Fontana-Masson, Warthin-Starry)
  - Differentiated with immunohistochemical stains (S100 and HMB-45)
- Lipofuscin: Fine yellow-brown "wear and tear" pigment granules within macrophages; common in liver, kidney, heart, adrenals, and neurons
  - Not birefringent with polarized light, negative with Prussian blue
  - Positive for Sudan black B
- Dystrophic calcifications: Variably sized with irregular edges, can be eosinophilic or basophilic, often seen in cardiac valves and areas of trauma; can resemble bacterial cocci
  - Refractile and positive with Von Kossa stain (calcium)
  - Negative with GMS, Gram

- **Exogenous pigments** can occur in specific anatomic sites (e.g., dermal tattoo ink, thyroid with minocycline) or following tissue processing (formalin, gross room ink)
  - Formalin: Birefringent using polarized light, extracellular
  - Carbon (anthracotic pigment): Variably sized intra- and extracellular granules, often in macrophages in lungs and lymph nodes; appears black on most stains

Nonspecific Staining

- AFB stains (Ziehl-Neelsen, Fite-Faraco)
  - Stain precipitate or nonspecific staining can be mistaken for mycobacteria, which should appear rod-shaped (bacillary) with smooth contours and regular caliber, in appropriate inflammatory background
  - Environmental mycobacteria or those used in control slides can contaminate tissue slides, often on edge of tissue sections or out of plane of focus
  - Mast cell granules stain purple with AFB stains
- Gram stain (Brown and Brenn): Stain precipitate can resemble gram-positive cocci
- Warthin-Starry stain highlights melanocyte dendrites, which resemble spirochetes but lack thin delicate corkscrew morphology
- Bacterial immunohistochemistry frequently cross reacts between species and genera due to similarities in cellular components, requiring careful attention to morphology, clinical context, cultures, and molecular testing

Challenging Morphology

- Antimicrobials can alter expected morphology and staining pattern: Gram-positive cocci may appear larger and gram negative
- Rows of cocci may appear rod-like if reviewed at low magnification
- Filamentous bacilli may be mistaken for fungal hyphae if width of organisms are overestimated
- Gram-positive yeast (e.g., *Candida* spp.) may be mistaken for gram-positive cocci if size is underestimated
- Correlation with cultures, clinical scenario, and use of confirmatory molecular testing can be helpful

VIRAL PITFALLS AND ARTIFACTS

Koilocyte Mimics

- True koilocytes are mature squamous cells infected with human papillomavirus (HPV) with large, sharply demarcated halo (filled with viral proteins) and enlarged, hyperchromatic nucleus with irregular contours
- Inflammatory changes associated with other infections (*Trichomonas vaginalis*) can mimic koilocytes but are distinguished by their smaller, less well-demarcated perinuclear halo and lack of cytologic atypia
- Pregnancy-related navicular cells distinguished by yellow-brown glycogen vacuoles and lack of cytologic atypia

Herpes Simplex and Varicella-Zoster Virus Mimics

- Reactive endocervical cells can mimic herpes simplex virus (HSV)- or varicella-zoster virus (VZV)-infected cells with multinucleation and nuclear molding but lack characteristic ground-glass chromatin and chromatin margination

Melamed-Wolinska Bodies

- Variably sized eosinophilic inclusions seen in urothelial cells in urine cytology are nonspecific cytoplasmic globules
- Can be differentiated from viral inclusions by their cytoplasmic location and lack of associated viral-induced nuclear changes

Nuclear Pseudoinclusions

- Invaginations of cytoplasm into nucleus; can be confused with true viral inclusions
- Generally nonspecific but can be seen in certain pathologic entities (papillary thyroid carcinoma, meningioma, usual ductal hyperplasia)

Electron Microscopy

- Normal cellular structures misidentified as viral particles: Clathrin-coated vesicles, multivesicular bodies, and rough endoplasmic reticulum reported as SARS-CoV-2

FUNGAL PITFALLS AND ARTIFACTS

Corpora Amylacea

- Variably sized eosinophilic structures found in prostate, brain, and, occasionally, lung
- Round to elliptical (30-200 μm) with dense corse and laminated appearance
- Typically highlighted by GMS and PAS stains but distinguished from yeast by lack of budding and stereotypical appearance

Gamna-Gandy Bodies

- Variably sized yellow-brown objects consisting of elastic fibers encrusted with calcium and iron (organization of small hemorrhages)
- Can be confused with fungal hyphae; usually negative by GMS but may be PAS positive
- Iron will stain positively with Prussian blue

Hamazaki-Wesenberg Bodies

- Small, round to oval ceroid bodies in lymph node sinuses
- Can resemble yeasts in lymph nodes; stain positively with GMS, PAS, and Fontana-Masson and sometimes appear to have budding forms

- Distinguished by yellow-brown color on H&E, size variability, and lack of host immune response

Myospherulosis

- Lipogranulomatous foreign body reaction to endogenous (breast, skin) or exogenous (medications, ointments, lubricated gauze) lipids
- Cyst-like structure with outer fibrous tissue filled with irregular variably sized eosinophilic spherules (up to 150 µm); resembles endosporulating organisms (*Coccidioides* spp., *Rhinosporidium seeberi*)
- Differentiated by pleomorphic appearance and lack of staining with GMS and PAS

Plant Material

- Undigested vegetable fibers can resemble fungal hyphae
- Often found in GI or abdominal specimens, distinguished by repeating square segments with rigid cell walls (cellulose)

Host Cells and Tissues

- Connective tissue: Collagen and elastin fibers may mimic fungal hyphae but have wavy appearance with greater size differentiation; may stain positively with GMS (in heavy preparations); negative PAS, positive trichrome
- RBCs may mimic yeasts but show no budding or capsule formation; can be GMS positive in heavy preparations
- Intracellular debris within phagocytic WBCs may stain positively with GMS or PAS and mimic intracellular organisms (e.g., *Histoplasma* spp., *Leishmania* spp.)

Environmental Contaminants

- Fungal spores and pollen granules are ubiquitous in atmosphere and may contaminate specimens throughout collection and processing
- Can be distinguished by presence on single slide, location at or away from tissue edge, out-of-focus plane
- Pollen granules are round or ovoid (6-100 µm) with double wall, outer wall can be smooth or rough; may resemble yeasts or endospores of *Coccidioides* spp. but distinguished by lack of budding and absence of specific pathogen characteristics
- Microalgae diatoms (2-200 µm) can be circular, elliptical, or triangular in shape; may occur via water contamination during processing, also associated with drowning
- Fiber contaminants from cotton swabs, hair, Cytobrush bristles, and tampons can be present in cytologic samples and confused with fungal hyphae

PARASITE PITFALLS AND ARTIFACTS

Melanosomes in Vitreous Fluid

- Can resemble *Toxoplasma gondii* and amastigotes of *Leishmania;* may be distinguished by immunohistochemistry (S100 and HMB-45 positive)

Liesegang Rings

- Round to oval laminated structures (5-1000 µm) with dense central core and fine radial striations; resembles parasite eggs (*Taenia* spp.) and *Echinococcus* spp. protoscoleces
- Associated with benign cysts and inflammatory tissue in variety of organs (kidney, breast, pleura, pericardium)
- Nonrefractile, stain positive with many stains (H&E, Pap, AFB, Gram stain, Masson trichrome, keratin, and epithelial membrane antigen)
- Negative GMS, PAS, von Kossa, Congo red, and iron stains

Uric Acid Crystals

- Can be lemon- or diamond-shaped (30-100 µm) and resemble eggs of *Schistosoma hematobium* when found in urine specimens
- Distinguished by lack of internal nuclei, fractured appearance with variation in shape and size, and presence of "points" on both ends
- Refractile and birefringent with polarized light

Foreign Bodies

- Splinters, plant materials, or embolic materials may resemble parasites in tissue
- Can usually be distinguished from roundworms by lack of internal structures (gut, testes, ovaries)
- Elastin stain may be useful to identify outline of blood vessel wall surrounding embolic materials

Curschmann Spirals

- Inspissated mucus forming cast-like structure in small bronchi and bronchioles can be confused as parasitic larvae or adult worm

Plant Material

- Seeds or pollen grains may be confused with parasitic eggs (e.g., *Enterobius vermicularis* in cervicovaginal smears)
  - *E. vermicularis* eggs distinguished by characteristic thick, double-contoured birefringent shell with internal granular embryo or bright orange-staining larvae
  - Pollen grains have 2 layers, including outer rough layer with warts or troughs
- Seeds and grains can have variable internal structures, including bright red globular spherules or repeating rectangles
  - Legume grains contain starch granules and are vaguely reminiscent of *Coccidioides* spp. spherules
  - Seeds are often found in GI specimens, particularly appendices

SELECTED REFERENCES

1. Issin G et al: Seeds or parasites? Clinical and histopathological features of seeds and parasites in the appendix. Turk Patoloji Derg. 39(1):42-54, 2023
2. Bullock HA et al: Difficulties in differentiating coronaviruses from subcellular structures in human tissues by electron microscopy. Emerg Infect Dis. 27(4):1023-31, 2021
3. Baker C et al: Pattern of cross-reactivity between mycobacterial immunohistochemical stain and normal human eosinophils: a potential pitfall in the diagnosis of cutaneous mycobacterial infections. Am J Dermatopathol. 42(5):368-71, 2020
4. Muzarath S et al: Contaminants and mimickers in cytopathology. J Cytol. 37(3):131-5, 2020
5. Razzano D et al: Disease, drugs, or dinner? Food histology can mimic drugs and parasites in the gastrointestinal tract. Virchows Arch. 477(4):593-5, 2020
6. Almarzooqi S et al: Artifacts and organism mimickers in pathology: case examples and review of literature. Adv Anat Pathol. 17(4):277-81, 2010
7. Ip YT et al: Nuclear inclusions and pseudoinclusions: friends or foes of the surgical pathologist? Int J Surg Pathol. 18(6):465-81, 2010
8. Martínez-Girón R et al: Erythrocytes as funguslike artifacts in pulmonary cytology. Acta Cytol. 51(2):247-8, 2007
9. Martínez-Girón R et al: Worm-like artifacts in exfoliative cytology. Diagn Cytopathol. 34(9):636-9, 2006
10. van Hoeven KH et al: Prevalence, identification and significance of fiber contaminants in cervical smears. Acta Cytol. 40(3):489-95, 1996

Corpora Amylacea Mimicking Fungal Yeast

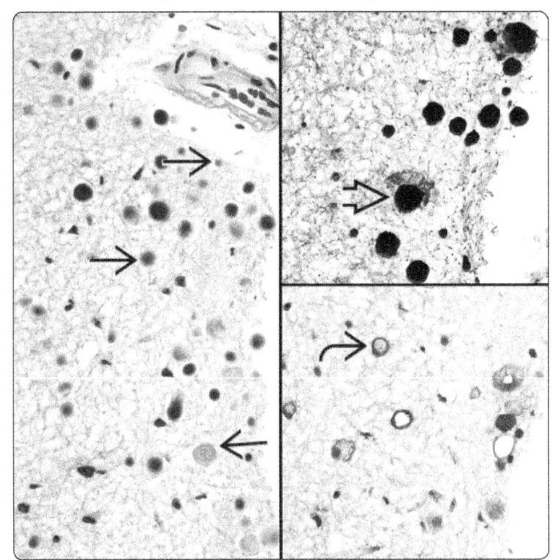

Melanin Pigment

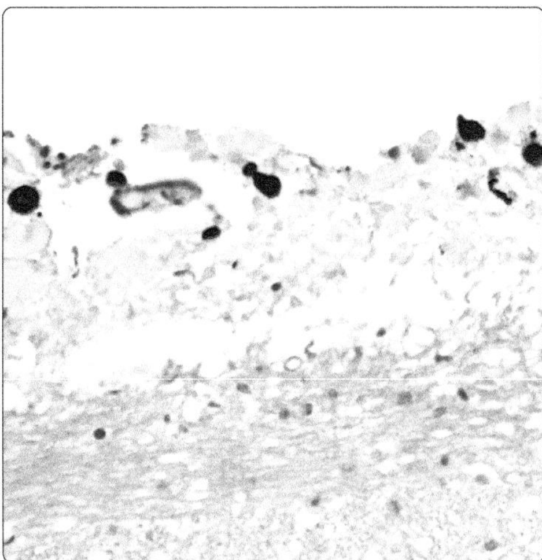

(Left) *Corpora amylacea are round, eosinophilic, variably sized structures with a dense core and laminated appearance ➙ that stain positive with GMS ➙ and PAS ➙ but can be differentiated from yeast by lack of budding and stereotypical appearance.* **(Right)** *Melanin pigment can be stained by silver stains (mimicking bacteria or fungi) and can be confused with positive IHC staining mimicking viral infection. The latter can be easily distinguished by identification of brown pigment on H&E stains.*

Lentil vs. Coccidiomycosis

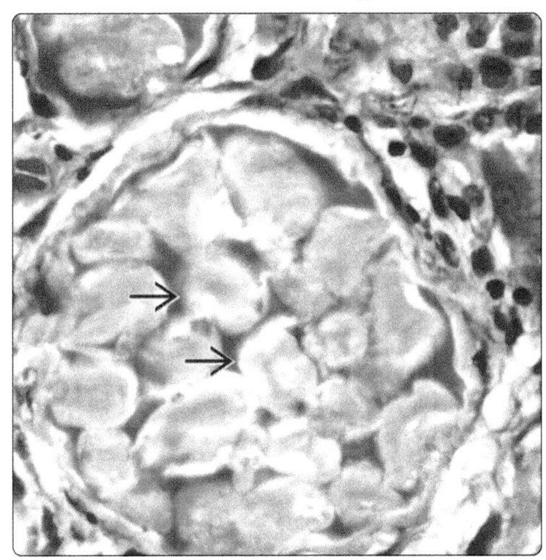

Plant Material Mimicking Fungi/Parasites

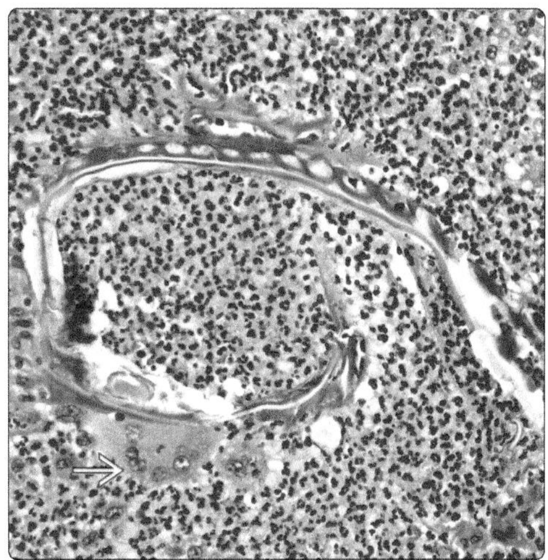

(Left) *Legume grains contain large starch granules ➙ and may mimic the spherules with endospores of coccidiomycosis. The large size, lack of a refractile wall, and context (GI tract specimen) are useful in making the distinction. (Courtesy A. Velez Hoyos, MD.)* **(Right)** *Abundant acute inflammation with adjacent ➙ multinucleated giant cell is associated with a vegetable fiber, distinguished from fungal hyphae or parasite larvae by plant cell walls made of repeating squares and lack of septations or branching.*

Environmental Contaminants in Cytology

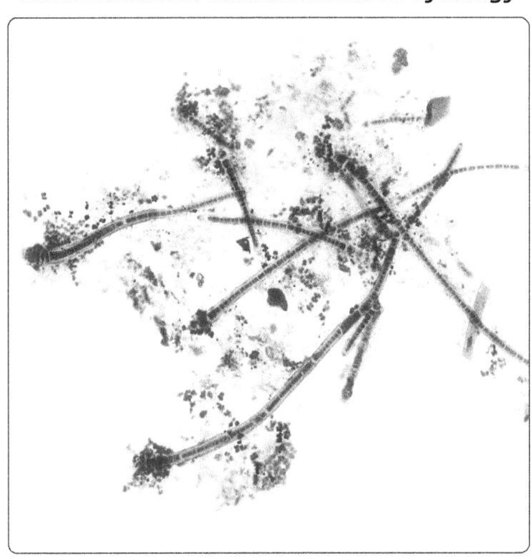

Cytology: Pollen Grains vs. Yeast

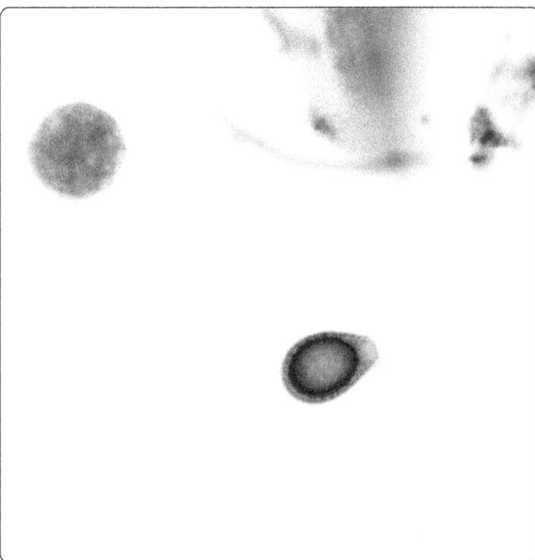

(Left) *This cytology specimen contains fibrils resembling fungal hyphae but favored to be an environmental contaminant compatible with plant material.* **(Right)** *Pollen grains are ubiquitous in the environment and can contaminate specimens throughout collection and processing. They can be distinguished from yeasts by their double cell wall and lack of budding.*

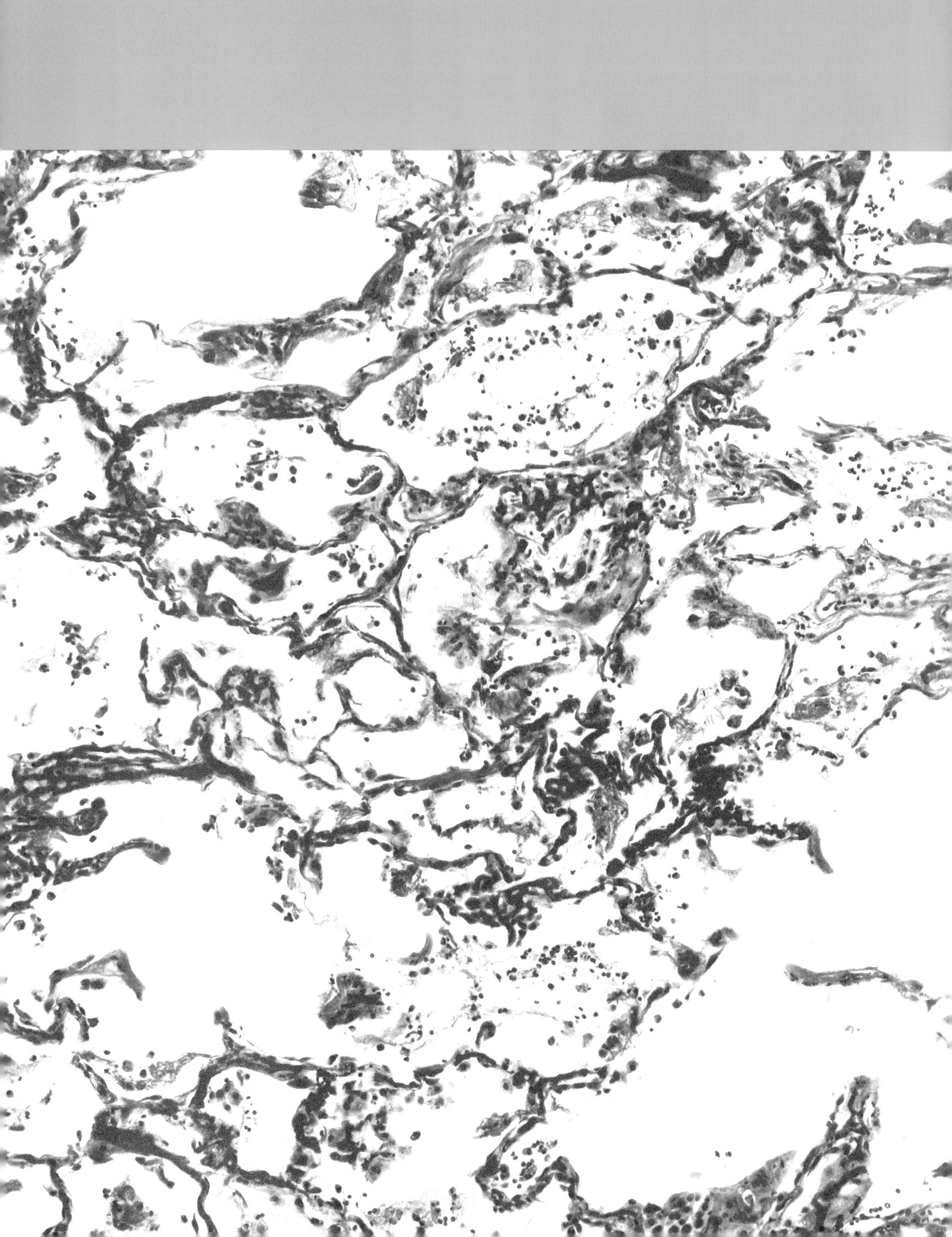

SECTION 2
Viral Infections

DNA Viruses

RNA Viruses

Herpes Simplex Virus 1 and 2 (HSV-1, HSV-2) Infections

KEY FACTS

ETIOLOGY/PATHOGENESIS

- Viral infections transmitted in vesicle fluid, saliva, and vaginal secretions; vertical transmission during childbirth

CLINICAL ISSUES

- > 80% of American/European adults have antibodies to herpes simplex virus 1 (HSV-1) (20% to HSV-2)
- Primary infections (oral or genital skin/mucosa) typically self-limited but can be life threatening with central nervous system/liver involvement
- Laboratory: IgM/IgG, PCR, direct antigen testing
- Treatment: Acyclovir for severe infections

MICROSCOPIC

- Skin: Epithelial vesicles; pustules with neutrophils
- Oral mucosa, esophagus: Ulceration, sloughed epithelial cells, neutrophilic infiltrate
- Liver: Coagulative necrosis with minimal inflammation
- Lung: Necrotizing pneumonia or diffuse interstitial pneumonitis
- Lymph nodes: Focal necrosis of interfollicular/paracortical regions
- Brain: Hemorrhage and necrosis predominantly in cortex
- Neonatal: Placenta typically normal; fetus with necrosis of liver, adrenal cortex, lungs, and brain
- Viral cytopathic effects include multinucleation, molding, and margination of chromatin; Cowdry type A inclusions

ANCILLARY TESTS

- HSV-1 and HSV-2 IHC performed as cocktail

TOP DIFFERENTIAL DIAGNOSES

- Varicella-zoster virus: Distinguish by IHC or PCR
- Cytomegalovirus: Larger cells with nuclear and cytoplasmic inclusions
- Adenovirus: Smudged nuclear inclusions
- Other viral and bacterial infections: Correlate with IHC, special stains, molecular testing, and cultures

(Left) *Transmission electron micrograph shows numerous spherical, enveloped virions measuring ~ 150 nm in diameter with icosahedral capsid, characteristic of herpes simplex viruses 1 and 2 (HSV-1, HSV-2). (Courtesy F. Murphy, DVM, PhD.)* **(Right)** *Photograph shows the lips of a patient with a herpes simplex lesion on the lower lip, on the 2nd day after onset, due to HSV-1. (Courtesy K. Hermann, MD, CDC/PHIL.)*

Ultrastructural Features

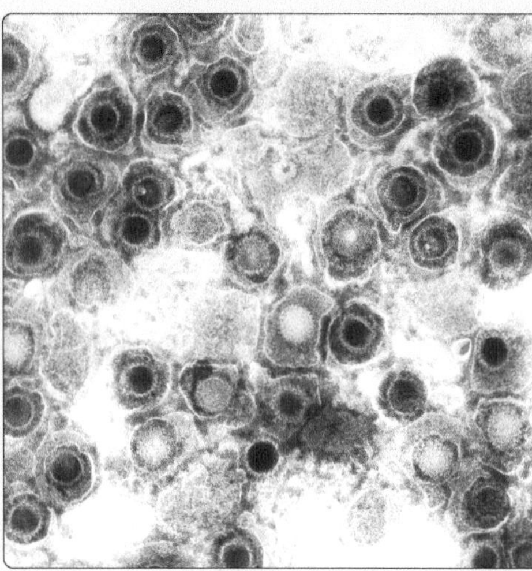

Herpes Labialis (Cold Sore)

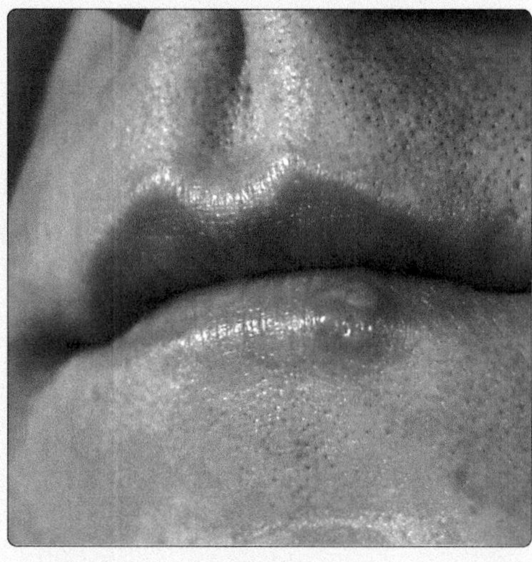

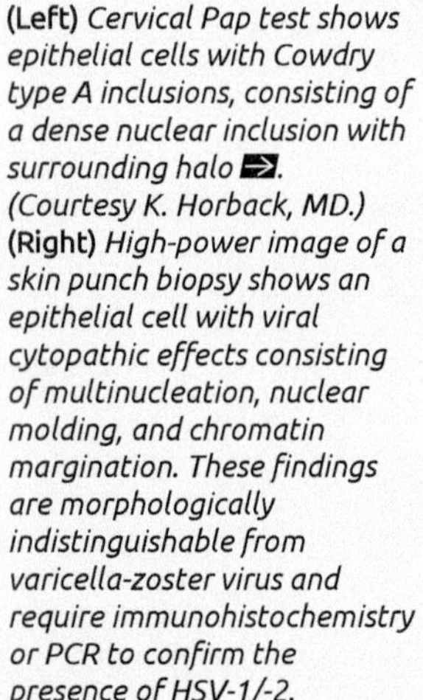

(Left) *Cervical Pap test shows epithelial cells with Cowdry type A inclusions, consisting of a dense nuclear inclusion with surrounding halo ➔. (Courtesy K. Horback, MD.)* **(Right)** *High-power image of a skin punch biopsy shows an epithelial cell with viral cytopathic effects consisting of multinucleation, nuclear molding, and chromatin margination. These findings are morphologically indistinguishable from varicella-zoster virus and require immunohistochemistry or PCR to confirm the presence of HSV-1/-2.*

HSV Cervicitis Cytology

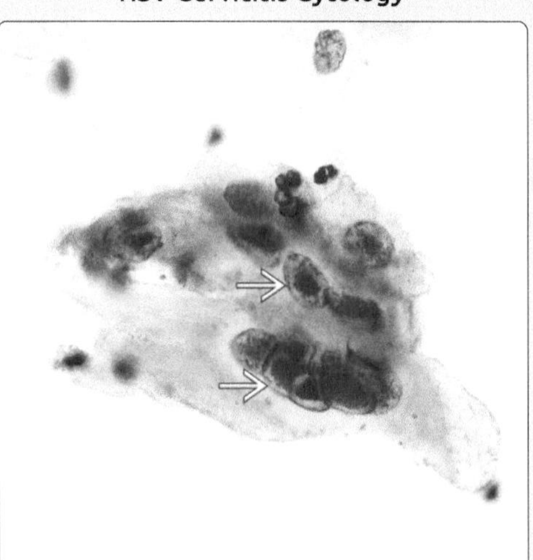

Viral Cytopathic Effects in Tissue

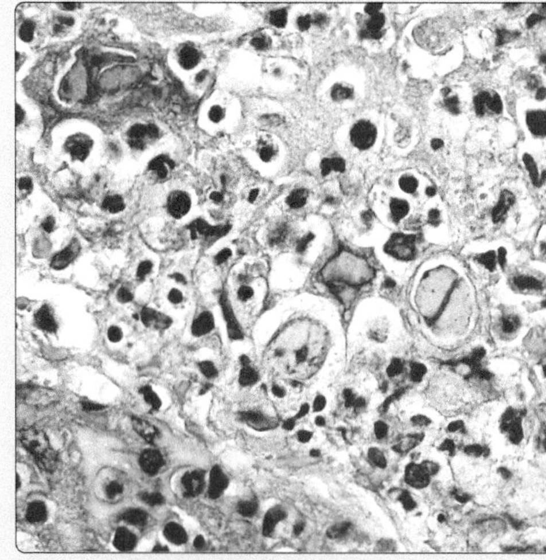

TERMINOLOGY

Synonyms

- *Human alphaherpesvirus 1*; herpes simplex virus 1 (HSV-1)
- *Human alphaherpesvirus 2*; herpes simplex virus 2 (HSV-2)
- Genital herpes, cold sore or fever blister, herpetic whitlow, herpes gladiatorum, ocular herpes, neonatal herpes, herpes encephalitis, Mollaret meningitis

Definitions

- *Herpesviridae* family: Derived from "herpein" (to creep)

ETIOLOGY/PATHOGENESIS

Infectious Agents

- Viral infections transmitted in vesicle fluid, saliva, and vaginal secretions, causing oral and genital lesions
- Virus also transmitted vertically during childbirth
- Entry into mucoepithelial cells by viral glycoprotein B (gB) binding to heparan sulfate, followed by nectin-1- and HveA-mediated fusion with plasma membrane, resulting in lytic infection
- Latency in neurons (e.g., trigeminal and sacral ganglia) with local reactivation in immunocompetent individuals and dissemination in immunosuppressed
- Virus modified for use as antitumor therapy (oncolytic HSV); T-VEC FDA approved for melanoma; trials underway for high-grade gliomas; risk for disseminated disease very low

CLINICAL ISSUES

Epidemiology

- Common human viruses affecting any age group
- > 80% of American/European adults have antibodies to HSV-1 (20% to HSV-2)
- Incidence increases with age/number of oral contacts and sex partners
- Most common cause of sporadic viral encephalitis

Site

- Oral skin/mucosa (HSV-1), nongenital skin (HSV-1 or -2), genital skin (HSV-2), brain temporal lobe(s) (HSV-1), eye, liver

Presentation

- Primary infection
  - Painful new lesions of mouth/genitalia
  - Severe headache with temporal lobe signs
  - New onset of rash with historical contact
  - Newborn ocular lesions (infected mother)
  - New onset of right upper quadrant pain ± jaundice
- Reactivation
  - Resurgence of painful lesions on mouth/genitalia
  - New onset of disseminated rash (immunosuppressed)

Laboratory Tests

- Serology: IgM (primary infection), IgG (ongoing, latent, reactivation)
- PCR (CSF, plasma, tissue): Qualitative for primary diagnosis or quantitative following immunosuppression
  - Both single and multiplex assays can result in false-negatives, and repeat testing is recommended for clinically suspected cases of encephalitis
- Direct antigen detection: Immunofluorescence

Natural History

- Primary infections typically self-limited but can be life threatening with central nervous system/liver involvement
- Lifelong latency with reactivation triggered by traumatic injury, surgery, exposure to extreme elements, menstruation, other infections

Treatment

- No vaccines currently available
- Antivirals: Acyclovir, valacyclovir, famciclovir, penciclovir, trifluridine (ocular lesions)
  - Antiviral treatment can reduce asymptomatic shedding
  - Foscarnet for acyclovir-resistant patients
- Cesarean section in infected mothers with active disease

Prognosis

- Lifelong infection with common reactivation within 1st year of infection
- Fulminant disease (encephalitis &/or hepatitis) is rapidly fatal without treatment
- Immunosuppression leads to more severe disease with reactivation

IMAGING

Radiographic Findings

- Lungs: X-ray/CT: Patchy ground-glass opacities and consolidation with pleural effusion; typically diffuse and bilateral
- Brain: MR shows hyperintensity in medial temporal and inferior frontal lobes, often with bilateral involvement; neonatal encephalitis can be multifocal involving any lobe

MICROBIOLOGY

Virus Features

- Enveloped, double-stranded DNA viruses
- 110- to 200-nm diameter, icosahedral capsid
- 152,000-155,000 nucleotide genomes (encoding > 70 proteins)

Culture

- High-quality swab or needle aspiration placed in viral transport media required
- Virus propagated in HeLa cells, human diploid fibroblasts, and other cell lines, producing characteristic cytopathic effects within 1-3 days
- Often overgrows slower growing viruses (i.e., adenovirus, varicella-zoster virus, and cytomegalovirus), making exclusion of coinfection difficult
- Subtyping by HSV-1- or HSV-2-specific antibodies

MACROSCOPIC

General Features

- Skin: Vesicles/pustules with erythematous base
- Oral mucosa/esophagus: Linear to irregular ulcers with purulent crust
- Brain: Temporal lobe necrosis, hemorrhage; resolved infections with atrophy, cystic encephalomalacia, and calcifications

MICROSCOPIC

Histologic Features

- Skin
  - Epithelial vesicles; pustules with neutrophils
  - Nuclear viral inclusions adjacent to vesicles and inflammatory lesions
  - Deep stromal infections may occur in absence of keratinocyte infection
- Oral mucosa, esophagus
  - Ulceration, sloughed epithelial cells with exudate, neutrophilic infiltrate
  - Nuclear viral inclusions in sloughed mucosa or at edge of ulcer
- Liver
  - Extensive nonzonal coagulative necrosis with minimal inflammation
  - Nuclear viral inclusions at interface of necrotic and viable areas
- Lung
  - Necrotizing pneumonia or diffuse interstitial pneumonitis resembling diffuse alveolar damage
  - Nuclear viral inclusions at edges of necrotic foci
- Lymph nodes
  - Focal necrosis of interfollicular/paracortical regions with infected cells
  - Nuclear viral inclusions in lymphocytes, histiocytes, endothelial and epithelial cells
  - Can occur simultaneously with lymphoma
- Brain
  - Hemorrhage and necrosis predominantly involving cortex with extension into subcortical white matter with intense neutrophilic and lymphocytic infiltrates involving leptomeninges
  - Pseudoischemic form in immunosuppressed consists of widespread "red-dead" neurons with minimal inflammation
  - Nuclear viral inclusions in neurons, astrocytes, oligodendrocytes
- Neonatal
  - Placenta typically normal; rarely necrotizing lymphoplasmacytic villitis or viral inclusions
  - Fetus with necrosis of liver, adrenal cortex, lungs, and brain

Cytologic Features

- Mildly enlarged cells with range of nuclear inclusions
  - Ground-glass nuclei with margination of chromatin
  - Multinucleation and molding common in mucocutaneous lesions
  - Variable Cowdry A inclusions: Eosinophilic nuclear inclusion with halo
- Tzanck test/smear
  - Sterilely unroofed vesicle is smeared onto clean slide
  - Air dried, fixed with methanol, stained with Giemsa, Wright stain, Diff-Quik, Field stain, or methylene blue
  - Identifies multinucleated cells with viral cytopathic effect

ANCILLARY TESTS

Immunohistochemistry

- HSV antigen targets
  - Glycoproteins (polyclonal preparations)
  - Thymidine kinase (monoclonal preparation)
- HSV-1 and HSV-2 performed as cocktail
  - No distinction required for treatment
  - Overlap of both virus types for all conditions as well as oncolytic viruses

DIFFERENTIAL DIAGNOSIS

Varicella-Zoster Virus

- May appear identical to HSV-1/2 with classic Cowdry type A nuclei
- IHC or PCR required to distinguish

Cytomegalovirus

- Markedly enlarged cells with nuclear clearing and large intranuclear inclusion ("owl's-eye" nucleus) as well as multiple eosinophilic cytoplasmic inclusions
- Infects variety of cell types, including stromal cells and endothelial cells

Adenovirus

- Nuclear inclusions are typically single and more smudged in appearance

Other Viral Infections (All Sites)

- RNA viruses resulting in necrosis ± inflammation
- Reference testing for confirmation of other viral infections is recommended
- Animal (rabies, lymphocytic choriomeningitis virus) and insect (arboviruses) exposure helpful to narrow cause of viral meningoencephalitis

Bacterial Infections (All Sites)

- Destructive necrotic lesions
- Demonstration of bacteria on Gram or silver stains
- Positive cultures of bacteria from sample

SELECTED REFERENCES

1. Beekman KE et al: Four cases of disseminated herpes simplex virus following talimogene laherparepvec injections for unresectable metastatic melanoma. JAAD Case Rep. 33:56-8, 2023
2. Lindström J et al: Assessment of the FilmArray ME panel in 4199 consecutively tested cerebrospinal fluid samples. Clin Microbiol Infect. 28(1):79-84, 2022
3. Krystel-Whittemore M et al: Deep herpes. Am J Surg Pathol. 45(10):1357-63, 2021
4. Ho DY et al: Herpesvirus infections potentiated by biologics. Infect Dis Clin North Am. 34(2):311-39, 2020
5. Hodgson YA et al: Herpes simplex necrotic lymphadenitis masquerading as Richter's transformation in treatment-naive patients with chronic lymphocytic leukemia. J Hematol. 8(2):79-82, 2019
6. Valerio GS et al: Ocular manifestations of herpes simplex virus. Curr Opin Ophthalmol. 30(6):525-31, 2019
7. Pinninti SG et al: Neonatal herpes simplex virus infections. Semin Perinatol. 42(3):168-75, 2018
8. Bradshaw MJ et al: Herpes simplex virus-1 encephalitis in adults: pathophysiology, diagnosis, and management. Neurotherapeutics. 13(3):493-508, 2016
9. Anderson NW et al: Light microscopy, culture, molecular, and serologic methods for detection of herpes simplex virus. J Clin Microbiol. 52(1):2-8, 2014
10. Hoyt B et al: Histological spectrum of cutaneous herpes infections. Am J Dermatopathol. 36(8):609-19, 2014

HSV Skin Lesion

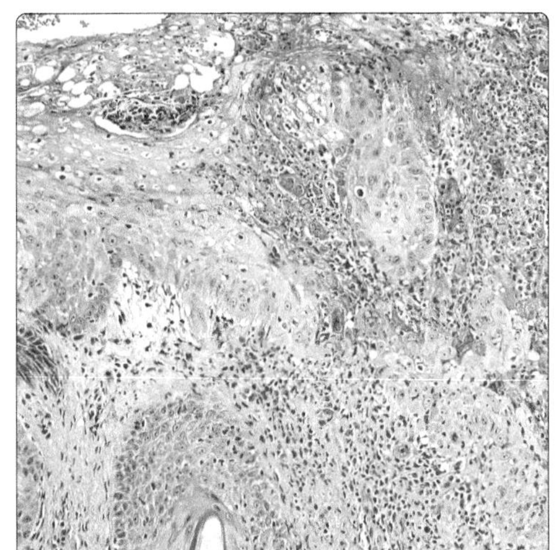

HSV Oral Mucosa Lesion

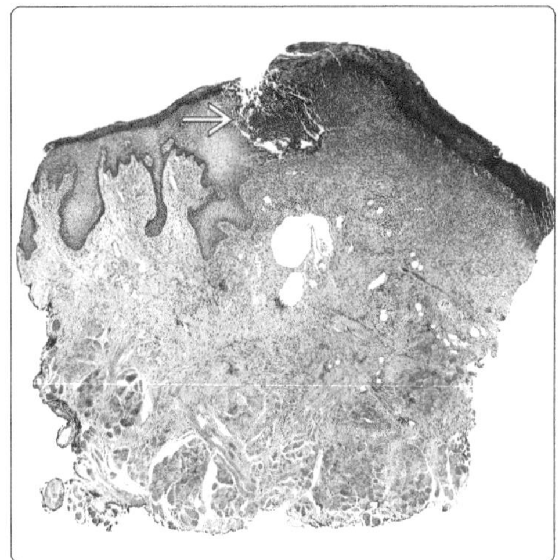

(Left) *Punch biopsy of a skin lesion on the buttock shows ulceration, acute and chronic inflammation, and necrosis.* **(Right)** *Low-power image of a punch biopsy of yellow-brown erosions on the anterior tongue reveal the presence of ulceration and necrosis ➡.*

HSV Oral Mucosa Lesion

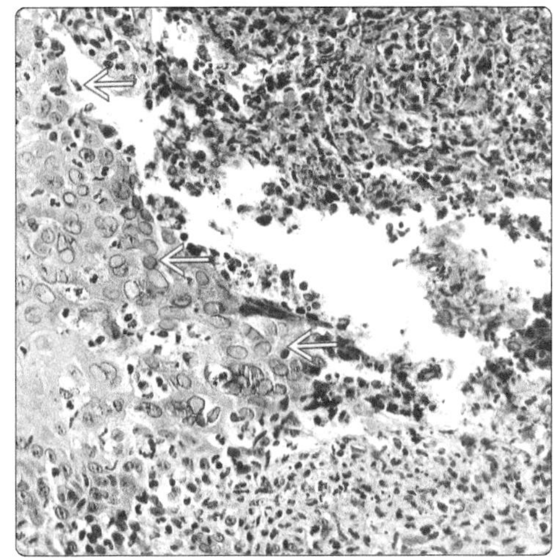

HSV Pneumonitis

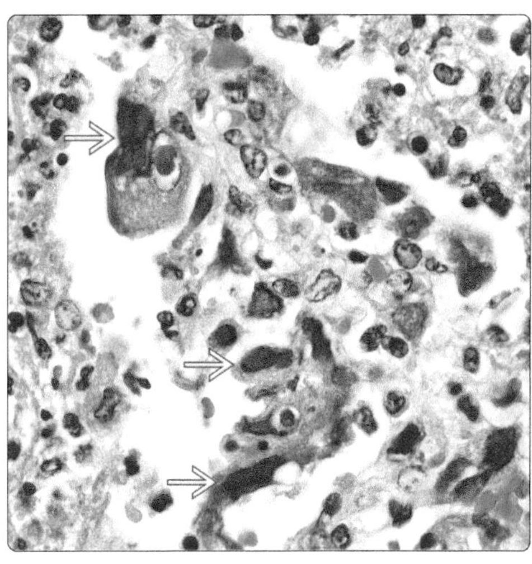

(Left) *Glassy nuclear inclusions ➡ are present in many epithelial cells adjacent to dense neutrophilic infiltrate in this anterior tongue biopsy.* **(Right)** *Autopsy lung section shows scattered multinucleated cells with molding and marginated chromatin ➡, features consistent with disseminated HSV infection.*

HSV Lymphadenitis: Histologic Features

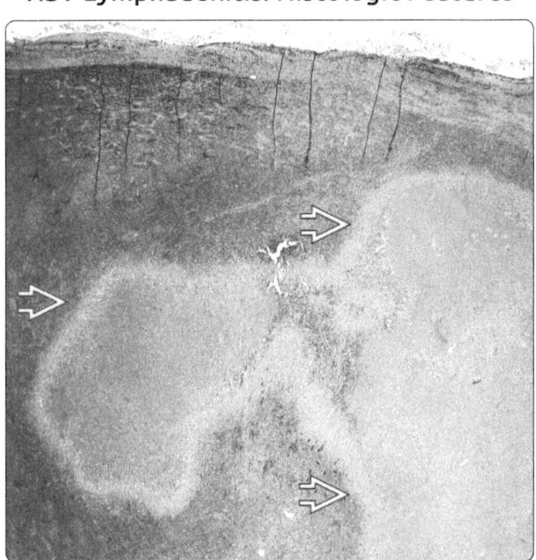

HSV Lymphadenitis: Immunohistochemistry

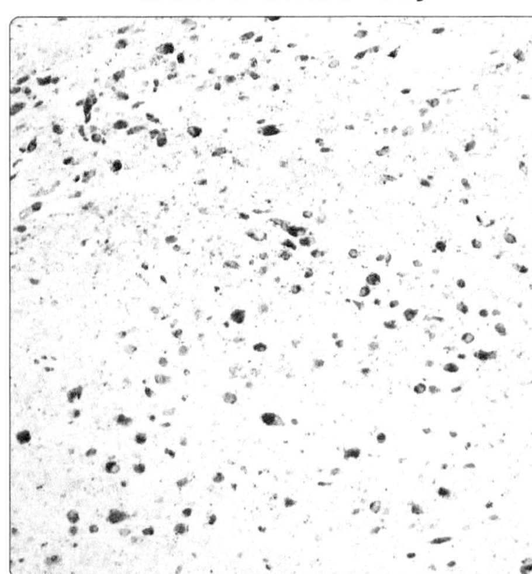

(Left) *Excisional biopsy of an inguinal lymph node shows a markedly enlarged lymph node with architecture effaced by chronic lymphocytic leukemia/small lymphocytic lymphoma containing large areas of coagulative necrosis ➡.* **(Right)** *HSV-1/2 immunohistochemistry from an inguinal lymph node demonstrates moderate to strong nuclear staining in scattered cells in the areas of geographic necrosis.*

(Left) *Esophageal biopsies show fragments of epithelium with dense inflammation containing cells that exhibit viral cytopathic effects →.* **(Right)** *Liver at autopsy from fulminant herpes simplex hepatitis shows geographic necrosis.*

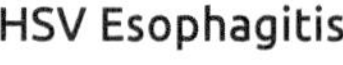

HSV Esophagitis

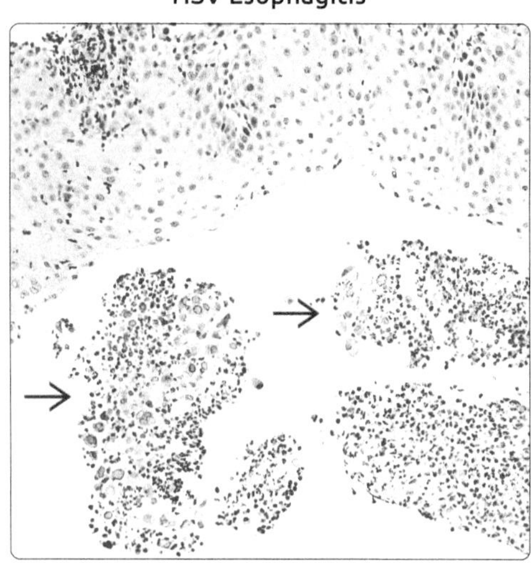

HSV Hepatitis: Gross Features

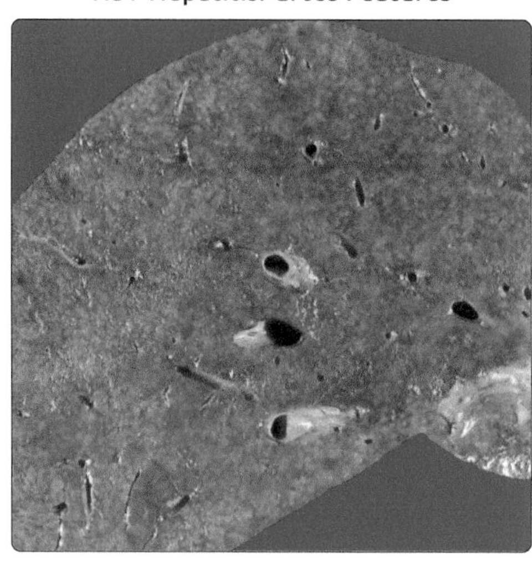

(Left) *Liver section from an autopsy of a patient who died of disseminated acute herpes simplex infection with fulminant hepatitis shows necrosis → adjacent to what appear to be viable cells →.* **(Right)** *HSV-1/2 immunohistochemistry from a fulminant hepatitis case demonstrates strong nuclear staining in infected viable cells as well as areas of necrosis.*

HSV Hepatitis: Histologic Features

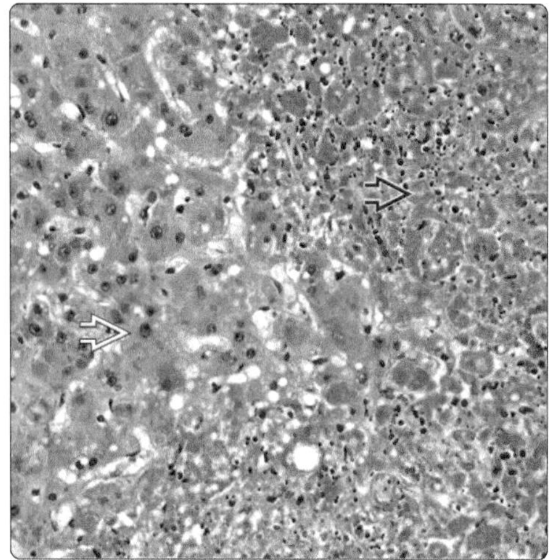

HSV Hepatitis: Immunohistochemistry

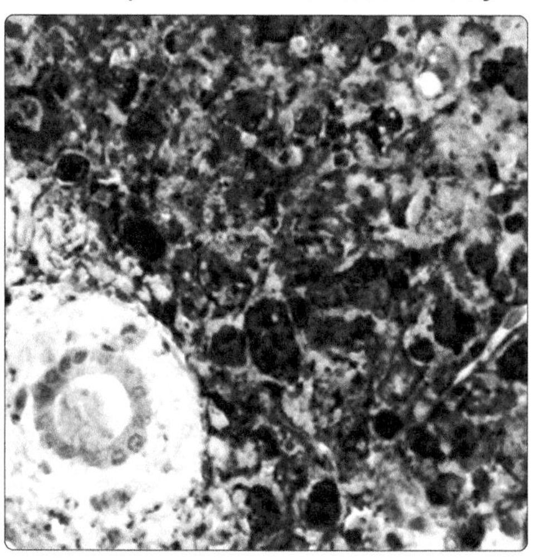

(Left) *Brain section from a fatal case of neonatal HSV-1 infection shows cells with viral cytopathic effect consisting of glassy nuclear inclusions and marginated chromatin →.* **(Right)** *HSV-1/2 immunohistochemistry from a neonatal HSV-1 case demonstrates strong staining in ependymal cells → as well as scattered cells in the choroid plexus →.*

Neonatal HSV Infection

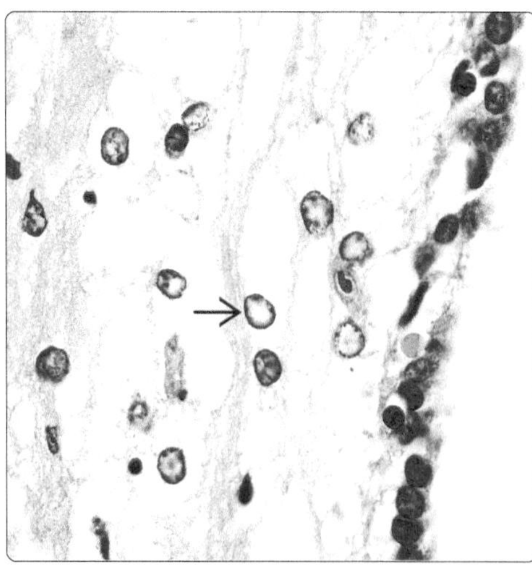

Neonatal HSV Infection: Immunohistochemistry

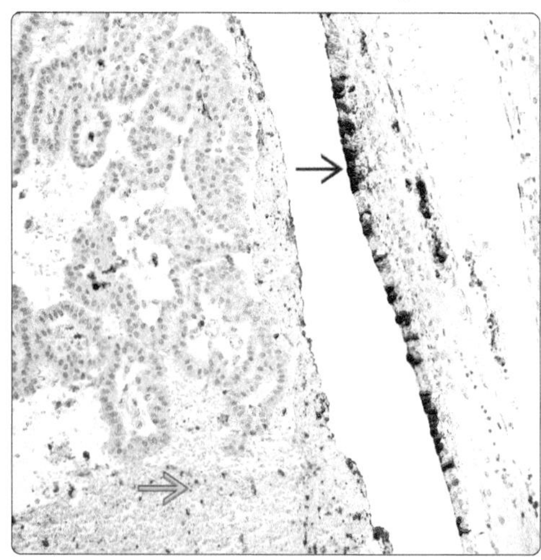

HSV Encephalitis: Radiographic Findings

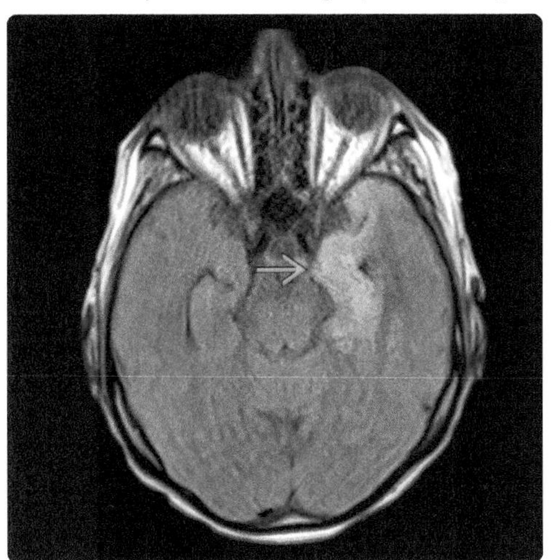

HSV Encephalitis: Gross Features

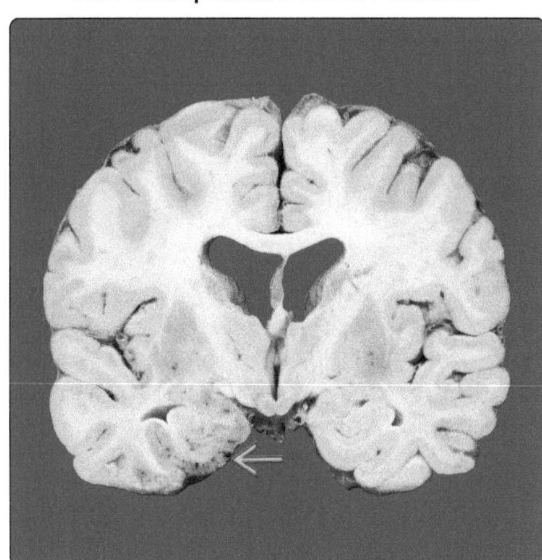

(Left) *FLAIR MR shows hyperintensity of the left temporal lobe ➡, a typical finding of HSV encephalitis. Bilateral involvement is often seen as well as the cingulate gyri and insular cortex with sparing of the basal ganglia.* **(Right)** *Photograph of a coronal brain section from a patient with fatal HSV-1 encephalitis shows discoloration in the left temporal lobe ➡, consistent with hemorrhage and necrosis.*

HSV Encephalitis: Histologic Features

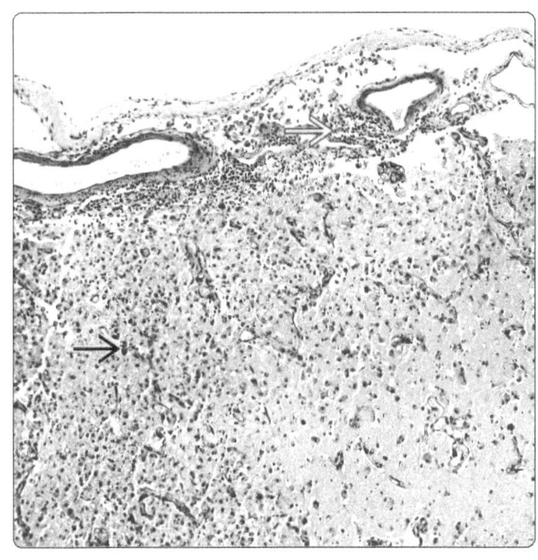

HSV Encephalitis: Immunohistochemistry

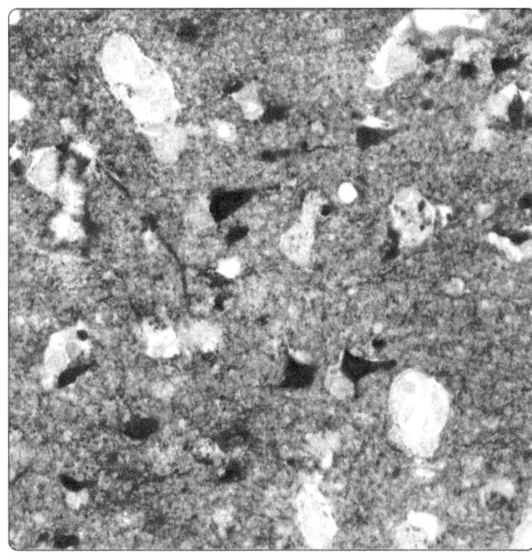

(Left) *Temporal lobe sections from a fatal case of HSV-1 encephalitis show necrotic, hypercellular cortex ➡ due to an influx of inflammatory cells. The overlying leptomeninges contain an infiltrate of lymphocytes and neutrophils ➡.* **(Right)** *HSV-1/2 immunohistochemistry from a temporal lobe section shows strong staining of cortical neurons, many of which are "red-dead" neurons simulating infarction.*

Resolved HSV Encephalitis

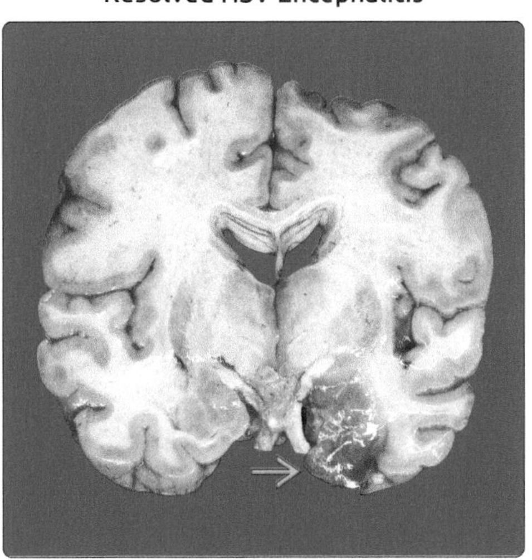

HSV Reactivation in Brain

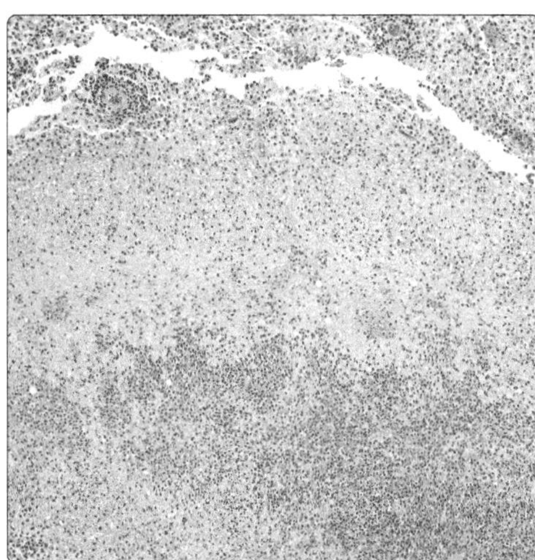

(Left) *Photograph shows a coronal section from a patient who died 10 years after surviving an episode of HSV encephalitis. The right temporal lobe exhibits atrophy and cystic encephalomalacia ➡.* **(Right)** *Inflammation and necrosis are shown in this autopsy brain section of a patient with a remote history of HSV encephalitis who developed new seizures during chemotherapy treatment. HSV immunohistochemistry highlighted rare positive cells suggestive of virus reactivation.*

Varicella-Zoster Virus (HHV-3) Infections

KEY FACTS

ETIOLOGY/PATHOGENESIS

- Transmission via airborne droplets or direct contact with lesions; latent virus reactivates in sensory nerve root ganglia and reaches skin by anterograde axonal transport

CLINICAL ISSUES

- Worldwide distribution; peak incidence in winter and spring in temperate climates
- Children < 1 year and adults are most at risk of complications and death
- Laboratory: RT-PCR, direct fluorescent antibody testing, serology (IgM, IgG)
- Vaccines for prevention of primary infection and reactivation; acyclovir and immunoglobulins for high risk

MACROSCOPIC

- Generalized vesicular rash (1-4 mm in diameter)
- Dermatomal distribution with reactivation

MICROSCOPIC

- Skin: Acantholysis or necrosis of epithelium, intraepidermal blister formation, lymphoid infiltrates, folliculitis
- CNS: Necrotizing vasculitis, small vessel vasculitis, encephalitis
- Cowdry type A eosinophilic intranuclear inclusions, ground-glass nuclei, syncytia formation

TOP DIFFERENTIAL DIAGNOSES

- HSV: VCPE indistinguishable from VZV; IHC, PCR, culture, or clinical correlation may be needed for diagnosis
- Monkeypox: Occasional Guarnieri bodies; confirm by IHC, PCR, and potential exposure history
- Hand, foot, and mouth disease: No distinctive VCPE; apoptosis of keratinocytes, edema, necrosis, and dyskeratosis; confirm by IHC, PCR
- Bullous pemphigoid: IgG and C3 basement membrane IF
- Pemphigus vulgaris: Epidermal intercellular IgG IF
- Contact dermatitis: Spongiosis with neutrophilic infiltrate

Ultrastructural Features

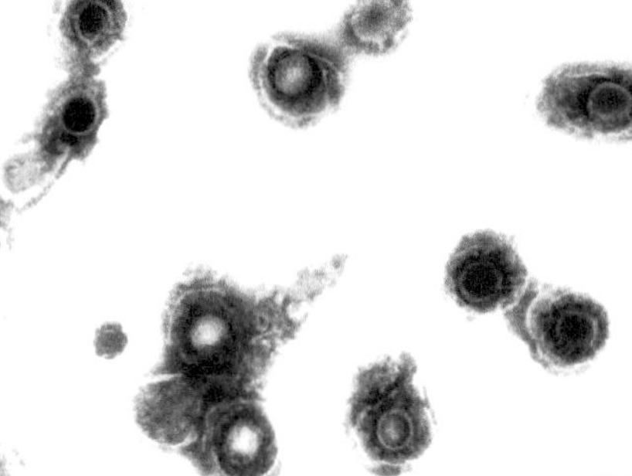

Chickenpox (Varicella)

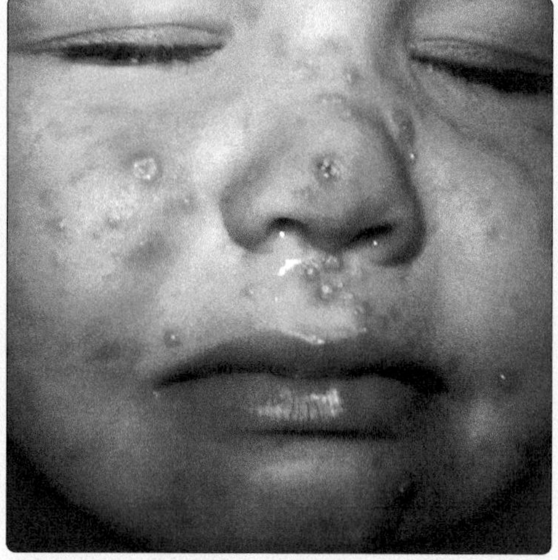

(Left) *Transmission electron micrograph from vesicle fluid shows spherical, enveloped particles measuring 180-200 nm in diameter, characteristic of varicella-zoster virus (VZV). (Courtesy E. Palmer, PhD, CDC/PHIL.)* **(Right)** *Clinical photograph depicts a number of vesicular chickenpox lesions on the face of a young child with primary VZV infection. (Courtesy J. Noble, Jr., MD, CDC/PHIL.)*

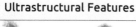

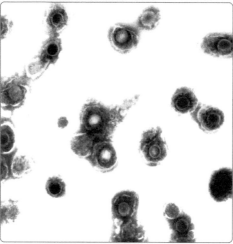

Skin Scraping: Tzanck Smear

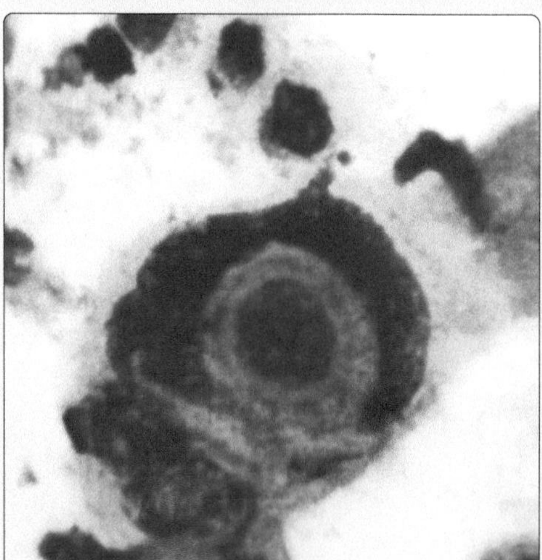

Viral Cytopathic Effects in Tissue Sections

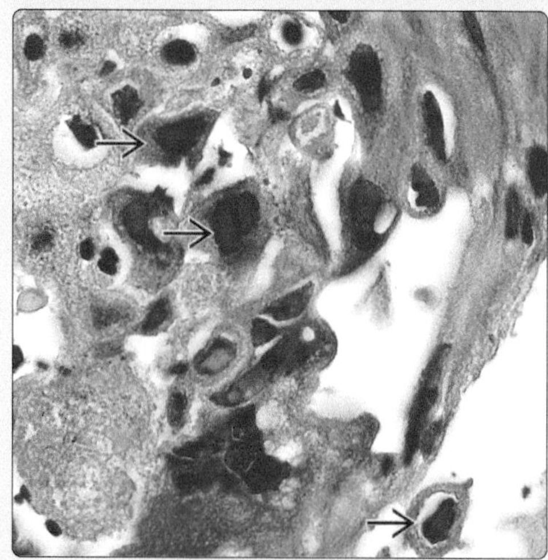

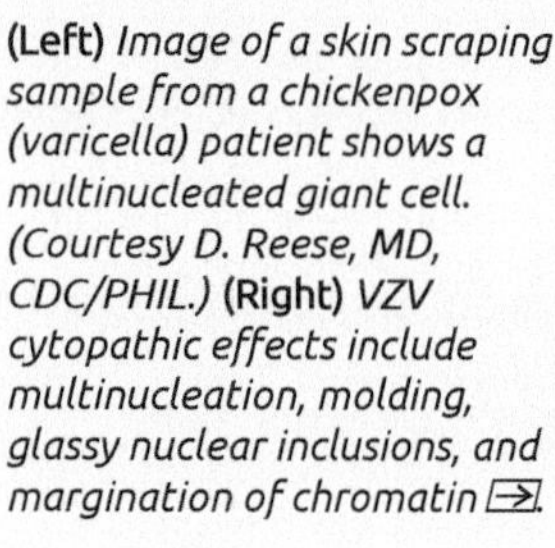

(Left) *Image of a skin scraping sample from a chickenpox (varicella) patient shows a multinucleated giant cell. (Courtesy D. Reese, MD, CDC/PHIL.)* **(Right)** *VZV cytopathic effects include multinucleation, molding, glassy nuclear inclusions, and margination of chromatin* ➙.

TERMINOLOGY

Synonyms

- Chickenpox virus, varicella virus, zoster virus
- Varicella-zoster virus (VZV)
- *Human alphaherpesvirus 3* (HHV-3)

Definitions

- Derived from New Latin term, "varicella" (diminutive of variola, denoting "speckled") and Greek term, "zoster" (belt)
- *Herpesviridae* family: Derived from "herpein" (to creep)

ETIOLOGY/PATHOGENESIS

Infectious Agents

- Viral infection spread via airborne droplets or direct contact with lesions; enters nasopharyngeal epithelium and conjunctiva, then spreads hematogenously
- Incubation period is 10-21 days; infectious from 1-2 days before rash until all blisters have formed scabs (5-7 days)
- Latent virus reactivates in sensory nerve root ganglia and reaches skin by anterograde axonal transport

CLINICAL ISSUES

Epidemiology

- Worldwide distribution; peak incidence in winter and spring in temperate climates
- USA: ~ 100% of population seropositive by adulthood; majority during first 4 years of life
- Prevaccine era (1995): 4 million cases annually, 12,000 hospital admissions, and 125 deaths; incidence, hospitalizations, and deaths decreased by > 90%

Presentation

- Primary infection (varicella, chickenpox): Mild prodrome followed by pruritic maculopapular then vesicular rash on head spreading to trunk and extremities
- Complications (infants, adults, immunocompromised) include secondary bacterial infection of skin lesions with bacteremia/sepsis, pneumonia, cerebellar ataxia, encephalitis, and hemorrhagic conditions
- Breakthrough varicella is milder form that can occur in vaccinated individuals
- Reactivation of latent virus (herpes zoster, shingles): Painful dermatomal vesicular rash, occasional ophthalmic nerve involvement leading to blindness (herpes zoster ophthalmicus), and dissemination to CNS, lungs, and liver

Laboratory Tests

- RT-PCR (skin lesions, CSF, bronchoalveolar lavage)
- Direct fluorescent antibody (DFA) testing of skin lesions
- Serology (IgM, 4-fold rise in IgG)
- Whole infected cell (wc) ELISA, purified glycoprotein ELISA (gpELISA), or fluorescent antibody to membrane antigen (FAMA) tests to detect seroconversion
- PCR genotyping to distinguish between wildtype or vaccine-type (Oka) strains

Treatment

- Primary prevention with live, attenuated vaccine; 2 doses (12-15 months, 4-6 years old)
- Recombinant zoster vaccine (RZV, Shingrix) licensed in 2017 by FDA; for adults > 50 years (> 18 if immunosuppressed); 2 doses 2-6 months apart
- Supportive treatment for uncomplicated children
- Acyclovir ± VZV immunoglobulin in immunocompromised, neonates, adults, and those with disseminated infection
- Gabapentin, amitriptyline, lidocaine, capsaicin, corticosteroids for shingles pain management

Prognosis

- Typically uncomplicated infections of 3- to 4-day duration
- Children < 1 year and adults are most at risk of complications: Bacterial infections, pneumonia, CNS infection, Reye syndrome, congenital varicella syndrome, herpes zoster (shingles), postherpetic neuralgia, and death

MICROBIOLOGY

Viral Features

- Enveloped, double-stranded DNA virus
- 180- to 200-nm diameter, icosahedral capsid
- 125,000 nucleotide genome [encoding > 70 open reading frames (ORFs)]

Culture

- Virus propagated in human foreskin fibroblasts, fetal kidney/lung cells, human lung carcinoma or human melanoma cell lines, and primary monkey kidney cells
- Cytopathic effect after 7-10 days (confirmed by PCR or DFA)

MACROSCOPIC

General Features

- Generalized vesicular rash: "Dew drop on rose petal" (1-4 mm in diameter)
- Dermatomal distribution with reactivation

MICROSCOPIC

Histologic Features

- Skin: Acantholysis or necrosis of epithelium, intraepidermal blister formation, lymphoid infiltrates, folliculitis
- CNS: Encephalitis, small vessel/necrotizing vasculitis
- Cowdry type A eosinophilic intranuclear inclusions, ground-glass nuclei, syncytia formation

ANCILLARY TESTS

Immunohistochemistry

- Anti-VZV Abs (red alkaline phosphatase preferred for skin)

DIFFERENTIAL DIAGNOSIS

Herpes Simplex Virus

- Viral cytopathic effects (VCPE) indistinguishable from VZV; IHC, PCR, culture, or clinical correlation may be needed for diagnosis

Monkeypox

- Occasional Guarnieri bodies; confirm by IHC, PCR, and potential exposure history

Hand, Foot, and Mouth Disease

- No distinctive VCPE; apoptosis of keratinocytes, edema, necrosis, and dyskeratosis; confirm by IHC, PCR

Impetigo, Eczema With Superimposed Infection, Bacterial Meningitis

- Neutrophilic infiltrate, positive Gram or silver stain demonstrating organisms

Bullous Pemphigoid

- IgG and C3 basement membrane IF

Pemphigus Vulgaris

- Epidermal intercellular IgG IF

Contact Dermatitis

- Spongiosis with neutrophilic infiltrate; clinical history/correlation important

SELECTED REFERENCES

1. Parameswaran GI et al: Increased stroke risk following herpes zoster infection and protection with zoster vaccine. Clin Infect Dis. 76(3):e1335-40, 2023
2. Bryant P et al: Vaccine strain and wild-type clades of varicella-zoster virus in central nervous system and non-CNS disease, New York State, 2004-2019. J Clin Microbiol. 60(4):e0238121, 2022
3. Dooling K et al: Clinical manifestations of varicella: disease is largely forgotten, but it's not gone. J Infect Dis. 226(Suppl 4):S380-4, 2022
4. Lenfant T et al: Neurological complications of varicella zoster virus reactivation: prognosis, diagnosis, and treatment of 72 patients with positive PCR in the cerebrospinal fluid. Brain Behav. 12(2):e2455, 2022
5. Marin M et al: Decline in severe varicella disease during the United States varicella vaccination program: hospitalizations and deaths, 1990-2019. J Infect Dis. 226(Suppl 4):S407-15, 2022
6. Tommasi C et al: The biology of varicella-zoster virus replication in the skin. Viruses. 14(5):982, 2022
7. Gershon AA et al: Varicella zoster virus infection. Nat Rev Dis Primers. 1:15016, 2015
8. Science M et al: Central nervous system complications of varicella-zoster virus. J Pediatr. 165(4):779-85, 2014
9. Leinweber B et al: Histopathologic features of cutaneous herpes virus infections (herpes simplex, herpes varicella/zoster): a broad spectrum of presentations with common pseudolymphomatous aspects. Am J Surg Pathol. 30(1):50-8, 2006

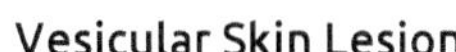

Vesicular Skin Lesion | **Immunohistochemistry: Skin Vesicle**

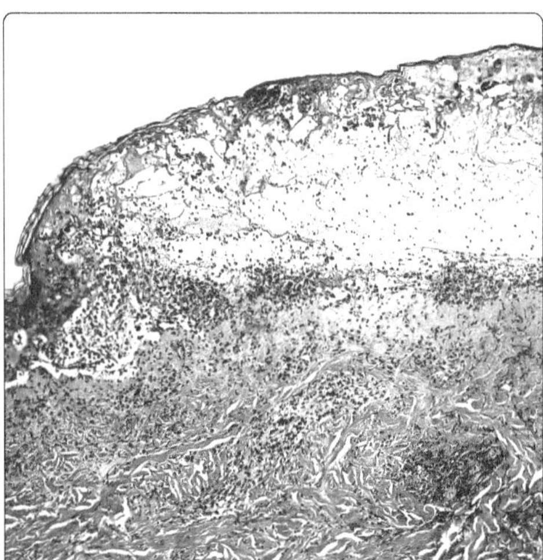

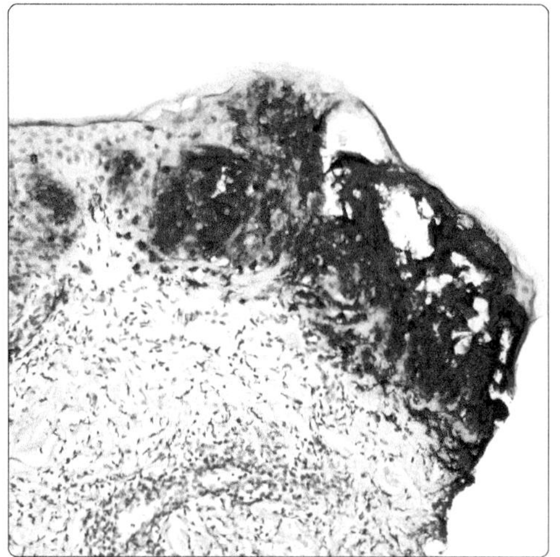

(Left) *H&E section through a vesicular lesion shows intraepidermal serous fluid with marked inflammation and scattered, acantholytic, virally infected cells.* **(Right)** *Immunohistochemical staining with anti-VZV antibody (red) shows numerous virally infected, intraepidermal epithelial cells.*

Folliculitis | **Immunohistochemistry: Folliculitis**

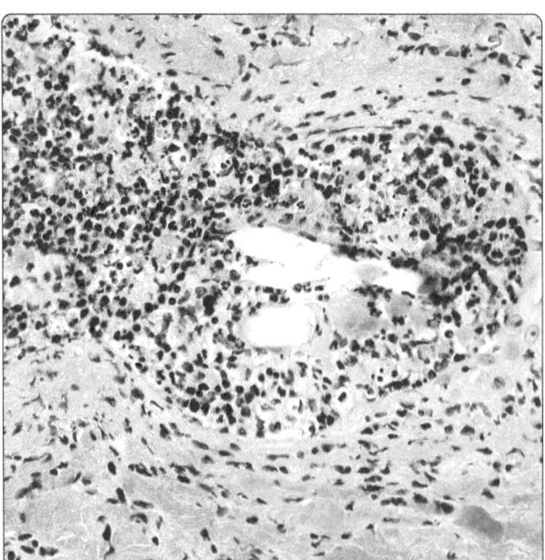

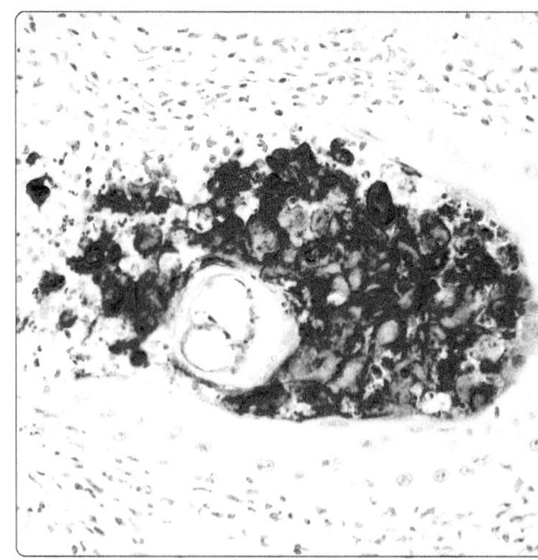

(Left) *Hair follicle involvement can be seen with VZV reactivation and is characterized by acantholysis, dyskeratosis, multinucleated keratinocytes, and necrosis of the hair follicle. Viral inclusions may not be readily apparent.* **(Right)** *Immunohistochemical staining with anti-VZV antibody (red) shows numerous virally infected hair follicle cells.*

Viral Cytopathic Effects

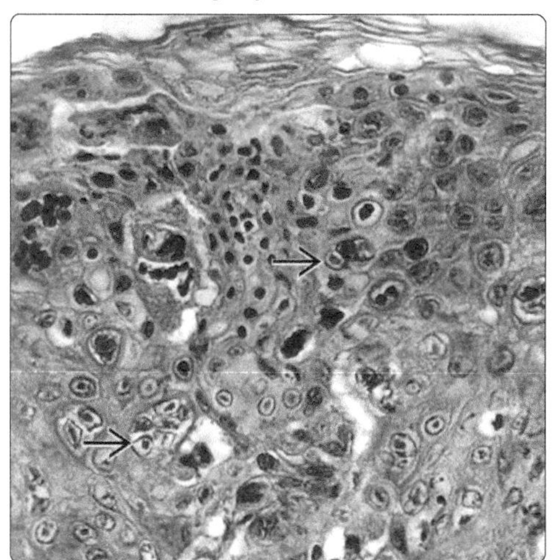

Shingles (Herpes Zoster)

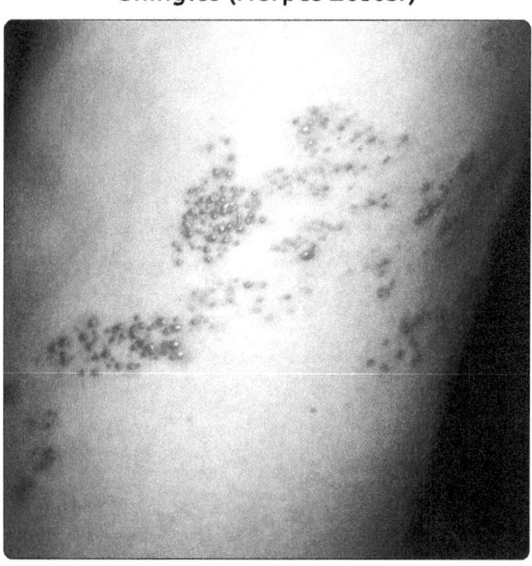

(Left) *Infected skin demonstrates the characteristic eosinophilic Cowdry type A nuclear inclusion bodies* ⮕. *(Courtesy Franz von Lichtenberg Collection of Infectious Disease Pathology, BWH.)* **(Right)** *This painful maculopapular rash is present at the T10-T11 dermatome, a pattern characteristic of VZV reactivation within a specific dorsal root ganglion. (Courtesy K. Herrmann, MD, CDC/PHIL.)*

Reactivation in Dorsal Root Ganglion

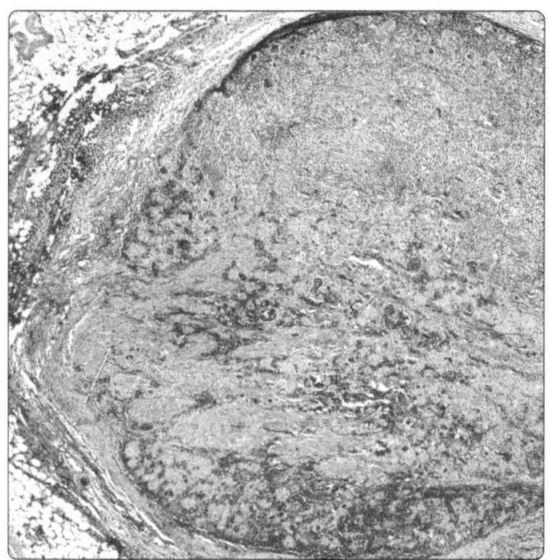

Reactivation in Dorsal Root Ganglion

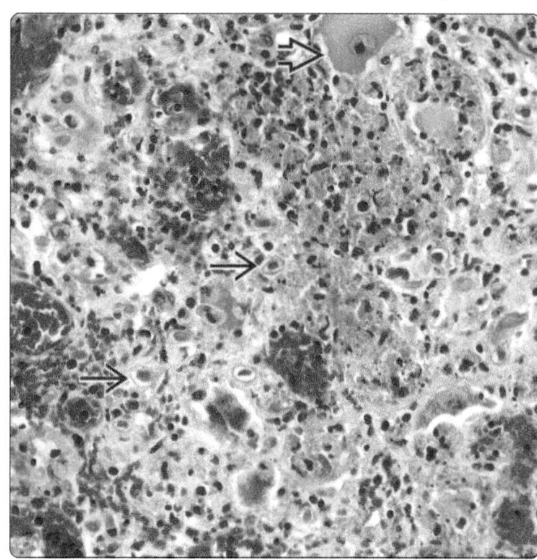

(Left) *Low-power H&E of a section of a dorsal root ganglion at autopsy in a patient with herpes zoster shows areas of hemorrhage and necrosis.* **(Right)** *High-power H&E of a dorsal root ganglion from a patient with herpes zoster shows necrosis, residual ganglion cells* ⮕*, and scattered, virally infected cells with Cowdry type A eosinophilic nuclear inclusions* ⮕.

MR of Trigeminal Neuralgia

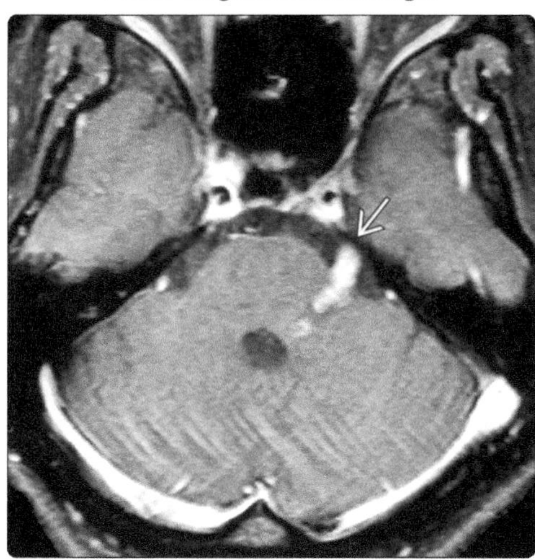

Mixed Ischemic-Demyelinative Lesions

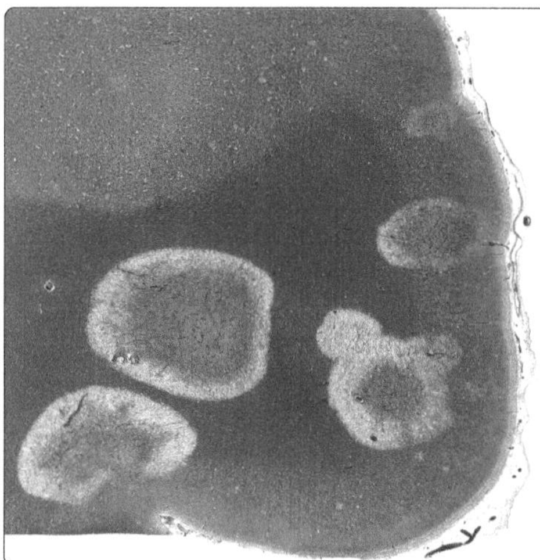

(Left) *Axial T1 C+ MR shows enhancement of CNV root entry zone* ⮕ *and brachium pontis in a patient with trigeminal neuralgia due to VZV infection. The most common form of cranial zoster involves the ophthalmic branch (V1). This usually develops in immunocompetent patients. (From DP: Neuro.)* **(Right)** *VZV spreading into CNS parenchyma may result in small vessel vasculitis and resultant ovoid mixed ischemic-demyelinative lesions concentrated at the gray-white junction. (From DP: Neuro.)*

Epstein-Barr Virus (HHV-4) Infection

KEY FACTS

ETIOLOGY/PATHOGENESIS

- Ubiquitous virus spread by oral/genital secretions; infects epithelial cells and B-lineage lymphocytes; latent infection with reactivation and numerous associated neoplasms

CLINICAL ISSUES

- 50% of children at 5 years and 95% of adults seropositive
- Infectious mononucleosis: Lymphadenopathy, hepatosplenomegaly ± jaundice, rash (less common)

MICROSCOPIC

- Infectious mononucleosis: Reactive lymph nodes, tonsillar tissue, hyperplastic spleen, and atypical lymphocytes
- Oral hairy leukoplakia: Parakeratosis, acanthosis, epithelial hyperplasia with eosinophilic balloon cells
- Posttransplant lymphoproliferative disorders (PTLDs): Plasmacytic hyperplasia, infectious mononucleosis-like hyperplasia, and reactive follicular hyperplasia, polymorphic PTLD, and lymphomas (B, T, NK)
- EBV mucocutaneous ulcer: Inflammatory infiltrate beneath ulcer with atypical lymphocytes
- Nasopharyngeal carcinoma: Undifferentiated, differentiated, and keratinizing types
- EBV-associated smooth muscle tumor: Well-circumscribed spindle cell tumor
- EBV-encoded RNA (EBER) ISH: Nuclear staining of EBV-infected nonneoplastic and tumor cells
- Latent membrane protein (LMP) IHC: Cytoplasmic and membranous staining of subset of infected cells

TOP DIFFERENTIAL DIAGNOSES

- CMV and HIV primary infections: Mononucleosis-like syndrome identical to EBV; distinguish by serology, PCR, CMV viral cytopathic effects, or IHC
- Non-EBV-related LPD/lymphomas: Similar clinical and histopathologic features but negative for EBV by ISH/IHC
- Other carcinomas/spindle cell tumors: Overlapping tumor histopathologic features but negative for EBV ISH/IHC

Ultrastructural Features

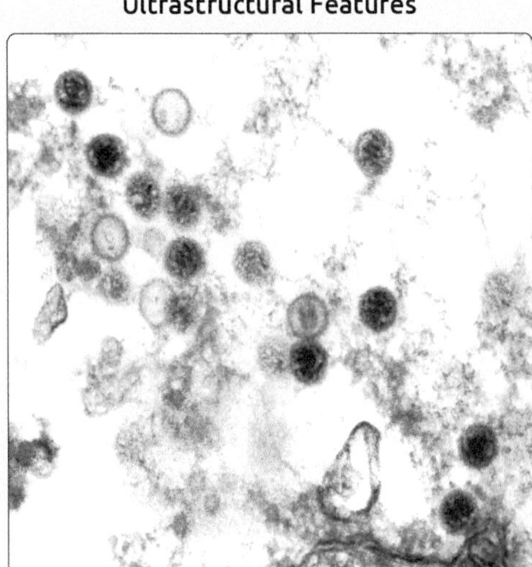

Atypical Lymphocytes in Peripheral Blood

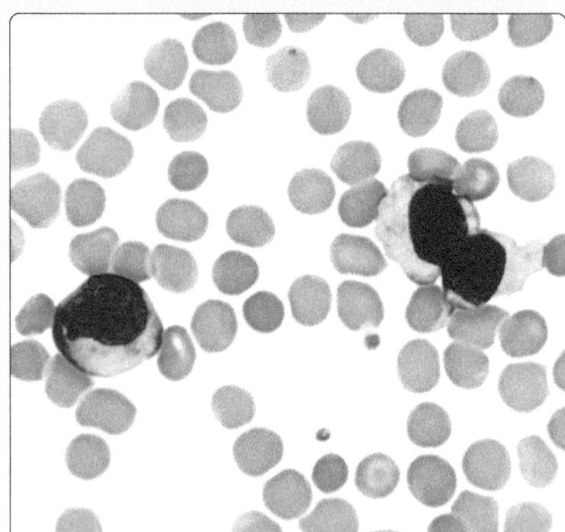

(Left) *Transmission electron microscopic image shows numerous 120- to 180-nm enveloped virions with icosahedral capsid, consistent with Epstein-Barr virus (EBV) virions. (Courtesy F. Murphy, DVM, PhD, CDC/PHIL.)* **(Right)** *Large, atypical lymphocytes are shown in a peripheral blood smear from a patient with acute EBV infection. The dark, open chromatin and nuclear morphology confirm the lymphocyte identity.*

EBV(+) DLBCL

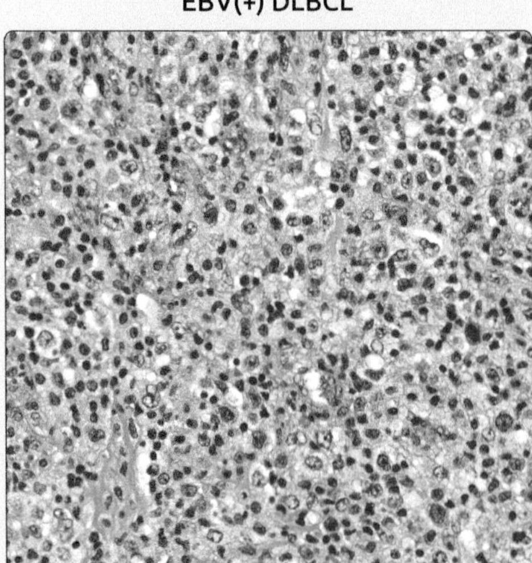

EBV(+) DLBCL: EBER ISH

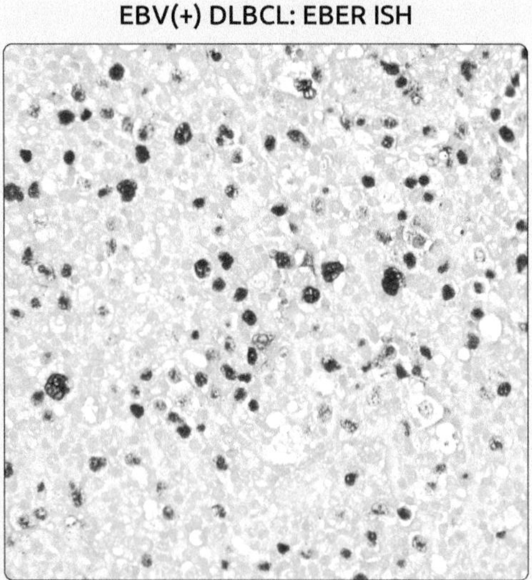

(Left) *Brain section shows florid inflammatory infiltrates containing scattered medium to large-sized atypical lymphoid cells with oval to irregular nuclei, dispersed and vesicular chromatin, variably prominent nucleoli, and scant to moderate amounts of cytoplasm, consistent with the diagnosis of monomorphic posttransplant lymphoproliferative disorder, EBV(+) DLBCL.* **(Right)** *ISH for EBV-encoded RNA (EBER) highlights atypical lymphoid cells in this case of EBV(+) DLBCL.*

TERMINOLOGY

Synonyms

- *Human gammaherpesvirus 4* (HHV-4); Epstein-Barr virus (EBV)
- Infectious mononucleosis (a.k.a. mono), glandular fever, Pfeiffer disease, kissing disease

Definitions

- EBV derived from M. A. Epstein and Y. Barr (University of Bristol and University of London, 1966)
- *Herpesviridae* family: Derived from "herpein" (to creep)

ETIOLOGY/PATHOGENESIS

Infectious Agents

- Ubiquitous virus spread by oral/genital secretions; infects oropharyngeal epithelial cells and B-lineage lymphocytes (via CD21); establishes persistent latent infection, which can reactivate and cause variety of neoplasms
- EBV DNA is linear in lytic cycle (predominantly involving epithelial cells); present as extrachromosomal episomes within nuclei of latently infected cells and tumor cells
- EBV-associated lymphoid proliferations and lymphomas classified by histologic diagnosis (i.e., hyperplasia, polymorphic lymphoproliferative disorder, mucocutaneous ulcer, lymphoma) and immune deficiency/dysregulation setting (i.e., inborn error of immunity, HIV infection, post transplant, autoimmune disease, iatrogenic/therapy related, and immune senescence)
- EBV infection also associated with multiple sclerosis, systemic lupus erythematosus, and rheumatoid arthritis; possible molecular mimicry between EBV and autoantigens

CLINICAL ISSUES

Epidemiology

- 50% of children at 5 years and 95% of adults seropositive

Site

- Infectious mononucleosis/reactivation involves lymph nodes, liver, spleen, tonsils, skin
- Malignant transformation can involve any body site

Presentation

- Initial infection is asymptomatic in most patients
- Infectious mononucleosis in older children/young adults (4- to 6-week incubation period, 1-2 weeks viral prodrome): Fatigue, lymphadenopathy, acute pharyngitis, hepatosplenomegaly, jaundice, rarely frank hepatitis, occasional maculopapular or palatal petechiae rashes
- Hepatitis in immunocompetent and immunocompromised: Elevated serum transaminase, alkaline phosphatase, bilirubin, hepatomegaly (10-15%), jaundice (5%)
- Oral hairy leukoplakia associated with HIV and smoking: White patches on tongue that cannot be scraped off
- EBV mucocutaneous ulcer: Age-related or iatrogenic immunosuppression; small (< 1-cm), well-circumscribed mucous or skin ulcers without associated masses that often resolve spontaneously
- Posttransplant lymphoproliferative disorders (PTLDs): Range from infectious mononucleosis-like to malignant lymphoma or plasma cell myeloma; 80% are EBV associated (lymph nodes > gastrointestinal tract, lungs, liver, skin, brain)
- EBV also associated with numerous types of lymphomas, including Burkitt, Hodgkin, diffuse large B-cell, extranodal NK-/T-cell, angioimmunoblastic T-cell, and peripheral T-cell and lymphomatoid granulomatosis
- Nasopharyngeal carcinoma: Masses arising in Rosenmüller fossa; high incidence in parts of Asia
- EBV-associated smooth muscle tumor: Rare circumscribed, solid or cystic 3- to 4-cm masses; predominantly in immunocompromised; high incidence in parts of Asia

Laboratory Tests

- Lymphocyte + monocyte count > 50%
- Transaminitis (with liver involvement)
- Viral capsid antigen (VCA): IgM appears early and disappears after 4-6 weeks; IgG peaks 2-4 months after acute infection and persists for life
- Early antigen (EA): IgG appears in acute phase of illness, then typically falls to undetectable levels after 3-6 months; detection may represent active infection or healthy individual
- EBV nuclear antigen (EBNA): Slowly appears 2-4 months after acute infection and persists for life
- Heterophil agglutination antibody test: Not recommended by CDC due to lack of sensitivity and specificity
- EBV PCR: Very high blood viral load suggests infectious stage; does not correlate well with PTLD

Treatment

- No effective antiviral drugs or vaccines currently available
- Surgery, chemotherapy, and decreased immunosuppression; supportive treatment with management of specific manifestations

Prognosis

- 95% of primary infections resolve without complications
- Rare complications of primary infection (< 5%) include meningoencephalitis, Guillain-Barré syndrome, myocarditis, fulminant hepatitis, splenic rupture, hemolytic anemia and other cytopenias, and hemophagocytic lymphohistiocytosis
- Lifelong viral infection with latency and risk of EBV-related malignancies with immunosuppression

IMAGING

General Features

- Brain: Nonspecific encephalitis; lymphomas involve periventricular white matter and deep gray nuclei as circumscribed masses or infiltrative growth with ring enhancement and restricted diffusion
- Chest: Pulmonary nodules with peripheral/basal predominance, bilateral airspace consolidation with visible air bronchograms, cavitation; pericardial or pleural effusions can occur
- Abdomen: Bowel wall thickening and aneurysmal dilatation, polypoid or eccentric masses, and intussusceptions; enlargement or masses in spleen and liver

MICROBIOLOGY

Virus Features

- Enveloped, lytic/latent, double-stranded DNA virus
- 120-180 nm, icosahedral capsid
- 192,000 bp genome (85 genes)

MICROSCOPIC

Histologic Features

- **Infectious mononucleosis**
  - Reactive lymph nodes/tonsillar tissue with paracortical hyperplasia and expansion of interfollicular areas with plasmalymphocytic cells; large atypical lymphocytes may have atypical contours and binucleation; sheet-like growth and necrosis
  - Spleen with immunoblastic hyperplasia, lymphocytic vasculitis, hypoplastic white pulp without germinal centers, apoptosis, necrosis, and hemorrhage
- **EBV hepatitis**: Lymphocytic infiltration of lined-up lymphocytes in sinusoids; scattered atypical lymphocytes, and small noncaseating epithelioid granulomas, minimal bile duct damage, and focal endotheliitis may be present
- **EBV enteritis**: Lymphoplasmacytic lamina propria infiltrate with immunoblast-like lymphocytes
- **EBV nephritis**: Lymphocytic-predominant interstitial inflammation with edema, tubulitis, epithelial cell nuclear atypia, and occasional mesangial hypercellularity
- **Oral hairy leukoplakia**: Irregular parakeratosis, acanthosis, epithelial hyperplasia, eosinophilic balloon cells with ground-glass intranuclear inclusions with margination and beading of chromatin; occasional *Candida* spp., minimal inflammation
- **PTLDs**: Plasmacytic hyperplasia, infectious mononucleosis-like hyperplasia, and reactive follicular hyperplasia, polymorphic PTLD, and lymphomas
- **EBV mucocutaneous ulcer**: Dense polymorphic inflammatory infiltrate beneath ulcer with Hodgkin and Reed-Sternberg-like cells; apoptosis, angioinvasion, and pseudoepitheliomatous hyperplasia may be present
- **Nasopharyngeal carcinoma**: Undifferentiated, differentiated, and keratinizing types
- **EBV-associated smooth muscle tumor**: Well-circumscribed storiform proliferation of spindle cells with pale cytoplasm and uniform, spindled nuclei, prominent vascularity, high mitotic activity

Cytologic Features

- Large, reactive lymphocytes with abundant cytoplasm; commonly seen in peripheral blood during acute infection
- No distinctive viral cytopathic effects

ANCILLARY TESTS

Immunohistochemistry/In Situ Hybridization

- EBV-encoded RNA (EBER) ISH: Nuclear staining of EBV-infected nonneoplastic and tumor cells
- Latent membrane protein (LMP) IHC: Cytoplasmic and membranous staining of subset of infected cells

Flow Cytometry

- Indicated in PTLD if mass lesion seen in resection specimen, lymph node biopsy, or tonsillectomy

Gene Rearrangements

- Gene rearrangement for immunoglobulins and T-cell receptors may be helpful for PTLD diagnosis

DIFFERENTIAL DIAGNOSIS

Cytomegalovirus Primary Infection

- May present with mononucleosis-like syndrome identical to EBV; distinguish by serology, PCR, CMV viral cytopathic effects, or IHC

Non-EBV-Related Lymphoproliferative Disorders and Lymphomas

- May present with similar clinical history, symptoms, histologic and immunophenotypical findings but negative for EBV by ISH/IHC

Other Carcinomas

- e.g., NUT carcinoma, sinonasal undifferentiated carcinoma, oropharyngeal nonkeratinizing carcinoma
- Some overlap with nasopharyngeal carcinoma tumor cytology, inflammatory components, and immunophenotype; negative for EBV ISH/IHC

Other Spindle Cell Tumors

- e.g., leiomyoma, leiomyosarcoma, solitary fibrous tumor, synovial sarcoma, PEComa
- Some overlap with EBV-associated smooth muscle tumor cytology, inflammatory components, and immunophenotype; negative for EBV ISH/IHC

SELECTED REFERENCES

1. Alaggio R et al: The 5th edition of the World Health Organization Classification of Haematolymphoid Tumours: lymphoid neoplasms. Leukemia. 36(7):1720-48, 2022
2. Almazyad A et al: Oral hairy leukoplakia: a series of 45 cases in immunocompetent patients. Oral Surg Oral Med Oral Pathol Oral Radiol. 132(2):210-16, 2021
3. Alruwaii ZI et al: Select Epstein-Barr virus-associated digestive tract lesions for the practicing pathologist. Arch Pathol Lab Med. 145(5):562-70, 2021
4. Chabay P: Advances in the pathogenesis of EBV-associated diffuse large B cell lymphoma. Cancers (Basel). 13(11):2717, 2021
5. Whaley RD et al: Epstein-Barr virus-associated smooth muscle tumors of larynx: a clinicopathologic study and comprehensive literature review of 12 cases. Head Neck Pathol. 15(4):1162-71, 2021
6. AbuSalah MAH et al: Recent advances in diagnostic approaches for Epstein-Barr virus. Pathogens. 9(3):226, 2020
7. Ikeda T et al: Clinicopathological analysis of 34 Japanese patients with EBV-positive mucocutaneous ulcer. Mod Pathol. 33(12):2437-48, 2020
8. Chen YP et al: Nasopharyngeal carcinoma. Lancet. 394(10192):64-80, 2019
9. Liu R et al: The clinicopathologic features of chronic active Epstein-Barr virus infective enteritis. Mod Pathol. 32(3):387-95, 2019
10. Fukayama M et al: Gastritis-infection-cancer sequence of epstein-barr virus-associated gastric cancer. Adv Exp Med Biol. 1045:437-57, 2018
11. Moretti M et al: Acute kidney injury in symptomatic primary Epstein-Barr virus infectious mononucleosis: Systematic review. J Clin Virol. 91:12-7, 2017
12. Ebell MH et al: Does this patient have infectious mononucleosis?: The rational clinical examination systematic review. JAMA. 315(14):1502-9, 2016

Ruptured Spleen

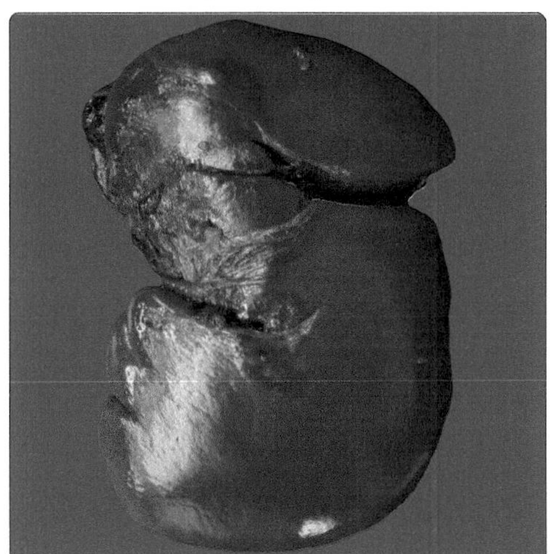

EBV Infection: Spleen

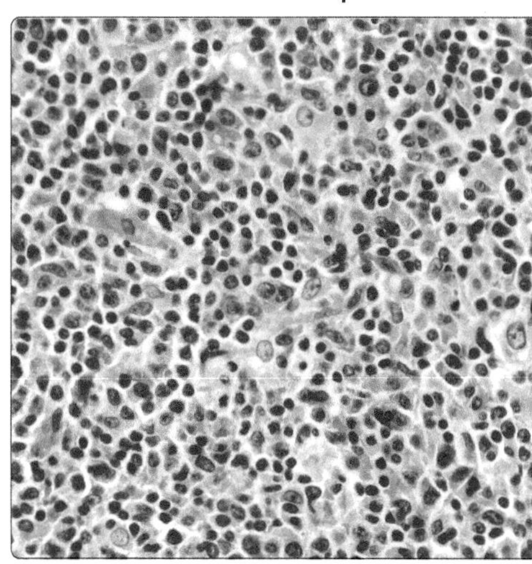

(Left) *Enlarged spleen from a 23-year-old patient with infectious mononucleosis and recent fall shows parenchymal hemorrhage and capsule disruption, consistent with splenic rupture.* **(Right)** *Section from an enlarged spleen shows intact white pulp containing predominantly small lymphocytes and scattered immunoblasts.*

EBV(+) Spleen: EBER ISH

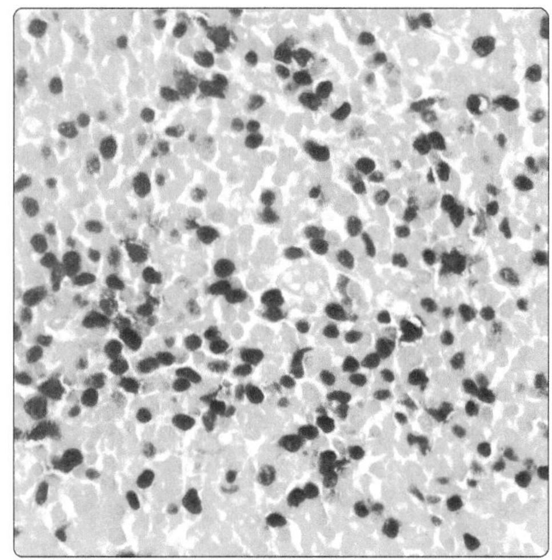

EBV Hepatitis

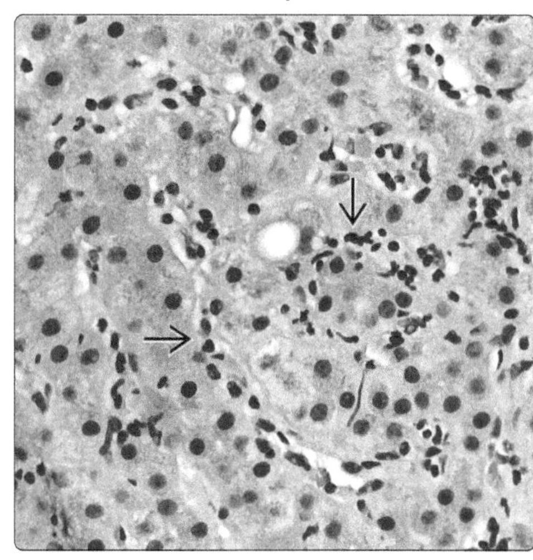

(Left) *ISH for EBER is positive in a significant subset of B cells within white pulp nodules. A stain for LMP1 is negative (not shown). The findings are consistent with splenic involvement by EBV infection.* **(Right)** *EBV hepatitis shows linear filing of lymphocytes ⮕ within the sinusoids.*

Oral Hairy Leukoplakia

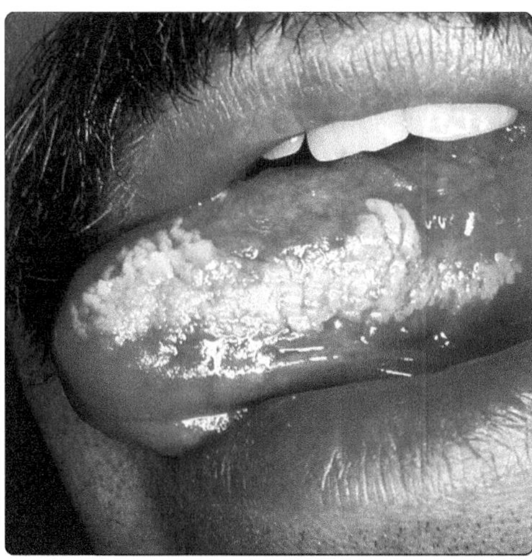

Oral Hairy Leukoplakia

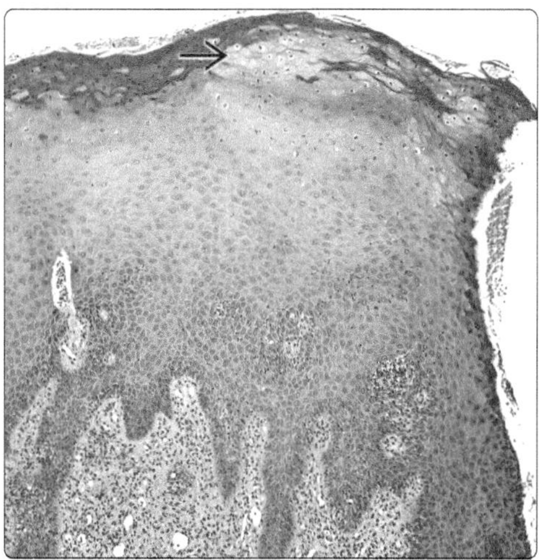

(Left) *Photograph from an HIV(+) patient shows white patches on the lateral border of the tongue, consistent with oral hairy leukoplakia. (Courtesy J. Greenspan, BDS and S. Silverman, Jr., DDS, CDC/PHIL.)* **(Right)** *Tongue biopsy from an 80-year-old shows superficial and deep acute and chronic inflammation, hyperkeratotic epithelium with balloon cells ⮕, consistent with oral hairy leukoplakia. A superficial fungal infection was identified by PAS-D staining (not shown). (Courtesy of J. Hanna, MD, PhD.)*

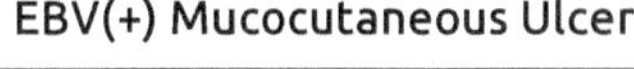

EBV(+) Mucocutaneous Ulcer

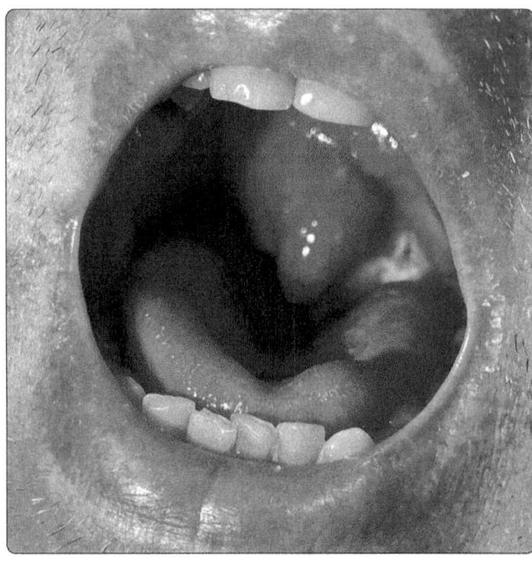

EBV(+) Mucocutaneous Ulcer

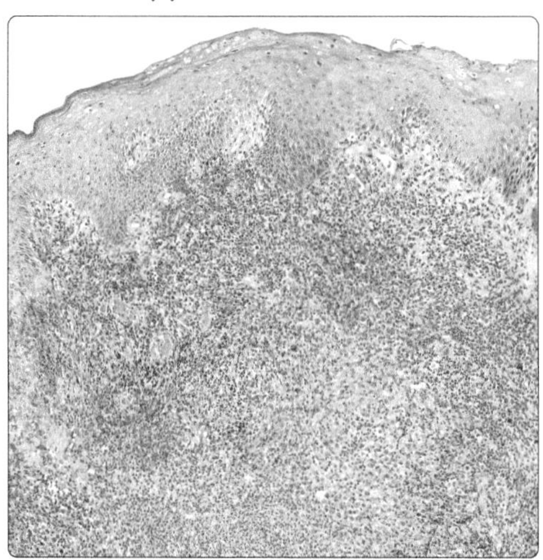

(Left) *This 50-year-old patient presented with a few-week history of sore throat and otalgia and was found to have left tonsillar erythema and firmness to palpation on physical examination.* **(Right)** *Tonsil section shows squamous mucosa with a polymorphous submucosal inflammatory infiltrate admixed with large, atypical cells with irregular frequently bilobed nuclei, open chromatin, prominent eosinophilic nucleoli, abundant eosinophilic cytoplasm, scattered mitoses, and focal necrosis.*

EBV(+) Mucocutaneous Ulcer: EBER ISH

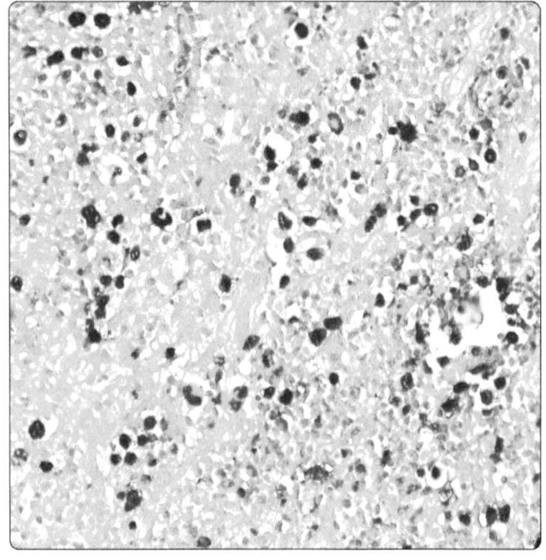

Burkitt Lymphoma

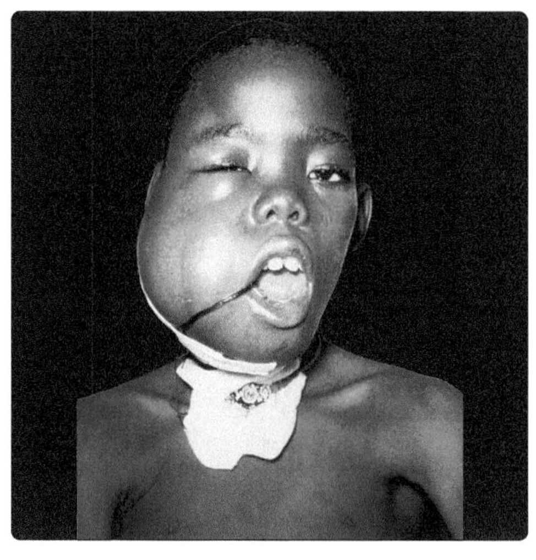

(Left) *ISH for EBER is positive in many of the large atypical cells that also exhibited weak staining for BSAP/PAX5. The overall features are compatible with an EBV(+) mucocutaneous ulcer, which frequently exhibits a self-limited indolent course.* **(Right)** *This large facial tumor in a child is due to Burkitt lymphoma, for which the majority of cases are associated with EBV. (Courtesy R. Craig, CDC/PHIL.)*

Burkitt Lymphoma

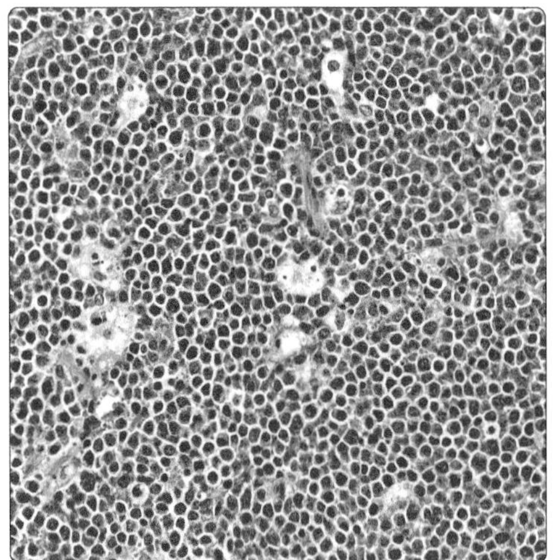

Burkitt Lymphoma: EBER ISH

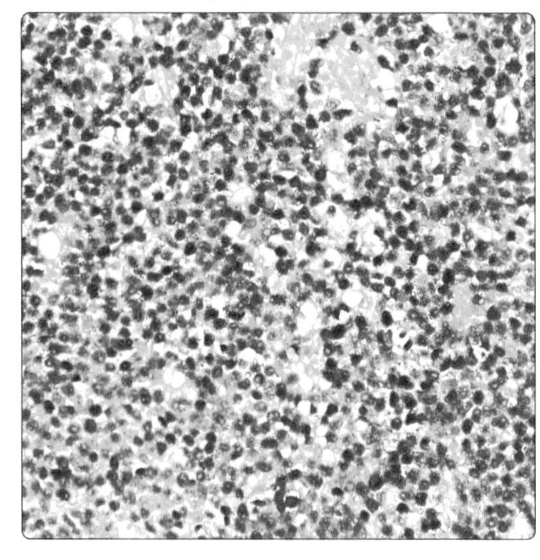

(Left) *Lymph node section shows an infiltrate of monotonous, intermediate-sized lymphoid cells with irregular nuclei, condensed chromatin, small basophilic nucleoli, and scant amphophilic cytoplasm with frequent mitoses, apoptotic bodies, and tingible body macrophages giving rise to a starry-sky appearance.* **(Right)** *EBER ISH is positive in the atypical cells, which also expressed CD20, CD10, BCL6, and MYC. Cytogenetic analysis identified a MYC rearrangement, consistent with Burkitt lymphoma.*

EBV(+) PTLD: Brain MR

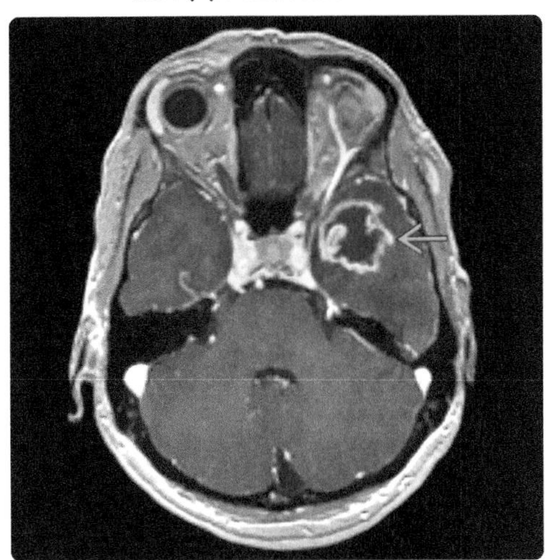

EBV(+) PTLD Involving Brain

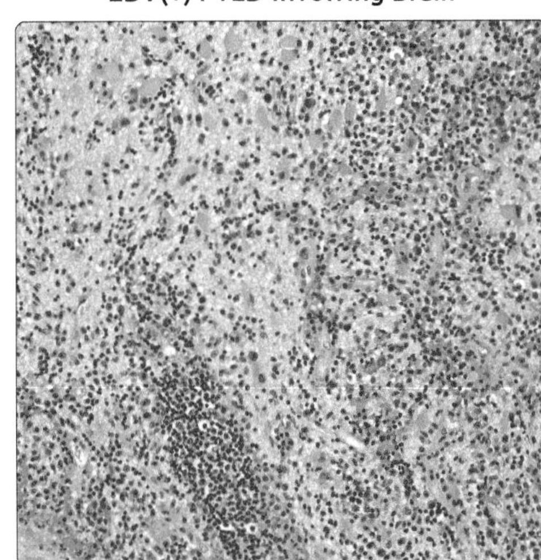

(Left) *Brain MR is from a 41-year-old woman with history of kidney transplants who presented with altered mental status and language difficulty and was found to have a left temporal rim-enhancing lesion ➡ with extensive vasogenic edema.* **(Right)** *Brain section shows florid nonneoplastic inflammatory infiltrates, scattered reactive astrocytes, and atypical lymphoid cells, consistent with EBV(+) DLBCL.*

Nasopharyngeal Carcinoma

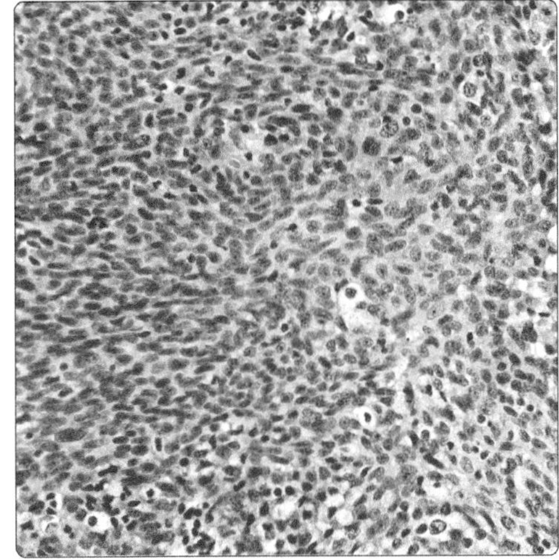

Nasopharyngeal Carcinoma: EBER ISH

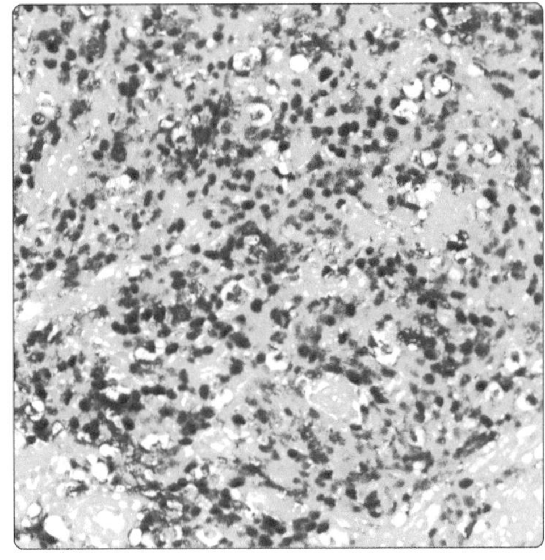

(Left) *Biopsy from a 72-year-old shows sheets of tumor cells positive for p40, consistent with nonkeratinizing nasopharyngeal carcinoma.* **(Right)** *Nasopharyngeal carcinoma cells are positive for EBER ISH. Tumor cells are typically positive for EBV-LMP, pancytokeratin, high molecular weight cytokeratin, p63, and p40.*

EBV-Associated Smooth Muscle Tumor

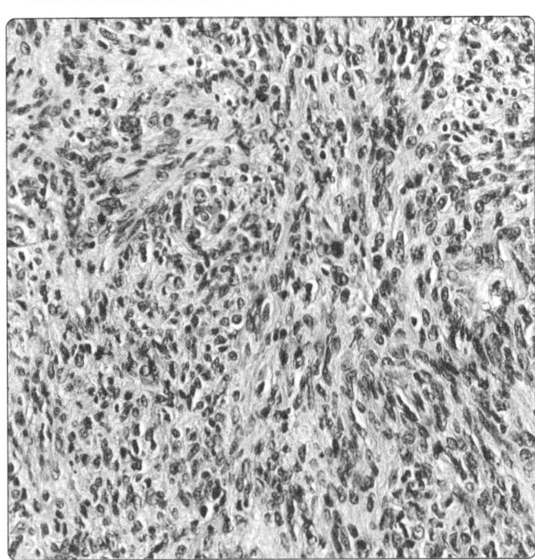

EBV-Associated Smooth Muscle Tumor: EBER ISH

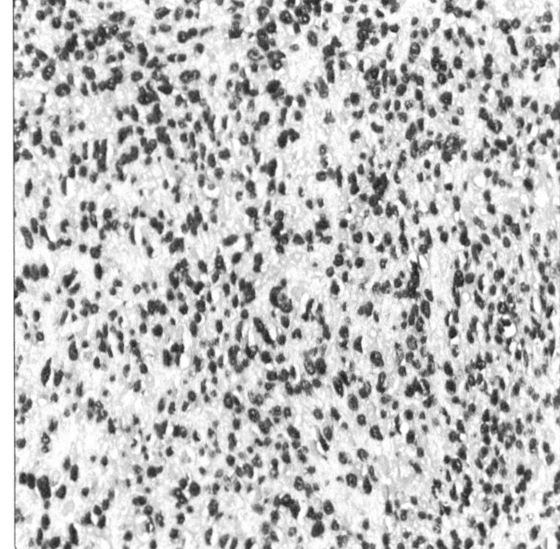

(Left) *Neck mass biopsy from a 41-year-old woman with HIV shows a storiform proliferation of spindle cells with pale cytoplasm and uniform, spindled nuclei, consistent with EBV-associated smooth muscle tumor.* **(Right)** *ISH for EBER is positive in tumor cells, which also expressed SMA and caldesmon. Desmin is occasionally positive but was negative in this case.*

Cytomegalovirus (HHV-5) Infections

KEY FACTS

ETIOLOGY/PATHOGENESIS

- Ubiquitous virus with asymptomatic latency in immunocompetent patients
- Loss of cell-mediated immunity (immunosuppression) can lead to viral reactivation and lytic cycle infection

CLINICAL ISSUES

- Mononucleosis-like initial presentation, TORCH infection in utero, and severe disease with HIV/low CD4 count, solid organ and bone marrow transplants
- Quantitative PCR on blood to follow immunosuppression but does not correlate with organ-specific disease

MICROSCOPIC

- Very large cells with "owl's-eye" nucleus and abundant cytoplasm ± distinctive red-purple granules
- Endothelial cells, stromal cells, and macrophages more commonly involved than epithelial cells
- Specific tissue patterns of injury include ischemia &/or necrosis (with vascular endothelial infection) and ulceration (gastrointestinal tract)
- May have minimal inflammation in severely immunocompromised patients

ANCILLARY TESTS

- Anti-CMV antibodies stain infected cells with and without VCPE observed on H&E

TOP DIFFERENTIAL DIAGNOSES

- HSV-1, HSV-2, VZV: Multinucleation, molding, and margination or chromatin; confirm by IHC, PCR, or serology
- Adenovirus: Smudgy basophilic nuclear inclusions
- RNA viruses: Necrosis ± inflammation; ± VCPE
- Bacterial infections: Destructive, necrotic lesions; organisms on Gram/silver stains
- Diffuse alveolar damage: CMV can directly lead to DAD, non-CMV-associated DAD can mimic CMV pneumonitis, and CMV can incidentally reactivate in DAD

Ultrastructural Features

CMV in Cytology Specimen

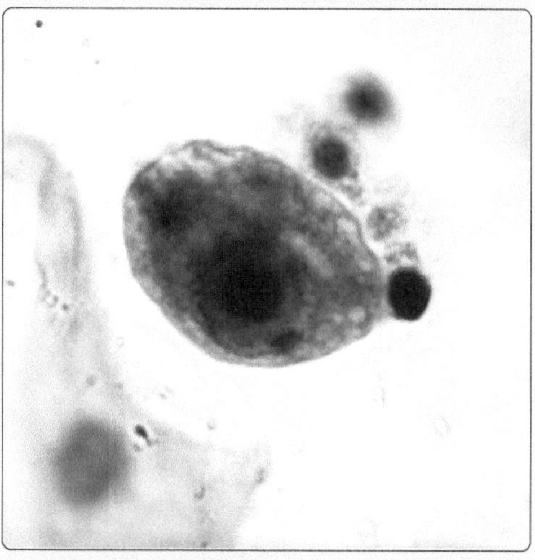

(Left) *Transmission electron microscopic (TEM) image depicts numbers of spherical particles 150-200 nm in diameter, characteristic of cytomegalovirus (CMV). (Courtesy S. Whitfield, MS, CDC/PHIL.)* **(Right)** *This image of a urine sample specimen shows a large nuclear "owl's-eye" inclusion and more subtle cytoplasmic inclusions, characteristic of a CMV infection. (Courtesy R. Haraszti, MD, CDC/PHIL.)*

Viral Cytopathic Effects in Tissue Sections

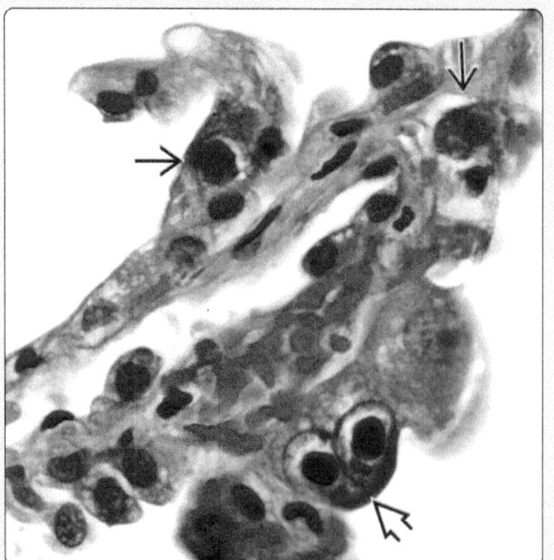

CMV IHC

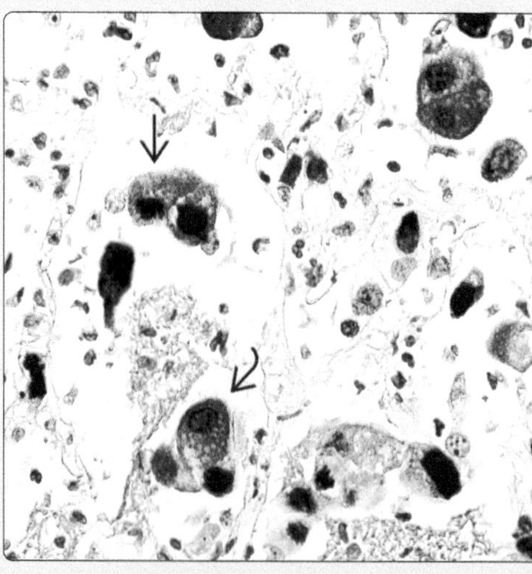

(Left) *A section of lung from a patient with CMV pneumonitis demonstrates multiple CMV-infected cells ⇒ with the classic "owl's-eye" nuclei ⇒ and enlargement of the infected cells.* **(Right)** *Nuclear ⇒ and cytoplasmic ⇒ staining of CMV-infected cells is shown in an immunocompromised patient with adjacent infected cells positive for antigen, which were not histologically suspicious cells.*

TERMINOLOGY

Synonyms

- *Human betaherpesvirus 5* (HHV-5); cytomegalovirus (CMV)

Definitions

- "CMV" from "cyto" (cell) and "megalo" (large)
- *Herpesviridae* family: Derived from "herpein" (to creep)

ETIOLOGY/PATHOGENESIS

Infectious Agents

- Ubiquitous virus able to infect many cell types; commonly found in saliva, urine, semen > other body fluids
- Initial infection route of entry is salivary glands with self-limited lytic infection
- Chronic infection: Asymptomatic latency in immunocompetent patients; viral shedding in infected hosts
- Loss of cell-mediated immunity (immunosuppression) can lead to viral reactivation and lytic cycle infection
- No direct evidence of oncogenesis but may work through oncomodulation to increase malignancy of tumors

CLINICAL ISSUES

Epidemiology

- Ubiquitous virus affecting all age groups; 36% in children rises to 91% of adults > 80 years
- Seropositivity rates depend on population and age: ~ 40% of population on average worldwide, 60% of adults in USA, and 90% of male homosexuals
- Transplant patients (20-60%) experience symptomatic infections

Site

- Immunocompetent patients: Lungs, liver, gastrointestinal tract, and brain; rarely, esophagus, salivary glands, kidneys, adrenals, pancreas
- Immunosuppressed patients: Any organ and many cell types

Presentation

- Primary infection (9-60 days) or reactivation of latency
- Range of clinical infections (mild to life threatening), including pneumonia, hepatitis, colitis, encephalitis
- Mononucleosis-like initial presentation (mimics Epstein-Barr virus infection) with lymphadenopathy, splenomegaly, and hepatitis in immunocompetent children and young adults
- In utero: TORCH (**t**oxoplasmosis, **o**ther infections, **r**ubella, **C**MV, **h**erpes simplex) organism
- Human immunodeficiency virus (HIV) infection with low CD4 count; coinfection with other opportunistic pathogens
- Solid organ transplants: Highest risk when donor is positive and recipient is negative
- Bone marrow transplants: Highest risk when donor is negative and recipient is positive

Laboratory Tests

- Serology (IgG &/or IgM)
- Direct or indirect immunofluorescence for CMV antigens (urine, saliva, blood, fluids)
- Culture from direct tissue sample > blood
- Qualitative PCR on blood
- Quantitative PCR on blood directly correlates with, and can be used to follow, immunosuppression but does not correlate with organ-specific disease
  - Example A: Patient with low CMV viral load may present with severe CMV pneumonia
  - Example B: Patient with high CMV viral load has no organ-specific symptoms or actual pathology
- CMV genes (e.g., *UL97*, *UL54*, *UL27*, and *UL56*) can be sequenced to detect mutations associated with resistance to ganciclovir, foscarnet, cidofovir, maribavir, and letermovir

Natural History

- Self-limited in immunocompetent patients
- Immunosuppressed patients may have moderate to severe organ-specific disease or severe disseminated disease

Treatment

- Prevention in immunosuppressed patients (prophylaxis) with valganciclovir (favored) or ganciclovir
- Treatment in immunosuppressed patients (all sites) with ganciclovir (1st line), foscarnet, cidofovir, or maribavir (2nd line) or CMV immunoglobulin (with ganciclovir for lung transplant patients)
- CMV retinitis treated with valganciclovir

Prognosis

- TORCH: Pregnancy loss to severe, long-term complications
- CMV organ-specific disease in immunosuppressed patients is better with preemptive treatment or prophylaxis and worse with unmonitored, acute-onset disease
- HIV-infected patients on highly active antiretroviral therapy (HAART) have better prognosis

MICROBIOLOGY

Virus Features

- Enveloped, lytic, double-stranded DNA virus
- 150-200 nm in size with icosahedral capsid
- 235,645 bp genome (largest of herpesviruses)

Culture

- Grows in human fetal fibroblasts (HFF) cell lines (1-2 weeks)
- Confirm by positive direct antigen visualization
- Shell-vial culture: Rapid, previral cytopathic effect detection by antibody

MACROSCOPIC

General Features

- Ulcerated lesions most common with well-circumscribed punched-out appearance

MICROSCOPIC

Histologic Features

- Very large cells (3-4x size of macrophages) with large, "owl's-eye" nucleus (red-purple inclusion within large, cleared nucleus), and abundant cytoplasm ± distinctive red-purple granules
- Endothelial cells, stromal cells, and macrophages more commonly involved than epithelial cells

- Specific tissue patterns of injury (in addition to viral cytopathic effect) include ischemia &/or necrosis (with vascular endothelial infection) and ulceration (gastrointestinal tract)
- May have minimal inflammation in severely immunocompromised patients

Cytologic Features

- Markedly enlarged mononuclear cells with basophilic, intranuclear inclusions and small, granular, cytoplasmic inclusions

ANCILLARY TESTS

Immunohistochemistry

- Anti-CMV antibodies stain infected ± viral cytopathic effects (VCPE) observed on H&E
- Should always be considered in concert with other herpesviruses and adenovirus without prior diagnosis
  - Example A: Patient with known positive CMV viral load = single IHC for confirmation of suspicious cells
  - Example B: Patient with new-onset, organ-specific symptoms and suspicious (but not diagnostic) VCPE on biopsy = panel of CMV and other herpesviruses

PCR

- Molecular detection of CMV DNA or RNA can be performed on fresh or formalin-fixed, paraffin-embedded tissue but is rarely needed

DIFFERENTIAL DIAGNOSIS

Other Viral Infections

- Herpes simplex virus 1 and 2 (HSV-1/HSV-2)
  - Viral infected cells exhibit multinucleation, molding, and margination or chromatin; classic Cowdry type A nuclei
  - Confirm by IHC, PCR, or serology
- Varicella-zoster virus (VZV)
  - Viral infected cells exhibit multinucleation, molding, and margination or chromatin; classic Cowdry type A nuclei
  - Confirm by IHC, PCR, or serology
- Adenovirus
  - Smudgy basophilic nuclear inclusions
  - Confirm by IHC, PCR, or serology
- RNA viruses resulting in necrosis ± inflammation
  - May exhibit VCPE (e.g., respiratory syncytial virus, human parainfluenza viruses, measles virus) or lack viral inclusions (e.g., influenza, severe acute respiratory syndrome coronavirus 2)
  - Correlated with CMV immune status, viral load, and IHC
  - Reference testing for confirmation of other viral infections is recommended
- When viral cytopathic effect is suspected, panel of HSV, VZV, CMV, and adenovirus IHC is advised

Bacterial Infections

- Destructive, necrotic lesions
- Demonstration of bacteria on Gram or silver staining
- Positive cultures or molecular detection of bacteria from sample

Diffuse Alveolar Damage

- Patients with acute respiratory distress syndrome (ARDS)
- Any condition leading to diffuse alveolar damage (DAD) can mimic CMV infection (and vice versa)
- CMV can lead directly to DAD
- CMV can reactivate in damaged lung tissue incidentally and not be root cause of DAD
- Reactive, degenerative cells may be suspicious for viral cytopathic effect
- Clinical history, culture, and IHC can exclude DAD of other causes

SELECTED REFERENCES

1. Schwartz M et al: Molecular characterization of human cytomegalovirus infection with single-cell transcriptomics. Nat Microbiol. 8(3):455-68, 2023
2. Goyal G et al: The trends of immunohistochemistry for tissue-invasive cytomegalovirus in gastrointestinal mucosal biopsies. Arch Pathol Lab Med. 146(3):360-5, 2022
3. Kotton CN et al: Cytomegalovirus in the transplant setting: where are we now and what happens next? A report from the International CMV Symposium 2021. Transpl Infect Dis. 24(6):e13977, 2022
4. Shih AR et al: Cytomegalovirus hepatitis in allograft livers may show histologic features of acute cellular rejection. Arch Pathol Lab Med. 147(6):655-64, 2022
5. Griffiths P et al: Pathogenesis of human cytomegalovirus in the immunocompromised host. Nat Rev Microbiol. 19(12):759-73, 2021
6. Ambelil M et al: The significance of so-called equivocal immunohistochemical staining for cytomegalovirus in colorectal biopsies. Arch Pathol Lab Med. 143(8):985-9, 2019
7. Lindholm K et al: Placental cytomegalovirus infection. Arch Pathol Lab Med. 143(5):639-42, 2019
8. Guo L et al: Routine hematoxylin and eosin stain is specific for the diagnosis of cytomegalovirus infection in gastrointestinal biopsy specimens. Int J Surg Pathol. 26(6):500-6, 2018
9. Wethkamp N et al: Identification of clinically relevant cytomegalovirus infections in patients with inflammatory bowel disease. Mod Pathol. 31(3):527-38, 2018
10. Zagórowicz E et al: Detection of cytomegalovirus by immunohistochemistry of colonic biopsies and quantitative blood polymerase chain reaction: evaluation of agreement in ulcerative colitis. Scand J Gastroenterol. 53(4):435-41, 2018
11. Juric-Sekhar G et al: Cytomegalovirus (CMV) in gastrointestinal mucosal biopsies: should a pathologist perform CMV immunohistochemistry if the clinician requests it? Hum Pathol. 60:11-5, 2017
12. Rawlinson WD et al: Congenital cytomegalovirus infection in pregnancy and the neonate: consensus recommendations for prevention, diagnosis, and therapy. Lancet Infect Dis. 17(6):e177-88, 2017
13. Teissier N et al: Cytomegalovirus-induced brain malformations in fetuses. J Neuropathol Exp Neurol. 73(2):143-58, 2014
14. Folkins AK et al: Diagnosis of congenital CMV using PCR performed on formalin-fixed, paraffin-embedded placental tissue. Am J Surg Pathol. 37(9):1413-20, 2013
15. Mills AM et al: A comparison of CMV detection in gastrointestinal mucosal biopsies using immunohistochemistry and PCR performed on formalin-fixed, paraffin-embedded tissue. Am J Surg Pathol. 37(7):995-1000, 2013

Severe CMV Colitis

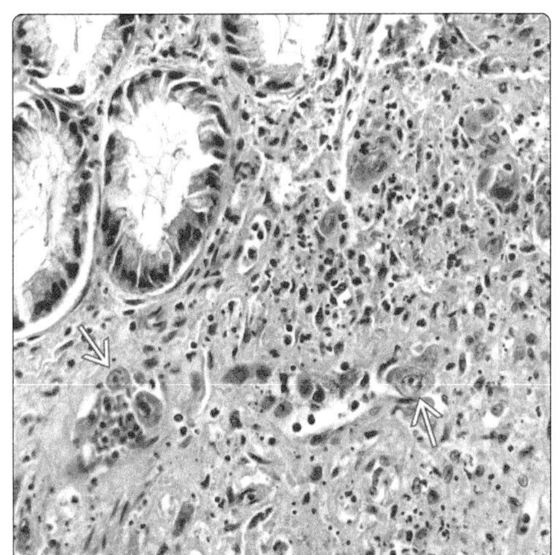

CMV Colitis

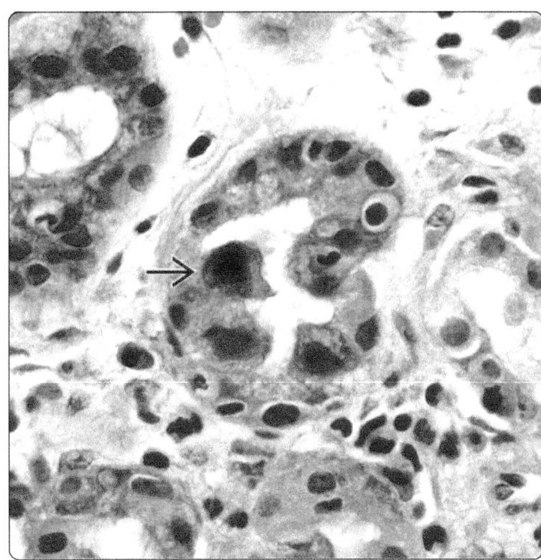

(Left) *Severe CMV colitis with numerous infected cells ➡, inflammation, and necrosis is shown.* **(Right)** *Colonic epithelium with reactive changes, degeneration of epithelial cells, and clear CMV viral cytopathic effect ➡ is shown. The scattered epithelial cells with pale pink cytoplasm are also infected with CMV.*

Intracytoplasmic CMV Inclusions

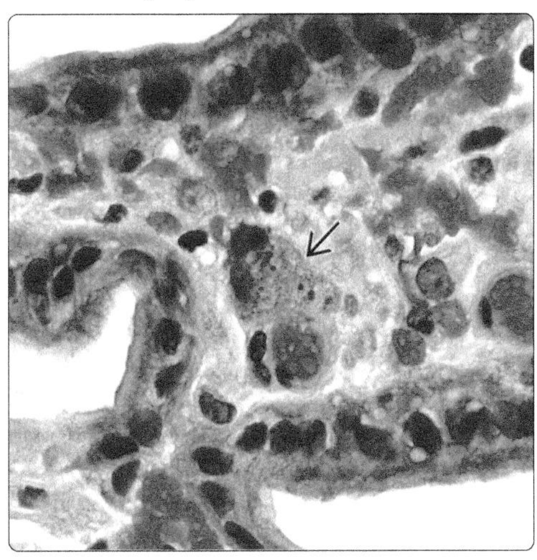

Subtle CMV Cytopathic Changes

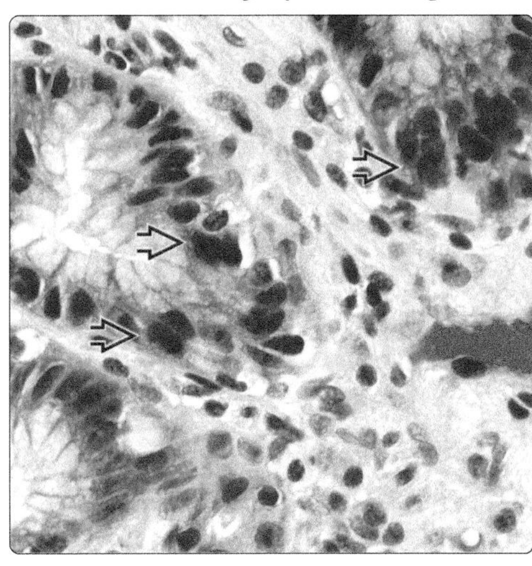

(Left) *Reactive and inflamed small bowel epithelium with hemorrhage contains an enlarged cell with prominent granules ➡. IHC was positive for CMV.* **(Right)** *Reactive and mildly inflamed colonic epithelium is shown with scattered cells suspicious for viral cytopathic effect ➡, which stained positive for CMV by IHC.*

CMV IHC

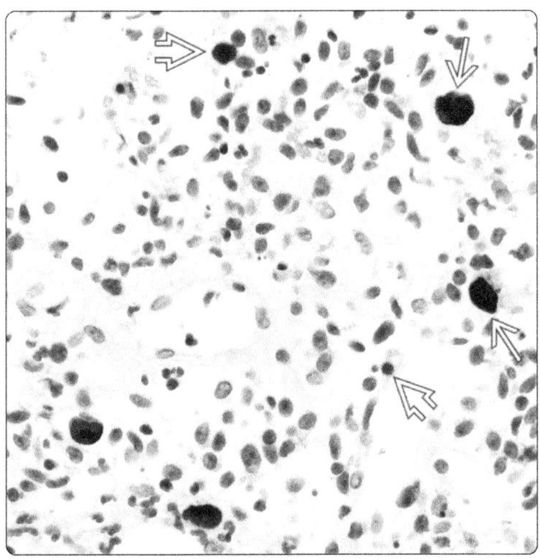

CMV Esophagitis

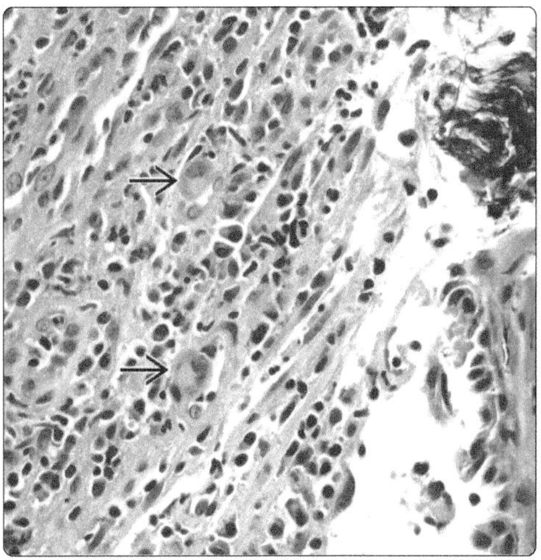

(Left) *The distinct morphology of CMV is usually sufficient to make a histologic diagnosis; however, when IHC for CMV is used, obviously infected cells ➡ and additional cells, which are infected ➡ but not yet classic in appearance, may be seen.* **(Right)** *Scattered cells ➡ in this ulcerated esophageal lesion exhibit large nuclear inclusions typical of CMV infection. In contrast to herpes simplex virus (HSV), CMV-infected cells tend to be deep in ulcer base rather than at edges.*

(Left) *Scattered CMV-infected cells are present in this lung section, which shows evidence of acute and chronic hemorrhage.* **(Right)** *Two CMV-infected cells are shown in an alveolus from a patient with severe CMV pneumonia. Note the purple granules in the cytoplasm of one cell and the "owl's-eye" nucleus of the other.*

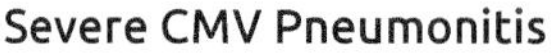

Severe CMV Pneumonitis

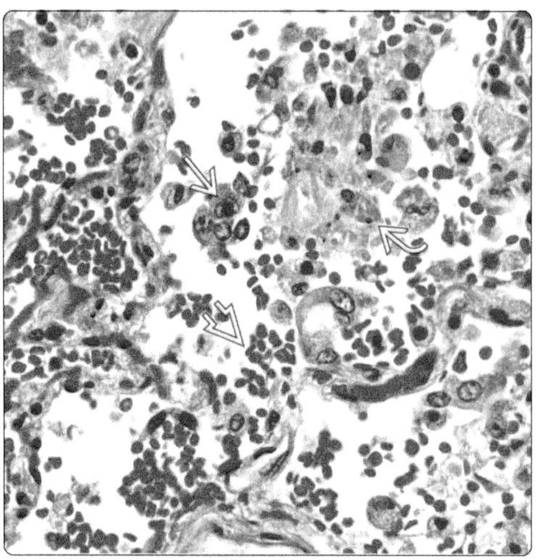

CMV Pneumonitis: Classic Viral Cytopathic Effects

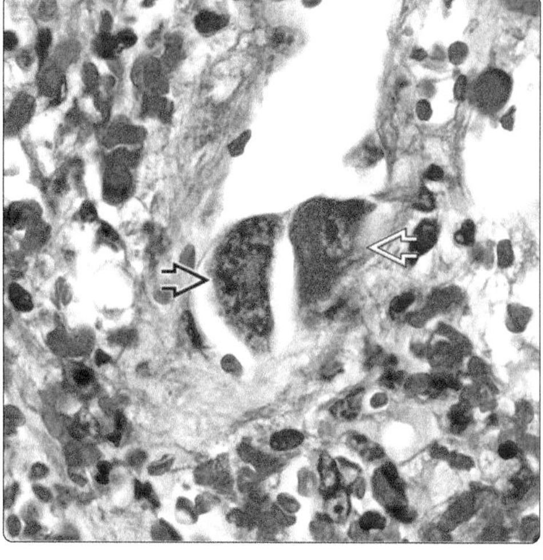

(Left) *Scattered CMV-infected cells, which are not massively enlarged, as is seen in the classic appearance, lead to a differential of other herpesvirus infections.* **(Right)** *Severe CMV pneumonia demonstrates predominantly nuclear staining for CMV antigens by IHC.*

CMV Pneumonitis: Uncertain Viral Cytopathic Effects

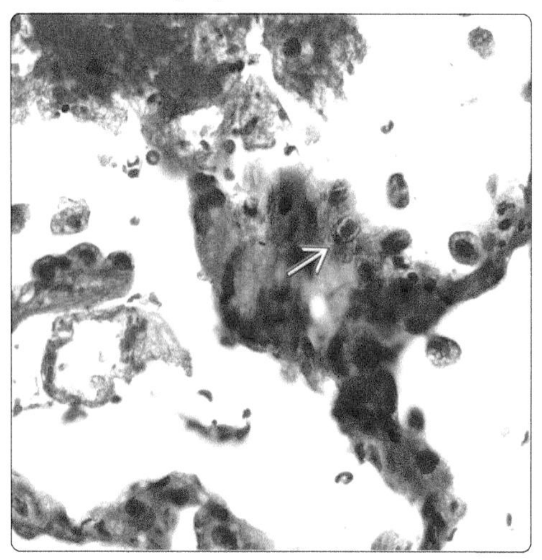

CMV Pneumonitis: IHC

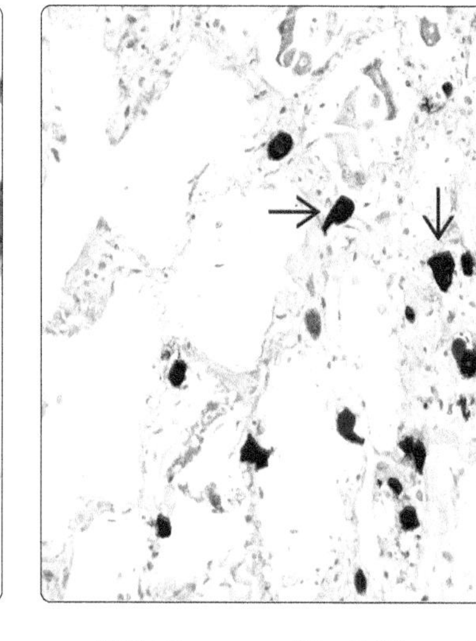

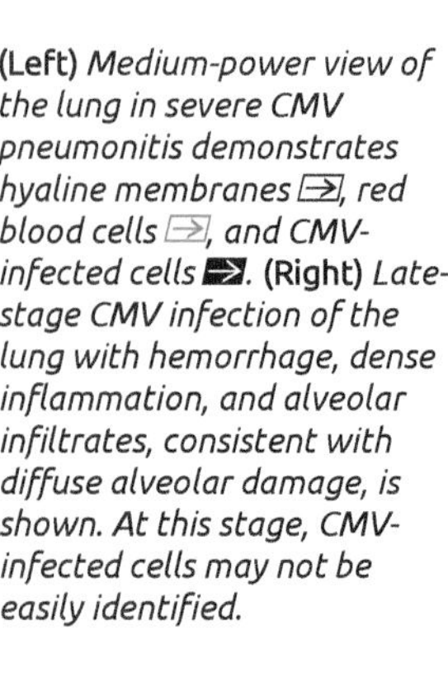

(Left) *Medium-power view of the lung in severe CMV pneumonitis demonstrates hyaline membranes, red blood cells, and CMV-infected cells.* **(Right)** *Late-stage CMV infection of the lung with hemorrhage, dense inflammation, and alveolar infiltrates, consistent with diffuse alveolar damage, is shown. At this stage, CMV-infected cells may not be easily identified.*

CMV Pneumonitis: Diffuse Alveolar Damage

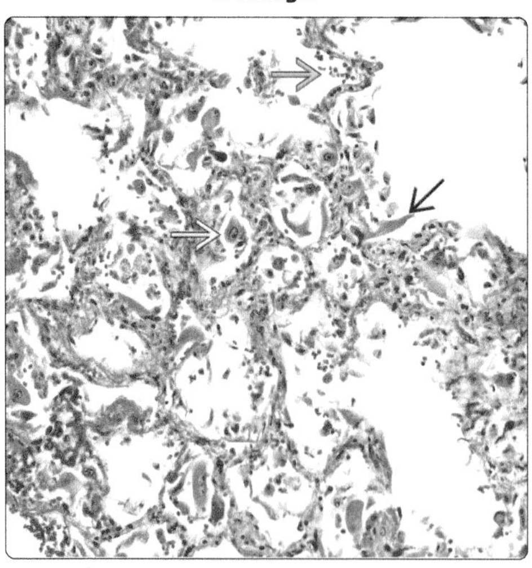

CMV Pneumonitis: Diffuse Alveolar Damage

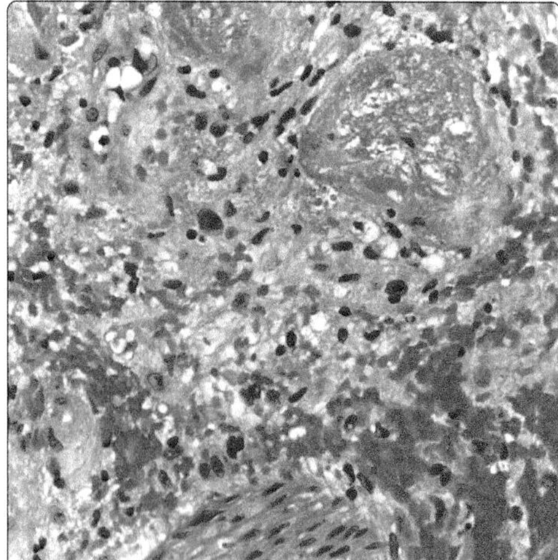

CMV Retinitis

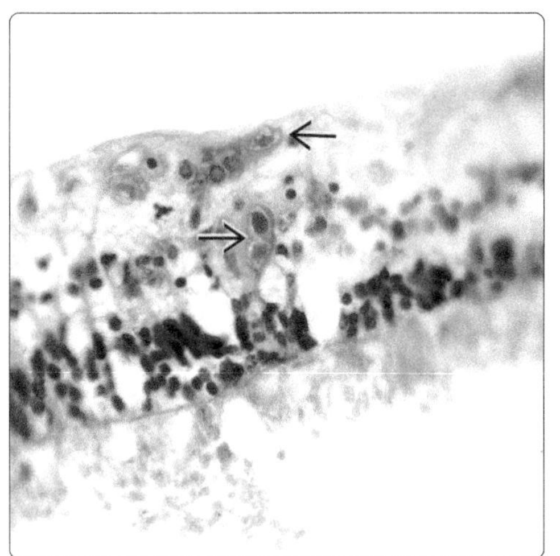

Fatal CMV Villitis

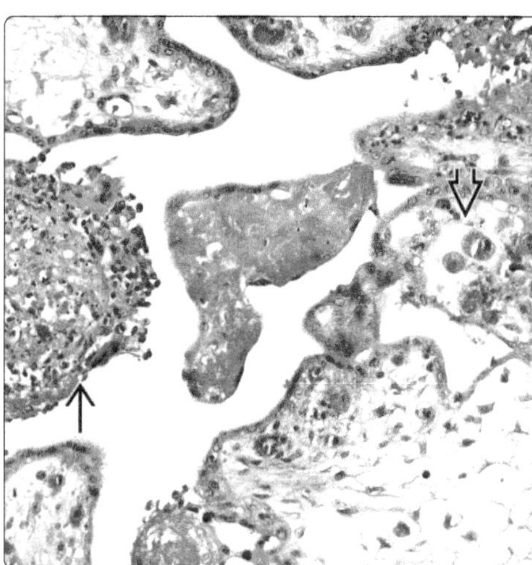

(Left) *CMV retinitis is often present in HIV-infected patients with CD4 counts < 50 cells/µL, which has significantly decreased with the widespread availability of antiretrovirals. Multiple large cells are present with typical CMV inclusions ⇒.* **(Right)** *Severe villitis in a case of fetal demise shows diffuse viral cytopathic effect with CMV ⇒ and severe inflammation with villous destruction ⇒.*

Congenital CMV Pneumonitis

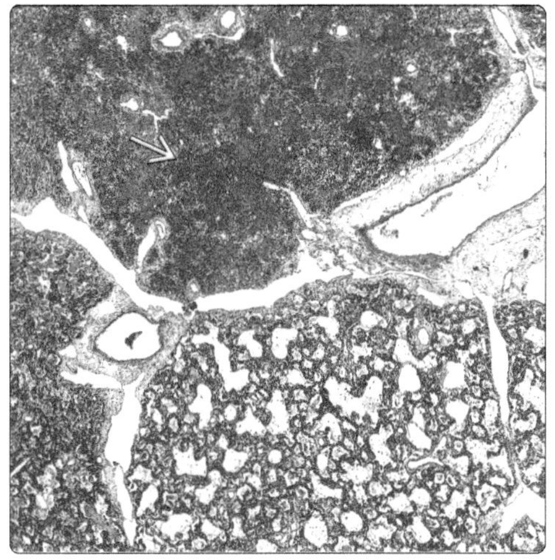

Congenital CMV Pneumonitis

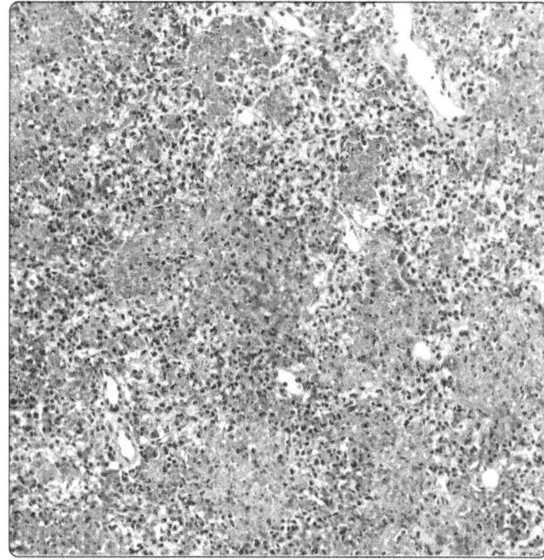

(Left) *Lungs from an infant with congenital CMV infection show dense, necrotic lesions ➡. CMV was found in most organs as well as the placenta.* **(Right)** *Higher magnification of CMV pneumonitis in congenital CMV infection demonstrates sheets of necrosis.*

Congenital CMV Encephalitis

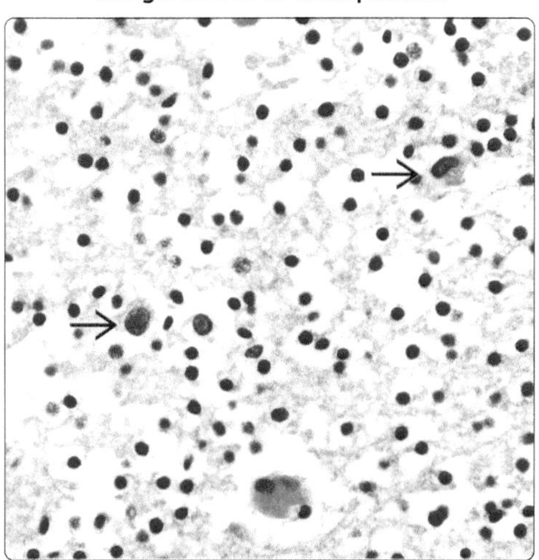

Congenital CMV Encephalitis: IHC

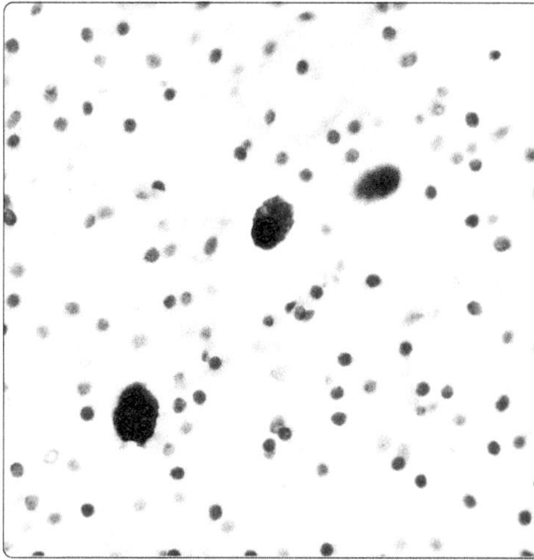

(Left) *Poorly preserved brain tissue from a case of fetal demise due to CMV infection shows scattered enlarged cells with nuclear inclusions typical for CMV ⇒.* **(Right)** *Scattered enlarged cells, some with distinct nuclear inclusions within the plane of section, are highlighted by CMV IHC in this case of fetal demise.*

Human Herpesvirus 6 and 7 (HHV-6, HHV-7) Infections

KEY FACTS

ETIOLOGY/PATHOGENESIS

- Viral infections transmitted person to person through infected saliva or respiratory secretions
- Replicates in lymphocytes, macrophages, histiocytes and endothelial, epithelial, and glial cells; causes lysis
- Latency in monocytes and cells in brain with reactivation in setting of impaired cell-mediated immunity (i.e., bone marrow and solid organ transplants)

CLINICAL ISSUES

- Peak incidence: 6-21 months of age; most children seropositive by 2 years of age
- Roseola infantum (primary infection): High fever, faint maculopapular rash involving back and trunk
- Reactivation: Fever, rash, bone marrow suppression, pneumonitis, meningitis, encephalitis
- Laboratory diagnosis: PCR, serology
- No vaccines available, decrease immunosuppression, antiviral benefit uncertain

IMAGING

- MR: T2/FLAIR hyperintensity in bilateral medial temporal lobes (hippocampus, amygdala, parahippocampal gyrus) and, occasionally, insular region and inferior frontal lobe

MICROSCOPIC

- HHV-6 encephalitis: Multifocal lymphohistiocytic inflammation of gray and white matter, subacute hippocampal sclerosis, and, occasionally, hemorrhage, necrosis, acute inflammation
- Viral inclusions typically not present

TOP DIFFERENTIAL DIAGNOSES

- Roseola infantum: Measles, enteroviruses, adenovirus, Epstein-Barr virus, rubella, parvovirus B19
- HHV-6 encephalitis: Enteroviruses, arboviruses, herpes simplex virus, paraneoplastic limbic encephalitis
- Alternative pathogens identified by histology, serology, PCR, or culture

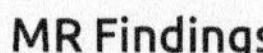

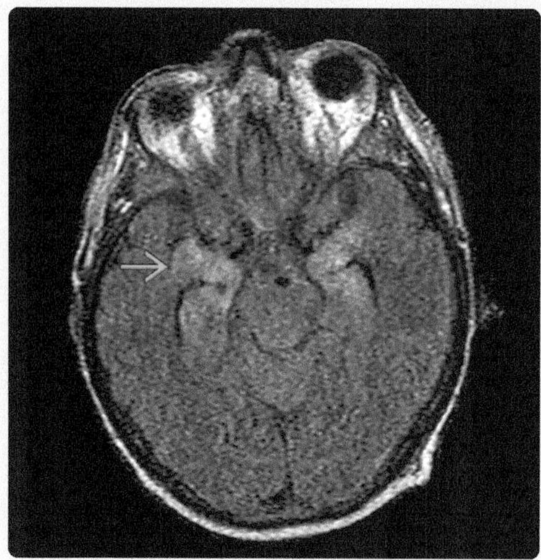

Ultrastructural Features

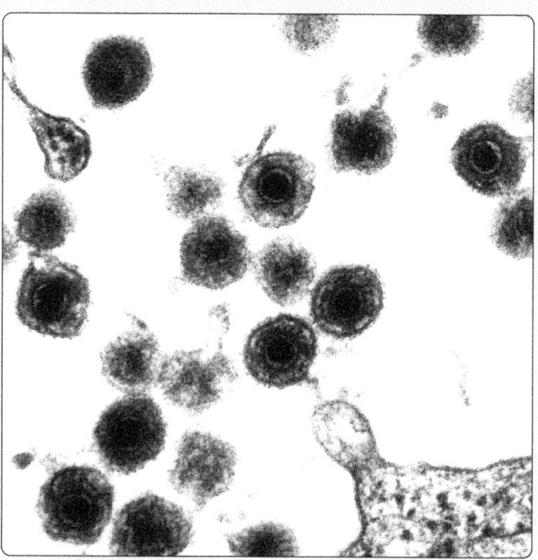

(Left) *MR shows T2/FLAIR hyperintensities of bilateral medial temporal lobes ➡ in a case of human herpesvirus 6b (HHV-6B) encephalitis.* **(Right)** *Electron micrograph shows multiple HHV-6 particles, which are spherical and enveloped with icosahedral capsids. (Courtesy B. Kramarsky, ScD.)*

Microglial Nodules

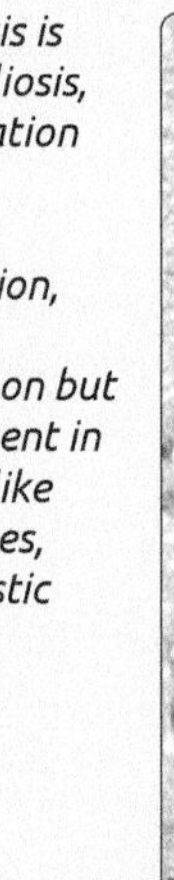

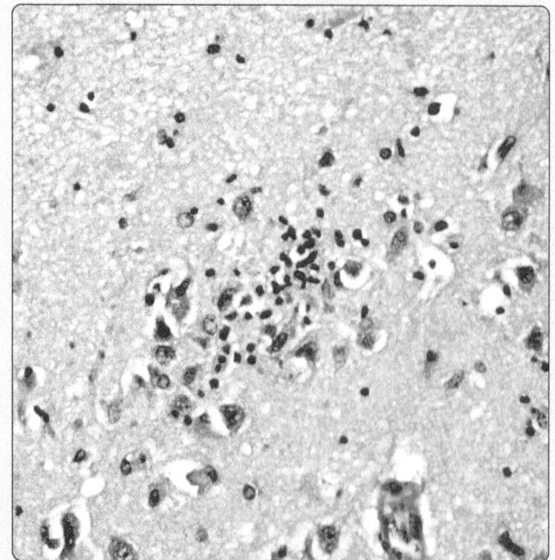

Perivascular Inflammation

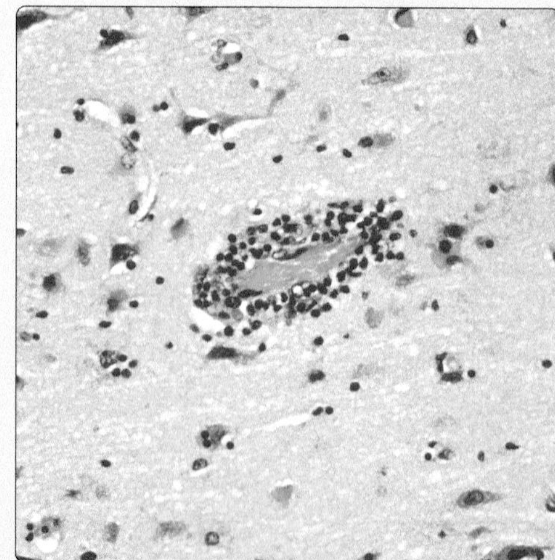

(Left) *HHV-6 encephalitis is associated with microgliosis, microglial nodule formation (seen here), and neuronophagia.* **(Right)** *Perivascular inflammation, largely consisting of lymphocytes, is a common but nonspecific finding present in HHV-6 encephalitis. Unlike many other herpesviruses, there are no characteristic viral cytopathic effects associated with HHV-6.*

TERMINOLOGY

Synonyms

- 6th disease, roseola infantum, exanthem subitum
- *Human betaherpesvirus 6A* (HHV-6A)
- *Human betaherpesvirus 6B* (HHV-6B)
- *Human betaherpesvirus 7* (HHV-7)

Definitions

- *Herpesviridae* family: Derived from "herpein" (to creep)

ETIOLOGY/PATHOGENESIS

Infectious Agents

- Viral infections transmitted person to person through infected saliva or respiratory secretions; also detected in breast milk, urine, and cervical secretions
- Replicates in lymphocytes, macrophages, histiocytes, endothelial cells, epithelial cells, and glial cells and causes direct cytolysis; cell receptors: CD46 (HHV-6A), CD134 (HHV-6B), and CD4 (HHV-7)
- Latency in monocytes and cells in brain with reactivation in setting of impaired cell-mediated immunity (i.e., bone marrow and solid organ transplants); HHV-6 may chromosomally integrate into genome
- Proposed roles in multiple sclerosis, Alzheimer disease, chronic fatigue syndrome/myalgic encephalomyelitis

CLINICAL ISSUES

Epidemiology

- Peak incidence: 6-21 months of age; most children seropositive by 2 years of age

Site

- Skin, brain, bone marrow, lungs

Presentation

- Primary infection: Febrile seizures, rarely meningitis or encephalitis, infectious mononucleosis-like syndrome
- Roseola infantum: High fever, faint maculopapular rash involving back and trunk, sparing face and distal extremities
- Reactivation in bone marrow and solid organ transplant recipients: Fever, rash, bone marrow suppression, pneumonitis, meningitis, encephalitis

Laboratory Tests

- PCR (blood, CSF): Qualitative and quantitative assays; high viral loads may indicate chromosomal integration
  - Incidental HHV-6 positivity requires clinical correlation
- Serology IgG/IgM: ELISA and immunofluorescence assay
- Viral culture (not routinely used): Requires coculture with peripheral blood mononuclear cells

Treatment

- No vaccines currently available
- Antivirals: Ganciclovir/valganciclovir, foscarnet, cidofovir
- Decrease immunosuppression

Prognosis

- Primary infections are generally self-limited
- Reactivation typically asymptomatic; HHV-6 encephalitis mortality > 50%

IMAGING

MR Findings

- T2/FLAIR hyperintensity in bilateral medial temporal lobes (hippocampus, amygdala, parahippocampal gyrus) and, occasionally, insular region and inferior frontal lobe

MICROBIOLOGY

Virus Features

- Enveloped, double-stranded DNA viruses
- 170- to 200-nm diameter, icosahedral capsid
- 145,000- to 170,000-nucleotide genome (~ 100 genes)

MACROSCOPIC

General Features

- HHV-6 encephalitis: Subacute hippocampal sclerosis and necrotic gray and white matter lesions may be visible

MICROSCOPIC

Histologic Features

- HHV-6 encephalitis: Multifocal lymphohistiocytic inflammation of gray and white matter, subacute hippocampal sclerosis, and, occasionally, hemorrhage, necrosis, acute inflammation
- Skin: Interface dermatitis, scattered necrotic keratinocytes, epidermal hyperplasia, lichenoid infiltrate

Cytologic Features

- No characteristic viral cytopathic effects

ANCILLARY TESTS

Immunohistochemistry

- HHV-6 (available at some reference laboratories): Positive in neurons, oligodendrocytes, and astrocytes

DIFFERENTIAL DIAGNOSIS

Other Causes of Rash and Fever in Children

- Measles, enteroviruses, adenovirus, Epstein-Barr virus, rubella, parvovirus B19
  - Identification by histology, serology, PCR, or culture

Other Causes of Meningoencephalitis Involving Temporal Lobes

- Enteroviruses, arboviruses, herpes simplex virus
  - Identification by histology, serology, PCR, or culture
- Paraneoplastic limbic encephalitis
  - Associated with extra-CNS tumors
  - Detection of autoantibodies in 60% of patients

SELECTED REFERENCES

1. Leung AKC et al: Roseola infantum: an updated review. Curr Pediatr Rev. ePub, 2022
2. Green DA et al: Clinical significance of human herpesvirus 6 positivity on the filmarray meningitis/encephalitis panel. Clin Infect Dis. 67(7):1125-8, 2018
3. Agut H et al: Update on infections with human herpesviruses 6A, 6B, and 7. Med Mal Infect. 47(2):83-91, 2017
4. Clark DA: Clinical and laboratory features of human herpesvirus 6 chromosomal integration. Clin Microbiol Infect. 22(4):333-9, 2016
5. Ongrádi J et al: Roseolovirus-associated encephalitis in immunocompetent and immunocompromised individuals. J Neurovirol. 23(1):1-19, 2016

Kaposi Sarcoma-Associated Herpesvirus (HHV-8) Infection

KEY FACTS

ETIOLOGY/PATHOGENESIS

- Viral infection with unclear mode of transmission associated with Kaposi sarcoma (KS), primary effusion lymphoma (PEL), and multicentric Castleman disease (MCD)

CLINICAL ISSUES

- Seroprevalence in adults ranges from 1-5% in USA, up to 80% in some African countries
- KS exists in 4 clinicoepidemiological forms: Classic indolent, endemic African, iatrogenic, epidemic
- Laboratory: PCR (tissue, CSF)
- Treatment: HAART, antivirals, chemotherapy, surgery

MACROSCOPIC

- KS: Pink, purple-red, or black patches, plaques, and nodules

MICROSCOPIC

- KS exhibits 3 well-defined stages of disease
  - Patch: Increased vascular spaces, chronic inflammation
  - Plaque: More extensive vascular proliferation, greater component of spindled cells, hyaline globules
  - Nodular: Well-circumscribed, intersecting fascicles of sieve-like vascular spaces and spindled cells, hyaline globules, frequent mitoses, mild cytologic atypia
- PEL composed of large lymphoid cells with irregular nuclei, prominent nucleoli, and abundant vacuolated cytoplasm
- MCD contains lymph nodes with sheets of polytypic plasma cells in interfollicular regions, with blurring of mantle zone border, and extensive vascular proliferation

ANCILLARY TESTS

- HHV-8 LANA-1 is sensitive and specific IHC marker

TOP DIFFERENTIAL DIAGNOSES

- KS: Angiosarcoma; hobnail, capillary, spindle cell, or tufted hemangioma; lymphangiomatosis
- PEL: DLBCL, plasmablastic lymphoma, Burkitt lymphoma
- MCD: Hyaline vascular variant CD, plasma cell variant CD, plasmacytoma

Ultrastructural Features

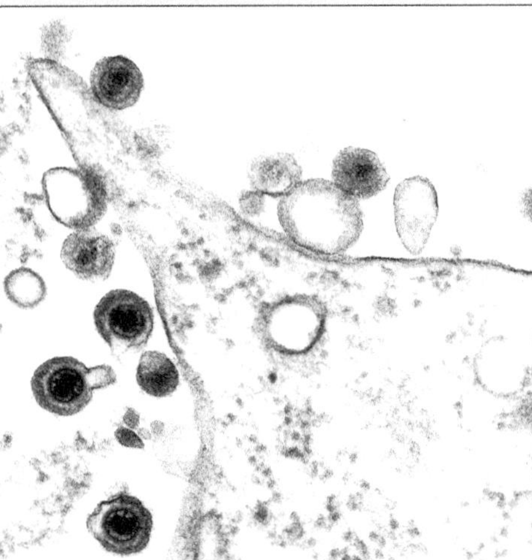

Kaposi Sarcoma

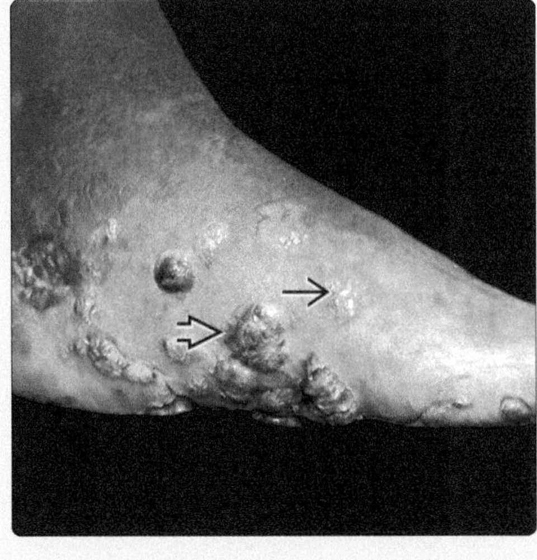

(Left) *EM of cultured cells shows several enveloped, spherical particles measuring ~ 120 nm in diameter, characteristic of human herpesvirus 8 (HHV-8). An inner nucleocapsid is surrounded by an envelope with a layer of tegument apposed to the envelope. (Courtesy C. Goldsmith, MS and J. Black, PhD, CDC.)* **(Right)** *A case of classic Kaposi sarcoma (KS) in an older man is shown. Although uncommon, both flat → and nodular lesions ⇨ are seen in this case. (From DP: Neoplastic Derm.)*

Kaposi Sarcoma

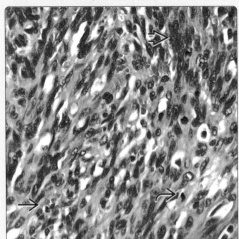

Kaposi Sarcoma: HHV-8 IHC

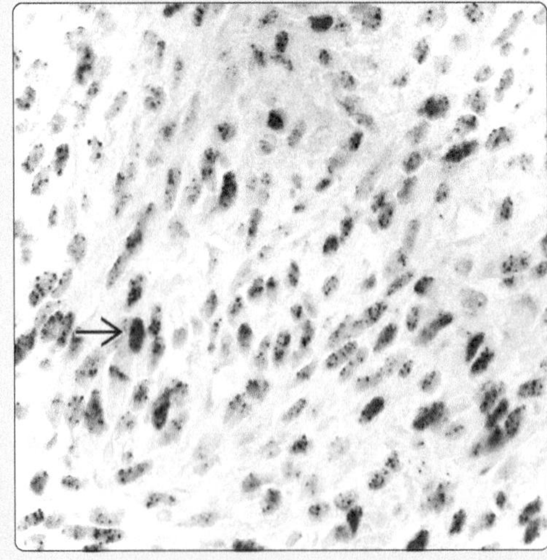

(Left) *High magnification of a KS lesion of the skin demonstrates the slit-like spaces filled with blood →, the spindle cell proliferation ⇨, and several mitoses ↷.* **(Right)** *Immunohistochemistry for HHV-8, the virus responsible for KS, reveals strong nuclear staining → within the KS lesion of the skin.*

TERMINOLOGY

Synonyms

- Kaposi sarcoma-associated herpesvirus (KSHV)
- *Human gammaherpesvirus 8* (HHV-8)

Definitions

- "Kaposi" from Moritz Kaposi (first described in 1872)
- *Herpesviridae* family: Derived from "herpein" (to creep)

ETIOLOGY/PATHOGENESIS

Infectious Agents

- Virus-associated diseases with unclear route of transmission (virus found in saliva and semen) leading to lifelong and latent infection; infection necessary but insufficient for development of Kaposi sarcoma (KS)
- Disease develops in immunocompromised; HIV/AIDS very common; HIV Tat transcription factor cross activates viral replication of HHV-8
- Virus evades host cytotoxic T-cell immunosurveillance by infecting B cells; in primary effusion lymphoma, B cells often coinfected with EBV
- HHV-8 encodes homologue of human IL-6 thought to contribute to development of multicentric Castleman disease (MCD); IL-6 regulates differentiation of B lymphocytes to plasma cells, T-cell function, and induces C-reactive protein production
- KSHV inflammatory cytokine syndrome displays MCD-like inflammatory symptoms but does not have pathologic findings of MCD

CLINICAL ISSUES

Epidemiology

- USA: Seroprevalence 1-5% in general population; up to 35% in HIV-positive men who have sex with men
- Worldwide: Seroprevalence ranges from 1-5% in Europe (10-20% in certain Mediterranean countries); up to 30-80% in parts of sub-Saharan Africa
- KS exhibits 4 clinicoepidemiological forms
  - Classic indolent
    - Affects older men of Eastern European or Mediterranean descent
    - Cutaneous lesions begin on extremities, enlarge and spread proximally
  - Endemic African
    - Affects children and young adults in sub-Saharan Africa
    - Variable clinical course: From indolent to locally infiltrative and aggressive
    - Generalized lymphadenopathy is common
  - Iatrogenic
    - Caused by medically induced immunosuppression
    - Male predilection
    - Involves mucocutaneous tissues, lymph nodes, and viscera
  - Epidemic AIDS associated
    - HIV-positive men who have sex with men at highest risk
    - Skin and visceral involvement can be extensive
    - Skin lesions have predilection for face and lower extremities
    - 50% of cases have visceral involvement
    - GI tract and lungs are 2 most frequent sites for visceral involvement
    - Lesions enlarge, multiply in number, and coalesce with decreasing CD4 count
- Primary effusion lymphoma rare; < 0.5% of all aggressive lymphomas in HIV-negative patients and ~ 4% of all HIV-related lymphomas
- MCD strongly associated with HIV-positive rates; becoming more common in era of highly active antiretroviral therapy

Site

- KS most commonly involves skin but can occur in any organ
- Primary effusion lymphoma typically involves pleural, peritoneal, &/or pericardial spaces; intracavitary mass in 25% of cases; extracavitary or solid variants do exist
- MCD can involve any lymph node group; spleen (80%), liver (50%), and bone marrow also commonly involved

Presentation

- KS
  - Primary presentation is purple to black flat, raised, or nodular skin lesions on any body surface
    - Chronic lesions may show severe crusting, erosion, ulceration, or superinfection
  - Internal organs may also be affected (most common in untreated HIV infection) and present with organ-specific symptoms
    - Liver involvement with transaminitis
    - Pulmonary involvement with hemoptysis
    - GI involvement with hematochezia, hematemesis, melena, or bright red blood per rectum
- Primary effusion lymphoma symptoms related to massive malignant effusion
  - Dyspnea due to compression from pleural or pericardial disease
  - Abdominal distension from peritoneal disease
- MCD associated with lymphadenopathy, hepatosplenomegaly, edema, body cavity effusions, and B symptoms (fever, night sweats, weight loss)

Laboratory Tests

- PCR (blood, tissue): Qualitative/quantitative for HHV-8 DNA
- Serology of limited clinical utility
- MCD: Elevated serum IL-6, erythrocyte sedimentation rate, lactate dehydrogenase levels, and hypergammaglobulinemia

Treatment

- Highly active antiretroviral therapy (HAART) for HIV-/AIDS-associated disease
- Some antiviral drugs (e.g., ganciclovir, cidofovir, foscarnet) and antiretroviral drugs (e.g., adefovir, lobucavir, nelfinavir) have anti-HHV-8 activity
- KS
  - Surgical resection typically reserved for solitary lesions
  - Systemic chemotherapy (vincristine) for severe, widespread, symptomatic, or rapidly progressive disease

- Local therapy, including topical chemotherapeutics, liquid nitrogen, and radiotherapy, for limited cutaneous disease or adjunct for progressive, chemotherapy unresponsive disease
- Primary effusion lymphoma: Intracavitary cidofovir; no consensus on additional chemotherapy
- MCD: Chemotherapy and steroids may have some effect

Prognosis

- KS survival varies by clinicoepidemiological form; very poor prognosis for late-stage KS in HIV-infected patients without treatment
- Poor prognosis (survival of months) in primary effusion lymphoma and MCD

IMAGING

Radiographic Findings

- KS
  - Pulmonary involvement: Nodular or reticular opacities with predilection for perihilar and lower lung fields
  - GI involvement: Nodular opacities
  - Lymphadenopathy may or may not be present
- Primary effusion lymphoma
  - Pleural (bilateral or unilateral), pericardial, or peritoneal effusion
  - Slight thickening of parietal pleura, pericardium, or peritoneum with absence of solid tumor or parenchymal involvement
- MCD
  - Nonspecific lymphadenopathy and hepatosplenomegaly
  - ~ 50% of lesions are FDG positive

MICROBIOLOGY

Viral Features

- Enveloped, double-stranded DNA virus
- 120-nm diameter, icosahedral capsid
- 160,000 nucleotide genome (encoding > 85 genes)
- 7 known subtypes based oK1 open reading frame (ORF-K1): A, B, C, D, E, F, and Z

Culture

- No routine use for clinical diagnosis

MACROSCOPIC

General Features

- KS
  - Patches, plaques, and nodules that vary in color from pink to purple-red to black
  - Mucocutaneous lesions may show associated lymphedema and scale
  - Wide variation in number and size of lesions

MICROSCOPIC

Histologic Features

- KS
  - Numerous described histologic variants: Anaplastic, lymphangioma-like, lymphangiectatic, hyperkeratotic, keloidal, micronodular
  - HIV-related cases may show more extensive dissecting vessels
  - Non-HIV cases may show greater anaplastic features and mitoses
  - Patch stage (histologic findings may be subtle)
    - Promontory sign: Vascular proliferation that dissects around skin adnexa and larger ectatic vessels (not pathognomonic of KS)
    - Proliferation of endothelial-lined vessels, with flat and uniform cells, present in dermis
    - Extravasated red blood cells and hemosiderin-laden macrophages
    - Sparse chronic inflammatory infiltrate: Lymphocytes and plasma cells
    - Rare spindled cell component
  - Plaque stage (represents exaggeration of patch stage)
    - Skin lesions involve most of dermis, may extend to subcutis
    - Greater component of spindled cells
    - Hyaline globules easily found (more frequent in AIDS-associated KS); eosinophilic material from fragments of erythrocytes present intra- or extracellularly
    - Chronic inflammatory infiltrate
  - Nodular stage
    - Well-circumscribed, intersecting fascicles of uniform spindled cells
    - Mitoses may be numerous
    - Mild cytologic atypia may be present
    - Slit-like vascular spaces with extravasated erythrocytes/hyaline globules
- Primary effusion lymphoma
  - Cytologic preparations of effusion fluid show large lymphoid cells with irregular nuclei, prominent nucleoli, and abundant vacuolated cytoplasm
  - Extracavitary/solid variants show sheets of large atypical cells with high mitotic activity and necrosis
- MCD
  - Lymph nodes show sheets of polytypic plasma cells in interfollicular regions, including immature and atypical forms, with lymphocyte depletion
  - Blurring of border between mantle zone and interfollicular area
  - Extensive vascular proliferation

Cytologic Features

- No characteristic viral inclusions

ANCILLARY TESTS

Histochemistry

- KS
  - Hyaline globules are positive for PAS
  - Iron stain highlights intra- and extracellular hemosiderin deposition

Immunohistochemistry

- HHV-8 antibodies targeting latency-associated nuclear antigen 1 (LANA-1)
  - Highly sensitive and specific marker for KS, primary effusion lymphoma, and MCD (mantle zones of follicles)
- KS

- Vascular channels and spindled cells are positive for vascular endothelial markers: CD31 and CD34 show membranous and cytoplasmic staining, while ERG and FLI-1 show nuclear positivity
- Lesional vascular spaces are not surrounded by SMA-positive pericytes

- Primary effusion lymphoma
  - Positive for CD45/LCA, pan-B cell markers (i.e., CD20, CD79a, PAX5), plasma cell-associated markers (i.e., CD138, MUM1)
  - Negative for CD10, BCL6, LMP1
  - Positive for EBER in majority of cases

Genetic Testing

- Primary effusion lymphoma
  - Monoclonal *IGH* rearrangements and somatic hypermutation of *IGH* variable regions
  - Usually complex karyotype
  - No recurrent chromosomal abnormalities identified and no rearrangements of *MYC, BCL2, BCL6, CCND1*
- MCD
  - Monoclonal *IGH* gene rearrangements occur in EBV- or HIV-positive cases

DIFFERENTIAL DIAGNOSIS

Kaposi Sarcoma

- Hobnail hemangioma
  - Solitary vascular lesions with biphasic growth and hobnail endothelial cells negative for HHV-8
  - Dilated vessels in superficial areas narrow with increasing dermal depth
- Capillary hemangioma
  - Lobular growth of narrow capillaries; negative for HHV-8
- Spindle cell hemangioma
  - KS-like features coincident with cavernous hemangioma-like features, scattered epithelioid tumor cells without increased mitoses, and negative for HHV-8
- Angiosarcoma
  - Anastomosing vascular structures with endothelial multilayering, prominent nuclear atypia, and negative for HHV-8
- Tufted hemangioma
  - Cannonball distribution of vascular tufts with endothelial cells surrounded by SMA-positive pericytes, crescent-shaped clefts, and negative for HHV-8
- Kaposiform hemangioendothelioma
  - Usually infants and young children with retroperitoneal and abdominal location
  - Infiltrative cellular lobules without increased mitoses; negative for HHV-8
- Lymphangiomatosis (of limbs)
  - Solitary, plaque-like lesions without increased mitoses or prominent inflammatory infiltrate; negative for HHV-8

Primary Effusion Lymphoma

- Diffuse large B-cell lymphoma
  - Can present as pleural mass in setting of longstanding chronic inflammation
  - Body cavity involvement can occur in systemic disease, often without history of immunosuppression
  - Large atypical B cells with immunoblastic or plasmacytoid differentiation
  - Negative for HHV-8
- Plasmablastic lymphoma
  - Immunoblastic (oral cavity and HIV-positive patients) and plasmablastic (nonoral sites) types
  - Weak or negative staining for CD45/LCA and CD20
  - Negative for HHV-8
- Burkitt lymphoma
  - Rarely exhibit plasmacytoid differentiation
  - Positive for CD10 and BCL6
  - MYC-associated translocations
  - Negative for HHV-8

Multicentric Castleman Disease

- Hyaline vascular variant
  - Large follicles with prominent hyaline vascular lesions
  - No atypical plasmablasts
  - Negative for HHV-8, EBV, and HIV
- Plasma cell variant
  - Single lymph node without mantle zone blurring
  - No monotypical plasma cells or IGH rearrangements
  - Negative for HHV-8, EBV, and HIV
- Plasmacytoma
  - Sheets of plasma cells replace lymph node architecture
  - Less vascularity in interfollicular region
  - Negative for HHV-8 and EBV

SELECTED REFERENCES

1. Calvani J et al: A comprehensive clinicopathologic and molecular study of 19 primary effusion lymphomas in HIV-infected patients. Am J Surg Pathol. 46(3):353-62, 2022
2. Carbone A et al: Castleman disease. Nat Rev Dis Primers. 7(1):84, 2021
3. Cesarman E et al: KSHV/HHV8-mediated hematologic diseases. Blood. 139(7):1013-25, 2021
4. Lopes AO et al: Update of the global distribution of human gammaherpesvirus 8 genotypes. Sci Rep. 11(1):7640, 2021
5. Cesarman E et al: Kaposi sarcoma. Nat Rev Dis Primers. 5(1):9, 2019
6. Katano H: Pathological features of Kaposi's sarcoma-associated herpesvirus infection. Adv Exp Med Biol. 1045:357-76, 2018
7. Narkhede M et al: Primary effusion lymphoma: current perspectives. Onco Targets Ther. 11:3747-54, 2018
8. Auten M et al: Human herpesvirus 8-related diseases: histopathologic diagnosis and disease mechanisms. Semin Diagn Pathol. 34(4):371-6, 2017
9. Schneider JW et al: Diagnosis and treatment of Kaposi sarcoma. Am J Clin Dermatol. 18(4):529-39, 2017
10. Rohner E et al: HHV-8 seroprevalence: a global view. Syst Rev. 3:11, 2014
11. Patel RM et al: Immunohistochemical detection of human herpes virus-8 latent nuclear antigen-1 is useful in the diagnosis of Kaposi sarcoma. Mod Pathol. 17(4):456-60, 2004
12. Hong A et al: Immunohistochemical detection of the human herpes virus 8 (HHV8) latent nuclear antigen-1 in Kaposi's sarcoma. Pathology. 35(5):448-50, 2003
13. Ioachim HL et al: Kaposi's sarcoma of internal organs. A multiparameter study of 86 cases. Cancer. 75(6):1376-85, 1995

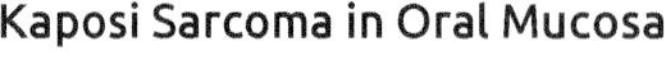

Kaposi Sarcoma in Oral Mucosa

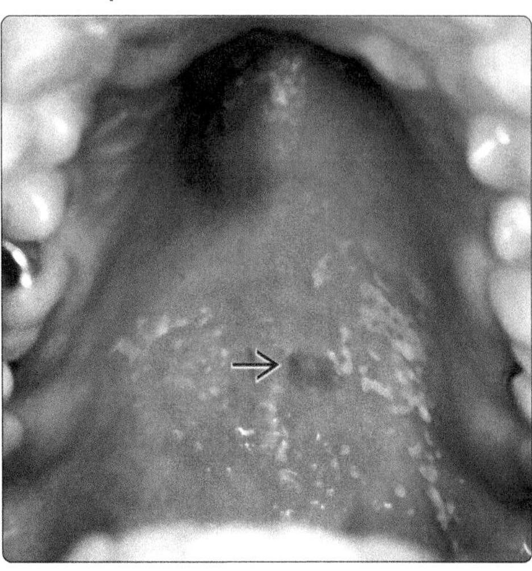

Kaposi Sarcoma in Eyelid

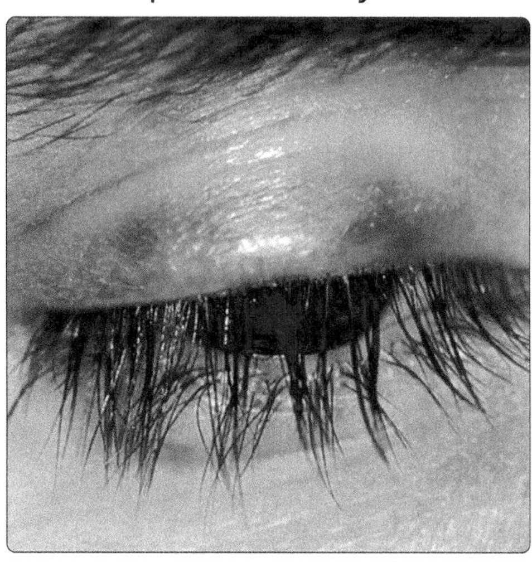

(Left) *KS lesions of the oral mucosa (hard palate) are shown, which may be difficult to detect. KS can involve any part of the body, and extensive internal disease has high mortality. (From DP: Head & Neck.)* **(Right)** *Patients with AIDS-related KS may present with lesions at unusual anatomic sites, as did this patient who developed small, reddish lesions on his upper eyelid. In patients with darker skin, lesions may be very subtle. (From DP: Neoplastic Derm.)*

Nodular Kaposi Sarcoma

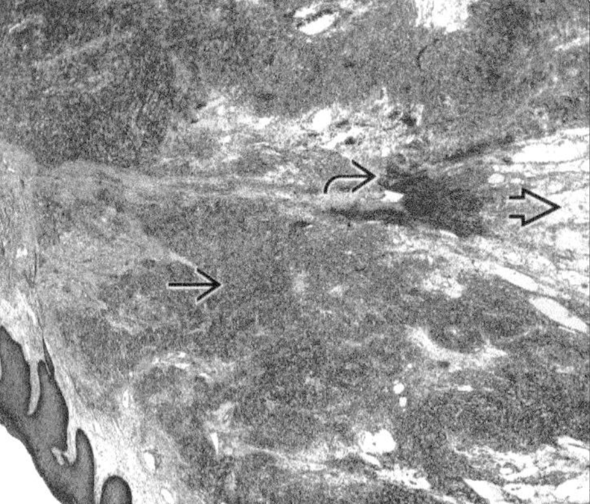

Kaposi Sarcoma: Hyaline Globules

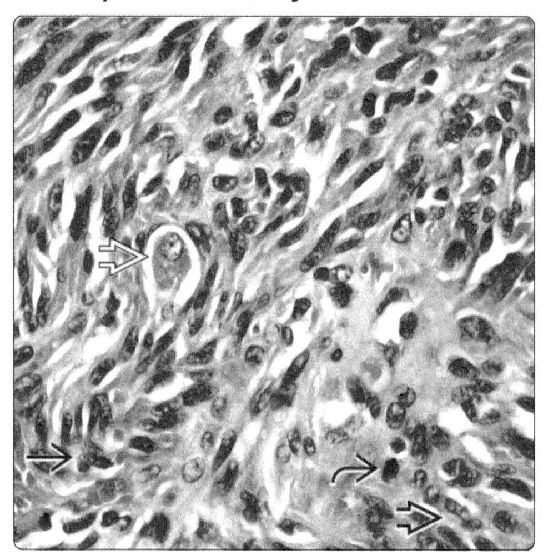

(Left) *Low magnification in a case of nodular KS in the skin demonstrates the tumor cells admixed with edema and areas of hemorrhage.* **(Right)** *High magnification of a KS lesion demonstrates the slit-like spaces filled with blood, the spindle cell proliferation, several mitoses, and conspicuous hyaline bodies within the cytoplasm, which are strongly PAS positive.*

Kaposi Sarcoma Patch Stage

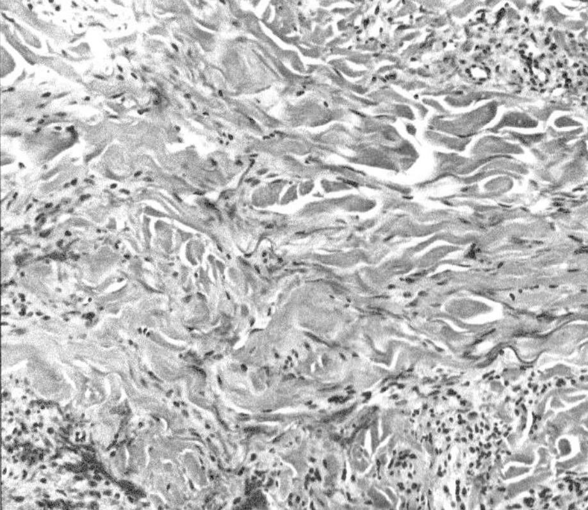

Kaposi Sarcoma Patch Stage: HHV-8 IHC

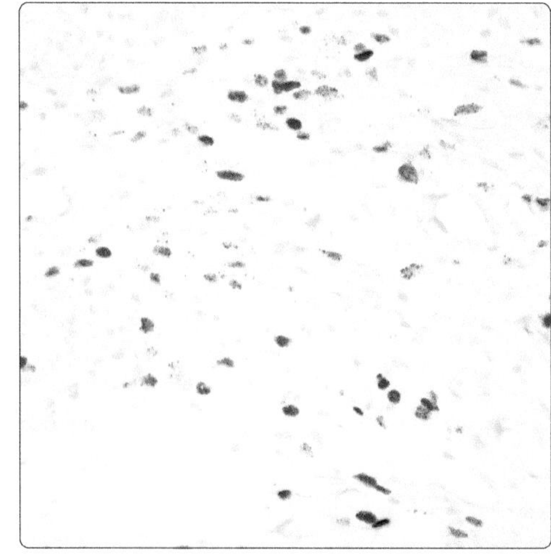

(Left) *Section shows a proliferation of endothelial-lined vessels with flat and uniform cells, extravasated red blood cells and hemosiderin-laden macrophages, and sparse chronic inflammatory infiltrate, features consistent with patch stage of KS. (Courtesy A. Laga, MD, MMSc.)* **(Right)** *HHV-8 immunohistochemistry highlights scattered positive cells with a dot-like staining pattern. (Courtesy A. Laga, MD, MMSc.)*

Multicentric Castleman Disease

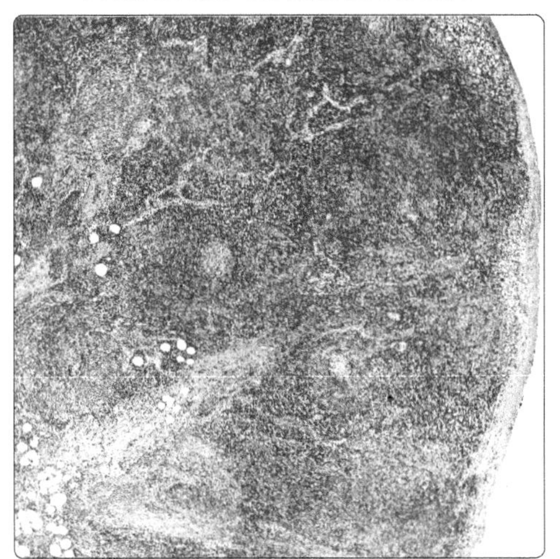

Multicentric Castleman Disease

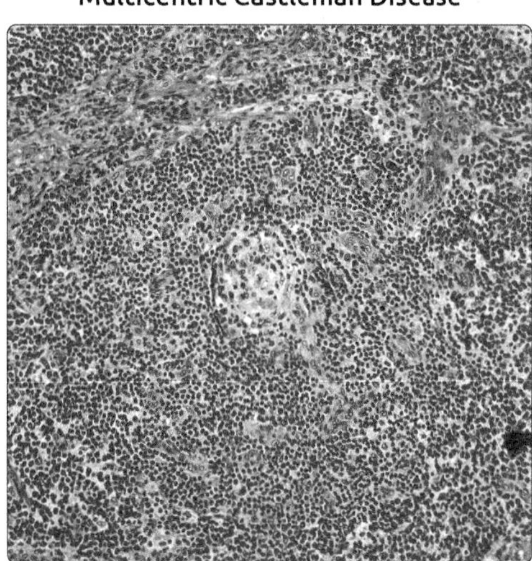

(Left) *Low-power image of an inguinal lymph node shows a thickened capsule with expansion of interfollicular plasma cells and prominent interfollicular vasculature.* **(Right)** *Medium-power image of an inguinal lymph node shows expansion of interfollicular plasma cells, prominent interfollicular vasculature, and follicles with features of regression and onion skinning.*

Multicentric Castleman Disease

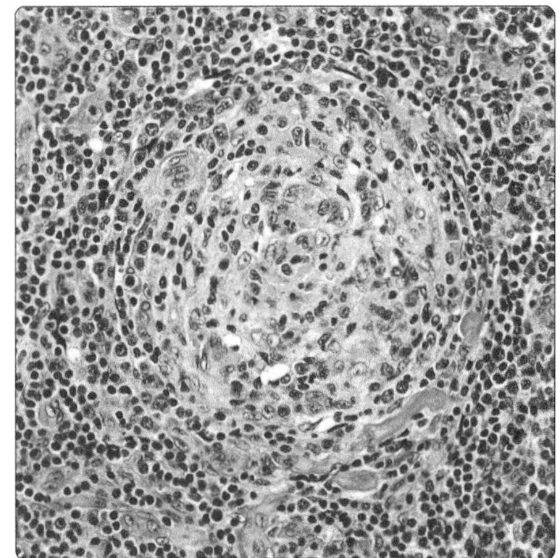

Multicentric Castleman Disease: HHV-8 IHC

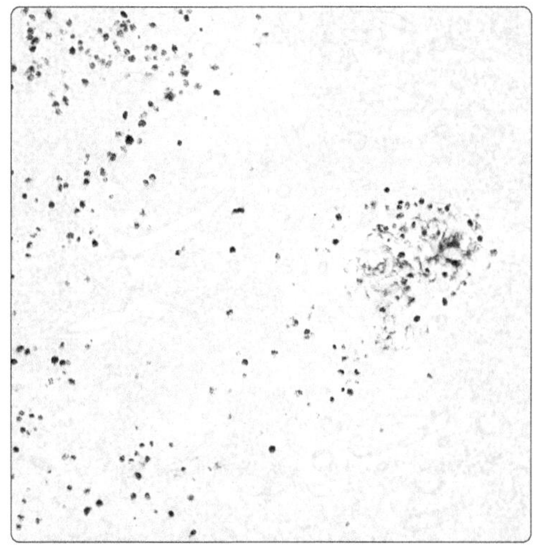

(Left) *High-power image of an inguinal lymph node shows a follicle with features of regression and onion skinning surrounded by numerous plasma cells and occasional eosinophils.* **(Right)** *HHV-8 immunostaining of an inguinal lymph node highlights scattered cells associated with atrophic germinal centers.*

Primary Effusion Lymphoma

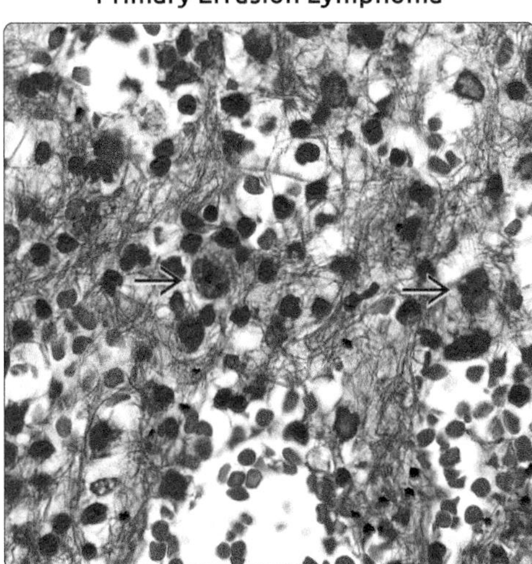

Primary Effusion Lymphoma: HHV-8 IHC

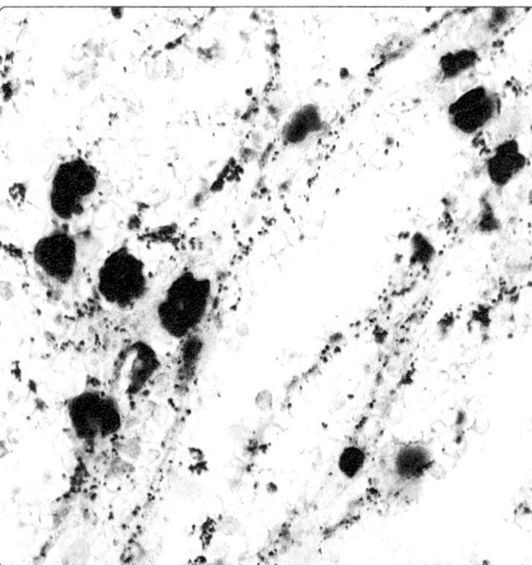

(Left) *Pleural fluid cell block from an HIV-positive individual with extensive KS skin lesions shows large cells with irregular nuclei, prominent nucleoli, and abundant cytoplasm ⊟.* **(Right)** *HHV-8 immunostaining of a pleural fluid cell block shows strong nuclear staining of scattered cells.*

Herpes B Virus Infection

KEY FACTS

ETIOLOGY/PATHOGENESIS

- Infections from bites or scratches from macaques or exposure to infectious materials entering though needle sticks or cuts

CLINICAL ISSUES

- Greatest risk for veterinarians, laboratory workers, and others who have close contact with Old World macaques or monkey cell cultures
- 50 documented human infections since 1932 (21 fatal)
- Symptoms include fever, headache, and vesicular skin lesions; can result in ascending myelitis, respiratory failure, and death
- Laboratory testing of exposed human and implicated macaque: RT-PCR, antibody detection, culture
- Classified as select agent; testing performed in biosafety level 4 (BSL-4) facility
- No vaccines are available; treat by cleaning wound and administration of oral or intravenous antivirals

MICROSCOPIC

- Cutaneous/mucosal: Ulceration, necrosis, ballooning degeneration
- CNS: Encephalomyelitis (upper cervical cord with extension to medulla and pons), hemorrhagic infarcts, edema, degeneration of motor neurons, gliosis, and astrocytosis
- Heart, liver, spleen, lungs, kidneys, and adrenals demonstrate congestion and focal necrosis
- Cowdry type A eosinophilic intranuclear inclusions rare

ANCILLARY TESTS

- Cross reactivity with some herpes simplex virus 1/2 (HSV-1/2) antibodies

TOP DIFFERENTIAL DIAGNOSES

- Varicella-zoster virus, HSV-1, or HSV-2 infections
  - Skin/mucosal lesions and histology may appear identical to herpes B virus; confirmation by IHC, PCR, serology, and correlation with macaque testing results

(Left) *Herpes B virus is characterized by spherical, enveloped particles with a diameter of ~ 200 nm, which are features similar to the herpes simplex virus (HSV) virions seen in this image. (Courtesy F. Murphy, PhD.)* **(Right)** *Herpes B virus is commonly found in macaque monkeys, which typically exhibit mild or no symptoms. Rhesus macaques are a common source of human transmission due to their extensive use in biomedical research. (Courtesy R. Broderson, DVM, PhD.)*

Ultrastructural Features

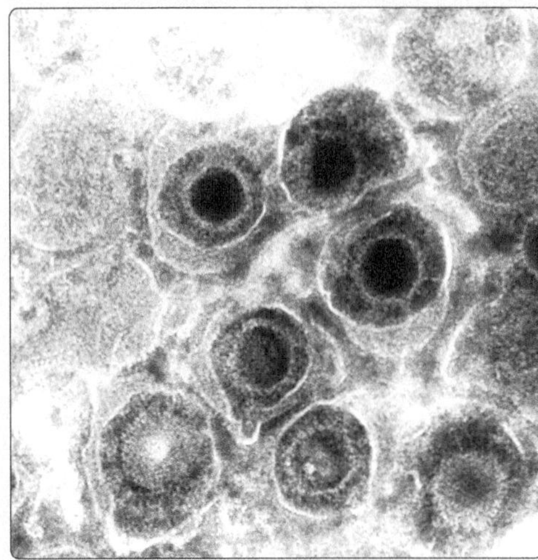

Rhesus Macaque (*Macaca mulatta*)

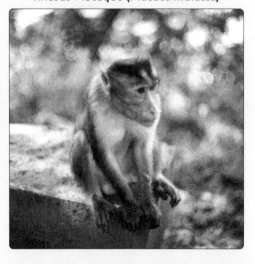

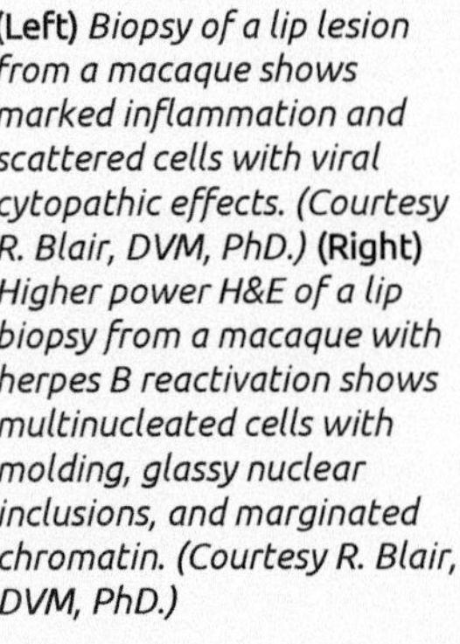

(Left) *Biopsy of a lip lesion from a macaque shows marked inflammation and scattered cells with viral cytopathic effects. (Courtesy R. Blair, DVM, PhD.)* **(Right)** *Higher power H&E of a lip biopsy from a macaque with herpes B reactivation shows multinucleated cells with molding, glassy nuclear inclusions, and marginated chromatin. (Courtesy R. Blair, DVM, PhD.)*

Lip Biopsy

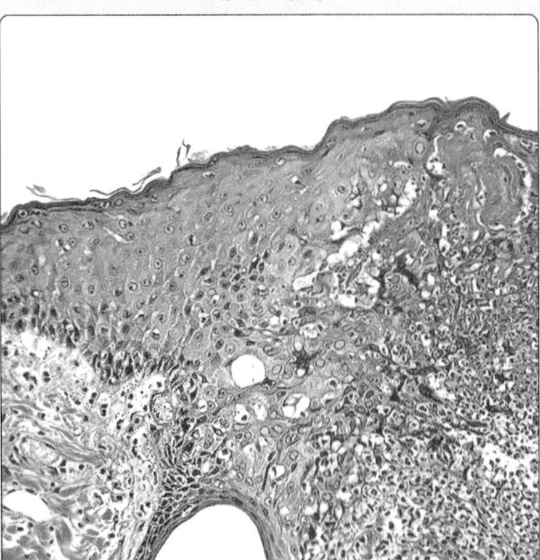

Viral Cytopathic Effects

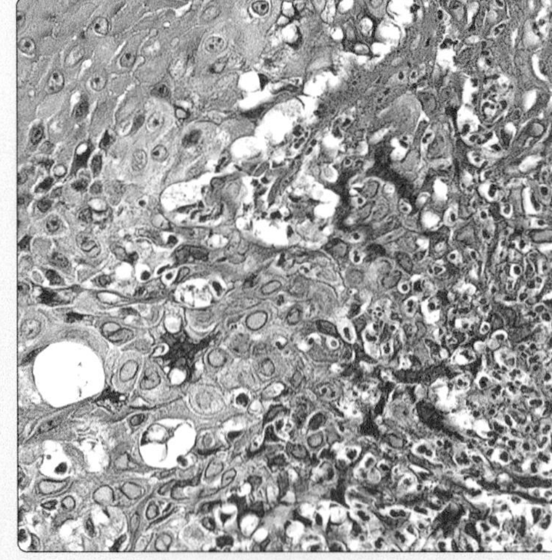

TERMINOLOGY

Synonyms

- B virus (BV), monkey B virus
- *Macacine alphaherpesvirus 1* (McHV-1); formerly *Cercopithecine herpesvirus 1, Herpesvirus simiae*

Definitions

- *Herpesviridae* family: Derived from "herpein" (to creep)

ETIOLOGY/PATHOGENESIS

Infectious Agents

- Macaques serve as natural host (virus can be present in saliva, feces, urine, or nervous tissue) and are usually symptom free or exhibit mild disease similar to herpes simplex virus (HSV) infection in humans
- Macaques housed in primate facilities usually become BV positive by time they reach adulthood; transmission during active viral shedding into mucosal surfaces following reactivation from latent state
- Infections result from animal bites/scratches, infectious materials entering broken skin through needlestick/cut, or mucosal splash exposure; minimal risk of human-to-human transmission
- Disease onset within 1 month of exposure (early as 3 days)
- Classified as select agent by United States Public Health Service, Department of Health and Human Services

CLINICAL ISSUES

Epidemiology

- 50 documented human infections since 1932 (21 fatal)
- Greatest risk for veterinarians, laboratory workers, and others who have close contact with Old World macaques or monkey cell cultures
- Possible risk of disease with exposure to Simian agent 8 (SA8; African Green monkeys), herpesvirus langur (HVL; langurs), or herpesvirus cercocebus (HVC; mangabeys)
- One suggested case of herpesvirus papio 2 (HVP-2; baboons) transmission

Presentation

- Initial symptoms include fever, headache, and vesicular skin lesions with numbness or paresthesia around site of inoculation; ocular involvement has been reported
- Ascending myelitis resulting in respiratory failure and death can occur 1 day to 3 weeks after symptom onset

Laboratory Tests

- Samples should be tested from exposed human and implicated macaque
- Testing performed at National B Virus Resource Laboratory located at Georgia State University
- RT-PCR (swabs, tissue, CSF) with sequencing verification
- Antibody detection (serum, CSF) by Western blot and confirmed by ELISA
- HSV-1/2 are not protective against BV infection and cause false-positive and false-negative results

Treatment

- No vaccines are available
- First aid prior to specimen collection: Thorough washing with soap, detergent, povidone iodine, or chlorhexidine followed by irrigation with water
- Prophylaxis: Oral valacyclovir or acyclovir for 14 days
- Treatment of infection: Intravenous acyclovir or ganciclovir

Prognosis

- Fatal in 70% of untreated patients
- Survivors may have no long-term effects or experience slow progressive neurologic decline

MICROBIOLOGY

Viral Features

- Enveloped, double-stranded DNA virus
- 200-nm diameter, icosahedral capsid
- ~ 160,000 nucleotide genome (encoding > 50 polypeptides)

Culture

- Performed on swabs, tissue, and CSF
- Virus grows in Vero cells; confirmed by PCR
- Requires biosafety level 4 (BSL-4) containment facility

MICROSCOPIC

Histologic Features

- Cutaneous/mucosal lesions include ulcers extending down to papillary layer of dermis with central area of necrosis surrounded by zone of ballooning degeneration
- CNS lesions include encephalomyelitis (primarily involving upper cervical cord with extension to medulla and pons): Hemorrhagic infarcts, prominent edema, degeneration of motor neurons, gliosis, and astrocytosis
- Heart, liver, spleen, lungs, kidneys, and adrenals demonstrate congestion and focal necrosis
- Cowdry type A eosinophilic intranuclear inclusions found in minority of cases

ANCILLARY TESTS

Immunohistochemistry

- Cross reactivity with some HSV-1/2 antibodies

DIFFERENTIAL DIAGNOSIS

Varicella-Zoster Virus and Herpes Simplex Virus 1 or 2 Infections

- Skin/mucosal lesions and histology may appear identical to herpes B virus
- Confirmation by IHC, PCR, serology, and correlation with macaque testing results

SELECTED REFERENCES

1. Centers for Disease Control and Prevention: B virus. Reviewed January 27, 2023. Accessed January 27, 2023. https://www.cdc.gov/herpesbvirus/index.html
2. Georgia State University: National B virus resource center. Reviewed January 27, 2023. Accessed January 27, 2023. https://biotech.gsu.edu/virology/
3. Eberle R et al: Questioning the extreme neurovirulence of monkey b virus (Macacine alphaherpesvirus 1). Adv Virol. 2018:5248420, 2018
4. Hilliard J et al: Monkey B virus. In Arvin A et al: Human Herpesviruses: Biology, Therapy, and Immunoprophylaxis. Cambridge: Cambridge University Press, 2007
5. Cohen JI et al: Recommendations for prevention of and therapy for exposure to B virus (cercopithecine herpesvirus 1). Clin Infect Dis. 35(10):1191-203, 2002

KEY FACTS

ETIOLOGY/PATHOGENESIS

- Ubiquitous DNA viruses spread via respiratory droplets
- Most adults have seropositivity to several serotypes; commonly found in respiratory tract and stools of children

CLINICAL ISSUES

- Range of clinical infections (mild to life threatening): Keratoconjunctivitis, tonsillitis, bronchiolitis, pneumonia, laryngotracheobronchitis, myocarditis, gastroenteritis, colitis, appendicitis, hepatitis, meningitis/encephalitis, nephritis, hemorrhagic cystitis
- Severe, life-threatening disease in immunosuppressed
- PCR on tissue sample, fluid, or blood; rising viral load correlates with risk of severe disease

MICROSCOPIC

- Classic viral cytopathic effects include glassy to smudged basophilic nuclear inclusions that must be differentiated from reactive cells by antiadenovirus IHC
- Lungs: Minimal inflammation to diffuse alveolar damage
- Liver: Focal to extensive necrosis with limited inflammation
- Gastrointestinal tract: Ulceration, inflammation, cell sloughing, and apoptosis
- Brain: Minimal inflammation to perivascular cuffing
- Heart: Limited mononuclear to dense inflammation with necrosis
- Kidneys: Acute necrotizing tubulointerstitial nephritis

TOP DIFFERENTIAL DIAGNOSES

- HSV-1/2, VZV: Multinucleation, margination of chromatin, and nuclear molding
- CMV: 2-4x size of adjacent cells, large "owl eye" nuclear inclusion
- Polyomavirus: Demyelinating (polyoma) vs. meningoencephalitis (adenovirus)
- DAD: Reactive, degenerative cells may be suspicious for viral cytopathic effect; any condition leading to DAD can mimic adenoviral infection (and vice versa)

Ultrastructural Features

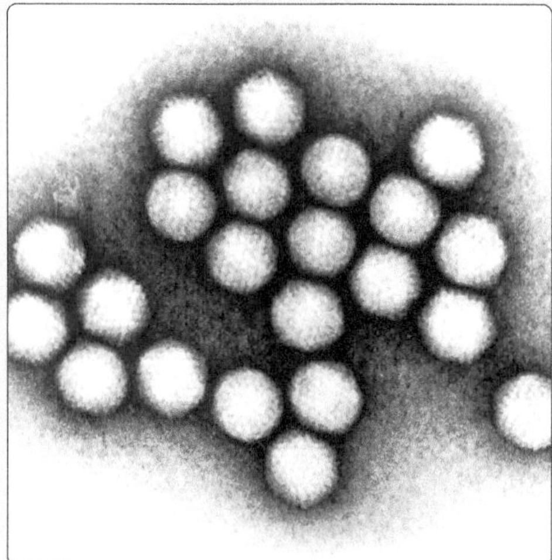

Severe Adenovirus Pneumonia

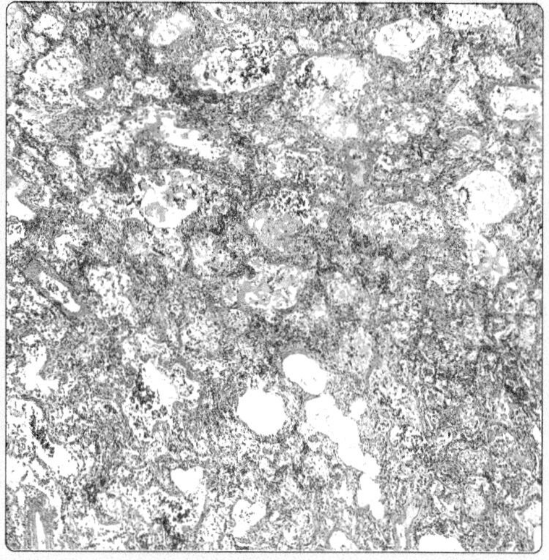

(Left) *Transmission electron micrograph demonstrates adenovirus particles with the characteristic icosahedral capsid, ~ 70-90 nm in diameter. (Courtesy G. W. Gary, Jr., CDC/PHIL.)* **(Right)** *Low-power view of severe pneumonia in an immunocompromised patient with adenovirus infection demonstrates diffuse alveolar damage (DAD). At this level, the features are consistent with DAD but not specific to adenovirus.*

Adenovirus Pneumonitis

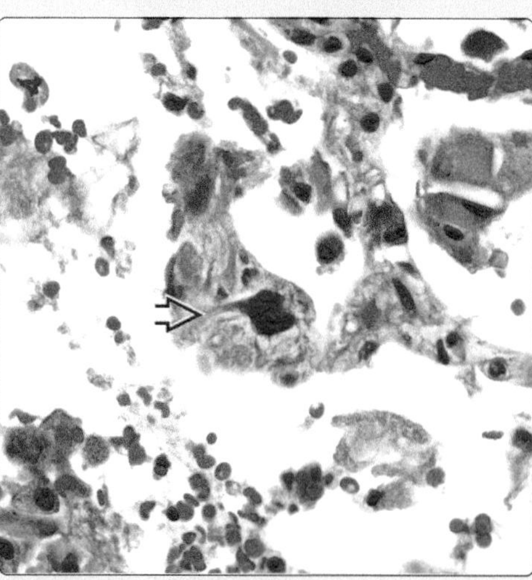

Adenovirus Pneumonia: IHC

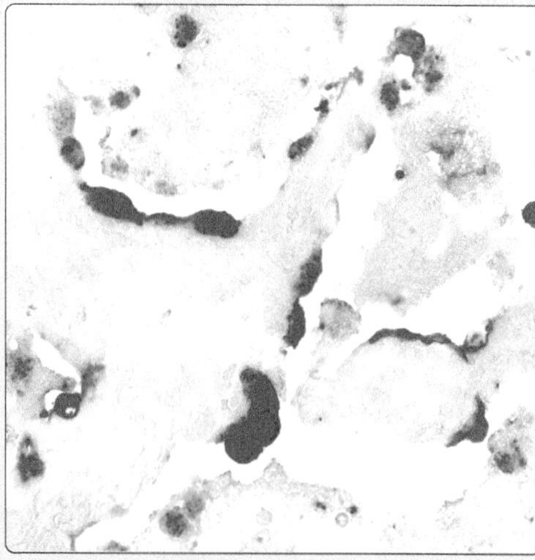

(Left) *An atypical smudged nucleus ➲ in the lung of an immunosuppressed patient is shown with minimal inflammation. Viral cytopathic effects need to be distinguished from reactive cells, which may be accomplished with immunohistochemistry.* **(Right)** *IHC for adenovirus antigens shows both nuclear and cytoplasmic staining in pneumonia with DAD.*

TERMINOLOGY

Synonyms

- Common "cold" (accounts for only 5%)

Definitions

- *Mastadenovirus* genus and *Adenoviridae* family: Derived from "mastos" (breast/mammal) and "adeno" (for adenoids where first isolated)
- Adenovirus (serovar #) = Ad#

ETIOLOGY/PATHOGENESIS

Infectious Agents

- Ubiquitous DNA viruses present in most vertebrates and able to infect many cell types; spread primarily via respiratory droplets as well as fecal routes and aerosols
- During initial infection (2-14 days incubation), virus enters epithelial cell via binding to CD46 or CAR adhesion receptor, replicates through entire lytic cycle, produces cytolysis ± inflammatory response (depending on patient)
- Chronic infection and reactivation of latency via unknown process occurring in various lymphoid tissues
- Oncogenic in animal models but not, to date, in humans
- Common tool for vaccine vectors and for development of novel cancer virotherapies

CLINICAL ISSUES

Epidemiology

- Ubiquitous viral family affecting all age groups
- Most adults have seropositivity to several serotypes
- Commonly found in respiratory tract and stool of children

Site

- Lungs, gastrointestinal tract, liver, heart, kidneys, brain, conjunctiva

Presentation

- Range of clinical infections (mild to life threatening)
- Keratoconjunctivitis (pink eye) &/or tonsillitis (Ad3, 4, 7, 8, 19, 37, 53, 54)
- Bronchiolitis &/or pneumonia (Ad3, 4, 7, 14, 21, 30)
- Laryngotracheobronchitis (Ad1, 2, 3, 5, 6, 7, 14)
- Myocarditis (chronic, leading to cardiomyopathy)
- Gastroenteritis, colitis, appendicitis (Ad40, 41)
- Hepatitis (Ad1-5, 7, 31): Fulminant, similar to herpesvirus
- Meningitis/encephalitis (Ad2, 7)
- Nephritis, hemorrhagic cystitis (Ad11, 21)

Laboratory Tests

- Serology is challenging to interpret unless serovar matched to symptoms
- Culture from direct tissue sample > blood
- Antigen detection: Stool for enteric (Ad40, Ad41)
- Direct fluorescence antigen detection &/or PCR on nasal swabs
- PCR: Molecular detection of virus DNA or RNA
  - Broad panels available for screening and diagnosis
  - Directly on tissue sample, fluid, or blood; most commonly used for enteric infection (stool) and CNS infection (CSF)
  - Qualitative or quantitative: Rising viral load correlates with risk of severe disease
  - Should be used with caution due to ubiquitous nature of virus

Treatment

- FDA-approved vaccine for Ad4/Ad7 (military use only)
- Supportive treatment for mild disease
- No specific antivirals available: IV ribavirin and cidofovir used in severe cases

Prognosis

- Most serovars: Self-limited infection, particularly in immunocompetent
- Immunocompromised (e.g., solid organ and bone marrow transplant recipients) at highest risk for severe disease: Mortality 50-80% in children and up to 70% in adults

IMAGING

Radiographic Findings

- Lungs: Pneumonia, bronchial wall thickening, hyperaeration
- Liver: Hypodense lesions on CT

MICROBIOLOGY

Virus Features

- Nonenveloped, lytic, double-stranded DNA virus
- 70-90 nm in size with icosahedral capsid
- 88 human serotypes divided into 7 species (groups A-G)
- 26,000- to 46,000-bp genome

Culture

- Grows in cell culture [e.g., HEK, HEp-2, A549 (laboratory diagnosis), Graham 293 (enteric adenovirus)] in 1-3 weeks
- Confirmed by cytopathic effect with positive direct antigen visualization

MACROSCOPIC

General Features

- Lungs: Heavy/edematous, congested mucosa, necrotic foci
- Liver: Hepatomegaly with foci of necrosis
- Gastrointestinal tract: Extensive mucosal ulcerations

MICROSCOPIC

Histologic Features

- Classic viral cytopathic effects include glassy to smudged basophilic nuclear inclusions that must be differentiated from reactive cells; nonspecific viral cytopathic effects are also common
- **Lungs**: Minimal inflammation to necrotizing bronchitis/bronchiolitis or acute necrotizing alveolitis resembling diffuse alveolar damage (DAD)
- **Liver**: Focal to extensive necrosis with limited inflammation
- **Gastrointestinal tract**: Increased lymphoplasmacytic and neutrophilic infiltrates in lamina propria; blunting and flattening of villous architecture; loss of nuclear orientation, sloughing, and apoptotic epithelial cells
- **Brain**: Minimal inflammation to perivascular cuffing and increased cellularity; necrosis is not a usually feature
- **Heart**: Limited mononuclear to dense lymphohistiocytic interstitial inflammation with necrosis

- **Kidneys**: Acute tubular injury and interstitial nephritis, focal necrosis of tubules, interstitial hemorrhage, edema, granulomas

Cytologic Features

- Medium to large cells with variable nuclear changes, nucleoli, smudged chromatin; background milieu may show necrosis or limited inflammation

ANCILLARY TESTS

Immunohistochemistry

- Antibodies targeting adenovirus antigens show nuclear and cytoplasmic staining
- Should always be considered in concert with herpesviruses without prior diagnosis

Immunofluorescence

- Performed on fresh, frozen, or FFPE tissue sections for confirmatory diagnosis

In Situ Hybridization

- Specific DNA probes for adenovirus target (available in reference laboratories)
- Use with caution due to ubiquitous nature of virus

PCR

- Molecular detection of virus DNA or RNA can be performed on tissue samples

Electron Microscopy

- Demonstration of icosahedral particles consistent with adenovirus

DIFFERENTIAL DIAGNOSIS

Herpesvirus Family (All Sites)

- HSV-1/2, varicella-zoster virus (VZV): Multinucleation, margination of chromatin, and nuclear molding
- Cytomegalovirus (CMV): 2-4x size of adjacent cells, large "owl's-eye" nuclear inclusion; smaller cytoplasmic inclusions
- When viral cytopathic effect is suspected in immunosuppressed patients, panel of HSV, VZV, CMV, and adenovirus IHC is advised

Polyomavirus (Cerebral Cortex, Kidney/Bladder)

- Demyelinating (polyoma) vs. meningoencephalitis (adenovirus); IHC for both agents is confirmatory

Other Viral Infections (All Sites)

- RNA viruses and others resulting in necrosis without inflammation; exclude adenovirus by IHC; reference tissue testing for confirmation of other viral infections is recommended

Bacterial Infection (All Sites)

- Destructive, necrotic lesions; demonstration of bacteria on Gram or silver staining with positive cultures

Diffuse Alveolar Damage (Lung)

- Reactive, degenerative cells may be suspicious for viral cytopathic effect
- Any condition leading to DAD can mimic adenoviral infection (and vice versa); clinical history, culture, and IHC can exclude DAD of other causes

SELECTED REFERENCES

1. Lynch JP 3rd et al: Adenovirus: epidemiology, global spread of novel types, and approach to treatment. Semin Respir Crit Care Med. 42(6):800-21, 2021
2. Shieh WJ: Human adenovirus infections in pediatric population - an update on clinico-pathologic correlation. Biomed J. 45(1):38-49, 2021
3. Wen S et al: The epidemiology, molecular, and clinical of human adenoviruses in children hospitalized with acute respiratory infections. Front Microbiol. 12:629971, 2021
4. Gu J et al: Adenovirus diseases: a systematic review and meta-analysis of 228 case reports. Infection. 49(1):1-13, 2020
5. Lamps LW: Infectious causes of appendicitis. Infect Dis Clin North Am. 24(4):995-1018, ix-x, 2010
6. Wong S et al: Detection of a broad range of human adenoviruses in respiratory tract samples using a sensitive multiplex real-time PCR assay. J Med Virol. 80(5):856-65, 2008
7. Dubberke ER et al: Acute meningoencephalitis caused by adenovirus serotype 26. J Neurovirol. 12(3):235-40, 2006

Adenovirus Hepatitis

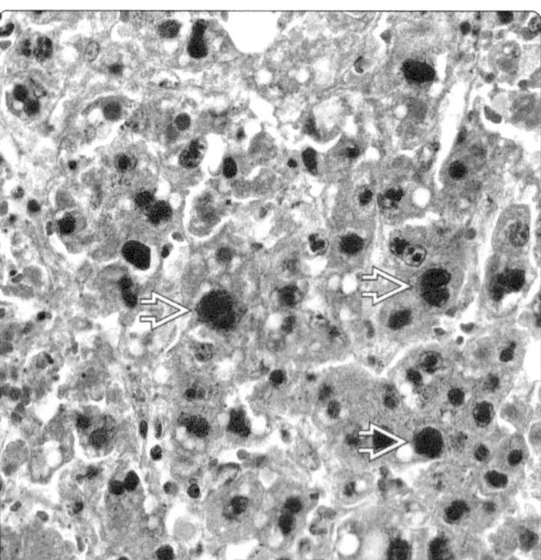

Adenovirus Hepatitis: IHC

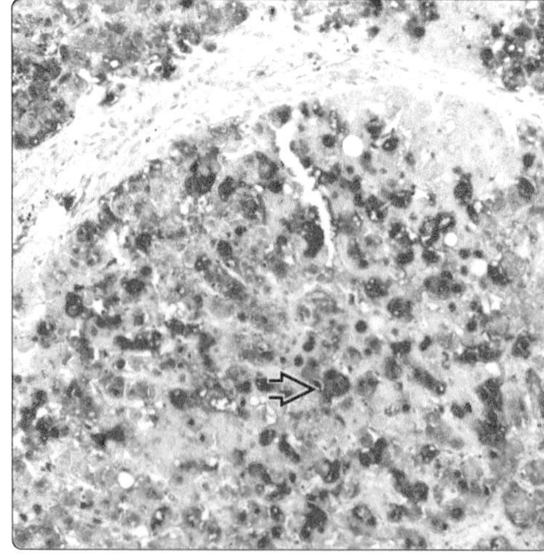

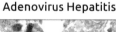

(Left) *Abnormal nuclei ➡ (smudged to Cowdry-like) are shown adjacent to the necrotic liver with no inflammation (fulminant adenovirus hepatitis), resulting in the death of an immunosuppressed patient.* **(Right)** *As in this case of adenovirus hepatitis, IHC will highlight cells (which may be numerous) that are positive for the virus that do not demonstrate viral cytopathic effect, although scattered cells may be suggestive of cytopathic effect ➡.*

Adenovirus Colitis

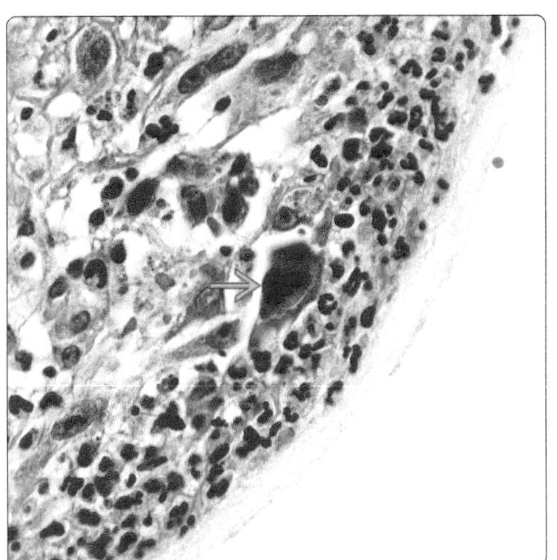

Adenovirus Colitis: IHC

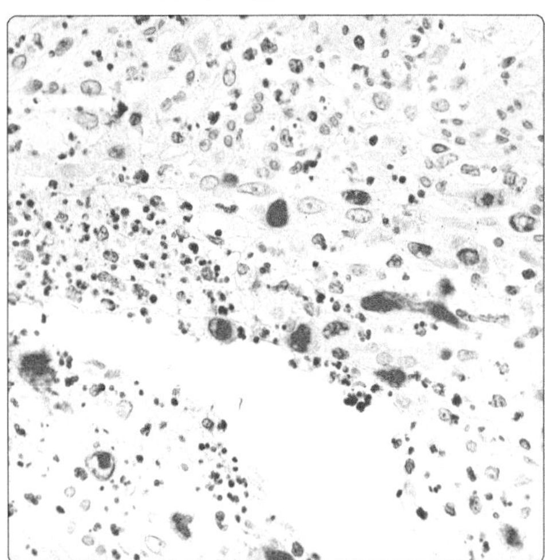

(Left) *A 39-year-old patient with Hodgkin lymphoma treated with bone marrow transplantation presented with rectal bleeding and abdominal pain and underwent colon resection for severe ulceration, which showed scattered cells with smudgy nuclear inclusions ➡.* **(Right)** *Antiadenovirus immunohistochemistry highlighted scattered epithelial cells near the ulcerated surface of the resected colon.*

Adenovirus Nephritis

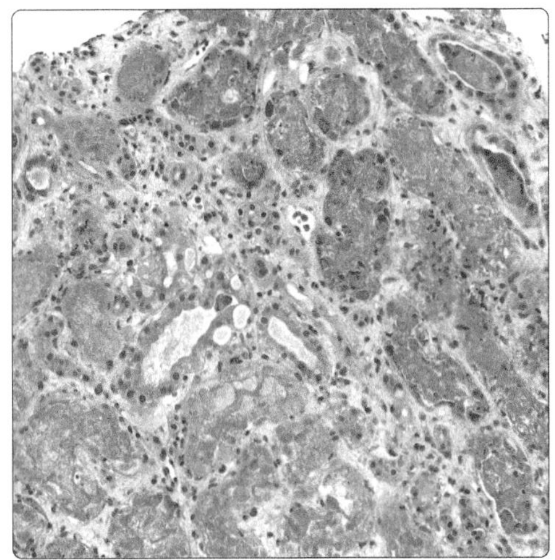

Adenovirus Nephritis: IHC

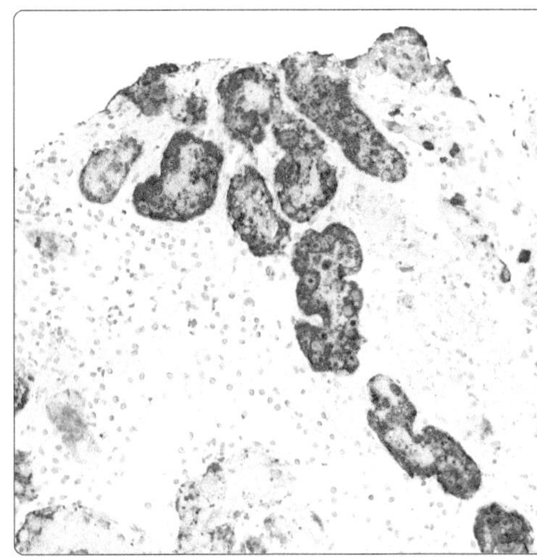

(Left) *Kidney biopsy shows tubules with extensive necrosis and degenerative changes of the nuclei, several of which show prominent viral inclusions.* **(Right)** *Antiadenovirus immunohistochemistry highlights necrotic material in tubules as well as several individual nuclei, confirming the cause of acute necrotizing tubulointerstitial nephritis in this patient.*

Brain MR: Adenovirus Infection

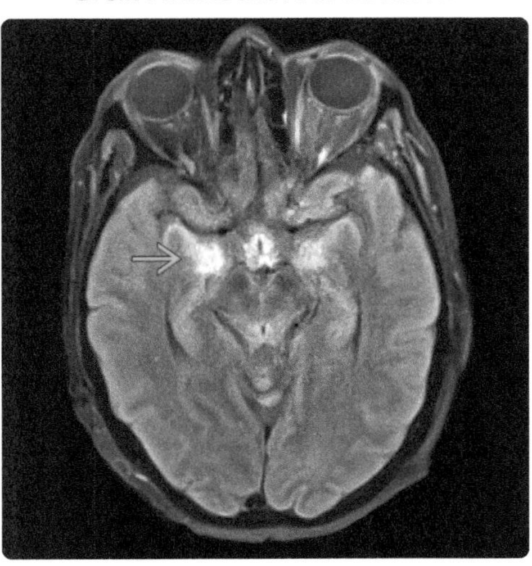

Adenovirus CNS Infection

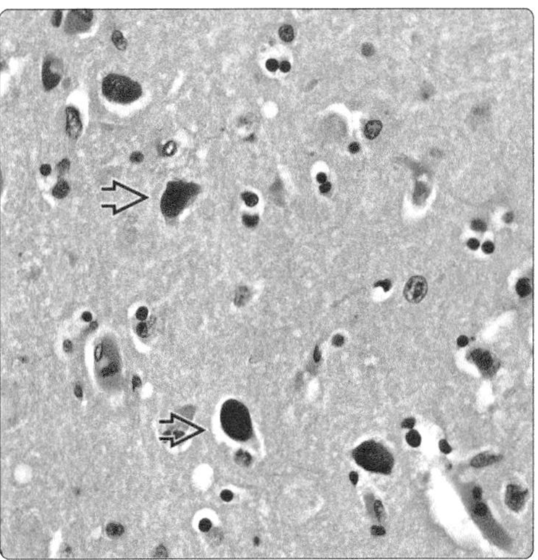

(Left) *A 58-year-old with T-cell prolymphocytic leukemia treated with allogeneic cord transplantation presented with fever and altered mental status and was found to have T2 hyperintensities in bilateral mesial temporal lobes ➡ and hypothalami. CSF PCR for adenovirus was markedly positive (~ 800,000 copies/mL).* **(Right)** *Adenovirus infection of the CNS involves cortical neurons ➡, which exhibit dark blue/purple smudged nuclei, red cytoplasm, and minimal reaction or inflammation.*

Hepatitis B and D Virus Infections

KEY FACTS

ETIOLOGY/PATHOGENESIS

- Viral infections transmitted through infected blood and body fluids
- Chronic infection associated with cirrhosis and hepatocellular carcinoma
- Hepatitis D virus (HDV) infection occurs as hepatitis B virus (HBV)-coinfection/superinfection

CLINICAL ISSUES

- 400 million people worldwide are chronically infected with HBV; 48 million people are infected with HDV
- Acute hepatitis B: HBsAg, anti-HBc IgM positive
- Chronic hepatitis B: HBsAg positive, anti-HBc IgM negative

MICROSCOPIC

- Acute hepatitis B: Hepatocytic swelling, mononuclear cell infiltrates, spotty necrosis, apoptotic bodies, confluent and bridging necrosis, collapse of hepatocytic cords, hepatocytic regeneration
- Chronic hepatitis B: Portal inflammation, interface hepatitis, lobular hepatitis, fibrosis
- Grading denotes inflammatory activity, whereas staging indicates degree of fibrosis
- IHC for HBV surface antigen (cytoplasmic staining) and core antigen (nuclear and cytoplasmic staining)

TOP DIFFERENTIAL DIAGNOSES

- Hepatitis A virus/hepatitis E virus (HAV/HEV): Acute lobular hepatitis; positive anti-HAV/HEV IgM or PCR
- Hepatitis C virus (HCV): Chronic hepatitis, portal inflammation and fibrosis, hepatocellular steatosis; positive HCV RNA
- Autoimmune hepatitis: Lobular hepatitis, portal/periportal plasma cells, positive autoimmune serologies
- Drug-/toxin-induced hepatitis: Similar to acute viral hepatitis; prominent eosinophils
- Primary biliary cirrhosis: Florid duct lesion (granuloma) destroying interlobular bile duct

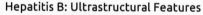

Hepatitis B: Ultrastructural Features

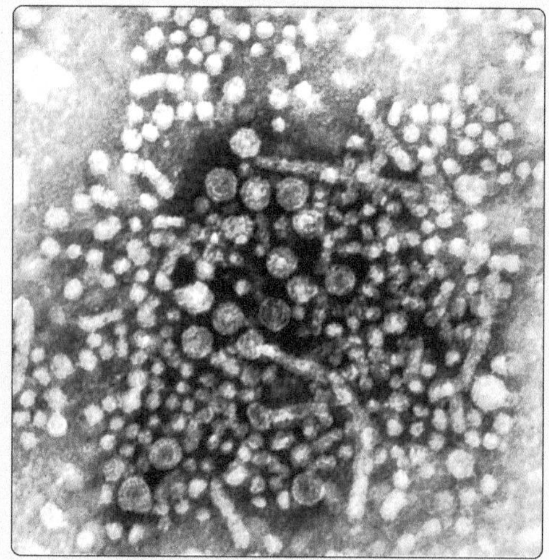

Hepatitis B: Morphology

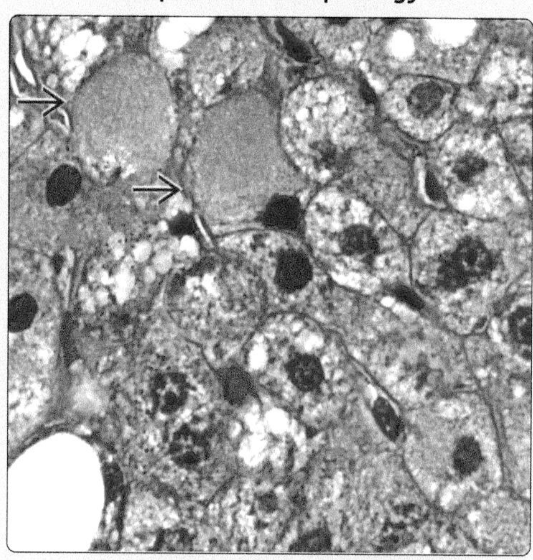

(Left) *This negative-stained transmission electron microscopic image reveals the presence of numerous spherical structures (a.k.a. Dane particles), consistent with hepatitis B virus virions. (Courtesy B. Partin, CDC/PHIL.)* **(Right)** *Ground-glass hepatocytes ➔ have glassy eosinophilic cytoplasm representing a proliferation of smooth ER in response to hepatitis B surface antigen (HBsAg).*

Hepatitis B: Nuclear Morphology

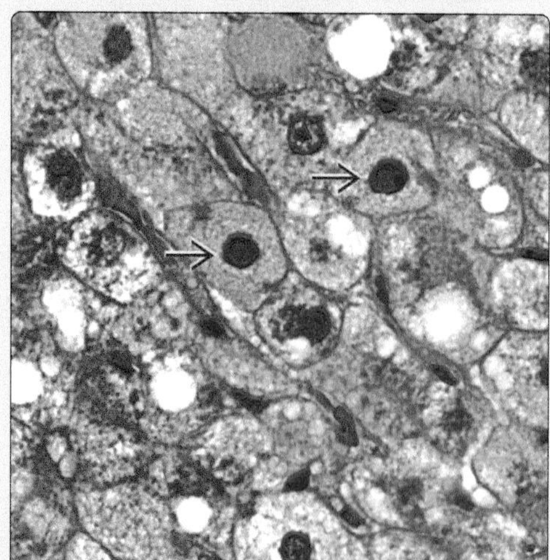

Hepatitis B: Lobar Inflammation

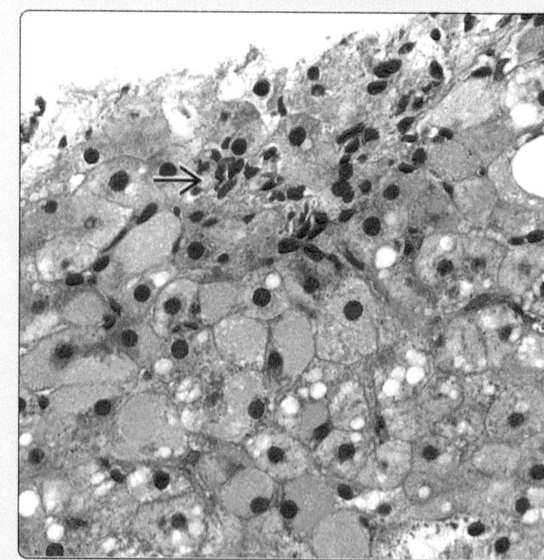

(Left) *Hepatitis B-infected hepatocytes have pale pink, finely granular intranuclear inclusions (sanded nuclei ➔) representing nuclear accumulation of hepatitis B core antigen (HBcAg).* **(Right)** *Hematoxylin and eosin section demonstrates a focus of lobular inflammation composed of lymphocytes and Kupffer cells ➔.*

TERMINOLOGY

Definitions

- Hepatitis B virus (HBV); *Hepatitis B virus*; *Hepadnaviridae* family from "Hepa" (of liver) and "DNA"
- Hepatitis D virus (HDV); *Deltavirus* genus; *Kolmioviridae* family from Finnish "kolmio" (triangle)

ETIOLOGY/PATHOGENESIS

Infectious Agents

- Viral infections transmitted through infected blood and body fluids, from mothers to newborn infants, between young children, and through sexual contact
- Virus gains entry into liver cells via NTCP bile transporter; liver injury appears to be immune mediated; HBV-specific T cells play key role in pathogenesis and viral clearance
- Increased risk of hepatocellular carcinoma (HCC); strongly associated with presence of cirrhosis but also occurs in absence of cirrhosis with high HBV viral loads
- HDV infection occurs as coinfection or superinfection of HBV infection

CLINICAL ISSUES

Epidemiology

- 400 million people worldwide are chronically infected with HBV
  - Africa and Asia have carrier rates of as high as 15%
  - North America has carrier rate of ~ 5%
  - HBV is uncommon in countries with highest standards of living
- Estimated 48 million people are infected with HDV
  - Most common in Southern and Eastern Europe, Mediterranean, Middle East, West and Central Africa, East Asia, and Amazon Basin

Site

- Liver

Presentation

- Acute hepatitis B
  - > 50% are asymptomatic
  - Symptoms include mild flu-like syndrome, nausea, vomiting, jaundice
  - < 1% develop fulminant liver failure leading to death or liver transplantation
  - Serum HBsAg and anti-HBc virus IgM Ab positive
- Chronic hepatitis B
  - Serum HBsAg positive and anti-HBc virus IgM Ab negative
- Hepatitis D coinfection or superinfection
  - Increase chance of liver failure in acute hepatitis B
  - More rapid progression to cirrhosis in chronic hepatitis B

Laboratory Tests

- Hepatitis B surface antigen (HBsAg; Australia antigen): Present in natural infection and vaccinated patients (4-24 weeks after infection)
- Hepatitis B core antigen (HBcAg): Only present in infected patients; not detected in routine clinical testing
- Hepatitis B early antigen (HBeAg): Only present in infected patients (5-14 weeks after infection)
- Anti-HBs: Present in natural infection late (32 weeks after infection) and in vaccinated patients (1-2 months after vaccination)
- Anti-HBc: IgM present 6-32 weeks after infection, disappears as anti-HBs appear, and not present in vaccinated patients
- Anti-HBe: Present 14 weeks after infection and persists indefinitely in naturally infected patients; not present in vaccinated patients
- Serum HBV DNA and viral load utilized to monitor response to therapy
- Anti-HDV IgG or IgM and serum HDV RNA to confirm diagnosis
- Albumin: Variable in acute infection; low in chronic infection implies cirrhosis
- Bilirubin: High in acute infection and stabilizes during chronic phase; high in chronic phase implies cirrhosis
- Prothrombin time (PT): Prolonged in chronic disease implies cirrhosis
- Alanine transaminase (ALT) and aspartate transaminase (AST): High in acute infection and stabilizes (borderline high) during chronic phase

Natural History

- 10% of infected individuals become chronically infected
- Lifelong risk of developing cirrhosis &/or HCC in chronic hepatitis B; viral genome can act as oncoprotein and integrate into host genome
- Coinfection with HIV and HCV is common, as they share transmission routes

Treatment

- Hepatitis B vaccine (HepB): 3-dose series at age 0, 1-2, and 6-18 years
- No vaccine available for HDV
- HBV vaccine and immune globulin (HBIG) for postexposure prophylaxis
- Drugs: Nucleoside analogue therapy with lamivudine, adefovir, entecavir; interferon
- Liver transplantation for cirrhosis and HCC; posttransplant recurrence of HBV is rare

Prognosis

- Viral clearance dependent on age when infected
  - Complete recovery in 95% of adults
  - Complete recovery in only 5% of infants; estimated lifetime risk of complications (cirrhosis or HCC) is 40%

MICROBIOLOGY

Viral Features

- HBV
  - Enveloped, partially double-stranded DNA virus
  - 42-nm spherical, icosahedral capsid
  - 3,200 nucleotide genome (C, P, S, and X genes)
  - 10 genotypes (A to J)
- HDV
  - Incomplete, small, circular, enveloped RNA virus
  - 36-nm spherical, nondistinct capsid structure
  - 1,700 nucleotide genome; can only propagate in presence of HBV
  - 8 genotypes (1-8)

Culture

- No routine role for culture in diagnosis

MACROSCOPIC

Cirrhosis

- Nodularity (macronodular or mixed macro- and micronodular) and scarring

MICROSCOPIC

Histologic Features

- Acute hepatitis B: Hepatocytic swelling, lymphoplasmacytic inflammatory cell infiltrates, apoptosis abundant with spotty necrosis, confluent or bridging necrosis, hepatocytic cord collapse (best seen on reticulin stain), regenerative changes in hepatocytes
- Chronic hepatitis B: Expanded portal tracts with lymphocytes, plasma cells, and Kupffer cells, interface hepatitis with apoptosis and inflammation beyond limiting plate, lobular hepatitis, fibrosis, ground-glass hepatocytes with sanded nuclei
- Fibrosis staging in biopsy has clinical treatment implications
    - Early: Portal regions
    - Mid: Beyond limiting plate
    - Late: Bridging (between portal and central regions)

Cytologic Features

- Balloon cell degeneration, pleomorphic hepatocytes with increased mitosis and binucleate forms, isolated hepatocyte necrosis, mononuclear inflammatory infiltrates, and Kupffer cell hyperplasia

ANCILLARY TESTS

Histochemistry

- Masson trichrome stain highlights reactive fibrosis and assists with staging

Immunohistochemistry

- HBV surface antigen: Cytoplasmic staining
- HBV core antigen: Nuclear and cytoplasmic staining

DIFFERENTIAL DIAGNOSIS

Other Viral Hepatitides

- Hepatitis A virus (HAV)
    - Food or travel associated
    - Acute lobular hepatitis without chronic phase
    - Positive anti-HAV IgM or HAV PCR
- Chronic hepatitis C virus (HCV)
    - Chronic hepatitis with predominantly portal inflammation and fibrosis; hepatocellular steatosis
    - Positive HCV RNA (serum)
- Hepatitis E virus (HEV)
    - Acute lobular hepatitis; chronic infection in immunosuppressed
    - Food or travel associated
    - Positive anti-HEV IgM or HEV PCR
- CMV hepatitis, EBV hepatitis, HSV hepatitis, yellow fever, Dengue fever, syphilitic hepatitis
    - Distinguish with serology, PCR, IHC/ISH

Autoimmune Hepatitis

- Positive autoimmune serologies (antinuclear antibodies, antismooth muscle antibodies, anti-liver-kidney-microsomal antibodies)
- Lobular hepatitis with portal and periportal hepatitis
- Prominent plasma cell infiltrates and fibrosis
- Responsive to immunosuppressive therapy

Drug-/Toxin-Induced Hepatitis

- Caused by toxic exposure to certain medications, vitamins, herbal remedies, or food supplements
- Hepatitis with eosinophils
- Self-limited and typically resolves with cessation of drug

Primary Biliary Cirrhosis

- Florid duct lesion (granuloma) destroying interlobular bile duct is diagnostic

Other Causes of Ground-Glass Cells

- Lafora disease
- Cyanamide toxicity
- Fibrinogen storage disease
- Glycogen pseudoground-glass cell change

SELECTED REFERENCES

1. Conners EE et al: Screening and testing for hepatitis B virus infection: CDC recommendations - United States, 2023. MMWR Recomm Rep. 72(1):1-25, 2023
2. Jeng WJ et al: Hepatitis B. Lancet. 401(10381):1039-52, 2023
3. Sulkowski MS: Hepatitis D virus infection: progress on the path toward disease control and cure. J Viral Hepat. 1:39-42, 2023
4. Matthews PC et al: Hepatitis B Virus: infection, liver disease, carcinogen or syndemic threat? Remodelling the clinical and public health response. PLOS Glob Public Health. 2(12):e0001359, 2022
5. Zheng Y et al: In situ analysis of hepatitis B virus (HBV) antigen and DNA in HBV-induced hepatocellular carcinoma. Diagn Pathol. 17(1):11, 2022
6. Gill US et al: Liver sampling: a vital window into HBV pathogenesis on the path to functional cure. Gut. 67(4):767-75, 2018
7. Goossens N et al: Effect of hepatitis B virus on steatosis in hepatitis C virus co-infected subjects: a multi-centre study and systematic review. J Viral Hepat. 25(8):920-9, 2018
8. Jiang XW et al: Hepatitis B reactivation in patients receiving direct-acting antiviral therapy or interferon-based therapy for hepatitis C: a systematic review and meta-analysis. World J Gastroenterol. 24(28):3181-91, 2018
9. Peeridogaheh H et al: Current concepts on immunopathogenesis of hepatitis B virus infection. Virus Res. 245:29-43, 2018
10. Wu CC et al: Hepatitis B virus infection: defective surface antigen expression and pathogenesis. World J Gastroenterol. 24(31):3488-99, 2018
11. Yuen MF et al: Hepatitis B virus infection. Nat Rev Dis Primers. 4:18035, 2018
12. Liang TJ: Hepatitis B: the virus and disease. Hepatology. 49(5 Suppl):S13-21, 2009
13. Mani H et al: Liver biopsy findings in chronic hepatitis B. Hepatology. 49(5 Suppl):S61-71, 2009
14. McMahon BJ: The natural history of chronic hepatitis B virus infection. Hepatology. 49(5 Suppl):S45-55, 2009
15. Goodman ZD: Grading and staging systems for inflammation and fibrosis in chronic liver diseases. J Hepatol. 47(4):598-607, 2007

Liver: Cirrhosis at Autopsy

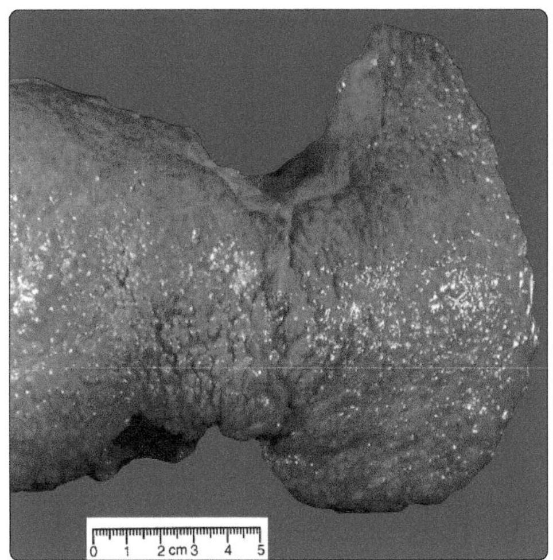

Hepatitis B: Portal Inflammation

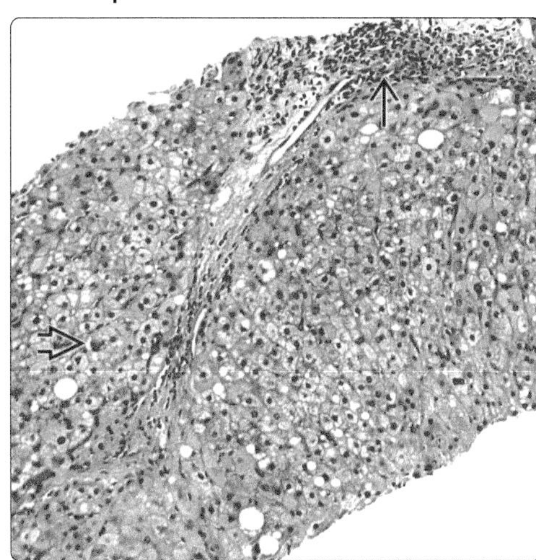

(Left) *Gross photograph of a liver at autopsy demonstrates end-stage cirrhosis with a distinctive nodular liver surface.* **(Right)** *Hematoxylin and eosin section illustrates chronic hepatitis B with portal inflammatory infiltrates ➙ and apoptotic bodies ➙ in the lobule.*

Hepatitis B: Chronic Inflammation

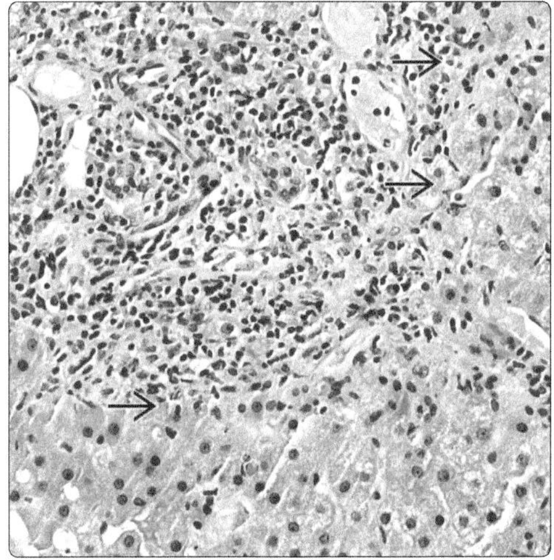

Hepatitis B: Trichrome Stain

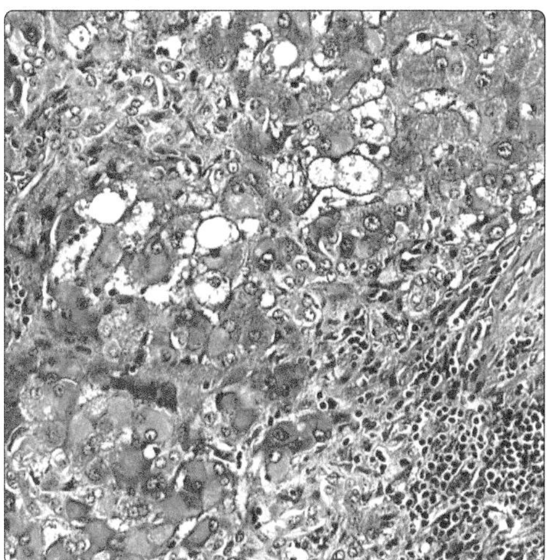

(Left) *Hematoxylin and eosin section shows interface hepatitis in chronic hepatitis B consisting of chronic inflammatory cells that extend beyond the limiting plate ➙ and replace dead hepatocytes.* **(Right)** *Masson trichrome stain shows collagen strands that extend beyond portal tracts to reach the central region and form bridging septa in chronic hepatitis B.*

Hepatitis B Virus Core Antigen: IHC

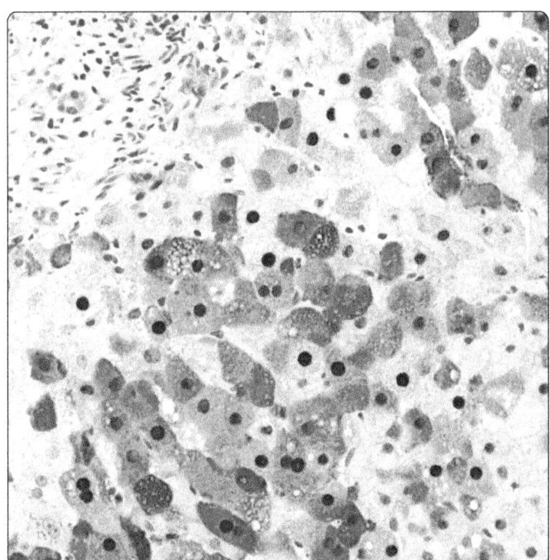

Hepatitis B Virus Surface Antigen: IHC

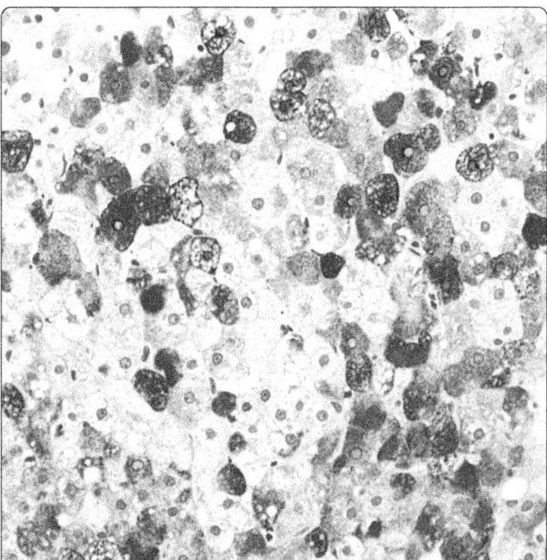

(Left) *Immunohistochemical stain for anti-HBc (core antigen) shows both cytoplasmic and nuclear staining.* **(Right)** *Immunohistochemical stain for anti-HBs (surface antigen) shows cytoplasmic staining.*

Parvovirus B19 Infection

KEY FACTS

ETIOLOGY/PATHOGENESIS

- Single-stranded DNA virus transmitted by respiratory droplets and replicates in erythroid precursor cells

CLINICAL ISSUES

- Erythema infectiosum: Stocking/glove rash and "slapped cheek"
- Fetal hydrops with 5-10% mortality for fetus
- Transient aplastic crisis: Anemia with symptoms
- Pure red cell aplasia: Chronic anemia in immunocompromised patients
- Viral myocarditis and dilated cardiomyopathy

MICROSCOPIC

- Placenta: Diffuse villous edema with increased nucleated red blood cells with intranuclear inclusions
- Fetus: Hypocellular bone marrow, liver with increased extramedullary hematopoiesis, hemosiderosis
- Peripheral blood: Normochromic/normocytic anemia
- Bone marrow: Severe erythroid hypoplasia; rare atypical giant cells with intranuclear inclusions
- Heart: Predominantly lymphocytic inflammatory infiltrate with myocyte necrosis

ANCILLARY TESTS

- Positive antiparvovirus B19 IHC or viral PCR is definitive

TOP DIFFERENTIAL DIAGNOSES

- Rubella: Lacks viral inclusions, PCR-based and serologic testing will differentiate
- Erythroblastosis fetalis: Immune-mediated hemolysis, lacks viral inclusions; may be clinical history of Rh factor incompatibility
- Chronic maternal-fetal transfusion: Fetal hydrops, no viral inclusions; fetal blood in intervillous blood space of placenta; positive Kleihauer-Betke stain on maternal blood

Ultrastructural Features

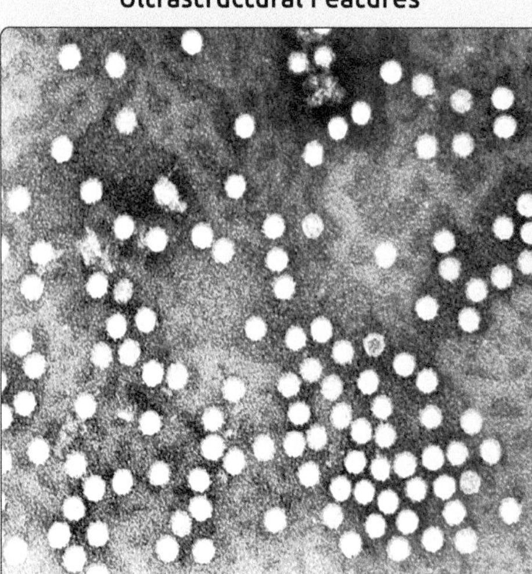

Viral Inclusions

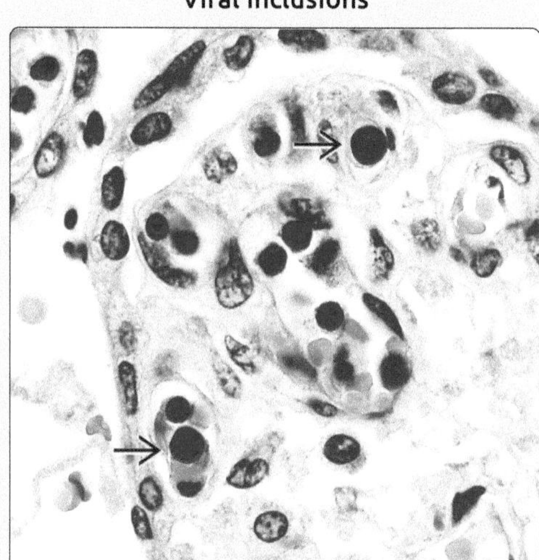

(Left) *Transmission electron micrograph shows numerous spherical, nonenveloped virions measuring 22-24 nm in diameter, characteristic of parvoviruses. (Courtesy R. Regnery, PhD, CDC PHIL.)* **(Right)** *Viral cytopathic effects of parvovirus B19 include glassy intranuclear inclusions ➙ in nucleated red blood cells.*

Hydrops Fetalis

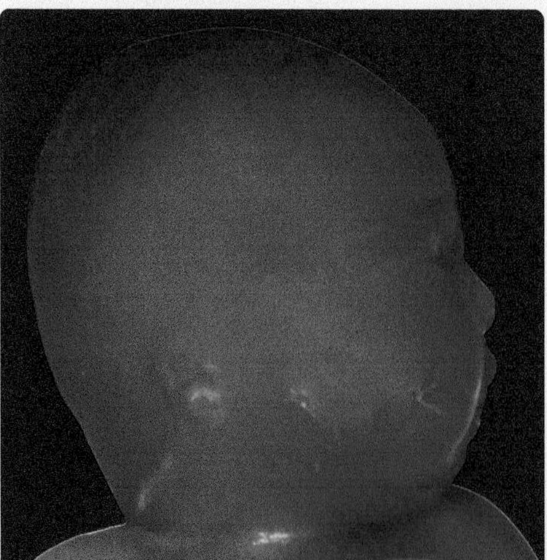

Erythema Infectiosum (5th Disease)

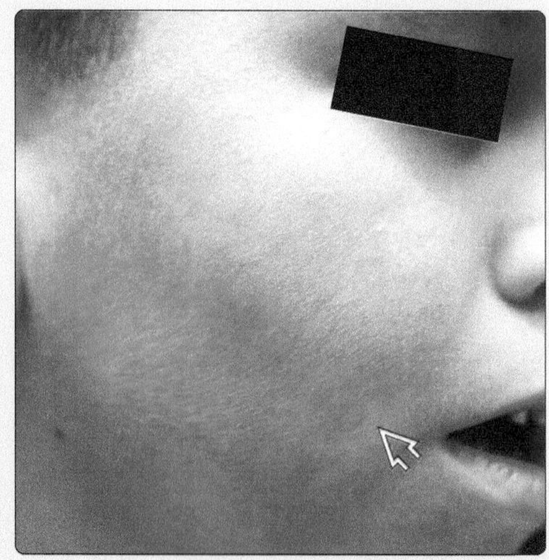

(Left) *Previable fetus with hydrops secondary to parvovirus infection is shown. (From DP: Placenta.)* **(Right)** *Clinical photograph shows the red "slapped-cheek" ➲ rash characteristic of erythema infectiosum or 5th disease. (Courtesy P. Brachman, MD, CDC PHIL.)*

TERMINOLOGY

Synonyms

- Erythema infectiosum, 5th disease, "slapped-cheek" disease
- *Primate erythroparvovirus 1*; parvovirus B19

Definitions

- *Parvoviridae* family: Derived from "parvum" (small, tiny)

ETIOLOGY/PATHOGENESIS

Infectious Agents

- Viral infection transmitted by respiratory droplets, vertically from mother to fetus, through stem cell/solid organ transplants and blood transfusion products (4- to 14-day incubation)
- Globoside (erythrocyte P) antigen required for infection of host cells; expressed on erythrocyte precursors, placental syncytiotrophoblasts and cytotrophoblasts, megakaryocytes, endothelial cells, and myocardium; virus propagates in erythroid precursors and is cytotoxic

CLINICAL ISSUES

Epidemiology

- Common in childhood; 80% of adults have been exposed
- More common in winter/spring; epidemics every 3-4 years

Presentation

- Erythema infectiosum (5th disease)
  - Children: Prodrome (fever, chills, malaise, headache), followed by slapped-cheek appearance with stocking/glove maculopapular rash and spread to trunk that disappears after 1-3 weeks
  - Adults: Often asymptomatic; may have rash or arthritis
- Congenital infection (33% of women with primary infection during pregnancy): Nonimmune hydrops 4 weeks after infection; severe anemia (fetus is highly susceptible to viral infection of erythroid precursors) and high cardiac output that can lead to fetal death
- Transient aplastic crisis: Hypoproliferative anemia that occurs in setting of coincident hemolytic anemia (hereditary spherocytosis, thalassemia, autoimmune hemolytic anemia); varying degree of neutropenia and thrombocytopenia
- Pure red cell aplasia due to chronic infection in immunocompromised patients
- Viral myocarditis and dilated cardiomyopathy

Laboratory Tests

- Serology: IgM (2 weeks after infection, persists for 3-6 months); IgG follows and persists for life
- PCR: May detect early infection prior to appearance of serum IgM (preferred for immunocompromised patients)

Treatment

- No specific antiviral therapy or vaccine is available
- IVIG may resolve anemia in immunocompromised patients
- Transfusions in patients with severe anemia (intrauterine transfusion for fetal anemia)

Prognosis

- Erythema infectiosum and aplastic anemia in immunocompetent typically self-limiting
- 5-10% of in utero cases will result in lethal hydrops fetalis (2nd trimester holds greatest risk)

MICROBIOLOGY

Virus Features

- Nonenveloped, single-stranded DNA virus
- 22- to 24-nm spherical, icosahedral capsid
- 5,596 nucleotide genome (VP1, VP2, NS1, etc.)
- 3 genotypes (subtypes 1a, 1b, 2, 3a, 3b)

Culture

- Does not grow in standard cell culture system

MACROSCOPIC

Fetal Hydrops

- Fetus with edema, pallor, cardiomegaly, hepatomegaly, and thick, pale, friable placenta

MICROSCOPIC

Histologic Features

- Placenta: Diffuse villous edema with increased nucleated red blood cells with intranuclear inclusions
- Fetus: Hypocellular bone marrow, liver with increased extramedullary hematopoiesis, hemosiderosis
- Peripheral blood: Normochromic/normocytic anemia
- Bone marrow: Severe erythroid hypoplasia; rare atypical giant cells with intranuclear inclusions
- Heart: Predominantly lymphocytic inflammatory infiltrate with myocyte necrosis

Cytologic Features

- Glassy intranuclear inclusions with marginated chromatin

ANCILLARY TESTS

Immunohistochemistry

- Antiparvovirus B19 antibodies stain nuclear inclusions

DIFFERENTIAL DIAGNOSIS

Rubella

- Lacks viral inclusions; differentiated by PCR and serology

Erythroblastosis Fetalis

- Immune-mediated hemolysis; lacks viral inclusions
- May have clinical history of Rh factor incompatibility

Chronic Maternal-Fetal Transfusion

- Fetal hydrops; no viral inclusions
- Fetal blood in intervillous blood space of placenta
- Positive Kleihauer-Betke stain on maternal blood

SELECTED REFERENCES

1. Bichicchi F et al: Next generation sequencing for the analysis of parvovirus B19 genomic diversity. Viruses. 15(1), 2023
2. Attwood LO et al: Identification and management of congenital parvovirus B19 infection. Prenat Diagn. 40(13):1722-31, 2020
3. Qiu J et al: Human parvoviruses. Clin Microbiol Rev. 30(1):43-113, 2017
4. Verdonschot J et al: Relevance of cardiac parvovirus B19 in myocarditis and dilated cardiomyopathy: review of the literature. Eur J Heart Fail. 18(12):1430-41, 2016

(Left) *Section of placenta from a case of fetal hydrops shows diffuse villous edema.* (Right) *Liver section from a case of fetal hydrops shows extramedullary hematopoiesis beyond what is expected for gestational age with increased erythroblasts.*

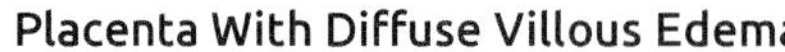

Placenta With Diffuse Villous Edema

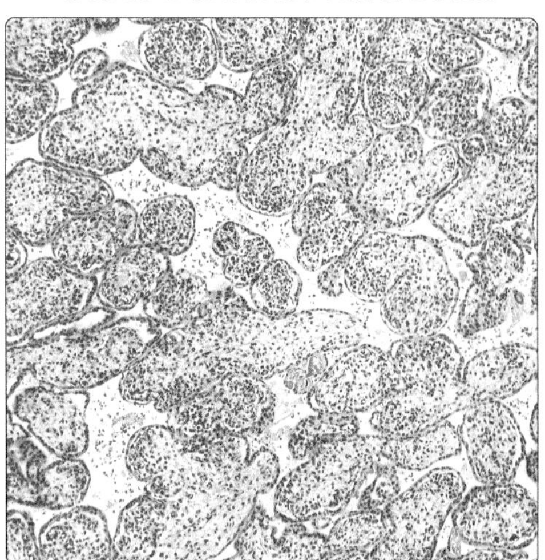

Extramedullary Hematopoiesis in Fetal Liver

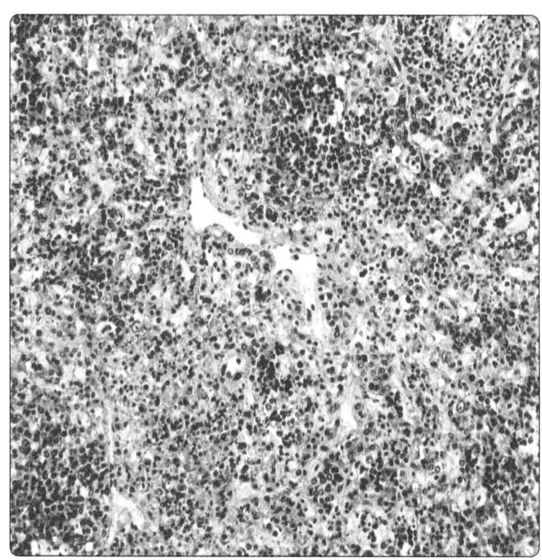

(Left) *Higher power image of placenta from a case of fetal hydrops shows numerous nucleated red blood cells containing parvovirus B19 nuclear inclusions* ➔. (Right) *Scattered parvovirus B19 nuclear inclusions* ➔ *are present in this higher power image of the liver from a case of fetal hydrops. Iron is diffusely present, which is indicative of increased turnover.*

Viral Inclusions in Placenta

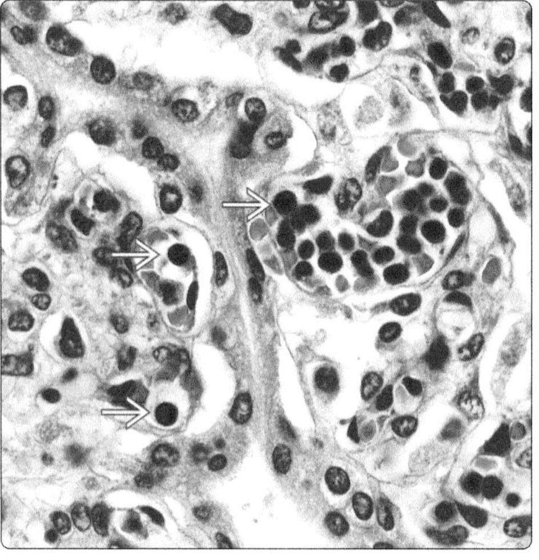

Viral Inclusions in Fetal Liver

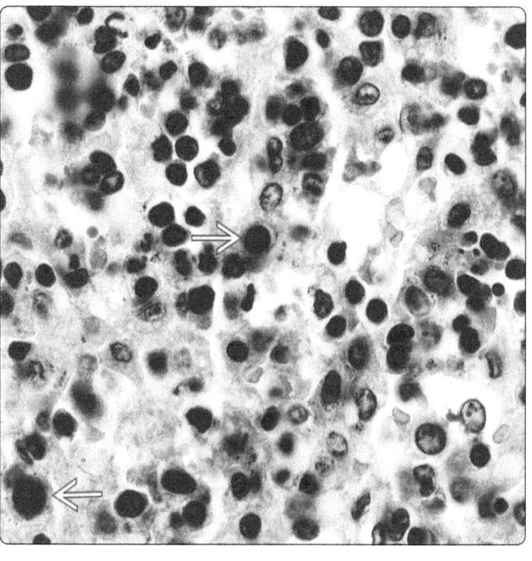

(Left) *Immunohistochemical staining for parvovirus B19 (brown) in the placenta highlights numerous positive nucleated red blood cells.* (Right) *Immunohistochemical staining for parvovirus B19 (brown) in the fetal liver highlights numerous positive nucleated red blood cells.*

Viral Immunostaining in Placenta

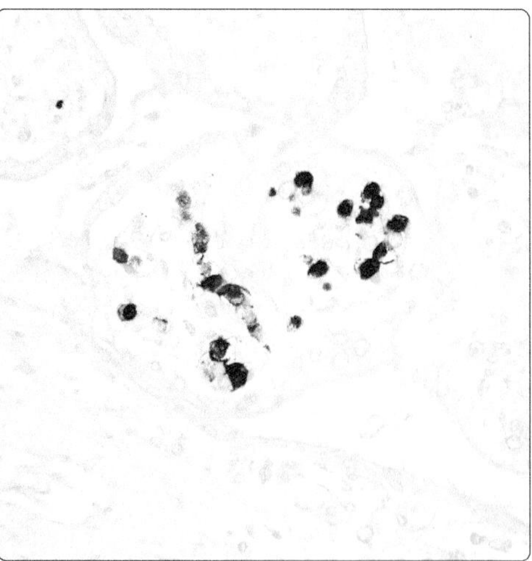

Viral Immunostaining in Fetal Liver

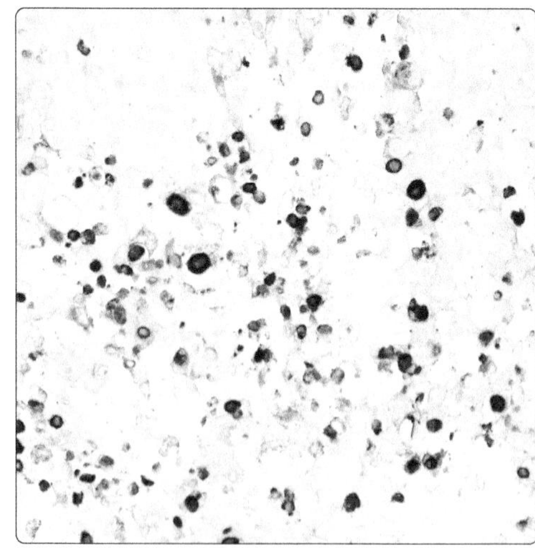

Fetal Bone Marrow

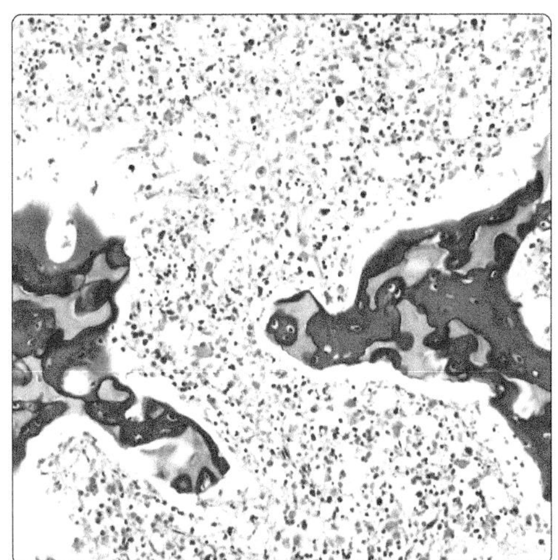

Bone Marrow Aspirate Smear

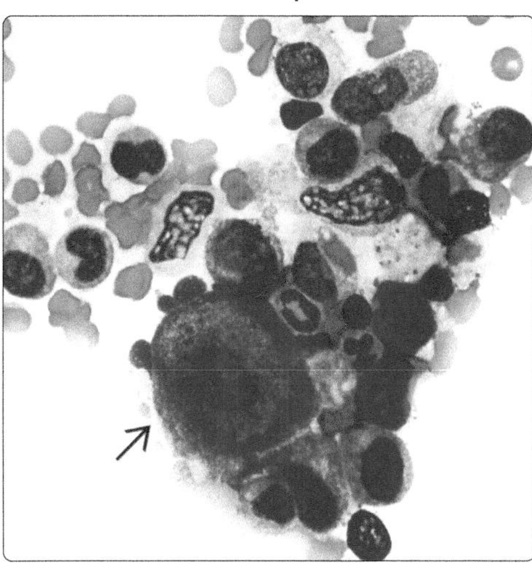

(Left) *Bone marrow from a fetus infected with parvovirus B19 shows marked hypocellularity.* **(Right)** *A giant proerythroblast ⇒ ("lantern" cell) is shown in a bone marrow aspirate smear from a patient with parvovirus B19 infection and hereditary spherocytosis. A nuclear viral inclusion is present with minimal erythroid maturation. (From DP: Nonneoplastic Pediatrics.)*

Bone Marrow Biopsy

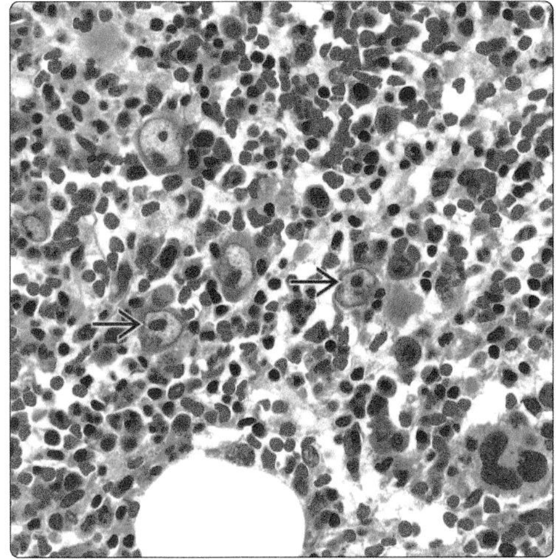

Viral Inclusions in Bone Marrow

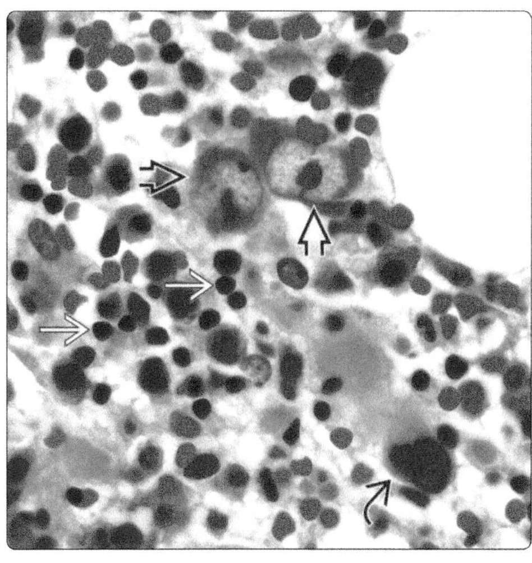

(Left) *Giant proerythroblasts ⇒ containing prominent eosinophilic nuclear inclusions are present in this bone marrow biopsy from a patient with HIV/AIDS. (From DP2: Blood and Bone Marrow.)* **(Right)** *Viral nuclear inclusions are present in proerythroblasts ⇒ in a bone marrow biopsy from a patient with HIV/AIDS. More mature erythroid precursors are observed ➡. HIV-related megakaryocytic atypia ⇒ is also present. (From DP2: Blood and Bone Marrow.)*

Lymphocytic Myocarditis

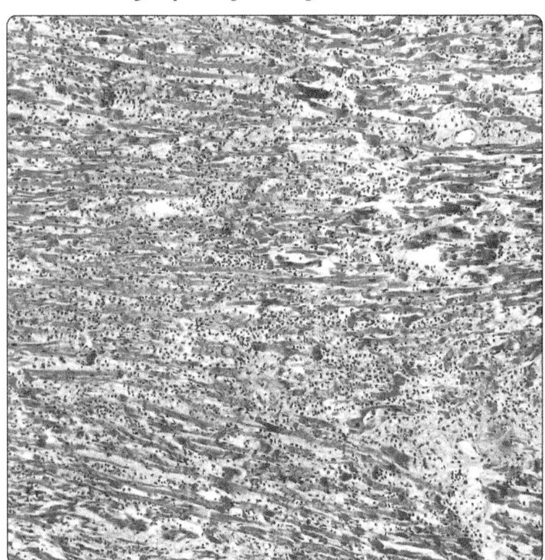

Myocyte Necrosis

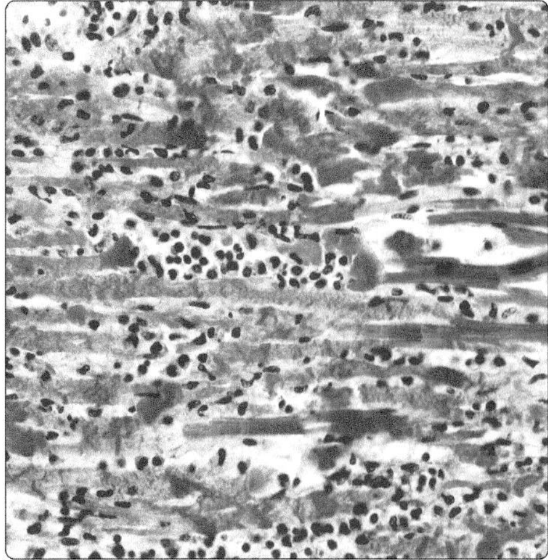

(Left) *Section of the heart in a 15-year-old with parvovirus B19 infection demonstrates a diffuse interstitial infiltrate, predominantly consisting of lymphocytes involving the ventricles and interventricular septum. There is extensive accompanying coagulative necrosis with minimal interstitial fibrosis.* **(Right)** *Higher power image in a case of fatal parvovirus B19 myocarditis shows a diffuse interstitial inflammatory infiltrate with extensive coagulative necrosis and minimal interstitial fibrosis. No viral inclusions were identified.*

JC Virus, BK Virus, and Other Polyomavirus Infections

KEY FACTS

ETIOLOGY/PATHOGENESIS

- Ubiquitous viruses that reactivate in immunosuppressed states and have varying oncogenic properties

CLINICAL ISSUES

- Polyomavirus nephropathy (BK virus, JC virus): Acute renal failure, hemorrhagic cystitis, and uretal obstruction
- Merkel cell carcinoma (MCC): Rapidly growing, nontender, red to violaceous, firm intradermal nodule ± positive lymph nodes and distant metastases
- Progressive multifocal leukoencephalopathy (JC virus): Weakness, vision loss, impaired speech, and cognitive deterioration
- Laboratory testing: BK virus (urine PCR, decoy cell in cytology); JC virus (CSF, brain tissue PCR)
- Decrease immunosuppression for PVN and PML; surgery/radiation for MCC; no direct antiviral treatment available

MICROSCOPIC

- PVN: Interstitial mononuclear inflammation, tubulitis; intranuclear inclusions in tubular epithelium
- MCC: Dermal nodule of small round blue cells with large, prominent nuclei, scant cytoplasm, diffusely dispersed chromatin, and numerous mitoses
- PML: Multifocal demyelination with relative axon sparing, loss of oligodendrocytes, and macrophages in area of demyelination; enlarged, glassy, dark-staining inclusions

ANCILLARY TESTS

- Antipolyomavirus antibodies (large T antigen)

TOP DIFFERENTIAL DIAGNOSES

- PVN: Acute tubulointerstitial rejection, adenovirus, acute tubular necrosis, acute interstitial nephritis
- MCC: Small cell lung cancer, small cell malignant melanoma, cutaneous lymphoma, Ewing sarcoma
- PML: Multiple sclerosis, infarct, high-grade glioma

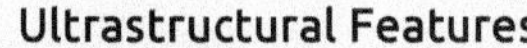

Ultrastructural Features

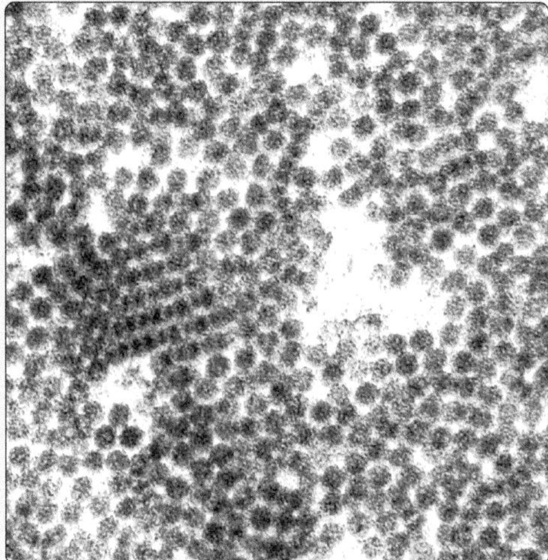

Decoy Cells: BK Virus

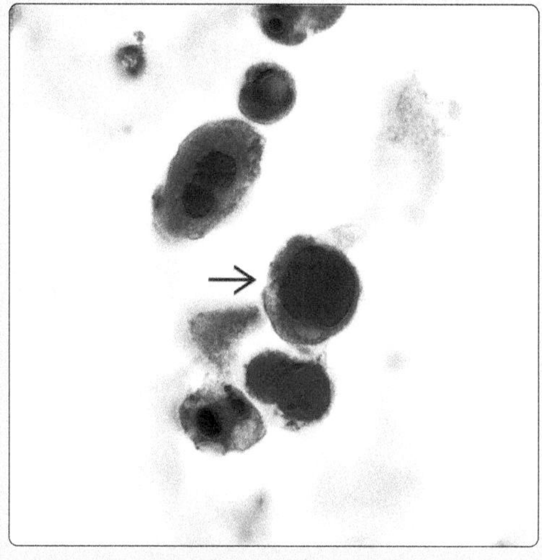

(Left) *Transmission electron micrograph of a tubular epithelial cell nucleus shows numerous nonenveloped icosahedral particles measuring ~ 50 nm, characteristic of polyomaviruses. (From DP: Kidney.)* **(Right)** *Decoy cells → seen in urine cytology specimens are nonneoplastic tubular epithelial cells infected with BK virus, characterized by enlarged nuclei with glassy basophilic nuclear inclusions.*

JC Virus-Infected Oligodendrocytes

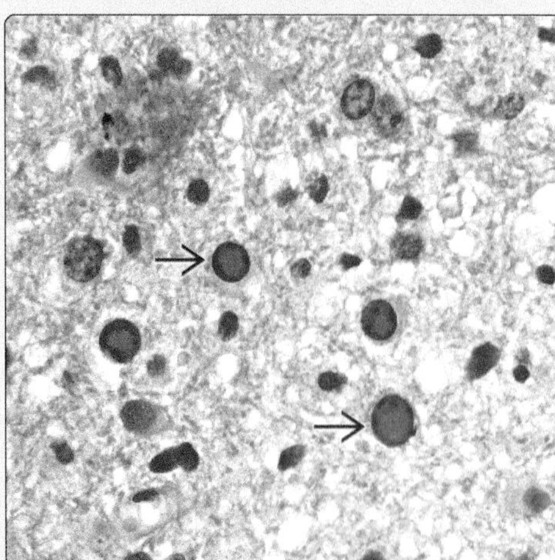

MCPyV IHC in Merkel Cell Carcinoma

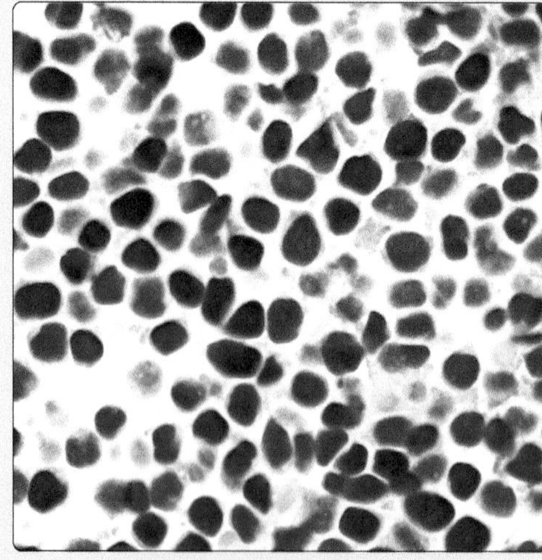

(Left) *Glassy nuclear inclusions → characteristic of JC virus are present in scattered oligodendrocytes from a patient with progressive multifocal leukoencephalopathy.* **(Right)** *Merkel cell polyomavirus (MCPyV) large T-cell antigen immunohistochemistry shows strong nuclear staining in Merkel cell carcinoma tumor cells in ~ 80% of cases.*

TERMINOLOGY

Definitions

- *Polyomaviridae* derived from "poly" many and "oma" tumors
- Species numbered sequentially (e.g., *Human polyomavirus 1*)
- Virus names derived from patient initials (e.g., JC and BK) or location (e.g., Washington University)

ETIOLOGY/PATHOGENESIS

Infectious Agents

- Ubiquitous dsDNA viruses that spread person to person
- BK polyomavirus (BK virus, BKPyV) reactivation in tubular epithelial cells causes 80% of polyomavirus-associated nephropathy (PVN); hemorrhagic cystitis
- JC polyomavirus (JC virus, JCPyV) reactivation in oligodendrocytes resulting in demyelination and causes progressive multifocal leukoencephalopathy (PML); 20% of PVN cases
- Merkel cell polyomavirus (MCPyV): Clonal integration of virus with large T tumor antigen (LT) and small tumor antigen (sT) target tumor suppressor genes in Merkel cells causes 80% of Merkel cell carcinoma (MCC) cases
- Human polyomaviruses 6 and 7 (HPyV6, HPyV7) associated with rare, pruritic skin eruptions
- Trichodysplasia spinulosa-associated polyomavirus (TSPyV): Trichodysplasia spinulosa, pilomatrix dysplasia
- No known disease association with Karolinska Institute polyomavirus (KIPyV), Washington University polyomavirus (WUPyV), human polyomavirus 9 (HPyV9), Malawi polyomavirus (MWPyV), St. Louis polyomavirus (STLPyV), human polyomavirus 12 (HPyV12), New Jersey polyomavirus (NJPyV), or Lyon IARC polyomavirus (LIPyV)
- Conflicting data on role of Simian virus 40 (SV40) in human disease

CLINICAL ISSUES

Epidemiology

- Seropositivity in 20-99% of individuals (variation with specific virus and population)
- 5% of kidney transplant patients with tacrolimus/mycophenolate develop PVN
- MCC: 0.79 per 100,000; 2:1 M:F ratio, 25x greater in White population; risk increases with sun exposure, age (median: 75-79 years), and immunosuppression
- PML: Immunosuppression due to HIV/AIDS, solid organ transplant, monoclonal antibodies (i.e., natalizumab, rituximab)

Presentation

- Primary infection: Mild respiratory infection and fever or asymptomatic
- PVN: Acute renal failure, hemorrhagic cystitis, uretal obstruction
- MCC: Rapidly growing, nontender, red to violaceous, firm intradermal nodule ± positive lymph nodes and distant metastases
- PML: Weakness, vision loss, impaired speech, and cognitive deterioration

Laboratory Tests

- JC virus: PCR (urine, plasma, CSF, brain tissue)
- BK virus: PCR (urine, plasma), decoy cells (urine cytology)

Treatment

- No direct antiviral treatment available
- PVN
  - Decrease immunosuppression
  - Cidofovir, leflunomide
- MCC
  - Wide local excision, ± sentinel node biopsy, fractionated radiation
  - Limited role for chemotherapy
  - Monoclonal antibodies avelumab (PD-L1 inhibitor) and pembrolizumab (PD-1 inhibitor) FDA approved for treatment of advanced disease
- PML
  - HAART, decrease immunosuppression
  - Plasma exchange for monoclonal antibodies
  - PD1 inhibitors nivolumab and pembrolizumab may provide some benefit

Prognosis

- PVN
  - Graft loss dependent on stage at diagnosis
  - Residual impairment of renal function common
  - Increased risk of urothelial carcinoma
- MCC
  - Local recurrence and distant metastasis common
  - 5-year disease-associated mortality is 46%
  - MCPyV-positive cases reported to behave less aggressively
- PML
  - Stability or improvement with HAART
  - Residual deficits depending on location of lesions

MICROBIOLOGY

Virus Features

- Nonenveloped, circular, double-stranded DNA virus
- 40-45 nm, icosahedral
- ~ 5,200 bp genome (6 genes)

MACROSCOPIC

Polyomavirus Nephropathy

- Streaky fibrosis of renal medulla and circumscribed cortical scars

Merkel Cell Carcinoma

- Tumor fills entire dermis with sparing of epidermis

Progressive Multifocal Leukoencephalopathy

- Small, demyelinating lesions at cortical gray matter-white matter junction that coalesce to occupy large volume of white matter

MICROSCOPIC

Histologic Features

- PVN
  - Interstitial mononuclear inflammation
  - Tubulitis and tubular injury
  - Intranuclear inclusions in tubular epithelium
- MCC

- Expansile dermal nodule with subepidermal aggregates of tumor cells
- Solid (most common), trabecular, and diffuse growth patterns
- Small round blue cells with large, prominent nuclei and scant cytoplasm
- Nuclei with diffusely dispersed chromatin and numerous mitoses

- PML
  - Multifocal demyelination with relative axon sparing, loss of oligodendrocytes, and macrophages in area of demyelination
  - Enlarged, glassy, dark-staining inclusions in oligodendrocytes or cerebellar granule neurons
  - Creutzfeldt cells: Multinucleated reactive astrocytes
- Other JC virus disease patterns have been reported in brain
  - JC virus granule cell neuronopathy (JCV GCN): Infection of cerebellar granule cell neurons resulting in cerebellar atrophy
  - JC virus encephalopathy (JCVE): Infection of cortical pyramidal neurons with minimal demyelination
  - JC virus meningitis (JCVM): Infection of leptomeningeal and choroid plexus cells in absence of white matter lesions

Cytologic Features

- Decoy cells (urine): Enlarged nuclei with basophilic nuclear inclusion

ANCILLARY TESTS

Immunohistochemistry

- Antipolyomavirus antibodies targeting LT
  - SV40, BK virus, and JC virus typically cross react; weak staining of normal-sized cells may be incidental reactivation
  - MWPyV can distinguish MCC from other tumors with neuroendocrine differentiation
- MCC
  - Positive: Cytokeratin (AE1/AE3, CAM5.2, CK20) and neuroendocrine markers (INSM1, synaptophysin, chromogranin A, NSE)
  - Negative: Thyroid transcription factor 1, S100, CEA, and lymphocyte markers

In Situ Hybridization

- PML: JC virus detectable in infected oligodendrocytes

Immunofluorescence

- PVN: Granular staining of tubular basement membranes for IgG, C3, and C4d

Electron Microscopy

- PVN: Virus particles (40-50 nm diameter) in epithelial cell nuclei and cytoplasm

DIFFERENTIAL DIAGNOSIS

Polyomavirus Nephropathy

- Acute tubulointerstitial rejection (type 1)
  - Prominent interstitial inflammation and tubulitis with negative polyomavirus IHC
- Adenovirus tubulointerstitial nephritis
  - Prominent interstitial inflammation, viral cytopathic effect, and necrosis with negative polyomavirus IHC
- Acute tubular necrosis
  - Nuclear enlargement and reactive atypia of tubular epithelium, no prominent interstitial inflammation, no inclusions, and negative polyomavirus IHC
- Acute interstitial nephritis
  - Marked interstitial inflammation, no intranuclear inclusions, and negative polyomavirus IHC

Merkel Cell Carcinoma

- Small cell lung cancer
  - IHC positive for TTF-1 and negative for CK20
- Small cell malignant melanoma
  - IHC positive for S100 and negative for cytokeratin
- Cutaneous lymphoma
  - IHC positive for lymphocyte markers and negative for cytokeratin
- Ewing sarcoma
  - IHC positive for CD99; FISH positive for t(11;22)(90%)

Progressive Multifocal Leukoencephalopathy

- Multiple sclerosis
  - No viral inclusions, IHC negative for JC virus, more likely to affect spinal cord, optic nerve, and immediate periventricular region
- Infarct
  - No viral inclusions, ischemic neurons, loss of axons and myelin, more cortical based
- High-grade glioma
  - No viral inclusions, demyelination with macrophage influx rare, cellular atypia more abundant

SELECTED REFERENCES

1. Lewis DJ et al: Merkel cell carcinoma. Dermatol Clin. 41(1):101-15, 2023
2. Gauci ML et al: Diagnosis and treatment of Merkel cell carcinoma: European consensus-based interdisciplinary guideline - update 2022. Eur J Cancer. 171:203-31, 2022
3. Bernard-Valnet R et al: Advances in treatment of progressive multifocal leukoencephalopathy. Ann Neurol. 90(6):865-73, 2021
4. Cortese I et al: Progressive multifocal leukoencephalopathy and the spectrum of JC virus-related disease. Nat Rev Neurol. 17(1):37-51, 2021
5. Harms PW et al: The biology and treatment of Merkel cell carcinoma: current understanding and research priorities. Nat Rev Clin Oncol. 15(12):763-76, 2018
6. Ambalathingal GR et al: BK polyomavirus: clinical aspects, immune regulation, and emerging therapies. Clin Microbiol Rev. 30(2):503-28, 2017
7. Moens U et al: Biology, evolution, and medical importance of polyomaviruses: An update. Infect Genet Evol. 54:18-38, 2017
8. Polyomaviridae study group of the International Committee on Taxonomy of Viruses. et al: a taxonomy update for the family Polyomaviridae. Arch Virol. 161(6):1739-50, 2016
9. Yan L et al: Polyomavirus large T antigen is prevalent in urothelial carcinoma post-kidney transplant. Hum Pathol. 48:122-31, 2016
10. Miskin DP et al: Novel syndromes associated with JC virus infection of neurons and meningeal cells: no longer a gray area. Curr Opin Neurol. 28(3):288-94, 2015

Polyomavirus Nephropathy

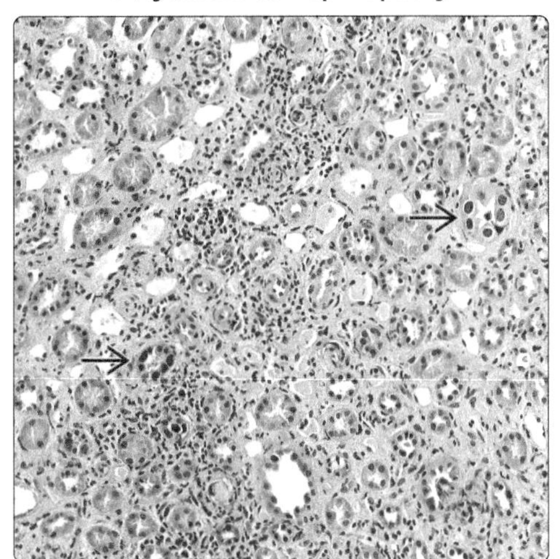

BK Virus Cytopathic Effects

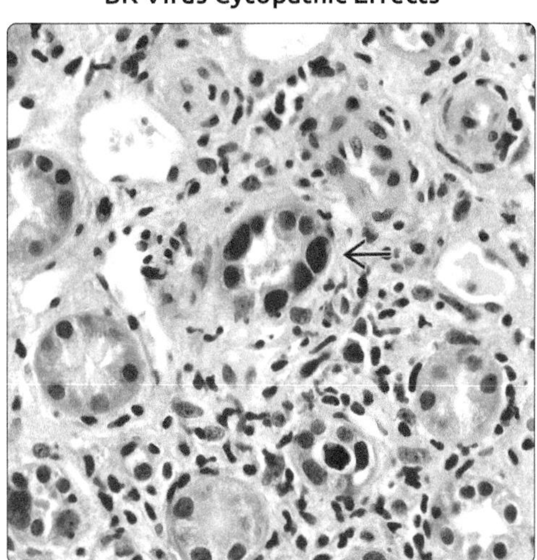

(Left) *Kidney biopsy from a renal transplant patient shows renal tubular epithelial cells with glassy nuclear inclusions ➞ indicative of BK virus (or JC virus) reactivation. Interstitial mononuclear inflammation is also present.* **(Right)** *High-power image of a renal transplant shows renal tubular epithelial cells with enlarged nuclei and glassy inclusions ➞.*

BK Virus Immunohistochemistry

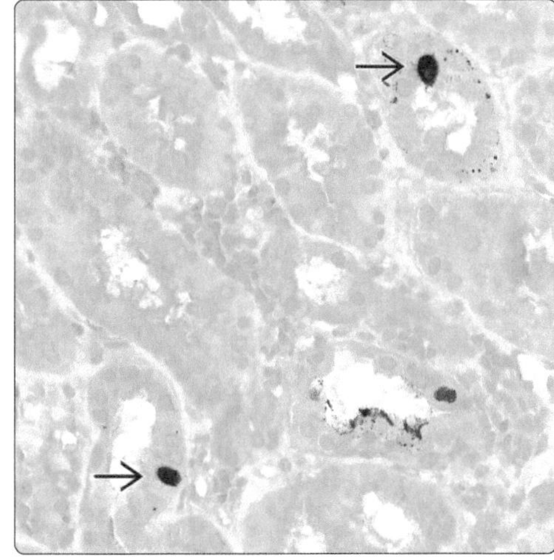

BK Virus Immunohistochemistry

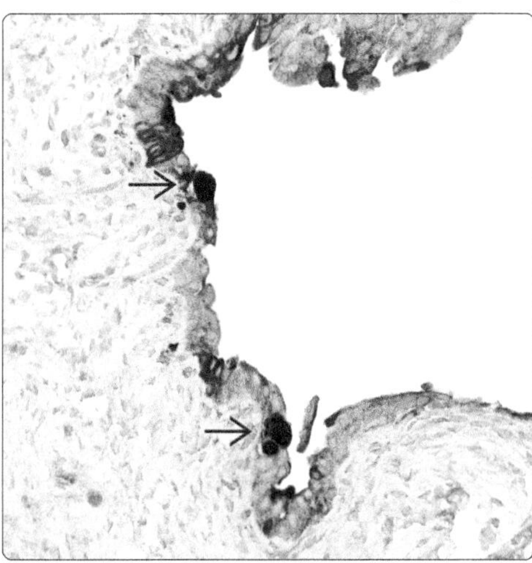

(Left) *Immunohistochemistry for polyomavirus antigen highlights occasional BK virus infected renal tubular epithelial cells with enlarged nuclei and glassy inclusions ➞.* **(Right)** *Immunohistochemistry for polyomavirus antigen highlights occasional BK virus-infected urothelial cells with enlarged nuclei and glassy inclusions ➞.*

Polyomavirus-Infected Urothelium

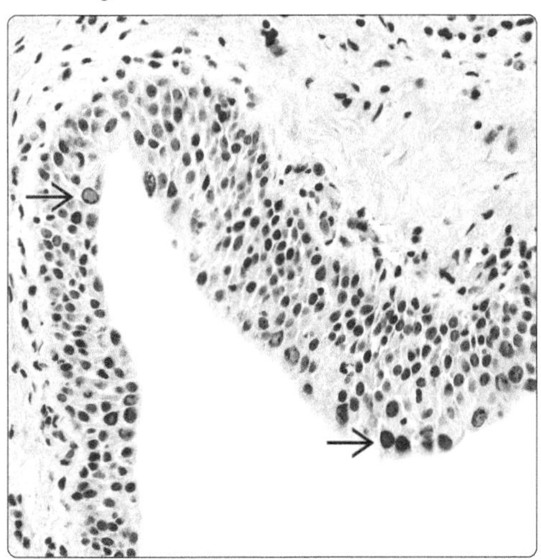

Polyomavirus-Associated Urothelial Carcinoma

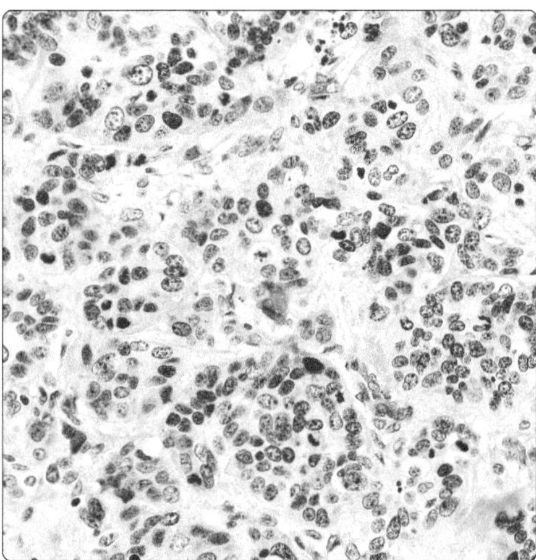

(Left) *Ureter section from a heart transplant patient shows urothelial cells with scattered glassy nuclear inclusions ➞, consistent with polyomavirus infection.* **(Right)** *This bladder section from a heart transplant patient shows invasive urothelial carcinoma. Polyomavirus IHC was positive in the majority of cells, supporting an oncogenic role for the virus in this tumor.*

(Left) *Clinical photograph of Merkel cell carcinoma shows a well-circumscribed, erythematous dermal nodule. (From DP: Neoplastic Derm.)* (Right) *Merkel cell carcinoma consists of expansile dermal nodules with subepidermal aggregates of tumor cells. The most common growth pattern is solid, followed by trabecular and diffuse.*

Merkel Cell Carcinoma: Skin

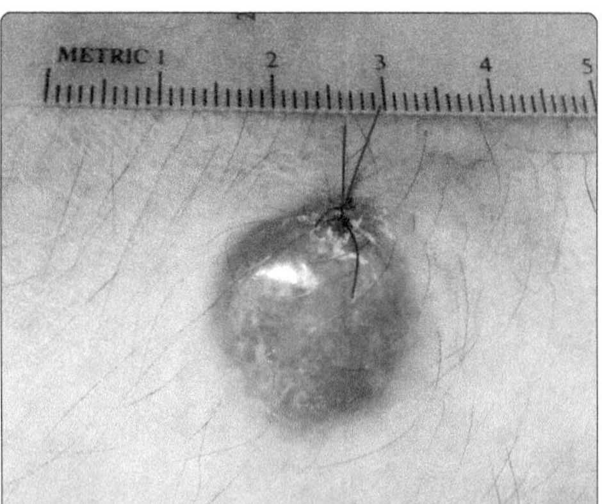

Merkel Cell Carcinoma

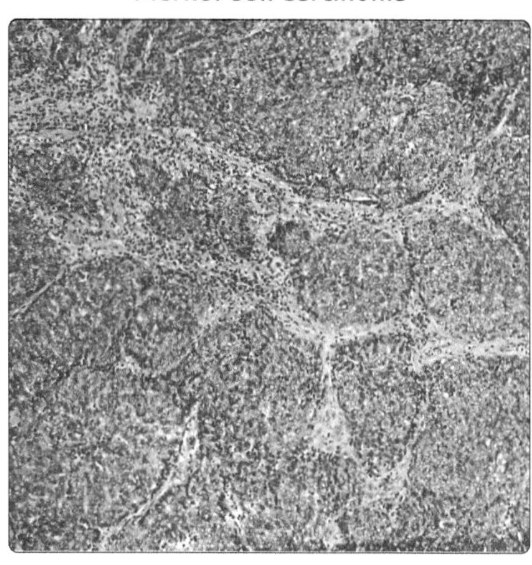

(Left) *Merkel cell carcinomas consist of small round blue cells with large, prominent nuclei, diffusely dispersed chromatin, scant cytoplasm, and frequent mitoses.* (Right) *Immunohistochemistry for MCPyV large T-cell antigen shows strong nuclear staining in Merkel cell carcinoma tumor cells, which helps distinguish from other tumors with neuroendocrine differentiation.*

Merkel Cell Carcinoma: Cytologic Features

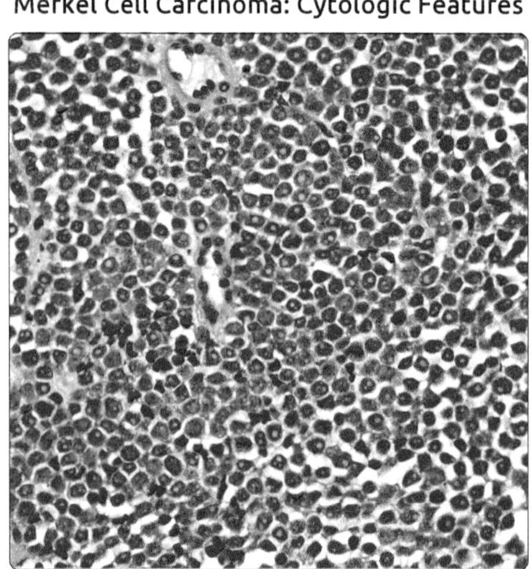

Merkel Cell Carcinoma: MCPyV IHC

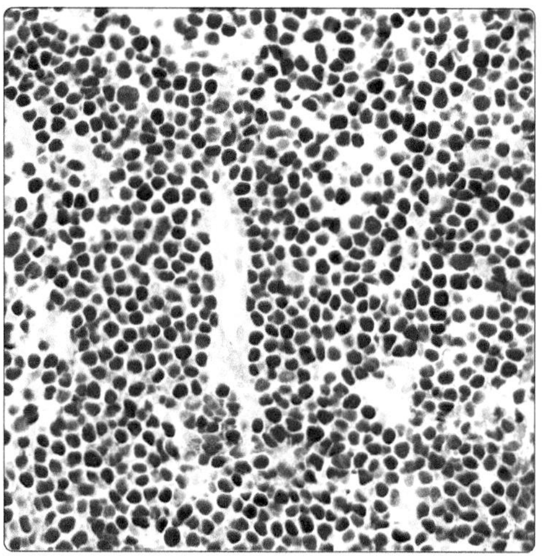

(Left) *Immunohistochemistry for CK20 shows strong perinuclear dot-like staining in Merkel cell carcinoma tumor cells and can help distinguish from metastatic small cell carcinoma of lung (typically CK20 negative and TTF-1 positive).* (Right) *Immunohistochemistry for INSM1 shows strong nuclear staining in Merkel cell carcinoma tumor cells and confirms neuroendocrine differentiation.*

Merkel Cell Carcinoma: CK20 IHC

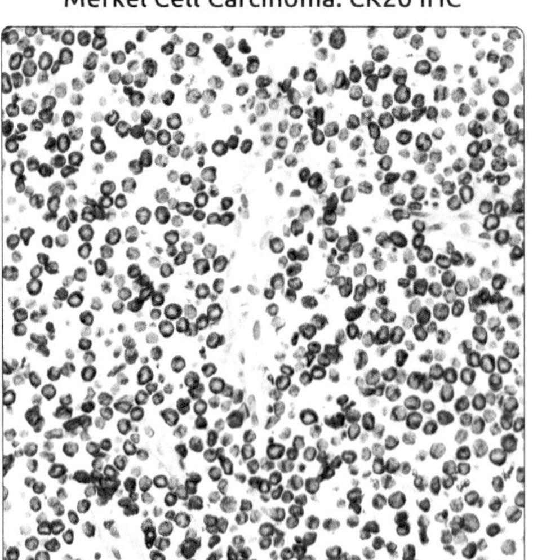

Merkel Cell Carcinoma: INSM1 IHC

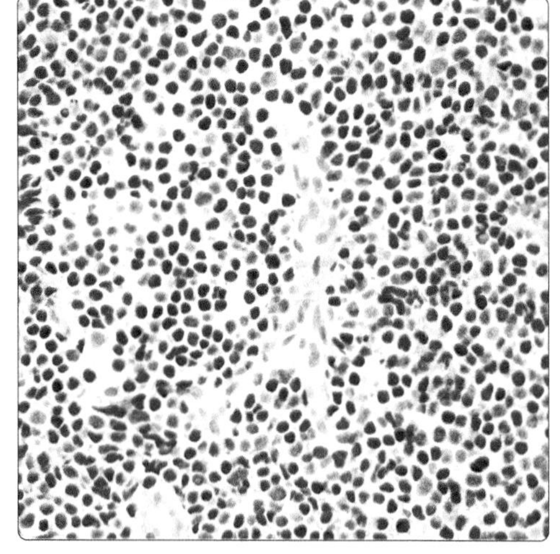

MR: Progressive Multifocal Leukoencephalopathy

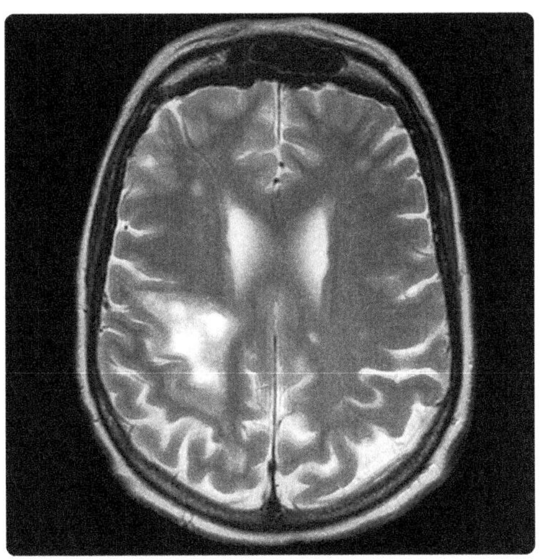

Gross Photograph: Progressive Multifocal Leukoencephalopathy

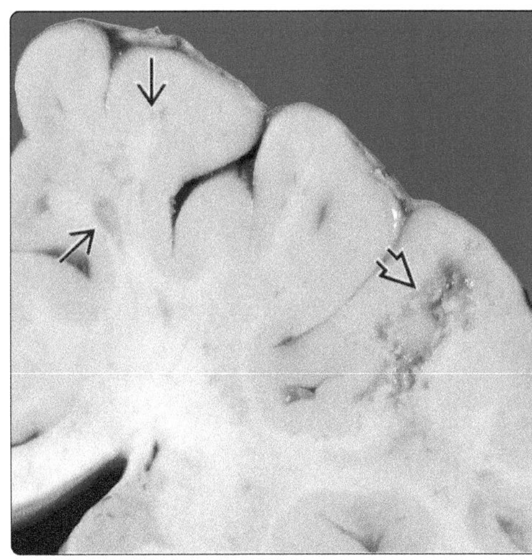

(Left) *Axial T2 MR from a patient with progressive multifocal leukoencephalopathy shows a focal area of hyperintensity with mild mass effect and patchy internal enhancement in the subcortical white matter of the posterior frontal lobe.* **(Right)** *Coronal section of the right posterior frontal lobe of an autopsied brain shows the biopsy site ⇨ as well as punctate and larger confluent gray plaques in the subcortical white matter ⇨ in progressive multifocal leukoencephalopathy. (Courtesy R. Folkerth, MD.)*

Histologic Features of Progressive Multifocal Leukoencephalopathy

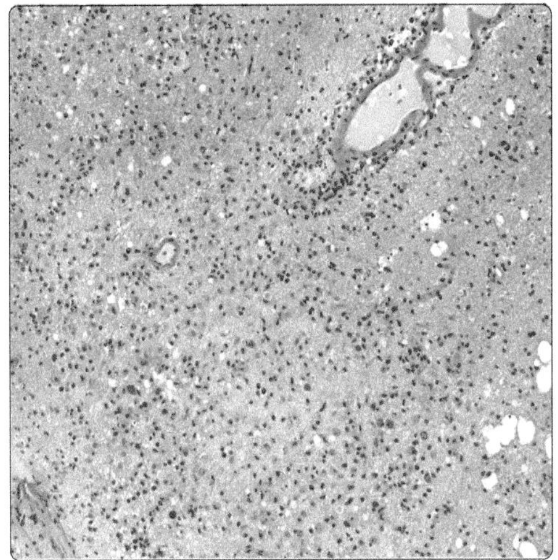

Histologic Features of Progressive Multifocal Leukoencephalopathy

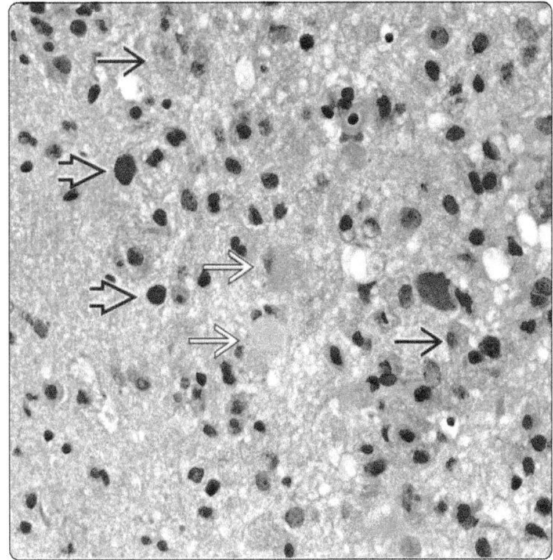

(Left) *Brain biopsy from a patient with progressive multifocal leukoencephalopathy shows a few perivascular lymphocytes, extensive macrophage infiltrates, and disruption of normal architecture. (Courtesy R. Folkerth, MD.)* **(Right)** *Macrophages ⇨ and glial cells contain "glassy" nuclear inclusions ⇨ in progressive multifocal leukoencephalopathy. Occasional enlarged and bizarre astrocytes ➡ are present. (Courtesy R. Folkerth, MD.)*

JC Virus Immunohistochemistry

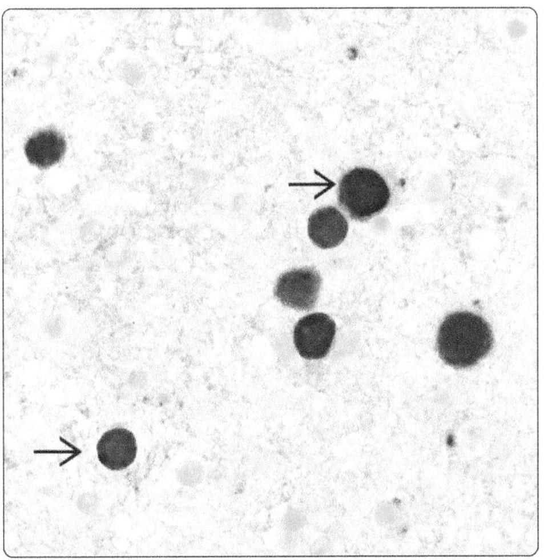

Demyelination in Progressive Multifocal Leukoencephalopathy

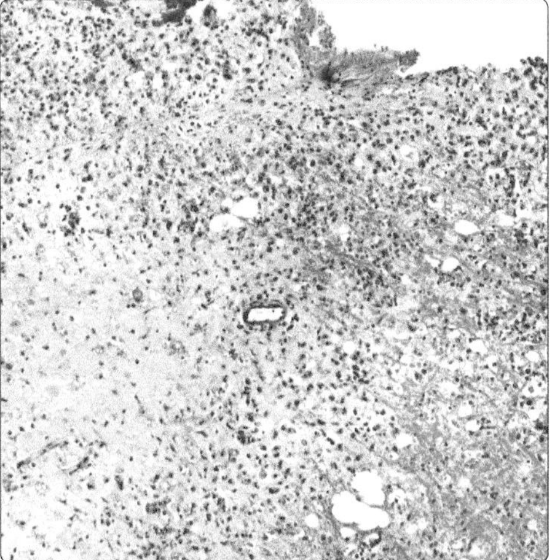

(Left) *Immunohistochemistry for polyomavirus antigen highlights oligodendrocyte with enlarged nuclei and glassy inclusions ⇨.* **(Right)** *Luxol fast blue (myelin) and PAS stain shows an area of myelin loss in progressive multifocal leukoencephalopathy. (Courtesy R. Folkerth, MD.)*

Human Papillomavirus Infection

KEY FACTS

ETIOLOGY/PATHOGENESIS

- Infection with human papilloma viruses (HPVs) via sustained direct skin-to-skin contact; > 200 HPV types identified with ~ 40 types cause cutaneous or mucosal infections
- Persistent infection with high-risk HPV types may progress to precancerous lesions and invasive cancer

CLINICAL ISSUES

- Most common sexually transmitted infection in world
- Associated with majority of cancers in cervix, vagina, anus, and in subset of cases in vulva, penis, oropharynx
- Prior infection with HPV does **not** provide immunity
- Bivalent (HPV 16, 18), tetravalent (6, 11, 16, 18), and 9-valent (6, 11, 16, 18, 31, 33, 45, 52, and 58) vaccines
- HPV DNA cotesting in women aged 30-65 years

MICROSCOPIC

- Warts: Acanthosis, prominent vascular cores, parakeratosis, hyperkeratosis (skin)
- LSIL: Koilocytic changes in superficial epithelial layers
- HSIL: Loss of epithelial maturation, frequent mitoses, high nuclear:cytoplasmic (N:C) ratio, irregular nuclear contour
- p16 is generally positive in HPV-associated precancerous and cancerous lesions

TOP DIFFERENTIAL DIAGNOSES

- Reactive epithelial changes: Squamous metaplasia, p16 negative
- Atrophy in cervix: Uniform nuclei, minimal nuclear pleomorphism or mitotic activity
- Radiation change in cervix: Uniformly spaced cells with enlarged nuclei, low N:C ratio, absence of mitosis
- Monkeypox: Reticular degeneration, epidermal necrosis, karyorrhexis, Guarnieri bodies
- Molluscum Contagiosum: Flesh-colored papules; Henderson-Patterson bodies
- Herpes simplex virus 1/2 and VZV: Distinctive viral cytopathic effects confirmed by IHC/PCR

Warts of Verruca Vulgaris

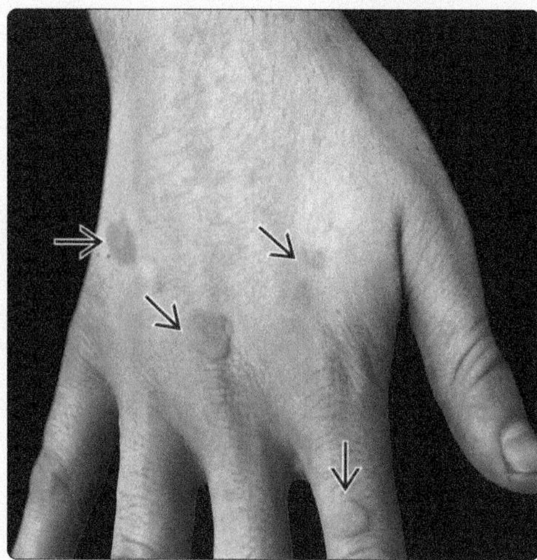

Verruca Vulgaris Histologic Features

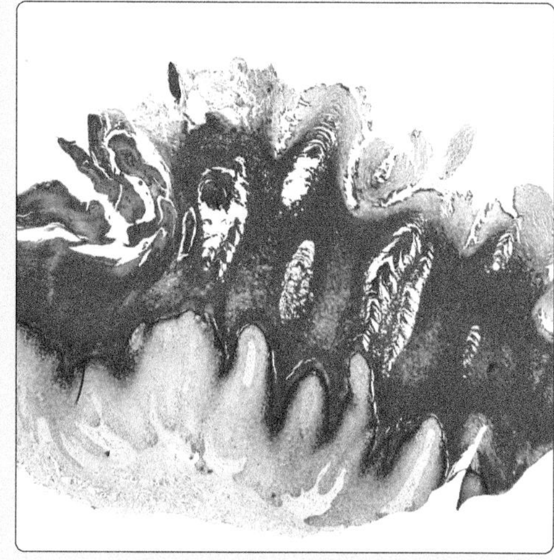

(Left) *Clinical photograph shows multiple pink flat, scaly papules ⇨ in areas of previously treated warts on hand dorsum. Histologic examination confirms recurrence of verruca vulgaris.* **(Right)** *Verruca vulgaris shows exophytic growth with marked hyperkeratosis, papillomatosis, and a prominent layer of stratum granulosum. The underlying squamous epithelium has bland cytologic features.*

Condyloma Acuminatum

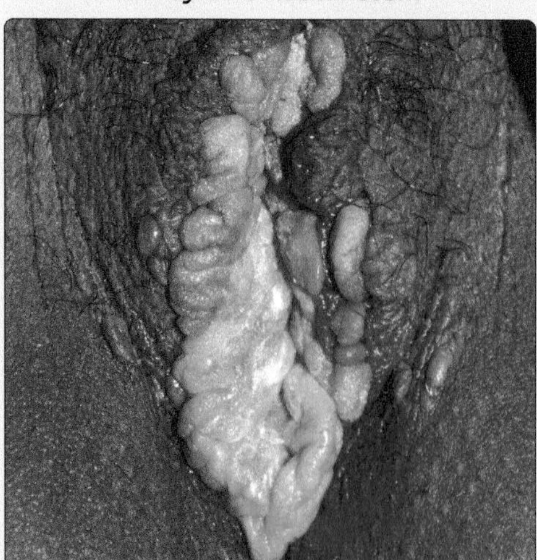

Condyloma Shows Histologic Features

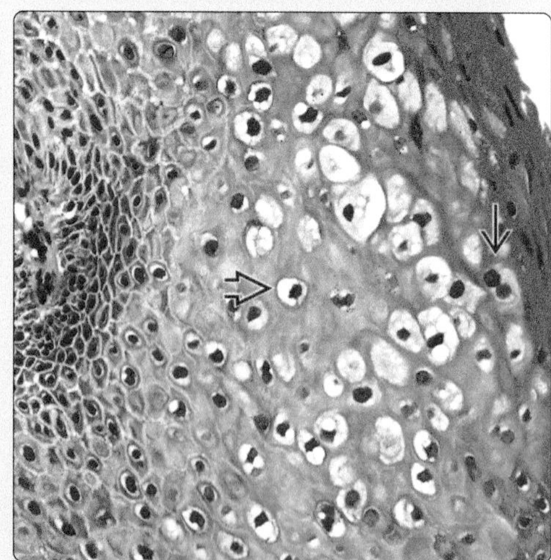

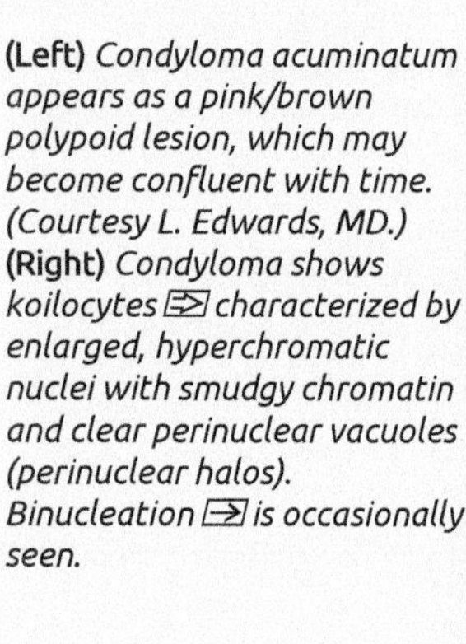

(Left) *Condyloma acuminatum appears as a pink/brown polypoid lesion, which may become confluent with time. (Courtesy L. Edwards, MD.)* **(Right)** *Condyloma shows koilocytes ⇨ characterized by enlarged, hyperchromatic nuclei with smudgy chromatin and clear perinuclear vacuoles (perinuclear halos). Binucleation ⇨ is occasionally seen.*

TERMINOLOGY

Definitions

- *Papillomaviridae* family from Latin "Papilla" (nipple) + "oma" (morbid growth, tumor)

ETIOLOGY/PATHOGENESIS

Infectious Agents

- Infection with human papilloma viruses (HPVs) via sustained direct skin-to-skin contact; productive infections only within stratified epithelia of skin, anogenital tract, and oral cavity
- > 200 HPV types identified (only infect humans); ~ 40 types cause cutaneous or mucosal infections based on tissue tropism; coinfection with multiple HPV types can occur
  - High-risk HPV types include 16, 18, 26, 31, 33, 35, 39, 45, 51, 52, 53, 56, 58, 59, 66, 68, 73, and 82
  - Low-risk HPV types include 6, 11, 40, 43, 44, 54, 69, 70, 71, and 74
  - Other vertebrate mammals have papillomavirus infections and associated tumors from different species-specific strains
- Virus infects basal cells in epithelium; early HPV genes *E1-E7* are expressed, and viral DNA replicates from episomal DNA
- Late genes *L1*, *L2*, and *E4* are expressed in upper epithelial layers; *L1* and *L2* encapsidate viral genomes to form progeny virions in nucleus, which are then shed to initiate new infections
- Persistent infection with high-risk HPV types may progress to precancerous lesions and invasive cancer
- Bethesda system squamous intraepithelial lesion (SIL) terminology for cytology &/or cervical biopsy diagnosis

CLINICAL ISSUES

Epidemiology

- Most common sexually transmitted infection in world; risk increased with unprotected sexual intercourse and increased number of lifetime and recent sex partners
- Primary and secondary immunodeficiency disorders, e.g., HIV infection, may predispose patients to HPV infections and to development of malignancies
- HPV prevalence increases following sexual debut, peaks at young reproductive age (~ 18-30 years), followed by age-related decline; HPV DNA detected in up to 99.7% of cervical cancers from all geographic areas
- Worldwide: > 600,000 new cases and 342,000 cervical cancer deaths in 2020; ~ 13,000 new cases 4,000 deaths in USA

Presentation

- Most infections are transient; studies suggest that 40-90% of cases clear within 1 year
- Benign cutaneous lesions include warts, flat condyloma and condylomata acuminata, verruca vulgaris, deep plantar warts, and verrucous cysts
- Benign mucosal lesions include recurrent respiratory papillomatosis and oropharyngeal papillomas
- HPV infection is associated with cancer development in majority of cases in cervix, vagina, and anus and in subset of cases in vulva, penis, oropharynx
- Epidermodysplasia verruciformis: Rare genetic disorder [*TMC6* (EVER1) and *TMC8* (EVER2) mutations] associated with persistent HPV infection; wart-like skin lesions in childhood with 50% risk of malignant transformation

Laboratory Tests

- Seroreactivity is not useful for diagnosis of HPV; can be negative despite HPV DNA positivity
- HPV typing for risk stratification

Treatment

- Small warts removed with local treatments (e.g., freezing)

Prognosis

- Most warts are benign but prone to recurrence
- HPV-associated anogenital lesions can be managed with screening, early detection, and removal
  - < 15% of low-grade SIL (LSIL) progress to high-grade SIL (HSIL)
  - ~ 10-20% HSIL progress to invasive cancer if left untreated
- HPV-associated oropharyngeal cancers have better prognosis than non-HPV-associated ones
- In immunocompromised patients, clinical course may be more aggressive

Prevention

- Prior infection with HPV does **not** provide immunity
- Bivalent (HPV types 16 and 18), tetravalent (HPV types 6, 11, 16, 18), and 9-valent (HPV types 6, 11, 16, 18, 31, 33, 45, 52, and 58) FDA-approved vaccines
- Vaccines safe and effective at preventing persistent infection and neoplastic lesions caused by targeted viruses; recommended before sexually active/HPV exposure

MICROBIOLOGY

Virus Characteristics

- Nonenveloped, double-stranded, circular DNA virus
- 55 nm in size, icosahedral capsid
- 10-200 virions per infected cell
- ~ 8,000 bp genome with multiple open reading frames producing 9 gene products: E1-E7 (viral regulatory proteins) and L1, L2 (viral capsid proteins)

Culture

- There is no role for culture in routine diagnosis of HPV

MACROSCOPIC

Gross Features

- Warts: Small (1- to 2-mm) to large (4-cm) lesions on any epithelial surface (most common is skin) with hard, horny to soft, ropy surface
- Dysplasia/SIL: Acetowhite lesion or leukoplakia on colposcopy
- Malignancy: Early lesions may be flat or slightly raised; large lesions can produce polypoid/fungating mass

MICROSCOPIC

Histologic Features

- Anogenital lesions

- Low-grade dysplasia/LSIL: Equivalent to condyloma, cervical intraepithelial neoplasia 1 (CIN 1), vaginal intraepithelial neoplasia 1 (VaIN 1), vulvar intraepithelial neoplasia 1 (VIN 1), penile intraepithelial neoplasia 1 (PIN 1), anal intraepithelial neoplasia 1 (AIN 1)
  - Koilocytic changes (enlarged, hyperchromatic nuclei with smudgy chromatin and perinuclear halos) in superficial epithelial layers
  - Cell maturation preserved in upper 2/3 of epithelium
  - Exophytic condyloma: Acanthosis with papillary or verrucous architecture, prominent vascular cores, parakeratosis, hyperkeratosis (skin)
- High-grade dysplasia/HSIL: Equivalent to CIN 2/3, VaIN 2/3, VIN 2/3, PIN 2/3, AIN 2/3
  - Loss of cellular maturation in lower 2/3 (grade 2) to full-thickness (grade 3) epithelium
  - Immature cells with high nuclear:cytoplasmic (N:C) ratio, irregular nuclear contour
  - Frequent mitoses; abnormal mitoses may be present
- Malignancies associated with HPV
  - Heterogeneity in cell type, growth type, and degree of differentiation, depending on cancer site and histologic subtype
  - e.g., cervix: Adenocarcinoma in situ and variants, adenocarcinoma (e.g., usual type, villoglandular type, endometrioid type), squamous cell carcinoma (SCC) and variants
  - e.g., anal/vaginal SCC, vulvar and penile SCC (basaloid and warty)

- HPV-associated oropharyngeal papillomas or cancers
  - Papilloma: Papillary fronds, fibrovascular cores; koilocytic changes may be present
  - Oropharyngeal SCC: Nonkeratinizing SCC is often causally related to HPV, while majority of keratinizing SCC is unrelated to HPV
- Skin lesion: Verruca vulgaris
  - Focal epidermal hyperplasia with hyperkeratosis, parakeratosis, papillomatosis, koilocytes in upper epithelial layers
  - Myrmecia (palmoplantar) warts show characteristic intracytoplasmic inclusions in association with ground-glass or basophilic nuclei in superficial keratinocytes

Cytologic Features

- LSIL: Nuclear enlargement > 3x size of normal nucleus, common multinucleation and variable nuclear hyperchromasia, koilocytosis
- HSIL: High N:C ratio and chromatin clumping, hyperchromatic clusters, syncytial-like aggregates, or single cells, nuclear hyperchromasia and variations in nuclear size and shape
- Nonkeratinizing SCC: Single cells or syncytial aggregates with poorly defined cell borders, coarsely clumped chromatin, nucleoli may be seen; tumor diathesis consisting of necrotic debris, old blood, and inflammatory cells
- Keratinizing SCC: Marked variation in nuclear pleomorphism, coarsely granular chromatin, nucleoli may be seen, tumor diathesis

ANCILLARY TESTS

Immunohistochemistry

- Condyloma acuminatum/exophytic LSIL: p16 weak or negative; Ki-67 (nuclear) positive in lower 2/3 of epithelium
- LSIL: p16 diffusely weak or strong staining in basal layer; Ki-67 (nuclear) positive in lower 2/3 of epithelium
- HSIL: p16 and Ki-67 (nuclear) positive in full-thickness epithelium
- Adenocarcinoma in situ and variants, cervix: p16 generally positive
- SCC, cervix: Positive for CK7, p63, and p16 (except verrucous variant)
- Adenocarcinoma, usual type, and other variants, cervix: p16 generally positive except gastric type (generally negative) and minimal deviation variant (positivity seen in ~ 30% of cases)
- HPV-associated oropharyngeal SCC: Positive for p16 and HPV in situ hybridization (ISH); significant minority of tumors are p16 positive and HPV ISH negative

In Situ Hybridization

- Useful for detecting HPV RNA/DNA in cytologic and histologic samples
- Can target individual HPV types or be pooled into high-risk and low-risk panels

HPV DNA Testing

- Cotesting (concurrent to Pap smear) in women aged 30-65 years

DIFFERENTIAL DIAGNOSIS

Reactive Epithelial Changes

- p16 negative, while LSIL/HSIL shows diffuse positivity for p16

Atrophy in Cervix

- Nuclei in atrophy shows uniform size and spacing with minimal nuclear pleomorphism or mitotic activity

Radiation Change in Cervix

- Uniformly spaced cells with enlarged nuclei, low N:C ratio, absence of mitosis

Monkeypox

- Reticular degeneration, epidermal necrosis, and karyorrhexis; Guarnieri bodies (type B viral inclusions); can be confirmed by IHC/PCR

Molluscum Contagiosum

- Skin lesions appear as raised flesh-colored 2- to 5-mm papules with central depression (umbilication)
- Henderson-Patterson bodies (molluscum bodies) are large eosinophilic to basophilic cytoplasmic inclusions

Human Herpesvirus Infections

- Herpes simplex virus 1/2 and VZV may produce scattered vesicles; distinctive viral cytopathic effects (i.e., nuclear molding, multinucleation, and margination of chromatin) that can be confirmed by IHC/PCR

Human Papillomavirus Types and Associated Lesions

Most Common Human Papillomavirus Type(s)	Disease Association
1, 2, 4, 63	Plantar warts (soles of feet; painful, deep)
2, 7, 22	Common warts (hands and palms)
3, 8, 10	Flat warts
2, 3, 5, 8, 9, 10, 12, 14, 15, 17; types 5, 8, and 14d are most commonly associated with malignant transformation	Epidermodysplasia verruciformis (*TMC6* and *TMC8* gene mutations lead to HPV susceptibility)
6, 11	Oropharyngeal papilloma
6, 11	Respiratory papillomatosis
16, 18	Oropharyngeal cancer
6, 11, 42, 44	Anogenital warts
6, 16, 18, 31, 53, 58	Anal dysplasia/intraepithelial lesion
16, 18	Anal cancer
6, 11	Condyloma acuminatum
16, 31, 6, 11	Low-grade squamous intraepithelial lesions
16, 18, 31, 52	High-grade squamous intraepithelial lesions
16, 18, 31, 45	Cervical, vulvar, penile cancers (squamous and adenocarcinoma): Highest risk; cervical adenocarcinoma; most strongly associated with HPV-18; cervical squamous cell carcinoma: Most strongly associated with HPV-16 and -18

HPV = human papillomavirus.

SELECTED REFERENCES

1. Lechner M et al: HPV-associated oropharyngeal cancer: epidemiology, molecular biology and clinical management. Nat Rev Clin Oncol. 19(5):306-27, 2022
2. McBride AA: Human papillomaviruses: diversity, infection and host interactions. Nat Rev Microbiol. 20(2):95-108, 2022
3. Van Doorslaer K: Revisiting papillomavirus taxonomy: a proposal for updating the current classification in line with evolutionary evidence. Viruses. 14(10), 2022
4. Rosenblum HG et al: Declines in prevalence of human papillomavirus vaccine-type infection among females after introduction of vaccine - United States, 2003-2018. MMWR Morb Mortal Wkly Rep. 70(12):415-20, 2021
5. Perkins RB et al: 2019 ASCCP risk-based management consensus guidelines for abnormal cervical cancer screening tests and cancer rrecursors. J Low Genit Tract Dis. 24(2):102-31, 2020
6. Ernstson A et al: Detection of HPV mRNA in self-collected vaginal samples among women at 69-70 years of age. Anticancer Res. 39(1):381-6, 2019
7. Tisi G et al: Role of HPV DNA, HPV mRNA and cytology in the follow-up of women treated for cervical dysplasia. APMIS. 127(4):196-201, 2019
8. Wang HY et al: Analytical performance evaluation of the HPV OncoCheck assay for detection of high-risk HPV infection in liquid-based cervical samples. Exp Mol Pathol. 106:149-56, 2019
9. Yang EJ: Human papilloma virus-associated squamous neoplasia of the lower anogenital tract. Surg Pathol Clin. 12(2):263-79, 2019
10. Akbari A et al: Validation of intra- and inter-laboratory reproducibility of the Xpert HPV assay according to the international guidelines for cervical cancer screening. Virol J. 15(1):166, 2018
11. Chen JY et al: The risk factors of residual lesions and recurrence of the high-grade cervical intraepithelial lesions (HSIL) patients with positive-margin after conization. Medicine (Baltimore). 97(41):e12792, 2018
12. Delgado Ramos GM et al: A pilot study on the identification of human papillomavirus genotypes in tongue cancer samples from a single institution in Ecuador. Braz J Med Biol Res. 51(11):e7810, 2018
13. Fiano V et al: Methylation in host and viral genes as marker of aggressiveness in cervical lesions: analysis in 543 unscreened women. Gynecol Oncol. 151(2):319-26, 2018
14. Goyal A et al: HPV test result monitoring of different Bethesda categories in gynaecologic cytology: a valuable quality assurance measure. Diagn Cytopathol. 46(11):914-8, 2018
15. Hosseini MS et al: Evaluation of anal cytology in women with history of abnormal Pap smear, cervical intraepithelial neoplasia, cervical cancer and high risk HPV for anogenital dysplasia Asian Pac J Cancer Prev. 19(11):3071-5, 2018
16. Palve V et al: Detection of high-risk human papillomavirus in oral cavity squamous cell carcinoma using multiple analytes and their role in patient survival. J Glob Oncol. 4:1-33, 2018
17. Schmitz M et al: Performance of a DNA methylation marker panel using liquid-based cervical scrapes to detect cervical cancer and its precancerous stages. BMC Cancer. 18(1):1197, 2018
18. Sun M et al: Meta-analysis on the performance of p16/Ki-67 dual immunostaining in detecting high-grade cervical intraepithelial neoplasm. J Cancer Res Ther. 14(Supplement):S587-93, 2018
19. Grønhøj Larsen C et al: Correlation between human papillomavirus and p16 overexpression in oropharyngeal tumours: a systematic review. Br J Cancer. 110(6):1587-94, 2014
20. Darragh TM et al: The lower anogenital squamous terminology standardization project for HPV-associated lesions: background and consensus recommendations from the College of American Pathologists and the American Society for Colposcopy and Cervical Pathology. Int J Gynecol Pathol. 32(1):76-115, 2013

LSIL: Pap Smear

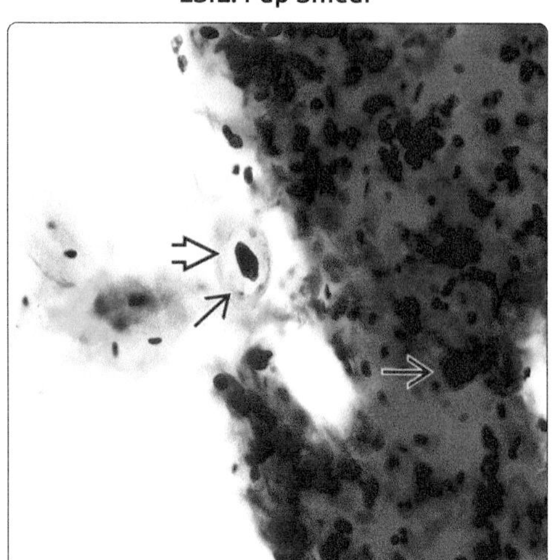

LSIL: Tissue Section

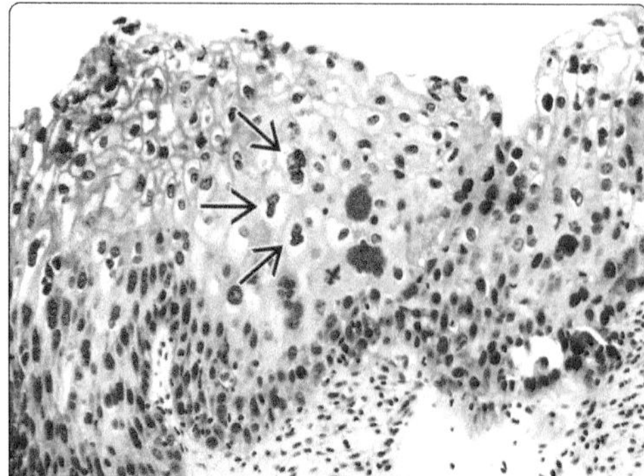

(Left) *Pap smear shows atypical squamous cells ⇒ with enlarged nuclei, irregular nuclear border, and hyperchromasia. One of the cells shows a distinct perinuclear halo ⇒. These findings are consistent with LSIL.* **(Right)** *Medium magnification of cervix shows LSIL characterized by enlarged, hyperchromatic nuclei with smudgy chromatin and perinuclear halos. Multinucleation ⇒ and increased cellular density are common. Cell polarity is generally well preserved at the base.*

HSIL: Pap Smear

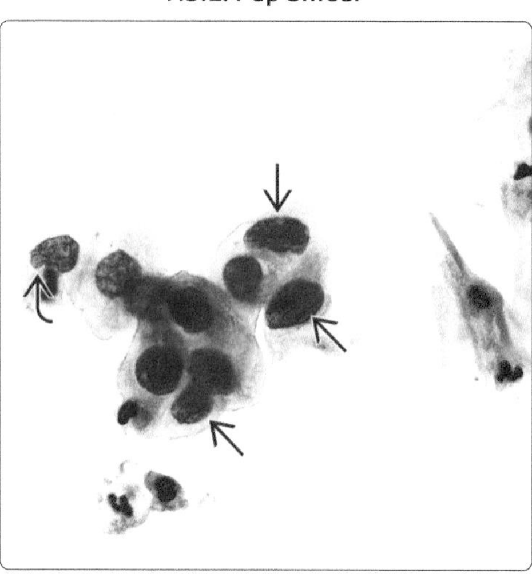

HSIL: Tissue Section

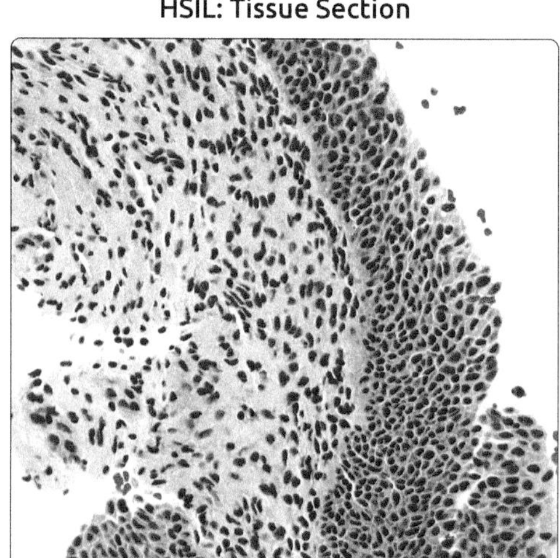

(Left) *High-magnification Pap smear shows atypical cells with high nuclear:cytoplasmic (N:C) ratio, hyperchromasia, coarse chromatin, and irregular nuclear membrane (occasional nuclear grooves ⇒ and indentation ⇒), consistent with high-grade squamous intraepithelial lesion (HSIL).* **(Right)** *Cervical biopsy shows crowded cells with cytologic atypia and loss of maturation through the full thickness of squamous epithelium, consistent with HSIL. The lesion would be diffusely positive for p16 and Ki-67 immunohistochemistry.*

HSIL: p16 Immunohistochemistry

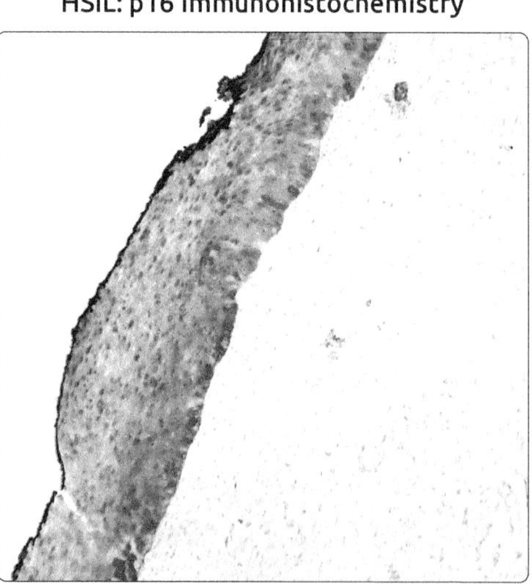

HSIL: Ki-67 Proliferative Activity

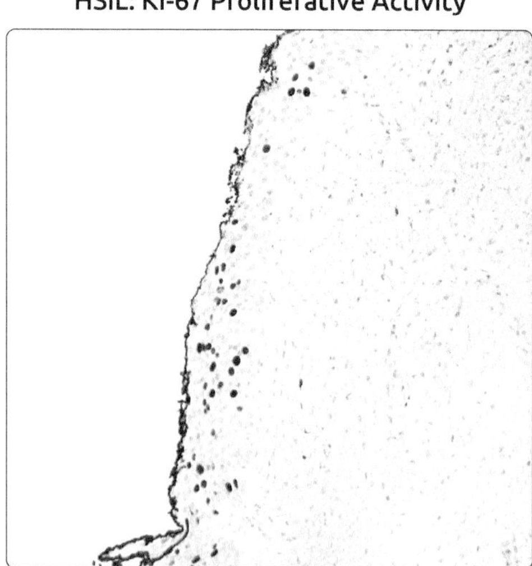

(Left) *p16 immunostain highlights the entire HSIL lesion in this cervical biopsy.* **(Right)** *HSIL cervical lesion characteristically exhibits proliferative activity through the full thickness of epithelium, which can be confirmed by positive Ki-67 stain. Both the p16 and Ki-67 immunostains are good tools to differentiate HSIL from its mimics, e.g., atrophy, when diagnosis is challenging on H&E sections.*

Condyloma Acuminatum

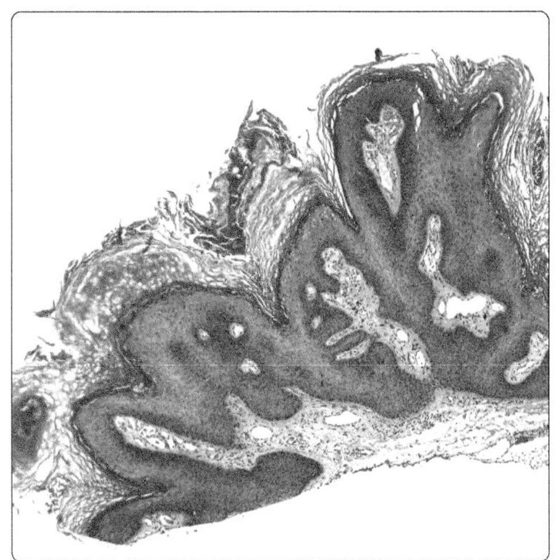

Condyloma Acuminatum: HPV 6/11 ISH

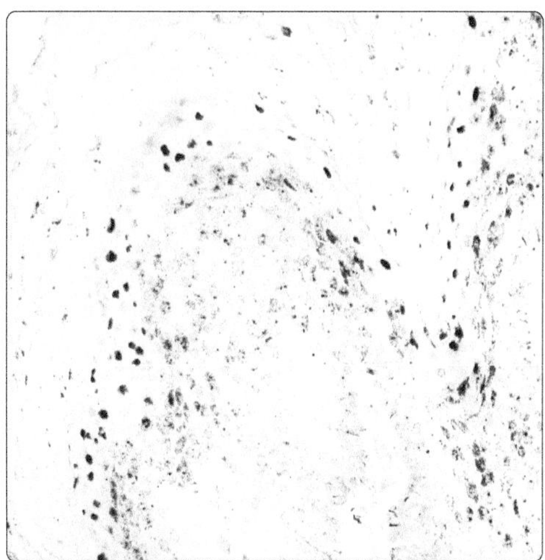

(Left) *This shave biopsy of a condyloma acuminatum shows hyperplastic papillary exophytic squamous epithelium.* **(Right)** *This section of a condyloma acuminatum shows positive staining for low-risk human papillomavirus (HPV) in cells within the upper portion of the epithelium by HPV 6/11 RNA in situ hybridization (ISH).*

Myrmecia Wart (Palmoplantar Wart)

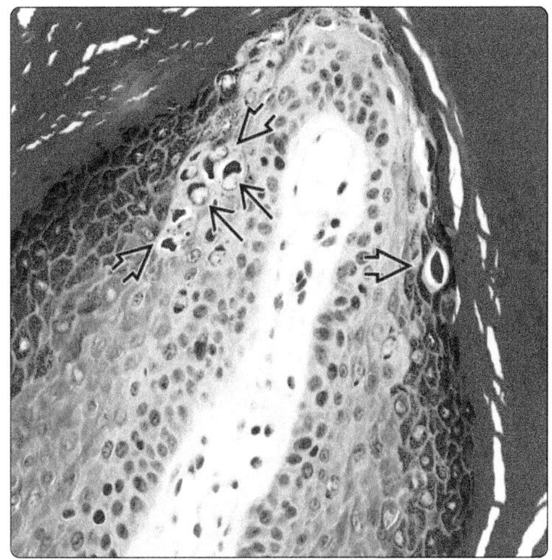

Vocal Cord Squamous Papilloma

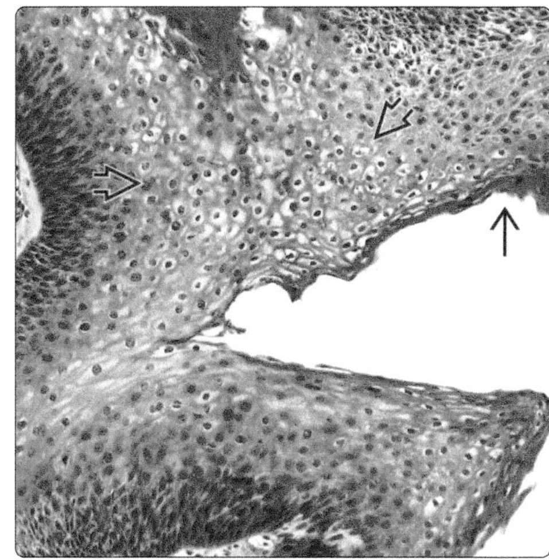

(Left) *High magnification of this myrmecia wart (palmoplantar wart) shows the characteristic large intracytoplasmic inclusions ➩ in association with ground-glass nuclei ➩ in the superficial keratinocytes.* **(Right)** *Resection of this vocal cord lesion reveals a squamous papilloma with hyperkeratosis ➩ and prominent koilocytic changes ➩, consistent with HPV viral cytopathic effect.*

Oropharyngeal Squamous Cell Carcinoma

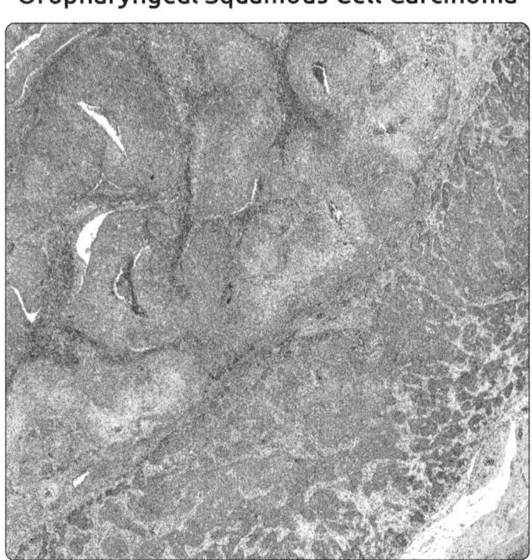

Squamous Cell Carcinoma: HPV 16/18 ISH

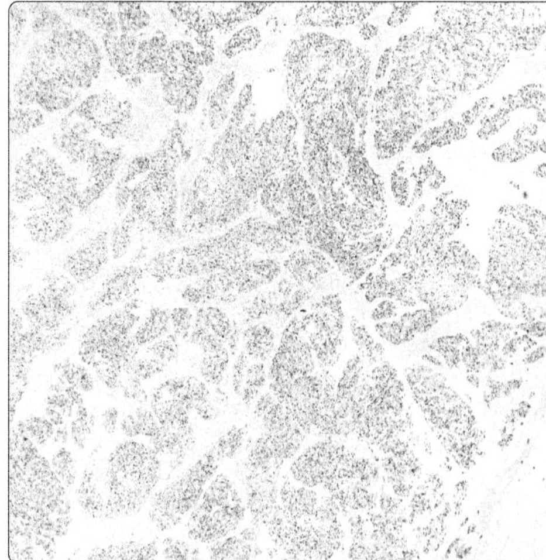

(Left) *This section of a mass originating at the base of the tongue shows invasive, nonkeratinizing squamous cell carcinoma that was positive for p16 and HPV16/18 RNA ISH.* **(Right)** *This section of a squamous cell carcinoma originating at the base of the tongue was positive for high risk HPV 16/18 by RNA ISH staining.*

Molluscum Contagiosum

KEY FACTS

ETIOLOGY/PATHOGENESIS

- *Molluscum contagiosum virus* (MCV) spreads through skin-to-skin contact or fomites and replicates within cytoplasm of epidermal cells

CLINICAL ISSUES

- Occurs worldwide, most commonly in children (< 10 years old) and immunosuppressed (e.g., HIV infected)
- Painless papules with depressed center in exposed areas of skin, including genitals, arms, legs, and face
- Resolves spontaneously in 6-12 months but can be treated with cryotherapy, topical creams, or cimetidine

MACROSCOPIC

- Skin lesions appear as raised flesh-colored 2- to 5-mm papules with central depression (umbilication)

MICROSCOPIC

- Hyperplasia of epidermis with necrosis of central cells creates cup-shaped lesion
- Henderson-Patterson bodies (molluscum bodies) are large eosinophilic to basophilic cytoplasmic inclusions
- Lack of inflammation unless lesions have been previously disturbed or disrupted

TOP DIFFERENTIAL DIAGNOSES

- Herpes simplex virus/varicella-zoster virus: May produce scattered vesicles; distinctive viral cytopathic effects can be confirmed by IHC
- Monkeypox: Reticular degeneration, epidermal necrosis, and karyorrhexis; Guarnieri bodies (type B viral inclusions)
- Hand, foot, and mouth disease: Apoptosis of keratinocytes, edema, necrosis, and dyskeratosis, no distinct viral cytopathic effects
- Other vesicle-forming skin diseases: History of exposure to vaccine, travel, or close contact; layer of separation in vesicle formation; ancillary tests for blistering disease (immunofluorescence)

Molluscum Papules

Ultrastructural Features

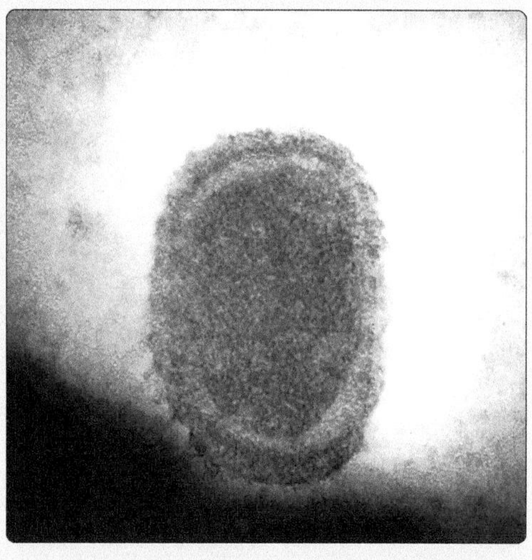

(Left) *Skin lesions in molluscum contagiosum are typically painless 2- to 5-mm flesh-colored papules with central depression. Papules may become inflamed, red, and swollen.* **(Right)** *Electron micrograph shows a large ovoid-shaped enveloped viral particle measuring ~ 320 nm in length and 250 nm in width with surface tubules and an electron-dense core, features characteristic of molluscum contagiosum virus. (Courtesy CDC/PHIL.)*

Molluscum: Histology

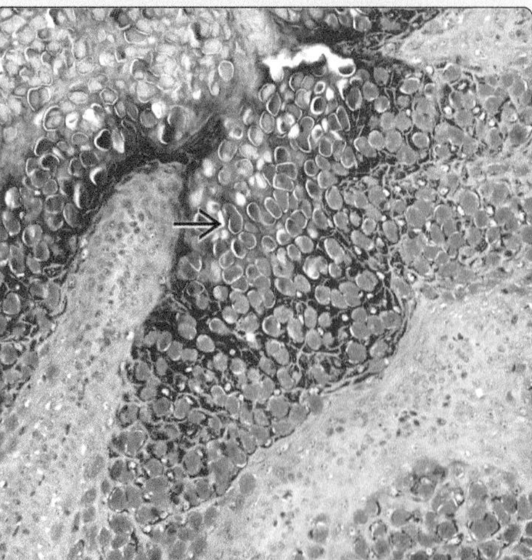

Disrupted Molluscum

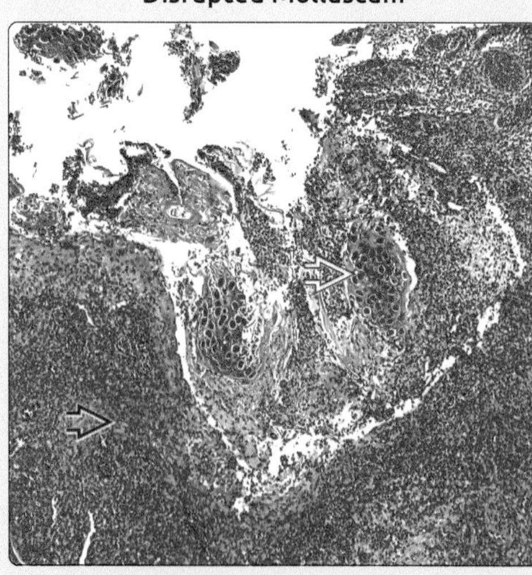

(Left) *A classic appearance of a molluscum contagiosum virus infection demonstrates Henderson-Patterson bodies, ghosts of epithelial cells with large cytoplasmic inclusions, coalescing collection within the epidermis.* **(Right)** *A medium magnification of a disrupted lesion of molluscum contagiosum demonstrates intense inflammation and remnants of the ghost cells. When disrupted, the lesions may be difficult to diagnose on biopsy if viral cytopathic effect is scarce.*

TERMINOLOGY

Synonyms

- *Molluscum contagiosum virus* (MCV)

Definitions

- *Molluscipoxvirus* genus: From Latin "molluscus" (soft) and "contagiosus" (contagious)
- *Poxviridae* family: From English/German "pox," "pock," or "pocc" (swell up, blow up)

ETIOLOGY/PATHOGENESIS

Infectious Agents

- Large DNA virus that spreads through skin-to-skin contact or fomites
- Infects human epidermal cells through plasma membrane fusion and macropinocytosis, then replicates entirely within cytoplasm of host cell (incubation period 2-6 months)

CLINICAL ISSUES

Epidemiology

- Occurs worldwide, most commonly in children (< 10 years old) and immunosuppressed (e.g., HIV infected)

Presentation

- Small fleshy painless papules (mollusca) with depressed center in exposed areas of skin, including genitals, arms, legs, and face (including eyelids)
- Spread may occur from contacted sites secondary to disruption

Laboratory Tests

- Rarely performed
- PCR (lesion crust, scab, skin material or swabs)

Treatment

- Cryotherapy, which may be painful but removes lesions
- Topical creams (not 100% effective)
- Cimetidine (children)
- Lesions can resolve spontaneously in 6-12 months

Prognosis

- Self-limited to diffuse skin dissemination
- May be difficult to eradicate but no mortality

MICROBIOLOGY

Viral Features

- Enveloped, linear, double-stranded DNA virus
- 320 x 250 x 200 nm, ovoid to brick-shaped
- 190 kb with 182 genes
- 4 subtypes (MCV-1 to MCV-4) with MCV-1 being most common

MACROSCOPIC

Skin lesions

- Pock or pox appears as raised 2- to 5-mm papule with central depression (umbilication) from necrosis of epithelial cells
- Usually distinct individual or clusters of lesions

MICROSCOPIC

Histologic Features

- Hyperplasia of epidermis with necrosis of central cells creates cup-shaped lesion
- Cellular changes include enlargement and pink to purple homogeneous nuclei
- Lack of inflammation unless lesions have been previously disturbed or disrupted

Cytologic Features

- Henderson-Patterson bodies (molluscum bodies) are large eosinophilic to basophilic cytoplasmic inclusions that push aside nucleus

DIFFERENTIAL DIAGNOSIS

Herpes Simplex Virus, Varicella-Zoster Virus

- Viral cytopathic effect in biopsy (classic herpetic changes) are distinct from MCV and confirmed by widely available anti-HSV or anti-VZV IHC
- May produce scattered vesicles to disseminated vesicles and pustules
- Usually occurs in immunosuppressed patients &/or unvaccinated children

Monkeypox

- Occasional Guarnieri bodies (type B viral inclusions), cytoplasmic eosinophilic inclusions
- Reticular degeneration, epidermal necrosis, and karyorrhexis
- Often with known clinical exposure

Hand, Foot, and Mouth Disease

- Skin in hand, foot, and mouth may show apoptosis of keratinocytes, edema, necrosis, and dyskeratosis
- No distinctive viral cytopathic effects

Other Vesicle-Forming Skin Diseases

- Clinical history of exposure to vaccine, travel, or close contact
- Ancillary tests for blistering disease (immunofluorescence)
- Layer of separation in vesicle formation

SELECTED REFERENCES

1. Han H et al: Molluscum contagiosum virus evasion of immune surveillance: a review. J Drugs Dermatol. 22(2):182-9, 2023
2. Yu CL et al: Interventions for molluscum contagiosum: a systematic review and network meta-analysis with normalized entropy assessment. J Am Acad Dermatol. 88(2):508-10, 2023
3. Creytens D: Melan A antibody cross-reactivity in molluscum contagiosum bodies. Int J Surg Pathol. 26(2):151-2, 2018
4. Rosner M et al: Periocular molluscum contagiosum: six different clinical presentations. Acta Ophthalmol. 96(5):e600-5, 2018
5. Azevedo T et al: Disseminated molluscum contagiosum lesions in an HIV patient. Cleve Clin J Med. 84(3):186-7, 2017
6. Kinoshita M et al: Case of disseminated molluscum contagiosum caused by ruxolitinib, a Janus kinase 1 and 2 inhibitor. J Dermatol. 43(11):1387-8, 2016
7. Chen X et al: Molluscum contagiosum virus infection. Lancet Infect Dis. 13(10):877-88, 2013
8. Connell CO et al: Congenital molluscum contagiosum: report of four cases and review of the literature. Pediatr Dermatol. 25(5):553-6, 2008
9. Brown J et al: Childhood molluscum contagiosum. Int J Dermatol. 45(2):93-9, 2006
10. Melquiot NV et al: Preparation and use of molluscum contagiosum virus from human tissue biopsy specimens. Methods Mol Biol. 269:371-84, 2004

Smallpox, Mpox, and Other Pox Virus Infections

KEY FACTS

ETIOLOGY/PATHOGENESIS

- Infection with dsDNA viruses in *Poxviridae* family
  - Orthopox group: Variola, vaccinia, monkeypox
  - Parapox group: Pseudocowpox, orf, bovine papular stomatitis virus
  - Yatapox group: Tanapox virus, Yaba monkey tumor virus

CLINICAL ISSUES

- Vaccinia vaccine protects against smallpox and monkeypox; associated with various VACV-related complications
- Eczema vaccinatum: Occurs in patients with history of eczema or atopic dermatitis
- Monkeypox endemic to Central Africa; 2022 global outbreak: Vesicular skin lesions (similar to smallpox) but with lymphadenopathy
- Orf virus: 2- to 3-cm ulcerative lesions or nodules on fingers, hands, or forearms
- RT-PCR (swab of lesion, lesion crusts), serology, electron microscopy, culture isolation
- Treatment with antivirals (tecovirimat, cidofovir, brincidofovir) and VACV immunoglobulin (VIg)

MICROSCOPIC

- Pocks of VACV, smallpox, monkeypox: Distinct, fluid-filled vesicle with increased inflammation
- Eosinophilic intracytoplasmic inclusions of smallpox, VACV, and monkeypox-infected epithelium (Guarnieri bodies)
- Orthopoxvirus antibodies highlight cytoplasm and inclusions

TOP DIFFERENTIAL DIAGNOSES

- VACV, monkeypox, smallpox within differential diagnoses of each other; distinguish based on exposure/vaccination history and molecular testing
- Molluscum contagiosum: Henderson-Patterson bodies (molluscum bodies)
- HSV, VZV: Vesicles and pustules, nuclear inclusions; can confirm with IHC, PCR

(Left) *This historic photograph of a child with smallpox shows the classic maculopapular rash with umbilicated pustules. (Courtesy, J. Noble, Jr., MD, CDC/PHIL.)* **(Right)** *This section shows a reduction in the normal thickness of the stratum corneum and ballooning degeneration of cells in the stratum spinosum, leading to rupture. Coalescence of ruptured cells forms microvesicles, causing outward growth of maculopapular lesions. (Courtesy R. Haraszti, MD, CDC/PHIL.)*

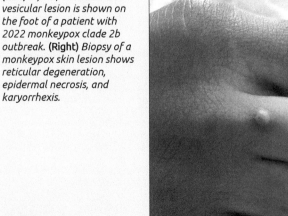

Smallpox

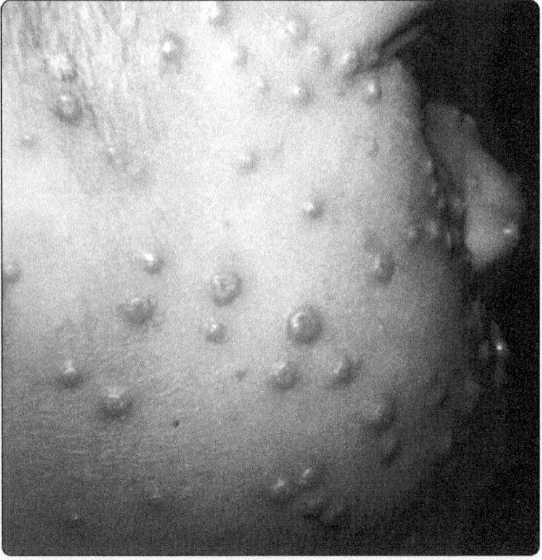

Smallpox Histology

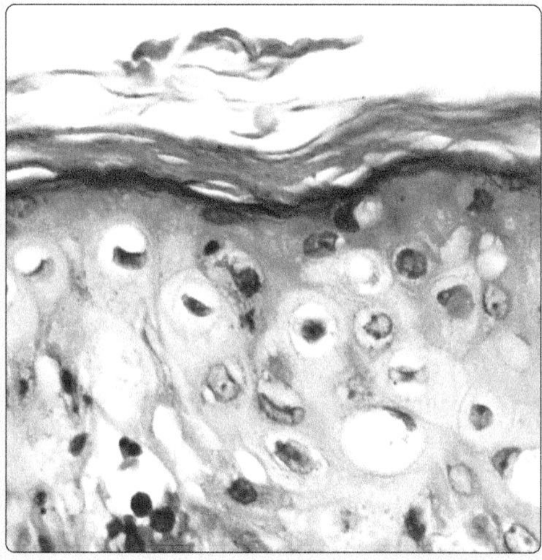

(Left) *A firm, circumscribed vesicular lesion is shown on the foot of a patient with 2022 monkeypox clade 2b outbreak.* **(Right)** *Biopsy of a monkeypox skin lesion shows reticular degeneration, epidermal necrosis, and karyorrhexis.*

Monkeypox

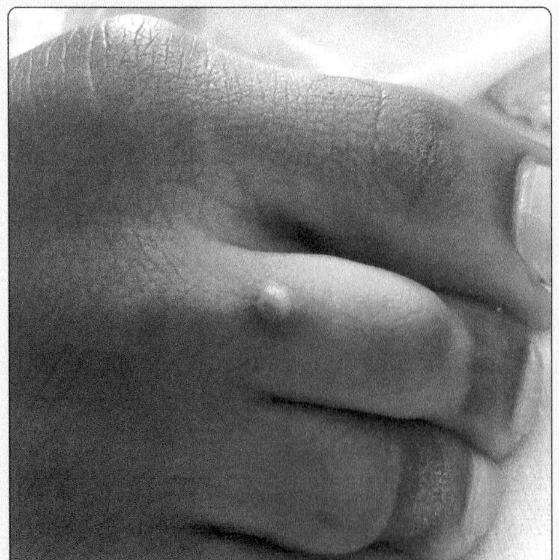

Monkeypox Histology

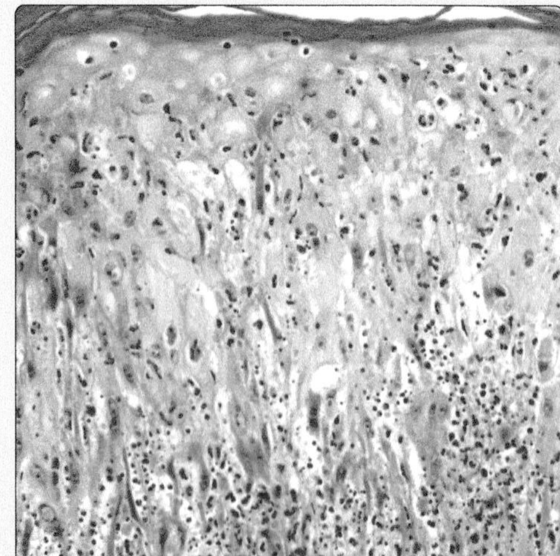

TERMINOLOGY

Synonyms

- Smallpox = variola, pox, red plague
- Monkeypox = Mpox

Definitions

- English/German: "Pox," from "pock" or "pocc" (swell up, blow up): Pus-filled, skin-eruptive swellings
- Latin: "Variola," "varius," or "varus" (spotted or pimple)

ETIOLOGY/PATHOGENESIS

Infectious Agents

- Infection with dsDNA viruses in *Poxviridae* family, which replicate within cytoplasm of host cell
  - Orthopox group
    - Smallpox virus (variola): Eradicated (1977)
    - Vaccinia virus (VACV or VV) (similar to cowpox)
    - Monkeypox virus (MPXV): 1st detected in research monkey colony
  - Parapox group
    - Pseudocowpox, orf, bovine papular stomatitis virus
  - Yatapox group
    - Tanapox virus, Yaba monkey tumor virus

CLINICAL ISSUES

Epidemiology

- VACV-related complications occur in those vaccinated for smallpox with VACV
- Monkeypox
  - Clade I (former Congo Basin/Central African clade)
  - Clade II (former West African clade)
    - Clade IIa: 2003 USA outbreak from African rodents imported into USA
    - Clade IIb: 2022 global outbreak (> 88,000 cases globally as of August 2, 2023)

Presentation

- VACV
  - Generalized vaccinia
    - Generalized pustular eruption of skin ~ 1 week following vaccination (rare)
  - Eczema vaccinatum
    - Severe widespread eruption of crusting skin rash
    - Follows exposure to vaccination or vaccinated individual
    - Occurs in patients with history of eczema or atopic dermatitis
  - Progressive vaccinia
    - Vaccinia gangrenosum or vaccinia necrosum
    - Progressive painless skin lesions with ulceration and necrosis (rare)
  - Roseola vaccinia
    - Postvaccination site erythematous halo
  - Jennerian pustule
    - Occurs at site of vaccination at 5 days post vaccination and becomes pustular at 10 days
    - Associated with fever and lymphadenopathy
    - Generates B- and T-cell responses, which are key to prevention of smallpox
    - Cross protection against cowpox and monkeypox
- Monkeypox
  - Incubation period after exposure is 10-14 days
  - Cutaneous eruption of vesiculopustules (similar to smallpox in appearance) but with lymphadenopathy
  - Genital and perianal lesions associated with sexual transmission; severe oropharyngeal or rectal pain common
  - Fever, chills, lymphadenopathy, fatigue, muscle aches, headache, respiratory symptoms
  - Exposure to infected animals by caretaking, slaughter/ingestion, or proximity
  - Human-to-human transmission occurs through direct contact with rash, scabs, bodily fluids, or respiratory secretions
  - Secondary bacterial skin infections (~ 20% in unvaccinated patients)
  - Concomitant sexually transmitted diseases (syphilis, gonorrhea, chlamydia) in 10-20% for clade IIb outbreak
- Orf: 2- to 3-cm ulcerative lesions or nodules on fingers, hands, or forearms

Laboratory Tests

- CDC RT-PCR (swab of lesion, lesion crusts) detects smallpox, monkeypox, vaccinia, orf, pseudocowpox, and bovine papular stomatitis virus (plus cowpox, sealpox, molluscum contagiosum, and tanapox virus in research capacity)
- CDC Poxvirus Serology (serum): IgM ELISA detects antibody response to orthopox infection

Treatment

- Vaccinia vaccine (smallpox vaccine)
  - ACAM2000: Live virus resulting in skin lesion ("take")
  - JYNNEOS (Imvamune; Imvanex): Nonreplicating live virus without "take"
  - Aventis Pasteur smallpox vaccine (APSV): Replication competent, not FDA approved
  - Available in USA from Strategic National Stockpile (SNS)
- Antivirals
  - Tecovirimat (TPOXX, ST-246); FDA approved in 2018
    - Inhibitor of orthopoxvirus VP37 envelope wrapping protein to block cellular transmission
  - Brincidofovir (Tembexa, CMX001); FDA approved in 2021
    - Lipid-conjugated cidofovir for intracellular release
  - Cidofovir; available through IND protocol for smallpox
- VACV immunoglobulin (VIg): for complications of smallpox vaccination
- No monkeypox virus-specific treatments
  - VIg
  - Tecovirimat, cidofovir, brincidofovir
  - Smallpox vaccines JYNNEOS and ACAM2000

Prognosis

- Eczema vaccinatum may be fatal if not recognized and treated immediately
- Monkeypox mortality may be 10% in low-resource settings but is usually nonfatal in developed nations, including 2022 Clade IIb outbreak

MICROBIOLOGY

Vaccinia Virus

- Enveloped, linear, double-stranded DNA virus
- 190 kb with 250 genes
- Agent used for smallpox eradication with > 10 strains used in research and vaccination settings

Monkeypox Virus

- Enveloped, linear, double-stranded DNA virus
- 197 kb with 190 genes
- Virus is very similar to smallpox virus

Culture

- Grow in many cultured cell lines (e.g., Vero, monkey kidney, HeLa and chick embryo fibroblast cell): Cytopathic effects appear as cell rounding with long cytoplasmic extensions
- Chorioallantoic membranes (CAMs) of 12-day-old chicken embryos: Orthopoxviruses produce pocks
- Routine culture not recommended for diagnosis of monkeypox virus

MACROSCOPIC

Cutaneous Pox

- Pox virus infections appear very similar clinically with distribution and history being important distinguishing factors
- "Pock" or "pox" appears as raised papule or pustule, sometimes with central umbilication
- In VACV/smallpox/monkeypox, evolution of lesion with loss of fluid and influx of neutrophils
- Smallpox/monkeypox may be disseminated

MICROSCOPIC

Histologic Features

- Type A viral inclusions (seen in cowpox among human infections): Large eosinophilic bodies appearing late in infection cycle composed of solitary protein (A type inclusion protein) that has embedded viral particles and provides environmental protection
- Type B (Guarnieri bodies): Eosinophilic intracytoplasmic inclusions of smallpox, VACV, and monkeypox-infected epithelium
- Pock of VACV, smallpox, parapox, and monkeypox
  - Endothelial cell activation with lymphocytes/histiocytes/plasma cell infiltrate
  - Progresses to dilated vessels, edema, and epithelial expansion (early vesicle)
  - Distinct, fluid-filled vesicle with increased inflammation
  - Becomes pustule when neutrophils infiltrate
  - Ulceration (loss of vesicle) with inflammation
  - Ends with reepithelialization and scarring

Cytologic Features

- Swollen squamous epithelial cells with large, glassy nuclei and eosinophilic intracytoplasmic inclusions (viral inclusions)

ANCILLARY TESTS

Immunohistochemistry

- Orthopoxvirus antibodies highlight cytoplasm and inclusions

Electron Microscopy

- Large enveloped viruses observed with negative staining methods
- Can distinguish between orthopoxviruses (brick-shaped) and parapoxviruses (ovoid) but not between species

DIFFERENTIAL DIAGNOSIS

Vaccinia Virus, Monkeypox, Smallpox

- These 3 entities are within differential diagnoses of each other
- Careful clinical history, including exposure and vaccination history, is paramount
- Electron microscopy, immunohistochemistry, and serology cannot distinguish monkeypox from smallpox; requires PCR/sequencing

Molluscum Contagiosum

- Molluscum contagiosum virus in *Molluscipoxvirus* genus
- Henderson-Patterson bodies (molluscum bodies) are large eosinophilic to basophilic cytoplasmic inclusions

Herpes Simplex Virus, Varicella-Zoster Virus

- May produce scattered vesicles to disseminated vesicles and pustules
- Usually occurs in immunosuppressed patients &/or unvaccinated children
- Viral cytopathic effect in biopsy (classic herpetic changes); can confirm with IHC

Other Vesicle-Forming Skin Diseases

- Clinical history of exposure to vaccine, travel, or close contact
- Ancillary tests for blistering disease (immunofluorescence)
- Layer of separation in vesicle formation

SELECTED REFERENCES

1. Birkhead M et al: Tanapox, South Africa, 2022. Emerg Infect Dis. 29(6):1206-9, 2023
2. Rodríguez-Cuadrado FJ et al: Clinical, histopathologic, immunohistochemical, and electron microscopic findings in cutaneous monkeypox: a multicenter retrospective case series in Spain. J Am Acad Dermatol. 88(4):856-63, 2023
3. MacNeill AL: Comparative pathology of zoonotic orthopoxviruses. Pathogens. 11(8), 2022
4. Thompson HJ et al: Orf Virus in humans: case series and clinical review. Cutis. 110(1):48-52, 2022
5. Thornhill JP et al: Monkeypox virus infection in humans across 16 countries - April-June 2022. N Engl J Med. 387(8):679-91, 2022
6. Yinka-Ogunleye A et al: Outbreak of human monkeypox in Nigeria in 2017-18: a clinical and epidemiological report. Lancet Infect Dis. 19(8):872-9, 2019
7. Grosenbach DW et al: Oral tecovirimat for the treatment of smallpox. N Engl J Med. 379(1):44-53, 2018
8. Eder I et al: Two distinct clinical courses of human cowpox, Germany, 2015. Viruses. 9(12), 2017
9. Cann JA et al: Comparative pathology of smallpox and monkeypox in man and macaques. J Comp Pathol. 148(1):6-21, 2013

Ultrastructural Features: Variola Virus

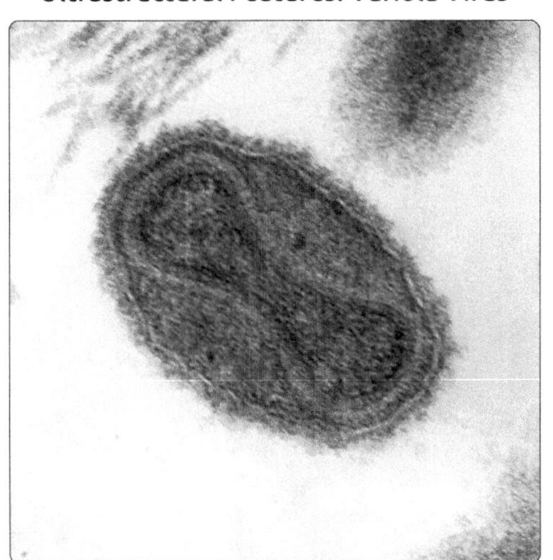

Ultrastructural Features: Vaccinia Virus

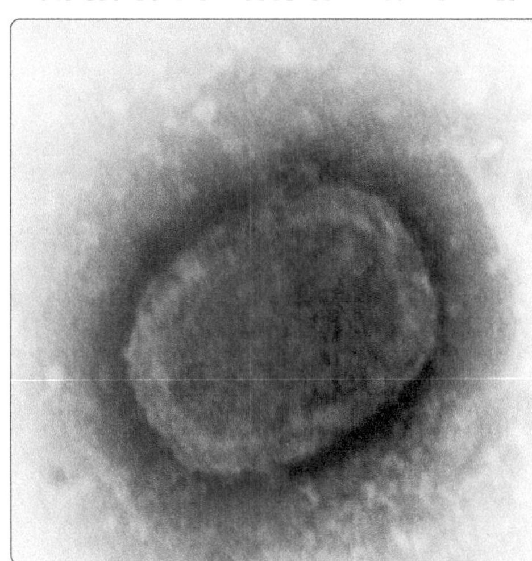

(Left) *This transmission electron micrograph shows a variola virus (smallpox) virion, containing a dumbbell-shaped structure corresponding to the viral core, features diagnostic of orthopoxviruses but not species specific. (Courtesy F. Murphy, DVM, PhD, S. Whitfield M.S., CDC/PHIL.)* **(Right)** *This transmission electron micrograph shows a large varicella virus virion, exhibiting the larger more electron-dense form with a capsule of complex structure referred to as C form. (Courtesy J. Nakano, PhD, CDC/PHIL.)*

Ultrastructural Features: Monkeypox Virus

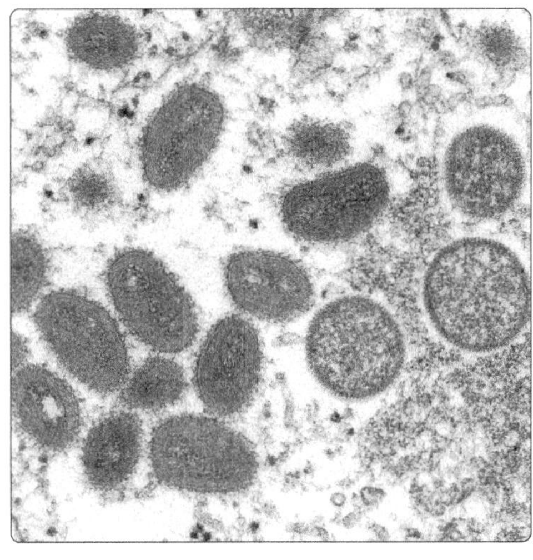

Ultrastructural Features: Orf Virus

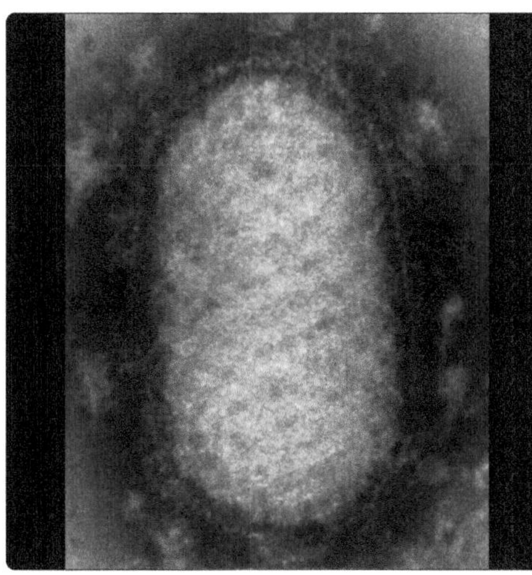

(Left) *This electron micrograph shows mature, oval-shaped virus particles measuring 200-250 nm (left) and crescents and spherical particles of immature virions (right). (Courtesy C. Goldsmith, MGS, CDC/PHIL.)* **(Right)** *This transmission electron micrograph shows an ovoid-shaped Orf virus virion with spirally arranged external tubular ridges, features characteristic of parapoxviruses. (Courtesy C. Goldsmith, MGS, CDC/PHIL.)*

Ultrastructural Features: Tanapox Virus

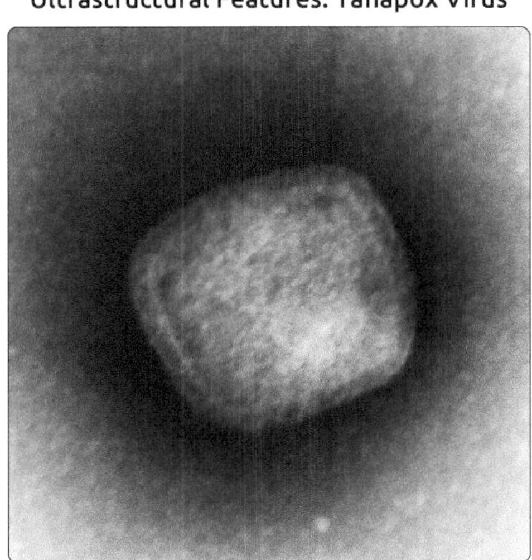

Ultrastructural Features: Yabapox Virus

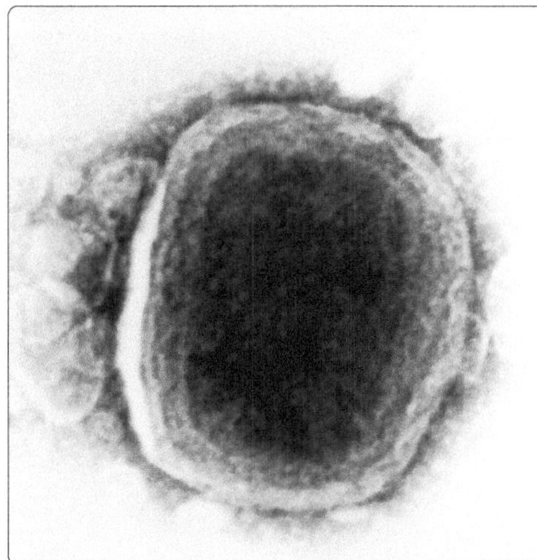

(Left) *This transmission electron micrograph shows a tanapox virus (Yatapox group) virion in C form with a capsular appearance of the virions' capsid or external protein coat. (Courtesy J. Nakano, PhD, CDC/PHIL.)* **(Right)** *This transmission electron micrograph shows a yabapox virus virion in C form with a capsular appearance of the virions' capsid or external protein coat. (Courtesy J. Nakano, PhD, CDC/PHIL.)*

Roseola Vaccinia

Vaccinia Necrosum

(Left) *This photograph of a young child following smallpox vaccination in the right shoulder shows an erythematous halo* ⇒ *surrounding the vaccination site. This child was subsequently diagnosed with roseola vaccinia. (Courtesy CDC/PHIL.)* **(Right)** *This photograph depicts the skin destruction, or vaccinia necrosum, on the upper left arm of a patient at the site of his smallpox vaccination. (Courtesy, R. Duma, MD, CDC/PHIL.)*

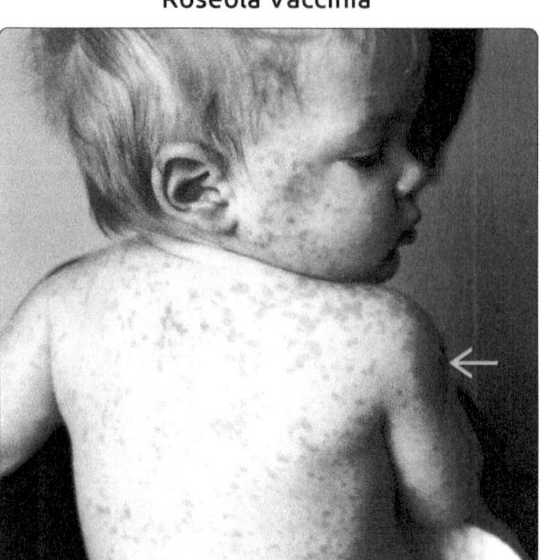

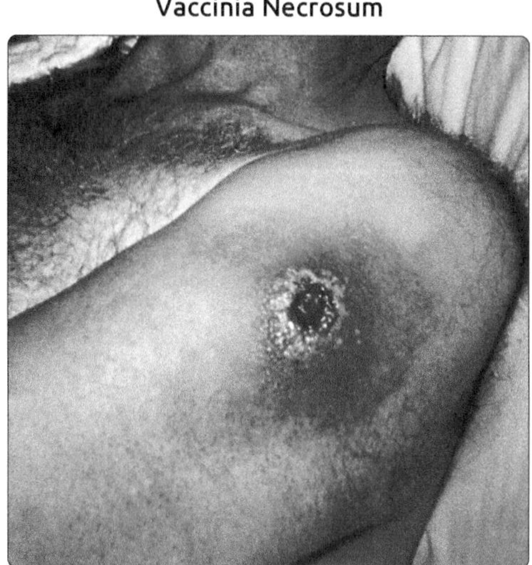

Eczema Vaccinatum

Eczema Vaccinatum Histology

(Left) *This photograph depicts the nape of a woman's neck, which displayed manifestations of a postsmallpox vaccination reaction known as eczema vaccinatum. This person had a known history of eczema. (Courtesy CDC/PHIL.)* **(Right)** *This skin section is from a patient with eczema vaccinatum lesion, manifesting after smallpox vaccination. (Courtesy J. Neff, MD, CDC/PHIL.)*

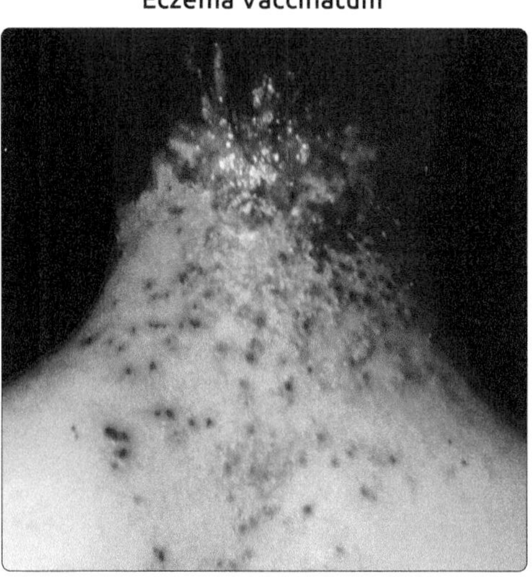

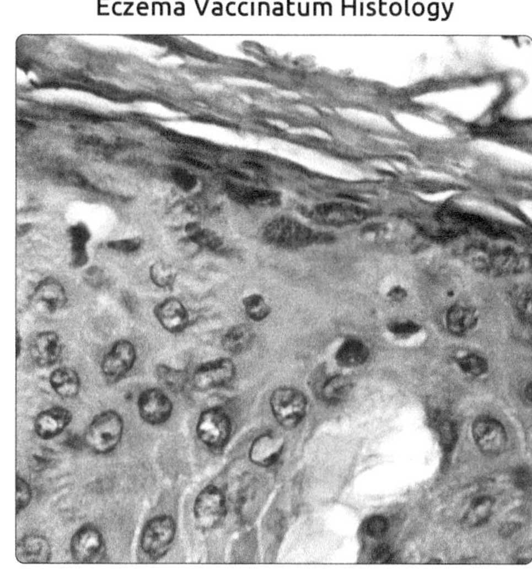

Monkeypox Histology

Monkeypox: Guarnieri Bodies

(Left) *At scanning magnification, reticular degeneration and epidermal necrosis with abundant karyorrhectic debris is noted in intact, fully developed vesicles.* **(Right)** *Biopsy of monkeypox skin lesions contains occasional Guarnieri bodies (type B viral inclusions), cytoplasmic eosinophilic blobs* ⇒*, in virus-infected epithelial cells.*

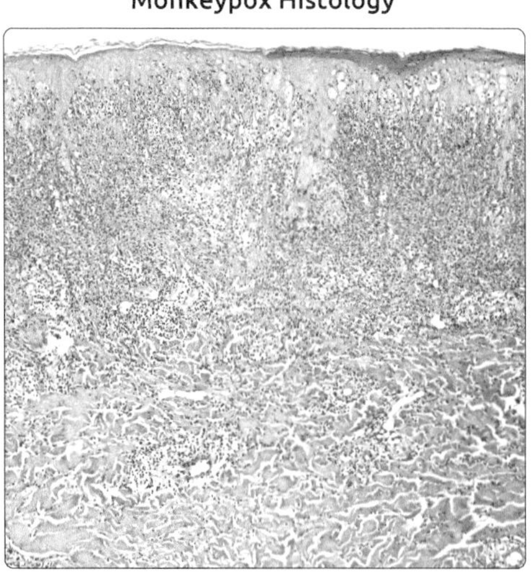

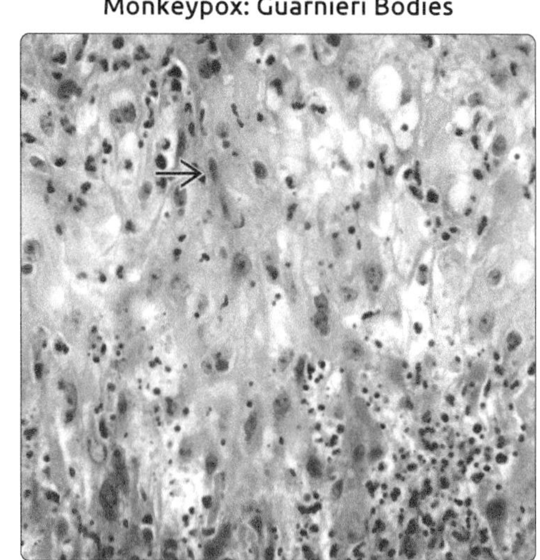

Monkeypox Immunohistochemistry

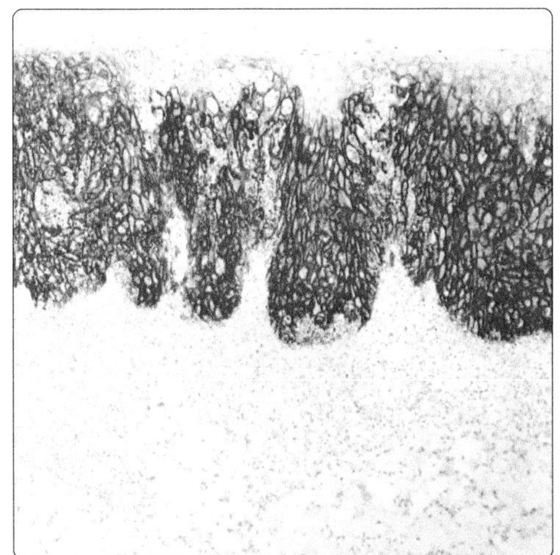

Monkeypox: Lymphadenopathy

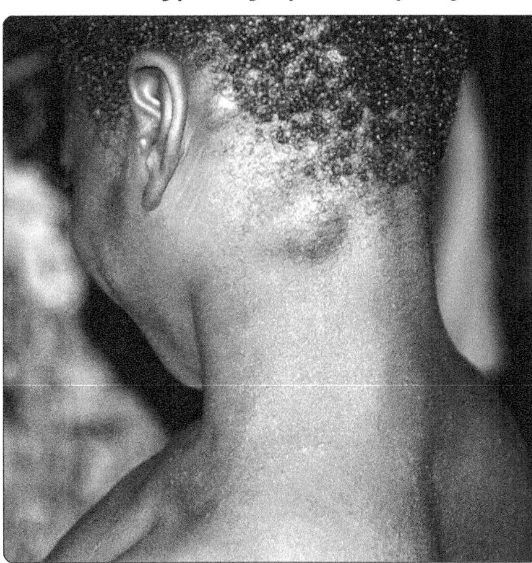

(Left) *Immunoperoxidase highlights abundant antigen within infected cells and is useful for rapid detection of Monkeypox in tissue sections.* **(Right)** *Prominent lymphadenopathy, shown here by cervical swelling, is a finding associated with monkeypox. (Courtesy B. Mahy, PhD, CDC/PHIL.)*

Monkeypox: Pox Mark Scars

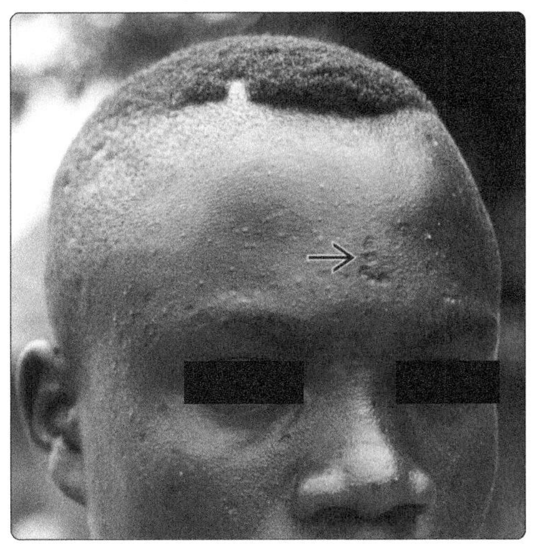

Orf Virus Lesions

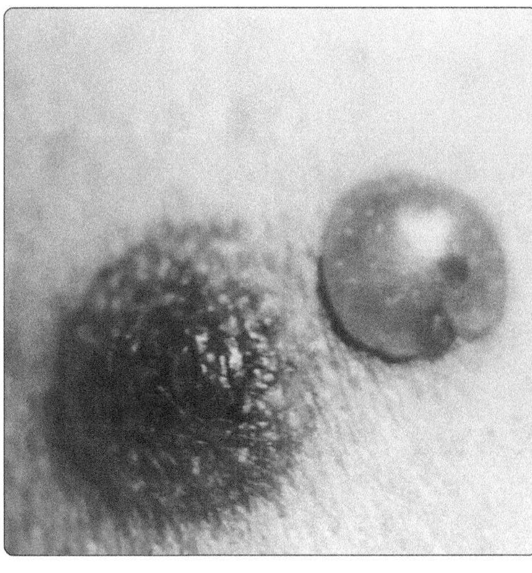

(Left) *Pox mark scars ➡ are shown on the face of a young man who recovered from a case of monkeypox. (Courtesy B. Mahy, PhD, CDC/PHIL.)* **(Right)** *This photograph from a patient with Orf virus infection shows a crust-type lesion on the left and a a fluid-filled, raised vesicular-type lesion on the right. (Courtesy J. Nakano, PhD, CDC/PHIL.)*

Ecthyma Contagiosum (Orf)

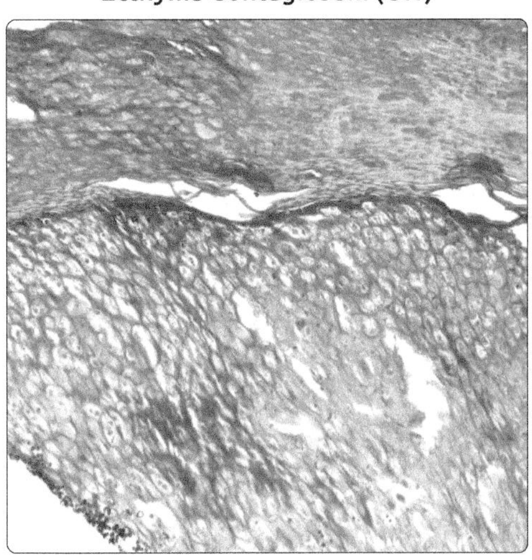

Ecthyma Contagiosum (Orf)

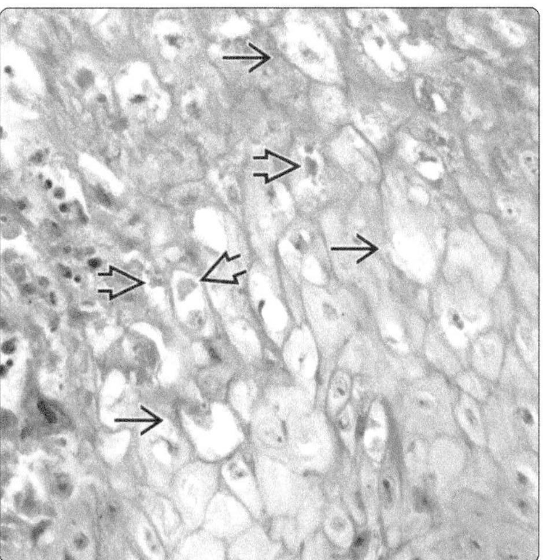

(Left) *Acral skin with diffuse necrosis that has an ischemic appearance at scanning magnification is shown in a finger biopsy from a patient with orf.* **(Right)** *Eosinophilic intracytoplasmic inclusions ➡ and ballooning degeneration ➡ of keratinocytes are shown in a biopsy from a patient with parapoxvirus infection.*

TERMINOLOGY

Definitions

- Arbovirus: Derived from "arthropod-borne virus"

ETIOLOGY/PATHOGENESIS

Infectious Disease

- Viral infections transmitted by arthropod vectors, such as mosquitos and ticks
- > 250 arboviruses; at least 80 cause human disease (e.g., hemorrhagic fever, encephalitis)
- Reservoir includes birds and mammals
- Majority not transmissible by humans due to low viremia (exceptions: Dengue fever, yellow fever, chikungunya disease)
- Onset 3-15 days after bite from infected mosquito or tick
- Symptomatic disease
  - New, nonimmune hosts encounters virus
  - Direct viral or host immune response leads to damage
  - Immunosuppressed patients may develop severe/fatal disease (e.g., rituximab maintenance therapy)

VIRUSES

Bunyavirales Order

- Named for Bunyamwera, village where virus first detected
- Viral features
  - Enveloped, single-stranded RNA viruses
  - 80-120 nm, pleomorphic, distinct surface projections, helical nucleocapsid
  - 10,500-22,700 nucleotide genomes
- *Peribunyaviridae* family
  - Batai virus (BATV): Europe and Asia
  - Bunyamwera virus (BUNV): Africa
  - Bwamba virus (BWAV): Africa
  - Cache Valley virus (CVV): North America
  - California encephalitis virus (CEV): North America
  - Jamestown Canyon virus (JCV): 276 cases reported in USA from 2013-2022
  - Keystone virus (KEYV): North America
  - La Crosse virus (LACV): 609 cases reported in USA from 2013-2022
  - Oropouche virus (OROV): Central and South America
  - Tahyna virus (TAHV): Europe, Asia, Africa
  - Tete virus (TETEV): Africa
- *Phenuiviridae* family
  - Bhanja virus (BHAV): Asia, Europe, and Africa
  - Heartland virus (HRTV): 60 cases reported in USA from 2009-2022
  - Severe fever with thrombocytopenia syndrome virus (SFTSV) : Asia
  - Alenquer virus (ALEV): South America
  - Adria virus (ADRV): Europe
  - Candiru virus (CDUV): Central and South America
  - Punta Toro virus (PTV): South America
  - Rift Valley fever virus (RVFV): Africa and Middle East
  - Sandfly fever Naples virus (SFNV): Europe and Asia
  - Sandfly fever Sicilian virus (SFSV): Europe and Asia
  - Toscana virus (TOSV): Europe
- *Nairoviridae* family
  - Crimean-Congo hemorrhagic fever virus (CCHFV): Africa, Asia, Europe
  - Dugbe virus (DUGV): Africa
  - Kasokero virus (KASV): Africa
  - Nairobi sheep disease virus (NSDV): Africa, Asia

Flaviviridae Family

- Derived from "flavus" (yellow); 1st virus identified
- Viral features
  - Enveloped, single-stranded RNA viruses
  - 40-60 nm, spherical, small surface projections, icosahedral nucleocapsid
  - 9,600-12,300 nucleotide genomes
- Family members
  - Dengue virus 1-4 (DENV-1-4); > 300 million cases worldwide annually
  - Japanese encephalitis virus (JEV): ~ 70,000 cases annually in Asia
  - Kyasanur forest disease virus (KFDV): India

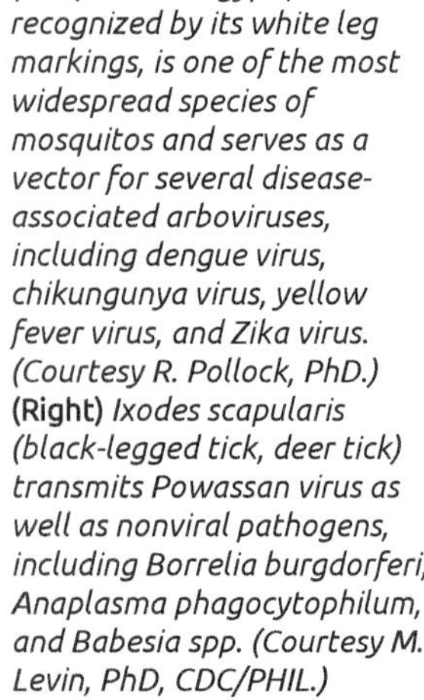

(Left) *Aedes aegypti, recognized by its white leg markings, is one of the most widespread species of mosquitos and serves as a vector for several disease-associated arboviruses, including dengue virus, chikungunya virus, yellow fever virus, and Zika virus. (Courtesy R. Pollock, PhD.)* **(Right)** *Ixodes scapularis (black-legged tick, deer tick) transmits Powassan virus as well as nonviral pathogens, including Borrelia burgdorferi, Anaplasma phagocytophilum, and Babesia spp. (Courtesy M. Levin, PhD, CDC/PHIL.)*

Aedes aegypti

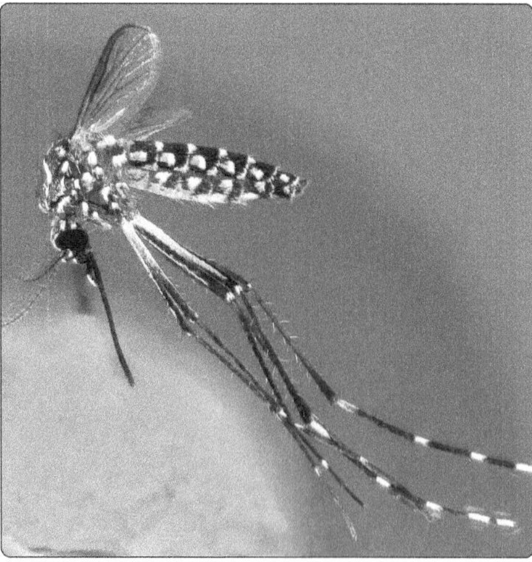

Ixodes scapularis

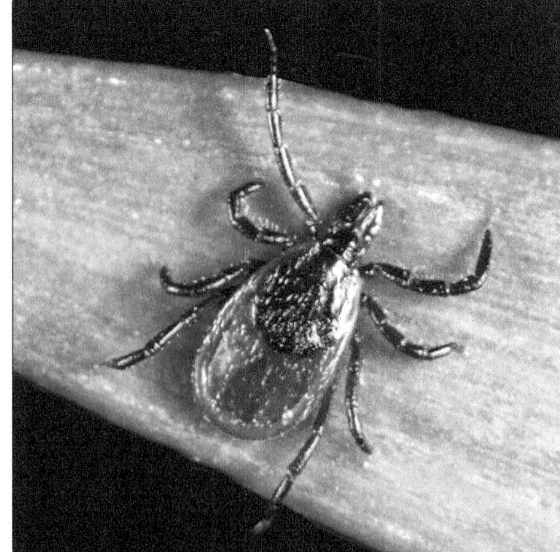

- Murray Valley encephalitis virus (MVEV): Australia, New Guinea
- Omsk hemorrhagic fever virus (OHFV): Russia
- Powassan virus (POWV): 239 cases reported in USA from 2013-2022
- Saint Louis encephalitis virus (SLEV): 143 cases reported in USA from 2013-2022
- Tick-borne encephalitis virus (TBEV): Europe, Russia
- Usutu virus (USUV): Africa, Europe
- West Nile virus (WNV): 19,481 cases (1,224 deaths) reported in USA from 2013-2022
- Yellow fever virus (YFVV): Central and South America, Africa
- Zika virus (ZIKV): 2015-2016 pandemic affecting > 90 countries/territories

Reovirales Order

- Derived from "respiratory enteric orphan" viruses
- Viral features
  - Nonenveloped, double-strand RNA viruses
  - 60-70 nm, wheel-shaped, icosahedral nucleocapsid
  - 18,200-30,500 nucleotide genomes
- *Sedoreoviridae* members
  - Banna virus (BAV): Asia
  - Great Island virus (GIV): Europe, Asia
- *Spinareoviridae* members
  - Colorado tick fever virus (CTFV): 59 cases reported in USA from 2010-2019
  - Eyach virus (EYAV): Europe

Togaviridae Family

- Derived from "toga" (garment covering), describing viral envelope
- Viral features
  - Enveloped, single-stranded RNA viruses
  - 60-70 nm, spherical/pleomorphic, distinct surface projections, icosahedral capsid
  - 10,000-12,000 nucleotide genomes
- Family members
  - Barmah Forest virus (BFV): Australia
  - Chikungunya virus (CHIKV): Worldwide (rare in USA)
  - Eastern equine encephalitis virus (EEEV): 97 cases reported in USA from 2013-2022
  - Mayaro virus (MAYV): South America
  - O'nyong'nyong virus (ONNV): Africa
  - Ross River virus (RRV): Australia and Pacific islands
  - Semliki Forest virus (SFV): Africa
  - Sindbis virus (SINV): Africa, Middle East, Australia
  - Venezuelan equine encephalitis virus (VEEV): South and North America
  - Western equine encephalitis virus (WEEV): North America

VECTORS

Mosquitos

- *Aedes*: Derived from "unpleasant"
  - Distinctive black and white markings on body/legs
  - > 700 spp., including *Aedes aegypti*, *Aedes albopictus*, *Aedes vexans*, *Aedes triseriatus*
  - Transmit: DENV, YFV, WNV, CHIKV, EEEV
- *Culex*: Latin term for "midge" or "gnat"
  - Drab monocolor mosquitoes
  - > 1,200 spp., including *Culex tritaeniorhynchus*, *Culex quinquefasciatus*, *Culex pipiens*
  - Transmit: WNV, JEV, SLEV, WEEV
- *Coquillettidia*
  - Large, yellowish mosquitos
  - 57 spp., including *Coquillettidia perturbans*
  - Transmit: WNV, EEEV

Ticks

- *Amblyomma americanum* (lone star tick)
  - Transmit: Heartland virus
- *Dermacentor andersoni* (Rocky Mountain wood tick)
  - Transmit: Colorado tick fever virus
- *Ixodes scapularis* (black-legged tick; deer tick), *Ixodes ricinus*, *Ixodes persulcatus*, *Ixodes cookei*
  - Transmit: TBEV, POWV

CLINICAL ISSUES

Presentation

- More common in warmer months when mosquitos and ticks are active
- Most infections are asymptomatic
- Mild cases with slight fever, headache, and body aches
- Severe infections with rapid onset, headache, high fever, disorientation, tremors, convulsions, paralysis, coma, or death
- Distinguishing features
  - Lymphadenopathy, rash: DENV, WNV
  - Arthralgia, rash: CHIKV, MAYV, RRV, BFV, SINV
  - Hemorrhagic signs: YFV, DENV, KFDV, OHFV, CHFV, DABV
  - Fever and CNS involvement: EEEV, WEEV, WNV, SLEV, VEEV, LACV, JEV, POWV, MVEV, KFDV, TBEV

Laboratory Tests

- EEG: Abnormalities (60-90% of cases)
- CSF: Pleocytosis
- CBC: Thrombocytopenia (DENV, DABV, HRTV)
- Virus-specific IgM, IgG and neutralizing antibodies (serum, CSF); may be negative in setting of B cell depletion (e.g., rituximab treatment)
- RT-PCR, metagenomic next-generation sequencing (mNGS) (serum, CSF, brain tissue)
- Virus culture

Treatment

- Primary prevention involves avoidance of mosquitos and ticks; minimization of exposed skin; use of insect repellents
- FDA-approved vaccines
  - DENV: CYD-TDV (Dengvaxia) live attenuated tetravalent chimeric vaccine for children with prior infection living in endemic areas; 3 doses over 6 months
  - JEV: Inactivated Vero cell culture-derived Japanese encephalitis vaccine (IXIARO): 2 doses (28 days apart)
  - TBEV: Inactivate virus (Ticovac); 3 doses over 12 months
  - YFV: 17D yellow fever vaccine (YF-Vax): 1 dose
  - Other vaccines (e.g., CHIKV, WNV, ZIKV) are in development
- Predominantly supportive care for symptomatic infections

- Intravenous immunoglobulin (IVIg) or steroids may provide some benefit
- Ribavirin for some hemorrhagic fever viruses (RVFV, CHFV)

Prognosis

- Full recovery in most cases; permanent neurologic symptoms and fatality in up to 20-30% of severe cases

IMAGING FINDINGS

MR

- Brain: T2 FLAIR hyperintensity (thalamus, basal ganglia, brainstem) and leptomeningeal contrast enhancement

MACROSCOPIC

Brain

- Features range from near normal to severe edema, hyperemia, and herniation
- No purulent material in meninges

MICROSCOPIC

Histologic Features

- Brain
  - Predominantly lymphocytic meningeal and perivascular inflammatory infiltrates (neutrophilic predominance may be seen with some viruses &/or early)
  - Liquefactive parenchymal necrosis
  - Microglial nodules: Clusters of activated microglial cells
  - Neuronophagia: Dying neuron within microglial nodule
  - Affects gray matter more than white matter
- Liver (DENV, YF)
  - Hepatic necrosis (without viral cytopathic effect)

Cytologic Features

- No characteristic nuclear inclusions

ANCILLARY TESTS

Immunohistochemistry

- CD68 highlights microglial clusters
- Virus-specific antibodies may be available commercially or at reference laboratories

In Situ Hybridization

- Viral specific probes may be available commercially or at reference laboratories

Molecular Testing

- Targeted RT-PCR ± sequencing
- mNGS: Nontargeted; can detect novel viruses

DIFFERENTIAL DIAGNOSIS

Other Viral Causes of Encephalitis

- Herpes simplex virus 1, herpes simplex virus 2, varicella-zoster virus, Epstein-Barr virus, cytomegalovirus, rabies virus, measles virus, JC polyomavirus, adenovirus
  - Characteristic nuclear inclusions or detection of virus by IHC with commercially available antibodies

Nonviral Causes of Encephalitis

- *Neisseria meningitidis*, *Borrelia* spp., *Treponema pallidum*, *Leptospira* spp., *Mycoplasma* spp., *Rickettsia rickettsii*, *Mycobacterium tuberculosis*, *Candida* spp., *Mucor* spp., *Cryptococcus neoformans*, *Toxoplasma gondii*, *Naegleria fowleri*, etc.
  - Organisms observed on H&E, Gram, AFB, MSS, or PAS-D stains
  - Neutrophilic or eosinophilic predominant infiltrates; granulomatous inflammation
- Autoimmune &/or immune-mediated encephalitides
  - Correlate with CSF/serum antibodies

Gliomas

- Infiltrating edge may appear modestly hypercellular with elongated tumor cell nuclei appearing microglial-cell-like; prominent perivascular lymphocytic cuffing can be present
- Increased cellularity, absence of microglial clusters, and cytologic atypia with hyperchromasia of tumor nuclei

KEY POINTS

Etiology

- Viral infections transmitted by arthropod vectors, such as mosquitos and ticks

Clinical Issues

- Incidence: Varies widely with virus and location
- Most infections are asymptomatic or are associated with slight fever, headache, and body aches
- Severe infections present with rapid onset, headache, high fever, and can progress to paralysis, coma, or death
- Laboratory tests: Serology, RT-PCR, mNGS, viral culture
- Treatment: Avoidance of mosquito and tick bites; vaccination (Japanese encephalitis, yellow fever); supportive therapy

Microscopic Pathology

- Predominantly lymphocytic meningeal and perivascular inflammatory infiltrates
- Microglial nodules and neuronophagia
- Identify specific virus by RT-PCR, IHC, ISH, viral culture, or serology

SELECTED REFERENCES

1. Bartholomeeusen K et al: Chikungunya fever. Nat Rev Dis Primers. 9(1):17, 2023
2. Hale GL: Flaviviruses and the traveler: around the world and to your stage. a review of West Nile, yellow fever, dengue, and Zika viruses for the practicing pathologist. Mod Pathol. 36(6):100188, 2023
3. Kapadia RK et al: Severe arboviral neuroinvasive disease in patients on rituximab therapy: a review. Clin Infect Dis. 76(6):1142-8, 2023
4. Bailey AL et al: Hepatopathology of flaviviruses. J Hepatol. 77(6):1711-3, 2022
5. Piantadosi A et al: Powassan virus encephalitis. Infect Dis Clin North Am. 36(3):671-88, 2022
6. Staples JE et al: Investigation of heartland virus disease throughout the United States, 2013-2017. Open Forum Infect Dis. 7(5):ofaa125, 2020
7. Wilson MR et al: Clinical metagenomic sequencing for diagnosis of meningitis and encephalitis. N Engl J Med. 380(24):2327-40, 2019
8. Turtle L et al: Japanese encephalitis - the prospects for new treatments. Nat Rev Neurol. 14(5):298-313, 2018
9. Kleinschmidt-DeMasters BK et al: West Nile virus encephalitis 16 years later. Brain Pathol. 25(5):625-33, 2015

West Nile Virus

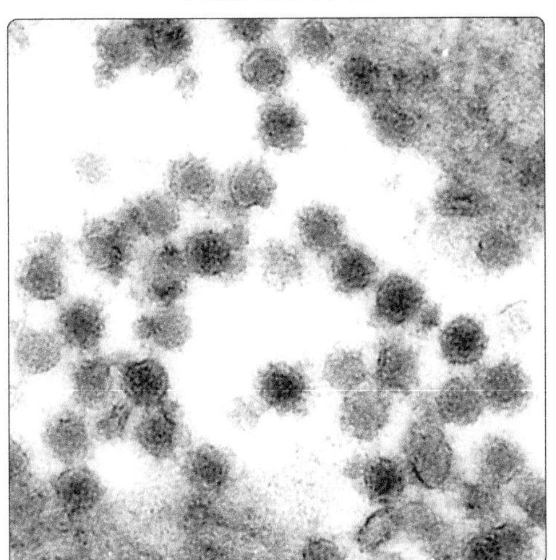

Saint Louis Encephalitis Virus

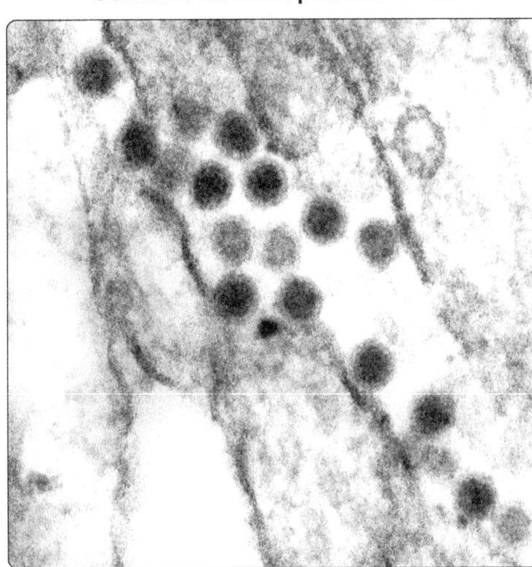

(Left) *Transmission electron micrograph of West Nile virus shows numerous spherical, enveloped particles, ~ 50 nm in diameter with small surface projections, features characteristic of flaviviruses. (Courtesy C. Goldsmith, MGS, CDC/PHIL.)* **(Right)** *Transmission electron micrograph of Saint Louis encephalitis virus shows several spherical, enveloped particles ~ 50 nm in diameter, features characteristic of flaviviruses. (Courtesy F. Murphy, DVM, PhD, CDC/PHIL.)*

Chikungunya Virus

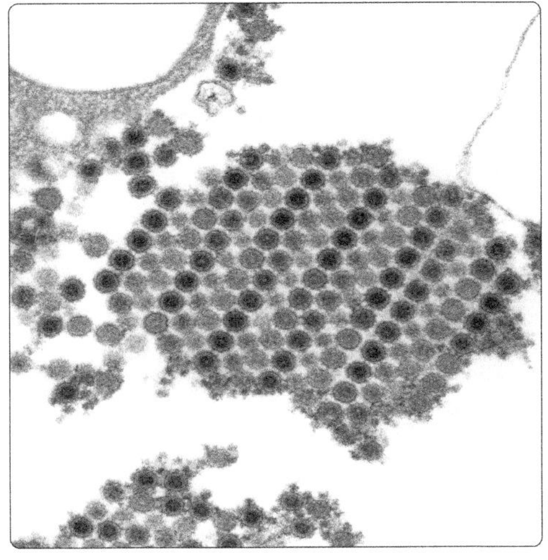

Eastern Equine Encephalitis Virus

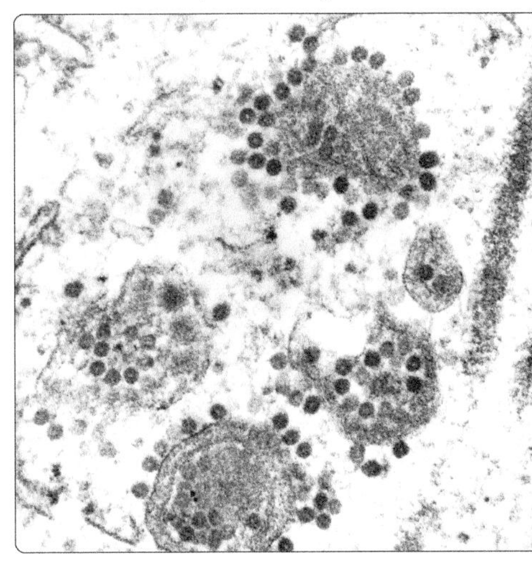

(Left) *Transmission electron micrograph of Chikungunya virus shows numerous spherical, enveloped particles measuring ~ 50 nm in diameter, features characteristic of togaviruses. (Courtesy C. Goldsmith, MGS, CDC/PHIL.)* **(Right)** *Transmission electron micrograph of eastern equine encephalitis virus shows numerous spherical, enveloped particles measuring ~ 50 nm in diameter, features characteristic of togaviruses. (Courtesy F. Murphy, DVM, PhD, CDC/PHIL.)*

Colorado Tick Fever Virus

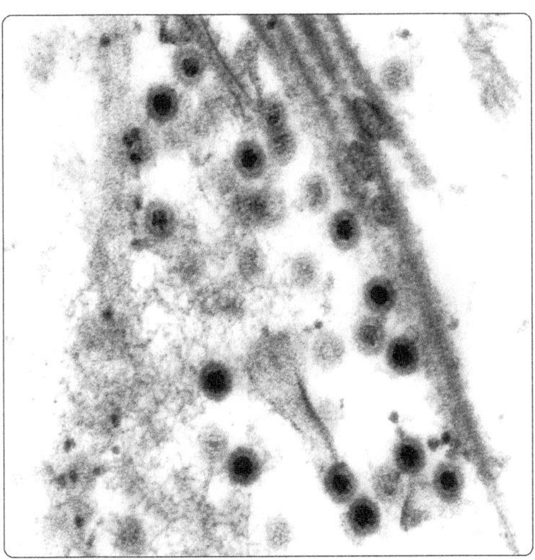

California Encephalitis Virus

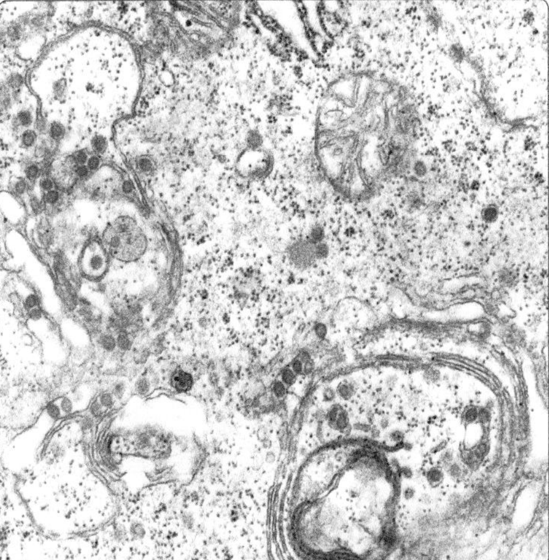

(Left) *Transmission electron micrograph of Colorado tick fever virus shows several spherical, nonenveloped, wheel-shaped particles measuring ~ 80 nm in diameter, features characteristic of rheoviruses. (Courtesy CDC/PHIL.)* **(Right)** *Transmission electron micrograph of California encephalitis virus shows several pleomorphic, enveloped particles measuring 80-100 nm in diameter, features characteristic of Bunyavirales order viruses. (Courtesy F. Murphy, DVM, PhD, CDC/PHIL.)*

(Left) *MR from a patient with eastern equine encephalitis shows T2/FLAIR hyperintensities of the thalamus, basal ganglia, and brainstem (not shown).* (Right) *MR from a patient with Powassan encephalitis shows marked edema of the cerebellum as well as leptomeningeal contrast enhancement.*

Eastern Equine Encephalitis: MR

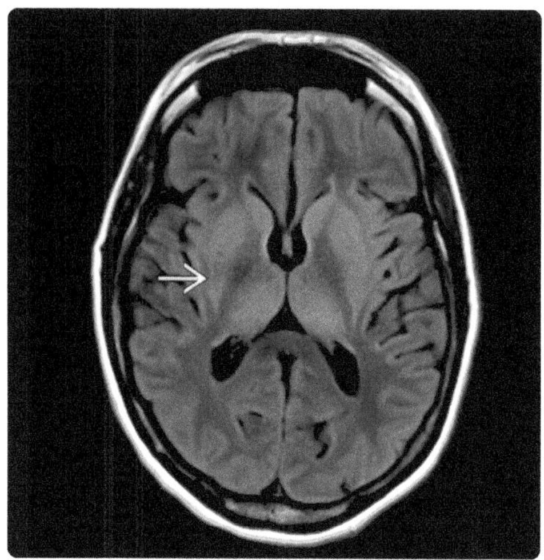

Powassan Encephalitis: MR

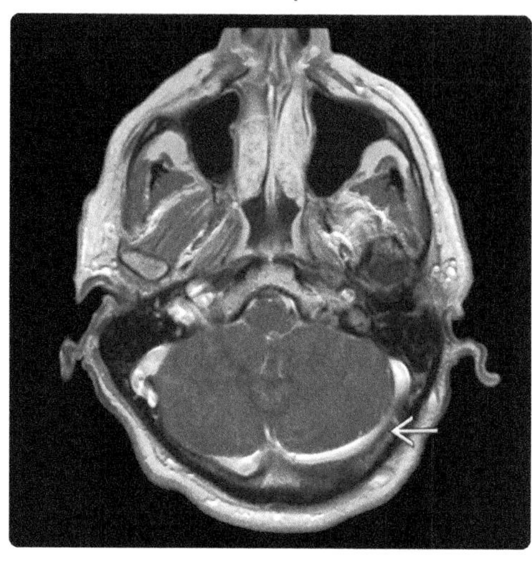

(Left) *Cerebellar biopsy from a patient with Powassan encephalitis shows marked loss of Purkinje neurons with Bergmann gliosis.* (Right) *Section of the cerebellum from a patient with Powassan encephalitis shows immunoreactivity for POWV antigen (red) in the remaining Purkinje cells and processes present in the molecular layer. (Courtesy S. Zaki, MD, PhD.)*

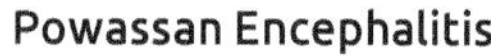

Powassan Encephalitis

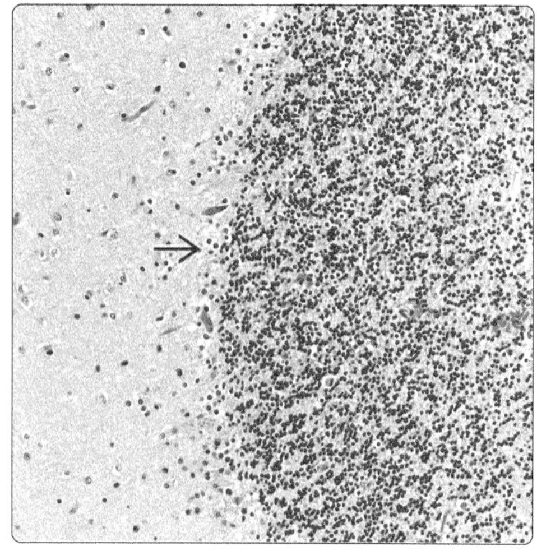

Powassan Virus: IHC

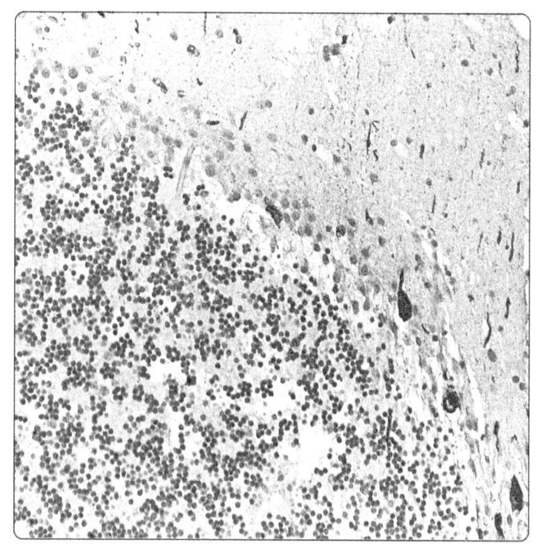

(Left) *Section of cerebral cortex from a patient with fatal eastern equine encephalitis shows a focus of liquefactive necrosis.* (Right) *Section of cerebral cortex from a fatal case of eastern equine encephalitis shows immunoreactivity for EEEV antigen (brown) in scattered cortical neurons.*

Eastern Equine Encephalitis

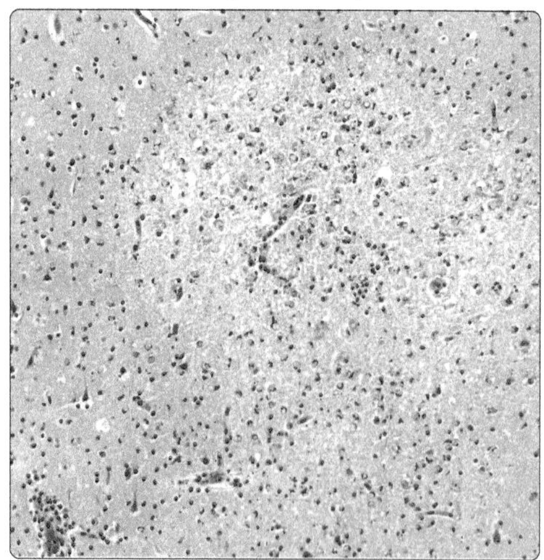

Eastern Equine Encephalitis Virus: IHC

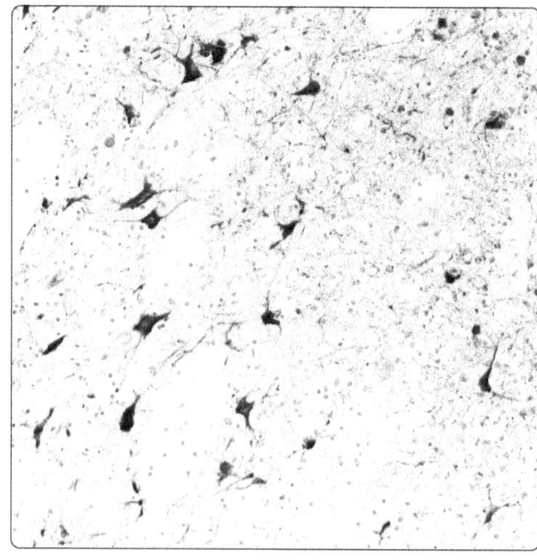

Jamestown Canyon Encephalitis

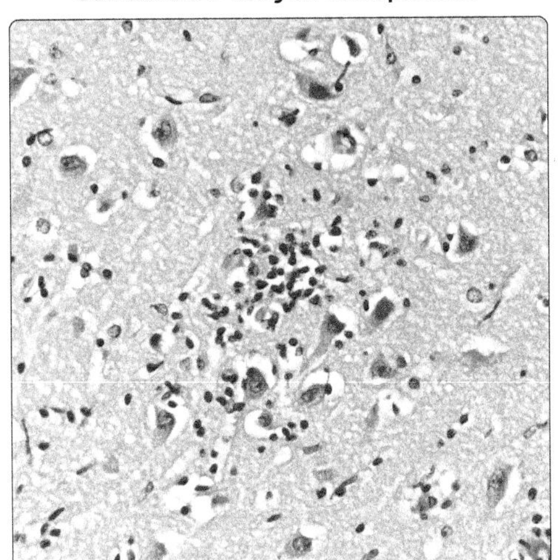

Jamestown Canyon Virus: ISH

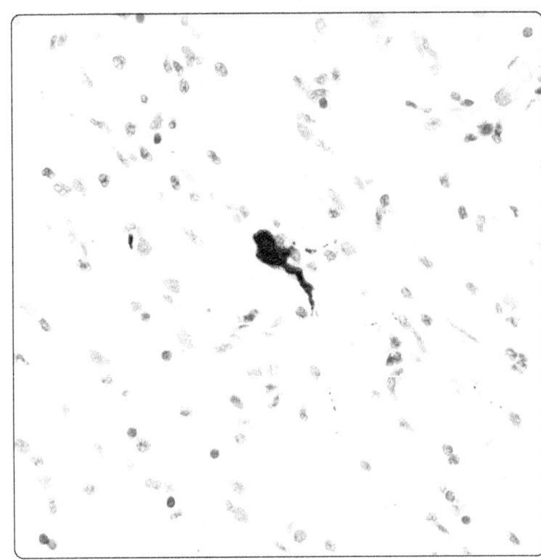

(Left) *Temporal lobe section from a patient with fatal Jamestown Canyon encephalitis shows a microglial nodule and neuronophagia.* **(Right)** *Section of the cerebral cortex from a rare fatal case of Jamestown canyon virus encephalitis shows stain for JCV RNA in situ hybridization (brown) in scattered cortical neurons.*

West Nile Encephalitis

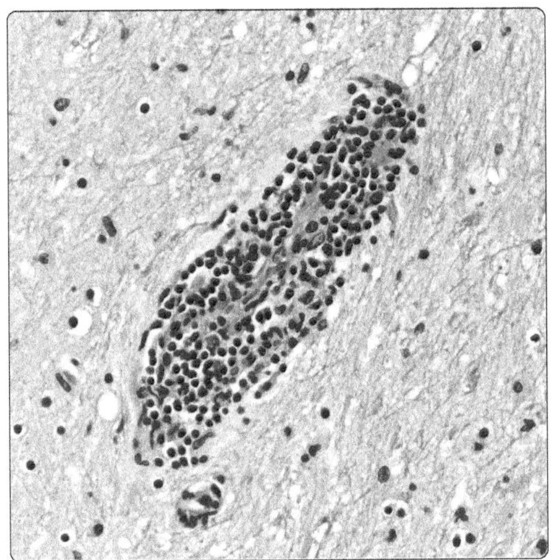

West Nile Virus: IHC

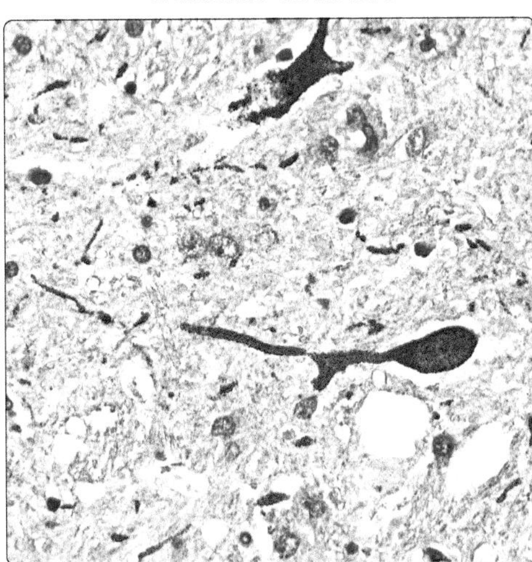

(Left) *Section from a fatal case of West Nile encephalitis shows a parenchymal blood vessel with perivascular chronic inflammation, consisting predominantly of lymphocytes.* **(Right)** *Section of an autopsied brain shows scattered neurons and processes positive for West Nile virus antigen (red). (Courtesy W. J. Shieh, MD, PhD and S. Zaki, MD, PhD, CDC/PHIL.)*

Japanese Encephalitis

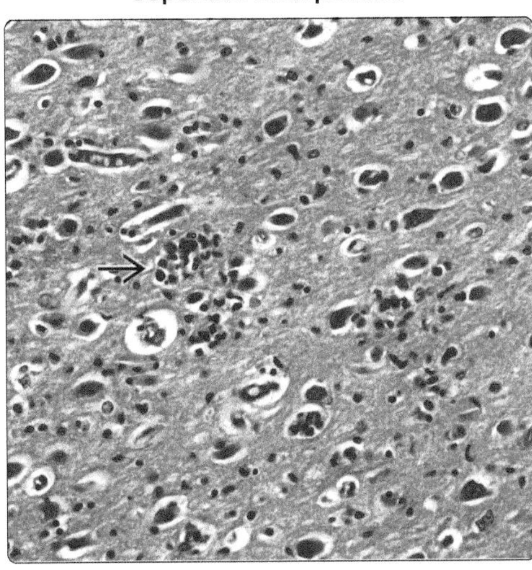

Japanese Encephalitis

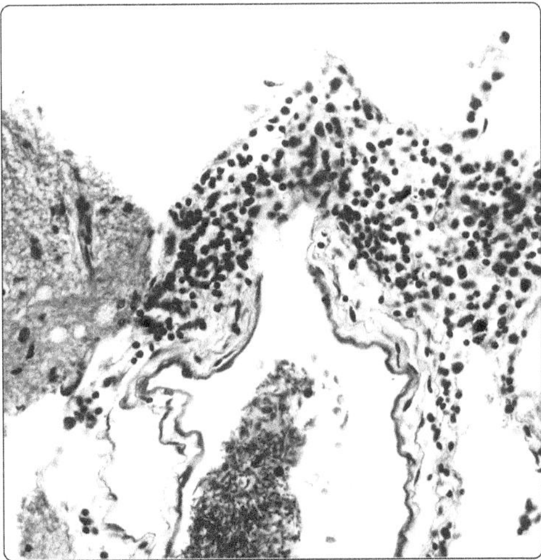

(Left) *Section from a fatal case of Japanese encephalitis shows a microglial nodule and neuronophagia involving the hippocampus* ➙. **(Right)** *Section from a fatal case of Japanese encephalitis shows leptomeningeal chronic inflammation composed predominantly of lymphocytes.*

Zika Virus Infection

KEY FACTS

ETIOLOGY/PATHOGENESIS

- Viral infection primarily transmitted by *Aedes* species mosquitos that can also be spread in utero or through sexual contact

CLINICAL ISSUES

- Most infections are asymptomatic (80%) or self-limited; hospitalization or death rare
- Mild symptoms include acute onset of fever, maculopapular rash, arthralgia, conjunctivitis
- Associated with microcephaly; loss of neuroprogenitor cells
- Laboratory testing: RT-PCR, serology
- Vaccines under development; treatment is supportive

IMAGING

- Ultrasound (in utero; late 2nd/early 3rd trimester): Microcephaly, calcifications, ventriculomegaly, cerebellar hypoplasia

MACROSCOPIC

- Microcephaly, micrencephaly, agyria, calcifications, lateral ventricle dilation, brainstem hypoplasia

MICROSCOPIC

- Fetal/neonatal brain: Dystrophic calcifications, microglial nodules, gliosis, cell degeneration and necrosis

ANCILLARY TESTS

- IHC (anti-ZIKV antibodies), RT-PCR, EM

TOP DIFFERENTIAL DIAGNOSES

- Viral infections with fever, rash, joint pain: Dengue and chikungunya (geographic overlap)
- Infectious causes of microcephaly: In utero exposure to toxoplasmosis, cytomegalovirus, varicella-zoster virus, rubella
- Noninfectious causes of microcephaly: Craniosynostosis, chromosomal abnormalities, fetal cerebral anoxia, severe malnutrition, exposure to drug, alcohol, or toxins in utero

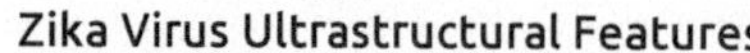

Zika Virus Ultrastructural Features

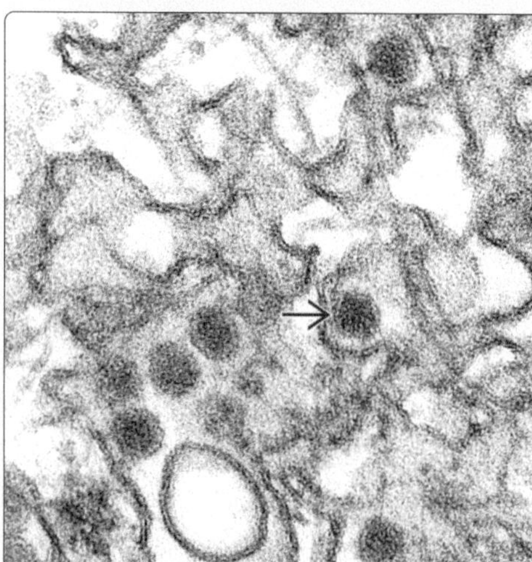

Aedes aegypti Mosquito

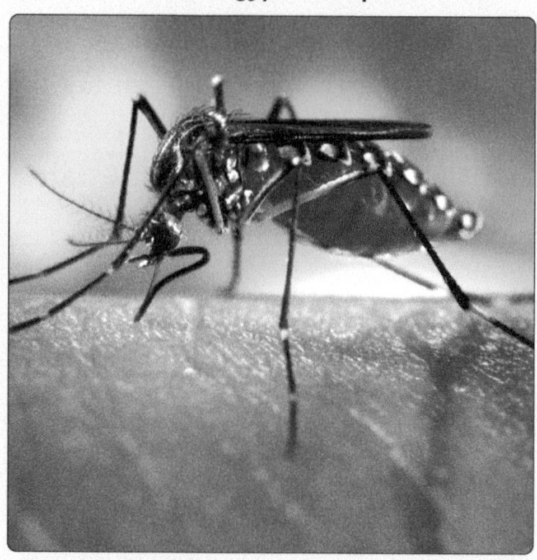

(Left) *This transmission electron micrograph shows scattered spherical, enveloped, viral particles ⇨ measuring 40-50 nm in diameter, features characteristic of Zika virus particles. (Courtesy C. Goldsmith, MGS.)* **(Right)** *This photograph depicts a female Aedes aegypti mosquito in the process of acquiring a blood meal. In addition to carrying Zika virus, A. aegypti serves as a vector for many other viruses, including dengue, chikungunya, and yellow fever. (Courtesy F. Collins, PhD.)*

Zika Virus Rash

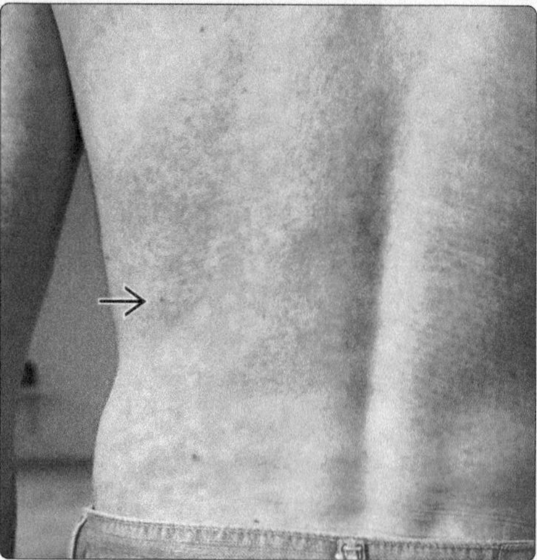

Zika Virus Microcephaly

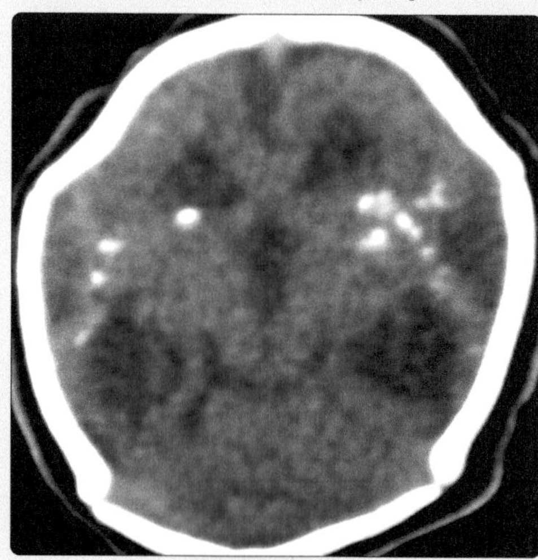

(Left) *Zika virus infections are typically asymptomatic but may include mild symptoms, including a blotchy rash ⇨, fever, joint pain, conjunctivitis, muscle pain, and headache. (Courtesy CDC/PHIL.)* **(Right)** *Axial NECT from an infant with in utero Zika virus infection shows periventricular and subcortical calcification with marked volume loss resulting in microcephaly (despite the presence of ventriculomegaly). (From DI: Pediatrics.)*

TERMINOLOGY

Definitions

- *Orthoflavivirus zikaense*; Zika virus (ZIKV) named for Zika Forest, Uganda where virus was first isolated (1947)
- *Flaviviridae* family: Derived from "flavus" (yellow)

ETIOLOGY/PATHOGENESIS

Infectious Agents

- Viral infection primarily transmitted by *Aedes* mosquitos (e.g., *Aedes aegypti* and *Aedes albopictus*); perinatal, in utero, sexual, and transfusion transmission events reported
- Infects keratinocytes and dendritic cells at inoculation site, then spreads via lymphatics and blood stream and crosses placenta to fetal circulation
- Virus RNA detected in semen, saliva, urine, breast milk, and donated whole blood
- Nonhuman primates most likely reservoir
- Incubation period is 3-7 days; symptoms last 4-7 days
- Virus remains in blood for ~ 7 days; unknown but longer time in semen and urine
- Associated with microcephaly; fetal loss due to direct fetal infection and neurotropism of virus; neuroprogenitor cells preferred target for ZIKV (possibly through AXL receptor), leading to apoptosis

CLINICAL ISSUES

Epidemiology

- 1st outbreak of ZIKV in Yap Island, Micronesia (2007); 49 confirmed cases; estimated 73% of population infected
- French Polynesian outbreak (2013-2014) spread to other Pacific Islands; 383 confirmed and 8,750 suspected cases; estimated 11% of population
- Worldwide outbreak starting in Brazil in May 2015 and spreading to > 90 countries/territories (> 1.5 million suspected or confirmed cases)
- USA: 5,790 symptomatic cases reported (2015-2021)
  - 231 locally acquired mosquito-borne cases (220 in Florida and 11 in Texas)
  - No local mosquito-borne ZIKV transmission reported in continental USA since 2018

Site

- Skin, eye, fetal/placental tissue

Presentation

- Most infections (80%) are asymptomatic
- Typically mild symptoms include acute onset of fever, maculopapular rash, arthralgia, nonpurulent conjunctivitis, myalgia, headache
- Neurologic complications may include Guillain-Barre syndrome, transverse myelitis, meningoencephalitis, sensory neuropathy, cerebrovascular complications, retinitis, and optic neuritis
- Congenital Zika syndrome (1st-trimester infections) includes microcephaly, ocular findings, contractures, and hypertonia

Laboratory Tests

- Recommended for specific groups
  - Symptomatic individuals
  - Pregnant women with exposure risk or suspicious prenatal ultrasound findings
  - Infants with maternal risk factors or suspicious clinical findings
- RT-PCR (single or multiplex with dengue and chikungunya viruses)
  - Serum, urine (< 14 days from onset of symptoms)
  - Amniotic fluid, placental tissue (if available)
  - Metagenomic sequencing under investigation as broad spectrum alternative
- Serology (IgM ELISA) (≥ 4 days after symptom onset)
  - Frequent cross reactivity with other flaviviruses (e.g., dengue)
  - Results confirmed by plaque-reduction neutralization testing (PRNT)
  - IgM antibodies can persist for months to years following infection

Treatment

- Primary prevention
  - No FDA-approved vaccines currently available
  - Multiple vaccine trials underway, including DNA vaccines, mRNA vaccines, purified inactivated virus vaccines, and viral vector-based vaccines
  - Avoid mosquitos in areas with active virus transmission
  - Avoid unprotected sex with infected partners if pregnant
- Presentation with symptoms
  - Supportive therapy only: Rest, fluids, acetaminophen
  - Avoid NSAIDs until dengue, chikungunya ruled out (bleeding risk)

Prognosis

- Typically self-limited; hospitalization uncommon and fatality rare
- Associated with Guillain-Barré syndrome
- Limited follow-up from microcephaly cases; neurologic symptoms likely permanent
- Men recommended to wait 3 months and women 2 months from last ZIKV exposure prior to attempting conception

IMAGING

Ultrasonographic Findings

- In utero (late 2nd/early 3rd trimester): Microcephaly, calcifications, ventriculomegaly, cerebellar hypoplasia

MICROBIOLOGY

Virus Features

- Enveloped, single-stranded RNA virus
- 40- to 50-nm diameter, icosahedral nucleocapsid
- ~ 10,800 nucleotide genome (polyprotein processed into capsid, precursor of membrane, envelope, and nonstructural proteins NS1, NS2A, NS2B, NS3 protease, NS4A, NS4B, and NS5 polymerase)
- Brazil 2015 outbreak most closely related to French Polynesian strains ("Asian lineage")

Culture

- Virus replicated in several cell lines, including Vero; cytopathic effects after 2-3 days

MACROSCOPIC

Fetal/Neonatal Abnormalities

- Microcephaly (occipitofrontal circumference < 3rd percentile)
- Micrencephaly (small brain), agyria, calcifications, lateral ventricle dilation
- Hypoplasia of brainstem and spinal cord

MICROSCOPIC

Histologic Features

- Skin
  - Mild to moderate perivascular lymphocytic dermal inflammation
- Fetal/neonatal brains
  - Widespread dystrophic calcifications (periventricular, cerebral parenchyma, thalami, basal ganglia)
    - Band-like pattern most prominent in frontal and parietal lobes and lateral ventricles
  - Cortical thinning with ventricular dilation; neuronal apoptosis/necrosis
  - Simplified gyral patterns (e.g., lissencephaly, pachygyria, agyria)
  - Cerebellar hypoplasia
  - Perivascular lymphocytic infiltrates, microglial proliferation and activation, and microglial nodules
- Placenta
  - Normal or chorionic villi with calcifications, fibrosis, fibrin deposition, and villitis

Cytologic Features

- No viral inclusions identified

ANCILLARY TESTS

Immunohistochemistry

- Anti-ZIKV antibodies available at some reference laboratories
  - Fetal/neonatal brain: Viral antigen detected in glial cells, endothelial cells, degenerating cortical neurons, and calcifications
  - 1st-trimester placenta: Viral antigen detected in Hofbauer cells, fetal endothelium, and maternal leukocytes

PCR

- Virus detected in brain and placental tissue (ZIKV NS5 gene)

DIFFERENTIAL DIAGNOSIS

Other Viral Infections With Fever, Rash, or Joint Pain

- Dengue and chikungunya
  - History of travel to endemic areas, exposure to mosquitos
  - Laboratory: Serology (cross reactive), PCR

Other Infectious Causes of Microcephaly (In Utero Exposures)

- Positive serology or PCR confirms diagnosis
- Cytomegalovirus (CMV)
  - Viral cytopathic effects (VCPE): Enlarged cells, "owl's-eye" nuclei, cytoplasmic inclusions
  - Necrotizing villitis
  - IHC: Anti-CMV antibodies
- Varicella-zoster virus (VZV)
  - VCPE: Glassy nuclear inclusions, multinucleated cells
  - Necrotizing villitis
  - IHC: Anti-VZV antibodies
- Rubella
  - No specific histologic findings
  - History of nonimmune mother
- *Toxoplasma gondii*
  - Parasites observed on H&E
  - IHC: Antitoxoplasma antibodies

Noninfectious Causes of Microcephaly

- Craniosynostosis
- Chromosomal abnormalities (i.e., Down syndrome)
- Fetal cerebral anoxia
- Severe malnutrition
- Exposure to drug, alcohol, or toxins in utero

SELECTED REFERENCES

1. Giraldo MI et al: Pathogenesis of Zika virus infection. Annu Rev Pathol. 18:181-203, 2023
2. Centers for Disease Control and Prevention: Zika virus. Updated November 2, 2022. Reviewed January 27, 2023. Accessed January 27, 2023. http://www.cdc.gov/zika.
3. Gomes JA et al: Molecular mechanisms of ZIKV-induced teratogenesis: a systematic review of studies in animal models. Mol Neurobiol. 60(1):68-83, 2023
4. Postler TS et al: Renaming of the genus Flavivirus to Orthoflavivirus and extension of binomial species names within the family Flaviviridae. Arch Virol. 168(9):224, 2023
5. Chauhan L et al: Nervous system manifestations of arboviral infections. Curr Trop Med Rep. 9(4):107-18, 2022
6. Melo NL et al: Microcephaly and associated risk factors in newborns: a systematic review and meta-analysis study. Trop Med Infect Dis. 7(10), 2022
7. Singh T et al: A Zika virus-specific IgM elicited in pregnancy exhibits ultrapotent neutralization. Cell. 185(25):4826-40.e17, 2022
8. Souza JVC et al: Viral metagenomics for the identification of emerging infections in clinical samples with inconclusive dengue, Zika, and Chikungunya viral amplification. Viruses. 14(9), 2022
9. Wang Y et al: Current advances in Zika vaccine development. Vaccines (Basel). 10(11), 2022
10. Paniz-Mondolfi AE et al: Cutaneous features of Zika virus infection: a clinicopathological overview. Clin Exp Dermatol. 44(1):13-9, 2019
11. Dirlikov E et al: Postmortem findings in patient with Guillain-Barré syndrome and Zika virus infection. Emerg Infect Dis. 24(1):114-7, 2018
12. Bhatnagar J et al: Zika virus RNA replication and persistence in brain and placental tissue. Emerg Infect Dis. 23(3):405-14, 2017
13. Ritter JM et al: Zika virus: pathology from the pandemic. Arch Pathol Lab Med. 141(1):49-59, 2017
14. Schwartz DA: Autopsy and postmortem studies are concordant: pathology of Zika virus infection is neurotropic in fetuses and infants with microcephaly following transplacental transmission. Arch Pathol Lab Med. 141(1):68-72, 2017
15. Martines et al: Pathology of congenital Zika syndrome in Brazil: a case series. Lancet. 388(10047):898-904, 2016
16. Mlakar J et al: Zika virus associated with microcephaly. N Engl J Med. 374(10):951-8, 2016

Zika Virus Microcephaly

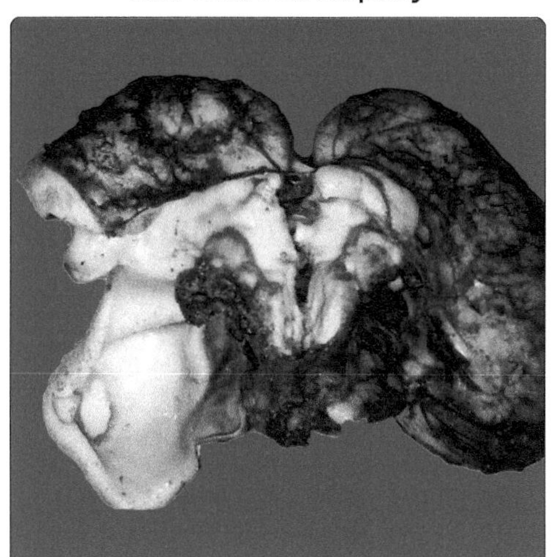

Zika Virus Cortical Degeneration

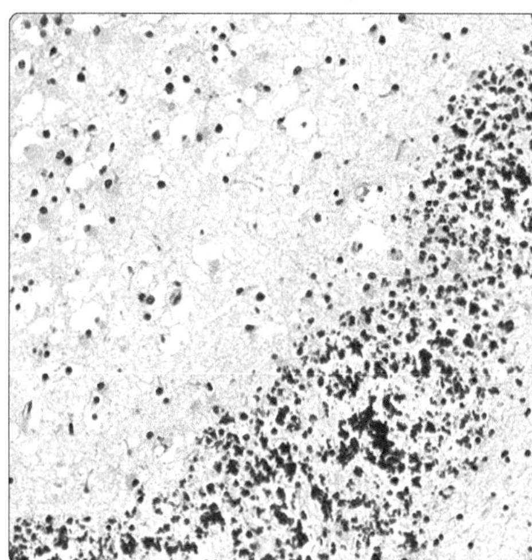

(Left) *Gross examination of the brain from a fatal case of congenital Zika virus infection shows 2 underdeveloped hemispheres with lissencephaly, ventriculomegaly of the lateral ventricle, and cerebellar hypoplasia. (Courtesy R.B. Martines, 2016.)* **(Right)** *Microscopic examination of the brain tissue from congenital Zika virus infection shows a subcortical band-like pattern of degenerating cells associated with calcifications. (Courtesy R.B. Martines, 2016.)*

Zika Virus Cortical Calcifications

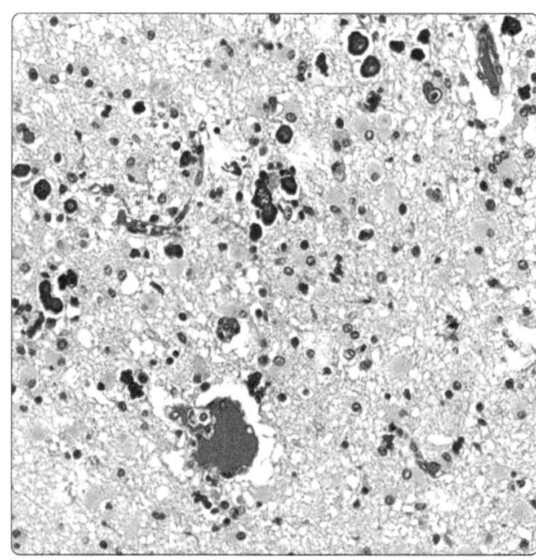

Zika Virus in Brain: IHC

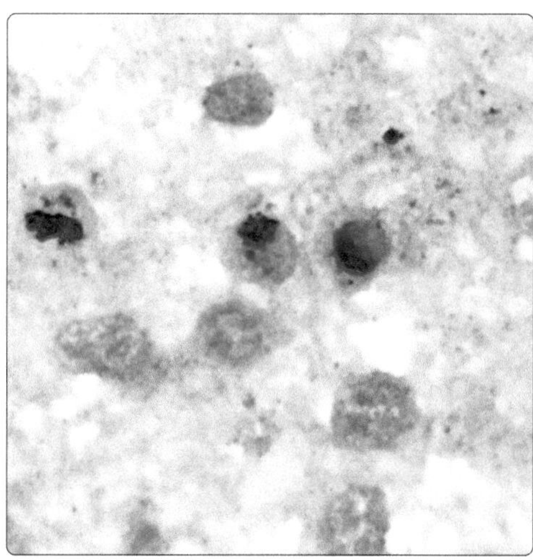

(Left) *Calcifications are distributed throughout the cortex in cases of fatal congenital Zika virus infection. (Courtesy R.B. Martines, 2016.)* **(Right)** *Zika viral antigens are detectable in glial cells (perinuclear staining), shown in this image, as well as in areas of calcifications and in degenerating neural cells. (Courtesy R.B. Martines, 2016.)*

Zika Virus Placenta

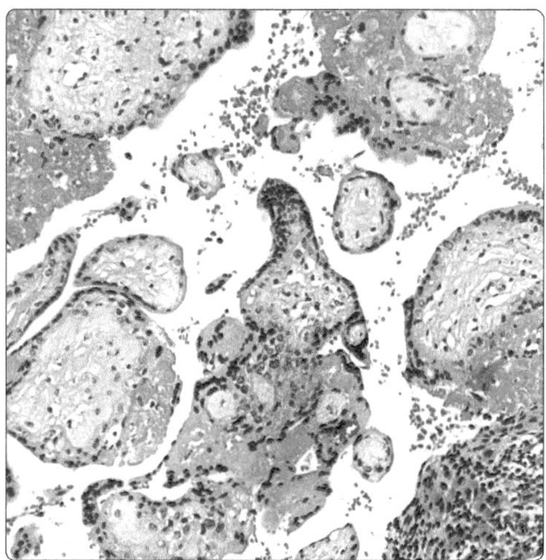

Zika Virus in Placenta: IHC

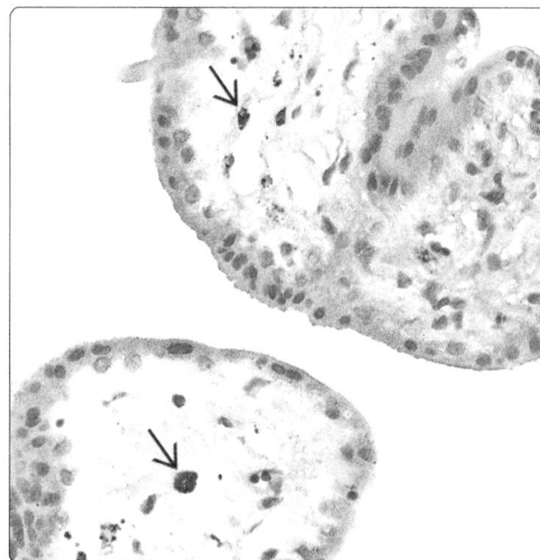

(Left) *This image from a spontaneously aborted 11-week placenta shows massive chronic intervillositis and fibrin deposition. (Courtesy R.B. Martines, 2016.)* **(Right)** *Zika virus antigen is detectable in Hofbauer cells ⮕ and in association with karyorrhectic debris of the chorionic villi. (Courtesy R.B. Martines, 2016.)*

Ebola, Marburg, and Other Hemorrhagic Fever Virus Infections

KEY FACTS

ETIOLOGY/PATHOGENESIS

- Viral infections in *Filoviridae* family, *Bunyavirales* order, and *Flaviviridae* family transmitted through direct contact with infected tissues or through animal vectors

CLINICAL ISSUES

- Incidence: Varies widely with virus and location
- Early infections present with flu-like symptoms
- Hemorrhagic symptoms in minority of patients (5-30%, depending on virus)
- Mortality up to 90% in some Ebola (EBOV) outbreaks
- Laboratory tests: Serology, PCR, viral culture
- Treatment: Avoidance of direct contact with infected material; some vaccines [i.e., yellow fever virus (YFV), EBOV] and specific treatments available [monoclonal antibodies (mAbs)]

MICROSCOPIC

- Hemorrhages, including petechiae, ecchymoses of skin, mucous membranes, visceral organs
- Multifocal necrosis (liver, spleen, kidneys) with minimal inflammatory response
- Virus specific immunohistochemistry available at some reference laboratories
- Electron microscopy can be used to confirm viral etiology for emerging infections

DIFFERENTIAL DIAGNOSIS

- EBOV and Marburg virus (MARV)
  - Infections with flu-like symptoms
    - Malaria, influenza, typhoid, meningitis, dengue virus (DENV), Lassa fever virus (LASV) fever
    - Lack of exposure history or travel to endemic areas; failure to develop rash
- Other hemorrhagic fever viruses
  - Systemic infectious disease
    - Typhoid fever, hepatitis, infectious mononucleosis, leptospirosis, rickettsioses, malaria
    - Identification of specific pathogen by PCR, serology, culture, or histologically

(Left) *Transmission electron micrograph of an Ebola virus virion demonstrates the filamentous structure that is characteristic of filoviruses. (Courtesy F. Murphy, DVM, PhD.)* **(Right)** *Bushmeat is raw or minimally processed meat that comes from wild animals (including bats, nonhuman primates, cane rats, and duiker), which is a potential source of Ebola and other infections and is illegal to import into the USA. (Courtesy E. Rothney, MPH, CDC/PHIL.)*

Ultrastructural Features of Ebola Virus

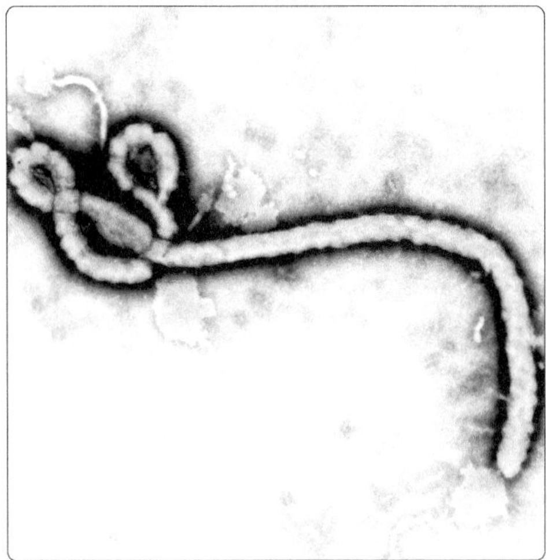

Bushmeat

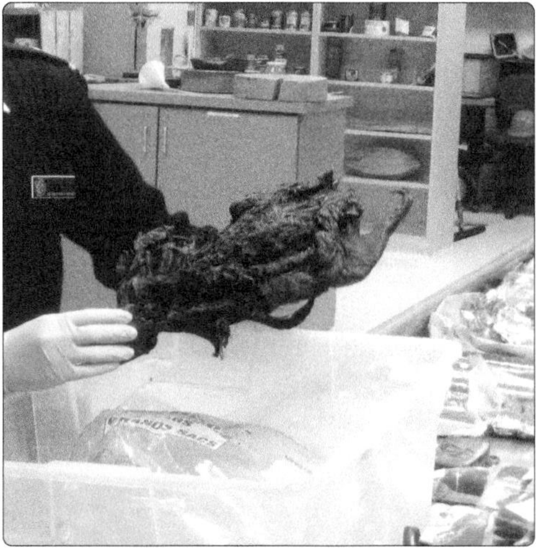

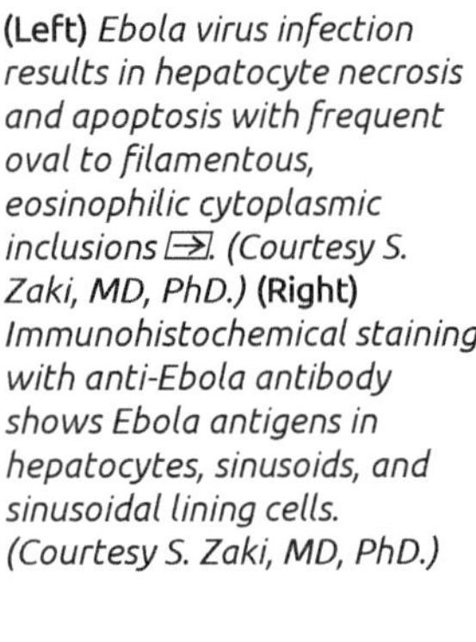

(Left) *Ebola virus infection results in hepatocyte necrosis and apoptosis with frequent oval to filamentous, eosinophilic cytoplasmic inclusions →. (Courtesy S. Zaki, MD, PhD.)* **(Right)** *Immunohistochemical staining with anti-Ebola antibody shows Ebola antigens in hepatocytes, sinusoids, and sinusoidal lining cells. (Courtesy S. Zaki, MD, PhD.)*

Histologic Features of Ebola Virus

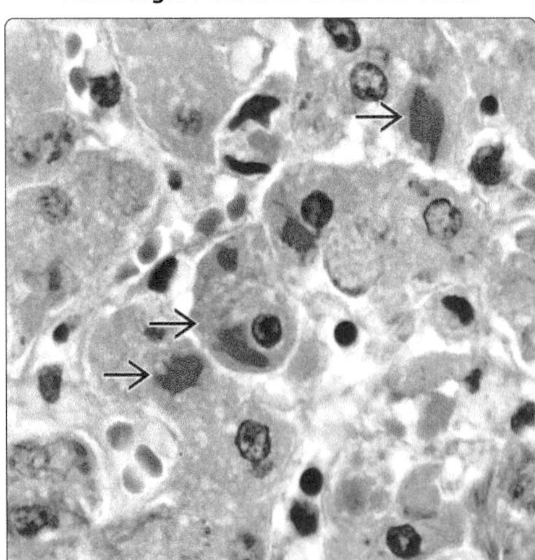

Ebola Virus Immunohistochemistry

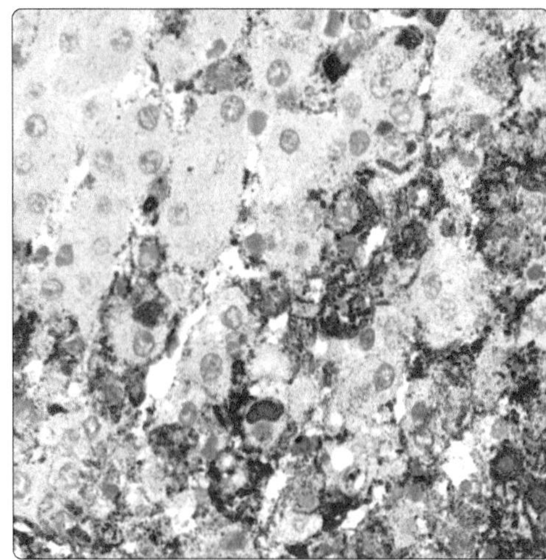

EBOLA AND MARBURG VIRUSES

TERMINOLOGY

- **Definitions**
  - *Filoviridae* family: Derived from "filo" (thread)
  - Virus names based on location 1st identified

ETIOLOGY/PATHOGENESIS

- **Infectious agents**
  - Viral infections transmitted through direct contact with infected tissues or bodily fluids (blood, saliva, sweat, mucus, vomit, urine, feces, breast milk, and semen), replicates in monocytes, macrophages, and dendritic cells, then disseminates to lymph nodes, liver, spleen
  - Index cases associated with animal exposure (nonhuman primates, pigs, bats) via hunting, butchering, processing meat from infected animals, and consuming "bushmeat"
  - *Rousettus aegyptiacus* (fruit bat) is reservoir for MARV; other fruit bats likely to be reservoir for EBOVs
  - Asymptomatic incubation period: 2-21 days (average: 8-10 days) after exposure
  - Infectious period: 21 days from onset of symptoms

CLINICAL ISSUES

- **Epidemiology**
  - Outbreaks originate in rural areas in tropical regions of Sub-Saharan Africa with occasional spread to larger cities and other countries via travel of infected individuals
    - MARV: 1st outbreaks during 1967 in Marburg and Frankfurt, Germany and Belgrade, Yugoslavia
    - EBOV: 1st outbreak during 1976 in Équateur province of Zaire
    - Sudan virus (SUDV): 1st outbreak 1976 in Nzara, Maridi, and surrounding areas in Sudan
    - Reston virus (RESTV): Discovered 1989 in monkey facility in Reston, Virginia; no reported disease in humans
    - Taï Forest virus (TAFV): Single known case in 1994 from Tai Forest in Côte d'Ivoire
    - Bundibugyo virus (BDBV): 1st outbreak in 2007 in Bundibugyo district of Uganda
    - Bombali virus (BOMV): 1st identified in 2018 in Bombali area of Sierra Leone; unclear if able to cause human disease
  - ~ 35,000 cases and 15,000 deaths reported for Ebola (EBOV, SUDV, TAFV, BDBV) from 1976-2022
  - ~ 475 cases and 379 deaths reported for MARV from 1967-2022
- **Presentation**
  - Early: Fever, headache, myalgia, diarrhea, vomiting, abdominal pain
  - Terminal state: Obtundation, tachypnea, anuria, shock, lowered body temperature
  - Hemorrhagic manifestations in 30% of patients
  - Petechial rash, conjunctival bleeding, epistaxis, melena, hematemesis
- **Laboratory tests**
  - ↓ WBC, lymphocytes, platelets; ↑ AST/ALT; ↑ PTT, TT
  - RT-PCR (blood)
  - Serology (antigen capture, IgM, IgG)
  - Virus isolation (blood)
- **Natural history**
  - Some have transient flu-like symptoms, mild coagulopathy, thrombocytopenia, leukocytosis, and full recovery
  - Majority develop severe illness, hemorrhage, disseminated intravascular coagulation (DIC), shock, and death (~ 10 days after onset of symptoms)
- **Treatment**
  - Primary prevention
    - Avoid direct contact with blood or body fluids from infected patients or animals
    - Vaccines for EBOV
      - rVSV-ZEBOV (ERVEBO): Replication-competent, live attenuated recombinant vesicular stomatitis virus vaccine FDA-approved in 2019
      - Available from CDC Strategic National Stockpile for preexposure prophylaxis for individuals with risk of occupational exposure
      - Duration of protection unclear; boosters may be administered on individual basis
  - Infected/symptomatic patients
    - Strict isolation and quarantine to contain outbreaks
    - Supportive care, including IV fluids, maintaining oxygen status and blood pressure, and treating additional infections
    - mAbs for EBOV
      - Atoltivimab/maftivimab/odesivimab-ebgn (Inmazeb): Combination of 3 mABs FDA approved in 2020
      - Ansuvimab (Ebanga): Single mAb FDA approved in 2020
- **Prognosis**
  - EBOV mortality rate: 25-90%
    - Survivors develop antibodies that last > 10 years
    - May have joint or vision problems
    - Virus may persist in semen for 9 or more months
  - MARV mortality rate: 23-90%

MICROBIOLOGY

- **Viral features**
  - Enveloped, single-stranded RNA viruses
  - 80 nm in diameter x 14,000 nm in length with helical nucleocapsid
  - 19,000 nucleotide genomes (7 proteins)
- **Culture**
  - Grows in Vero and Vero-E6 cells
  - Requires biosafety level 4 (BSL-4) facility

MACROSCOPIC

- **General features**
  - Petechiae, ecchymoses of skin, mucous membranes, visceral organs; large effusions

MICROSCOPIC

- **Histologic features**
  - Multifocal necrosis in liver, spleen, kidneys, testes, and ovaries with minimal inflammatory response
  - Liver: Hepatocyte necrosis, apoptosis, microvesicular steatosis, Kupffer cell hyperplasia
  - Eosinophilic oval/filamentous cytoplasmic inclusions (EBOV nucleoproteins)

ANCILLARY TESTS

- **Immunohistochemistry**
  - Anti-EBOV/anti-MARV antibodies at reference laboratories
- **In situ hybridization**
  - Virus RNA in macrophages and endothelial cells
- **Electron microscopy**
  - Filamentous virus particles

DIFFERENTIAL DIAGNOSIS

- Infections with flu-like symptoms
  - e.g., malaria, influenza, typhoid, meningitis, DENV, LASV fever
    - Lack of exposure history or travel to endemic areas; failure to develop rash
    - Identification of specific pathogen by PCR, serology, culture, or IHC

OTHER HEMORRHAGIC FEVER VIRUSES

TERMINOLOGY

- **Definitions**
  - *Bunyavirales* order: Named for Bunyamwera, which was location of 1st virus
  - *Flaviviridae* family: Derived from "flavus" (yellow)
  - Virus names typically based on location 1st identified

ETIOLOGY/PATHOGENESIS

- **Infectious agents**
  - Viral infections transmitted through mucous membranes, cutaneous wounds, aerosol, or animal bites
  - Viruses spread hematogenously and infect susceptible cells (i.e., hepatocytes, Kupffer cells)
  - Natural reservoirs and vectors include mosquitos, ticks, rodents, bats, and nonhuman primates
  - Potential for geographic spread determined by animal reservoirs/vectors and by transmissibility between humans

CLINICAL ISSUES

- **Epidemiology**
  - *Bunyavirales* order viruses
    - *Arenaviridae* family: Derived from "arena" (sandy)
      - Chapare virus (CHPV): Bolivia
      - Guanarito virus (GTOV): Venezuela
      - Junin virus (JUNV): Argentina
      - Lassa fever virus (LASV): West Africa
      - Lujo virus (LUJV): Zambia
      - Machupo virus (MACV): Bolivia
      - Sabia virus (SABV): Brazil
    - *Hantaviridae* family: Hantan River, South Korea
      - Andes virus (ANDV): North and South America
      - Choclo virus (CHOV): North and South America
      - Dobrava virus (DOBV): Europe
      - Hantaan virus (HTNV): Asia, Europe
      - Puumala virus (PUUV): Europe
      - Seoul virus (SEOV): Asia, Europe
      - Sin Nombre virus (SNV): North and South America
    - *Nairoviridae* family: Nairobi sheep disease
      - Crimean-Congo hemorrhagic fever virus (CCHFV): Africa, Europe, Asia
    - *Phenuiviridae* family
      - Rift Valley fever virus (RVFV): Africa and Arabian Peninsula
      - Severe fever with thrombocytopenia syndrome virus (SFTSV): China
    - Transmitted by rodents (ANDV, CHOV, DOBV, HTNV, PUUV, SEOV, SNV), mosquitos (RVFV), or ticks (CCHFV, SFTSV)
  - *Flaviviridae* family
    - Alkhurma virus (ALKV): Saudi Arabia
    - DENV: 4 serotypes; worldwide
    - Kyasanur forest disease virus (KFDV): India
    - Omsk hemorrhagic fever virus (OMFV): Russia
    - YFV: Central and South America, Africa
    - Transmitted by mosquitos (YFV, DENV) or ticks (OMFV)
- **Presentation**
  - Specific signs and symptoms vary by viral infection
  - DENV: Fever, myalgia, severe retroorbital headache, nausea, vomiting, conjunctival congestion, rash, lymphadenopathy, mild to severe hemorrhages, shock
  - LASV: Fever, malaise, weakness, headache, hemorrhage, respiratory distress, vomiting, facial swelling, chest, back, and abdominal pain, shock, hearing loss, tremors, and encephalitis
  - YFV: Fever, myalgia, nausea, vomiting, bradycardia, conjunctival congestion, followed by remission, then jaundice, hemorrhages, and renal failure
- **Laboratory tests**
  - RT-PCR (blood)
  - Serology (IgM, IgG)
  - Virus isolation (blood); may require BSL-4 facility
- **Natural history**
  - Mostly asymptomatic with only minority developing hemorrhagic fever, which is severe
- **Treatment**
  - Primary prevention
    - Avoidance of mosquitos, ticks, rodents; minimize exposed skin; use of insect repellents
    - Few FDA-approved vaccines available
      - YF-VAX: Live-attenuated yellow fever vaccine available since 1930s
      - CYD-TDV (Dengvaxia): Live attenuated tetravalent chimeric vaccine, approved for use only in previously infected individuals due to risk of more severe disease without prior infection
  - Symptomatic patients
    - Predominantly supportive case
    - Ribavirin for some hemorrhagic fever viruses (e.g., LFV)
- **Prognosis**
  - Typically full recovery; higher rates of mortality with some viruses and with suboptimal supportive care

MICROBIOLOGY

- **Viral features**
  - *Bunyavirales* order
    - Enveloped, single-stranded RNA viruses
    - Spherical, 80-130 nm, helical nucleocapsid
    - 10,500-22,700 nucleotides (4-6 proteins)
  - *Flaviviridae* family

Major Outbreaks of Ebola Virus Disease and Marburg Hemorrhagic Fever

Year	Location	Virus	Deaths	Cases	Fatality (%)
1967	Germany and Yugoslavia	MARV	7	31	23
1976	Zaire	EBOV	280	318	88
1976	Sudan	SUDV	151	284	53
1995	Zaire	EBOV	250	315	79
1998-2000	Democratic Republic of Congo	MARV	128	154	83
2000-2001	Uganda	SUDV	224	425	53
2002-2003	Republic of Congo	EBOV	128	143	89
2004-2005	Angola	MARV	227	252	90
2007	Democratic Republic of Congo	EBOV	187	264	71
2007	Uganda	BDBV	37	149	25
2014-2016	West Africa (Sierra Leone, Liberia, Guinea)	EBOV	11,323	28,646	40
2018-2020	Democratic Republic of Congo, Uganda	EBOV	2287	3470	66
2020	Democratic Republic of Congo	EBOV	55	130	42
2022	Uganda	SUDV	55	164	34

BDBV = Bundibugyo virus; EBOV = Ebola virus; MARV = Marburg virus; SUDV = Sudan virus.

- Enveloped, single-stranded RNA viruses
- Spherical, 37-50 nm, icosahedral nucleocapsid
- 9,600-12,300 nucleotides [1 open reading frame (ORF)]

MICROSCOPIC

- **Histologic features**
  - DENV
    - Gastrointestinal mucosa, skin, pulmonary alveoli, serosal surface hemorrhages
    - Infection of mononuclear phagocytes and hepatocytes
    - Liver necrosis with minimal inflammatory response
  - LASV
    - Liver and spleen necrosis and mononuclear phagocytic activation with minimal immune cell infiltrates or tissue damage
    - Viral antigen detected in hepatocytes, Kupffer cells, endothelial cells, macrophages, dendritic cells, mesothelial cells, breast ductal epithelium, adrenal cortical cells, ovarian theca and stromal cells, and placental trophoblastic cells
  - YFV
    - Liver and kidney show apoptosis, necrosis of hepatocytes, Kupffer cells, and tubular epithelial cells with minimal inflammatory response

ANCILLARY TESTS

- **Immunohistochemistry**
  - Viral-specific antibodies available commercially or at reference laboratories
- **Molecular testing**
  - Targeted RT-PCR ± sequencing
  - Unbiased metagenomic next-generation sequencing (mNGS) if no specific virus is suspected

DIFFERENTIAL DIAGNOSIS

- Systemic infectious disease
  - e.g., typhoid fever, hepatitis, infectious mononucleosis, leptospirosis, rickettsioses, malaria
    - Identification of specific pathogen by PCR, serology, culture, or histologically

SELECTED REFERENCES

1. Centers for Disease Control and Prevention: Ebola (Ebola virus disease). Updated January 27, 2023. Reviewed January 30, 2023. Accessed January 30, 2023. http://www.cdc.gov/vhf/ebola/
2. Dyal J et al: Risk factors for ebola virus persistence in semen of survivors - Liberia. Clin Infect Dis. 76(3):e849-56, 2022
3. Shieh WJ et al: Pathology and pathogenesis of Lassa fever: novel immunohistochemical findings in fatal cases and clinico-pathologic correlation. Clin Infect Dis. 74(10):1821-30, 2022
4. Wanninger TG et al: Macrophage infection, activation, and histopathological findings in ebolavirus infection. Front Cell Infect Microbiol. 12:1023557, 2022
5. Woolsey C et al: Natural history of Sudan ebolavirus infection in rhesus and cynomolgus macaques. Emerg Microbes Infect. 11(1):1635-46, 2022
6. Agbonlahor DE et al: 52 years of Lassa fever outbreaks in Nigeria, 1969-2020: an epidemiologic analysis of the temporal and spatial trends. Am J Trop Med Hyg. 105(4):974-85, 2021
7. McEntire CRS et al: Neurologic manifestations of the World Health Organization's list of pandemic and epidemic diseases. Front Neurol. 12:634827, 2021
8. Tomori O et al: Ebola virus disease: current vaccine solutions. Curr Opin Immunol. 71:27-33, 2021
9. Jacob ST et al: Ebola virus disease. Nat Rev Dis Primers. 6(1):13, 2020
10. Kuhn JH et al: New filovirus disease classification and nomenclature. Nat Rev Microbiol. 17(5):261-3, 2019
11. Domingo C et al: Yellow fever in the diagnostics laboratory. Emerg Microbes Infect. 7(1):129, 2018
12. Giang HTN et al: Dengue hemophagocytic syndrome: a systematic review and meta-analysis on epidemiology, clinical signs, outcomes, and risk factors. Rev Med Virol. 28(6):e2005, 2018
13. Basler CF: Molecular pathogenesis of viral hemorrhagic fever. Semin Immunopathol. 39(5):551-61, 2017
14. Raabe V et al: Laboratory diagnosis of Lassa fever. J Clin Microbiol. 55(6):1629-37, 2017
15. Martines RB et al: Tissue and cellular tropism, pathology and pathogenesis of Ebola and Marburg viruses. J Pathol. 235(2):153-74, 2015
16. Zaki SR et al: Viral hemorrhagic fevers. In: Connor DH et al: Pathology of Infectious Diseases. Appleton & Lange. 347-64, 1997

Ultrastructural Features of Marburg Virus

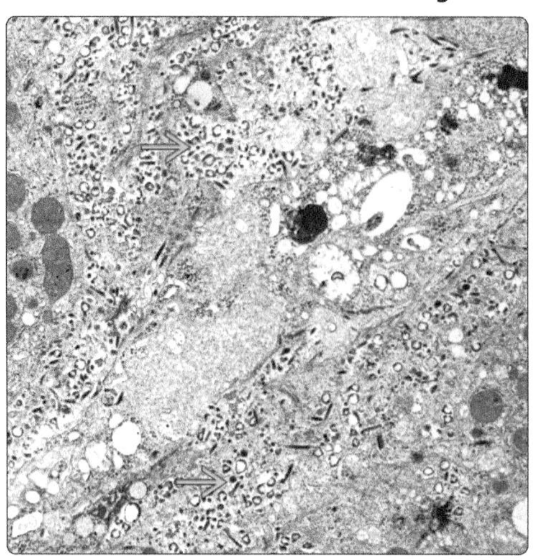

Histologic Features of Marburg Virus

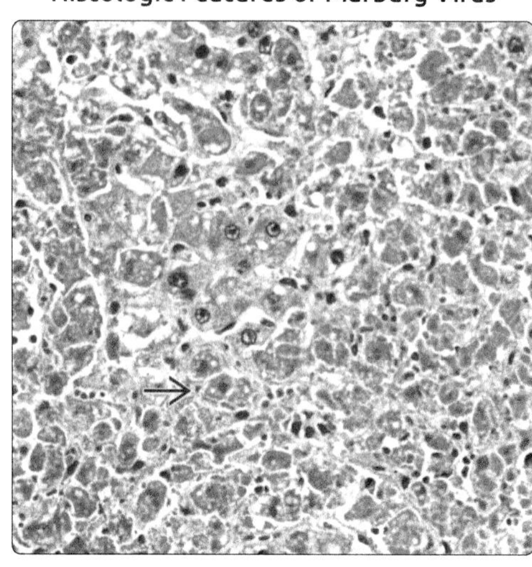

(Left) *Electron micrograph of the liver demonstrates Marburg virus particles ⇒ in the extracellular space. (Courtesy F. Murphy, DVM, PhD.)* **(Right)** *Marburg virus infection results in hepatocyte necrosis ⇒ and apoptosis but lacks distinct viral inclusions. (Courtesy S. Zaki, MD, PhD.)*

Marburg Virus Immunohistochemistry

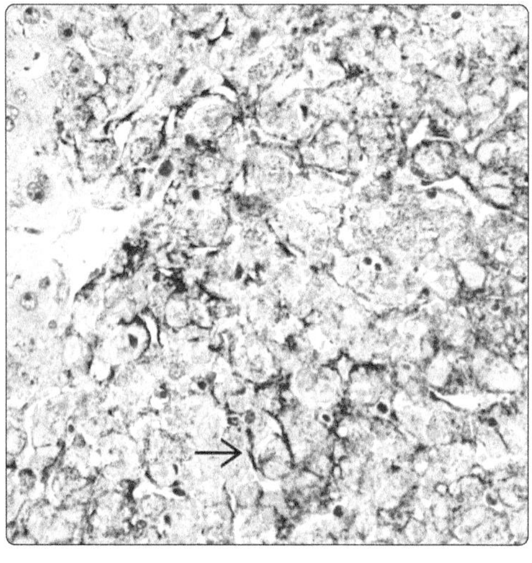

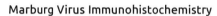

Ultrastructural Features of Lassa Virus

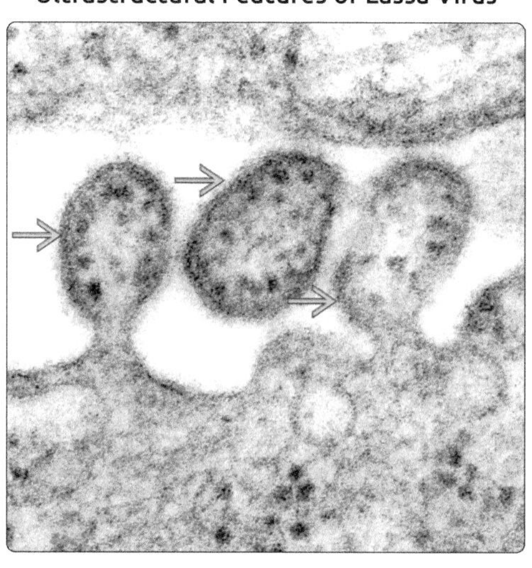

(Left) *Immunohistochemical staining with anti-Ebola virus antibody shows Marburg antigens in sinusoidal lining cells ⇒. (Courtesy S. Zaki, MD, PhD.)* **(Right)** *This electron micrograph shows 3 Lassa virus particles ⇒ in the process of budding. Lassa virus is a member of the Arenaviridae family. They are enveloped, spherical viruses with helical capsids. (Courtesy C. Goldsmith, MGS.)*

Histologic Features of Lassa Fever Virus

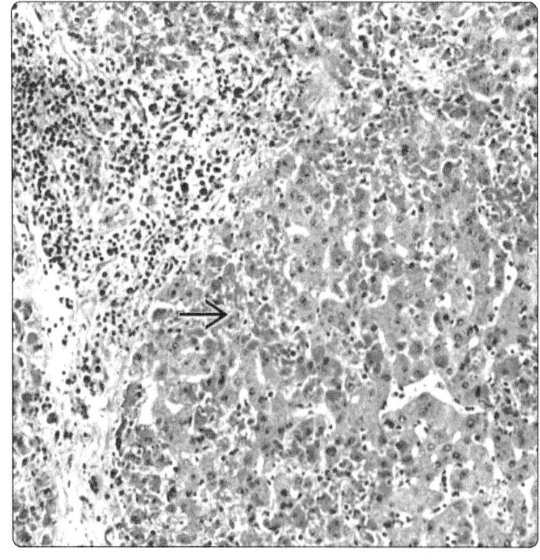

Lassa Fever Virus Immunohistochemistry

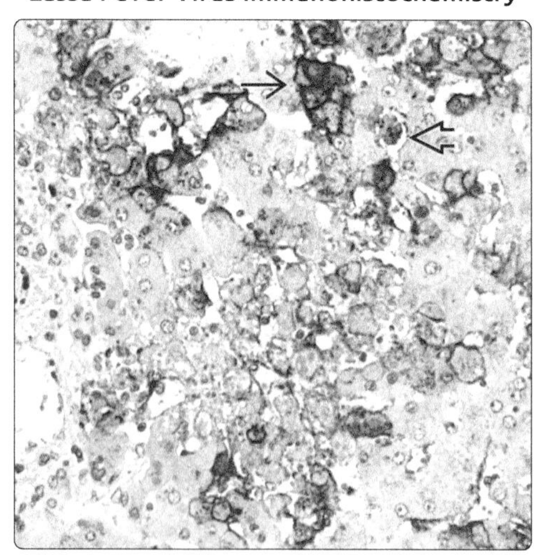

(Left) *Lassa fever virus infection is characterized by eosinophilic necrosis ⇒ of hepatocytes as well as larger foci of hepatocellular destruction. (Courtesy S. Zaki, MD, PhD.)* **(Right)** *Immunohistochemical staining with anti-Lassa antibody shows Lassa antigens in hepatocytes ⇒ and Kupffer cells ⇒. (Courtesy S. Zaki, MD, PhD.)*

Ultrastructural Features of Yellow Fever Virus

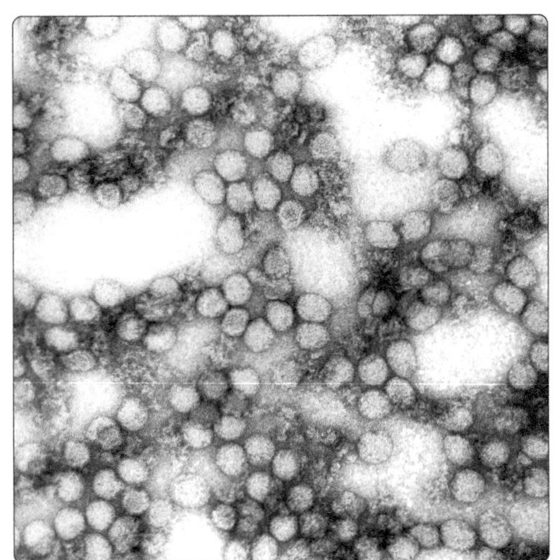

Histologic Features of Yellow Fever Virus

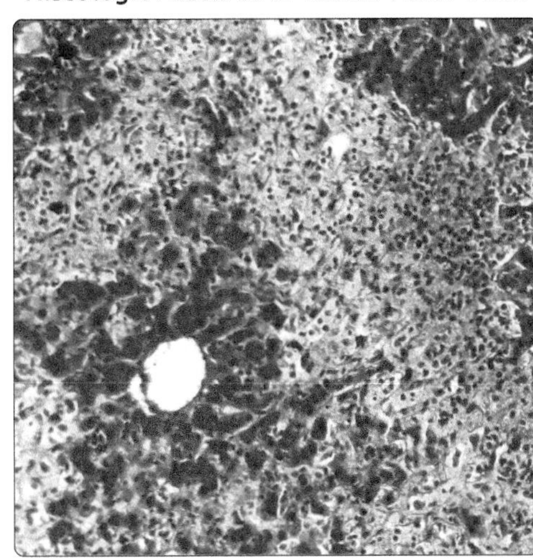

(Left) *This electron micrograph shows multiple virions of yellow fever virus, a member of the Flaviviridae family. They are enveloped, spherical viruses with icosahedral capsids. (Courtesy E. Palmer, PhD.)* **(Right)** *Yellow fever virus-infected liver shows characteristic midzonal hepatic necrosis. (Courtesy M. C. Williams, MBBS, CDC/PHIL.)*

Yellow Fever Virus: Councilman Bodies

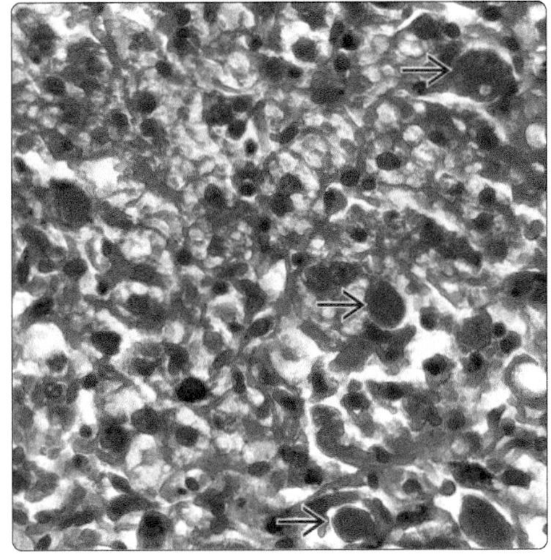

Ultrastructural Features of Dengue Virus

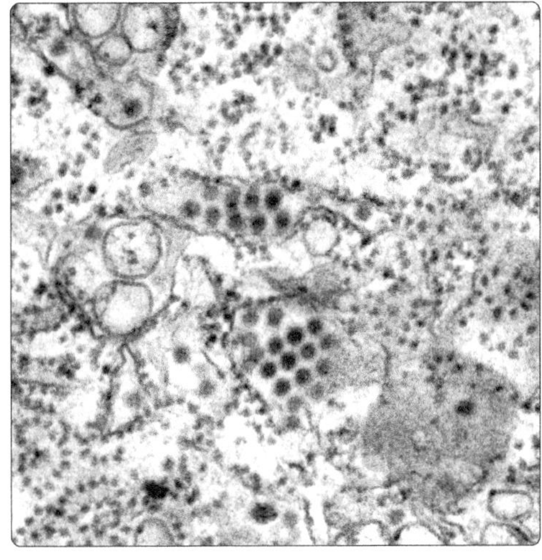

(Left) *Yellow fever virus infection of liver contains scattered eosinophilic Councilman bodies, or Councilman hyaline bodies* ⇨*, first identified in yellow fever but can be seen with other viral hemorrhagic fevers and viral hepatitis. (Courtesy M. C. Williams, MBBS, CDC/PHIL.)* **(Right)** *This transmission electron microscopic image depicts a number of round, dengue virus particles that were revealed in this tissue specimen. (Courtesy F. Murphy, DVM, PhD.)*

Ultrastructural Features of Rift Valley Fever Virus

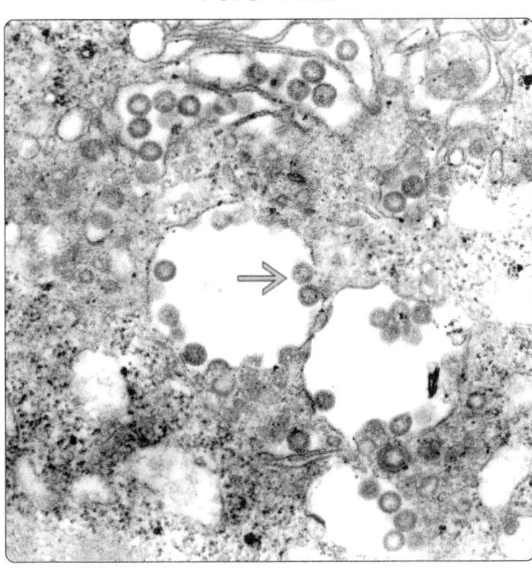

Ultrastructural Features of Chapare Virus

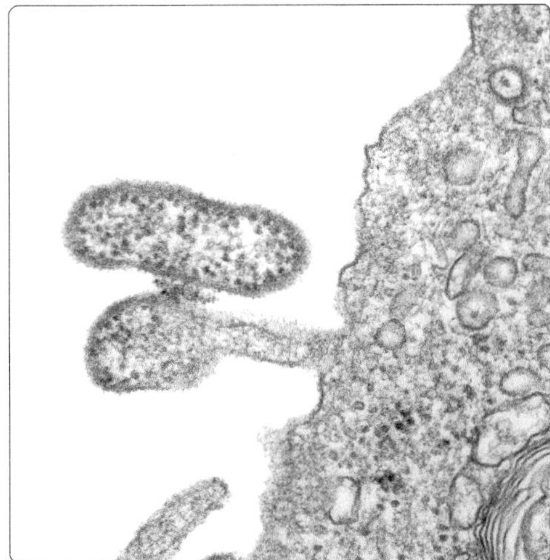

(Left) *This electron micrograph shows tissue infected with Rift Valley fever virus* ⇨*, a phlebovirus in the Bunyavirales order. They are enveloped, spherical viruses with helical capsids. (Courtesy F. Murphy, DVM, PhD.)* **(Right)** *This electron micrograph of Chapare virus-infected cells shows typical arenavirus morphology with pleomorphic virions containing ribosomes. (Courtesy C. Goldsmith, MGS and M. Morales-Betoulle, PhD, CDC/PHIL.)*

Enterovirus Infections

KEY FACTS

ETIOLOGY/PATHOGENESIS

- Viral infections transmitted via feces, secretions, or blister fluid; nondisinfected surfaces may transmit virus through touching and contact with mucous membranes

CLINICAL ISSUES

- 10-15 million infections per year (USA) with ~ 1% hospitalization rate
- Mostly asymptomatic infection or mild illness
- Hand, foot, and mouth disease, herpangina, conjunctivitis, meningitis, encephalitis, acute flaccid myelitis, myocarditis, pericarditis, neonatal sepsis
- PCR/sequencing of CSF, respiratory secretions, body fluids

MICROSCOPIC

- No specific viral cytopathic effects
- HFMD: Intraepidermal blister, apoptosis of keratinocytes, edema, necrosis, and dyskeratosis, neutrophilic or lymphocytic inflammation
- Meningoencephalitis: Lymphocytic inflammation, microglial nodules, neuronal loss
- Myocarditis: Lymphocytic inflammation with myocyte damage
- IHC: Anti-*Enterovirus* capsid protein (VP1) antibodies

TOP DIFFERENTIAL DIAGNOSES

- Other viral skin infections
  - VZV, HSV-1/2: Vesicles, multinucleated cells, nuclear molding, marginated chromatin; confirm with IHC
  - Monkeypox: Occasional Guarnieri bodies; IHC, PCR, and potential exposure history
  - Molluscum contagiosum: Henderson-Patterson bodies
- Other causes of meningoencephalitis
  - HSV-1/2: Prominent necrosis; HSV IHC
  - Arboviruses: Lack VCPE; viral IHC/ISH, PCR, serology
  - HIV: Multinucleated giant cells; HIV IHC, PCR, serology
- Other causes of lymphocytic myocarditis (e.g., parvovirus B19, adenovirus, HHV-6): confirm specific etiology by PCR

(Left) *Transmission electron microscopic image reveals numerous, spheroid-shaped 30-nm virions, consistent with enterovirus D68 (EV-D68). Note that some of the viral particles appear as if they were empty, missing their contents of single-stranded RNA. (Courtesy C. Goldsmith, MS, Y. Zhang, MSc, CDC/PHIL.)* **(Right)** *Enterovirus encephalitis shows perivascular lymphocytic inflammation with neuronal damage and scattered microglia.*

Enterovirus D68 Ultrastructural Features

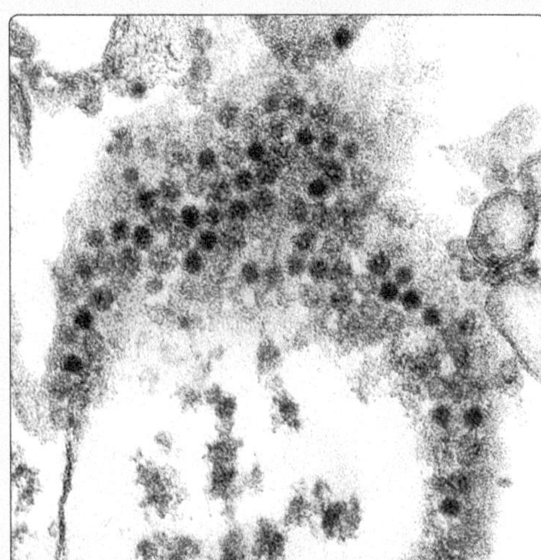

***Enterovirus* Encephalitis**

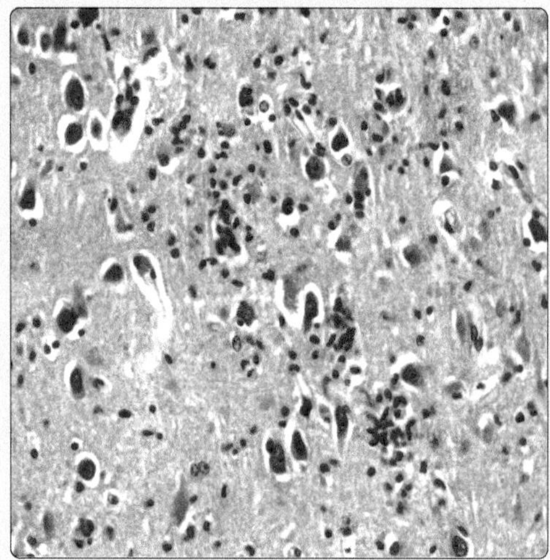

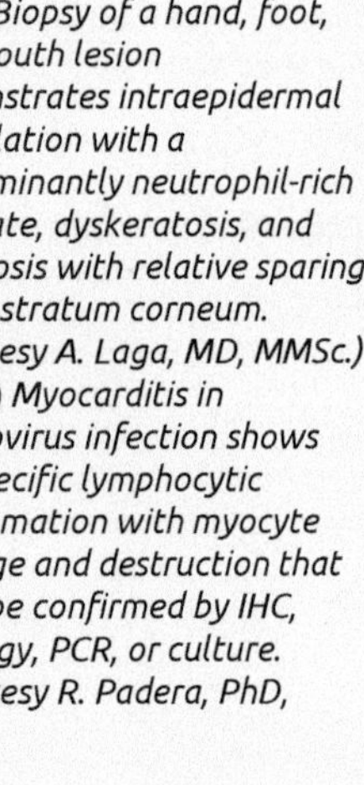

(Left) *Biopsy of a hand, foot, and mouth lesion demonstrates intraepidermal vesiculation with a predominantly neutrophil-rich infiltrate, dyskeratosis, and apoptosis with relative sparing of the stratum corneum. (Courtesy A. Laga, MD, MMSc.)* **(Right)** *Myocarditis in Enterovirus infection shows nonspecific lymphocytic inflammation with myocyte damage and destruction that must be confirmed by IHC, serology, PCR, or culture. (Courtesy R. Padera, PhD, MD.)*

Hand, Foot, and Mouth Disease

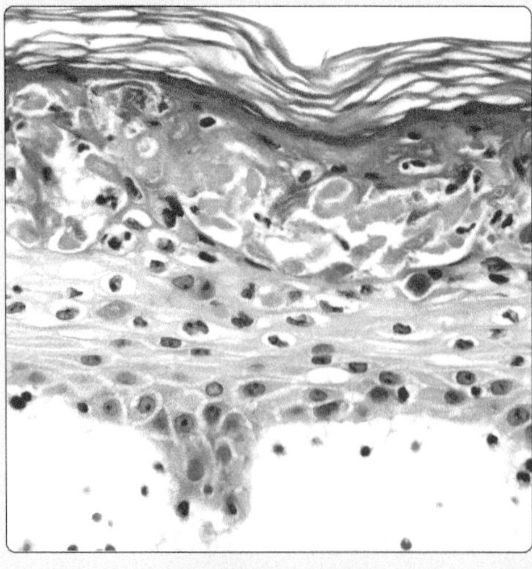

***Enterovirus* Myocarditis**

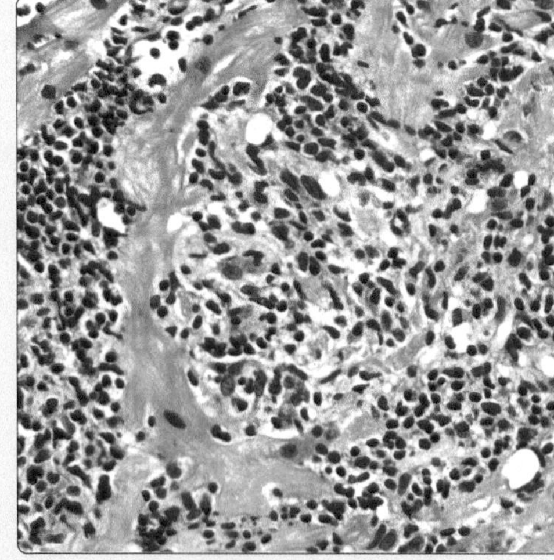

TERMINOLOGY

Definitions

- *Enterovirus* genus from Greek "enteron" (intestine)
- *Picornaviridae* family from "pico" (small) + "rna"
- "Enteric cytopathogenic human orphan" (ECHO)
- Coxsackie, NY: Location of 1st identification of virus

ETIOLOGY/PATHOGENESIS

Infectious Agents

- Viral infections transmitted via feces, secretions, or blister fluid; nondisinfected surfaces may transmit virus through touching and contact with mucous membranes
- *Enterovirus A*: Coxsackievirus A2-A8, A10, A12, A14, A16, enterovirus A71, A76, A89-A92, A114, A119-A125
- *Enterovirus B*: Coxsackievirus B1-B6, A9, echovirus 1-7, 9, 11-21, 24-27, 29-33, enterovirus B69, B73-B75, B77-B88, B93, B97, B98, B100, B101, B106, B107, B110-B114
- *Enterovirus C*: Poliovirus 1-3, coxsackievirus A1, A11, A13, A17, A19-A22, A24, enterovirus C95, C96, C99, C102, C104, C105, C109, C113, C116-C118
- *Enterovirus D*: Enterovirus D68, D70, D94, D111, D120
- *Rhinovirus A-C*: Large group of serotypes associated with common cold

CLINICAL ISSUES

Epidemiology

- Infections are more frequent in summer and fall; illness more likely to occur in children < 18 years of age, including infants and children
- 10-15 million infections per year (USA) with ~ 1% hospitalization rate

Presentation

- Mostly asymptomatic infection or mild illness with fever, runny nose, sneezing, cough, skin rash, mouth blisters, body and muscle aches
- Hand, foot, and mouth disease (coxsackievirus A16, A6, enterovirus A71)
- Herpangina (coxsackievirus A6, A10): Blisters of soft palate or tonsillar pillars
- Conjunctivitis (coxsackievirus A24, enterovirus D70)
- Aseptic meningitis, encephalitis, acute flaccid myelitis (enterovirus D68, A71)
- Myocarditis, pericarditis
- Severe neonatal sepsis

Laboratory Tests

- ECG with ST-segment elevation to heart block (myocarditis)
- Aseptic meningitis on CSF studies
- PCR/sequencing of CSF, respiratory secretions, body fluids to detect viral RNA

Treatment

- No vaccines available; treatment is supportive

Prognosis

- Most patients are asymptomatic or fully recover with rare instances of mortality or long-term morbidity, especially in encephalitis and paralysis cases

MICROBIOLOGY

Virus Features

- Nonenveloped, positive-sense single-stranded RNA viruses
- 30 nm in diameter, icosahedral capsid
- 7,200-8,500 nucleotide genomes
- Single open reading frame with 9-10 protein products

Culture

- Culture on cynomolgus or rhesus monkey kidney cells (< 5 days); cell lysis with no viral cytopathic effect

MICROSCOPIC

Histologic Features

- Necrosis and hemorrhage may be prominent with no viral cytopathic effect
- HFMD: Intraepidermal blister, apoptosis of keratinocytes, edema, necrosis, and dyskeratosis, neutrophilic or lymphocytic inflammation
- Meningoencephalitis: Nonspecific lymphocytic inflammation of leptomeninges and brain parenchyma, microglial nodules, neuronal loss
- Myocarditis: Lymphocytic inflammation with myocyte damage, including necrosis, vacuolization (Dallas criteria)

ANCILLARY TESTS

Immunohistochemistry

- Antibodies to *Enterovirus* capsid protein (VP1)

DIFFERENTIAL DIAGNOSIS

Other Viral Skin Infections

- VZV, HSV-1/2: Vesicles, multinucleated cells, nuclear molding, marginated chromatin; confirm by IHC
- Monkeypox: Occasional Guarnieri bodies; confirm by IHC, PCR, and potential exposure history
- Molluscum contagiosum: Henderson-Patterson bodies (large eosinophilic to basophilic cytoplasmic inclusions)

Other Causes of Meningoencephalitis

- HSV-1/2: Preferentially involve temporal lobes; prominent necrosis, confirm with IHC
- Arboviruses: Lack specific viral cytopathic effects; confirm specific etiology by IHC/ISH, serology, PCR/mNGS
- HIV: Multinucleated giant cells; confirm by IHC, PCR, serology

Other Causes of Lymphocytic Myocarditis

- e.g., parvovirus B19, adenovirus, HHV-6
- Similar lymphocytic inflammation and myocyte damage; confirm specific etiology by PCR

SELECTED REFERENCES

1. Ammirati E et al: State-of-the-art of endomyocardial biopsy on acute myocarditis and chronic inflammatory cardiomyopathy. Curr Cardiol Rep. 24(5):597-609, 2022
2. Murphy OC et al: Acute flaccid myelitis: cause, diagnosis, and management. Lancet. 397(10271):334-46, 2021
3. Laga AC et al: Atypical hand, foot and mouth disease in adults associated with coxsackievirus A6: a clinico-pathologic study. J Cutan Pathol. 43(11):940-5, 2016
4. Muehlenbachs A et al: Tissue tropism, pathology and pathogenesis of enterovirus infection. J Pathol. 235(2):217-28, 2015

KEY FACTS

ETIOLOGY/PATHOGENESIS

- Virus with fecal-oral route of infection
- Brief viremic stage rarely results in spread within nerve fiber pathways, replicating and destroying motor neurons
- Serum neutralizing antibodies correlate with disease protection

CLINICAL ISSUES

- Eradicated in USA in 1979; remains endemic in Afghanistan, and Pakistan
- Majority are asymptomatic, ~ 25% have mild illness, < 1% have permanent paralysis
- Primary prevention with inactivated polio vaccine (IPV) or live-attenuated oral polio vaccine (OPV)
    - OPV shed in feces of vaccines can revert to neurovirulence; circulating vaccine-derived virus (cVDPV) now responsible for majority of cases worldwide (1,113 cases in 2020)
- Diagnosis by cell culture and RT-PCR/genome sequencing to identify strain/origin
- Postpolio syndrome
    - New muscle pain, weakness, paralysis after 15-40 years

MICROSCOPIC

- Acute phase: Mononuclear inflammation of spinal gray matter with perivascular cuffing, neuronophagia, and meningeal inflammation
- Chronic phase: Loss of motor neurons, atrophy and fibrosis of anterior nerve root, and neurogenic muscle atrophy

TOP DIFFERENTIAL DIAGNOSES

- Paraneoplastic (autoimmune) encephalitis
    - Involves limbic system, brainstem, cerebellum, and spinal cord (less common); no detection of poliovirus
- Rasmussen encephalitis
    - Chronic inflammation, perivascular cuffing, microglial nodule formation, rarefaction (single hemisphere); no detection of poliovirus

Ultrastructural Features

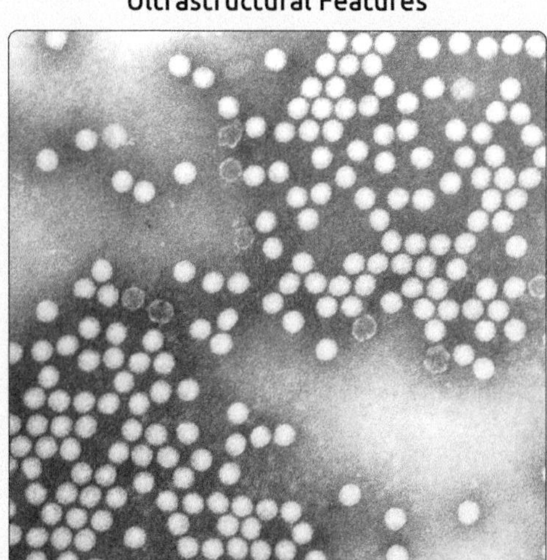

Poliomyelitis

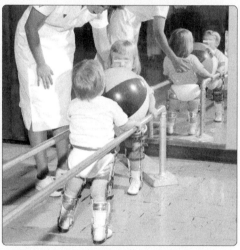

(Left) *This transmission electron micrograph shows numerous round, nonenveloped virions with icosahedral symmetry measuring 20-30 nm in diameter, characteristic of poliovirus. (Courtesy J. Esposito, MD.)* **(Right)** *This photograph shows a physical therapist assisting 2 children with lower limb exercises following infection with poliovirus. (Courtesy C. Farmer.)*

Acute Poliomyelitis

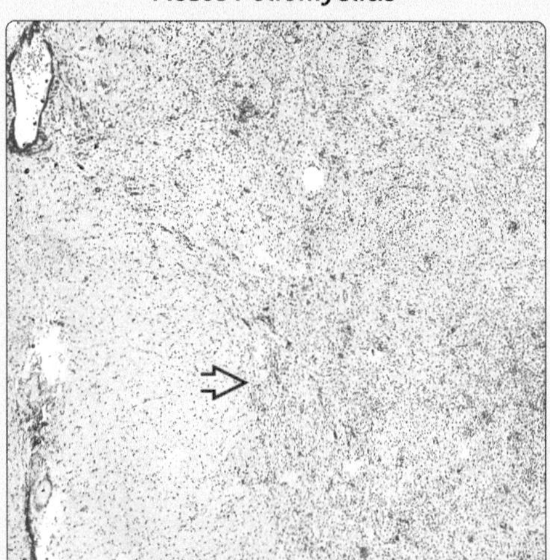

Chronic Poliomyelitis

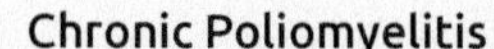

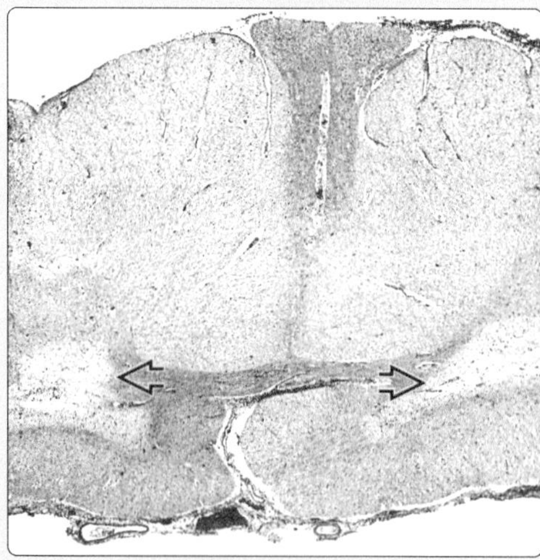

(Left) *Cresyl violet staining of the lumbar spinal cord in acute poliomyelitis shows infiltration with inflammatory cells and destruction of anterior horn ⇨.* **(Right)** *Autopsy section from the cervical cord in the chronic phase of poliomyelitis shows selective destruction of anterior horns ⇨, cavitation, gliosis, and complete destruction of motor neurons.*

TERMINOLOGY

Definitions

- Poliovirus: Derived from "polio" (gray) referring to gray matter of spinal cord
- Serotype of the species *Enterovirus C*
- *Picornaviridae* family: Derived from "pico" (small)

ETIOLOGY/PATHOGENESIS

Infectious Agents

- Fecal-oral route of infection; viral replication in tonsillar tissue and alimentary tract with shedding in feces
- Incubation period 6-20 days; infectivity occurs from 7-10 days before onset of symptoms
- Transient viremia with rare (5%) spread to brown fat, reticuloendothelial tissue, and muscle
- Rarely (1%), virus spreads within nerve fiber pathways, replicating in and destroying motor neurons
- Virus binds immunoglobulin-like receptor CD155 on cell surface of host cells

CLINICAL ISSUES

Epidemiology

- Mainly affects children < 5 years old; peaks in summer
- USA: Increasing outbreaks in early 20th century peaked in 1952 (57,000 cases, 21,000 with paralysis, 3,000 deaths); vaccine (IPV) approved in 1955; eradicated in USA in 1979
- Worldwide: Reported cases decreased > 99% from 1988 (~ 350,000) to 2020 (1,113 vaccine derived and 140 wildtype); Afghanistan and Pakistan are last endemic countries
- Live attenuated oral vaccine strain (OPV) can revert to neurovirulence and cause disease

Presentation

- Majority are asymptomatic; mild illness in ~ 25%, fever, fatigue, nausea, headache, flu-like symptoms, stiffness in neck/back, pain in limbs
- < 1% have permanent paralysis of limbs (usually legs)
- Majority of cases currently in immunocompromised patients (particularly B-cell deficiencies) and in regions with low vaccination coverage or still endemic for PV1

Laboratory Tests

- Cell culture (stool, pharyngeal swab, CSF)
- Intratypic differentiation (RT-PCR) and partial genome sequencing to distinguish serotypes, wildtype vs. vaccine derived, and likely geographic origin
- Serology (neutralizing antibodies)
- CSF: ↑ WBC (primarily lymphocytes) and mildly elevated protein (40-50 mg/100 mL)

Natural History

- 5-10% with paralysis will die from respiratory failure

Treatment

- Primary prevention
  - Inactivated polio vaccine (IPV): 4 doses (2, 4, 6-18 months, and 4-6 years)
  - Oral polio vaccine (OPV): No longer available in USA
- Presentation with symptoms; supportive therapy only

Prognosis

- Nonparalytic infections recover completely
- Some function regained in 4-6 weeks, but permanent paralysis (~ 50%) and death (5-10%) can occur
- Postpolio syndrome: New muscle pain, exacerbation of existing weakness, and development of new weakness/paralysis after 15-40 years

MICROBIOLOGY

Viral Features

- Single-stranded, positive sense, RNA virus; 7,500 bp genome (~ 10 viral proteins)
- 30-nm icosahedral, nonenveloped
- 3 serotypes (PV1-3)

Culture

- Cell lines: L20B (poliovirus specific) and RD or Hep2 (other enteroviruses)
- Viral cytopathic effects within 14 days
- Identification with neutralization tests or PCR

MACROSCOPIC

General Features

- Acute phase: Brain and spinal cord typically normal
- Chronic phase: Wasting of affected muscles; thinning and gray discoloration of anterior nerve roots

MICROSCOPIC

Histologic Features

- Acute phase: Mononuclear inflammation of spinal gray matter with perivascular cuffing, neuronophagia, leptomeningeal inflammation
- Chronic phase: Loss of motor neurons, atrophy and fibrosis of anterior nerve roots, neurogenic muscle atrophy

DIFFERENTIAL DIAGNOSIS

Paraneoplastic (Autoimmune) Encephalitis

- Involves limbic system, brainstem, cerebellum, and spinal cord (less common); no detection of poliovirus

Rasmussen Encephalitis

- Chronic inflammation, perivascular cuffing, microglial nodule formation, rarefaction (single hemisphere); no detection of poliovirus

Acute Flaccid Myelitis

- Similar clinical presentation to poliomyelitis but with other viral etiologies [nonpolio enteroviruses (EV-D68, EV-A71), flaviviruses (West Nile virus, Japanese encephalitis virus), herpesviruses, adenovirus]

SELECTED REFERENCES

1. Centers for Disease Control and Prevention: Polio: polio eradication. Reviewed December 5th, 2022. Accessed December 5th, 2022. http://www.cdc.gov/polio/
2. Alleman MM et al: Update on vaccine-derived poliovirus outbreaks - worldwide, July 2019-February 2020. MMWR Morb Mortal Wkly Rep. 69(16):489-95, 2020
3. Bao J et al: Polio - The old foe and new challenges: an update for clinicians. J Paediatr Child Health. 56(10):1527-32, 2020

Rabies Virus Infection

KEY FACTS

ETIOLOGY/PATHOGENESIS

- Zoonotic infection transmitted by animal bites (i.e., dogs, bats, raccoons)
- Virus replicates in muscle, spreads from peripheral nerves to central nervous system by retrograde axonal transport, then to salivary glands and other organs (1- to 3-month incubation)

CLINICAL ISSUES

- 59,000 deaths per year worldwide
- Presents with fever, pain, and paraesthesia at wound site; furious (70%) and paralytic (30%) forms
- Animals: Direct fluorescent antibody (dFA) test (gold standard)
- Antemortem testing in humans: Saliva (culture, RT-PCR), CSF/serum (serology), neck biopsy (RT-PCR, IF)
- Prevention: Rabies vaccine; monitor titre with rapid fluorescent focus inhibition test
- Prophylaxis: Wound treatment, vaccine, ± immunoglobulin

MICROSCOPIC

- Mild leptomeningeal and perivascular lymphocytic inflammatory infiltrate, neuronophagia, and microglial nodules (Babès nodules)
- Cytoplasmic Negri bodies (not required for diagnosis)
- Antirabies virus IHC (available at some reference laboratories)

TOP DIFFERENTIAL DIAGNOSES

- Other infectious causes of encephalitis
  - Arboviruses, measles virus, Nipah virus
    - May have cytoplasmic, Negri body-like inclusions (measles/Nipah)
    - Lack of detection of rabies viral antigen by immunofluorescent staining or nucleic acids
    - Prolonged clinical stability or improvement
- Guillain-Barré syndrome: Lack of detection of viral antigen or nucleic acids; sensory involvement, lack of fever, absence of encephalitic signs

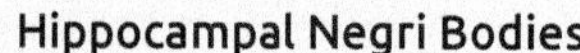

Hippocampal Negri Bodies

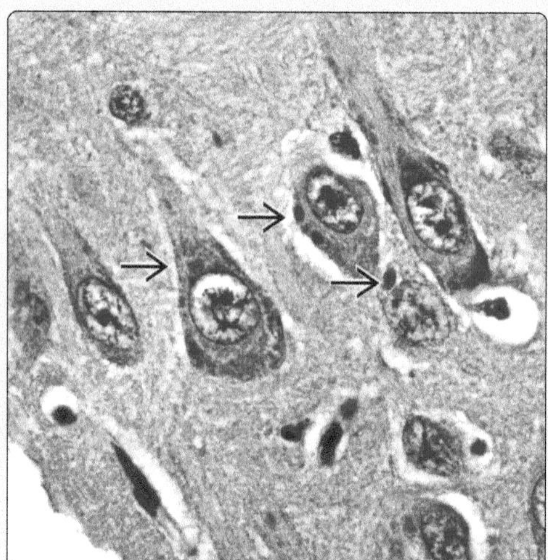

Ultrastructural Features

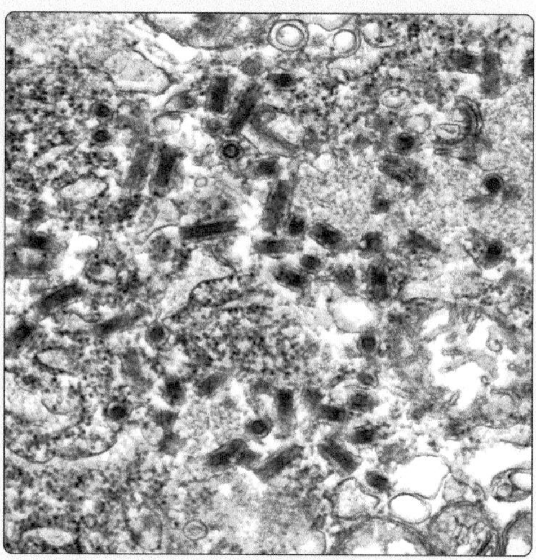

(Left) *Hippocampal pyramidal neurons from a raccoon contain Negri bodies ⇒, pathognomonic cytoplasmic eosinophilic inclusions characteristic (but not required for diagnosis) of rabies encephalitis.* **(Right)** *Rabies virus particles have a bullet-shaped morphology seen on thin-section electron microscopy. (Courtesy G. Nielsen, MD.)*

Purkinje Cell Negri Bodies

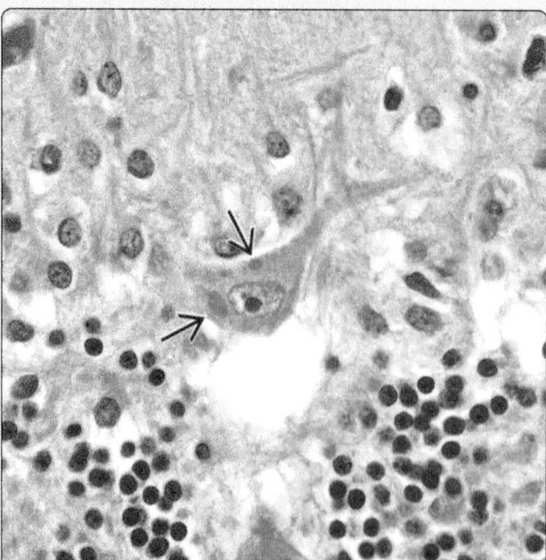

Microglial Nodule

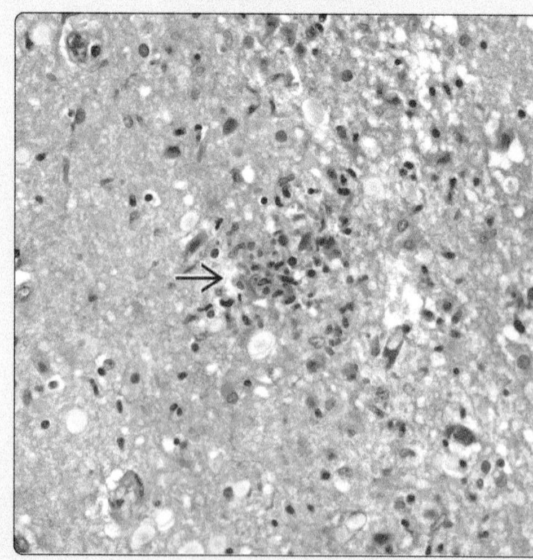

(Left) *Eosinophilic cytoplasmic Negri bodies ⇒ are present in a cerebellar Purkinje cell from a lethal case of rabies.* **(Right)** *A microglial reaction to nerve cell necrosis ⇒ is present in rabies encephalitis, also referred to as a Babès nodules.*

TERMINOLOGY

Synonyms

- *Rabies lyssavirus*; rabies virus (RV)

Definitions

- Derived from Latin "rabies" (rage, madness)
- Lyssavirus genus: Derived from "Lyssa" (Greek goddess of madness, rage, and frenzy)
- *Rhabdoviridae* family: Derived from "rhabdos" (rod)

ETIOLOGY/PATHOGENESIS

Infectious Agents

- Zoonotic viral infection transmitted by bites from infected animals (dogs > bats > other mammals)
- Virus replicates in muscle, spreads from peripheral nerves to central nervous system by retrograde axonal transport, then to salivary glands and other organs (incubation period: 1-3 months; longer with more distal bites)

CLINICAL ISSUES

Epidemiology

- 59,000 deaths per year (primarily Asia and Africa)
- Most common in children < 15 years of age

Site

- Skin, muscle, central nervous system

Presentation

- Initial symptoms of fever and pain and paraesthesia at wound site, early onset of autonomic dysfunction (often overlooked), and excess salivation may be evident
- Furious rabies (70%): Hyperactivity, excited behavior, hydrophobia, and aerophobia with progression to death by cardiorespiratory arrest (days)
- Paralytic rabies (30%): Gradual muscle paralysis starting at wound site, coma development, and eventual death (more prolonged time course)

Laboratory Tests

- Direct fluorescent antibody (dFA) test (brain tissue)
- RT-PCR (saliva, skin biopsy)
- Antibodies (serum, CSF)
- Animal testing performed by public health services

Natural History

- Progressive fatal inflammation of brain and spinal cord

Treatment

- Primary prevention
  - Human diploid cell vaccine (HDCV) or purified chick embryo cell vaccine (PCECV)
  - Rapid fluorescent focus inhibition test (RFFIT) for RV neutralizing antibody serum level
- Postexposure prophylaxis
  - Local treatment of wound (i.e., soap and water, detergent, or povidone iodine)
  - Nonimmunized: Human rabies immune globulin (HRIG) and HDCV or PCECV
  - Previously Immunized: HDCV or PCECV
- Presentation with symptoms
  - Palliative therapy
  - Aggressive therapy with rare survival (i.e., rabies vaccine, HRIG, ribavirin, IFN-α, and ketamine)

Prognosis

- Typically fatal once symptoms develop

MICROBIOLOGY

Virus Features

- Enveloped, single-stranded, RNA virus
- Bullet shape 180 nm x 75 nm, helical nucleocapsid
- 11,600-12,000 nucleotide genome (5 genes)

Culture

- Virus detectable by immunofluorescence in mouse neuroblastoma cells (MNA) or baby hamster kidney (BHK) cells 5 hours to 5 days post inoculation

MICROSCOPIC

Histologic Features

- Leptomeningeal and perivascular lymphocytic inflammatory infiltrate (often mild)
- Neuronophagia and microglial nodules (Babès nodules)

Cytologic Features

- Negri bodies: Eosinophilic cytoplasmic inclusions (2-10 μm) in neurons (not required for diagnosis)
  - Magenta with Mann, Giemsa, and Sellers stains with basophilic interior granules

ANCILLARY TESTS

Immunohistochemistry

- Anti-RV antibodies (nucleocapsid)

Electron Microscopy

- Bullet-shaped virions; Negri bodies with budding virus

DIFFERENTIAL DIAGNOSIS

Other Infectious Causes of Encephalitis

- Arboviruses, measles virus, Nipah virus
  - May have cytoplasmic, Negri body-like inclusions (measles/Nipah)
  - Lack of detection of rabies viral antigen by immunofluorescent staining or nucleic acids
  - Prolonged clinical stability or improvement

Guillain-Barré Syndrome

- Lack of detection of viral antigen or nucleic acids
- Sensory involvement, lack of fever, absence of encephalitic signs

SELECTED REFERENCES

1. Centers for Disease Control and Prevention. Rabies. Updated December 8, 2022. Reviewed February 3, 2023. Accessed February 3, 2023. www.cdc.gov/rabies
2. Nadin-Davis SA et al: Ampliseq for illumina technology enables detailed molecular epidemiology of rabies lyssaviruses from infected formalin-fixed paraffin-embedded tissues. Viruses. 14(10), 2022
3. Whitehouse ER et al: Human rabies despite post-exposure prophylaxis: a systematic review of fatal breakthrough infections after zoonotic exposures. Lancet Infect Dis. 23(5):e167-74, 2022
4. Fisher CR et al: The spread and evolution of rabies virus: conquering new frontiers. Nat Rev Microbiol. 16(4):241-55, 2018
5. Fooks AR et al: Rabies. Nat Rev Dis Primers. 3:17091, 2017

Lymphocytic Choriomeningitis Virus Infection

KEY FACTS

ETIOLOGY/PATHOGENESIS

- Viral infection transmitted by exposure to infected rodents (predominantly *Mus musculus*), during pregnancy, or through solid organ transplantation

CLINICAL ISSUES

- Human seroprevalence is 2-5%
- Biphasic febrile illness (8-13 days incubation): Flu-like symptoms (3-5 days), recovery (~ 4 days), then fever, meningitis, &/or encephalitis
- CSF: ↑ protein, ↑ WBC, ↓ glucose
- Self-limited (mortality < 1%); fetal loss and birth defects common; high mortality in solid organ transplants

MICROSCOPIC

- Brain: Predominantly lymphohistiocytic infiltrate involving meninges, choroid plexus, and ependyma, cerebromalacia, glial proliferation, and perivascular edema
- Fetus: Lymphocytic myocarditis, extramedullary hematopoiesis

ANCILLARY TESTS

- IHC highlights infected neurons as well as various cell types in transplanted organs

TOP DIFFERENTIAL DIAGNOSES

- Viral infections with aseptic meningitis
  - e.g., enteroviruses, herpes simplex, mumps, HIV, arboviruses, measles, parainfluenza, adenovirus, varicella, Epstein-Barr, cytomegalovirus, influenza, rubella, rotavirus
    - Confirmation by histology, IHC, serology, or PCR
- Perinatal infections with congenital malformations (TORCH infections)
  - e.g., toxoplasmosis, cytomegalovirus, herpes simplex, varicella, syphilis, mumps, parvovirus, HIV
    - Confirmation by histology, IHC, serology, or PCR

Ultrastructural Features

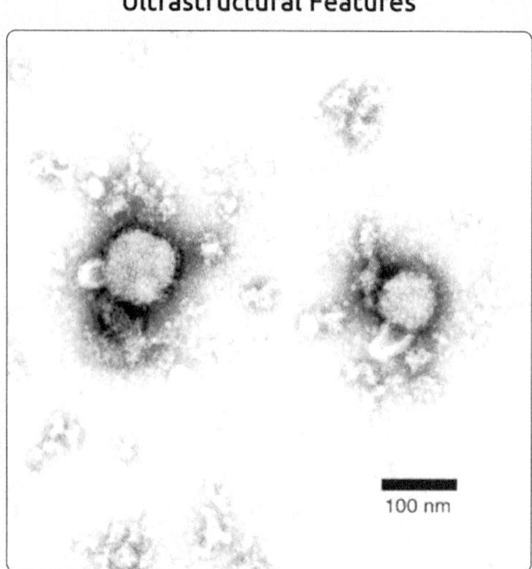

Lung From LCMV-Infected Donor

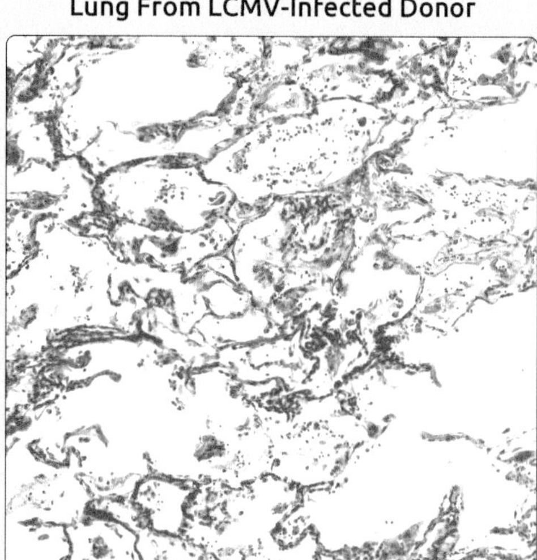

(Left) *This electron micrograph shows spherical virions measuring ~ 100 nm in diameter with envelope spikes, projections, and sandy viral inclusions, characteristic of lymphocytic choriomeningitis virus infection (LCMV). (Courtesy E. Foster, MD.)* **(Right)** *This section of transplanted lung from an asymptomatic LCMV-infected donor shows exudative diffuse alveolar damage, and the presence of a viral antigen was confirmed by IHC.*

Perivascular Inflammation

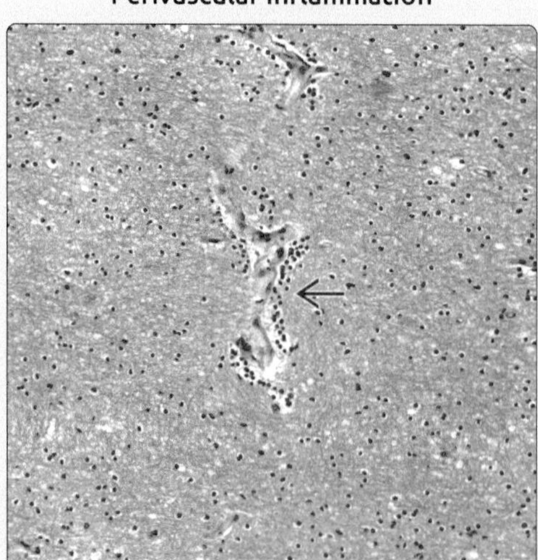

Leptomeningeal Inflammation

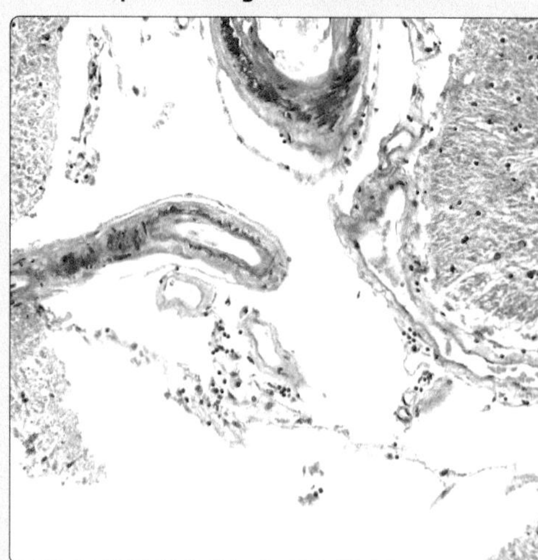

(Left) *This section from a fatal case of LCMV infection transmitted through a lung transplantation shows a mild perivascular, predominantly lymphocytic pattern of inflammation ⇒, consistent with a mild encephalitis.* **(Right)** *Only scant lymphocytic meningeal inflammation is present in a section from a fatal case of LCMV transmitted by lung transplantation.*

TERMINOLOGY

Synonyms

- *Lymphocytic choriomeningitis mammarenavirus* (LCMV)

Definitions

- *Arenaviridae* family: Derived from "arena" (sand), describing grainy particles (ribosomes) seen by electron microscopy

ETIOLOGY/PATHOGENESIS

Infectious Agents

- Viral infection transmitted by exposure to fresh urine, droppings, saliva, or nesting materials from infected rodents (incubation period: 8-13 days)
- Virus can also be transmitted from mother to fetus during pregnancy and from human to human through solid organ transplant
- Primary viremia with extra-CNS seeding followed by secondary viremia with CNS involvement
- Symptoms due to natural killer cell and cytotoxic T-cell production of interferon and other inflammatory mediators

CLINICAL ISSUES

Epidemiology

- *Mus musculus* (house mouse) is predominant carrier (up to 5% infected)
- Cases reported in Europe, North America, South America, Australia, and Japan
- Prevalence of LCMV antibodies in human population ranges from 2-5%
- Seasonal peak in fall and winter

Site

- Brain, spinal cord

Presentation

- Typically asymptomatic or mild febrile illness
- Biphasic febrile illness
  - Initial phase (3-5 days): Fever, anorexia, headache, myalgia, malaise, nausea, and vomiting
  - Recovery (~ 4 days)
  - Final phase: Fever, meningitis, encephalitis, acute hydrocephalus, myelitis (rare)
- Fetal involvement: Hydrocephalus, ventriculomegaly, chorioretinitis, intracerebral hemorrhage

Laboratory Tests

- CBC: Leukopenia and thrombocytopenia
- CSF: Increased protein and WBC; decreased glucose
- IgM and IgG antibodies (serum, CSF)
- PCR or virus isolation (CSF)

Treatment

- Primary prevention through avoidance of contact with wild mice and precautions when handling pet rodents
- Treatment is supportive; ribavirin used in some cases

Prognosis

- Mortality from meningitis or encephalitis rare (< 1%); permanent neurologic damage may occur
- In utero infection may result in fetal loss (35%) or birth defects (hydrocephalus, chorioretinitis, intellectual disability)
- Infection in transplant recipients often results in death

MICROBIOLOGY

Virus Features

- Enveloped, single-stranded RNA virus
- 60-300 nm in size, with helical nucleocapsid
- 10,600-nucleotide genome

Culture

- Forms plaques in Vero cells after 4 days

MICROSCOPIC

Histologic Features

- Brain: Predominantly lymphohistiocytic infiltrate involving meninges, choroid plexus, and ependyma, cerebromalacia, glial proliferation, and perivascular edema
- Fetus: Lymphocytic myocarditis, extramedullary hematopoiesis
- Transplanted organs may show minimal inflammation

ANCILLARY TESTS

Immunohistochemistry

- Anti-LCMV and anti-Lassa fever virus antibodies (available at some reference laboratories) highlight infected neurons as well as various cell types in transplanted organs

DIFFERENTIAL DIAGNOSIS

Viral Infections With Aseptic Meningitis

- Enteroviruses, herpes simplex, mumps, HIV, arboviruses, measles, parainfluenza, adenovirus, varicella, Epstein-Barr, cytomegalovirus, influenza, rubella, rotavirus
  - Presence of characteristic inclusions or detection by immunohistochemistry, serology, or PCR
  - Negative for LCMV serology, viral protein, or RNA

Perinatal Infections With Congenital Malformations (TORCH Infections)

- Toxoplasmosis, cytomegalovirus, herpes simplex, varicella, syphilis, mumps, parvovirus, HIV
  - Negative for LCMV serology, viral protein, or RNA

SELECTED REFERENCES

1. Sironi M et al: Mammarenavirus genetic diversity and its biological implications. Curr Top Microbiol Immunol. 439:265-303, 2023
2. Pencole L et al: Congenital lymphocytic choriomeningitis virus: a review. Prenat Diagn. 42(8):1059-69, 2022
3. Anesi JA et al: Arenaviruses and West Nile virus in solid organ transplant recipients: Guidelines from the American Society of Transplantation Infectious Diseases Community of Practice. Clin Transplant. 33(9):e13576, 2019
4. Basavaraju SV et al: Encephalitis caused by pathogens transmitted through organ transplants, United States, 2002-2013. Emerg Infect Dis. 20(9):1443-51, 2014
5. Centers for Disease Control and Prevention: Lymphocytic choriomeningitis (LCM). Updated May 6, 2014. Reviewed February 21, 2023. Accessed February 21, 2023. http://www.cdc.gov/vhf/lcm/
6. Macneil A et al: Solid organ transplant-associated lymphocytic choriomeningitis, United States, 2011. Emerg Infect Dis. 18(8):1256-62, 2012
7. Fischer SA et al: Transmission of lymphocytic choriomeningitis virus by organ transplantation. N Engl J Med. 354(21):2235-49, 2006

Measles Virus Infection

KEY FACTS

ETIOLOGY/PATHOGENESIS

- Highly contagious viral infection transmitted by respiratory droplets

CLINICAL ISSUES

- 9 million cases worldwide in 2021 (128,000 deaths)
- Officially eradicated from USA in 2000; outbreaks in unvaccinated (13-1,274 cases/year)
- Prodrome with mild to moderate fever, cough, coryza, conjunctivitis, and Koplik spots; maculopapular rash and high fever (> 40°C)
- Typically self-limited but 1 per 1,000 die from respiratory or neurologic complications; subacute sclerosing panencephalitis after 7-10 years (rare)

MICROSCOPIC

- Histologic features
  - Skin: Spongiotic epidermis with vesiculation; keratinocytes with degenerative changes
  - Lymph nodes: Follicular hyperplasia
  - Lungs: Bronchiolitis, pneumonia, diffuse alveolar damage
  - Brain: Perivascular inflammation, gliosis, loss of neurons; eosinophilic nuclear inclusions
- Cytologic features
  - Eosinophilic cytoplasmic inclusions and intranuclear inclusions with clear halo
  - Warthin-Finkeldey giant cells
- Antimeasles virus IHC (at reference laboratories)

TOP DIFFERENTIAL DIAGNOSES

- Infections presenting with fever and rash [e.g., rubella, scarlet fever (*Streptococcus pyogenes*), erythema infectiosum (parvovirus B19), meningococcemia, typhoid fever, varicella]: Lack of Koplik spots or serum measles IgM
- Giant cell-associated viral infections (e.g., cytomegalovirus, herpes simplex virus, varicella-zoster virus, respiratory syncytial virus human parainfluenza viruses): Lack of staining by antimeasles immunohistochemistry

Measles Rash

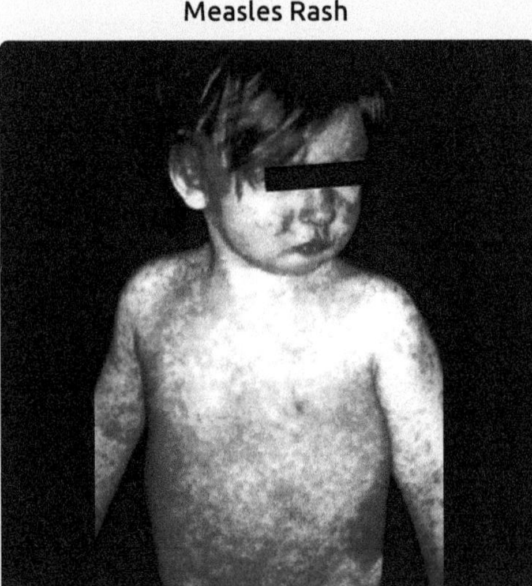

Ultrastructural Features

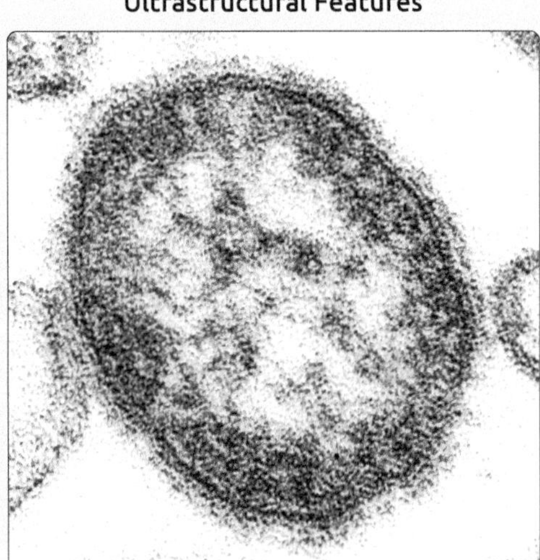

(Left) *Clinical photograph shows the characteristic maculopapular rash of measles, which appeared on the 4th day of infection and spread from the face to involve the neck, trunk, and arms. (Courtesy B. Rice, CDC PHIL.)* **(Right)** *Transmission electron micrograph shows an enveloped virion measuring 100-200 nm in diameter, characteristic of the measles virus. (Courtesy C. Goldsmith, CDC PHIL.)*

Measles Pneumonia

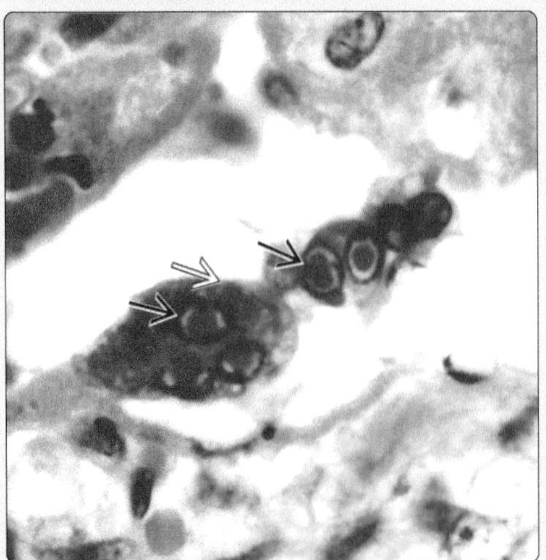

Subacute Sclerosing Panencephalitis

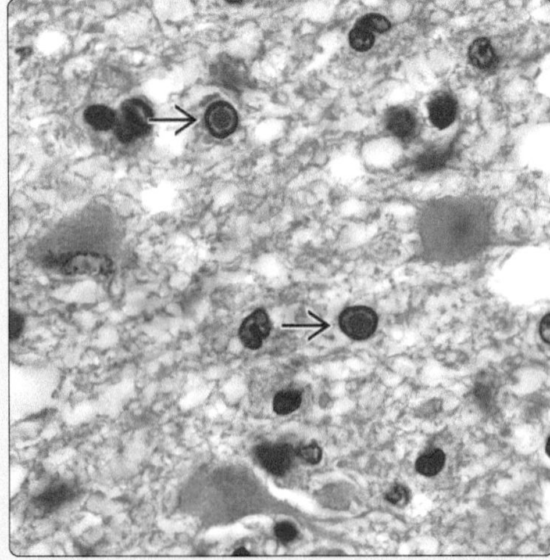

(Left) *This section of a lung autopsy shows multinucleated cells containing eosinophilic cytoplasmic ➡ and nuclear ⇨ inclusions with perinuclear halos that are characteristic of measles virus infection.* **(Right)** *Glassy nuclear viral inclusions ⇨ are typical in brain tissue in subacute sclerosing panencephalitis.*

TERMINOLOGY

Synonyms

- Rubeola, morbilli, English measles
- *Measles morbillivirus* (MeV), measles virus (MV)

Definitions

- "Masel" (Middle Dutch): "Pustule"
- *Paramyxoviridae* family: Derived from "para-" (beyond) and "myxo-" (mucus)

ETIOLOGY/PATHOGENESIS

Infectious Agents

- Highly contagious: 90% of nonimmune will become infected when exposed to respiratory droplets
- Infects dendritic cells in alveoli, then lymph node lymphocytes, then hematologic spread to skin, lung, liver, spleen, and brain (incubation period: 7-21 days)
- Cell receptors: CD46 (all nucleated cells) and CD150/signaling lymphocyte activation molecule (SLAM) (activated T and B lymphocytes)
- Contagious period: Duration of rash plus 4 days before and after rash is visible

CLINICAL ISSUES

Epidemiology

- Worldwide: ~ 9 million cases in 2021 (~ 128,000 deaths)
- USA: 13-1,274 cases per year (2010-2022); 3-4 million cases per year (~ 500 deaths) (pre-1963)

Presentation

- Prodrome: Mild to moderate fever, cough, coryza, conjunctivitis, and Koplik spots (pathognomonic) on buccal mucosa
- Maculopapular rash spreading from face to trunk and extremities (14 days after exposure) and high fever (> 40°C)
- Common complications: Otitis media, diarrhea, bronchopneumonia, and laryngotracheobronchitis
- Acute encephalitis (1 per 1,000)
- Subacute sclerosing panencephalitis (SSPE): 7-10 years following infection

Laboratory Tests

- Serology (IgG and IgM)
- Culture from direct tissue sample
- RT-PCR (oropharyngeal, nasal, nasopharyngeal swab; urine)
- Distinguish vaccine strain from wildtype by genotyping

Treatment

- Primary prevention: Measles, mumps, rubella (MMR) vaccine (doses at 12-15 months and 4-6 years)
- Postexposure prophylaxis for nonimmune: MMR (within 72 hours); IgG (< 6 days)
- Active infection: Supportive care

Prognosis

- Symptoms typically resolve after 7-10 days
- 1-2 per 1,000 die from respiratory and neurologic complications; higher risk < 5 or > 20 years old, pregnant women, and immunocompromised
- SSPE: Progressive neurologic decline and death (1-2 years)

MICROBIOLOGY

Virus Features

- Enveloped, single-stranded RNA virus
- 100-300 nm in size with helical nucleocapsid
- 15,894 nucleotides encoding 6 genes (7 proteins)
- 8 clades with 24 genotypes based on hemagglutinin (H) and nucleoprotein (N) gene sequences
- N-450 (nucleoprotein C-terminal 150 amino acid-encoding nucleotides) targeted for genotyping

Culture

- Grows in VERO/hSLAM or B95a cells (1-2 weeks)
- Confirmed by immunofluorescence staining

MACROSCOPIC

Oral Mucosa

- Koplik spots (3 days before rash)

Skin

- Generalized maculopapular erythematous eruption

MICROSCOPIC

Histologic Features

- Skin: Spongiotic epidermis with vesiculation; keratinocytes with degenerative changes
- Lymph nodes: Follicular hyperplasia
- Lungs: Bronchiolitis to pneumonia and diffuse alveolar damage
- Brain: Perivascular inflammation, gliosis, loss of neurons; eosinophilic nuclear inclusions

Cytologic Features

- Eosinophilic cytoplasmic inclusions and intranuclear inclusions with clear halo
- Warthin-Finkeldey giant cells

ANCILLARY TESTS

Immunohistochemistry

- Antimeasles antibodies at some reference laboratories

DIFFERENTIAL DIAGNOSIS

Infections Presenting With Fever and Rash

- Rubella, scarlet fever (*Streptococcus pyogenes*), erythema infectiosum (parvovirus B19), meningococcemia, typhoid fever, varicella
  - Lack of Koplik spots or serum measles IgM

Giant Cell-Associated Viral Infections

- Cytomegalovirus, herpes simplex virus, varicella-zoster virus, respiratory syncytial virus, parainfluenza
  - Lack of staining by antimeasles immunohistochemistry

SELECTED REFERENCES

1. Klassen-Fischer MK et al: The reemergence of measles. Am J Clin Pathol. 159(1):81-8, 2023
2. Minta AA et al: Progress toward regional measles elimination - worldwide, 2000-2021. MMWR Morb Mortal Wkly Rep. 71(47):1489-95, 2022
3. Khetsuriani N et al: High risk of subacute sclerosing panencephalitis following measles outbreaks in Georgia. Clin Microbiol Infect. 26(6):737-42, 2020

Mumps Virus Infection

KEY FACTS

ETIOLOGY/PATHOGENESIS

- Highly contagious virus transmitted through direct contact with respiratory secretions

CLINICAL ISSUES

- Incidence: 154-6,369 cases per year in USA; primarily in outbreaks with peaks in late winter and spring
- Fever, headache, malaise, anorexia, myalgia, parotitis, orchitis, mastitis, meningitis, encephalitis
- Diagnose with RT-PCR (buccal/oral swab, serum), serology (IgM), or culture; biopsy rarely indicated
- Whole-genome sequencing to track outbreaks
- Symptoms typically resolve after 1-2 weeks
- Primary prevention with MMR vaccine

MICROSCOPIC

- Salivary gland: Hemorrhage, necrosis, chronic inflammatory infiltrate
- Testes: Edema, mixed interstitial inflammation and lymphoid aggregation, congestion of tunica vasculosa, necrosis of spermatogenic cells (Sertoli cells spared)

TOP DIFFERENTIAL DIAGNOSES

- Other causes of parotitis
  - Viral infections: Bilateral; lobular architecture maintained; no evidence of mumps
  - Bacterial infections: Unilateral; ascending with adjacent cellulitis; acinar degeneration, mixed inflammation, microabscesses
  - Calculus induced: Unilateral; radiopaque stone in parotid duct
- Other causes of orchitis
  - Ascending genitourinary tract bacterial infections
    - Unilateral, spread from epididymis; improvement with antibiotics; no evidence of mumps

Parotitis

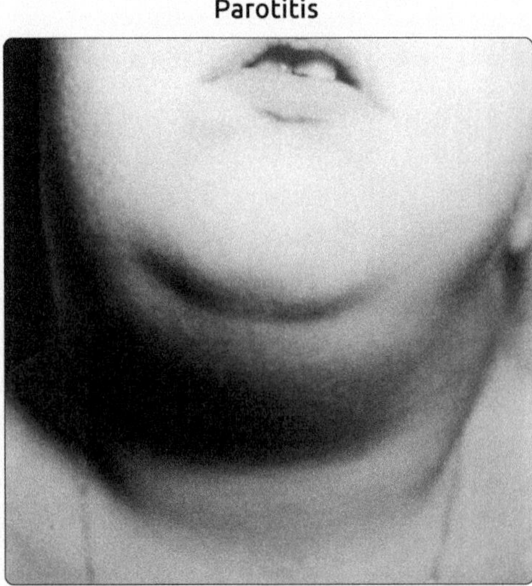

Ultrastructural Features

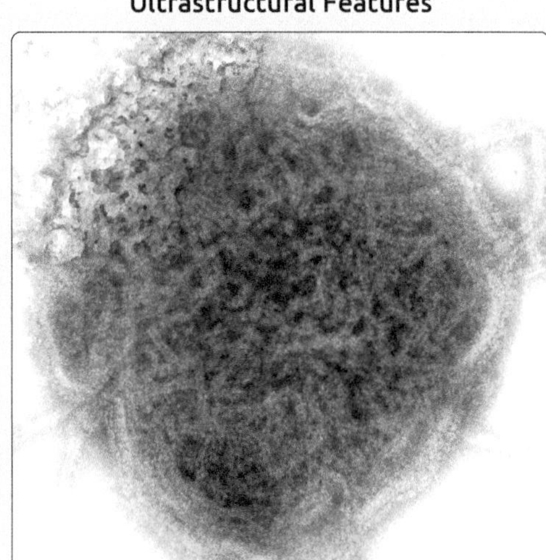

(Left) *This photograph depicts the anterior neck of a young child, which displays the characteristic cervical swelling due to enlargement of the submaxillary salivary glands brought on by a mumps infection. (Courtesy CDC PHIL.)* **(Right)** *This transmission electron micrograph shows an enveloped pleomorphic virion measuring ~ 200 nm in diameter, characteristic of mumps virus. (Courtesy F. Murphy, CDC PHIL.)*

Orchitis

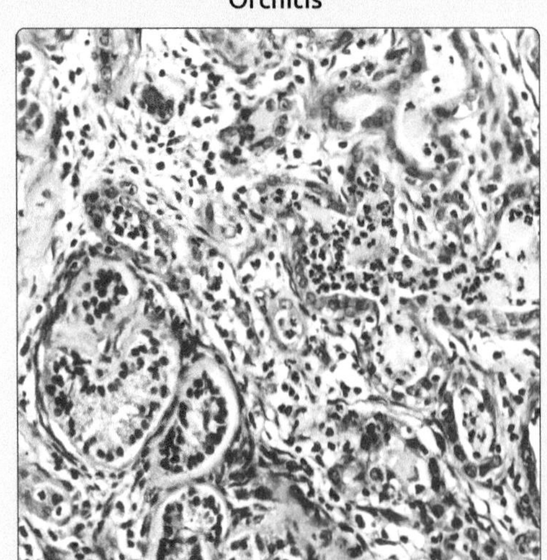

Subpial Demyelination

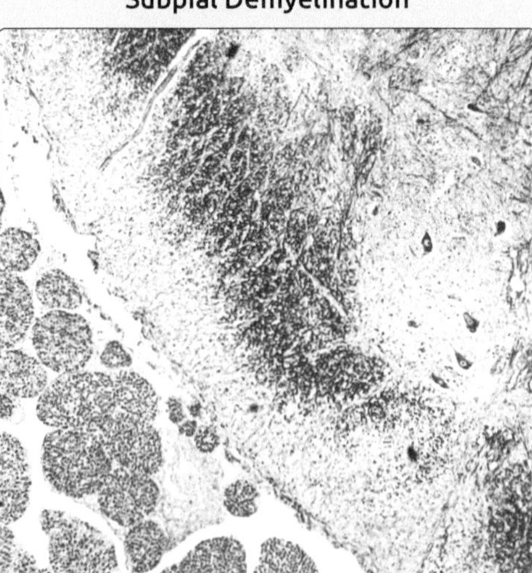

(Left) *Necroinflammatory debris and degeneration of the seminiferous tubules are present in this case of mumps orchitis. (Courtesy L. Rorke-Adams, MD.)* **(Right)** *Luxol fast blue-cresyl violet staining shows subpial demyelination in the spinal cord of a child with mumps. (Courtesy L. Rorke-Adams, MD.)*

Mumps Virus Infection

TERMINOLOGY

Synonyms

- *Mumps orthorubulavirus*, mumps virus (MuV)

Definitions

- *Paramyxoviridae* family: Derived from "para" (beyond) and "myxo" (mucus)
- Mumps from "mump" (grimace; most likely referring to painful difficulty in swallowing)

ETIOLOGY/PATHOGENESIS

Infectious Agents

- Transmitted through direct contact with respiratory secretions
- Virus replicates in upper respiratory tract, regional lymphoid tissue, then systemic dissemination (incubation period: 12-25 days)
- Infectious period: 1-2 days before until 5 days after onset of parotitis

CLINICAL ISSUES

Epidemiology

- USA: 186,000 cases per year (prevaccination era: 1949); 154-6,369 cases per year from 2010 to 2022 (varies with number and severity of outbreaks)
- Occurs year-round with peaks in late winter and spring

Site

- Salivary glands, brain, spinal cord, testicles, ovaries, breasts

Presentation

- Fever, headache, malaise, anorexia, myalgia, swollen salivary glands (parotitis) (30-40%)
- Complications: Orchitis (12-66%), mastitis (31%), meningitis (10%), oophoritis (5%), pancreatitis (3.5%), encephalitis (0.3%), sensorineural hearing loss (1 per 20,000 cases)

Laboratory Tests

- RT-PCR (buccal/oral swab, serum, urine, cerebrospinal fluid)
- Serology (IgM or increased IgG)
- Viral whole-genome sequencing may be needed to track outbreaks and to rule out vaccine strains

Natural History

- Symptoms typically resolve after 1-2 weeks

Treatment

- Primary prevention: MMR vaccine (12-15 months and 4-6 years of age)
- Presentation with symptoms: Symptomatic treatment only

Prognosis

- Typically self-limited
- Permanent neurological sequelae and deaths are rare (1 per 5,000 cases prevaccine)

IMAGING

Parotid

- Enlarged parotid glands with surrounding fat stranding

Testes

- Enlarged, hyperemic testis on color Doppler US

MICROBIOLOGY

Virus Features

- Enveloped, single-stranded RNA virus
- 200 nm in size, helical nucleocapsid
- 15,384 nucleotide genome (7 genes)
- 12 WHO recognized genotypes (A-D, F-L, N)

Culture

- Grow in primary monkey kidney cells and Vero cells
- Detection of virus with immunofluorescent antibody staining or RT-PCR

MICROSCOPIC

Histologic Features

- Salivary gland
  - Hemorrhage, necrosis, chronic inflammatory infiltrate
- Testes
  - Edema, mixed interstitial inflammation and lymphoid aggregation, congestion of tunica vasculosa
  - Necrosis of spermatogenic cells (Sertoli cells spared)

DIFFERENTIAL DIAGNOSIS

Other Causes of Parotitis

- Viral infections (parainfluenza, influenza, Coxsackie A and B, echovirus, lymphocytic choriomeningitis virus)
  - Bilateral; lobular architecture maintained with interstitial subacute infiltrate
  - No detection of mumps antibodies or nucleic acids
- Bacterial infections (*Staphylococcus aureus, Streptococcus, Haemophilus, Escherichia coli*, anaerobes)
  - Typically unilateral; usually due to ascending infection; may result from adjacent cellulitis
  - Acinar degeneration with mixed inflammatory infiltrate; microabscesses with necrotic amorphous debris and neutrophils
- Calculus induced
  - Unilateral with radiopaque stone in parotid duct

Other Causes of Orchitis

- Ascending genitourinary tract infections: *S. aureus, E. coli, Chlamydia, Treponema pallidum, Mycobacterium tuberculosis, Pseudomonas, Klebsiella, Proteus mirabilis*
  - Unilateral; secondary spread from adjacent epididymis
  - Improvement with antibiotics
  - No detection of mumps antibodies or nucleic acids

SELECTED REFERENCES

1. Centers for Disease Control and Prevention: Mumps. Updated January 6, 2023. Reviewed February 1. 2023. Accessed February 1, 2023. https://www.cdc.gov/mumps/outbreaks.html
2. Gokhale DV et al: Disentangling the causes of mumps reemergence in the United States. Proc Natl Acad Sci U S A. 120(3):e2207595120, 2023
3. Bryant P et al: Streamlined whole-genome sequencing of mumps virus for high-resolution outbreak analysis. J Clin Microbiol. 60(1):e0084121, 2022
4. Kubota M et al: Unique tropism and entry mechanism of mumps virus. Viruses. 13(9), 2021
5. Wu H et al: Mumps orchitis: clinical aspects and mechanisms. Front Immunol. 12:582946, 2021

Rubella Virus Infection

KEY FACTS

ETIOLOGY/PATHOGENESIS

- Virus transmitted by respiratory droplets; spreads hematogenously and crosses placenta

CLINICAL ISSUES

- Rare in USA post 2004 eradication
- Light red rash spreads from face to body; low fever, lymphadenopathy
- Perinatal morbidity/mortality decreases with later gestational age at time of maternal infection
- Congenital rubella syndrome (CRS): Deafness, cataracts, and heart defects
- Diagnosis: RT-PCR, serology, or viral culture
- Primary prevention: MMR vaccine

MICROSCOPIC

- Placenta: Noninflammatory necrosis in epithelium of chorion and in endothelial cells; immature villous pattern with villous hypoplasia
- Infant/fetus: Necrotizing chorioretinitis, myocardial necrosis, interstitial pneumonitis, swelling and vacuolization of liver cells, chronic inflammation of leptomeninges, lung, and uveal tract of eye
- Blueberry muffin lesion: Foci of erythrocyte precursors within dermis and subcutis

TOP DIFFERENTIAL DIAGNOSES

- Infections presenting with fever and rash
  - Measles, scarlet fever (*Streptococcus pyogenes*), erythema infectiosum (parvovirus B19), meningococcemia, typhoid fever, varicella
    - Negative for rubella serology, viral protein or RNA
- Perinatal infections presenting with rash and ocular findings (TORCH infections)
  - Toxoplasmosis, cytomegalovirus, herpes simplex, varicella, syphilis, mumps, parvovirus, HIV
    - Negative for rubella serology, viral protein, or RNA

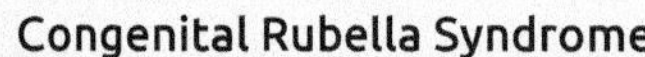

Congenital Rubella Syndrome

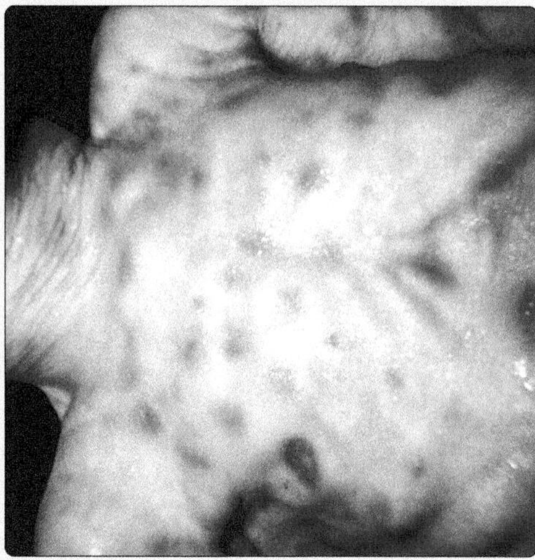

Ultrastructural Features

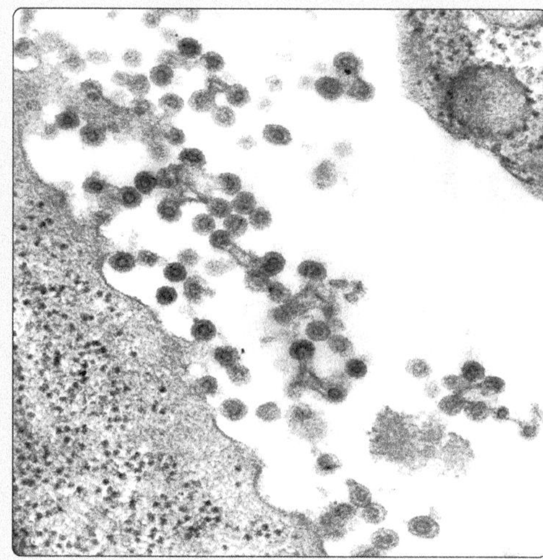

(Left) *"Blueberry muffin" lesions consist of foci of erythrocyte precursors within the dermis and subcutis and are characteristic of infants with congenital rubella syndrome. (Courtesy L. Rorke-Adams, MD.)* **(Right)** *This transmission electron micrograph shows multiple spherical enveloped virions, measuring 50-70 nm in diameter, budding from the host cell surface, characteristic of rubella virus. (Courtesy F. Murphy, CDC PHIL.)*

Cataracts

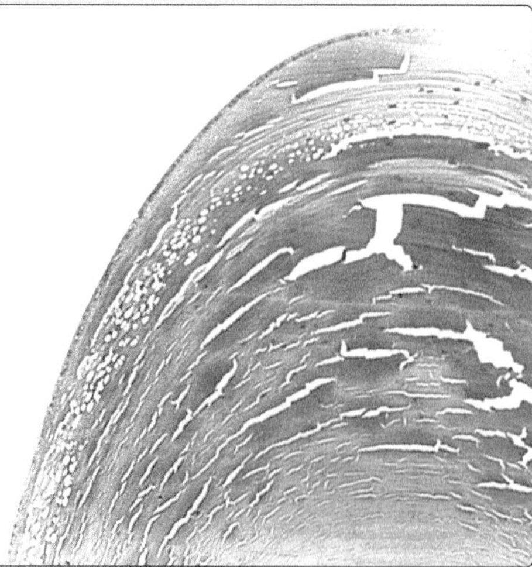

Brain Lesions

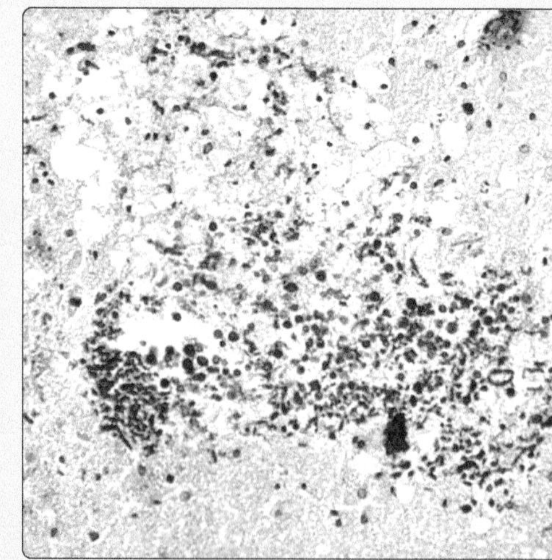

(Left) *Sensorineural deafness, heart defects, and nuclear cataracts (shown here) are typical features of congenital rubella syndrome. [Courtesy H. Wainwright, MBChB, FFPath (SA).]* **(Right)** *Focal necrosis is present in the centrum semiovale in congenital rubella syndrome. (Courtesy L. Rorke-Adams, MD.)*

TERMINOLOGY

Synonyms

- German measles; 3-day measles
- *Rubivirus rubellae;* rubella virus (RuV)

Definitions

- Rubella: Derived from Latin ("little red")
- *Matonaviridae* family: Named after George de Maton, who first distinguished rubella from measles and scarlet fever

ETIOLOGY/PATHOGENESIS

Infectious Agents

- Virus transmitted by respiratory droplets, replicates in nasopharynx and lymph nodes, and spreads hematogenously
- Incubation period: 12-23 days
- Contagious period: From 7 days before until 7 days after appearance of rash
- Virus crosses placenta, then kills or prevents replication of cells (risk decreases with increasing gestational age at time of maternal infection)

CLINICAL ISSUES

Epidemiology

- Mostly affects children 5-9 years old; peaks in spring; epidemics every 6-9 years
- USA: 12.5 million cases (1964-1965 epidemic) with 11,250 therapeutic or spontaneous abortions; 2,100 neonatal deaths; and 20,000 infants with congenital rubella syndrome (CRS); currently < 10 cases reported/year
- Worldwide: 100,000 infants with CRS annually

Site

- Skin, respiratory tract, lymph nodes

Presentation

- Children: Pink or light red rash that begins in face and spreads to rest of body (fades after 3 days), low fever (< 38.3°C), posterior cervical lymphadenopathy
- Adults: Prodrome of low-grade fever, headache, malaise, mild coryza, and conjunctivitis; arthralgia or arthritis (70% of women)
- Neonates: Miscarriage, fetal death/stillbirth, and "blueberry muffin" skin lesions
- CRS: Sensorineural deafness, cataracts, heart defects (patent ductus arteriosus, interventricular septal defects, and pulmonic stenosis)

Laboratory Tests

- RT-PCR: Oropharyngeal/nasopharyngeal swab, urine, blood, CSF, amniotic fluid
- Molecular genotyping to track source of infection (E1 protein coding region, nucleotides 8731-9469)
- IgM detectable 4-30 days after onset of rash; false-positives due to rheumatoid factors
- IgG detectable ~ 8 days after infection; increased levels in 2nd specimen or low avidity indicates recent infection
- Culture: Can be used to rule out infectivity in CRS patients

Natural History

- Mild, self-limited infection; often asymptomatic
- CRS patients may shed virus for up to 1 year after birth

Treatment

- Primary prevention: Measles, mumps, rubella (MMR) vaccine; screening recommended prior to conception
- Active infection: Supportive therapy
- Congenital infection: Management of complications

Prognosis

- Acquired: Complete recovery
- Congenital: Varies with severity of complications; neurologic symptoms typically permanent

MICROBIOLOGY

Virus Features

- Single-stranded, positive-sense RNA virus
- 50- to 70-nm enveloped icosahedral capsid
- 9,762 bp genome (5 proteins)
- 13 genotypes recognized in 2 clades (1A-J, 2A-C)

Culture

- Immunofluorescence in Vero cells (1-2 weeks)

MACROSCOPIC

Skin

- Generalized maculopapular erythematous eruption

MICROSCOPIC

Histologic Features

- Placenta: Noninflammatory necrosis in epithelium of chorion and in endothelial cells; immature villous pattern with villous hypoplasia
- Infant/fetus: Necrotizing chorioretinitis, myocardial necrosis, interstitial pneumonitis, swelling and vacuolization of liver cells, chronic inflammation of leptomeninges, lung, and uveal tract of eye
- "Blueberry muffin" lesion: Foci of erythrocyte precursors within dermis and subcutis

DIFFERENTIAL DIAGNOSIS

Infections Presenting With Fever and Rash

- Measles, scarlet fever (*Streptococcus pyogenes*), erythema infectiosum (parvovirus B19), meningococcemia, typhoid fever, varicella
  - Negative for rubella serology, viral protein or RNA

Perinatal Infections Presenting With Rash and Ocular Findings (TORCH Infections)

- Toxoplasmosis, cytomegalovirus, herpes simplex, varicella, syphilis, mumps, parvovirus, HIV
  - Negative for rubella serology, viral protein, or RNA

SELECTED REFERENCES

1. Winter AK et al: Rubella. Lancet. 399(10332):1336-46, 2022
2. Zimmerman LA et al: Progress toward rubella and congenital rubella syndrome control and elimination - worldwide, 2012-2020. MMWR Morb Mortal Wkly Rep. 71(6):196-201, 2022
3. Centers for Disease Control and Prevention: Rubella (German measles, three-day measles). Updated December 31, 2020. Reviewed February 1, 2023. Accessed February 1, 2023. http://www.cdc.gov/rubella
4. Bouthry E et al: Rubella and pregnancy: diagnosis, management and outcomes. Prenat Diagn. 34(13):1246-53, 2014

Human Immunodeficiency Virus Infection

KEY FACTS

ETIOLOGY/PATHOGENESIS

- HIV-1/HIV-2 spread via sexual contact, contaminated blood and needles, or from mother to child
- AIDS leads to opportunistic infections and cancers

CLINICAL ISSUES

- Primary HIV infection: 50% of patients report fever, lethargy, fatigue, rash, myalgias, and headache
- PCR for diagnosis (qualitative) or viral load (quantitative) predicts long-term prognosis
- Highly active antiretroviral therapy (HAART) tailored to virus genotype and viral load; preexposure prophylaxis (PrEP) highly effective in preventing infection

MICROSCOPIC

- Persistent lymphadenopathy: Florid lymphoid hyperplasia of lymph nodes with prominent germinal centers
- HIV encephalitis: Perivascular microglial nodules, p24(+) multinucleated giant cells, focal necrosis
- HIV-associated nephropathy: Focal segmental glomerulosclerosis, segmental and global collapse of capillaries, hypertrophy and hyperplasia of podocytes, and tubulointerstitial disease
- Opportunistic infections: Wide range of organisms; inflammation may be absent to severe

TOP DIFFERENTIAL DIAGNOSES

- Overlap with primary infection: Syphilis (rash), EBV mononucleosis, CMV mononucleosis-like disease (mono), enteroviral meningitis (meningitis)
- Other causes of lymphadenopathy: Lymphoma/leukemia (clonal proliferation; EBV or HHV8), cat-scratch disease [stellate necrosis; gram(-) bacilli]
- Other causes of nephropathy: Similar changes with parvovirus B19 and pamidronate
- Other causes of encephalitis: Specific virus identified by VCPE, IHC, serology, or molecular testing; autoimmune/paraneoplastic

(Left) *This transmission electron micrographic image reveals the presence of multiple 100-nm diameter, enveloped virions of the HIV in a tissue sample. (Courtesy A. Harrison, P. Feorino; E. Palmer, CDC/PHIL.)* **(Right)** *Malignancy associated with an HIV infection is a continuing problem despite the wide availability of HAART. Cervical cancer secondary to HPV infection (seen here with p16 staining) ➡ is a major challenge in low- and middle-income countries. (From DP: Molecular Oncology.)*

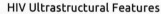

HIV Ultrastructural Features

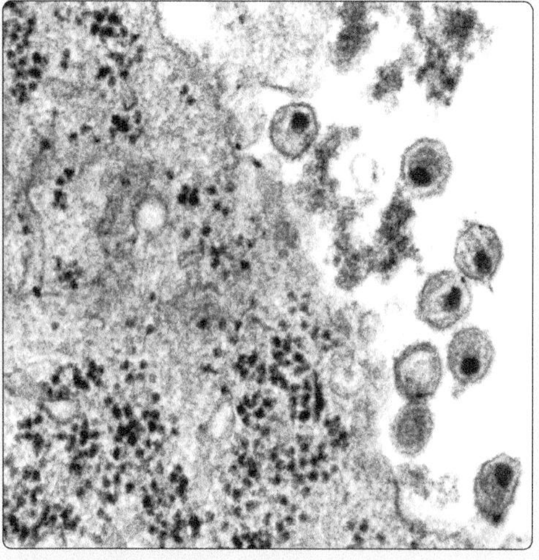

HIV-Related Cancers

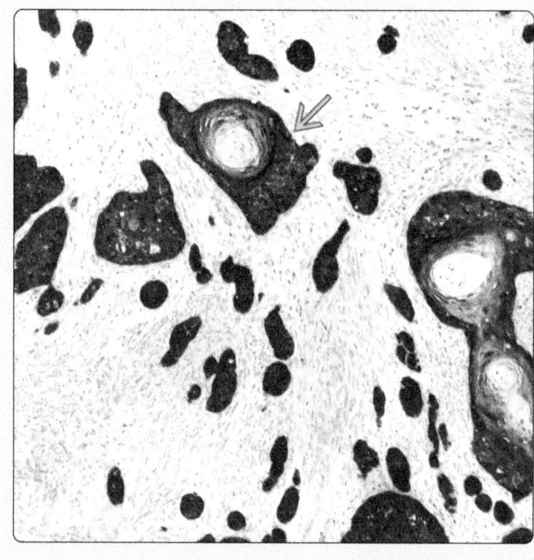

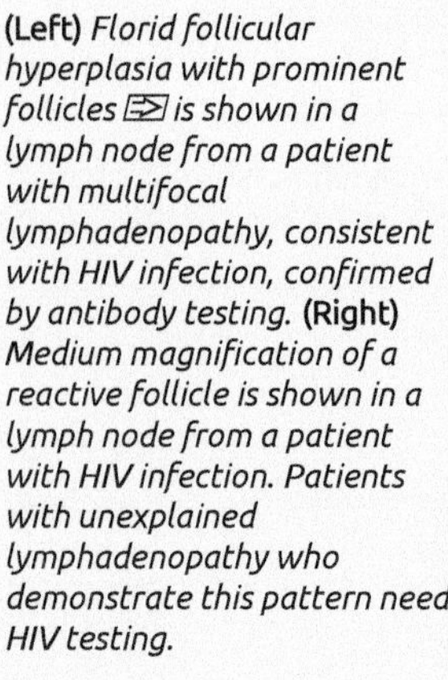

(Left) *Florid follicular hyperplasia with prominent follicles ➡ is shown in a lymph node from a patient with multifocal lymphadenopathy, consistent with HIV infection, confirmed by antibody testing.* **(Right)** *Medium magnification of a reactive follicle is shown in a lymph node from a patient with HIV infection. Patients with unexplained lymphadenopathy who demonstrate this pattern need HIV testing.*

HIV Lymphadenopathy

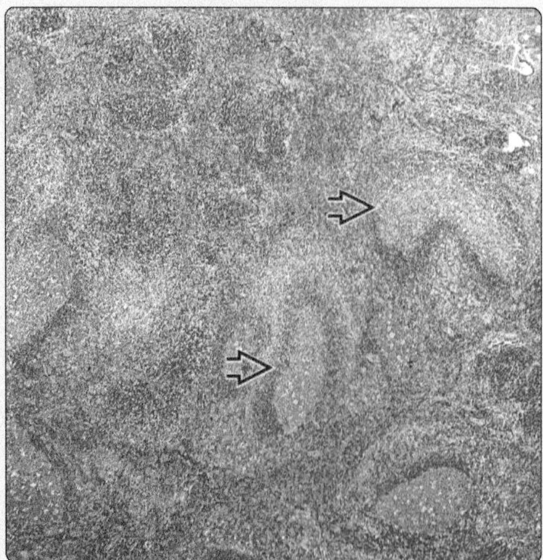

HIV Lymphadenopathy

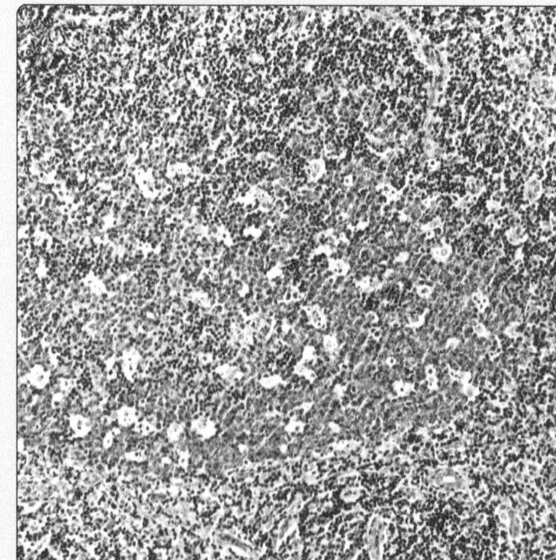

TERMINOLOGY

Definitions

- *Human immunodeficiency virus 1* (HIV-1) and HIV-2
- *Lentivirus* genus derived from Latin "lentus" (slow)
- *Retroviridae* family derived from Latin "retro" (backwards) referring to reverse transcriptase

ETIOLOGY/PATHOGENESIS

Infectious Agents

- Infection with with HIV-1/HIV-2 spread via sexual contact, contaminated blood and needles, or from mother to child
- Virus infects CD4(+) T cells and macrophages/microglia; RNA genome is converted to DNA provirus
- AIDS develops with severe cell-mediated immunodeficiency and consequent opportunistic infections and cancers

CLINICAL ISSUES

Epidemiology

- Estimated > 80 million people have been infected with > 33 million associated deaths
- HIV-1 most common worldwide (B type); HIV-2 more limited geography with less severe disease in AIDS

Presentation

- Primary HIV infection: 50% of patients report fever, lethargy, fatigue, rash, myalgias, and headache
- Latent phase: Patient remains asymptomatic [variable viral load (VL) and CD4 count]; may present with persistent lymphadenopathy, HIV encephalitis, or HIV-associated nephropathy
- AIDS: Uncontrolled VL, low CD4 count, opportunistic infections

Laboratory Tests

- HIV serologic antibodies for primary diagnosis
- Traditionally confirmed by Western blot
- PCR for diagnosis (qualitative) or VL (quantitative; blood, CSF) predicts long-term prognosis
- CD4 count to stage immune system

Treatment

- Highly active antiretroviral therapy (HAART) tailored to virus genotype and VL; reactivation will occur following cessation of HAART
- No FDA-licensed vaccine available
- Preexposure prophylaxis (PrEP) highly effective

Prognosis

- With HAART therapy, excellent long-term prognosis
- Immune restoration inflammatory syndrome (IRIS) may occur following initiation of antiretroviral treatment
- Mechanisms underlying accelerated aging and HIV-associated neurocognitive disorders (HAND) unclear (HIV effect vs. HAART effect)

MICROBIOLOGY

Virus Characteristics

- Enveloped, single-stranded RNA retrovirus
- 100-nm diameter, icosahedral capsid
- 9,700 nucleotide genome, 3 open reading frames (ORFs) (*gag, env, pol*)

Culture

- Phytohemagglutinin-stimulated peripheral blood mononuclear cells from seronegative donors

MICROSCOPIC

Histologic Features

- Persistent lymphadenopathy: Florid lymphoid hyperplasia of lymph nodes with prominent germinal centers
- Lymphoid tissues progress from hyperplasia to involution to atrophy
- HIV encephalitis: Microglial nodules in/around vessels with multinucleated giant cells [p24 IHC(+)], focal necrosis
- HIV-CD8 encephalitis: Dense infiltrate of CD8 lymphocytes; p24 IHC(-) and no multinucleated giant cells
- HIV-associated nephropathy: Focal segmental glomerulosclerosis with segmental and global collapse of capillaries, hypertrophy and hyperplasia of podocytes, and tubulointerstitial disease
- > 150 known opportunistic infections/complications
  - MTB, *Mycobacterium avium* complex, *Salmonella* sepsis
  - Cryptococcosis, *Pneumocystis* pneumonia, candidiasis, histoplasmosis, coccidioidomycosis
  - Progressive multifocal leukoencephalopathy (polyomavirus), Kaposi sarcoma, herpes simplex, herpes zoster, hairy leukoplakia, CMV, human papillomavirus-related cancers, EBV-related lymphomas
  - Toxoplasmosis, malaria, cryptosporidiosis, cystoisosporiasis

DIFFERENTIAL DIAGNOSIS

Overlap With Primary HIV Infection Symptoms

- Syphilis (rash), EBV mononucleosis, CMV mononucleosis-like disease (mono), enteroviral meningitis (meningitis)

Other Causes of Lymphadenopathy

- Lymphoma/leukemia: Clonal proliferation; EBV or HHV8
- Cat-scratch disease: Stellate necrosis late; bacilli stain with Warthin-Starry or IHC

Other Causes of Nephropathy

- Similar histologic changes seen in parvovirus B19 infection and pamidronate treatment

Other Causes of Encephalitis

- Specific viral infections confirmed by VCPE, IHC, serology, or molecular testing
- Autoimmune/paraneoplastic encephalitis may appear similar to CD8 encephalitis; serum/CSF antibodies

SELECTED REFERENCES

1. Lucas S: Historical and current issues in HIV encephalitis, and the role of neuropathology in HIV disease: a pathological perspective. J Neurol. 270(3):1337-45, 2022
2. Sneller MC et al: Combination anti-HIV antibodies provide sustained virological suppression. Nature. 606(7913):375-81, 2022
3. Fauci AS et al: Four decades of HIV/AIDS - much accomplished, much to do. N Engl J Med. 383(1):1-4, 2020
4. Nelson AM et al: Immune reconstitution inflammatory syndrome (IRIS): what pathologists should know. Semin Diagn Pathol. 34(4):340-51, 2017
5. Lucas S et al: HIV and the spectrum of human disease. J Pathol. 235(2):229-41, 2015

(Left) *A section of brain tissue from a patient with HIV encephalitis demonstrates perivascular inflammation and microglial nodule formation.* **(Right)** *A section of brain tissue from a patient with HIV encephalitis demonstrates perivascular giant cells, which are the hallmark of the disease.*

HIV Encephalitis

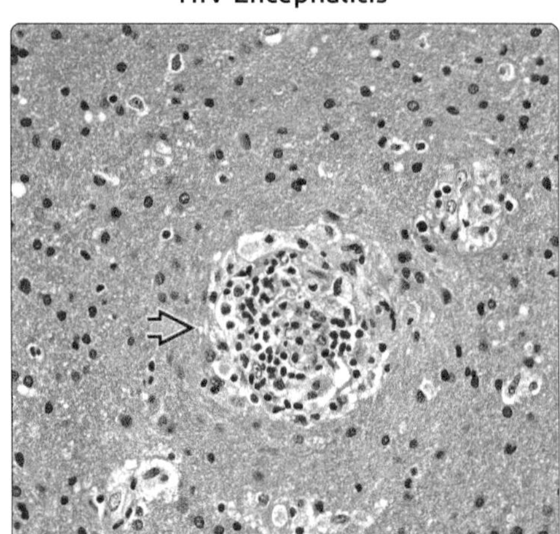

Giant Cells: HIV Encephalitis

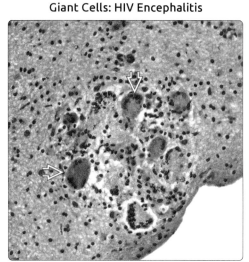

(Left) *An IHC stain for HIV p24 antigen shows the giant cells of HIV encephalitis to be diffusely positive for the protein.* **(Right)** *A single acid-fast bacillus within a giant cell is shown from a case of tuberculosis (TB). TB affects both HIV-positive and HIV-negative patients but has a higher mortality in the former.*

HIV Encephalitis: p24 IHC

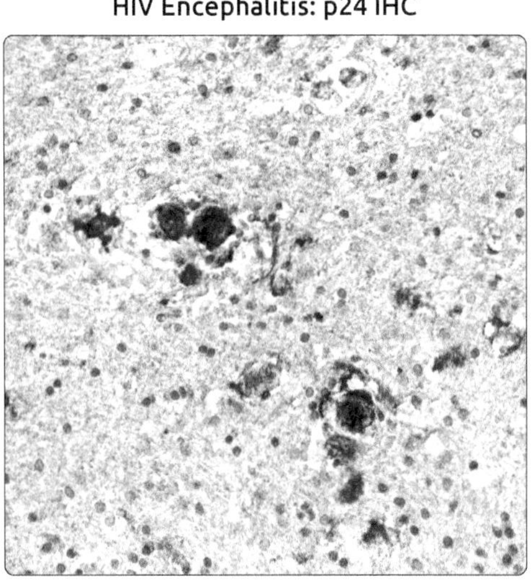

Tuberculosis in HIV Infection

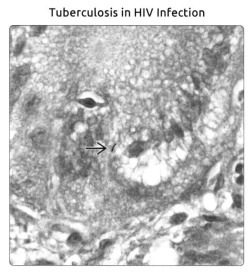

(Left) *A small bowel biopsy demonstrates cryptosporidiosis, which causes watery diarrhea in untreated HIV patients. Note the lack of inflammation and subtle intracytoplasmic surface coccidian parasites.* **(Right)** *A large cryptococcoma caused by Cryptococcus neoformans, which presented as a large abdominal mass in an undiagnosed HIV patient, is shown with sheets of fungi spaced by the mucoid capsule and no inflammation. The patient died within days of surgery.*

Cryptosporidium in HIV Infection

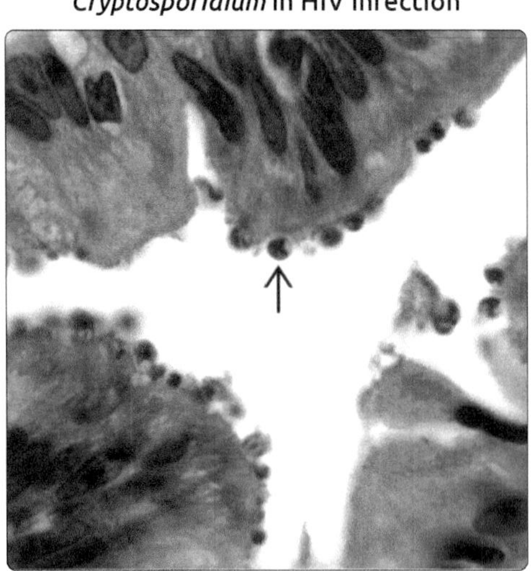

Cryptococcus in HIV Infection

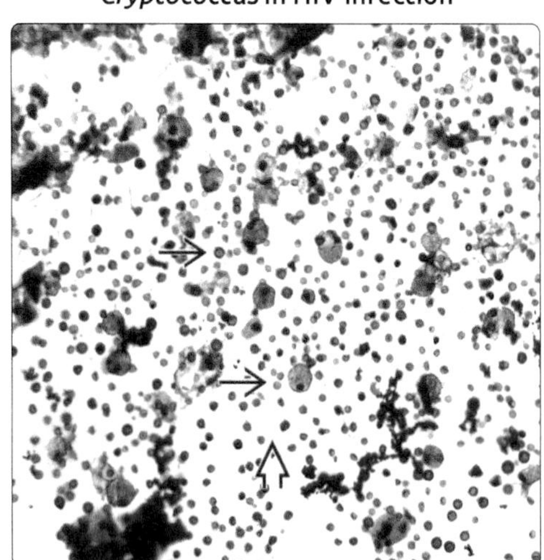

Candida in HIV Infection

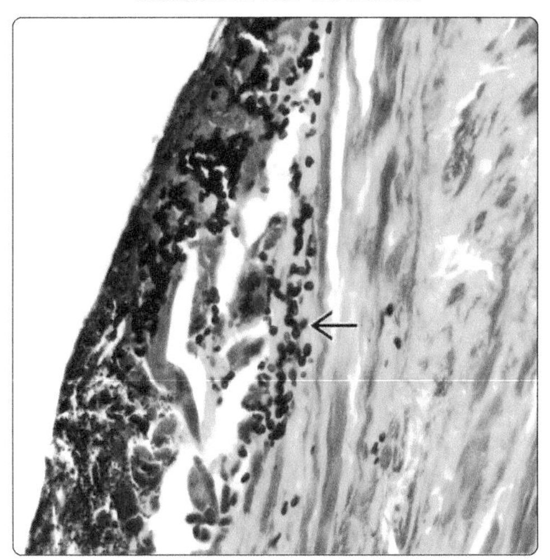

Kaposi Sarcoma in HIV Infection

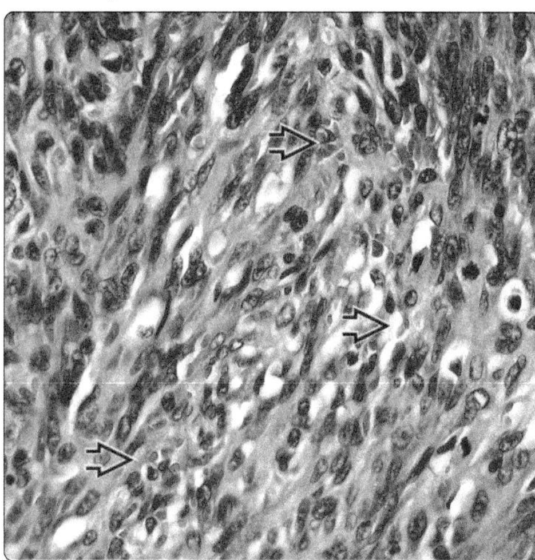

(Left) *Candida infections (most commonly Candida albicans ➡) can occur in HIV-infected patients before they have low CD4 counts or other signs of clinical AIDS. The appearance is typical of other Candida infections, although inflammation may be limited.* **(Right)** *Kaposi sarcoma caused by human herpesvirus 8 [Kaposi sarcoma-associated herpesvirus (KSHV)] demonstrates typical slit-like spaces ➡ filled with blood. The KSHV virus is cross activated by the HIV Tat/Rev transcription complex.*

Cytomegalovirus in HIV Infection

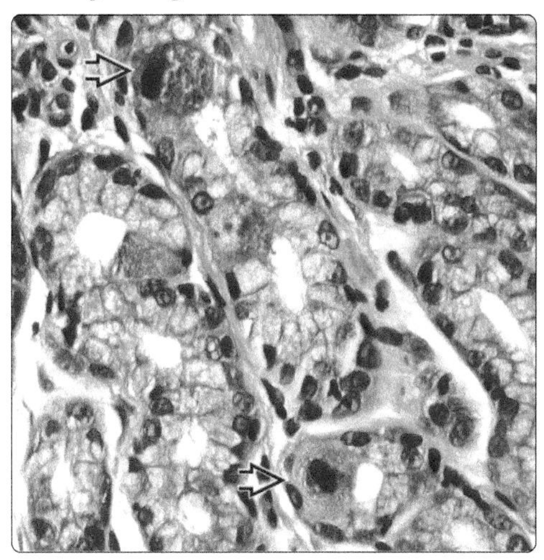

High-Burden Nontuberculous Mycobacteria

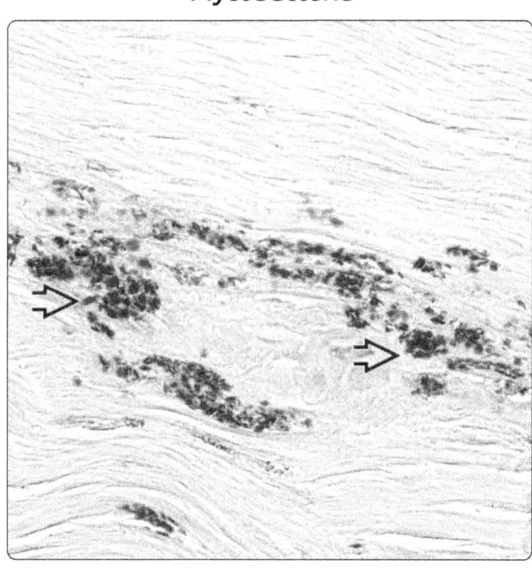

(Left) *Cytomegalovirus is a common reactivating infection in patients with untreated HIV, which can affect any organ. As seen here, there is no inflammatory reaction associated with the viral inclusion ➡.* **(Right)** *Mycobacterial infections in HIV patients may include TB, Mycobacterium avium complex, or several other rare pathogens, including Mycobacterium gordonae and Mycobacterium kansasii. Unlike TB, organism burden ➡ may be very high, as seen here in non-TB mycobacterial disease.*

EBV-Associated Lymphoma in HIV Infection

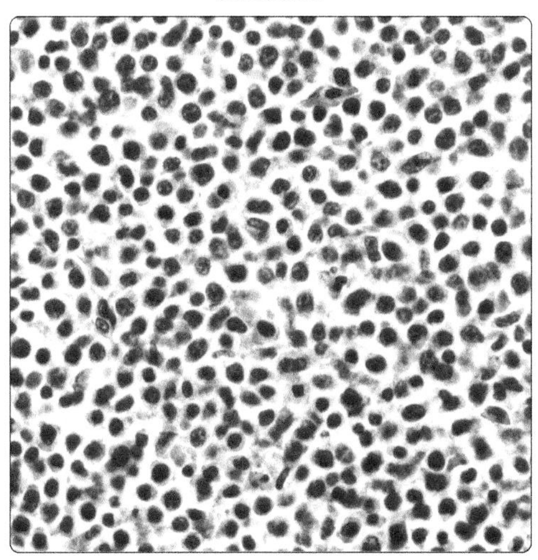

Toxoplasma Cyst in HIV Infection

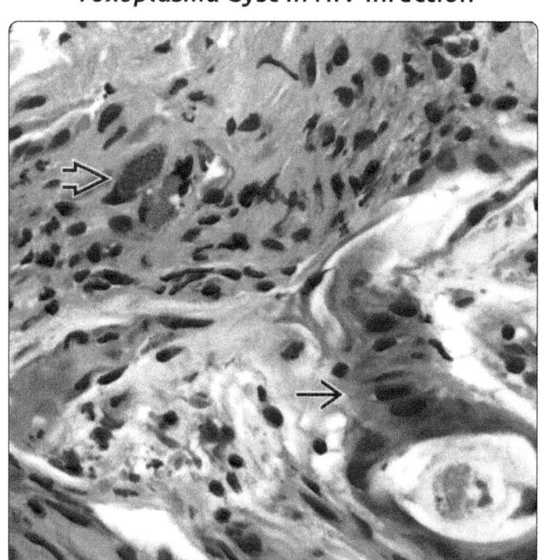

(Left) *Diffuse large B-cell lymphoma (DLBCL) associated with Epstein-Barr virus (EBV) infection is a common fatal complication of untreated HIV infection, although it may also occur in patients on therapy. Features are identical to DLBCL occurring in other hosts except that EBV in situ hybridization is more often positive.* **(Right)** *A Toxoplasma cyst ➡ is seen in the small bowel of an HIV patient with clinical diarrhea, mucosal distortion ➡, and no inflammation.*

KEY FACTS

ETIOLOGY/PATHOGENESIS

- Viral infection with tropism for CD4(+) T cells with integration into cellular DNA as provirus

CLINICAL ISSUES

- Estimated 5-10 million people infected worldwide; prevalence ranges from 1-30%
- Presentation: Adult T-cell leukemia/lymphoma (ATLL), HTLV-1-associated myelopathy/tropical spastic paraparesis, uveitis, and other neurologic manifestations
- Laboratory: Serology, PCR
- Treatment: Chemotherapy, bone marrow transplantation (malignancy); antivirals, immunosuppression

MICROSCOPIC

- Lymphomatous involvement (ATLL)
  - Medium to large pleomorphic cells with prominent nucleoli
- Cutaneous involvement (ATLL)
  - Pautrier-like microabscesses (similar to mycosis fungoides)
- Cloverleaf or flower-shaped nuclei in peripheral blood

ANCILLARY TESTS

- ATLL cells are positive for CD2, CD3, CD4, CD5, CD25, TCR-αβ, and FOXP3
- ATLL cells are negative for CD7, CD8, CD10, CXCL13, TCL1, and ALK1

TOP DIFFERENTIAL DIAGNOSES

- Other T-cell neoplasms/conditions
  - Mycosis fungoides/Sézary syndrome: Cerebriform cells in peripheral blood
  - Anaplastic large cell lymphoma: Strong, uniform expression of CD30, bizarre (horseshoe, embryoid) forms; perforin (+), granzyme-B (+), ALK1[(+) variable]
  - Angioimmunoblastic T-cell lymphoma: Expanded follicular dendritic cell network, increased vascularity; CD10(+), PD1(+), CXCL13(+)

Ultrastructural Features

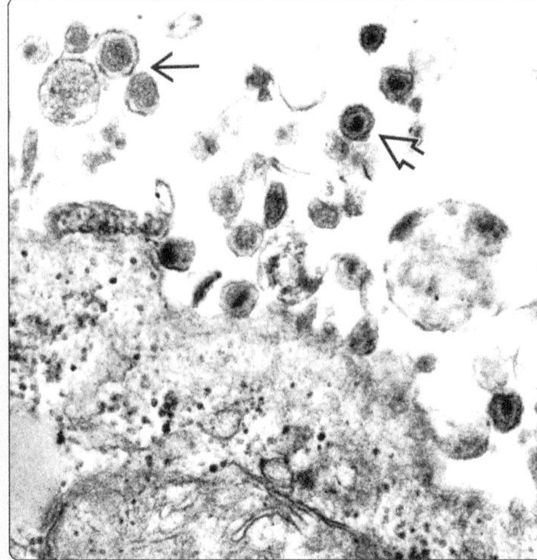

ATLL Skin Infiltration

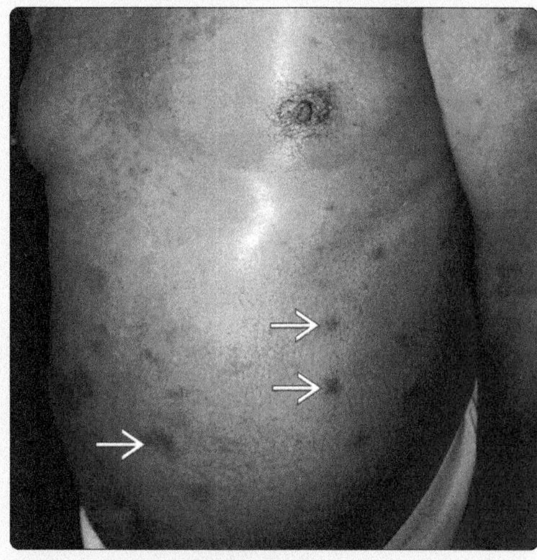

(Left) *Transmission electron microscopy demonstrates the presence of both the human T-cell leukemia type 1 virus (HTLV-1) ➡ (a.k.a. the human T-lymphotropic virus type 1 virus) and the human immunodeficiency virus (HIV) ➡. (Courtesy C. Goldsmith, MGS, CDC/PHIL.)* **(Right)** *The torso of a patient with HTLV-1-associated adult T-cell leukemia lymphoma (ATLL) demonstrates multiple skin lesions ➡, consistent with tumor involvement. (Courtesy D. Fisher, MD.)*

ATLL in Peripheral Blood

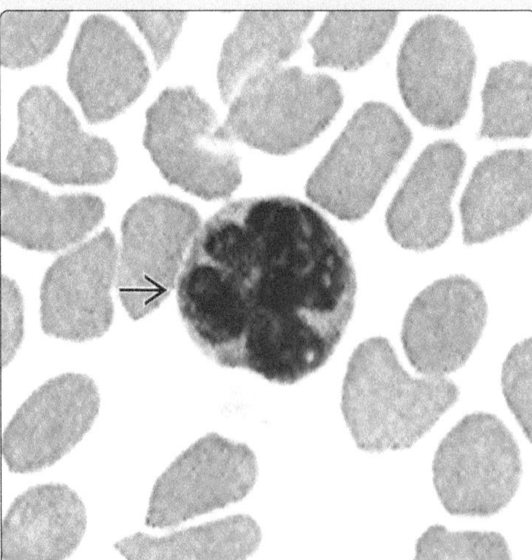

ATLL Histologic Features

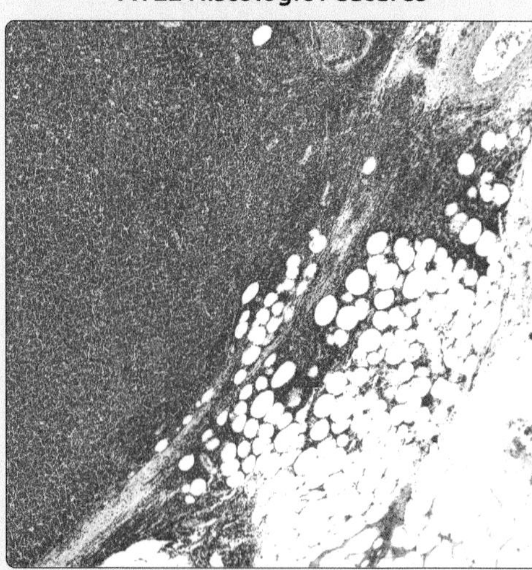

(Left) *Peripheral blood smear from a patient with ATLL shows a classic cloverleaf or flower cell ➡, which is highly suggestive of the disease. (Courtesy E. Morgan, MD.)* **(Right)** *Skin biopsy from a patient with ATLL with HTLV-1 demonstrates dense tumor infiltrates in the dermis and spilling into subcutaneous adipose tissue.*

TERMINOLOGY

Synonyms

- *Primate T-lymphotropic virus 1*
- Human T-lymphotropic virus type 1 (HTLV-1)

Definitions

- *Retroviridae* family: Derived from "retro" (backward)

ETIOLOGY/PATHOGENESIS

Infectious Agents

- Viral infection transmitted by breastfeeding, sexual intercourse, transfusion of blood products, sharing contaminated needles, and organ transplantation
- Tropism is for CD4(+) T cells [similar to human immunodeficiency virus (HIV)]; and virus integrates into cellular DNA by reverse transcription and subsequently exists as provirus
- Important viral oncoprotein is Tax (transcription factor)

CLINICAL ISSUES

Epidemiology

- Estimated 5-10 million people infected worldwide; prevalence in affected populations ranges from 1-30%
- Endemic in Japan, sub-Saharan Africa, Caribbean, parts of South America, Middle East, and Australo-Melanesia
- High rates of infections in intravenous drug users

Presentation

- 95% of infected individuals are asymptomatic
- Adult T-cell leukemia lymphoma (ATLL): Lymphadenopathy, cutaneous lesions, hepatosplenomegaly, paraneoplastic hypercalcemia, and opportunistic infections
  - Acute (55%), lymphomatous (20%), chronic (20%), and smoldering (5%) types
- HTLV-1-associated myelopathy/tropical spastic paraparesis: Chronic myelopathy with autonomic dysfunction
- Other neurologic manifestations: Uveitis, encephalomyelitis, polymyositis, inclusion body myositis, peripheral neuropathy

Laboratory Tests

- Elevated WBC, eosinophilia, hypercalcemia
- CSF: Mild leukocytosis, moderately raised protein, detectable anti-HTLV-1 antibodies
- Serology: Screening EIA/ELISA; confirmation by line immunoassay (LIA) or Western blot
- PCR: Quantitative; distinguishes HTLV-1/HTLV-2

Treatment

- Malignancies: Chemotherapy, bone marrow transplantation
- Antiviral approaches: Valproic acid with zidovudine

Prognosis

- Opportunistic infections (e.g., strongyloidiasis) in infected individuals and coinfection with other viruses (e.g., HIV, Hep C) usually lead to morbidity and mortality

MICROBIOLOGY

Virus

- Enveloped, positive-sense RNA retrovirus (80-100 nm)
- 8.5 kb with 9 proteins/polyproteins producing 16 functional products
- Seven main molecular genotypes of HTLV-1 (a-g)

MICROSCOPIC

Histologic Features

- ATLL
  - Diffuse infiltration of lymph nodes and other organs (early lesions may show paracortical expansion)
  - Variable morphology, typically medium to large cells with coarse chromatin and prominent nucleoli
  - Large to medium-sized cells with glassy basophilic cytoplasm, multilobed nuclei, coarse chromatin, and prominent nucleoli
  - Eosinophilia and background Reed-Sternberg-like cells may be present
- Cutaneous
  - Pautrier-like microabscesses (similar to mycosis fungoides)
  - Dermal and epidermotropic infiltrates that are perivascular &/or extending as nodules into fat

Cytologic Features

- Cloverleaf or flower-shaped nuclei in peripheral blood

ANCILLARY TESTS

Immunohistochemistry

- Viral antigen/RNA highlighted by IHC/ISH
- ATLL cells are positive for CD2, CD3, CD4, CD5, CD25, TCR-αβ, and FOXP3
- ATLL cells are negative for CD7, CD8, CD10, CXCL13, TCL1, and ALK1

DIFFERENTIAL DIAGNOSIS

Other T-Cell Neoplasms/Conditions

- Mycosis fungoides/Sézary syndrome: Cerebriform cells in peripheral blood; may be impossible to distinguish on histologic basis
- Anaplastic large cell lymphoma: Strong, uniform expression of CD30, bizarre (horseshoe, embryoid) forms (may be present in anaplastic variant of ATLL); perforin (+), granzyme-B (+), ALK1 [(+) variable]
- Angioimmunoblastic T-cell lymphoma: Expanded follicular dendritic cell network, increased vascularity; CD10(+), PD1(+), CXCL13(+)

SELECTED REFERENCES

1. Bangham CRM: HTLV-1 persistence and the oncogenesis of adult T cell leukemia/lymphoma. Blood. 141(19):2299-306, 2023
2. Ye L et al: Human T-cell lymphotropic virus type 1 and strongyloides stercoralis co-infection: a systematic review and meta-analysis. Front Med (Lausanne). 9:832430, 2022
3. Araujo A et al: Management of HAM/TSP: systematic review and consensus-based recommendations 2019. Neurol Clin Pract. 11(1):49-56, 2021
4. Takatori M et al: A new diagnostic algorithm using biopsy specimens in adult T-cell leukemia/lymphoma: combination of RNA in situ hybridization and quantitative PCR for HTLV-1. Mod Pathol. 34(1):51-8, 2021
5. Matsuura E et al: Visualization of HTLV-1-specific cytotoxic T lymphocytes in the spinal cords of patients with HTLV-1-associated myelopathy/tropical spastic paraparesis. J Neuropathol Exp Neurol. 74(1):2-14, 2015

Influenza Virus Infections

KEY FACTS

ETIOLOGY/PATHOGENESIS

- Viral infections transmitted by respiratory droplets
- Mutations in hemagglutinin (HA) and neuraminidase (NA) result in antigenic drift
- Reassortment of *HA* and *NA* genes (antigenic shift) can lead to pandemics

CLINICAL ISSUES

- Millions hospitalized yearly with seasonal influenza A and B
- Abrupt onset of fever, myalgia, headache, malaise, nonproductive cough, sore throat, and rhinitis
- Complications include viral pneumonia or secondary bacterial pneumonia, encephalopathy, transverse myelitis, myositis, myocarditis, and pericarditis
- Annual vaccine recommended for influenza; antivirals can decrease symptoms
- Laboratory testing includes rapid antigen testing, viral culture, direct or indirect fluorescent antibody staining, and nucleic acid amplification testing (single or multiplex assay)

MICROSCOPIC

- Seasonal influenza A and B: Diffuse, superficial, necrotizing tracheobronchitis with sloughing of ciliated respiratory epithelium
- Pandemic influenza A (H1N1): Inflammation of large airways and diffuse alveolar damage and hemorrhage
- No viral inclusions detectable by light microscopy

ANCILLARY TESTS

- Antiinfluenza A/B antibodies available at some reference laboratories

TOP DIFFERENTIAL DIAGNOSES

- Other respiratory viral or bacterial infections, including respiratory syncytial virus, human metapneumovirus, parainfluenza viruses, rhinoviruses, coronaviruses, *Mycoplasma pneumoniae*, and *Legionella* species
- Noninfectious causes of diffuse alveolar damage, including drugs, inhaled toxins, shock, sepsis, and collagen vascular disease

Acute Influenza Infection

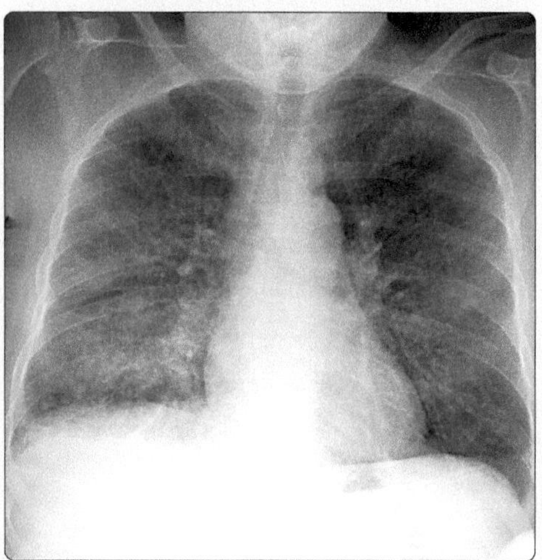

Ultrastructural Features

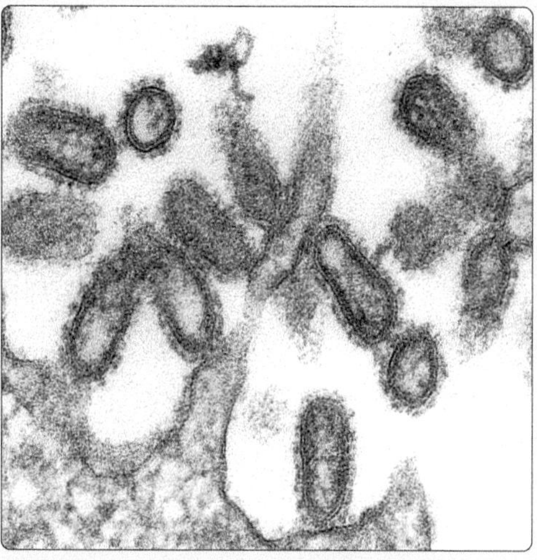

(Left) *Chest radiograph of a 61-year-old man with chronic lymphocytic leukemia and an acute influenza infection shows bilateral asymmetric, patchy airspace and interstitial opacities. (From DI: Chest.)* **(Right)** *Transmission electron micrograph of 1918 influenza virus virions shows prominent surface projections composed of hemagglutinin and neuraminidase glycoproteins, surrounding a helical nucleocapsid. (Courtesy C. Goldsmith MGS, CDC/PHIL.)*

H1N1 Influenza A Severe Lung Disease

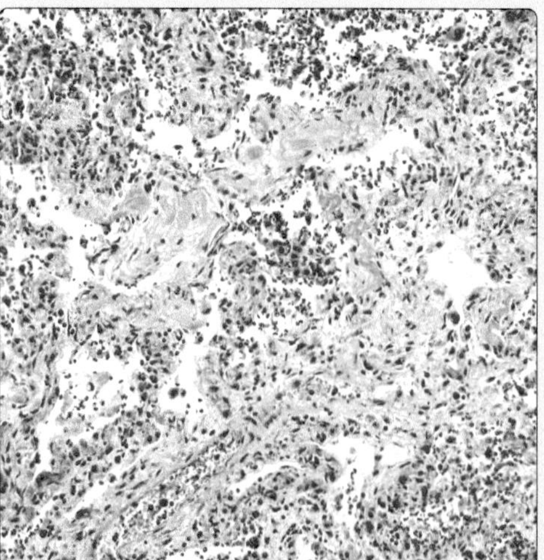

Influenza B Tracheobronchitis

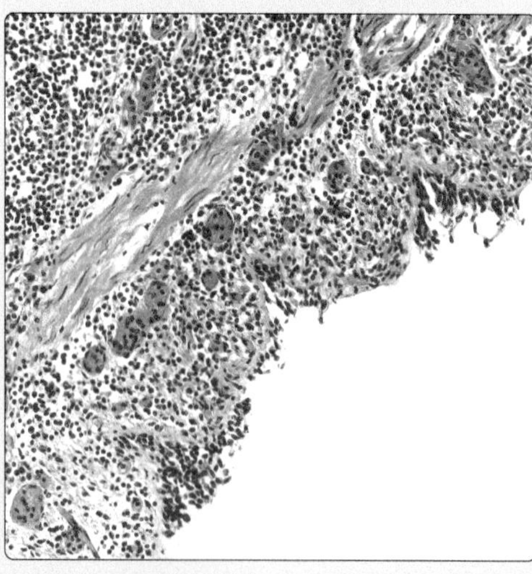

(Left) *Autopsy lung section from a fatal case of H1N1 influenza shows severe acute and organizing lung injury, a nonspecific pattern requiring clinical, laboratory, or IHC correlation for definitive diagnosis.* **(Right)** *Section of large airway from a patient with influenza B shows loss of ciliated columnar respiratory epithelium and dense inflammatory infiltrate.*

TERMINOLOGY

Synonyms

- *Influenza A virus* (IAV); genus *Alphainfluenzavirus*
- *Influenza B virus* (IBV); genus *Betainfluenzavirus*
- *Influenza C virus* (ICV); genus *Gammainfluenzavirus*
- "The flu"

Definitions

- *Orthomyxoviridae* family: Derived from "ortho" (straight) and "myxo" (mucus)

ETIOLOGY/PATHOGENESIS

Infectious Agents

- Viral infections transmitted person to person via respiratory droplets; incubation period is 1-4 days, and infectious period is 1 day before until 5 days after onset of symptoms
- Virus hemagglutinin (HA) binds sialic acids on cell surface, causing viral uptake into host cells, while neuraminidase (NA) enzymatically removes sialic acids, promoting viral release from infected cells
- Antigenic drift: Production of new viral strains by mutations in *HA* and *NA* genes
- Antigenic shift: Development of new combinations of *HA* and *NA* genes due to reassortment of viral genome subunits; can result in pandemics
- Virus family members
  - Influenza A: Infects humans, birds, and pigs
    - 18 HA and 11 NA serotypes
  - Influenza B: Primarily infects humans
    - 1 HA and 1 NA serotype
    - 2 lineages (Victoria-like and Yamagata-like)
  - Influenza C: Infects humans and pigs
    - HA-esterase fusion antigen

CLINICAL ISSUES

Epidemiology

- Seasonal influenza A and B
  - Worldwide: 3-5 million hospitalizations and 290,000-650,000 deaths per year
  - USA: 9-41 million illnesses, 140,000-710,000 hospitalizations, and 12,000-52,000 deaths per year (2010-2020)
- Pandemic influenza A
  - 1889: H3N8 Russian influenza (1 million deaths worldwide)
  - 1918: H1N1 Spanish influenza (50 million deaths worldwide; 675,000 in USA)
  - 1957: H2N2 Asian influenza (2 million deaths worldwide; 69,800 in USA)
  - 1968: H3N2 Hong Kong influenza (1 million deaths worldwide; 33,800 in USA)
  - 2009: H1N1 swine flu (284,000 deaths worldwide)
- Avian IAVs
  - Highly pathogenic stains (e.g., H5N1, H5N6, and H7N9): Exposure to birds in Asia; associated with high mortality but no sustained person-to-person transmission
  - Low pathogenic strains (e.g., H9N2): Observed in children exposed to poultry; mild upper respiratory tract illness, conjunctivitis; severe pneumonia and death in few cases
- Swine influenza/variant IAVs
  - Exposure to pigs; generally associated with mild symptoms; no sustained person-to-person transmission
  - H1N1v, H3N2v, and H1N2v: 491 cases in USA from 2010-2022

Site

- Upper and lower respiratory tracts

Presentation

- Abrupt onset of fever, myalgia, headache, malaise, nonproductive cough, sore throat, and rhinitis

Laboratory Tests

- Best samples: Nasopharyngeal or nasal swab, nasal aspirate or wash (collect with 4 days of onset of illness)
- Rapid antigen assays (≤ 15 minutes); 50-70% sensitive and > 90% specific; no subtype information
- Viral culture (3-10 days); essential for strain determination and surveillance
- Immunofluorescence, direct or indirect fluorescent antibody staining (1-4 hours)
- RT-PCR (1-6 hours); single or multiplexed assays with other respiratory virus panels (e.g., respiratory syncytial virus, parainfluenza viruses, and adenovirus)

Natural History

- Self-limited infection that resolves after 3-7 days (cough and malaise can last for > 2 weeks)
- Complications include viral pneumonia or secondary bacterial pneumonia, encephalopathy, transverse myelitis, myositis, myocarditis, and pericarditis

Treatment

- Influenza vaccine: Recommended annually for all persons > 6 months old
  - Traditionally produced by egg-based methods; cell-based and recombinant vaccines approved by FDA in 2012 and 2013
  - Quadrivalent formulations containing HA antigen of 2 influenza A strains (i.e., H1N1 and H3N2) and 2 influenza B strains (Victoria and Yamagata)
  - Formulations are updated yearly to match antigenically circulating strains according to WHO predictions; estimated yearly effectiveness ranged 19-60% from 2009-2022
  - Universal influenza vaccines currently under development
- Antivirals
  - NA inhibitors: Oseltamivir (oral), zanamivir (inhaled), peramivir (intravenous)
  - Inhibitor of cap-dependent endonuclease: Baloxavir (oral)
  - M2 protein inhibitors: Amantadine and rimantadine not currently recommended for use due to resistance

Prognosis

- Uncommonly fatal in immunocompetent patients (H1N1, avian flu, influenza B in pediatric patients with myocarditis)

- Highest risk at age > 65, children, pregnant women, and those with underlying health conditions (morbid obesity, diabetes, underlying respiratory illness)

IMAGING

General Features

- CXR: Normal in uncomplicated disease; diffuse infiltrates, mottled densities, and consolidations in severe disease
- Pleural effusions are suggestive of bacterial coinfection

MICROBIOLOGY

Viral Features

- Enveloped, single-stranded RNA viruses
- Spherical and filamentous (100- to 200-nm diameter) with helical nucleocapsid
- HA and NA surface spikes (10-12 nm in length)
- 14,000 nucleotide segmented genome (10 proteins)

Culture

- Grows in several cell lines (e.g., Vero and MDCK)
- Detectable by immunofluorescence after 4-8 days

MACROSCOPIC

General Features

- Fatal cases: Heavy, congested, edematous lungs; mucosal surfaces of trachea and bronchi hyperemic and swollen
- Purulent luminal debris, abscess/empyema, hemorrhage in bacterial coinfections

MICROSCOPIC

Histologic Features

- Seasonal influenza A and B
  - Diffuse, superficial, necrotizing tracheobronchitis
  - Sloughing of ciliated respiratory epithelium
- Pandemic influenza A (H1N1)
  - Inflammation of large airways and diffuse alveolar damage and hemorrhage
  - Squamous metaplasia of bronchoalveolar lining cells
- No viral inclusions detectable by light microscopy
- Secondary infection by pyogenic bacteria
- Extra pulmonary manifestations include myocarditis, cerebral edema, and rhabdomyolysis

ANCILLARY TESTS

Immunohistochemistry and In Situ Hybridization

- Available at some reference laboratories
- Seasonal influenza A and B: Respiratory epithelial cells in distal trachea and bronchi
- Pandemic influenza A (H1N1): Upper and lower airways

PCR

- RT-PCR (fresh or formalin-fixed tissue) more sensitive for prolonged illness or with extensive necrosis

DIFFERENTIAL DIAGNOSIS

Other Respiratory Viral Infections

- Measles, respiratory syncytial virus, human metapneumovirus, parainfluenza viruses, adenovirus
  - Significant overlap in histology, which may include necrotizing tracheobronchitis, interstitial pneumonia, or diffuse alveolar damage
  - Presence of characteristic nuclear or cytoplasmic viral inclusions
  - Confirmation by culture, direct fluorescent antibody and rapid antigen assays, serology, PCR, or IHC
- Rhinovirus, coronaviruses, enteroviruses
  - Significant overlap in histologic features and lacks associated viral inclusions
  - Confirmation by culture, direct fluorescent antibody and rapid antigen assays, serology, PCR, or IHC

Bacterial Infections

- *Mycoplasma pneumoniae, Legionella* species, etc.
  - Organisms may be visualized by Gram, Warthin-Starry, or IHC stains
  - Confirmation by culture, serology, or PCR

Noninfectious Causes of Diffuse Alveolar Damage

- Drugs, inhaled toxins, shock, sepsis, collagen vascular disease
  - Similar severe histology as pandemic influenza
  - Exclusion of infectious etiology via appropriate laboratory testing

SELECTED REFERENCES

1. Centers for Disease Control and Prevention: Influenza (flu). Updated March 2, 2023. Reviewed March 8, 2023. Accessed March 8, 2023. http://www.cdc.gov/flu/
2. Shi J et al: Alarming situation of emerging H5 and H7 avian influenza and effective control strategies. Emerg Microbes Infect. 12(1):2155072, 2023
3. Nealon J et al: Looking back on 50 years of literature to understand the potential impact of influenza on extrapulmonary medical outcomes. Open Forum Infect Dis. 9(8):ofac352, 2022
4. Uyeki TM et al: Influenza. Lancet. 400(10353):693-706, 2022
5. Li Y et al: The epidemiology of swine influenza. Anim Dis. 1(1):21, 2021
6. Wei CJ et al: Next-generation influenza vaccines: opportunities and challenges. Nat Rev Drug Discov. 19(4):239-52, 2020
7. Oxford JS et al: Unanswered questions about the 1918 influenza pandemic: origin, pathology, and the virus itself. Lancet Infect Dis. 18(11):e348-54, 2018
8. Bhatnagar J et al: Localization of pandemic 2009 H1N1 influenza A virus RNA in lung and lymph nodes of fatal influenza cases by in situ hybridization: new insights on virus replication and pathogenesis. J Clin Virol. 56(3):232-7, 2013
9. Paddock CD et al: Myocardial injury and bacterial pneumonia contribute to the pathogenesis of fatal influenza B virus infection. J Infect Dis. 205(6):895-905, 2012
10. Shieh WJ et al: 2009 pandemic influenza A (H1N1): pathology and pathogenesis of 100 fatal cases in the United States. Am J Pathol. 177(1):166-75, 2010

H1N1 Influenza Autopsy Lung

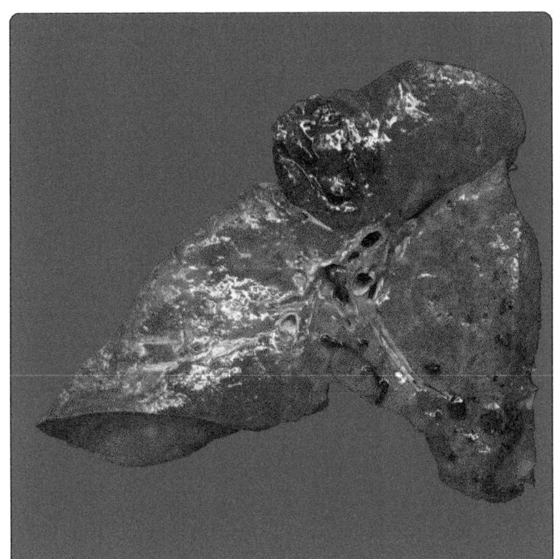

Diffuse Alveolar Damage (H1N1)

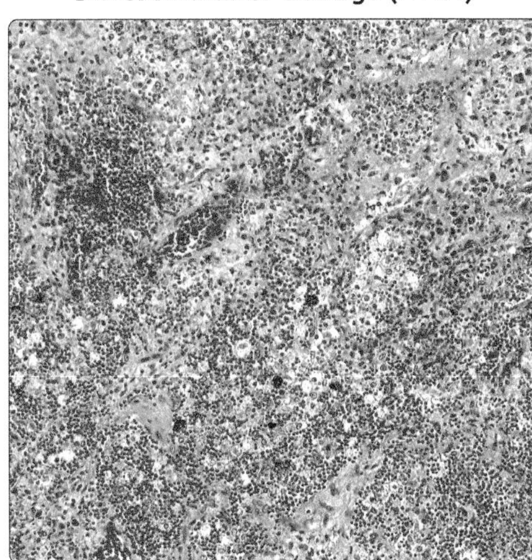

(Left) *Lungs from a fatal case of H1N1 influenza are large (3x upper limit of normal weight) and diffusely hemorrhagic.* **(Right)** *Section from a fatal case of H1N1 influenza shows acute and organizing lung injury, consistent with a diffuse alveolar damage pattern of injury with intraalveolar hemorrhage and hemosiderosis.*

Hyaline Membrane Formation (H1N1)

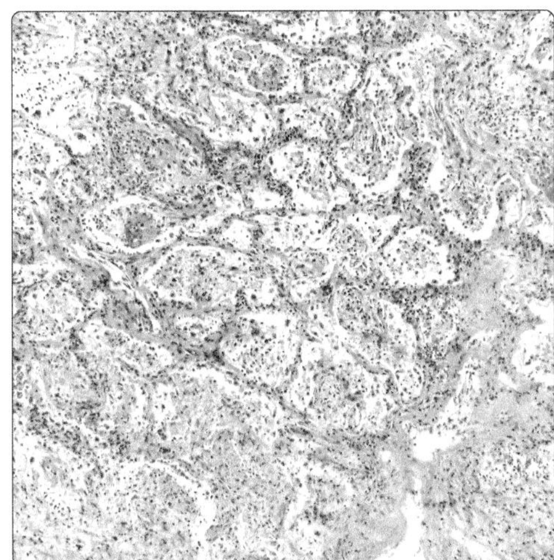

Pandemic Influenza A Infection

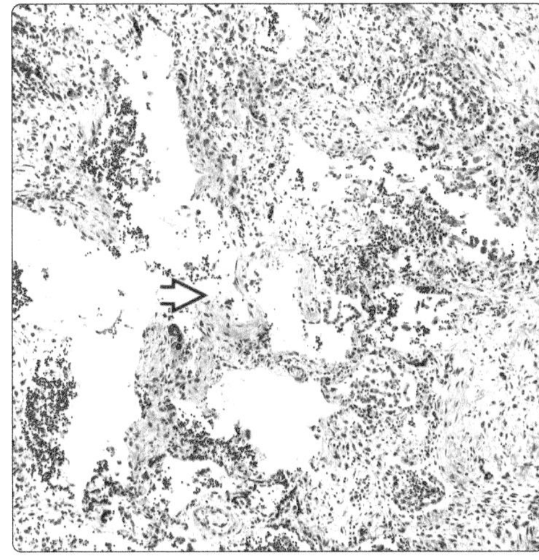

(Left) *Section from a fatal case of H1N1 influenza exhibits a diffuse alveolar damage pattern with hyaline membrane formation and increased collagen within the alveolar walls.* **(Right)** *Hyaline membrane formation ⇨ and increased collagen within alveolar walls are typical findings of fatal pandemic influenza infection.*

Abscess Formation in H1N1 Influenza

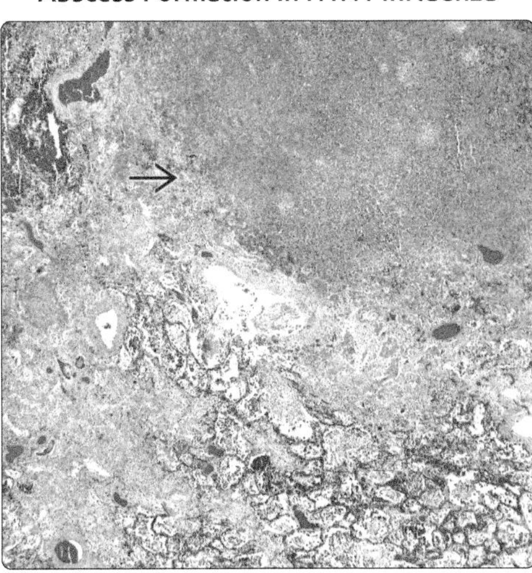

Immunohistochemistry

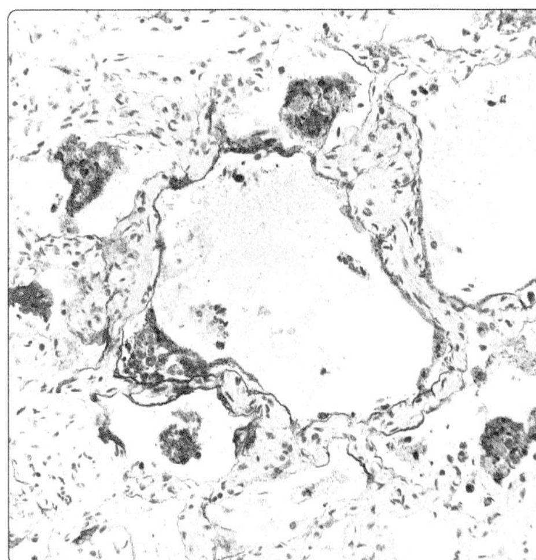

(Left) *Cavitating abscess formation ⇨ of at least several weeks duration is present in this section of lung from a fatal case of H1N1 influenza with bronchopneumonia.* **(Right)** *Immunohistochemical staining for influenza A/B can be performed at some reference laboratories and typically highlights scattered respiratory cells in the distal trachea and bronchi.*

Parainfluenza Virus Infections

KEY FACTS

ETIOLOGY/PATHOGENESIS

- Viral infections transmitted person to person via respiratory droplets

CLINICAL ISSUES

- 70,000 hospital admissions per year in USA
- Fever, rhinorrhea, cough, laryngotracheobronchitis (croup), bronchitis, bronchiolitis, pneumonia
- Laboratory: RT-PCR (respiratory secretions), viral culture, antigen detection, serology
- No vaccines or specific antiviral treatments available; hospitalization for respiratory distress, stridor, or severe dehydration

MACROSCOPIC

- Heavy, congested, hemorrhagic, and edematous lungs

MICROSCOPIC

- Mild tracheobronchitis to interstitial pneumonitis with mononuclear cell infiltrates and diffuse alveolar damage
- Multinucleated giant cells with eosinophilic cytoplasmic inclusions
- IHC: Viral antigen detected in alveolar lining cells, multinucleated cells, and respiratory epithelium

TOP DIFFERENTIAL DIAGNOSES

- Respiratory syncytial virus infection: Multinucleated syncytial giant cells with eosinophilic cytoplasmic inclusions; confirm by PCR, antigen testing
- Human metapneumovirus infection: Eosinophilic nuclear and cytoplasmic inclusions; confirm by PCR, antigen testing
- Measles virus infection: Eosinophilic cytoplasmic inclusions, intranuclear inclusions with clear halo; Warthin-Finkeldey giant cells; confirm by PCR, culture, serology
- Influenza virus infection: No specific viral cytopathic effects; confirm by PCR, IHC, antigen testing
- Coronavirus disease 2019: No specific viral cytopathic effects; confirm by PCR, IHC, serology, antigen testing

Radiographic Features: Croup

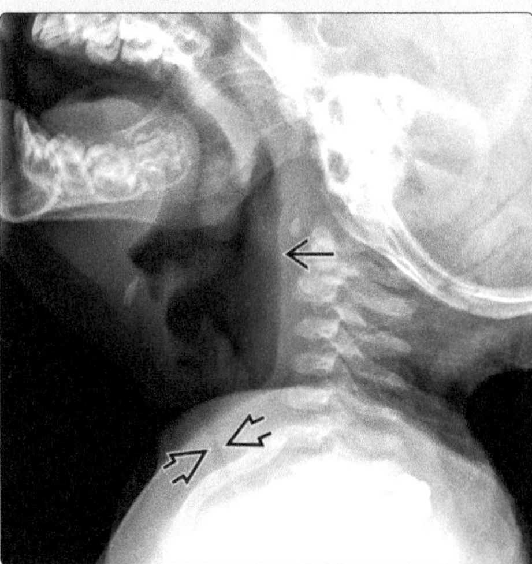

Ultrastructural Features

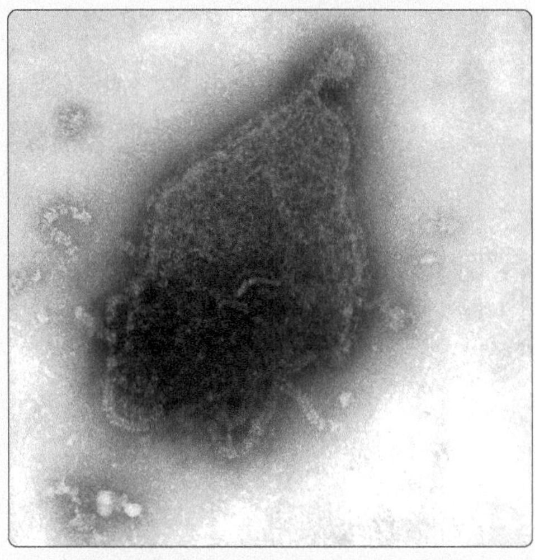

(Left) *Lateral neck radiograph of a young child with croup shows marked subglottic airway narrowing ➙, overdistension of the hypopharynx ➙, and a normal-appearing epiglottis. (From DI: Pediatrics.)* **(Right)** *This transmission electron micrograph shows an enveloped, irregularly shaped virion measuring 150-250 nm in diameter, characteristic of human parainfluenza virus, type 4a (HPIV-4a). (Courtesy F. Murphy, DVM, PhD, CDC/PHIL.)*

Viral Cytopathic Effects

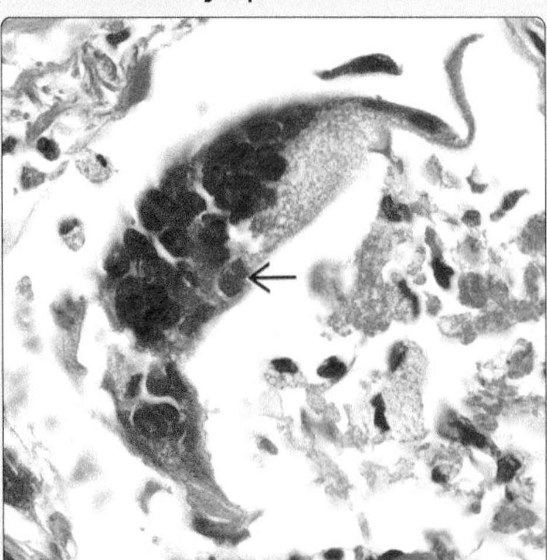

Infection of Respiratory Epithelium

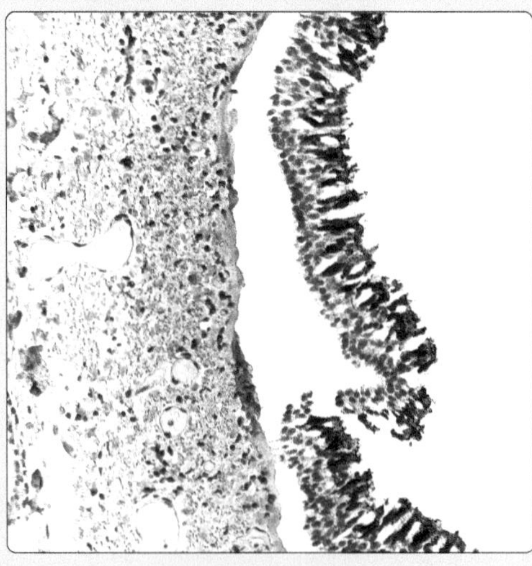

(Left) *This section from a fatal case of HPIV-3 pneumonia exhibits multinucleated giant cells with eosinophilic cytoplasmic inclusions ➙.* **(Right)** *Immunohistochemical staining for a parainfluenza antigen shows positive staining in infected respiratory epithelial cells (red).*

TERMINOLOGY

Synonyms

- *Human respirovirus 1*; human parainfluenza virus 1 (HPIV-1)
- *Human rubulavirus 2*; human parainfluenza virus 2 (HPIV-2)
- *Human respirovirus 3*; human parainfluenza virus 3 (HPIV-3)
- *Human rubulavirus 4*; human parainfluenza virus 4 (HPIV-4)

Definitions

- *Paramyxoviridae* family: Derived from "para" (beyond) and "myxo" (mucus)

ETIOLOGY/PATHOGENESIS

Infectious Agents

- Viral infections transmitted person to person via respiratory droplets (2- to 7-day incubation period); hemagglutinin-neuraminidase-mediated attachment and cell uptake

CLINICAL ISSUES

Epidemiology

- 70,000 hospital admissions per year in USA (2nd highest after respiratory syncytial virus); HPIV-1 and HPIV-2 peak in fall; HPIV-3 peak in spring/summer
- Common in infants/children (antibodies by age 5)

Site

- Upper and lower respiratory tracts

Presentation

- Fever, rhinorrhea, cough, laryngotracheobronchitis/croup (HPIV-1 and HPIV-2); bronchitis, bronchiolitis, pneumonia (HPIV-3); mild to severe respiratory illness (HPIV-4)

Laboratory Tests

- RT-PCR (respiratory secretions)
- Viral culture
- Direct viral antigen tests using immunofluorescence or enzyme immunoassay
- Serology (IgM or rise in IgG)

Treatment

- No FDA-approved vaccines available
- Primary prevention through avoidance of sick individuals and good hand hygiene
- No specific antiviral treatments available; symptomatic, supportive treatment, rest and rehydration; hospitalization for respiratory distress, stridor, or severe dehydration

Prognosis

- Typically self-limited; resolves within 7-10 days
- Mortality rare in immunocompetent

IMAGING

Radiographic Findings

- Chest x-ray: For evaluation of croup (classic steeple sign), epiglottitis, or pneumonia

MICROBIOLOGY

Viral Features

- Enveloped, single-stranded RNA viruses
- 150-250 nm with helical capsid
- 15,000 nucleotide genome (6 proteins)
- 5 types (HPIV-1, HPIV-2, HPIV-3, HPIV-4a, HPIV-4b)

Culture

- Grows in primary monkey kidney and LLC-MK2 cells
- Detection by hemadsorption with guinea pig erythrocytes within 3-10 days

MACROSCOPIC

General Features

- Heavy, congested, hemorrhagic, and edematous lungs

MICROSCOPIC

Histologic Features

- Vary from mild tracheobronchitis to interstitial pneumonitis with mononuclear cell infiltrates, diffuse alveolar damage

Cytologic Features

- Multinucleated giant cells with eosinophilic cytoplasmic inclusions

ANCILLARY TESTS

Immunohistochemistry

- Anti-HPIV antibodies stain viral antigen in alveolar lining cells, multinucleated cells, and respiratory epithelium

DIFFERENTIAL DIAGNOSIS

Respiratory Syncytial Virus Infection

- Multinucleated syncytial giant cells with eosinophilic cytoplasmic inclusions; confirm by PCR, antigen testing

Human Metapneumovirus Infection

- Eosinophilic nuclear and cytoplasmic inclusions; confirm by PCR, antigen testing

Measles Virus Infection

- Eosinophilic cytoplasmic inclusions, intranuclear inclusions with clear halo; Warthin-Finkeldey giant cells; confirm by PCR, culture, serology

Influenza Virus Infection

- No specific viral cytopathic effects; confirm by PCR, IHC, antigen testing

Coronavirus Disease 2019

- No specific viral cytopathic effects; confirm by PCR, IHC, serology, antigen testing

SELECTED REFERENCES

1. Centers for Disease Control and Prevention: Human parainfluenza viruses (HPIVs). Updated November 18, 2022. Reviewed February 23, 2023. https://www.cdc.gov/parainfluenza/index.html
2. de Zwart A et al: Respiratory syncytial virus, human metapneumovirus, and parainfluenza virus infections in lung transplant recipients: a systematic review of outcomes and treatment strategies. Clin Infect Dis. 74(12):2252-60, 2022
3. Hetrich MK et al: Epidemiology of human parainfluenza virus type 3 (HPIV-3) and respiratory syncytial virus (RSV) infections in the time of COVID-19: findings from a household cohort in Maryland. Clin Infect Dis. 76(8):1349-57, 2022
4. DeGroote NP et al: Human parainfluenza virus circulation, United States, 2011-2019. J Clin Virol. 124:104261, 2020

Coronavirus Disease 2019 (COVID-19)

KEY FACTS

ETIOLOGY/PATHOGENESIS

- Infection with SARS-CoV-2 via respiratory droplets
- Predominant circulating variants change over time

CLINICAL ISSUES

- Presentation: Fever, headache, myalgias, cough, dyspnea
- CT: Bilateral multiple lobar consolidation or ground-glass opacity with subsegmental areas of consolidation
- Labs: Antigen, PCR, serology; culture not recommended
- Vaccine, monoclonal antibodies, antivirals

MICROSCOPIC

- Lungs: Diffuse alveolar damage, edema, hyaline membranes, lymphocytic infiltration, microthrombosis
- SARS-CoV-2 antinucleocapsid and antispike antibodies and viral RNA ISH stain cytoplasm of infected cells
- Brain: Acute hypoxic ischemic injury, diffuse microgliosis, minimal lymphocytic inflammation, hemorrhage, occasional thrombi/infarcts, rare demyelinating lesions
- Other organs rarely exhibit virally infected cells; changes due to hypoxia, inflammation, coagulopathy, etc.
- Bacterial and fungal (e.g., aspergillosis and mucormycosis) coinfections common
- Placenta: Histiocytic intervillositis, perivillous fibrin deposition, and trophoblast necrosis
- Postacute/long COVID-19 under investigation

TOP DIFFERENTIAL DIAGNOSES

- Other respiratory viral infections (e.g., other coronaviruses, influenza A or B, RSV, CMV, HSV): Confirmation by viral cytopathic effects, IHC, PCR, cultures, serology
- Bacterial, mycobacterial, and fungal infections (e.g., *Mycoplasma pneumoniae*, *Mycobacterium avium* complex, *Cryptococcus* spp.): Positive stains, PCR, cultures, serology
- Noninfectious DAD: Transplantation complications, connective tissue diseases, idiopathic pulmonary fibrosis exacerbations, drugs, radiation therapy, acute interstitial pneumonia; negative viral serology, PCR, cultures

SARS-CoV-2

Ultrastructural Features

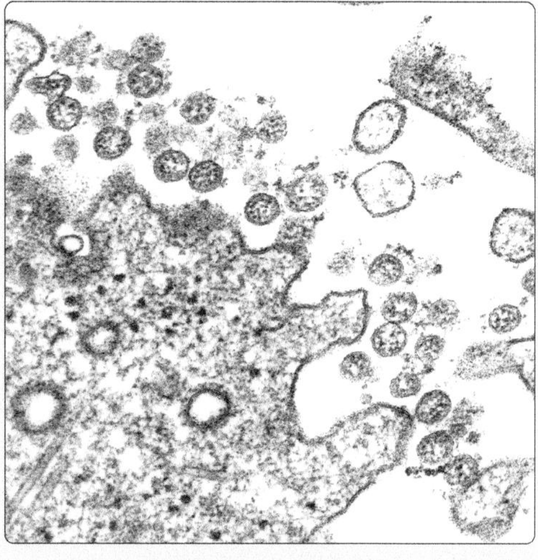

(Left) *This graphic of severe acute respiratory syndrome coronavirus 2 (SARS-CoV-2) shows surface spikes (red) giving a halo appearance, which is incorporated into the name "corona." (Courtesy A. Eckert, MSMI, D. Higgins, MAMS, CDC/PHIL.)* **(Right)** *This transmission electron micrograph shows spherical extracellular particles with surface spikes and cross sections through the viral genome (black dots), features characteristic of SARS-CoV-2. (Courtesy C. Goldsmith, MS, A. Tamin, PhD, CDC/PHIL.)*

Histopathologic Features

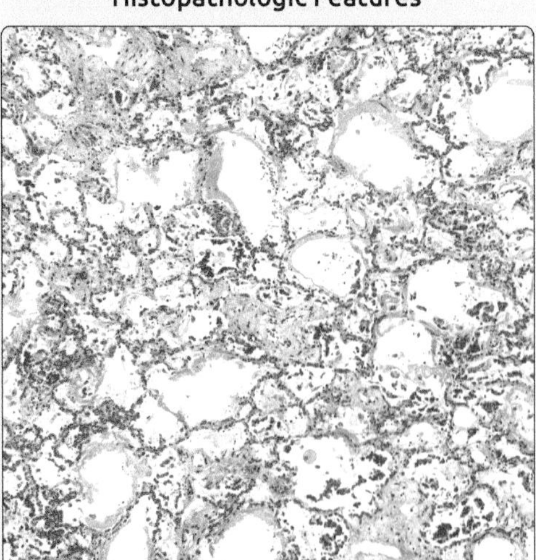

SARS-CoV-2 Spike Immunohistochemistry

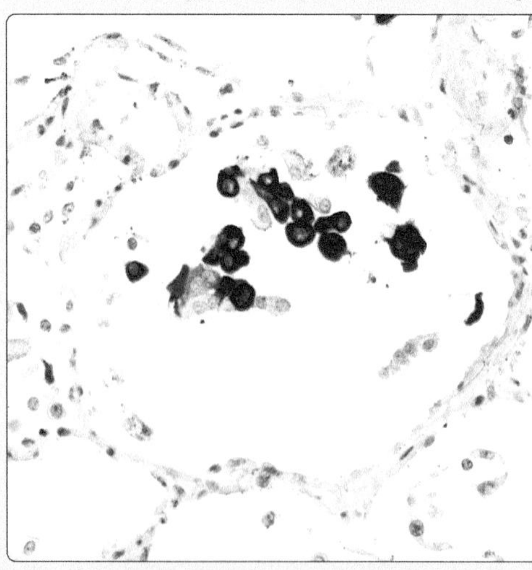

(Left) *This autopsy lung section shows hyaline membranes, interstitial edema and inflammation, and squamous metaplasia, features consistent with diffuse alveolar damage. Confirmation of SARS-CoV-2 infection requires IHC, ISH, and PCR. (Courtesy R. Padera, Jr., MD, PhD.)* **(Right)** *SARS-CoV-2 spike protein immunohistochemistry highlights several cells (pneumocytes and alveolar macrophages) in this autopsy lung section of a patient who died from COVID-19.*

TERMINOLOGY

Definitions

- Initially referred to as 2019 novel coronavirus (2019-nCoV)
- *Coronaviridae* family: "Corona" (crown, halo) ultrastructural appearance

ETIOLOGY/PATHOGENESIS

Infectious Agents

- Infection with severe acute respiratory syndrome coronavirus 2 (SARS-CoV-2) via human-to-human transmission by respiratory droplets; risk for intrauterine vertical transmission
- *Betacoronavirus* genus; virus sequences similar to bat coronaviruses and SARS-CoV
- Angiotensin-converting enzyme 2 (ACE2) used for cellular entry and serine protease TMPRSS2 used for spike protein priming
- Neuropilin-1 (NRP1) is additional host cell entry factor that binds furin-cleaved S1 fragment of spike protein
- Organ damage likely due to combination of cytokine storm, microthrombosis, hypoxemia, and ischemia
- Mechanisms underlying multisystem inflammatory syndrome in children and long COVID (postacute sequelae of SARS CoV-2 infection) under active study

CLINICAL ISSUES

Epidemiology

- Initial animal source of virus is unknown (likely bats)
- 1st identified cases linked to seafood and animal market in Wuhan, China
- Declared pandemic by World Health Organization on 3/11/2020; end of public health emergency of international concern declared on 5/5/2023
- Current variant(s) of concern (VOC): Omicron (B.1.1.529 and descendant lineages)
- > 750 million confirmed cases and ~ 6.9 million deaths worldwide (as of 8/28/2023)
  - > 100 million cases and > 1.1 million deaths in USA (as of 8/28/2022)
- Majority of cases in adults; severe cases relatively uncommon in pediatric population

Presentation

- Infections may be asymptomatic or associated with mild symptoms
- Incubation period: 2-14 days; contagious period: 2-3 days before and 8 days after symptom onset
- Severe respiratory illness more common in unvaccinated population
- Common symptoms include fever, cough, dyspnea, chills, myalgia, headache, sore throat, and new loss of taste or smell; variable skin manifestations also reported
- Laboratory abnormalities include leukopenia, leukocytosis, lymphopenia, thrombocytopenia, elevated alanine aminotransferase and aspartate aminotransferase levels

Laboratory Tests

- Antigen: Rapid test (15-30 minutes) that can be performed at home; lower sensitivity than PCR
- PCR: Gold standard (1 hour to multiple days for results); may be incorporated into multiplex assay with other respiratory viruses
- Serology: Used for public health surveillance and diagnosis of subacute, chronic, or resolved infections
- Validated sample types vary with assay: Upper respiratory [nasopharyngeal (NP), oropharyngeal, nasal midturbinate, anterior nares, and NP wash/aspirate] vs. lower respiratory (bronchoalveolar lavage, tracheal aspirate, and sputum)

Treatment

- USA FDA-authorized vaccines
  - mRNA vaccines: Pfizer-BioNTech/Comirnaty, Moderna/Spikevax
  - Multivalent vaccines and retargeting may be required as circulating strains change
  - Protein subunit vaccine: Novavax
- Antiviral
  - Paxlovid (nirmatrelvir/ritonavir): PO within 5 days of symptom onset
  - Lagevrio (molnupiravir): PO within 5 days of symptom onset
  - Veklury (remdesivir): IV within 7 days of symptom onset
- Monoclonal antibodies
  - Actemra (tocilizumab): Interleukin-6 inhibitor
  - Olumiant (baricitinib): Janus kinase inhibitor
  - Kineret (anakinra): Interleukin-1 receptor antagonist
  - Gohibic (vilobelimab): C5a inhibitor

Prognosis

- Complications include acute respiratory distress syndrome, viremia, acute cardiac injury, and secondary infection
- Higher risk in older adults, individuals living in nursing homes or long-term care facilities, and individuals of any age with severe underlying conditions (e.g., cardiovascular disease, diabetes, pulmonary disease, liver disease, chronic kidney disease, and severe obesity)
- 80% of deaths reported in individuals > 65 years of age; worst outcomes in individuals > 85 years of age

IMAGING

Radiographic Findings

- CT: Bilateral multiple lobar consolidation (ICU cases) or ground-glass opacity (non-ICU cases) with subsegmental areas of consolidation

MICROBIOLOGY

Virus Features

- Enveloped, single-stranded RNA virus
- 60-140 nm in size, helical nucleocapsid, 9- to 12-nm surface projections (spikes)
- ~ 30,000-nucleotide genome (encoding nonstructural proteins as well as spike, envelope, membrane, and nucleocapsid)

Culture

- Virus isolated in human airway epithelial cells and Vero-CCL81, Vero E6, and Huh-7 cell lines
- Cytopathic effects observed after 4-6 days
- Not recommended for diagnosis due to biosafety considerations

MACROSCOPIC

General Features

- Heavy edematous lungs

MICROSCOPIC

Histologic Features

- Lungs: Diffuse alveolar damage (DAD) with edema, hemorrhage, hyaline membranes, interstitial lymphocytic infiltrates, pneumocyte damage, fibrin thrombi, capillary megakaryocytes, vasculitis, pulmonary thrombosis, acute bronchopneumonia
- Heart: Variable myocyte necrosis, degeneration, lymphocytic myocarditis, edema
- Liver: Periportal lymphocytic inflammation, patchy necrosis, hepatocytes with ballooning degeneration, nuclear glycogen accumulation
- Spleen: Depletion of white pulp (lymphoid hypoplasia, lymphocytic depletion); red pulp congestion, hemorrhage
- Kidneys: Acute tubular injury, endothelial injury, microthrombi, collapsing glomerulopathy
- Adrenal glands: Hemorrhagic necrosis, cortical lipid degeneration, focal inflammation
- Testis: Lymphocytic infiltration, germ cell destruction, edema
- Placenta: Histiocytic intervillositis, perivillous fibrin deposition, and trophoblast necrosis
- Skin: Parakeratosis, acanthosis, dyskeratotic/necrotic keratinocytes, acantholytic clefts, superficial and deep lymphocytic infiltration
- Brain: Acute hypoxic ischemic injury, diffuse microgliosis, minimal lymphocytic inflammation, hemorrhage, occasional thrombi/infarcts, rare acute disseminated encephalomyelitis (ADEM)-like demyelinating lesions
- Coinfections
  - COVID-19-associated pulmonary aspergillosis (CAPA)
  - Rhino-orbital-cerebral mucormycosis
- Histopathology of postacute/long COVID-19 under investigation

Biosafety Considerations

- Autopsies should be performed in negative pressure rooms, using standard personal protective equipment and N95 respirator or higher with avoidance of bone saws or other aerosol-generating procedures
- Routine cleaning and disinfection procedures are considered appropriate
- Frozen sections should be avoided to prevent cryostat-generated aerosols
- Routine formalin fixation and heating during paraffin infiltration inactivate virus

ANCILLARY TESTS

Immunohistochemistry

- Antinucleocapsid and antispike antibodies stain cytoplasm of infected cells

In Situ Hybridization

- Viral RNA can be detected with targeted probes

Electron Microscopy

- Viral particles reported in lung (type I and type II pneumocytes), trachea (epithelial cells and extracellular mucus), kidney (tubular epithelium and endothelial cells), and large intestines
- Spherical particles (60-140 nm in diameter) with some pleomorphism and distinctive spikes (9-12 nm)

DIFFERENTIAL DIAGNOSIS

Other Coronavirus Infections

- HCoV 229E, NL63, OC43, and HKU1; MERS-CoV, SARS-CoV
  - Confirmation by molecular testing or serology

Other Respiratory Viral Infections

- Influenza A or B, respiratory syncytial virus, cytomegalovirus, herpes simplex virus, etc.
  - Confirmation by histology, IHC, molecular testing, or serology

Bacterial, Mycobacterial and Fungal Infections

- *Mycoplasma pneumoniae*, *Mycobacterium avium* complex, *Cryptococcus* infections, etc.
  - Positive Gram, MSS, or AFB stains, molecular testing, culture results, or serology

Noninfectious Causes of Diffuse Alveolar Damage

- Complications of transplantation, connective tissue diseases, acute exacerbation of idiopathic pulmonary fibrosis, drugs, radiation therapy, acute interstitial pneumonia
  - Negative viral serology, molecular testing, and cultures

SELECTED REFERENCES

1. Altmann DM et al: The immunology of long COVID. Nat Rev Immunol. ePub, 2023
2. Lucas F et al: Hematopathology of severe acute respiratory syndrome coronavirus 2 infection and coronavirus disease-19. Surg Pathol Clin. 16(2):197-211, 2023
3. Shih AR et al: COVID-19: gastrointestinal and hepatobiliary manifestations. Hum Pathol. 132:39-55, 2023
4. Dittmayer C et al: Continued false-positive detection of SARS-CoV-2 by electron microscopy. Ann Neurol. 92(2):340-1, 2022
5. Jeganathan K et al: Vertical transmission of SARS-CoV-2: a systematic review. Obstet Med. 15(2):91-8, 2022
6. Jonigk D et al: Organ manifestations of COVID-19: what have we learned so far (not only) from autopsies? Virchows Arch. 481(2):139-59, 2022
7. Krasemann S et al: Assessing and improving the validity of COVID-19 autopsy studies - a multicentre approach to establish essential standards for immunohistochemical and ultrastructural analyses. EBioMedicine. 83:104193, 2022
8. Reagan-Steiner S et al: Detection of SARS-CoV-2 in neonatal autopsy tissues and placenta. Emerg Infect Dis. 28(3):510-7, 2022
9. Stram MN et al: Neuropathology of pediatric SARS-CoV-2 infection in the forensic setting: novel application of ex vivo imaging in analysis of brain microvasculature. Front Neurol. 13:894565, 2022
10. Bryce C et al: Pathophysiology of SARS-CoV-2: the Mount Sinai COVID-19 autopsy experience. Mod Pathol. 34(8):1456-67, 2021
11. Martines RB et al: Pathology and pathogenesis of SARS-CoV-2 associated with fatal coronavirus disease, United States. Emerg Infect Dis. 26(9):2005-15, 2020
12. Puelles VG et al: Multiorgan and renal tropism of SARS-CoV-2. N Engl J Med. 383(6):590-2, 2020
13. Rockx B et al: Comparative pathogenesis of COVID-19, MERS, and SARS in a nonhuman primate model. Science. 368(6494):1012-5, 2020
14. Solomon IH et al: Neuropathological features of Covid-19. N Engl J Med. 383(10):989-92, 2020

Chest Radiograph

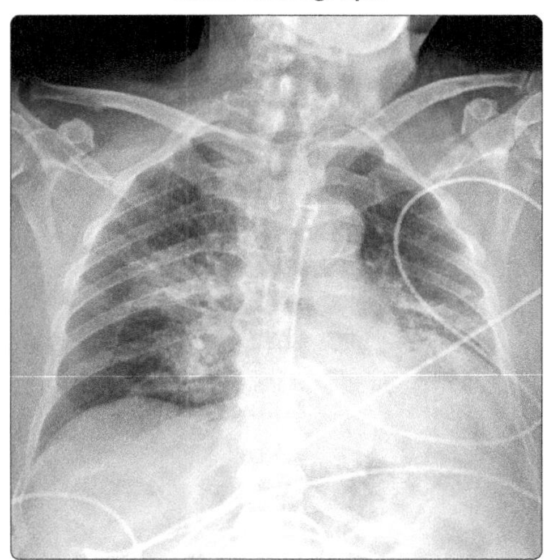

Gross Features

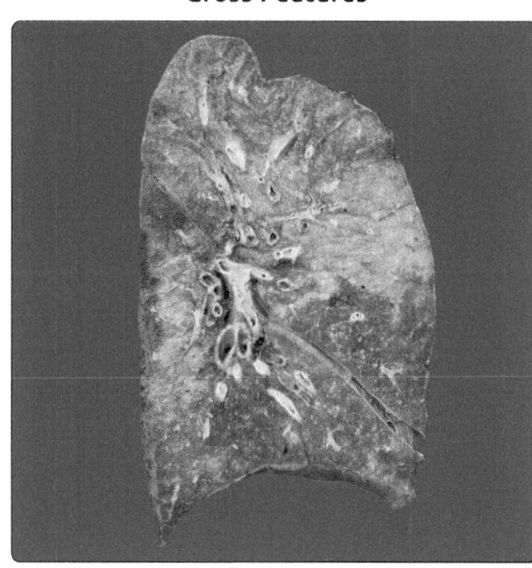

(Left) *This portable chest radiograph shows parenchymal opacities with asymmetric distribution, consolidation in the right perihilar region, and opacity in left lung base, findings consistent with COVID-19 pneumonia.* **(Right)** *This section of lung from a fatal case of COVID-19 shows areas of red congested and edematous parenchyma, consistent with diffuse alveolar damage. (Courtesy R. Padera, Jr., MD, PhD.)*

Hyaline Membranes

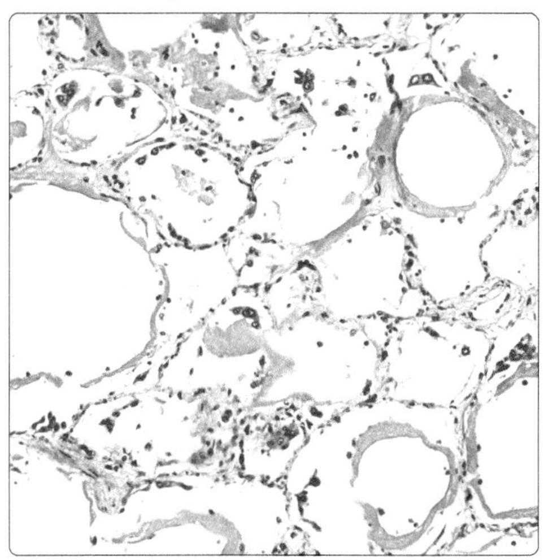

Hyaline Membranes: SARS-CoV-2 Spike IHC

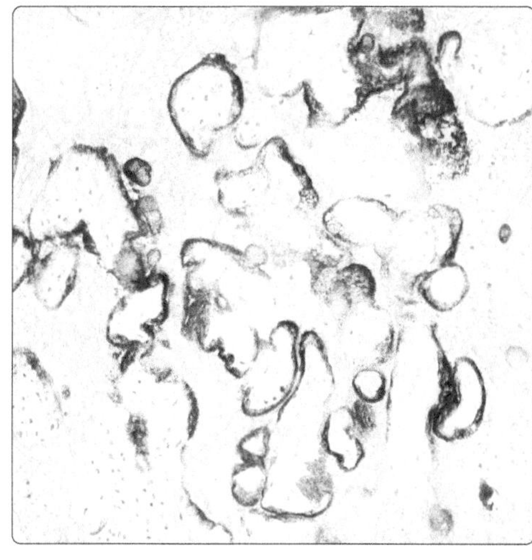

(Left) *Early histologic findings in COVID-19 pneumonia include eosinophilic hyaline membranes, consistent with exudative (acute) diffuse alveolar damage. (Courtesy R. Padera, Jr., MD, PhD.)* **(Right)** *SARS-CoV-2 spike immunohistochemistry highlights hyaline membranes in this autopsy lung section.*

Interstitial Inflammation and Edema

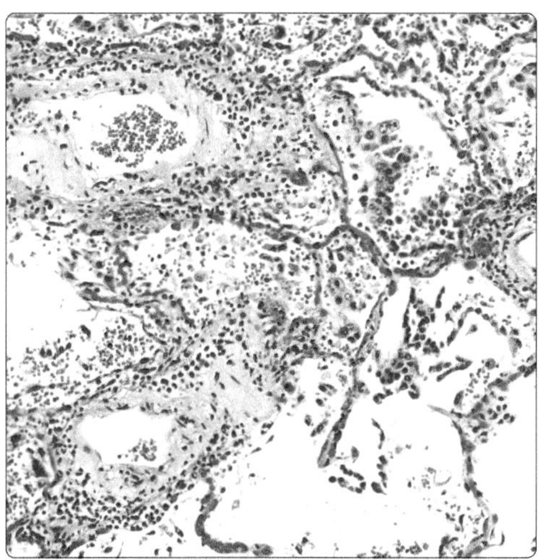

SARS-CoV-2 Spike In Situ Hybridization

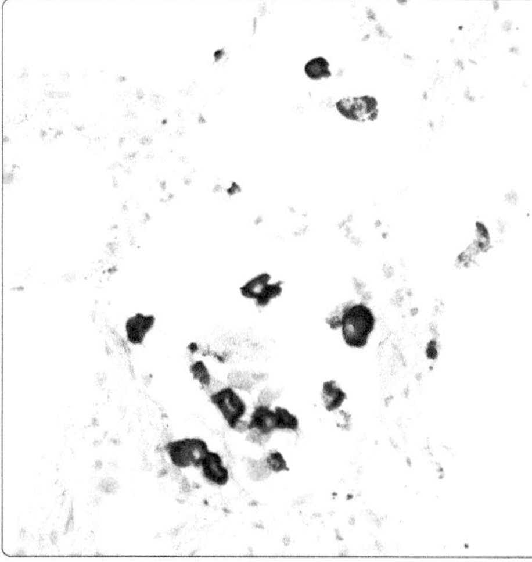

(Left) *COVID-19 pneumonia includes variable amounts of interstitial and perivascular chronic inflammation and edema. (Courtesy R. Padera, Jr., MD, PhD.)* **(Right)** *SARS-CoV-2 spike RNA in situ hybridization highlights viral RNA in infected pneumocytes and alveolar macrophages, confirming the diagnosis of COVID-19 in this autopsy lung section.*

(Left) *Multinucleated giant cells with prominent reactive-appearing nucleoli are variably present in COVID-19 pneumonia* → *. (Courtesy R. Padera, Jr., MD, PhD.)* **(Right)** *Fibrin thrombi involving small vessels are occasionally present in COVID-19 pneumonia. (Courtesy R. Padera, Jr., MD, PhD.)*

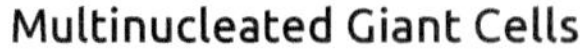

Multinucleated Giant Cells

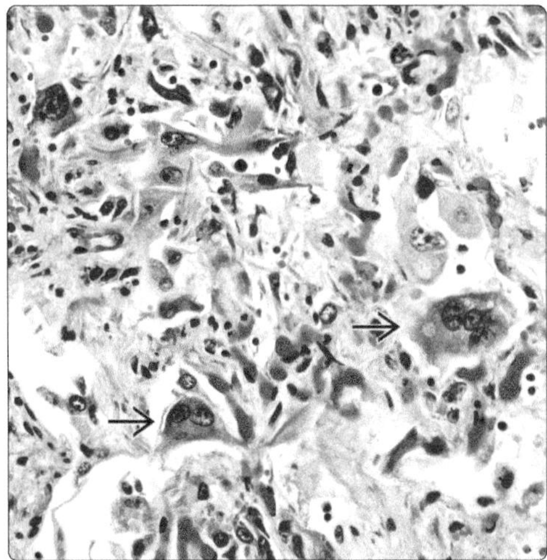

Fibrin Thrombi

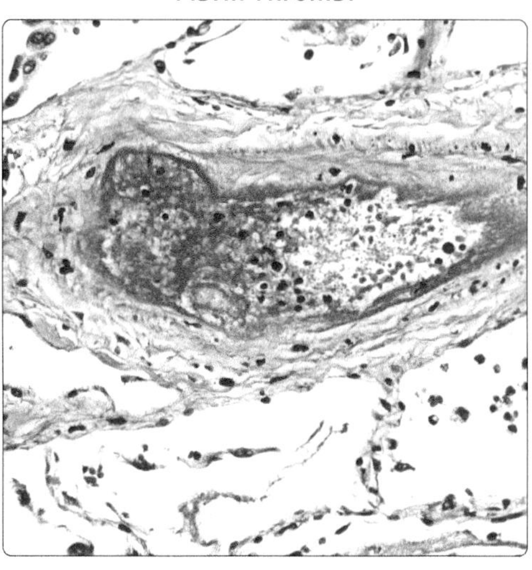

(Left) *Squamous metaplasia is frequently present in the lungs in COVID-19 pneumonia and can exhibit significant cytologic atypia. (Courtesy R. Padera, Jr., MD, PhD.)* **(Right)** *Later changes in COVID-19 pneumonia include proliferation of pneumocytes and fibroblasts to form loose organizing connective tissue. (Courtesy R. Padera, Jr., MD, PhD.)*

Squamous Metaplasia

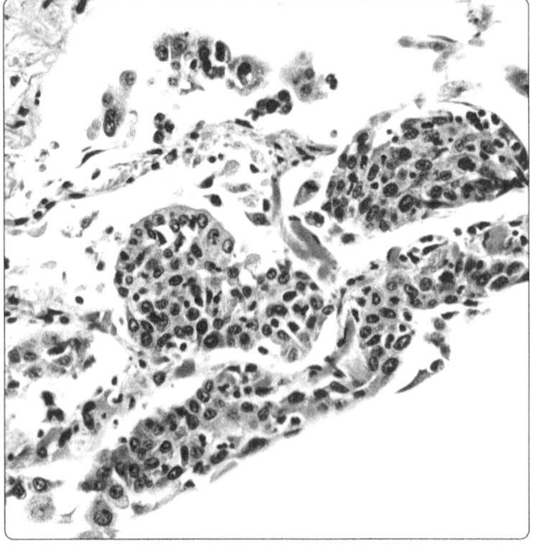

Proliferative (Organizing) Phase

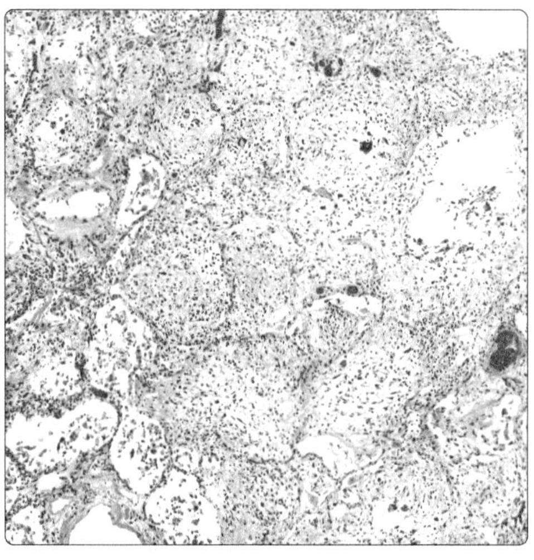

(Left) *Fibroblast proliferation and collagen production in alveolar spaces reflect organized alveolar damage. (Courtesy R. Padera, Jr., MD, PhD.)* **(Right)** *Coinfections with bacteria, fungi, and other respiratory viruses are common with COVID-19. This section shows multiple collections of basophilic bacteria* → *embedded in intraalveolar neutrophils. (Courtesy R. Padera, Jr., MD, PhD.)*

Fibroblast Proliferation

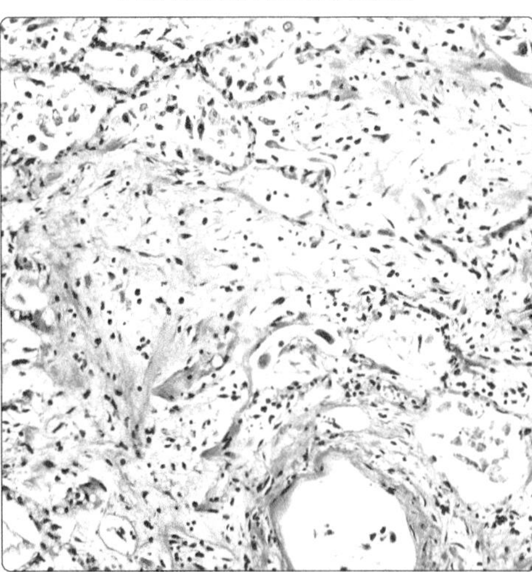

Bacterial Bronchopneumonia

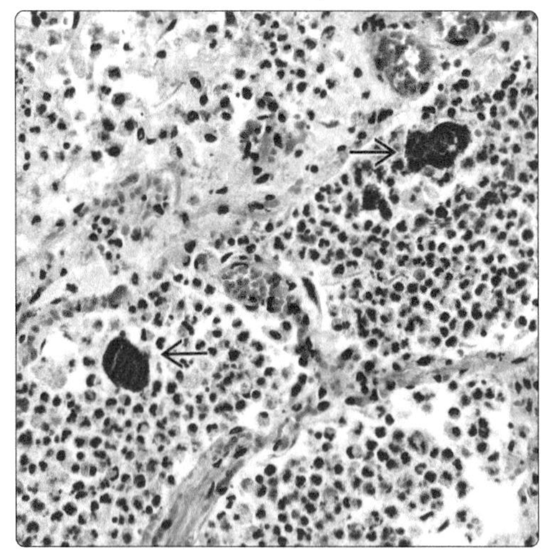

Large Airway Involvement

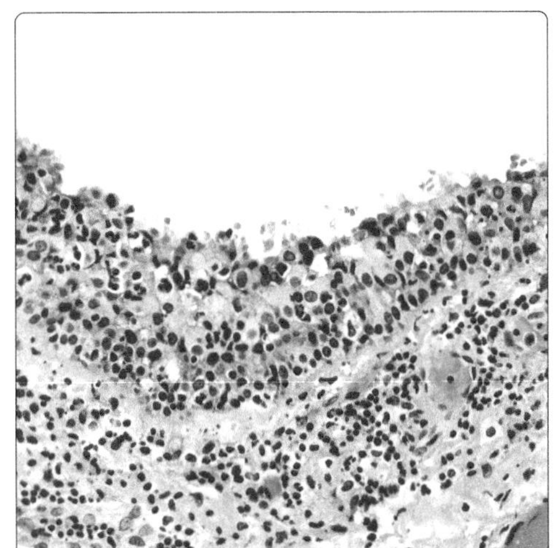

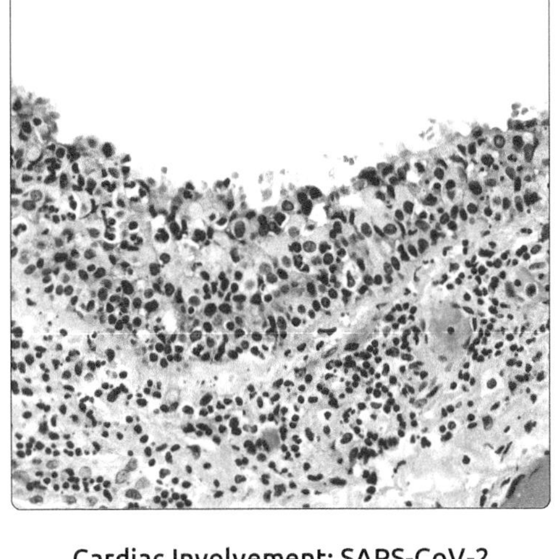

Large Airway Involvement: SARS-CoV-2 Nucleocapsid IHC

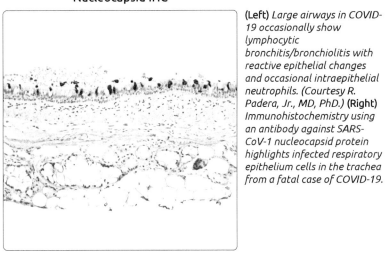

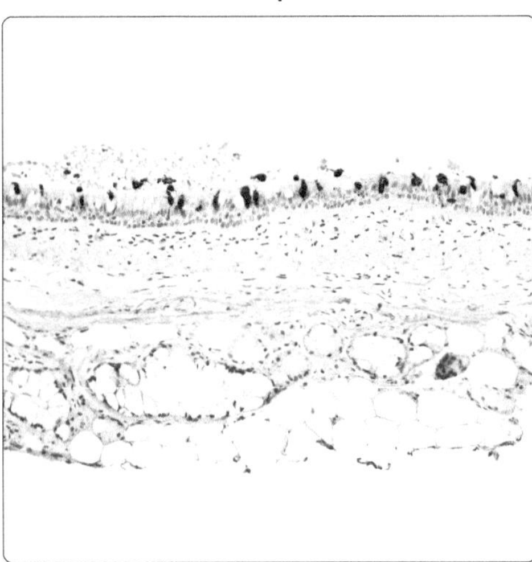

(Left) *Large airways in COVID-19 occasionally show lymphocytic bronchitis/bronchiolitis with reactive epithelial changes and occasional intraepithelial neutrophils. (Courtesy R. Padera, Jr., MD, PhD.)* **(Right)** *Immunohistochemistry using an antibody against SARS-CoV-1 nucleocapsid protein highlights infected respiratory epithelium cells in the trachea from a fatal case of COVID-19.*

Cardiac Involvement: SARS-CoV-2 Nucleocapsid IHC

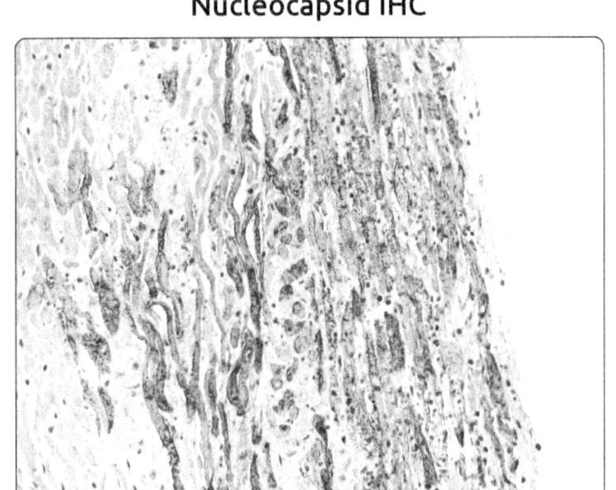

Gastrointestinal Involvement: SARS-CoV-2 Nucleocapsid IHC

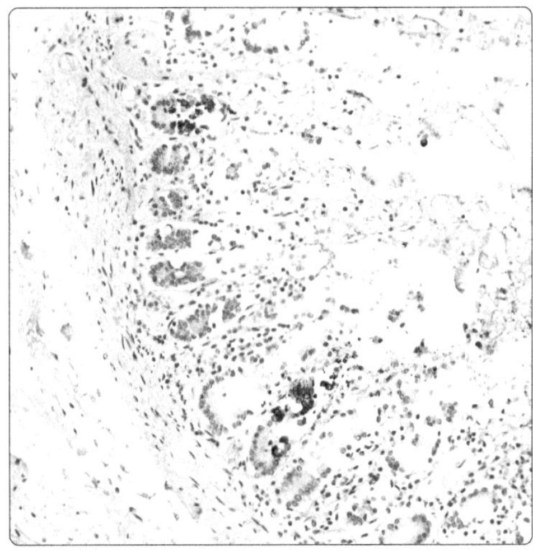

(Left) *Cardiac involvement is an uncommon finding in COVID-19 and is typically associated with severe immunosuppression. In this section, cardiac myocytes are demonstrated to be infected by expression of SARS-CoV-2 nucleocapsid protein.* **(Right)** *Involvement of the gastrointestinal tract, including stomach, small intestine, large intestine, and liver, is also uncommon and is demonstrated in this duodenal section by SARS-CoV-2 nucleocapsid immunohistochemistry.*

Brain Involvement

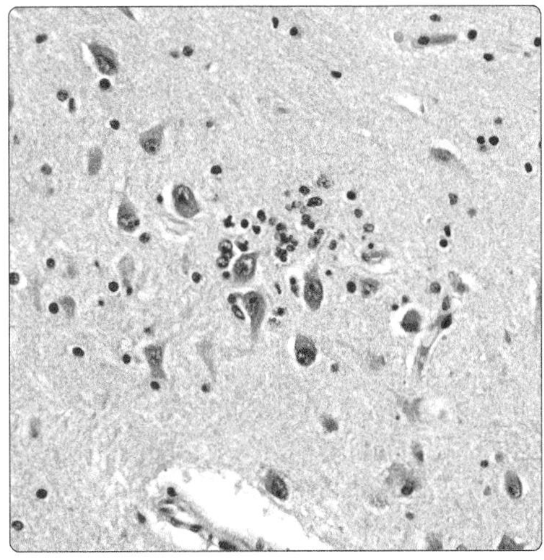

Placental Involvement

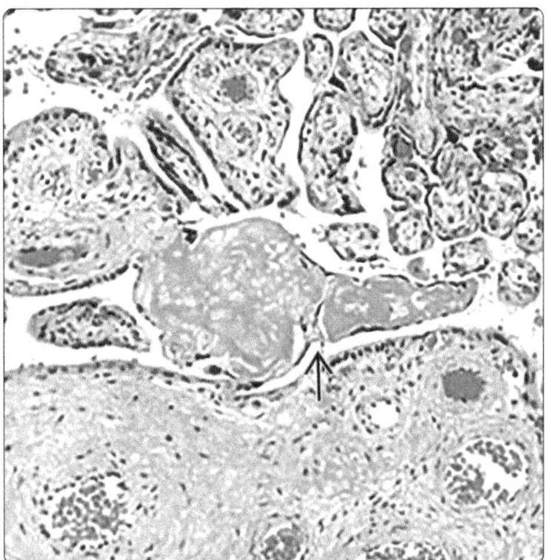

(Left) *SARS-CoV-2 has not been detected in significant levels in fatal cases of COVID-19, and neuropathological changes (e.g., hypoxic-ischemic changes and rare microglial nodules) can be accounted for by severe lung disease and system inflammation.* **(Right)** *Placenta from a neonatal autopsy following 2nd-trimester maternal COVID-19 demonstrates fibrinoid necrosis →. [Courtesy Reagan-Steiner et al. Emerg Infect Dis. 2022;28(3):510-517.]*

Severe Acute Respiratory Syndrome (SARS), Middle East Respiratory Syndrome (MERS), and Other Coronavirus Infections

KEY FACTS

ETIOLOGY/PATHOGENESIS

- Viral infections transmitted by respiratory droplets

CLINICAL ISSUES

- No cases of severe acute respiratory syndrome (SARS) since 2004
- Occasional outbreaks of Middle East respiratory syndrome (MERS) since 2012
- Seasonal endemic infections with other HCoVs: HCoV-NL63, HCoV-229E, HCoV-OC43, HCoV-HKU1
- Presentation: Fever, headache, myalgias, cough, dyspnea; radiographically confirmed pneumonia
- Rare reports of neuroinvasive disease
- Labs: Serology, RT-PCR, viral isolation
- Supportive therapy; no vaccines or targeted therapies
- Overall fatality: ~ 10% in SARS and 30-40% in MERS

MICROSCOPIC

- SARS: Lungs with diffuse alveolar damage (DAD)
- MERS: Necrotizing pneumonia, pulmonary DAD, acute kidney injury, portal and lobular hepatitis, myositis
- No viral inclusions

ANCILLARY TESTS

- Anti-SARS-CoV-1 IHC: Positive staining in alveolar epithelial cells and macrophages
- Anti-MERS-CoV IHC: Positive staining in pneumocytes and epithelial syncytial cells

TOP DIFFERENTIAL DIAGNOSES

- Other respiratory viral infections (e.g., influenza A or B, RSV, CMV, HSV): Confirmed by IHC, PCR, etc.
- Bacterial, mycobacterial, and fungal infections: Organisms identified with special stains, PCR, cultures, etc.
- Noninfectious causes of DAD (e.g., complications of transplantation, connective tissue diseases, acute exacerbation of idiopathic pulmonary fibrosis, drugs, radiation therapy, and acute interstitial pneumonia): Negative viral serology, molecular testing, and cultures

(Left) *Chest x-ray (CXR) shows diffuse, bilateral, ground-glass opacities ➡ in a patient with severe acute respiratory syndrome (SARS). Focal lower lung opacities are the most common finding, but radiographs are normal in 20% of symptomatic patients. (From DI: Chest.)* **(Right)** *Section of a lung in a patient with SARS shows diffuse alveolar damage and a multinucleated giant cell with no conspicuous viral inclusions ➡. (Courtesy S. Zaki, MD, PhD.)*

Chest X-Ray: SARS

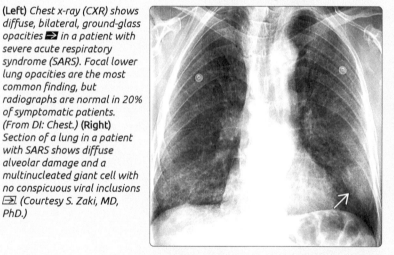

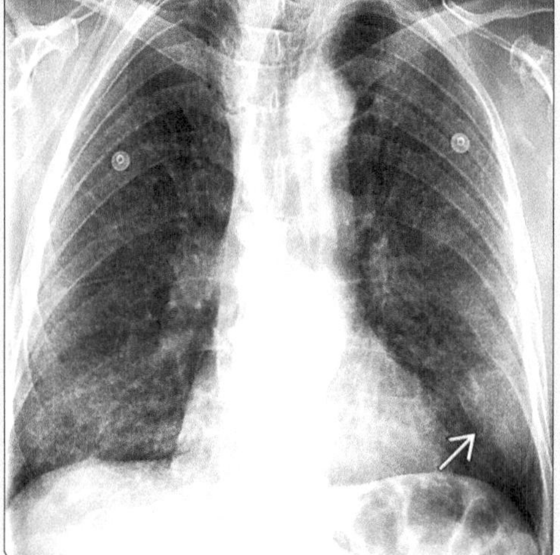

Histopathology: SARS

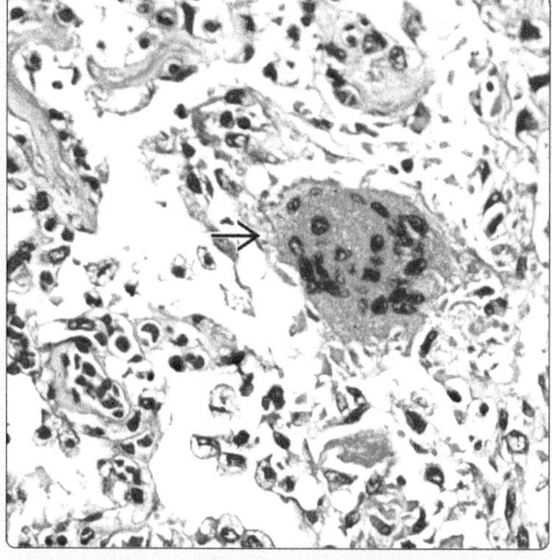

(Left) *Transmission electron micrograph (EM) shows numerous spherical, enveloped virions with surface projections (corona or halo) measuring ~ 80 nm in diameter, characteristic of SARS-associated coronavirus (CoV). (Courtesy C. Humphrey, PhD, T. Ksiazek, DVM.)* **(Right)** *Transmission EM shows spherical, viral particles measuring 50-150 nm in diameter with surface spike projections, characteristic of Middle East respiratory syndrome-associated CoV (MERS-CoV). (Courtesy M. Metcalfe MS, A. Tamin, PhD.)*

Ultrastructural Features: SARS-Associated Coronavirus

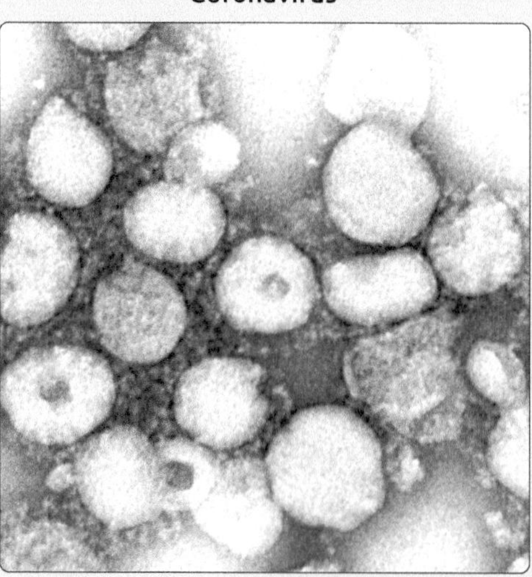

Ultrastructural Features: MERS-Associated Coronavirus

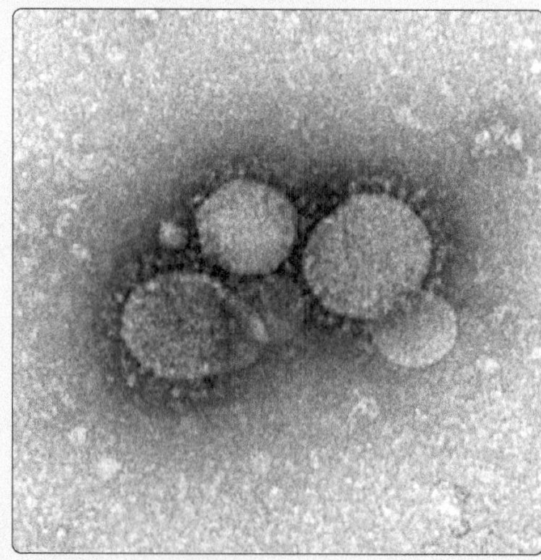

Severe Acute Respiratory Syndrome (SARS), Middle East Respiratory Syndrome (MERS), and Other Coronavirus Infections

TERMINOLOGY

Definitions

- *Coronaviridae* family: "Corona" (crown, halo) ultrastructural appearance

ETIOLOGY/PATHOGENESIS

Infectious Agents

- Viral illness with human-to-human transmission by respiratory droplets; bat reservoir with palm civet and dromedary camel intermediary hosts
- Incubation period: 2-10 days; contagious period from start of symptoms until 10 days after resolution
- Spike protein subunit S1 recognizes host cell receptors (e.g., angiotensin-converting enzyme 2), which vary in tissue distribution for each virus
- Severe acute respiratory syndrome coronavirus 1 (SARS-CoV-1)
- Middle East respiratory syndrome coronavirus (MERS-CoV)
- Other human coronaviruses (HCoV): HCoV-NL63, HCoV-229E, HCoV-OC43, HCoV-HKU1

CLINICAL ISSUES

Epidemiology

- SARS: 2002-2003 outbreak originating in Asia resulted in > 8,000 cases and 916 deaths in 29 countries worldwide; no reported cases since 2004
- MERS: Outbreaks starting in 2012 originating in Arabian peninsula; > 2,600 cases and 935 deaths in 27 countries
- Other HCoVs: Global distribution; seasonal transmission; 0.6-2.5% of adult community-acquired pneumonia

Presentation

- SARS predominantly in young healthy individuals, while MERS seen mostly in adults > 50 years with preexisting chronic illnesses
  - Present with fever, cough, myalgia, shortness of breath, sore throat, and occasional diarrhea/vomiting; acute kidney injury common; shock
- Other HCoVs: Typically mild to moderate upper respiratory tract illnesses, severe lower respiratory tract infections occur in neonates, older adults, and immunosuppressed patients; rare reports of meningoencephalitis

Laboratory Tests

- Serology: Enzyme immunoassay (EIA)
- RT-PCR (respiratory samples, stool, plasma, serum)

Treatment

- No vaccines or targeted therapies currently available
- Primarily supportive (antipyretics, oxygen, ventilation)

Prognosis

- Overall fatality: ~ 10% in SARS and 30-40% in MERS

IMAGING

Radiographic Findings

- Nonspecific findings with airspace opacities most commonly seen in SARS and ground-glass opacities and consolidation most commonly seen in MERS

MICROBIOLOGY

Virus Features

- Enveloped, single-stranded RNA viruses
- 50-150 nm in size, helical nucleocapsid, surface projections
- 27,000-30,000 nucleotide genomes (6-14 proteins)

Culture

- Grows in Vero-E6 cells (requires biosafety level 3 facility)

MICROSCOPIC

Histologic Features

- SARS: Lungs with diffuse alveolar damage (DAD): Edema, hyaline membranes, alveolar collapse, desquamation of alveolar epithelial cells, fibrous tissue in alveolar space
  - Interstitial/airspace fibrosis and pneumocyte hyperplasia after 10-14 days
- MERS autopsy: Necrotizing pneumonia, pulmonary DAD, acute kidney injury, portal and lobular hepatitis, and myositis with muscle atrophic changes; unremarkable brain and heart
- No viral inclusions observed

ANCILLARY TESTS

Immunohistochemistry

- Anti-SARS-CoV antibodies stain alveolar epithelial cells and macrophages
- Anti-MERS-CoV antibodies stain pneumocytes and epithelial syncytial cells

DIFFERENTIAL DIAGNOSIS

Other Respiratory Viral Infections

- Influenza A or B, respiratory syncytial virus, cytomegalovirus, herpes simplex virus, etc.
  - Confirmation by histology, IHC, molecular testing, or serology

Bacterial, Mycobacterial, and Fungal Infections

- *Mycoplasma pneumoniae*, *Mycobacterium avium* complex, *Cryptococcus* infections, etc.
  - Positive Gram, MSS, or AFB stains, molecular testing, culture results, or serology

Noninfectious Causes of Diffuse Alveolar Damage

- Complications of transplantation, connective tissue diseases, acute exacerbation of idiopathic pulmonary fibrosis, drugs, radiation therapy, acute interstitial pneumonia
  - Negative viral serology, molecular testing, and cultures

SELECTED REFERENCES

1. Ruiz-Aravena M et al: Ecology, evolution and spillover of coronaviruses from bats. Nat Rev Microbiol. 20(5):299-314, 2022
2. Alsaad KO et al: Histopathology of Middle East respiratory syndrome coronovirus (MERS-CoV) infection - clinicopathological and ultrastructural study. Histopathology. 72(3):516-24, 2018
3. Morfopoulou S et al: Human coronavirus OC43 associated with fatal encephalitis. N Engl J Med. 375(5):497-8, 2016
4. Gu J et al: Pathology and pathogenesis of severe acute respiratory syndrome. Am J Pathol. 170(4):1136-47, 2007
5. Goldsmith CS et al: Ultrastructural characterization of SARS coronavirus. Emerg Infect Dis. 10(2):320-6, 2004

Respiratory Syncytial Virus Infection

KEY FACTS

ETIOLOGY/PATHOGENESIS

- Viral infection transmitted by respiratory droplets and contact with contaminated surfaces

CLINICAL ISSUES

- Majority of children infected by 2 years of age; hospitalization rare in healthy patients
- Lower respiratory symptoms in 25-40% of cases; upper respiratory less common
- Laboratory: RT-PCR, antigen testing
- Treatment: Supportive; palivizumab for high-risk infants

MACROSCOPIC

- Heavy congested lungs with areas of consolidation and expansion, and plugging of small airways

MICROSCOPIC

- Airway epithelium with inflammation, ulceration, necrosis, and sloughing/obstruction, diffuse alveolar damage, and regenerative changes (e.g., squamous metaplasia)
- Multinucleated syncytial giant cells with eosinophilic cytoplasmic inclusions lining bronchi, bronchioles, and alveoli

TOP DIFFERENTIAL DIAGNOSES

- Human parainfluenza virus infection: Multinucleated giant cells with eosinophilic cytoplasmic inclusions; confirm by PCR, antigen testing
- Human metapneumovirus infection: Eosinophilic nuclear and cytoplasmic inclusions; confirm by PCR, antigen testing
- Measles virus infection: Eosinophilic cytoplasmic inclusions, intranuclear inclusions with clear halo; Warthin-Finkeldey giant cells; confirm by PCR, culture, serology
- Influenza virus infection: No specific viral cytopathic effects; confirm by PCR, IHC, antigen testing
- Asthma: Detached epithelium, eosinophilic plugging, smooth muscle hyperplasia, marked inflammatory infiltrate

(Left) *Radiograph of an infant with respiratory syncytial virus (RSV) demonstrates hyperinflation and diffuse interstitial markings with flattened diaphragm and blunting of the costophrenic angles. (From DP: Pediatric Neoplasms.)* **(Right)** *Transmission electron micrograph shows an irregularly shaped, enveloped virion with glycoprotein spikes, measuring 120-300 nm in diameter, characteristic of RSV. (Courtesy E. Palmer, CDC/PHIL.)*

Radiographic Findings

Ultrastructural Features

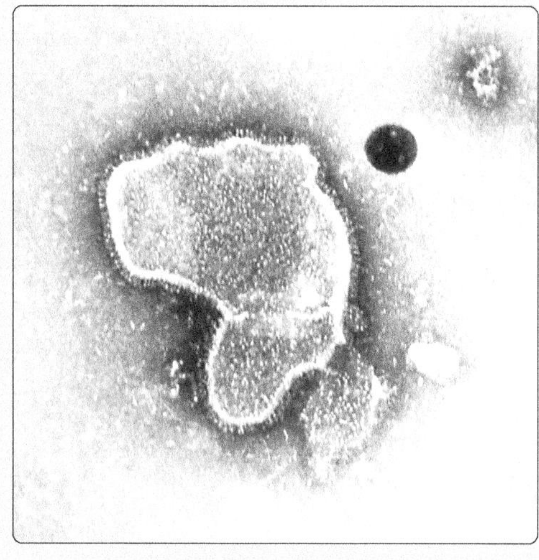

(Left) *Section from a fatal case of RSV pneumonia shows diffuse alveolar damage, intraalveolar hemorrhage, interstitial inflammation, and occasional multinucleated, giant syncytial cells →.* **(Right)** *A giant syncytial cell is present in the lung of a fatal case of RSV pneumonia. The cell contains multiple nuclei and an eosinophilic cytoplasmic inclusion →.*

Severe Lung Disease

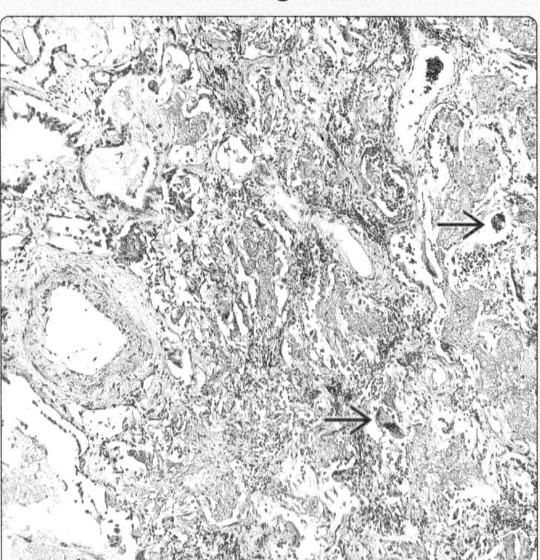

Viral Cytopathic Effects

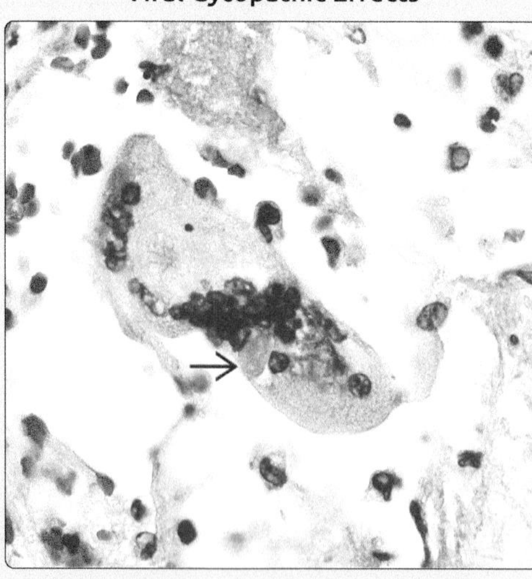

TERMINOLOGY

Synonyms

- *Human orthopneumovirus*; respiratory syncytial virus (RSV)

Definitions

- Syncytial: Derived from Latin "syn" (together) and "cyt" (cell)
- *Pneumoviridae* family: Derived from "pneumo" (lung)

ETIOLOGY/PATHOGENESIS

Infectious Agents

- Viral infection transmitted by respiratory droplets and contact with contaminated surfaces; incubation period: 2-8 days; infectious period: 5 days to 3 weeks
- Infection of respiratory epithelium results in inflammation/necrosis and formation of "plugs" of mucus, fibrin, and necrotic material in smaller airways
- F proteins cause cell membrane fusion to form syncytia

CLINICAL ISSUES

Epidemiology

- Worldwide: ~ 64 million infections/year (160,000 deaths)
- Most common in fall, winter, and spring in temperate climates but can vary annually
- Affects 70% of infants by 1 year of age and ~ 100% of infants by 2 years of age (peak infection: 2-3 months)

Presentation

- Lower respiratory tract infections (bronchiolitis or pneumonia) occur in 25-40% of cases
- Upper respiratory tract infections (croup, otitis media, rhinitis, tracheobronchitis, fever) are less common
- Secondary asthma exacerbations and coinfections with bacteria, fungi, or other viruses also occur
- High-risk factors: HIV infection, stem cell transplantation, prematurity, and congenital heart disease

Laboratory Tests

- RT-PCR (individual or multiplex assay)
- Antigen testing in nasopharyngeal specimens 80-90% sensitive in young children but lower for adults
- Serology and cell culture less commonly used

Treatment

- No FDA-approved vaccines or specific antiviral treatments
- Palivizumab (monoclonal anti-RSV protein F antibody) for high-risk infants (5 monthly injections)
- Supportive treatment ± ribavirin for severe cases

Prognosis

- Low mortality in previously healthy patients (0.3-1.0%)
- Up to 40% mortality in very young infants, preterm infants, and patients with HIV or other immunodeficiency or underlying pulmonary or cardiac disease
- Repeated infections may increase risk for asthma

IMAGING

Radiographic Findings

- Hyperinflation, diffuse interstitial markings, and peribronchial thickening

MICROBIOLOGY

Viral Features

- Enveloped, negative-sense, single-stranded RNA virus
- 120- to 200-nm, irregularly shaped, helical capsid
- 15.2 kb nucleotide genome; 10 genes (*NS1*, *NS2*, *N*, *P*, *M*, *SH*, *G*, *F*, *M2*, and *L*) (11 proteins)

Culture

- Grows in HEp-2 cells; syncytia formation after 3-7 days

MACROSCOPIC

General Features

- Heavy congested lungs with areas of consolidation and expansion and plugging of small airways

MICROSCOPIC

Histologic Features

- Airway epithelium with inflammation, ulceration, necrosis, and sloughing/obstruction, diffuse alveolar damage, and regenerative changes (e.g., squamous metaplasia)

Cytologic Features

- Multinucleated giant syncytial cells with eosinophilic cytoplasmic inclusions lining airways

ANCILLARY TESTS

Immunohistochemistry

- anti-RSV antibodies highlight cytoplasm of infected epithelial cells

DIFFERENTIAL DIAGNOSIS

Human Parainfluenza Virus Infection

- Multinucleated giant cells with eosinophilic cytoplasmic inclusions; confirm by PCR, antigen testing

Human Metapneumovirus Infection

- Eosinophilic nuclear and cytoplasmic inclusions; confirm by PCR, antigen testing

Measles Virus Infection

- Eosinophilic cytoplasmic inclusions, intranuclear inclusions with clear halo; Warthin-Finkeldey giant cells; confirm by PCR, culture, serology

Influenza Virus Infection

- No specific viral cytopathic effects; confirm by PCR, IHC, antigen testing

Asthma

- Detached epithelium, eosinophilic plugging, smooth muscle hyperplasia, marked inflammatory infiltrate

SELECTED REFERENCES

1. Mazur NI et al: Respiratory syncytial virus prevention within reach: the vaccine and monoclonal antibody landscape. Lancet Infect Dis. 23(1):e2-1, 2023
2. Centers for Disease Control and Prevention: Respiratory syncytial virus infection (RSV). Updated October 28, 2022. Reviewed February 26, 2023. Accessed February 26, 2023. https://www.cdc.gov/rsv/index.htm
3. Johnson JE et al: The histopathology of fatal untreated human respiratory syncytial virus infection. Mod Pathol. 20(1):108-19, 2007

Rhinoviruses, *Human Metapneumovirus*, and Other Respiratory Virus Infections

KEY FACTS

ETIOLOGY/PATHOGENESIS

- Viral infections spread person to person via respiratory droplets [rhinoviruses and *Human metapneumovirus* (HMPV)] or via aerosolized droplets from infected rodents (hantaviruses)

CLINICAL ISSUES

- Rhinoviruses cause mild upper respiratory tract infections; lower tract disease increasingly recognized
- HMPV affects both upper and lower respiratory tracts; severe disease in premature infants/older adults
- Hantaviruses can cause hantavirus pulmonary syndrome (HPS) with high mortality
- Laboratory: RT-PCR, antigen detection, serology

MICROSCOPIC

- Rhinoviruses: Minimal damage to nasal epithelium, mild inflammatory infiltrate; bronchiolitis
- HMPV: Intraluminal, sloughed epithelial cells and debris, interstitial edema/inflammation, alveolitis, and eosinophilic nuclear and cytoplasmic inclusions
- Hantaviruses: Fibrinous pulmonary edema, hyaline membranes, immunoblastic proliferation involving reticuloendothelial system

ANCILLARY TESTS

- IHC positive in nasal/airway epithelium (rhinoviruses, HMPV) or endothelial cells (hantaviruses)

TOP DIFFERENTIAL DIAGNOSES

- Other viral causes of tracheobronchitis, pneumonia, and giant cell pneumonia (e.g., measles, influenza, adenoviruses, coxsackieviruses, respiratory syncytial virus, varicella-zoster virus, herpes simplex virus): Detection virus by culture, PCR, IHC, etc.
- Allergic rhinitis: Associated with specific allergens; may be seasonal or perennial; improves with steroids and allergen avoidance

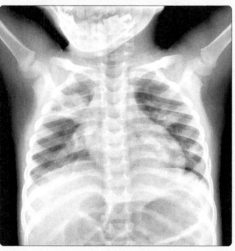

Human metapneumovirus | **Human metapneumovirus**

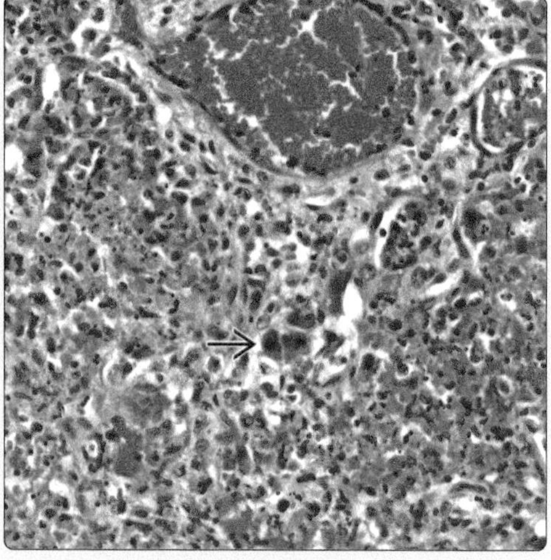

(Left) *This chest radiograph demonstrates perihilar infiltrates, peribronchial cuffing, and lobar infiltrates, findings characteristic of, but not specific for, human metapneumovirus infection. (From DP: Nonneoplastic Pediatrics.)* **(Right)** *This lung section demonstrates alveolitis and interstitial inflammation with multinucleated giant cells showing eosinophilic nuclear and cytoplasmic inclusions →, typical of human metapneumovirus infection. (From DP: Nonneoplastic Pediatrics.)*

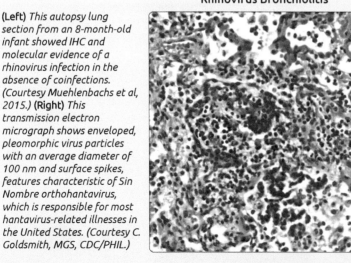

Rhinovirus Bronchiolitis | **Hantavirus Ultrastructural Features**

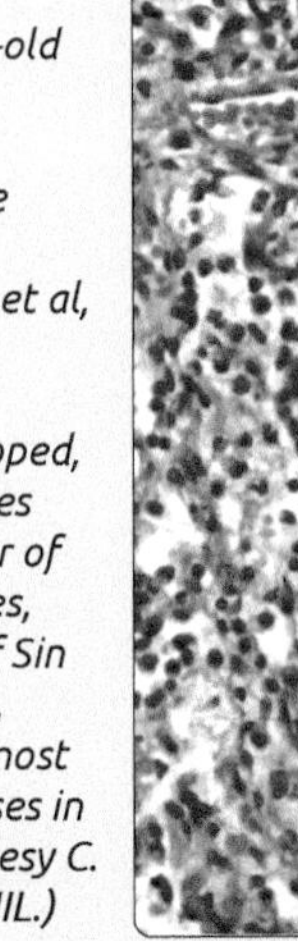

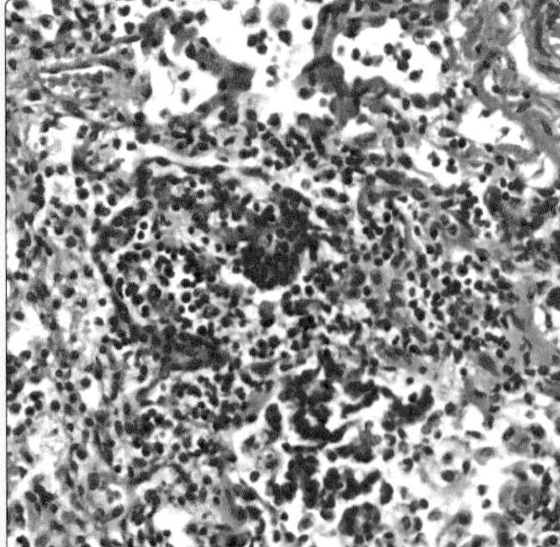

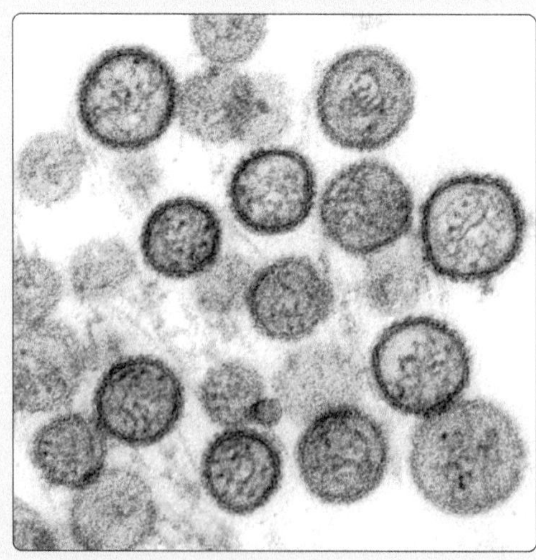

(Left) *This autopsy lung section from an 8-month-old infant showed IHC and molecular evidence of a rhinovirus infection in the absence of coinfections. (Courtesy Muehlenbachs et al, 2015.)* **(Right)** *This transmission electron micrograph shows enveloped, pleomorphic virus particles with an average diameter of 100 nm and surface spikes, features characteristic of Sin Nombre orthohantavirus, which is responsible for most hantavirus-related illnesses in the United States. (Courtesy C. Goldsmith, MGS, CDC/PHIL.)*

Rhinoviruses, *Human Metapneumovirus*, and Other Respiratory Virus Infections

TERMINOLOGY

Definitions

- *Rhinovirus A, B, C*: Derived from "rhino" (nose); *Picornaviridae* family [derived from "pico" (small) and "RNA"]
- *Human metapneumovirus* (HMPV): Derived from "meta" (after) and "pneumo" (lung); *Pneumoviridae* family
- Hantaviruses, *Orthohantavirus* (genus): Named for Hantan River in South Korea; *Hantaviridae* family

ETIOLOGY/PATHOGENESIS

Infectious Agents

- Rhinoviruses spread person to person via respiratory droplets; binds ICAM-1/CD54 receptors on respiratory epithelial cells and replicates between 33-35°C (intranasal temperature); incubation period: 2-3 days, symptoms last ~ 7 days
- HMPV spreads person to person via respiratory droplets; infects airway epithelium via glycoprotein (G) protein-glycosaminoglycan interactions
- Hantaviruses spread by inhalation of aerosolized droplets of urine, saliva, or respiratory sections from infected rodents; incubation period is 2-4 weeks

CLINICAL ISSUES

Epidemiology

- Rhinoviruses: 30-50% of common cold (~ 20-33 million cases per year in USA); most common in fall and spring
- HMPV: ~ 25% of childhood respiratory tract infections (peak for hospitalizations: 6-12 months); most common in late winter and spring
- Hantavirus outbreaks due to number of different species reported worldwide; 833 cases reported in USA from 1993-2020; most commonly due to *Sin Nombre orthohantavirus*

Presentation

- Rhinoviruses typically cause mild upper respiratory tract infections; increasingly associated with lower respiratory tract disease, including wheezing, asthma exacerbations, and pneumonia
- HMPV associated with bronchiolitis, pneumonia, croup, and exacerbation of reactive airways disease; severe disease in premature infants, immunocompromised, and adults > 65 years
- Hantaviruses can cause hantavirus pulmonary syndrome (HPS); 36% mortality

Laboratory Tests

- RT-PCR (single target or multiplex)
- Antigen detection: Enzyme immunoassay (EIA), direct fluorescent antibody (DFA) tests
- Serology (IgM or rise in IgG)
- 5-point blood smear screen for HPS: Thrombocytopenia, elevated hemoglobin/hematocrit, neutrophil left shift, absence of neutrophilic toxic granulations, and > 10% immunoblasts/plasma cells

Treatment

- No FDA-approved vaccines or specific antiviral treatments
- Supportive/symptomatic treatment; hospitalization for respiratory distress, stridor, or severe dehydration

MICROBIOLOGY

Viral Features

- Rhinoviruses
  - Nonenveloped, single-stranded RNA viruses
  - Spherical, 30 nm in diameter, icosahedral nucleocapsid
  - 7,200-8,500 nucleotide genomes (1 open reading frame)
  - 3 species (A, B, C); > 160 types based on VP1 gene
- HMPV
  - Enveloped, single-stranded RNA virus
  - Pleomorphic, 150- to 200-nm, helical nucleocapsid
  - ~ 13,000 nucleotide genome (9 proteins)
- Hantaviruses
  - Enveloped, singe-stranded RNA virus
  - Pleomorphic, 100-nm, helical nucleocapsid; 6-nm spikes
  - ~ 12,000 nucleotide genome (3 segments)

Culture

- Cytopathic effects detectable in multiple cell lines

MICROSCOPIC

Histologic Features

- Rhinoviruses: Minimal damage to nasal epithelium, mild inflammatory infiltrate (lymphocytes and eosinophils), neutrophils abundant in nasal lavage fluids; bronchiolitis
- HMPV: Intraluminal, sloughed epithelial cells and debris, loss of ciliated epithelium, interstitial edema, alveolitis, interstitial inflammation, and eosinophilic nuclear and cytoplasmic inclusions
- Hantaviruses: Fibrinous pulmonary edema, hyaline membranes, immunoblastic proliferation involving reticuloendothelial system

ANCILLARY TESTS

Immunohistochemistry

- Antigen detectable in nasal/airway epithelium (rhinoviruses, HMPV) or endothelial cells (hantaviruses)

DIFFERENTIAL DIAGNOSIS

Other Viral Causes of Tracheobronchitis, Pneumonia, and Giant Cell Pneumonia

- e.g., measles, influenza, adenoviruses, coxsackieviruses, respiratory syncytial virus, varicella-zoster virus, herpes simplex virus
- Detection of specific pathogen by culture, DFA, serology, PCR, histochemical stains, or IHC

Allergic Rhinitis

- Associated with specific allergens; may be seasonal or perennial; improves with steroids and allergen avoidance

SELECTED REFERENCES

1. Esneau C et al: Understanding rhinovirus circulation and impact on illness. Viruses. 14(1):141, 2022
2. Jesse ST et al: Zoonotic origins of human metapneumovirus: a journey from birds to humans. Viruses. 14(4), 2022
3. Perez A et al: Respiratory virus surveillance among children with acute respiratory illnesses - New Vaccine Surveillance Network, United States, 2016-2021. MMWR Morb Mortal Wkly Rep. 71(40):1253-9, 2022
4. Joyce AK et al: Hantavirus disease and COVID-19. Am J Clin Pathol. 157(3):470-5, 2021

KEY FACTS

ETIOLOGY/PATHOGENESIS

- Viruses transmitted by fecal-oral route
- Infects and replicates in enterocytes of small intestine villi; symptoms due to malabsorption/secretory mechanisms
- Viral shedding starts before onset of symptoms and stops several days after resolution

CLINICAL ISSUES

- Endemic viruses with worldwide distribution
- Rotavirus causes 150,000 deaths worldwide/year; norovirus causes 50,000 deaths; astrovirus has less severe disease
- Mild to severe gastroenteritis with vomiting, watery diarrhea, and low-grade fever lasting 3-8 days
- Laboratory testing: ELISA, immunochromatography, or RT-PCR (stool)
- Rotavirus vaccines available; supportive treatment (oral or IV rehydration)

MICROSCOPIC

- Small intestine: Reactive and degenerative epithelium, villous blunting, increased crypt depth, increased intraepithelial lymphocytes

TOP DIFFERENTIAL DIAGNOSES

- Gluten-sensitive enteropathy (celiac disease)
  - Clinical suspicion &/or serologic correlation with celiac disease-associated antibodies (tTG, EMA, DGP)
- *Helicobacter pylori*-associated duodenitis
  - Commonly occurs in setting of *H. pylori* gastritis; organisms seen in associated gastric biopsies
- Adenovirus, sapovirus, coronavirus, echovirus, enterovirus, and other viral infections
  - Identification of specific, active viral infection by PCR, culture, serology, or IHC
  - Most likely infection varies with age, geographic location, and immune status

Ultrastructural Features of Rotavirus

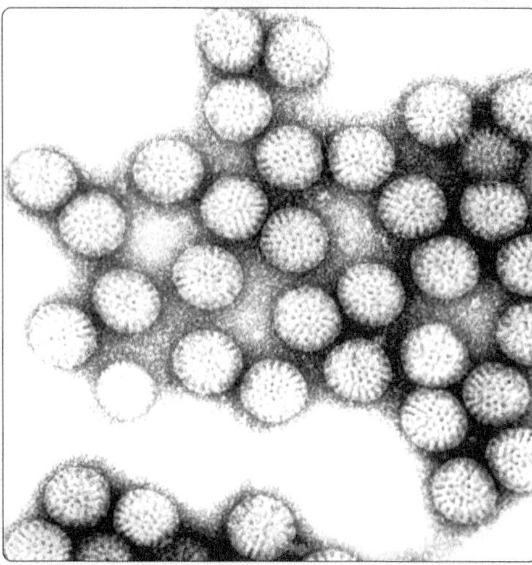

Ultrastructural Features of Norovirus

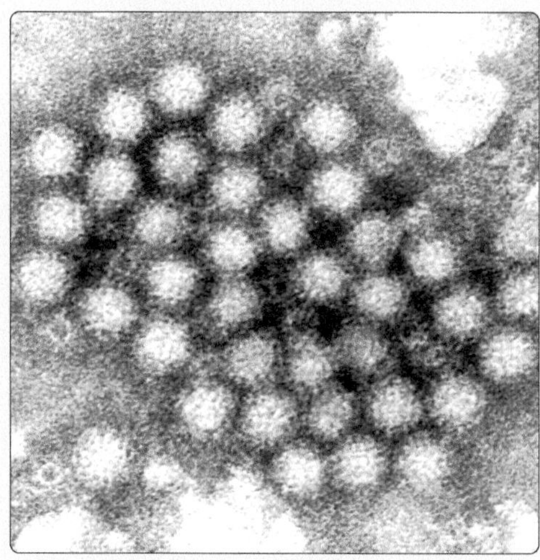

(Left) *This transmission electron micrograph shows spherical, nonenveloped particles exhibiting a wheel-like appearance and measuring 70-75 nm in diameter, characteristic of rotavirus. (Courtesy E. Palmer, PhD.)* **(Right)** *This transmission electron micrograph shows spherical, nonenveloped, viral particles measuring 27-40 nm in diameter, features characteristic of norovirus. (Courtesy C. Humphrey, PhD.)*

Viral Gastroenteritis

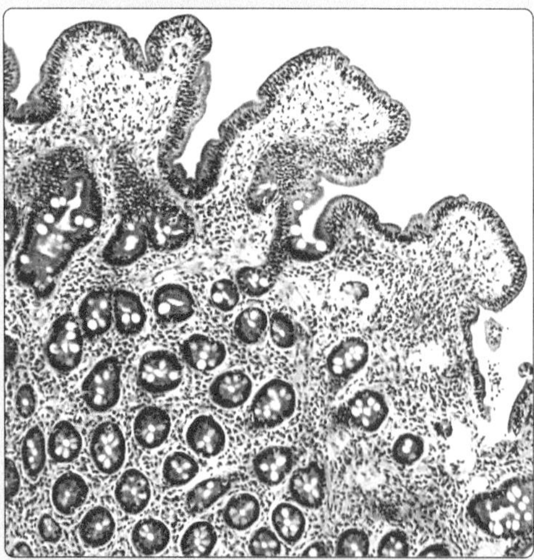

Rotavirus Infection

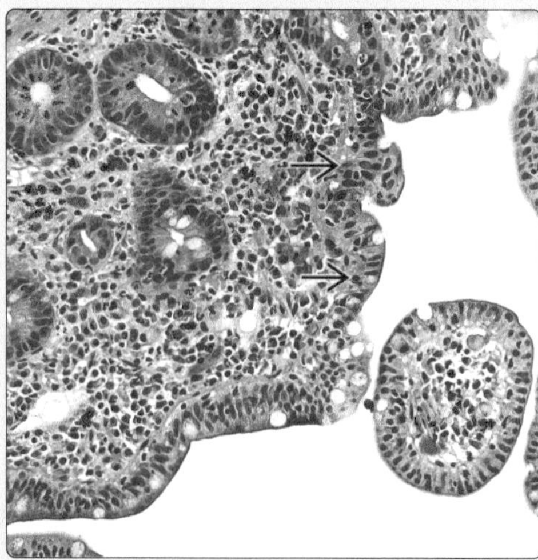

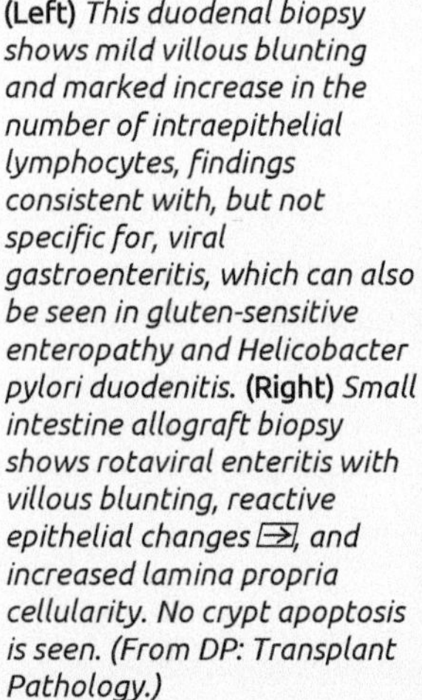

(Left) *This duodenal biopsy shows mild villous blunting and marked increase in the number of intraepithelial lymphocytes, findings consistent with, but not specific for, viral gastroenteritis, which can also be seen in gluten-sensitive enteropathy and Helicobacter pylori duodenitis.* **(Right)** *Small intestine allograft biopsy shows rotaviral enteritis with villous blunting, reactive epithelial changes →, and increased lamina propria cellularity. No crypt apoptosis is seen. (From DP: Transplant Pathology.)*

Rotavirus, *Norovirus*, and *Astrovirus* Infections

TERMINOLOGY

Synonyms

- Winter vomiting disease, stomach flu, stomach bug

Definitions

- *Rotavirus* (genus) derived from "rota" (wheel); member of *Reoviridae* family (**r**espiratory **e**nteric **o**rphan viruses)
- *Norovirus* (genus); *Norwalk virus* (species) named for Norwalk, OH where virus was identified; member of *Caliciviridae* family [derived from "calyx" (cup/goblet) due to cup-shaped depressions]
- *Astrovirus* (genus) derived from "astro" (star); member of *Astroviridae* family

ETIOLOGY/PATHOGENESIS

Infectious Agents

- Viruses transmitted by fecal-oral route (very low infectious dose required for norovirus)
- Infects and replicates in enterocytes of villi of small intestine causing diarrhea through malabsorptive and secretory mechanisms
- Incubation period 2 days; contagious period starts before symptom onset and ends several days after resolution

CLINICAL ISSUES

Epidemiology

- Endemic viruses with high seroprevalence by late childhood; seasonal variation in incidence
- Rotaviruses cause ~150,000 deaths worldwide/year in developing countries without vaccine programs (predominantly children < 5 years old)
- Noroviruses affect all ages and is leading cause of outbreaks of acute gastroenteritis; 685 million cases worldwide annually and 50,000 child deaths
- Astroviruses cause 5-10% of viral gastroenteritis in children with less severe disease than rotavirus or norovirus

Presentation

- Mild to severe gastroenteritis with vomiting, watery diarrhea, and low-grade fever lasting 3-8 days
- Astroviruses rarely associated with meningoencephalitis in immunocompromised patients

Laboratory Tests

- Enzyme-linked immunosorbent assay (ELISA) or immunochromatography (stool)
- RT-PCR (stool) (single and multiplex assays)

Treatment

- Rotavirus vaccines (oral): RotaTeq, Rotarix
- No FDA-approved vaccines for norovirus or astrovirus
- Supportive treatment; rehydration (oral or IV)

Prognosis

- Viral gastroenteritis is generally self-limited, but death can occur without adequate rehydration

MICROBIOLOGY

Virus Features

- *Rotavirus* species
  - Nonenveloped, double-stranded RNA viruses
  - 70-75 nm in diameter, 3-layered icosahedral capsid
  - 18,500 nucleotide genome (11 genes, 12 proteins)
  - *Rotavirus A* serotypes defined by glycoprotein VP7 and protease-sensitive protein VP4 [e.g., G1P(8)]
- *Norovirus* species
  - Nonenveloped, single-stranded RNA virus
  - 27-40 nm in diameter, icosahedral capsid
  - 7,500-7,700 nucleotide genome (3 ORFs)
  - Classified into VP1 genogroups/genotypes and RdRp P-types (e.g., GI.6[P6])
- *Astrovirus* species
  - Nonenveloped, single-stranded RNA virus
  - 38-41 nm in diameter, icosahedral capsid
  - 6,200-7,700 nucleotide genome (3 ORFs)
  - 8 serotypes (human astrovirus types 1-8)

Culture

- Not routinely used for diagnosis

MICROSCOPIC

Histologic Features

- Small intestine: Reactive and degenerative epithelium, villous blunting, increased crypt depth, increased intraepithelial lymphocytes

ANCILLARY TESTS

Immunohistochemistry

- Commercial antibodies available but not routinely used
- Antigen detectable in epithelial cells, lamina propria, and lymphoid cells

DIFFERENTIAL DIAGNOSIS

Gluten-Sensitive Enteropathy (Celiac Disease)

- Clinical suspicion &/or serologic correlation with celiac disease-associated antibodies (tTG, EMA, DGP)

Helicobacter pylori-Associated Duodenitis

- Commonly occurs in setting of *H. pylori* gastritis; organisms seen in associated gastric biopsies

Adenovirus, Sapovirus, Coronavirus, Echovirus, Enterovirus, and Other Viral Infections

- Identification of specific, active viral infection by PCR, culture, serology, or IHC
- Most likely infection varies with age, geographic location, and immune status

SELECTED REFERENCES

1. Hissong E et al: Histologic and clinical correlates of multiplex stool polymerase chain reaction assay results. Arch Pathol Lab Med. 146(12):1479-85, 2022
2. Omatola CA et al: Rotaviruses: from pathogenesis to disease control-a critical review. Viruses. 14(5), 2022
3. White AE et al: Foodborne illness outbreaks reported to national surveillance, United States, 2009-2018. Emerg Infect Dis. 28(6):1117-27, 2022
4. Abbas A et al: Viral enteritis in solid-organ transplantation. Viruses. 13(10), 2021
5. Cortez V et al: Astrovirus biology and pathogenesis. Annu Rev Virol. 4(1):327-48, 2017
6. Karandikar UC et al: Detection of human norovirus in intestinal biopsies from immunocompromised transplant patients. J Gen Virol. 97(9):2291-300, 2016

Hepatitis A and E Virus Infections

KEY FACTS

ETIOLOGY/PATHOGENESIS

- Viral infections transmitted by fecal-oral route as well as person-to-person, food-borne, and zoonotic transmission resulting in acute hepatitis

CLINICAL ISSUES

- Hepatitis A virus (HAV): Increasing outbreaks in USA in post-vaccine era (since 1995); 114 million cases/year worldwide
- Hepatitis E virus (HEV): 20 million cases/year worldwide; chronic infection in immunosuppressed patients
- Presentation: Fever, malaise, abdominal pain, jaundice, fatigue, anorexia, right upper quadrant pain, hepatomegaly
- Increased ALT, bilirubin; positive anti-HAV or anti-HEV IgM
- HAV vaccine, immune globulin for prophylaxis

MICROSCOPIC

- Diffuse, lobular, predominantly lymphocytic inflammation, hepatocyte swelling, necrosis, and regeneration, Kupffer cell hyperplasia
- Mild portal or periportal inflammation, confluent hepatocyte necrosis (severe cases), and canalicular cholestasis may be present

TOP DIFFERENTIAL DIAGNOSES

- HBV: Predominant lobular injury in acute phase; positive for HBsAg, HBeAg, HBV DNA, or anti-HBcAg IgM
- HCV: Acute infection rarely biopsied; positive viral RNA
- HDV: In setting of HBV; severe necroinflammatory activity, rapid disease progression
- EBV: Liver involvement in 90% of infectious mononucleosis; portal/periportal inflammation; positive EBER ISH
- CMV: Similar to EBV hepatitis; viral inclusions positive by IHC
- Autoimmune hepatitis: Lobular hepatitis, portal/periportal plasma cell-rich inflammation, positive autoimmune serologies
- Drug-/toxin-induced hepatitis: Similar to acute viral hepatitis; prominent eosinophils

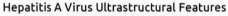

Hepatitis A Virus Ultrastructural Features

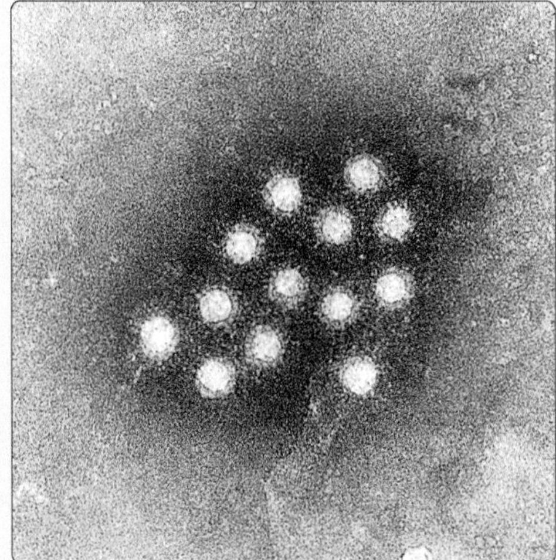

Acute Hepatitis A Virus Infection

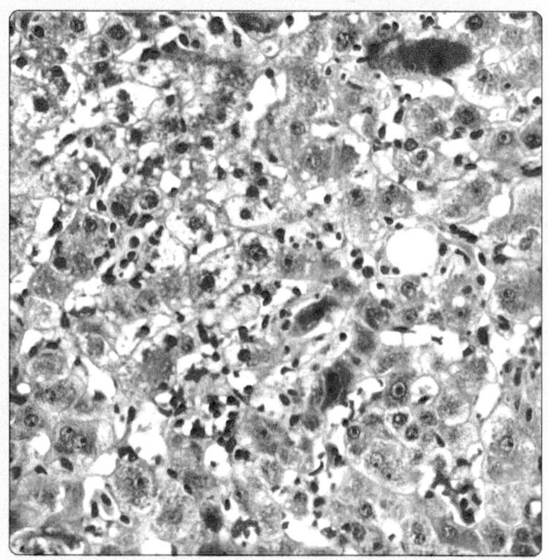

(Left) *This transmission electron micrograph shows several spherical, nonenveloped viral particles measuring ~ 27 nm in diameter, characteristic of hepatitis A virus (HAV). (Courtesy B. Partin, CDC PHIL.)* **(Right)** *Liver biopsy from acute HAV infection shows extreme hepatocellular disarray with features of a lobular hepatitis as well as a cholestatic hepatitis. (Courtesy M. Pittman, MD.)*

Hepatitis E Virus Ultrastructural Features

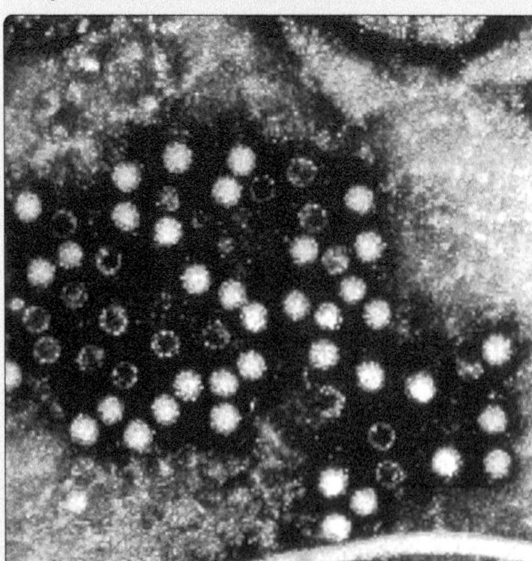

Acute Hepatitis E Virus Infection

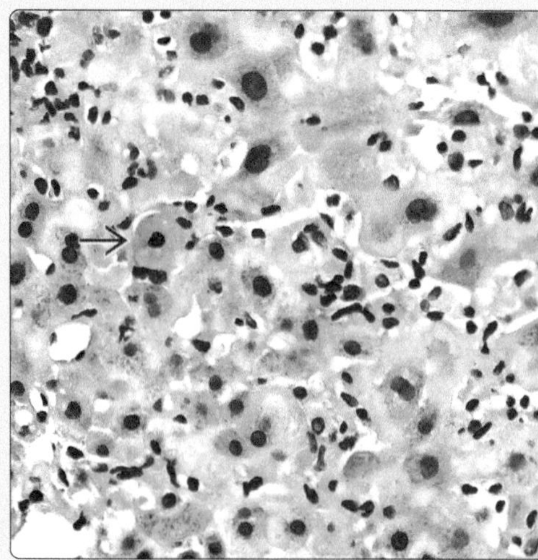

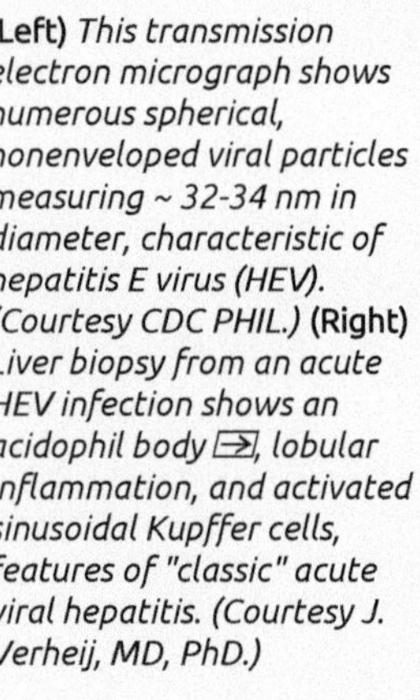

(Left) *This transmission electron micrograph shows numerous spherical, nonenveloped viral particles measuring ~ 32-34 nm in diameter, characteristic of hepatitis E virus (HEV). (Courtesy CDC PHIL.)* **(Right)** *Liver biopsy from an acute HEV infection shows an acidophil body ⇒, lobular inflammation, and activated sinusoidal Kupffer cells, features of "classic" acute viral hepatitis. (Courtesy J. Verheij, MD, PhD.)*

TERMINOLOGY

Definitions

- Hepatitis A virus (HAV); *Hepatovirus A*; *Picornaviridae* family: from "pico" (small) and "RNA"
- Hepatitis E virus (HEV); *Orthohepevirus A*: *Hepeviridae* family: from "**hep**atitis **E**"

ETIOLOGY/PATHOGENESIS

Infectious Agents

- Viral infections transmitted by fecal-oral route, vertically, parenterally, or through consumption of raw or undercooked meat of infected animals
- HEV animal reservoirs include pigs, deer, and rodents
- Virus enters bloodstream following ingestion, then infects and multiplies in liver hepatocytes and Kupffer cells and is secreted in bile and shed in stool
- Symptoms due to immunopathologic response to infected hepatocytes (incubation period is 3-6 weeks; infectious period is 2 weeks before to 1 week after symptom onset)

CLINICAL ISSUES

Epidemiology

- Account for majority of enterically transmitted viral hepatitis
- HAV
  - Worldwide: 114 million infections and 11,000 deaths annually; most common in low- and middle-income countries with poor sanitary conditions and hygienic practices
  - USA: 9,952 total cases reported (19,900 estimated) in 2020; declined 95% following HAV vaccine (1995) but increased due to large outbreaks with person-to-person transmission (27,354 hospitalizations and 421 deaths from 2016 to March 2023)
- HEV
  - Worldwide: 20 million infections and 44,000 deaths annually
  - USA: Uncommon; typically result of travel to endemic region
  - Genotype 1: Asia and Africa; waterborne fecal-oral person-to-person transmission, outbreaks commons
  - Genotype 2: Mexico and West Africa; waterborne fecal-oral transmission with smaller scale outbreaks
  - Genotype 3: Developed countries; food-borne, zoonotic transmission; associated with older adults, immunocompromised; chronic Infections
  - Genotype 4: China, Taiwan, Japan; food-borne, zoonotic transmission

Site

- Liver; less commonly, pancreas and kidneys

Presentation

- Fever, malaise, abdominal pain, jaundice, fatigue, anorexia, right upper quadrant pain, hepatomegaly
- Likelihood of symptomatic infection increases with age; young children often asymptomatic

Laboratory Tests

- Presence of anti-HAV IgM in patient with hepatitis symptoms and jaundice, elevated total bilirubin (≥ 3.0 mg/dL), or elevated alanine transaminase (ALT) (>200 IU/L) is diagnostic of acute HAV infection
- Anti-HAV IgG persists for life and confers protection
- Presence of anti-HEV IgM is diagnostic of acute HEV infection; often diagnosis of exclusion
- PCR (blood, stool)

Natural History

- Generally self-limited infections (~ 2 months for HAV; 1-4 weeks for HEV)
- Chronic HEV infection in immunosuppressed patients
- No progression to chronic hepatitis with HAV infection
- Acute liver failure in 1% of HAV and 0.1-4.0% of HEV infections

Treatment

- HAV vaccine: 2 doses (6 months apart)
  - Recommended for children (> 1 year old), international travelers, men who have sex with men, illegal drug users, occupational exposure, close contact with international adoptees, homeless, chronic liver disease, HIV
- No FDA-licensed HEV vaccine
- HAV preexposure prophylaxis with immune globulin
- HAV postexposure prophylaxis: HAV vaccine (within 2 weeks) and immune globulin
- No specific treatment; avoid acetaminophen and other hepatotoxic medications
- Liver transplant for acute liver failure

Prognosis

- 0.1-2.0% overall mortality with HAV infection; increased in patients with chronic liver disease and > 40 years old
- 1-4% overall mortality with HEV infection; increased mortality in pregnant women (20%)

IMAGING

Ultrasonographic Findings

- Hepatosplenomegaly and edema; decreased liver echogenicity
- Increased echogenicity of portal venous walls (starry-sky appearance)
- Periportal hypoechoic area (hydropic swelling of hepatocytes)
- Thickening of gallbladder wall

MR Findings

- Increase in T1 and T2 relaxation times in liver
- Periportal hyperintensity (fluid, lymphedema)

CT Findings

- Hepatomegaly; gallbladder wall thickening
- Periportal hypodensity (fluid, lymphedema)
- Heterogeneous parenchymal enhancement

MICROBIOLOGY

Virus Features

- HAV
  - Nonenveloped, single-stranded RNA virus

- 27-nm spherical, icosahedral capsid
- 7,474-nucleotide genome; 1 open reading frame (ORF) (11 proteins)
- 6 genotypes (IA, IB, IIA, IIB, IIIA, IIIB)
- HEV
  - Nonenveloped, single-stranded RNA virus
  - 32- to 34-nm spherical, icosahedral capsid
  - 7,300-nucleotide genome; 3 ORFs (9 proteins)
  - 5 genotypes (1-4, 7)

Culture

- No routine role for culture in diagnosis

MACROSCOPIC

Liver

- Homogeneously enlarged and congested
- Cut surface is reddish brown (bright yellow or green with cholestasis)
- Shrinks and softens due to extensive necrosis in fulminant hepatitis

MICROSCOPIC

Histologic Features

- Acute lobular hepatitis
  - Diffuse, mixed (predominantly lymphocytic) inflammatory cell infiltrate; mild portal and periportal inflammation may be present
  - Spotty (lytic) necrosis: Small foci of lymphocytes and macrophages surrounding individual, damaged hepatocytes or fragments of dead hepatocytes; areas of confluent hepatocyte necrosis in severe cases
  - Numerous apoptotic bodies (acidophilic bodies), hepatocyte swelling and regeneration, and Kupffer cell hyperplasia
  - Canalicular cholestasis present in some cases
- Chronic hepatitis: Dense portal lymphocytic inflammation with variable interface activity; variable fibrosis

ANCILLARY TESTS

Immunohistochemistry

- HEV pORF2 shows cytoplasmic and nuclear staining

Histochemical Stains

- Trichome and reticulin show parenchymal collapse
- Periodic acid-Schiff shows pigment-laden macrophages

DIFFERENTIAL DIAGNOSIS

Other Viral Hepatitides

- Hepatitis B virus (HBV)
  - Acute hepatitis with predominant lobular injury seen in acute infection, during disease flares, and with hepatitis D virus (HDV) superinfection
  - Most biopsies exhibit chronic hepatitis with predominantly portal inflammation and fibrosis
  - Cytoplasmic ground-glass hepatocyte inclusions
  - Positive hepatitis B surface antigen (HBsAg), markers of virus replication (HBeAg, HBV DNA), &/or antihepatitis B core antigen IgM (anti-HBcAg)
- Hepatitis C virus (HCV)
  - Acute infection rarely biopsied
  - Chronic hepatitis with predominantly portal inflammation and fibrosis; hepatocellular steatosis
  - Positive HCV RNA (serum)
- HDV
  - Only occurs in setting of acute or chronic HBV infection
  - More severe necroinflammatory activity and more rapid disease progression
  - Sanded hepatocyte nuclei
  - Positive antihepatitis D virus IgM (anti-HDV)
- Epstein-Barr virus (EBV)
  - Liver involvement in > 90% of cases of infectious mononucleosis
  - Portal and periportal lymphocytic infiltrate with occasional larger immunoblastic cells
  - Minimal liver cell ballooning; hepatocyte regeneration, canalicular cholestasis, and Kupffer cell hyperplasia
  - Areas of necrosis infiltrated by mononuclear cells creating granulomatous appearance
  - Detection of EBV by in situ hybridization for EBV-encoded RNA or by PCR
- Cytomegalovirus
  - Accounts for 8% of cases of infectious mononucleosis-like syndrome with hepatic involvement
  - Similar histologic findings as EBV hepatitis
  - Amphophilic nuclear inclusions surrounded by halo

Autoimmune Hepatitis

- Positive autoimmune serologies (antinuclear antibodies, antismooth muscle antibodies, anti-liver-kidney-microsomal antibodies)
- Lobular hepatitis with portal and periportal hepatitis
- Prominent plasma cell infiltrates and fibrosis
- Responsive to immunosuppressive therapy

Drug-/Toxin-Induced Hepatitis

- Caused by toxic exposure to certain medications, vitamins, herbal remedies, or food supplements
- Histologically similar to acute viral hepatitis
- Eosinophils may be prominent
- Self-limited and typically resolves with cessation of drug

SELECTED REFERENCES

1. Abravanel F et al: Diagnostic and management strategies for chronic hepatitis E infection. Expert Rev Anti Infect Ther. 21(2):143-8, 2023
2. Peron JM et al: The pressing need for a global HEV vaccine. J Hepatol. 79(3):876-80, 2023
3. Qian Z et al: Prevalence of hepatitis E virus and its association with adverse pregnancy outcomes in pregnant women in China. J Clin Virol. 158:105353, 2023
4. Foster MA et al: Widespread hepatitis A outbreaks associated with person-to-person transmission - United States, 2016-2020. MMWR Morb Mortal Wkly Rep. 71(39):1229-34, 2022
5. Pisano MB et al: Hepatitis E virus infection in the United States: seroprevalence, risk factors and the influence of immunological assays. PLoS One. 17(8):e0272809, 2022
6. Ramachandran S et al: Changing molecular epidemiology of hepatitis A virus infection, United States, 1996-2019. Emerg Infect Dis. 27(6):1742-5, 2021
7. Lenggenhager D et al: Clinicopathologic features and pathologic diagnosis of hepatitis E. Hum Pathol. 96:34-8, 2020
8. Kamar N et al: Hepatitis E virus infection. Nat Rev Dis Primers. 3:17086, 2017
9. Lefkowitch JH: The pathology of acute liver failure. Adv Anat Pathol. 23(3):144-58, 2016

Lobular Hepatitis in Hepatitis A Virus Infection

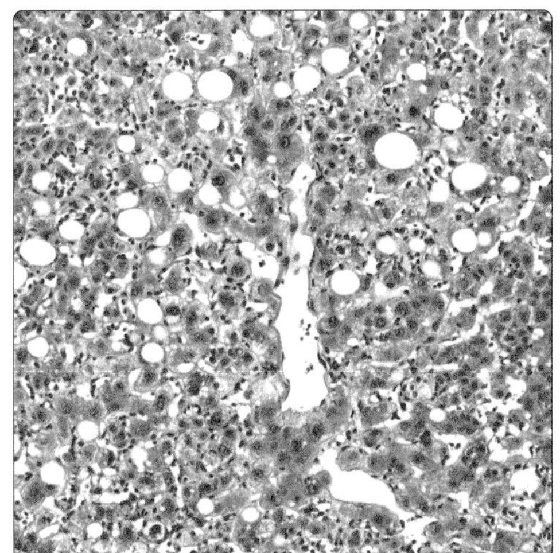

Cholestasis in Hepatitis A Virus Infection

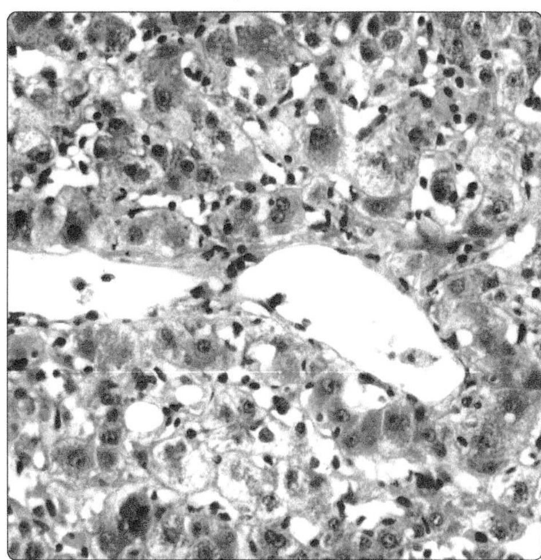

(Left) *Acute HAV infections exhibit relatively nonspecific findings. Zones 2 and 3 show lobular hepatitis with marked lobular disarray, multiple foci of spotty necrosis, and prominent anisonucleosis. (Courtesy M. Pittman, MD.)* **(Right)** *Acute HAV infection shows zone 3 cholestasis with bile plugs. The central vein (terminal hepatic venule) does not appear to be damaged. (Courtesy M. Pittman, MD.)*

Severe Hepatocellular Necrosis in Hepatitis A Virus Infection

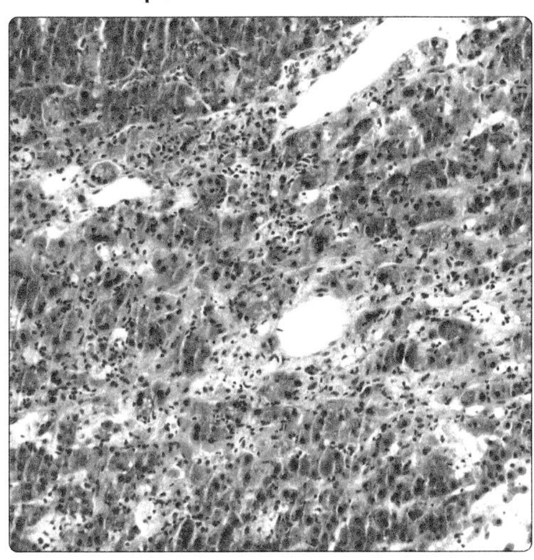

Panlobular Hepatitis in Hepatitis E Virus Infection

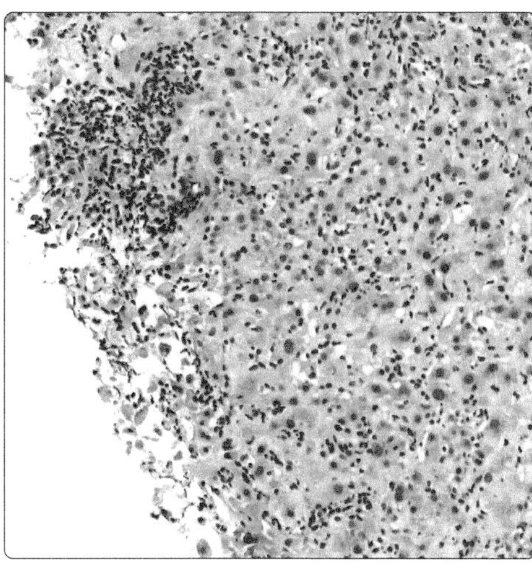

(Left) *A severe episode of acute HAV infection shows a cholestatic pattern of injury around the central vein with severe hepatocellular necrosis, the so-called "feathery" degeneration, characteristic of biliary injury. (Courtesy M. Pittman, MD.)* **(Right)** *Acute HEV infections exhibit panlobular hepatitis. There is clear interface hepatitis in the small portal tract with hepatocellular disarray and an inflammatory infiltrate throughout the lobule. (Courtesy J. Verheij, MD, PhD.)*

Interface Hepatitis in Hepatitis E Virus Infection

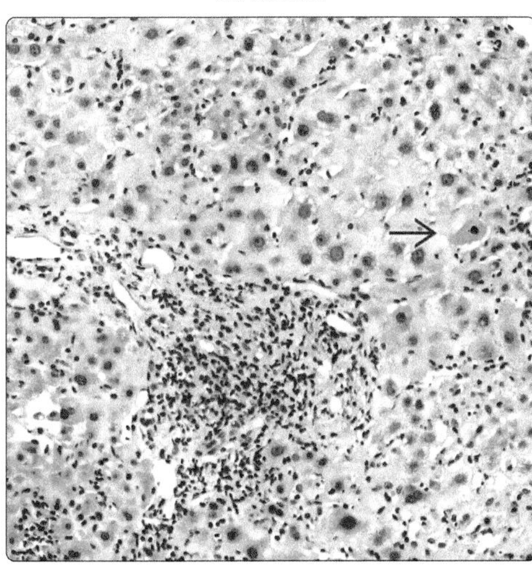

Acidophil Bodies in Hepatitis E Virus Infection

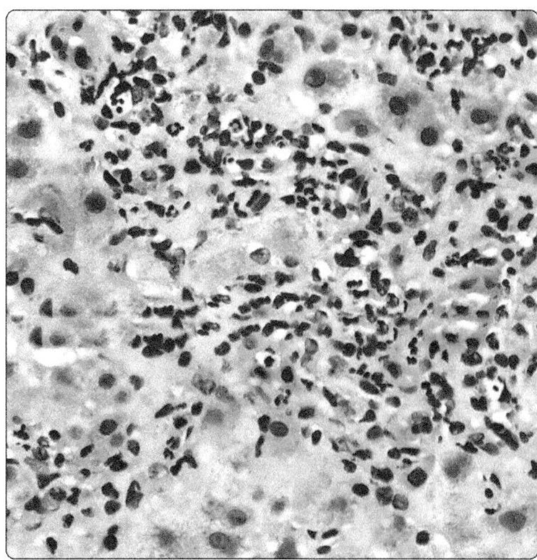

(Left) *Acute HEV infection shows interface hepatitis with a mixed chronic inflammatory infiltrate with surrounding swollen hepatocytes. An acidophil body is identified in the lobule ⮕ next to a dilated canaliculus with a pale bile plug. (Courtesy J. Verheij, MD, PhD.)* **(Right)** *Acute HEV infection is characterized by nonspecific features, including acidophil bodies, lobular inflammation, and activated sinusoidal Kupffer cells. (Courtesy J. Verheij, MD, PhD.)*

Hepatitis C Virus Infection

KEY FACTS

ETIOLOGY/PATHOGENESIS

- Parenterally transmitted virus that causes liver fibrosis and cirrhosis due to active yet ineffective immune response, which damages liver tissue but fails to eradicate virus

CLINICAL ISSUES

- 58 million people worldwide are estimated to be chronically infected (2.4 million in USA)
- Serology for anti-HCV IgG antibodies with enzyme immunoassay and confirm with hepatitis C virus (HCV) RNA PCR
- 30% develop chronic HCV infection, 15-30% cirrhosis, 1-5% annual risk of hepatocellular carcinoma with established cirrhosis
- Direct acting antivirals achieve sustained viral response in 95% of patients

MICROSCOPIC

- Acute hepatitis: Ballooning degeneration, apoptosis, cholestasis, macrophage aggregates
- Chronic hepatitis: Lymphoid aggregates in portal tracts and steatosis, interface hepatitis in more severe cases with inflammation extending to periportal parenchyma, and cirrhosis with regenerative nodules of hepatocytes with intervening bands of fibrosis
- Grading of disease is based on inflammation; staging is based on fibrosis
- Cryoglobulinemia: Dense deposits are seen in glomeruli via immunofluorescence or electron microscopy

TOP DIFFERENTIAL DIAGNOSES

- Viral hepatitis: Serologic discrimination between hepatitis A, B, D, and E (HAV, HBV, HDV, and HEV); travel and food contamination (HAV/HEV); parenteral infection without steatosis (HBV/HDV)
- Autoimmune hepatitis: Serologic discrimination (i.e., ANA, SMA, LKM-1) and lack of exposure history
- Drug-induced hepatitis: Drug history and presence of eosinophils

(Left) *Electron micrograph of hepatitis C virus (HCV) purified from cell culture shows a spherical, enveloped virion ~ 50 nm in diameter. (Courtesy M. Catanese, PhD; Center for the Study of Hepatitis C, The Rockefeller University.)* **(Right)** *Liver section from an autopsy of a patient with end-stage liver disease demonstrates macronodular cirrhosis ⇨ with prominent fibrosis ➡. Careful examination for potential nodules of hepatocellular carcinoma is required, especially when borders appear infiltrative or distinct.*

Ultrastructural Features

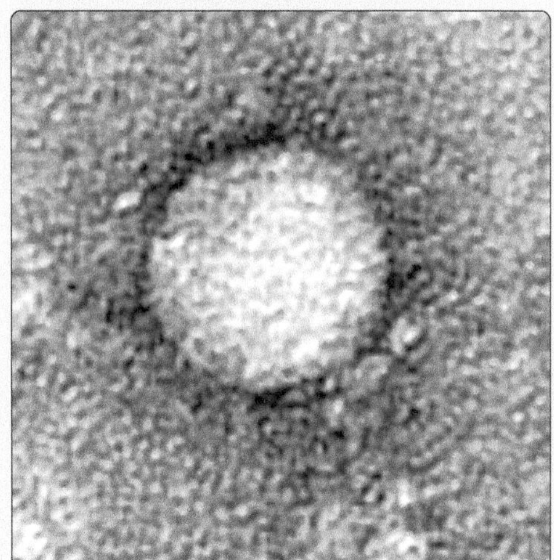

Macronodular Cirrhosis

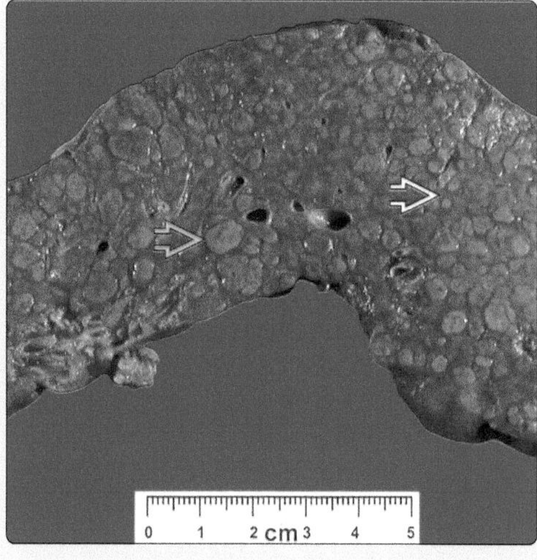

(Left) *Macrovesicular steatosis ⇨ is characteristic, but not diagnostic, of chronic HCV infection. (Courtesy Franz von Lichtenberg Collection of Infectious Disease Pathology, BWH.)* **(Right)** *Periportal lymphoid aggregates ⇨ and adjacent interface hepatitis ⇨ are shown with bile duct infiltration ➡, characteristic of HCV. Patients are often asymptomatic at this stage.*

Steatosis

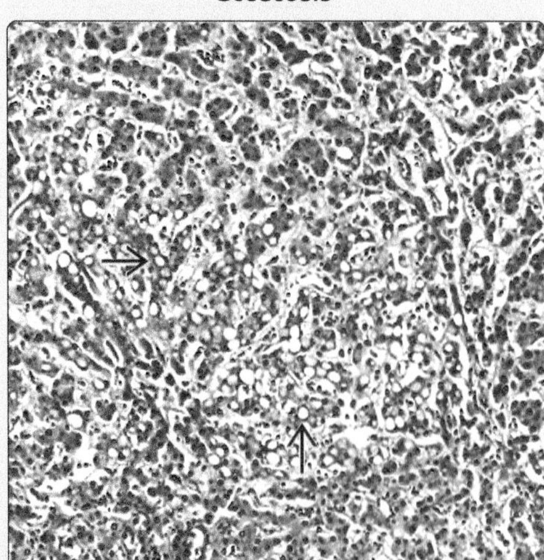

Lymphoid Aggregates/Interface Hepatitis

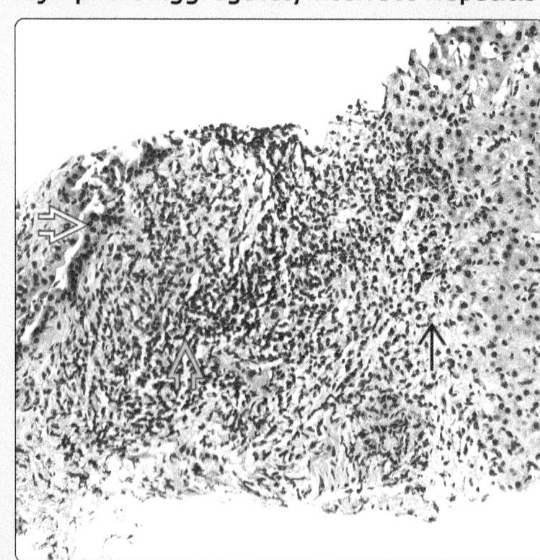

TERMINOLOGY

Abbreviations

- Hepatitis C virus (HCV)

Definitions

- *Hepacivirus hominis*; *Flaviviridae* family: From "flavus" (yellow); non-A, non-B hepatitis

ETIOLOGY/PATHOGENESIS

Infectious Agents

- Viral infection transmitted parenterally by IV drug use, contaminated blood transfusion products, and organ transplants (prior to screening), occupational needle stick injury (0.1% risk); rare vertical or sexual transmission
- Liver fibrosis and cirrhosis are due to active yet ineffective immune response, which damages liver tissue but fails to eradicate virus
- Immune complex-mediated glomerular injuries

CLINICAL ISSUES

Epidemiology

- 58 million people worldwide are estimated to be infected chronically with HCV; 1.5 million new infections per year and 290,000 deaths (2019)
- 2.4 million infected in USA with > 15,000 deaths/year

Site

- Liver, kidneys

Presentation

- Acute hepatitis C: Majority are asymptomatic; minority have vague symptoms, including fatigue, nausea, abdominal discomfort; rarely, fulminant hepatic failure
- Chronic hepatitis C: Often incidentally noted as elevated transaminases with subsequent finding of HCV positivity; rarely, may present as decompensated liver cirrhosis
- Extrahepatic manifestations include cryoglobulinemia, glomerulonephritis, lichen planus, lymphoproliferative disorders, Sjögren syndrome
- Can also be detected in peripherally circulating monocytes, which are thought to be major source of recurrence in liver transplant recipients

Laboratory Tests

- Serology for anti-HCV IgG antibodies with enzyme immunoassay (EIA)
- Confirm positive antibody test by HCV RNA PCR
- Liver function tests may show transaminitis

Treatment

- No vaccines currently available
- Direct acting antivirals (e.g., glecaprevir/pibrentasvir, sofosbuvir/velpatasvir) achieves sustained viral response (SVR) in 95% of patients
- Liver transplant for cirrhosis

Prognosis

- 30% will develop chronic HCV infection, 15-30% will develop cirrhosis over 20 years, 1-5% annual risk of hepatocellular carcinoma with cirrhosis
- Reinfection of donor liver following transplant, often with accelerated course to cirrhosis

MICROBIOLOGY

Virus Features

- Enveloped, positive-stranded RNA virus
- 50- to 60-nm spherical, icosahedral capsid
- 9,600 nucleotide genome; 1 open reading frame (ORF) (10 proteins)
- 6 major genotypes; guides therapy

Viral Culture

- No routine role for culture in diagnosis

MICROSCOPIC

Histologic Features

- Acute hepatitis: Ballooning degeneration, apoptosis, cholestasis, macrophage aggregates
- Chronic hepatitis
  - Lymphoid aggregates in portal tracts and steatosis, interface hepatitis in more severe cases with inflammation extending to periportal parenchyma
  - Deposition of fibrous tissue, beginning in portal tracts and leading to septal fibrosis
  - Cirrhosis: Regenerative nodules of hepatocytes with intervening bands of fibrosis
  - Staging based on degree of fibrosis (Metavir scale); grading based on level of necroinflammatory activity (Batts-Ludwig grading scale)
- Cryoglobulinemia: Dense deposits are seen in glomeruli via immunofluorescence or electron microscopy

DIFFERENTIAL DIAGNOSIS

Viral Hepatitis

- Serologic discrimination between hepatitis A, B, D, and E (HAV, HBV, HDV, and HEV)
- HAV/HEV associated with travel and food contamination
- HBV/HDV also associated with parenteral infection but lack steatosis

Autoimmune Hepatitis

- Serologic discrimination; antinuclear antibodies (ANA), antismooth muscle antibodies (SMA), antiliver kidney microsome type 1 antibodies (LKM-1)
- Lack of exposure history

Drug-Induced Hepatitis

- Drug history; presence of eosinophils

SELECTED REFERENCES

1. Jain D et al: Evolution of the liver biopsy and its future. Transl Gastroenterol Hepatol. 6:20, 2021
2. Ghany MG et al: Hepatitis C guidance 2019 update: American Association for the Study of Liver Diseases-Infectious Diseases Society of America recommendations for testing, managing, and treating hepatitis C virus infection. Hepatology. 71(2):686-721, 2020
3. Pol S et al: Hepatitis C virus and the kidney. Nat Rev Nephrol. 15(2):73-86, 2018
4. Manns MP et al: Hepatitis C virus infection. Nat Rev Dis Primers. 3:17006, 2017
5. Whitcomb E et al: Biopsy specimens from allograft liver contain histologic features of hepatitis C virus infection after virus eradication. Clin Gastroenterol Hepatol. 15(8):1279-85, 2017

(**Left**) *Macrovesicular hepatosteatosis* ⇨ *is characteristic of, but not pathognomonic for, chronic HCV infection. Note the lymphocytic inflammatory cells around the portal regions and extending into the parenchyma. (Courtesy Franz von Lichtenberg Collection of Infectious Disease Pathology, BWH.)* (**Right**) *Periportal inflammation in an HCV liver biopsy demonstrates steatosis* ⇨ *and dense lymphocytic inflammation in the periportal region* ➡.

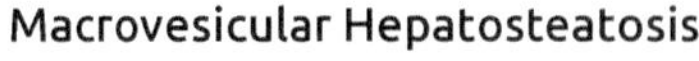

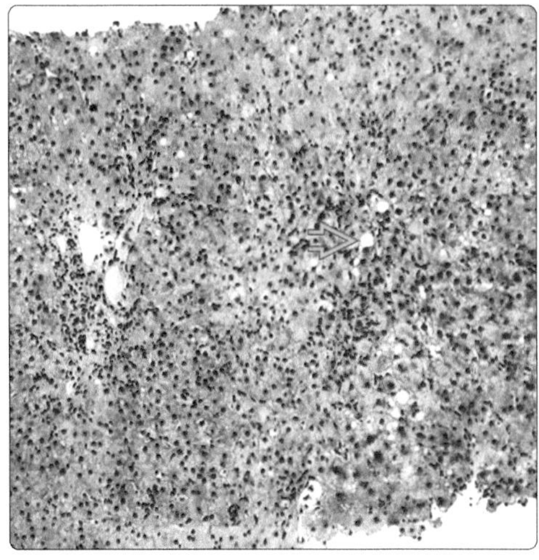

Steatosis

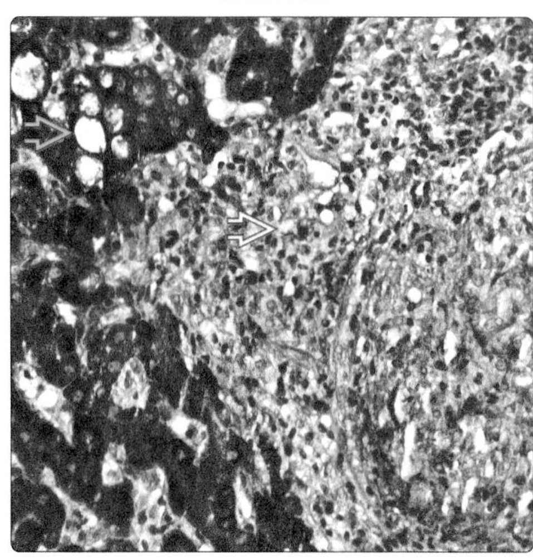

(**Left**) *Graphic illustrates the grading of chronic hepatitis. Upper left is minimal activity (grade 1), upper right is mild (grade 2), lower left is moderate (grade 3), and lower right is severe (grade 4).* (**Right**) *Chronic lymphocytic inflammation* ⇨ *in the periportal region of a liver shows damage with loss of hepatocytes* ➡ *and scattered areas of macrovesicular steatosis* →.

Grading of Chronic Hepatitis

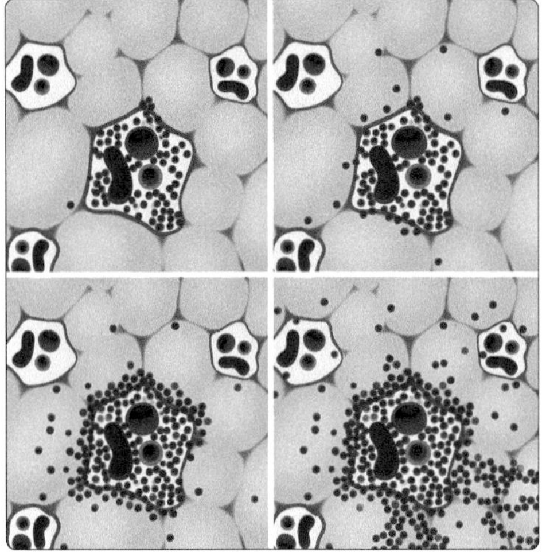

Periportal Inflammation

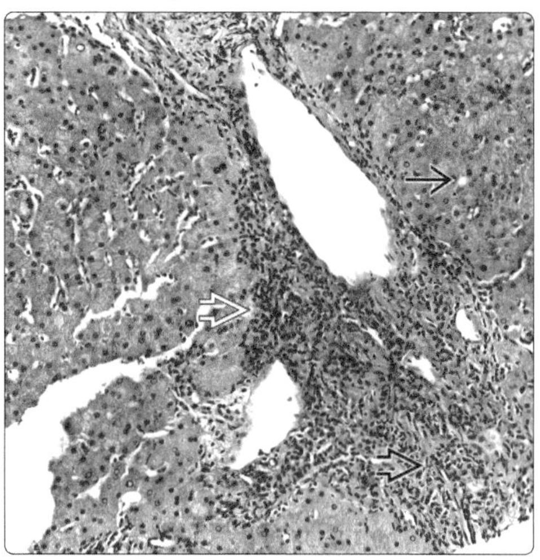

(**Left**) *Graphic illustrates the staging of fibrosis. Upper left is portal fibrosis (stage 1), upper right is periportal (stage 2), lower left is bridging (stage 3), and lower right is cirrhosis (grade 4).* (**Right**) *Trichrome stain of a liver with chronic HCV infection demonstrates cirrhosis seen as bands of bridging fibrosis* ⇨ *with intervening regenerative hepatic nodules* ➡.

Staging of Fibrosis

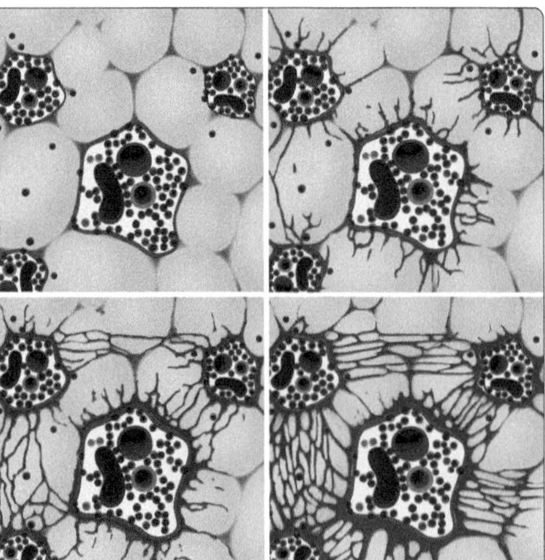

Bridging Fibrosis

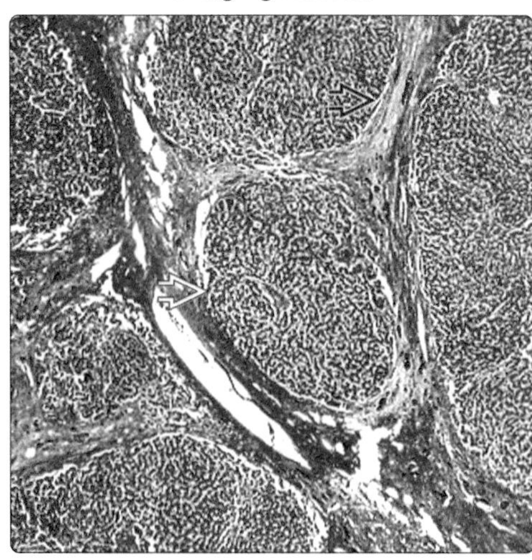

Micronodular Cirrhosis

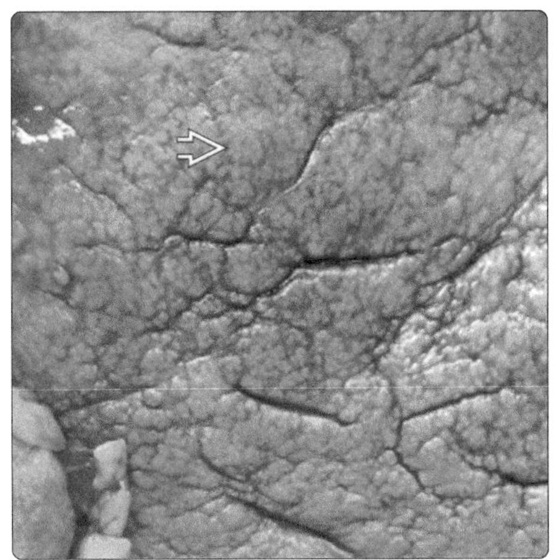

Transplant Recurrence

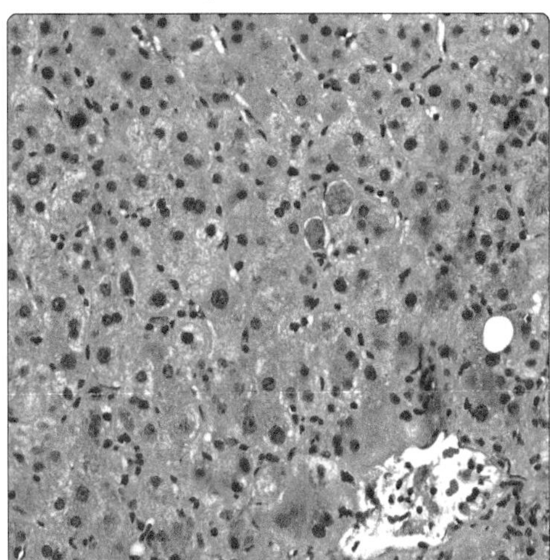

(Left) *Autopsied liver of a patient with end-stage liver disease demonstrates micronodular cirrhosis ➡ without distinctively suspicious areas for hepatocellular carcinoma.* **(Right)** *Lobular inflammation and numerous acidophil bodies are seen in a case of early, recurrent HCV after liver transplantation. Acute infection is rarely biopsied in native livers, but an early/acute phase is often recognized with recurrence after liver transplantation. (From DP: Hepatobiliary and Pancreas.)*

Hepatocellular Carcinoma

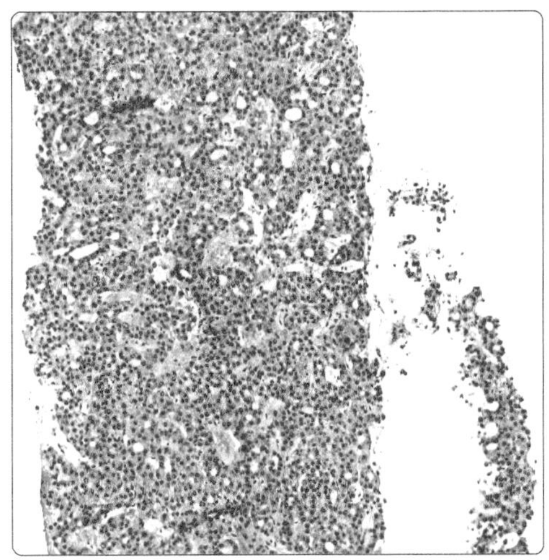

Hepatocellular Carcinoma

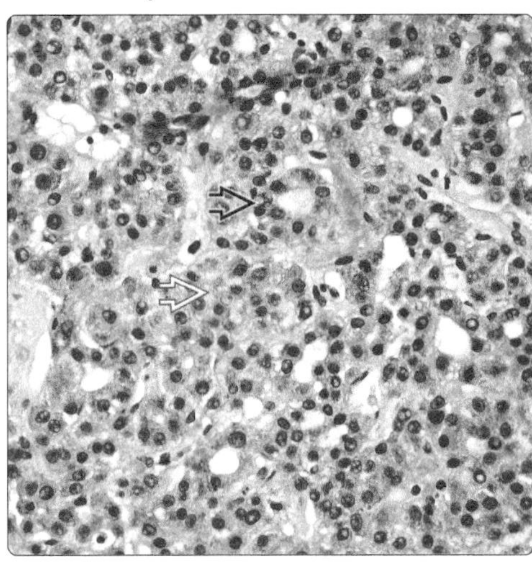

(Left) *A liver core biopsy from a patient with longstanding HCV demonstrates a pseudoglandular pattern, lack of portal triads, and cords of hepatocytes > 2 layers thick, consistent with hepatocellular carcinoma.* **(Right)** *The pseudoglandular pattern ⇨ and thick cords of hepatocytes ➡ seen here are consistent with hepatocellular carcinoma.*

Hepatitis C Virus-Associated Cryoglobulinemia: Immunofluorescence

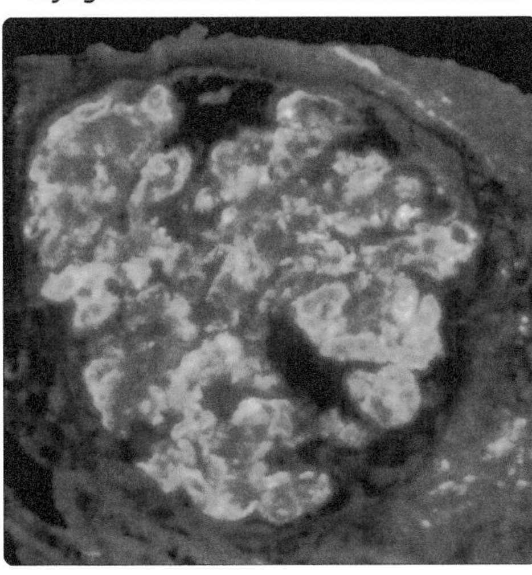

Hepatitis C Virus-Associated Cryoglobulinemia: Electron Microscopy

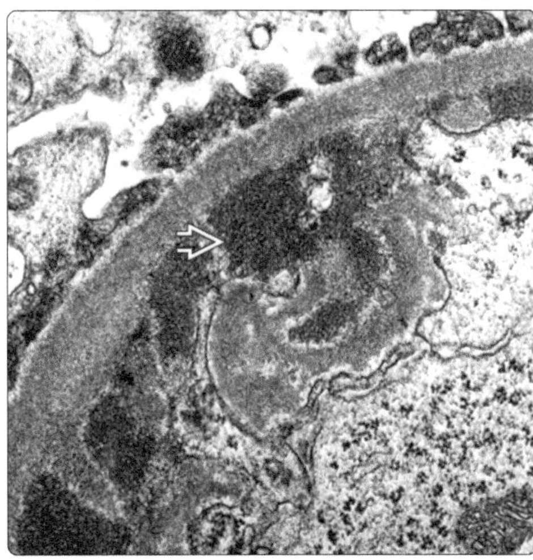

(Left) *Immunofluorescence demonstrates glomerular dense deposits in the kidney as a result of HCV-associated cryoglobulinemia. (Courtesy Franz von Lichtenberg Collection of Infectious Disease Pathology, BWH.)* **(Right)** *Electron micrograph demonstrates glomerular dense deposits as a result of HCV-associated cryoglobulinemia ➡. (Courtesy Franz von Lichtenberg Collection of Infectious Disease Pathology, BWH.)*

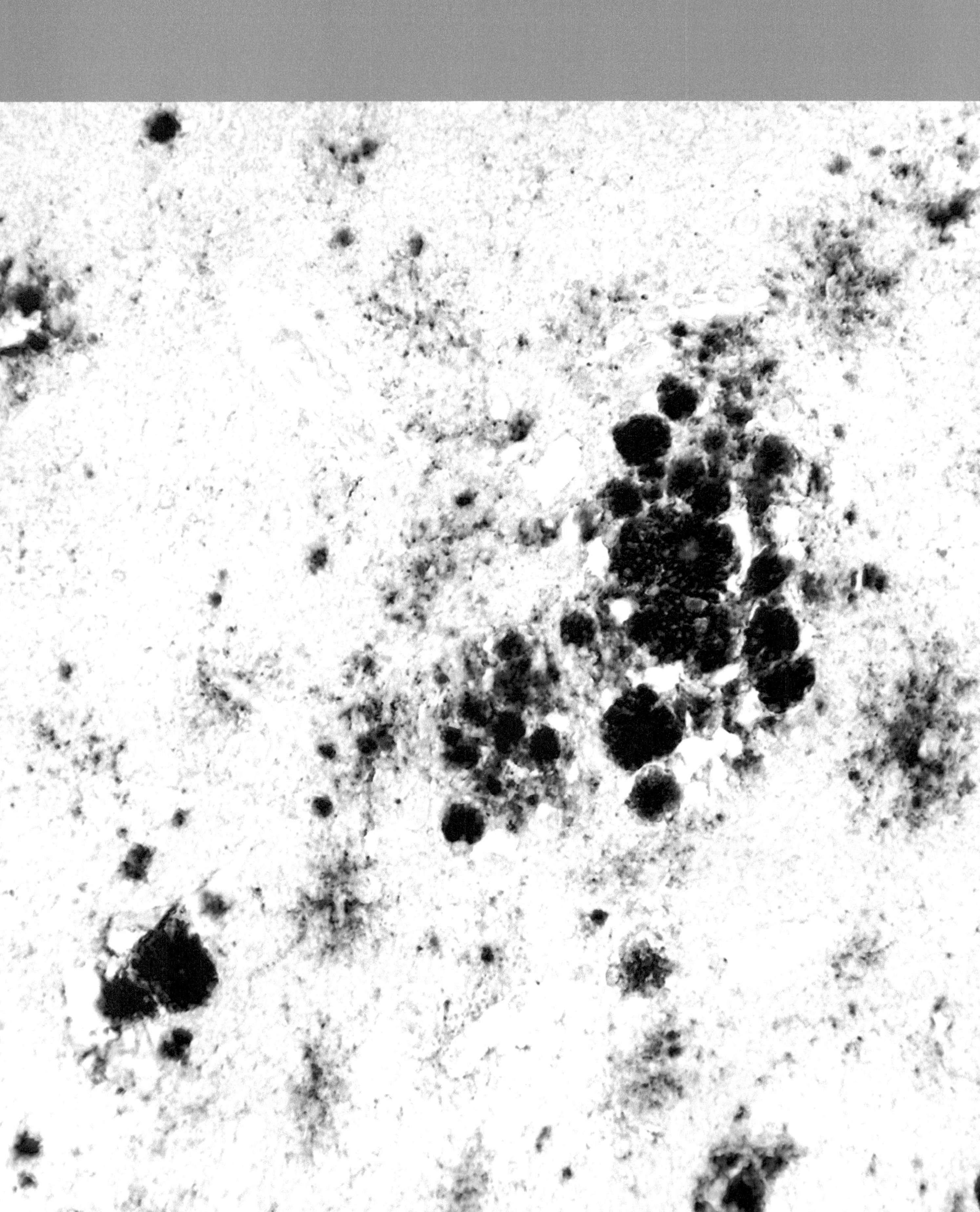

SECTION 3

Prion Diseases

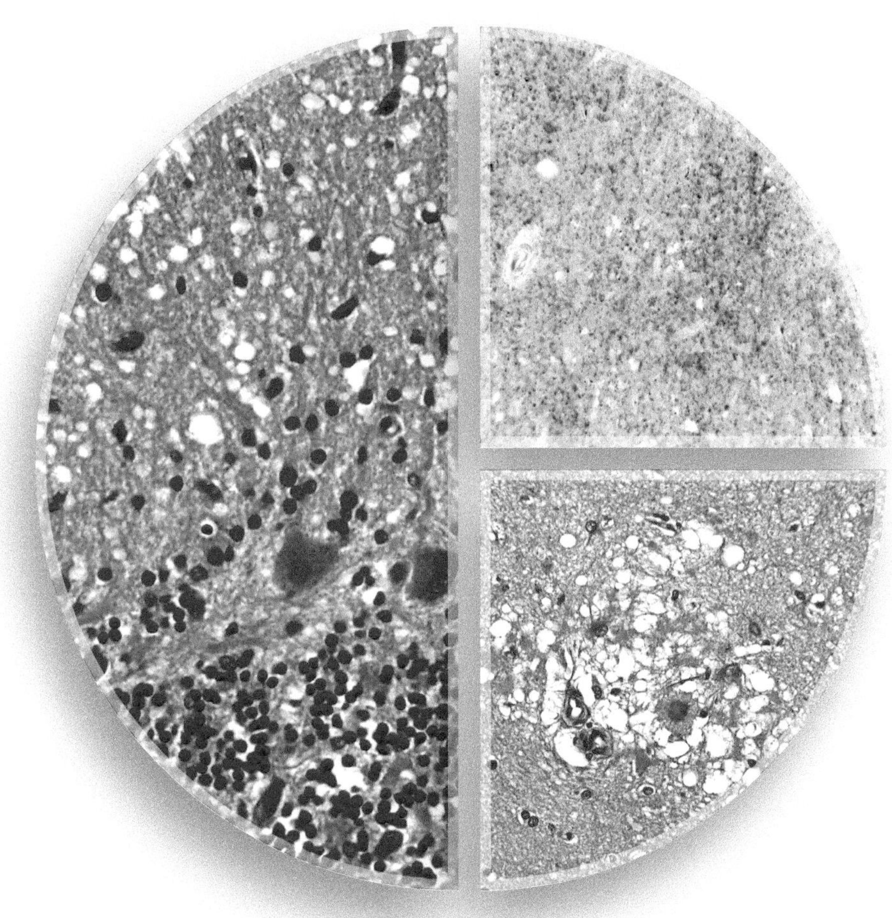

Transmissible Spongiform Encephalopathies

KEY FACTS

ETIOLOGY/PATHOGENESIS

- Prions are infectious proteinaceous molecules that replicate through self-templated refolding mechanism [PrP(C) →PrP(Sc)] and cause symptoms through neuronal dysfunction and cell death

CLINICAL ISSUES

- Incidence: ~ 1 per million/year; 85% of cases are sporadic Creutzfeldt-Jakob disease (sCJD), 10-15% of cases are familial CJD (fCJD) (Gerstmann-Sträussler-Scheinker syndrome, fatal familial insomnia), and < 5% of cases are infectious [kuru, variant CJD (vCJD)] or iatrogenic CJD
- Presentation: Rapidly progressive dementia, ataxia, myoclonus, cortical blindness, sleep disturbances (order and severity vary with specific disease and strain)
- CSF testing (14-3-3 and tau proteins, RT-QuIC), MR (DWI and FLAIR), EEG
- Brain tissue necessary for definitive diagnosis; biopsy only to rule out potentially treatable conditions
- Treatment/prognosis: No effective treatments or cures; death typically occurs within 1 year of onset of symptoms

MICROSCOPIC

- Spongiform degeneration, marked neuronal loss, and reactive gliosis (distribution varies with disease and strain)
- IHC: Aggregates stain with anti-PrP antibody 3F4

ANCILLARY TESTS

- Western blot: Proteinase K-resistant fragments
- Sequencing: *PRNP* disease-associated mutations

TOP DIFFERENTIAL DIAGNOSES

- Altered mental status with vacuoles (e.g., fixation artifact, cerebral edema, and status spongiosis)
  - Vacuoles lack discrete round to oval-shaped, punched-out appearance of spongiform degeneration
  - Lacks protein aggregates stained by PrP IHC, protease-resistant bands on Western blot

MR of Sporadic Creutzfeldt-Jakob Disease

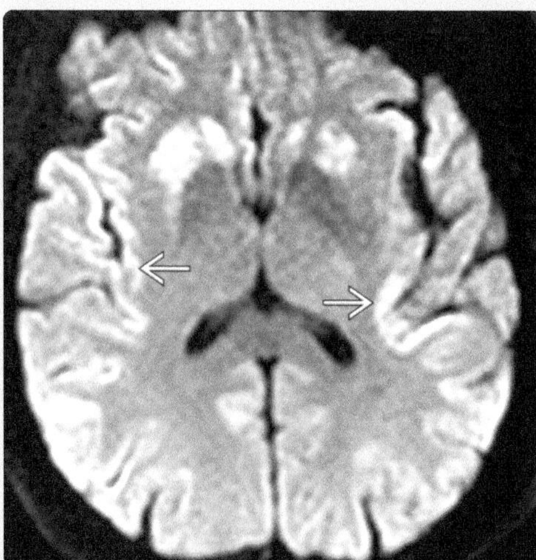

Western Blot With Proteinase K Digestion

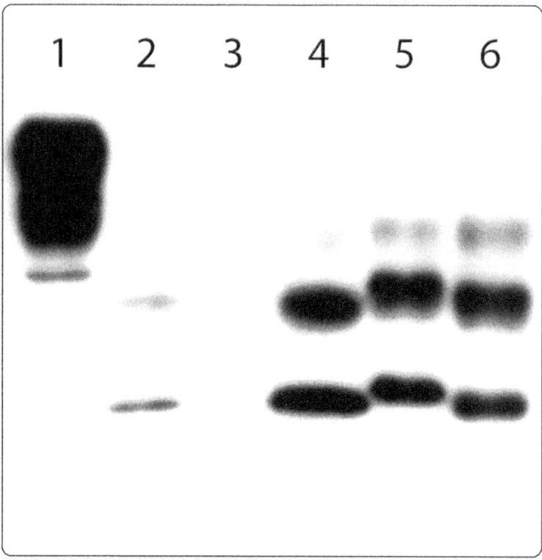

(Left) *Axial DWI MR shows asymmetric diffusion restriction in the caudate nuclei and putamen. Asymmetric hyperintensity is present in the frontal and temporal lobe cortical ribbons ➡, typical of sporadic Creutzfeldt-Jakob Disease (sCJD). (Courtesy N. Fischbein, MD.)* **(Right)** *Western blot from a patient with VV2 sCJD shows proteinase K-resistant fragments, diagnostic of CJD [predigestion (lane 1), dilutions post digestion (lanes 2-4), type 1 control (lane 5), and type 2 control (lane 6)]. (Courtesy M. Cohen, MD.)*

Histologic Findings in Sporadic Creutzfeldt-Jakob Disease

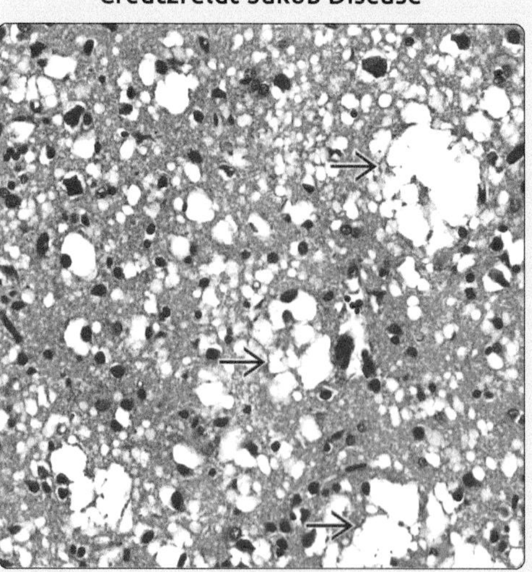

Anti-PrP IHC With Sporadic Creutzfeldt-Jakob Disease

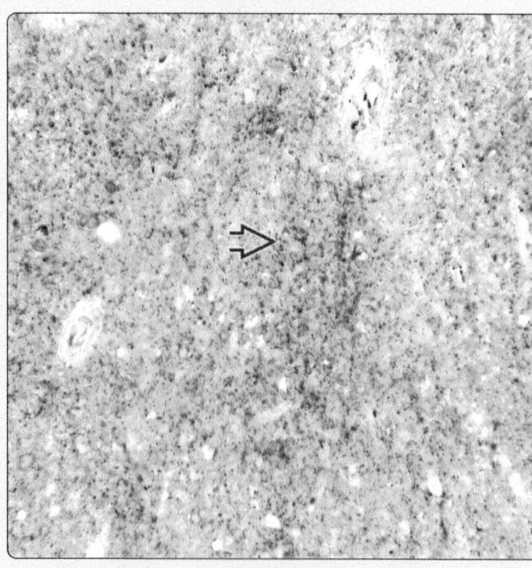

(Left) *Severe spongiform degeneration ➡, marked neuronal loss, and reactive gliosis are present in the cerebral cortex of a patient with sCJD.* **(Right)** *Immunohistochemical staining with anti-PrP antibody (3F4) shows a fine, granular synaptic pattern ➡, characteristic of sCJD MM1 and MV1. (Courtesy M. Cohen, MD.)*

TERMINOLOGY

Definitions

- Prion: Derived from term proteinaceous infectious particle

ETIOLOGY/PATHOGENESIS

Infectious Agents

- Prions are infectious proteinaceous molecules devoid of coding nucleic acids
- Replication is by self-templated refolding mechanism: α-helical, protease-sensitive, endogenously expressed, "cellular" prion protein [PrP(C)] is transformed into β-sheet-rich, protease-resistant, disease-associated "scrapie" isoform [PrP(Sc)]
- Initial molecule of PrP(Sc) either forms sporadically or due to autosomal dominant mutations in *PRNP* gene, or it is acquired through exposure to prion-infected tissues or improperly decontaminated instruments (incubation period is years to decades)
- PrP(Sc) &/or soluble intermediates cause symptoms through neuronal dysfunction and cell death

CLINICAL ISSUES

Epidemiology

- Overall incidence: 1 per million/year (worldwide)
- Human prion diseases include Creutzfeldt-Jakob disease (CJD), variant CJD (vCJD), Gerstmann-Sträussler-Scheinker syndrome (GSS), fatal familial insomnia (FFI), and kuru
- 85% of cases are sporadic (sCJD); average: 60 years old
  - Phenotypes determined by strain (type 1, type 2) and codon 129 genotype (MM, VV, MV)
  - Majority present with rapidly progressive dementia (MM1, MV1; ~ 2/3) or ataxia (VV2, MV2; ~ 1/3)
- 10-15% of cases are familial (fCJD, GSS, FFI); 40-50 years old
  - > 20 disease-associated mutations identified (point mutations, premature stop codons, and octapeptide repeat insertions)
  - M129V polymorphism determines FFI or fCJD phenotype, respectively, in context of D178N mutation
- < 5% of cases are infectious (kuru, vCJD) or iatrogenic (iCJD)
  - Consumption of prion-infected tissues; exposure to prion-contaminated growth hormones, corneal transplants, dural grafts, or inadequately sterilized surgical instruments
  - All cases of vCJD are codon 129MM; 20-30 years old
- Animal prion diseases include bovine spongiform encephalopathy (BSE) (mad cow disease), chronic wasting disease (deer, elk), and scrapie (sheep)

Presentation

- Rapidly progressive dementia, ataxia, myoclonus, cortical blindness, sleep disturbances
- Order of presentation and severity of symptoms vary with specific prion disease and strain

Laboratory Tests

- EEG: Periodic sharp wave complexes triphasic or sharp wave bursts every 0.5-2.0 seconds
- CSF: 14-3-3 and tau proteins (ELISA); real-time quaking-induced conversion (RT-QuIC) (sensitivity 90% and specificity 98.5%)
- Urine and nasal brushings and skin punch biopsies have also been evaluated by RT-QuIC &/or protein misfolding cyclic amplification in research settings
- National Prion Disease Pathology Surveillance Center (NPDPSC) offers most current guidelines

Natural History

- Progressive fatal neurodegenerative illness

Treatment

- No effective treatments or cures
- Anti-PrP(c) monoclonal antibodies piloted in human subjects

Prognosis

- Death typically within 1 year of onset of symptoms

IMAGING

MR

- Diffusion-weighted imaging: Hyperintensity of cerebral cortex (cortical ribboning), striatum, and thalamus (high sensitivity and specificity for sCJD)
- Fluid-attenuated inversion recovery imaging: Pulvinar sign (most sensitive for vCJD)

MICROBIOLOGY

Prion Features

- Aggregates of β-sheet-rich isoform of *PRNP* gene product PrP(Sc) arranged in amyloid fibers and plaques
- Strains have identical protein sequences but differ in affected brain areas, incubation times, and biochemical properties
- Differences in protein sequences and structures (species barrier) determines whether prion can spread from 1 species to another (e.g., BSE → vCJD)

MACROSCOPIC

Brain

- Can be grossly normal or exhibit atrophy of cerebral cortex, neostriatum, and cerebellar cortex

MICROSCOPIC

Biosafety Guidelines

- Brain biopsy only undertaken to rule out other potentially treatable conditions
- Treat formalin-fixed surgical or autopsy tissue with formic acid prior to processing and paraffin embedding

Histologic Features

- sCJD MM1/MV1: Fine, full-thickness spongiform degeneration with astrocytosis throughout neocortex and basal ganglia, most severe in occipital lobes; spares hippocampus
- sCJD VV2/MV2: Cortical spongiform degeneration in deep laminae (layers 5 and 6); hippocampal involvement; corpus striatum, substantia nigra, and cerebellar degeneration

- Kuru: Gross cerebellar atrophy, absence of inflammation, intraneuronal vacuoles in medial frontal lobes, corpora striatum, thalami, and cerebellum; amyloid plaques with starburst morphology within granular cell layer of cerebellum
- vCJD: Florid plaques consisting of kuru plaque-like stamen surrounded by spongiform petals in cerebellar and cerebral cortices; severe spongiform degeneration within corpora striata and marked neuronal loss with gliosis in posterior thalami
- GSS: Multicentric amyloid plaques within both cerebral and cerebellar cortices

ANCILLARY TESTS

Immunohistochemistry

- Monoclonal anti-PrP antibody 3F4
- sCJD MM1/MV1: Fine, granular reactivity with synaptic pattern
- sCJD VV2/MV2: Kuru plaques within granule cell layer; plaque-like reactivity in neocortex, basal ganglia, cerebellum, and substantia nigra; perineuronal pattern in hippocampus and cerebral cortex

Electron Microscopy

- Fibrils and plaques (limited diagnostic utility)

Western Blot

- Fresh brain tissue (gold standard)
- Strain and familial mutation information gained from banding pattern of proteinase K-resistant fragments

DNA Sequencing

- Identifies *PRNP* disease-associated mutations and M129V genotype

DIFFERENTIAL DIAGNOSIS

Rapidly Progressive Dementia

- Autoimmune/paraneoplastic encephalitis, primary angiitis of nervous system, and lymphomatous CNS disease (primary and intravascular)
  - May present with rapidly progressive dementia, elevated CSF 14-3-3 protein
  - Lacks spongiform degeneration, protein aggregates stained by PrP IHC, or protease-resistant bands on Western blot

Dementia With Protein Aggregates

- Alzheimer disease, Parkinson disease, Huntington disease, frontotemporal dementia, tauopathies, etc.
  - May present with dementia, ataxia, or sleep disturbances
  - Typically longer time course (years to decades), characteristic gross/radiologic signs of atrophy, disease-specific protein aggregates (i.e., β-amyloid, tau, α-synuclein, TDP-43)
  - Lacks spongiform degeneration, protein aggregates stained by PrP IHC, or protease-resistant bands on Western blot

Altered Mental Status With Vacuoles

- Fixation artifact, cerebral edema, and status spongiosis
  - Vacuoles lack discrete round to oval-shaped, punched-out appearance of spongiform degeneration
  - Lacks protein aggregates stained by PrP IHC, protease-resistant bands on Western blot

STAGING

Centers for Disease Control Diagnostic Criteria for Creutzfeldt-Jakob Disease (2018)

- sCJD
  - Definite: Diagnosed by standard neuropathologic techniques, IHC, Western blot confirmed protease-resistant PrP, or presence of scrapie-associated fibrils
  - Probable
    - Neuropsychiatric disorder plus positive RT-QuIC (CSF or other tissues)
    - **Or** rapidly progressive dementia and ≥ 2 of 4 clinical features: Myoclonus, visual, or cerebellar signs, pyramidal/extrapyramidal signs, akinetic mutism
    - **And** ≥ 1 positive laboratory test: EEG, 14-3-3, or MR
    - **And** no alternative diagnoses from routine work-up
  - Possible
    - Progressive dementia and ≥ 2 of 4 clinical features
    - **And** 0 positive laboratory tests: EEG, 14-3-3, or MR
    - **And** duration of illness < 2 years
    - **And** no alternative diagnoses from routine work-up
- iCJD
  - Progressive cerebellar syndrome in recipient of human cadaveric-derived pituitary hormone or sCJD with recognized exposure risk
- fCJD
  - Definite or probable CJD plus definite or probable CJD in 1st-degree relative
  - Neuropsychiatric disorder plus *PRNP* gene mutation

SELECTED REFERENCES

1. Hermann P et al: Application of real-time quaking-induced conversion in Creutzfeldt-Jakob disease surveillance. J Neurol. 1-13, 2023
2. Kortazar-Zubizarreta I et al: Analysis of a large case series of fatal familial insomnia to determine tests with the highest diagnostic value. J Neuropathol Exp Neurol. 82(2):169-79, 2023
3. The National Prion Disease Pathology Surveillance Center. Reviewed February 5, 2023. Accessed February 5, 2023. https://case.edu/medicine/pathology/divisions/prion-center
4. Appleby BS et al: Genetic aspects of human prion diseases. Front Neurol. 13:1003056, 2022
5. Mead S et al: Prion protein monoclonal antibody (PRN100) therapy for Creutzfeldt-Jakob disease: evaluation of a first-in-human treatment programme. Lancet Neurol. 21(4):342-54, 2022
6. Pritzkow S: Transmission, strain diversity, and zoonotic potential of chronic wasting disease. Viruses. 14(7), 2022
7. Centers for Disease Control and Prevention: Diagnostic Criteria for Creutzfelt-Jakob Disease (CJD), 2018 Updated October 18, 2021. Reviewed February 5, 2023. Accessed February 5, 2023. https://www.cdc.gov/prions/cjd/diagnostic-criteria.html
8. Ritchie DL et al: Variant CJD: reflections a quarter of a century on. Pathogens. 10(11), 2021
9. Bizzi A et al: Evaluation of a new criterion for detecting prion disease with diffusion magnetic resonance imaging. JAMA Neurol. 77(9):1141-9, 2020
10. Mammana A et al: Detection of prions in skin punch biopsies of Creutzfeldt-Jakob disease patients. Ann Clin Transl Neurol. 7(4):559-64, 2020
11. Appleby BS et al: A practical primer on prion pathology. J Neuropathol Exp Neurol. 77(5):346-52, 2018
12. Chitravas N et al: Treatable neurological disorders misdiagnosed as Creutzfeldt-Jakob disease. Ann Neurol. 70(3):437-44, 2011
13. Rutala WA et al: Guideline for disinfection and sterilization of prion-contaminated medical instruments. Infect Control Hosp Epidemiol. 31(2):107-17, 2010
14. Prusiner SB: prions. Proc Natl Acad Sci U S A. 95(23):13363-83, 1998

Sporadic Creutzfeldt-Jakob Disease With Grossly Normal Brain

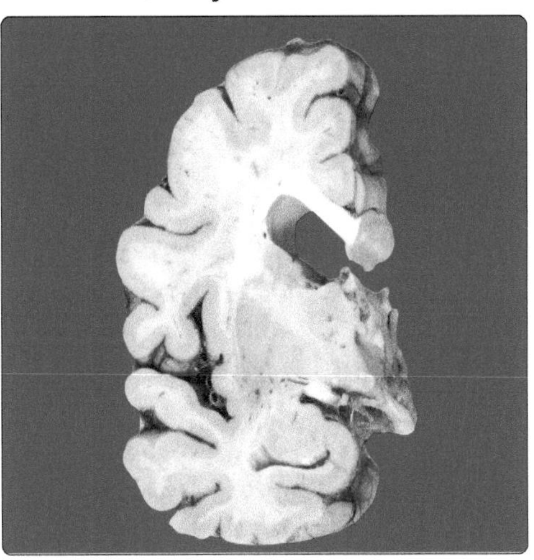

Spongiform Degeneration in Sporadic Creutzfeldt-Jakob Disease

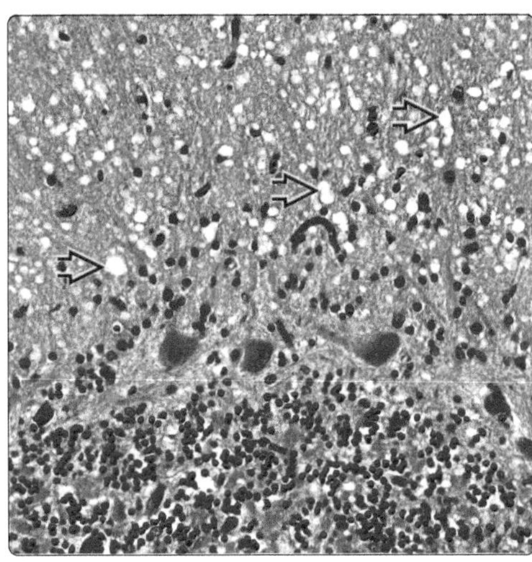

(Left) *Although no specific gross pathologic features are associated with CJD, generalized cerebral atrophy may be seen in individuals with a prolonged clinical course.* **(Right)** *Moderate to severe spongiform degeneration ⇨ is present in the molecular layer of the cerebellum, characterized by round to oval vacuoles with a sharply demarcated, punched-out appearance, typical of sCJD.*

Florid Plaques in Variant Creutzfeldt-Jakob Disease

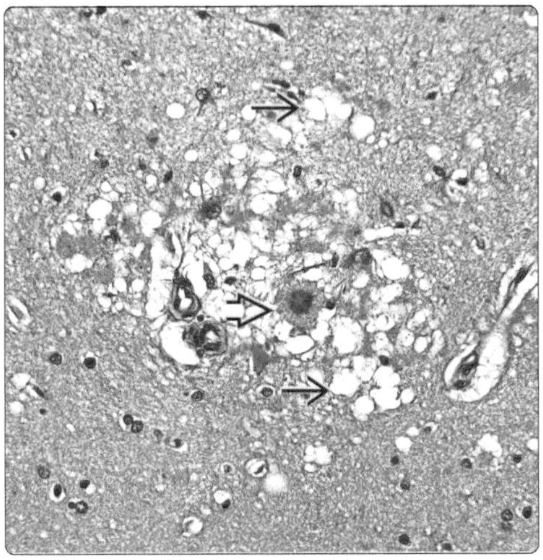

Anti-PrP IHC in Variant Creutzfeldt-Jakob Disease

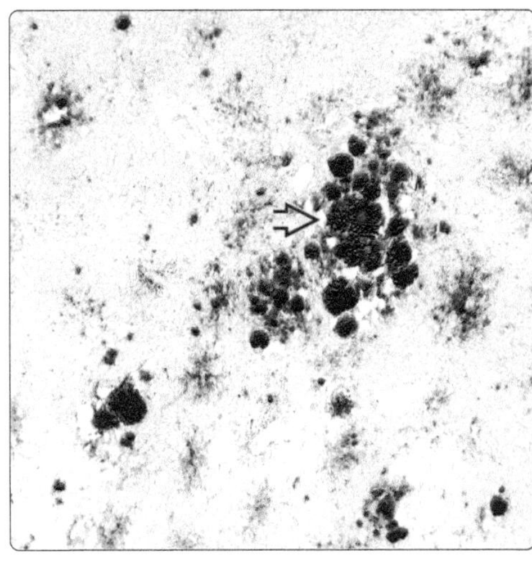

(Left) *Florid plaques ⇨, severe spongiform degeneration →, marked neuronal loss, and gliosis are characteristic features of variant CJD (vCJD). (Courtesy M. Cohen, MD.)* **(Right)** *Immunohistochemical staining with anti-PrP antibody (3F4) highlights florid plaques ⇨ of vCJD. (Courtesy M. Cohen, MD.)*

Kuru

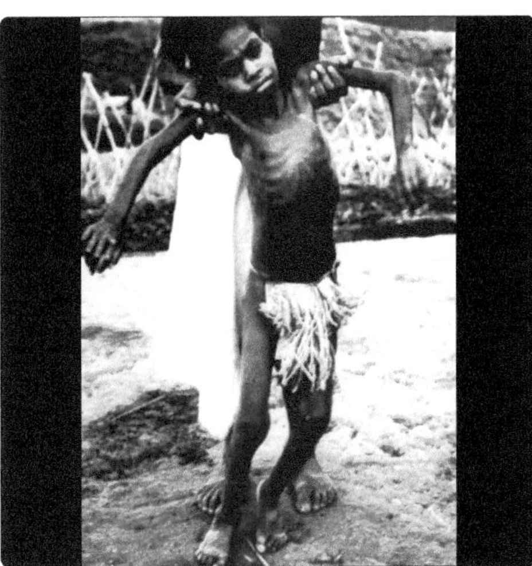

Bovine Spongiform Encephalopathy

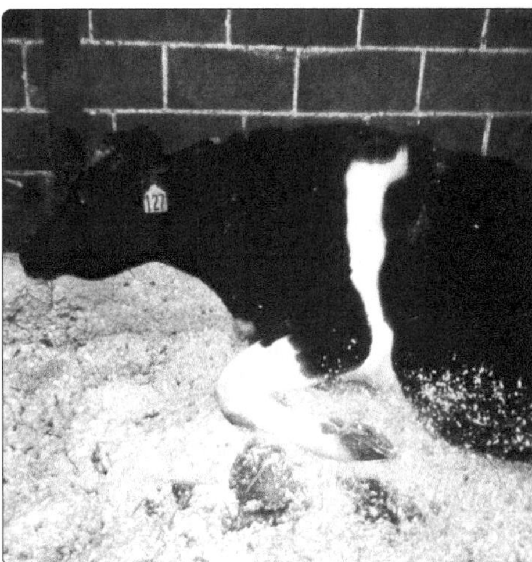

(Left) *Clinical photograph shows a child with advanced kuru who could neither stand nor sit without support. (Courtesy C. Gajdusek, Open-i.)* **(Right)** *Photograph shows a cow affected by bovine spongiform encephalopathy with progressive degeneration of the nervous system resulting in nervousness/aggression, weakness, ataxia, weight loss, and death. (Courtesy A. Davis, USDA/APHIS.)*

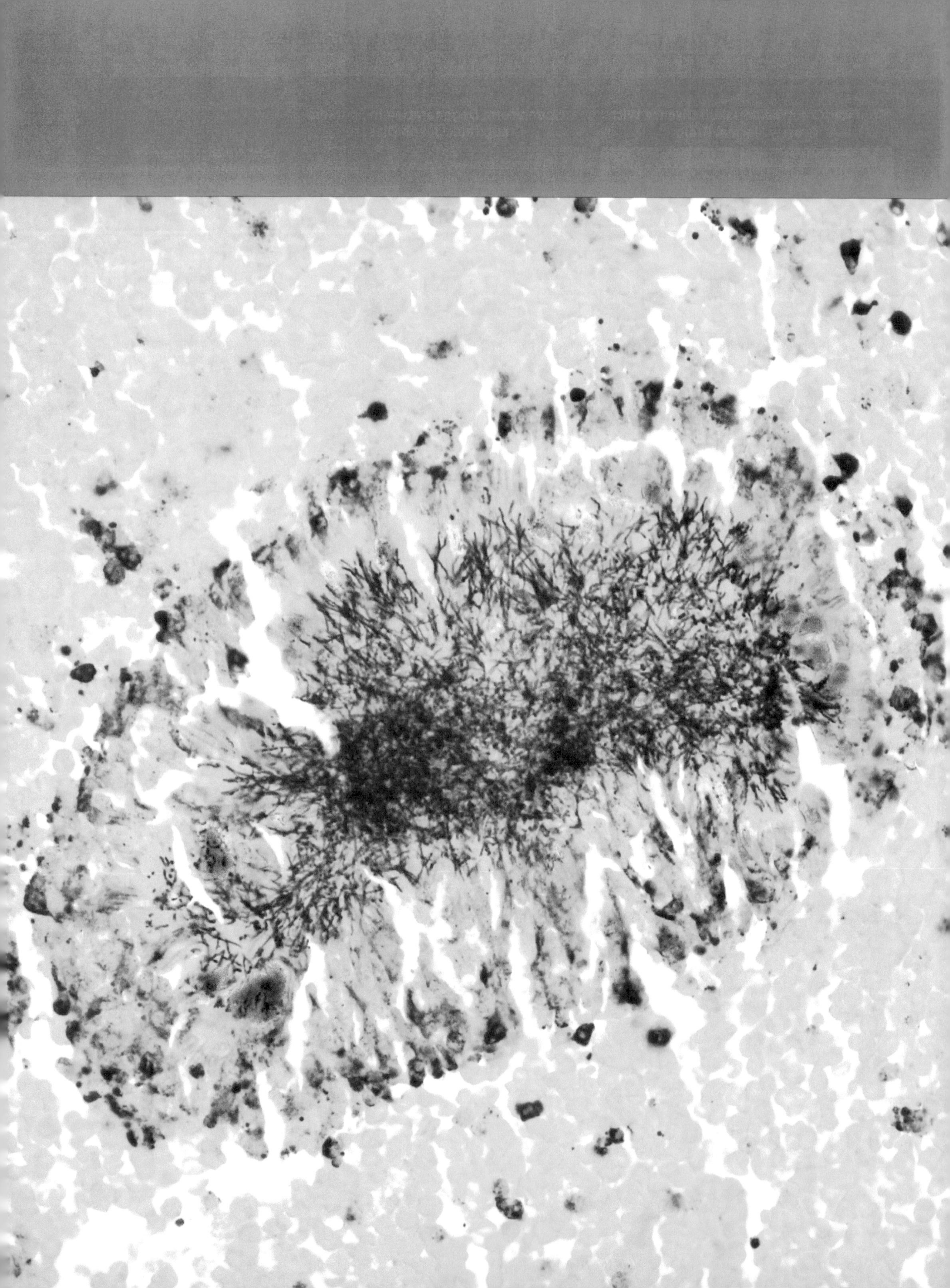

SECTION 4

Bacterial Infections

Gram-Positive Bacteria

Gram-Negative Bacteria

Acid-Fast Bacteria

TERMINOLOGY

Definitions

- Gram positive
  - Cell is bounded by inner lipid membrane surrounded by thick layer of peptidoglycan
  - Purple on Gram stain due to retention of crystal violet
- Gram negative
  - Cell is bounded by inner lipid membrane, surrounded by thin layer of peptidoglycan and outer lipid membrane
  - Uniquely associated with lipopolysaccharide (LPS) in outer membrane
  - Appears red on Gram stain due to safranin counterstain and lack of retention of crystal violet
- Spirochete
  - Cell is bounded by inner lipid membrane, surrounded by thin layer of peptidoglycan and outer lipid membrane
  - Characteristic spiral shape is due to periplasmic (between inner and outer membrane) location of flagella
  - Requires dark-field microscopy, Warthin-Starry stain, or immunohistochemistry for visualization
- Acid-fast bacterium
  - Cell is bounded by inner lipid membrane, surrounded by thin layer of peptidoglycan and outer lipid membrane
  - Peptidoglycan is complexed with arabinogalactan and long-chain mycolic acids, which impart characteristic waxy, acid-fast properties of cell
  - Appears red on carbol fuchsin-based Ziehl-Neelsen and Kinyoun stains; mycolic acids resist decolorization with acid or alcohol
- Aerobe: Requires oxygen for energy production
- Anaerobe
  - Obligate anaerobe: Poisoned by oxygen; must be cultured in anaerobic jar, chamber, or bottle
  - Facultative anaerobe: Use oxygen when available but can produce energy anaerobically
  - Microaerophilic: Requires lower concentration than atmospheric oxygen; must be cultured in low-oxygen environment

Bacterial Phylogenetic Tree Derived From 16s Sequence

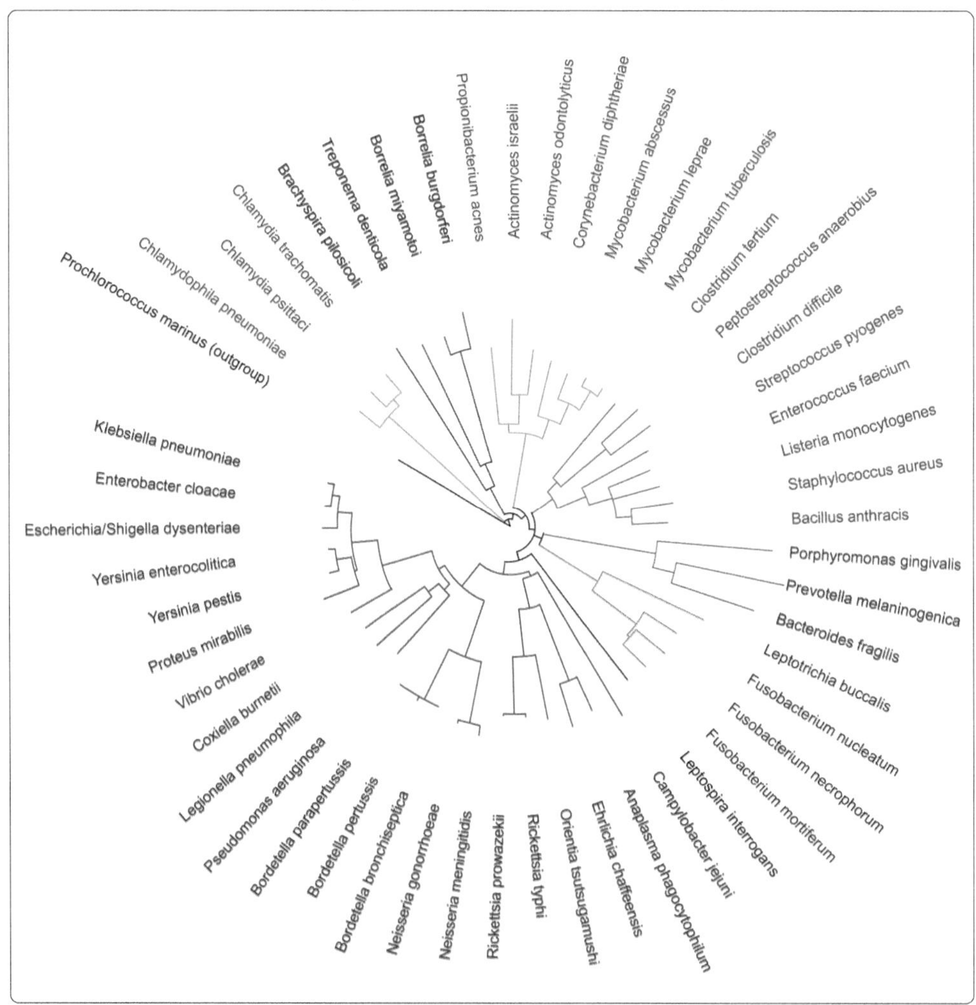

Phylogenetic tree is based on 16S sequence. Type sequences from the Ribosomal Database Project (www.rdp.org) is visualized using the ITOL viewer (itol.emble.de). Aqua: Chlamydiae; purple: Spirochetes; green: Actinobacteria; red: Firmicutes; magenta: Bacteroidetes; orange: Fusobacteria, blue: Proteobacteria.

TAXONOMY

Prokaryotic Phyla

- Firmicutes: Mainly gram-positive pathogens (both rods and cocci) with exception of Mollicutes
  - Clostridia (*Clostridium, Peptostreptococcus*, etc.)
  - Mollicutes (*Mycoplasma, Ureaplasma*)
  - Bacilli: Bacillales (*Bacillus, Listeria, Staphylococcus*, etc.) and Lactobacillales (*Lactobacillus, Enterococcus, Streptococcus*, etc.)
- Bacteroidetes: Gram-negative, rod-shaped organisms; both aerobic and anaerobic
  - Bacteroidia (*Bacteroides, Porphyromonas, Prevotella*)
  - Flavobacteria (*Capnocytophaga*, etc.)
  - Sphingobacteria (*Sphingobacterium*, etc.)
- Fusobacteria: Gram-negative, rod-shaped, obligate anaerobes
  - *Fusobacteria, Leptotrichia*, and *Streptobacillus*
- Proteobacteria: Gram-negative, rod-shaped, obligate anaerobes
  - α (*Rickettsia, Bartonella, Brucella*, etc.), β (*Neisseria, Burkholderia*, etc.), γ (*Enterobacteriaceae, Pseudomonas, Vibrio*, etc.), δ (*Desulfovibrio*, etc.), ε (*Campylobacter*, etc.)
- Actinobacteria: Gram-positive pathogens, high G+C content
  - *Corynebacterium, Nocardia, Mycobacterium, Propionibacterium, Rhodococcus*, etc.
- Chlamydiae: Obligate intracellular pathogens
  - *Chlamydia* (*Chlamydia trachomatis*, etc.) and *Chlamydophila* (*Chlamydophila pneumoniae, Chlamydophila psittaci*, etc.)
- Spirochetes: Spiral or helical-shaped pathogens
  - *Borrelia, Leptospira, Treponema*, etc.

ETIOLOGY/PATHOGENESIS

Colonizers

- Indigenous flora, composed of commensals (benefit without harm) and pathogens (disease in certain contexts, e.g., immunocompromised host or breach of epithelium)
- Respiratory flora (nares and upper airway): *Staphylococcus*, α-hemolytic *Streptococcus, Moraxella, Neisseria*, etc.
- Oral: *Streptococcus* (α-hemolytic), *Fusobacterium, Neisseria, Rothia, Veillonella, Gemella*, etc.
- Gastrointestinal: Many members of Bacteroidetes and Firmicutes phyla, also some Proteobacteria, and others
- Genitourinary (female): *Lactobacillus* and other anaerobes
- Skin: *Staphylococcus, Corynebacterium, Propionibacterium*

Pathogens

- Not associated with indigenous flora; can cause disease in normal (uncompromised) host
- Foodborne: Pathogenic *Escherichia coli, Shigella, Campylobacter, Salmonella* (nontyphoidal), *Listeria, Yersinia enterocolitica, Aeromonas, Bacillus cereus*
- Droplet/airborne: *Legionella pneumophila, Chlamydia pneumoniae, Mycoplasma pneumoniae, Francisella tularensis, Bordetella, Nocardia, Mycobacterium*
- Sexually transmitted: *Neisseria gonorrhoeae, C. trachomatis, Treponema pallidum, Haemophilus ducreyi*
- Vector borne: Anaplasmosis and ehrlichiosis, *Borrelia* spp., *F. tularensis, Rickettsia* spp., *Yersinia pestis*

Virulence Factors

- Toxin mediated: Disease caused by effects of toxin, which may disseminate widely from point of infection
- Capsule/biofilm mediated: Capsular polysaccharides can aid in immune evasion and contribute to formation of biofilms
- Adhesions: Mediate attachment to host cells and assist in invasion
- Intracellular survival: Organisms may escape from phagosome or inhibit phagolysosomal fusion
- Quorum sensing: Pathogens express genes in population-density-dependent manner
- Invasion: Organisms may induce uptake by host cells
- Nutrient acquisition: Scavenging limited resources in host environment (e.g., iron via siderophore binding)

DIAGNOSTIC APPROACHES

Histopathology

- Organisms can be detected with H&E and special stains; reported descriptively (e.g., gram-positive cocci)
- Most useful for identification of bacterial etiology prior to culture positivity as well as confirmation of tissue infection vs. surface colonization or contamination (i.e., in setting of unexpected culture or molecular results)
- Immunohistochemistry highly sensitive but frequent cross reactivity with related organisms
- In situ hybridization is highly sensitive and specific but not widely used for clinical diagnosis

Culture

- Most clinically relevant pathogens can be cultured on appropriate media ± anaerobic conditions
- Growth is typically 1-2 days, but some organisms may take weeks (e.g., *Mycobacterium tuberculosis*)
- Growth on selective and differential agars can partially identify pathogen, but biochemical assays or MALDI MS are usually required to make species level identification

Serology/Antigen Testing

- Fastidious/unculturable organisms may be best diagnosed using serology (e.g., *Borrelia, Coxiella*)
- Enzyme-linked immunoassays (EIA) exist for rapid diagnosis of select pathogens via antigen detection

Molecular

- Targeted PCR or probe-based assays are often assay of choice for fastidious pathogens
- Assays may be individual or part of multiplexed panels organized around syndromes that include fungal, viral, and parasitic targets as well
- Broad-range PCR targeting 16s ribosomal RNA region can be used on cultured isolates, FFPE tissue, and primary specimens but may require reference laboratory

SELECTED REFERENCES

1. Bennett JE et al: Mandell, Douglas, and Bennett's Principles of Infectious Diseases. 8th ed. Saunders Elsevier, 2015
2. Jorgensen JH et al: Manual of Clinical Microbiology. 11th ed. American Society for Microbiology Press, 2015
3. Buchan BW et al: Emerging technologies for the clinical microbiology laboratory. Clin Microbiol Rev. 27(4):783-822, 2014
4. Grice EA et al: The human microbiome: our second genome. Annu Rev Genomics Hum Genet. 13:151-70, 2012
5. Woese CR: Bacterial evolution. Microbiol Rev. 51(2):221-71, 1987

Botryomycosis

KEY FACTS

ETIOLOGY/PATHOGENESIS

- Caused by response to nonfilamentous bacteria, most commonly *Staphylococcus aureus*, as well as gram-negative *Proteus* spp., *Escherichia coli*, and *Pseudomonas aeruginosa*

CLINICAL ISSUES

- More common among immunocompromised patients
- Can involve skin with primary or secondary visceral disease
- Successful treatment depends on site of lesion and immune status of host

MICROSCOPIC

- Abscess containing basophilic granules composed of nonfilamentous bacteria, surrounded by granulomatous reaction with frequent giant cells
- Granules surrounded by eosinophilic material (Splendore-Hoeppli phenomenon)
- Gram ± Warthin-Starry stains to classify bacteria
- Cultures or 16S rRNA sequencing to identify specific causative agent

TOP DIFFERENTIAL DIAGNOSES

- Actinomycetoma: Colored grains with fine (≤ 1-μm) radially oriented filaments highlighted by Gram ± mAFB stains
  - Caused by *Nocardia* spp., *Actinomadura* spp., *Streptomyces* spp., etc.
- Eumycetoma: Colored grains with septate hyphae (2-6 μm in diameter) accompanied by numerous chlamydoconidia and swollen cells highlighted by GMS and PAS-D stains;
  - Caused by at least 30 hyaline and pigmented species of fungi, including *Madurella mycetomatis*, *Leptosphaeria senegalensis*, and *Scedosporium boydii*
- Cysts: Epidermal cysts ± communication and contain keratin or fluid; no granules or bacteria identified
- Carcinoma: Visceral disease may mimic carcinoma (and vice versa); no granules or bacteria identified

Botryomycosis Granule

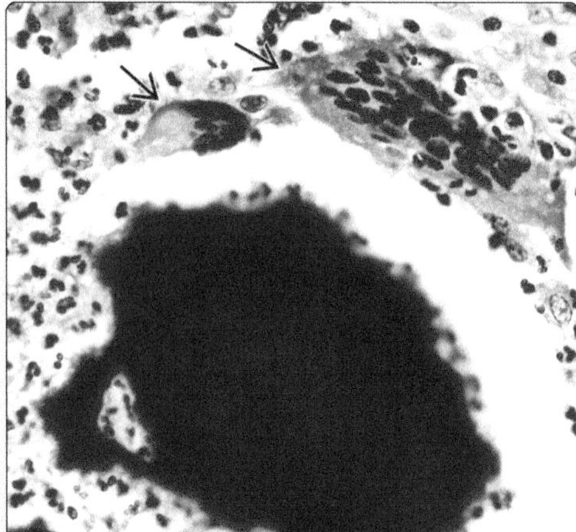

Cutaneous Botryomycosis

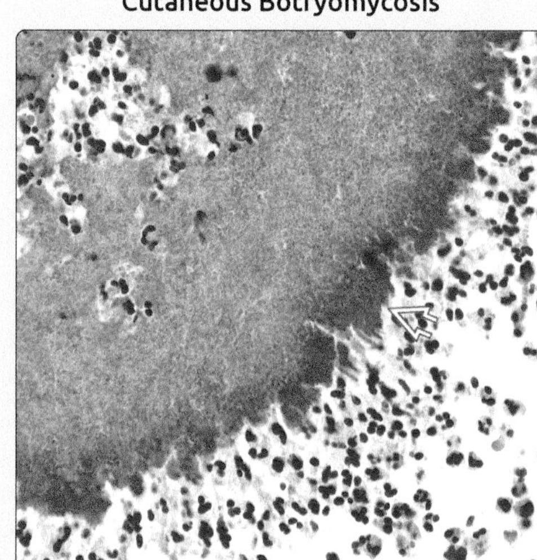

(Left) *This section shows a granule containing a dense collection of basophilic cocci surrounded by multinucleated giant cells ⇨ and embedded in a neutrophilic abscess.* **(Right)** *Biopsy from a 50-year-old woman who presented with tender leg nodules showed abscess with scattered granules. The edge of this granule shows a dense eosinophilic matrix (Splendore-Hoeppli material) ➡.*

Gram Stain

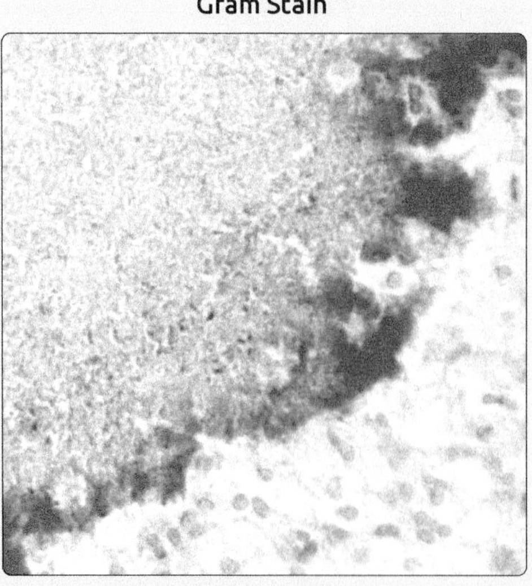

Warthin-Starry Stain

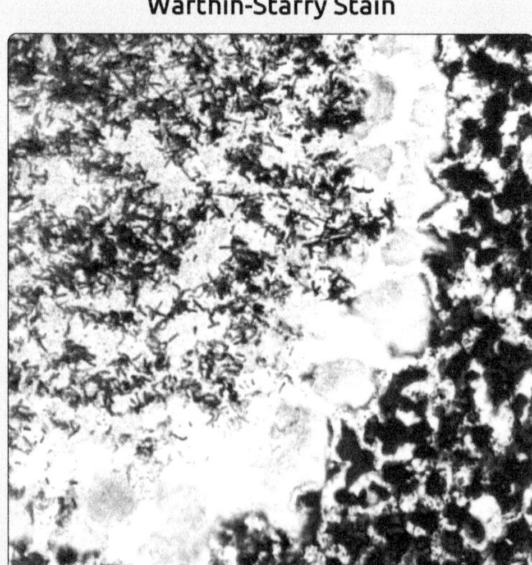

(Left) *Gram staining (in conjunction with mAFB and GMS stains) helps to determine the type of organisms composing Botryomycosis granules. In this case, the lack of Gram staining is consistent with a gram-negative bacillus.* **(Right)** *Warthin-Starry staining can be used to confirm the presence of gram-negative bacilli in botryomycosis cases caused by Escherichia coli, Pseudomonas aeruginosa, Proteus spp., and others.*

TERMINOLOGY

Synonyms

- Pyoderma vegetans, bacterial pseudomycosis

Definitions

- "Botrys" is Latin term for "bunch of grapes"

ETIOLOGY/PATHOGENESIS

Infectious Agents

- Unusual host response to several nonfilamentous bacteria which form granules surrounded by matrix of antigen-antibody complexes (Splendore-Hoeppli phenomenon); exact pathogenesis remains unknown
- Culture-proven lesions are often due to *Staphylococcus aureus* (gram-positive cocci)
- Gram-negative organisms, such as *Proteus* spp., *Escherichia coli*, and *Pseudomonas aeruginosa*, among others, have been reported

CLINICAL ISSUES

Epidemiology

- ~ 200 reported cases
- Occurs in all age groups; M > F

Presentation

- More common among immunocompromised patients involving skin &/or viscera
- In cutaneous disease, patients present with mass or plaques, abscesses, and ulcers with draining sinuses, which can mimic mycetoma or other fungal causes (eumycetoma)
- Botryomycosis of oral cavity is rare and present on tongue, tonsils, and palate
- Visceral disease can be primary (e.g., lung, liver, vulva, heart, etc.) and can mimic carcinoma
- Visceral diseases can be secondary when infection spreads to internal organs from cutaneous lesion

Treatment

- Long-term antibiotic therapy and surgical debridement

Prognosis

- Cutaneous botryomycosis usually responds better than visceral form to antibiotic therapy
- Successful treatment depends on site of lesion and immune status of host

MICROBIOLOGY

Bacterial Culture

- Gold standard to isolate/identify strain and perform susceptibility testing
  - Aerobic and anaerobic should be performed

MACROSCOPIC

General Features

- Draining sinuses may show granules
- Cut sections may show deep-seated granules

MICROSCOPIC

Histologic Features

- Abscess containing numerous basophilic granules composed of nonfilamentous bacteria, surrounded by granulomatous reaction with frequent giant cells
- Granules are surrounded by eosinophilic material (Splendore-Hoeppli phenomenon), which may be absent in severely immunosuppressed patients

Cytologic Features

- Granules may demonstrate bacterial forms at edges if smeared

ANCILLARY TESTS

Histochemistry

- Gram ± Warthin-Starry stains to determine if it is gram-positive or gram-negative bacteria
- Periodic acid-Schiff stain to stain granule

PCR

- 16S rRNA sequencing to identify specific causative agent

DIFFERENTIAL DIAGNOSIS

Actinomycetoma

- Colored grains with fine (≤ 1-μm) radially oriented filaments highlighted by Gram ± mAFB stains
- Caused by traumatic inoculation of filamentous bacteria (e.g., *Nocardia* spp., *Actinomadura* spp., *Streptomyces* spp.) through contact with contaminated materials

Eumycetoma

- Colored grains with septate hyphae (2-6 μm in diameter) accompanied by numerous chlamydoconidia and swollen cells highlighted by GMS and PAS-D stains
- Caused by at least 30 hyaline and pigmented species of fungi (e.g., *Madurella mycetomatis, Magnaporthe grisea, Leptosphaeria senegalensis*, and *Scedosporium boydii*) through contact with contaminated materials

Cysts

- Epidermal cysts ± communication and contain keratin or fluid; no granules or bacteria identified

Carcinoma

- Visceral disease may mimic carcinoma (and vice versa); no granules or bacteria identified

SELECTED REFERENCES

1. Corrêa DG et al: Magnetic resonance imaging and histopathological aspects of botryomycosis. Rev Soc Bras Med Trop. 55:e0646, 2022
2. Shimagaki H et al: Case of cutaneous botryomycosis in an 8-year-old immunocompetent boy with a review of the published work. J Dermatol. 47(5):542-5, 2020
3. Bender-Saebelkampf S et al: Cutaneous and pulmonary botryomycosis. Lancet Infect Dis. 19(6):670, 2019
4. DeWitt JP et al: Extensive cutaneous botryomycosis with subsequent development of nocardia-positive wound cultures. J Cutan Med Surg. 1203475418755762, 2018
5. Gupta K et al: Cardiac botryomycosis: an autopsy report. J Clin Pathol. 61(8):972-4, 2008

Malakoplakia

KEY FACTS

ETIOLOGY/PATHOGENESIS

- Defective digestion of bacteria in phagolysosomes (e.g., *Escherichia coli, Proteus, Klebsiella, Staphylococcus aureus, Mycobacterium, Rhodococcus equi*)

CLINICAL ISSUES

- More prevalent in females and immunocompromised populations
- Most frequent site of involvement: Urinary tract, especially bladder
- Surgery is best curative therapy; ideal for localized/unilateral disease

MACROSCOPIC

- Yellow-brown, soft plaques and nodules
- Umbilicated centers

MICROSCOPIC

- Sheets of von Hansemann cells: Eosinophilic histiocytes with eccentric nuclei
- Michaelis-Gutmann bodies: 5- to 10-μm basophilic structures composed of mineralized bacterial fragments
- Histologic evidence of bacteria may or may not be present
- Acute and chronic inflammation
- Late lesions may show marked fibrosis

ANCILLARY TESTS

- von Hansemann cells: Positive for CD68, α-chymotrypsin; negative for S100
- Michaelis-Gutmann bodies stain positive on periodic acid-Schiff, Prussian blue, and von Kossa stains

TOP DIFFERENTIAL DIAGNOSES

- Langerhans cell histiocytosis: Positive for S100, langerin, and CD1a
- Granular cell tumor: Positive for S100
- Xanthogranuloma: Macrophages foamy and lipid laden
- Malignancy: Positive for cytokeratins/lineage markers

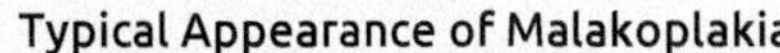

Michaelis-Guttman Bodies

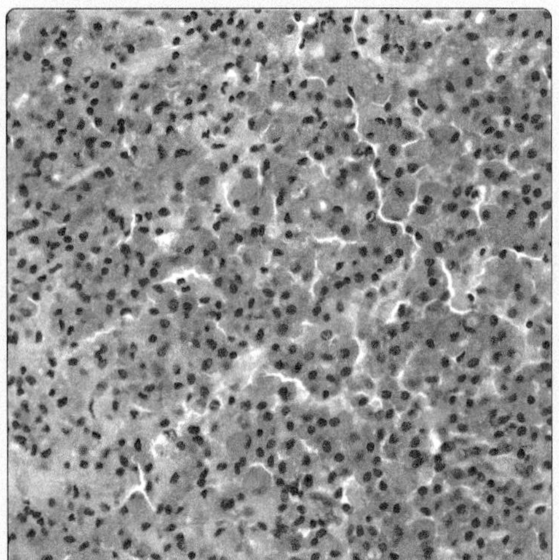

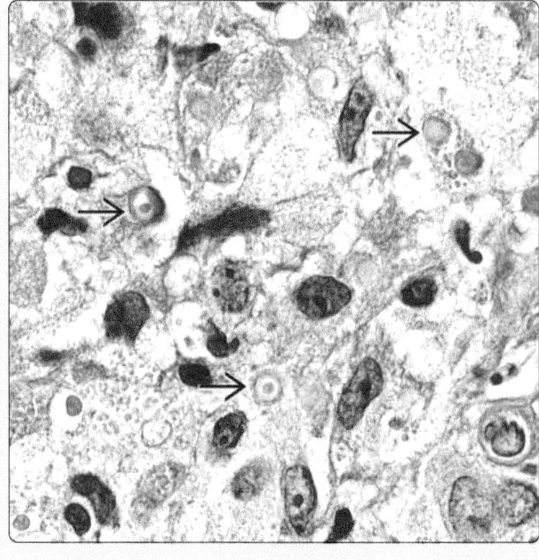

(Left) *Malakoplakia is characterized by sheets of histiocytes with eccentric, bland nuclei and brightly eosinophilic granular cytoplasmic (a.k.a. von Hansemann) cells.* **(Right)** *In this colon biopsy, intracytoplasmic inclusions, known as Michaelis-Guttman bodies* ➡*, are identified, which are pathognomonic for malakoplakia. They are smaller than the nuclei of von Hansemann cells, round/targetoid, and basophilic.*

Periodic Acid-Schiff Stain

von Kossa Stain

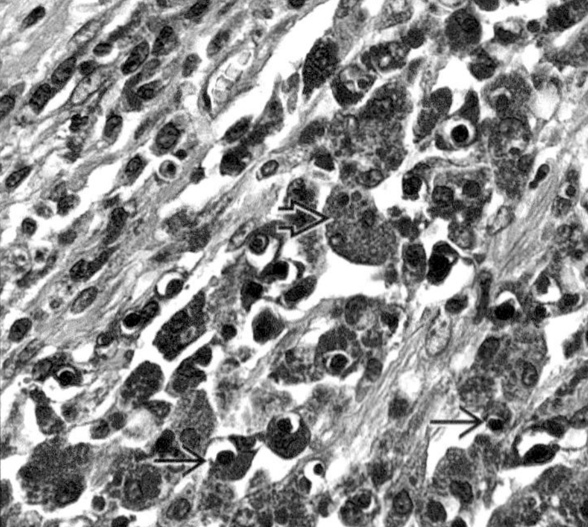

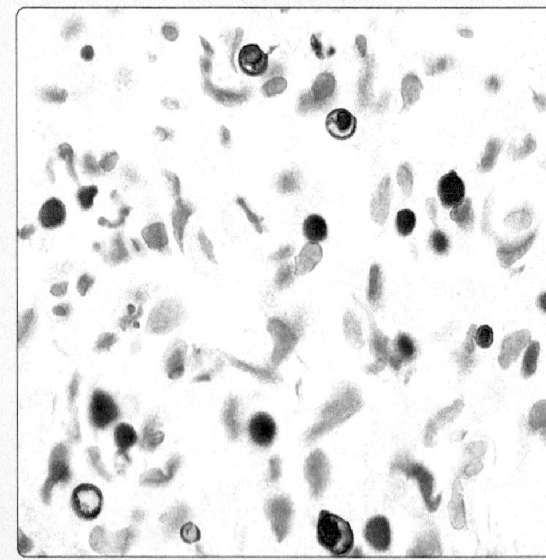

(Left) *Periodic acid-Schiff stain of renal malakoplakia highlights the granular cytoplasm of macrophages known as von Hansemann cells* ➡ *and intensely stains the characteristic Michaelis-Gutmann bodies* ➡*.* **(Right)** *Mineralized calcium within Michaelis-Gutmann bodies is highlighted by a von Kossa stain.*

TERMINOLOGY

Definitions

- Malakoplakia: From Greek term meaning "soft plaques"

ETIOLOGY/PATHOGENESIS

Acquired/Infectious

- Defective intracytoplasmic digestion of bacteria in phagolysosomes in setting of chronic/indolent infections
  - *Escherichia coli, Proteus, Klebsiella, Staphylococcus aureus, Mycobacterium, Rhodococcus equi*
- Cellular and extracellular accumulation of partially digested bacteria becomes trapped in lysosomal components

CLINICAL ISSUES

Epidemiology

- Age: Adults; peak incidence in 5th decade
- Sex: More common in females
- More prevalent in immunocompromised populations
  - HIV/AIDS and inherited immune disorders as well as posttransplant patients
  - Chronic steroid use and chronic alcohol abuse
  - Uncontrolled diabetes

Site

- Urinary tract: Most frequently involved organ system
  - Associated with chronic coliform cystitis
  - Bladder more common than ureters and kidneys
- Gastrointestinal tract, lungs, thyroid, prostate, salivary glands, colon, testes, skin less common

Presentation

- Urinary tract lesions
  - Urinary bladder: Frequency, urgency, dysuria, hematuria
  - Ureters: Obstructive renal failure
  - Kidneys: Hematuria, proteinuria
- Gastrointestinal tract: Diarrhea, obstruction, pain or clinically silent
- Skin: Subcutaneous nodule with sinus tract formation
- Salivary glands: Enlarging mass ± lymph node involvement

Treatment

- Surgery is best curative therapy; ideal for localized/unilateral disease
- Drugs: Antibiotics, vitamin C, bethanechol

Prognosis

- Varies by site, extent, associated disease conditions, and therapeutic options

MACROSCOPIC

Gross Features

- Yellow-brown, soft plaques and nodules
- Umbilicated centers

MICROSCOPIC

Histologic Features

- Sheets of von Hansemann cells
  - Histiocytes with eccentric nuclei and brightly eosinophilic cytoplasm
- Michaelis-Gutmann bodies
  - Basophilic, concentric, targetoid, or owl's-eye structures composed of mineralized bacterial fragments trapped in lysosomal components
  - 5-10 µm in diameter (smaller than nuclei of von Hansemann cells) that present within von Hansemann cells or in extracellular spaces
  - Pathognomonic but not necessary for diagnosis; may not be present in early or late lesions
- Histologic evidence of bacteria may or may not be present
- Inflammation with lymphocytes, neutrophils, plasma cells; late lesions may show marked fibrosis

ANCILLARY TESTS

Histochemistry

- von Hansemann cells: Positive on periodic acid-Schiff stain
- Michaelis-Gutmann bodies: Positive on periodic acid-Schiff, Prussian blue, and von Kossa stains

Immunohistochemistry

- von Hansemann cells: Positive for CD68, α-chymotrypsin; negative for S100

Electron Microscopy

- Curved membrane-bound phagolysosomes that contain fragments of bacterial organisms

DIFFERENTIAL DIAGNOSIS

Langerhans Cell Histiocytosis

- Large cells with notched/kidney bean-like nuclei
- Cells positive for S100, langerin, and CD1a

Granular Cell Tumor

- Large cells with abundant eosinophilic granular cytoplasm
- Cells positive for S100

Xanthogranuloma

- Macrophages foamy and lipid laden
- Lacks Michaelis-Gutman bodies

Malignancy

- e.g., renal cell carcinoma, urothelial carcinoma, prostatic carcinoma
- Cells positive for cytokeratins and lineage specific markers
- Lacks Michaelis-Gutman bodies

SELECTED REFERENCES

1. Acosta AM et al: Prostatic malakoplakia: clinicopathological assessment of a multi-institutional series of 49 patients. Histopathology. 81(4):520-8, 2022
2. Manini C et al: Mimickers of urothelial carcinoma and the approach to differential diagnosis. Clin Pract. 11(1):110-23, 2021
3. Ahumada VH et al: Pulmonary malakoplakia by Rhodococcus equi in an HIV-infected patient in Mexico: a case report. Case Rep Infect Dis. 2020:3131024, 2020
4. Ho L et al: Renal malakoplakia mimicking a malignancy and diagnosed by fine-needle aspiration: a case report. Diagn Cytopathol. 48(11):1093-7, 2020
5. Jung YS et al: Ultrastructural evidence of the evolutional process in malakoplakia. Histol Histopathol. 35(2):177-84, 2020
6. Lee M et al: Malakoplakia of the gastrointestinal tract: clinicopathologic analysis of 23 cases. Diagn Pathol. 15(1):97, 2020
7. Zhang Y et al: Gastrointestinal malakoplakia: clinicopathologic analysis of 26 cases. Am J Surg Pathol. 44(9):1251-8, 2020

Actinomycosis

KEY FACTS

ETIOLOGY/PATHOGENESIS

- *Actinomyces* spp. are among predominant inhabitants of oral cavity, also commonly found in gut, genitourinary tract, and skin; associated with disease following mucosal disruption
- > 25 spp. isolated from humans; *Actinomyces israelii* is most common pathogenic spp.
- Risk factors include chronic steroid use, leukemia, HIV, organ transplantation, prolonged intrauterine device (IUD) use

CLINICAL ISSUES

- Orocervicofacial (most common site of infection): Fever, pain, and localized swelling that may be mistaken for neoplastic process
- Thoracic (aspiration of oropharyngeal secretions), abdominopelvic (ruptured appendix, prolonged IUD use), central nervous system abscess (direct extension or hematogenous)

MICROSCOPIC

- Basophilic filamentous branching bacterial forms highlighted by Gram stain and GMS stains; negative modified acid-fast stains
- Sulfur granules: Core of bacteria with eosinophilic periphery (Splendore-Hoeppli phenomenon)
- Tissue necrosis, abscess formation, acute and chronic inflammation, ± sinus tract formation

TOP DIFFERENTIAL DIAGNOSES

- Nocardiosis: Gram-positive, partially acid-fast filamentous bacteria that may form granules
- Eumycetoma: Fungal mycetoma with hyphae
- Botryomycosis: Clumps of nonfilamentous bacteria highlighted by Gram or Warthin-Starry stains
- Pseudoactinomycotic radiate granules: Found in endometrial biopsies and curettings from IUD users; refractile without dense core, negative for organisms

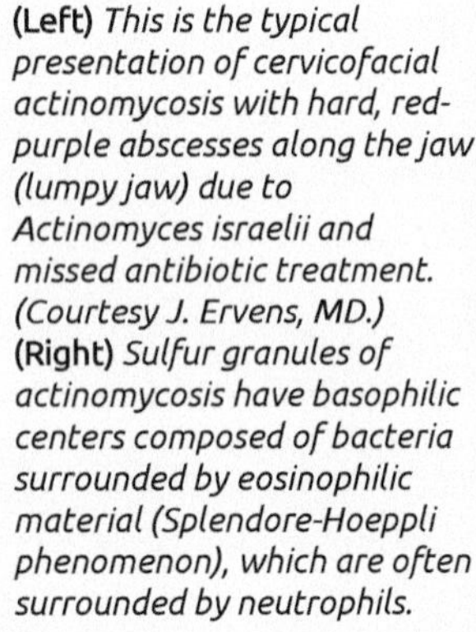
(Left) *This is the typical presentation of cervicofacial actinomycosis with hard, red-purple abscesses along the jaw (lumpy jaw) due to Actinomyces israelii and missed antibiotic treatment. (Courtesy J. Ervens, MD.)* **(Right)** *Sulfur granules of actinomycosis have basophilic centers composed of bacteria surrounded by eosinophilic material (Splendore-Hoeppli phenomenon), which are often surrounded by neutrophils.*

Lumpy Jaw: *Actinomyces israelii*

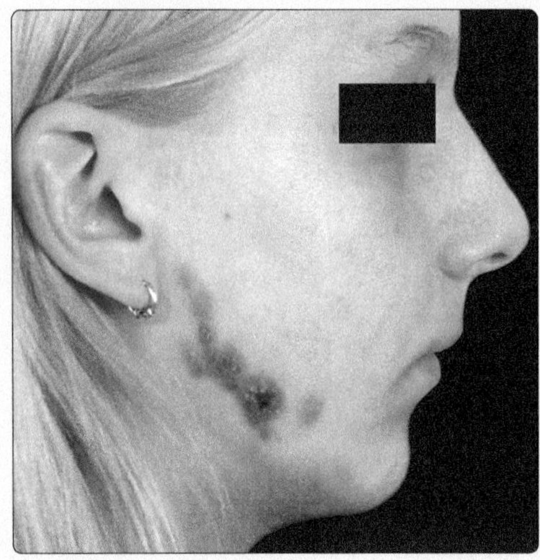

Actinomycosis: Sulfur Granule

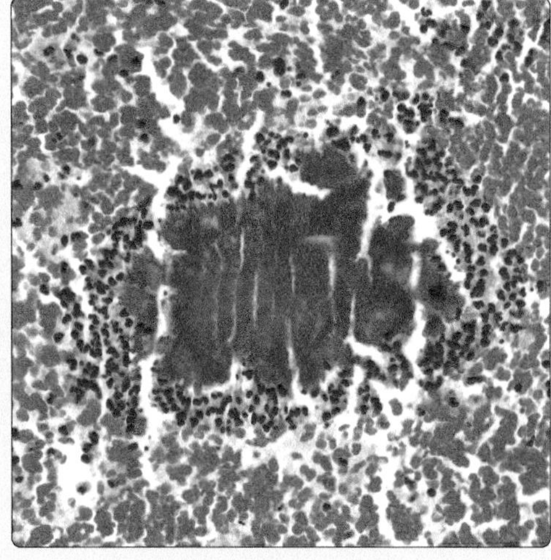

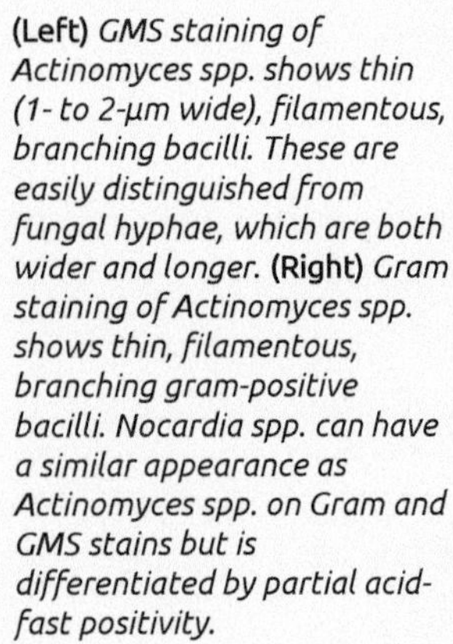
(Left) *GMS staining of Actinomyces spp. shows thin (1- to 2-µm wide), filamentous, branching bacilli. These are easily distinguished from fungal hyphae, which are both wider and longer.* **(Right)** *Gram staining of Actinomyces spp. shows thin, filamentous, branching gram-positive bacilli. Nocardia spp. can have a similar appearance as Actinomyces spp. on Gram and GMS stains but is differentiated by partial acid-fast positivity.*

Actinomycosis: GMS Stain

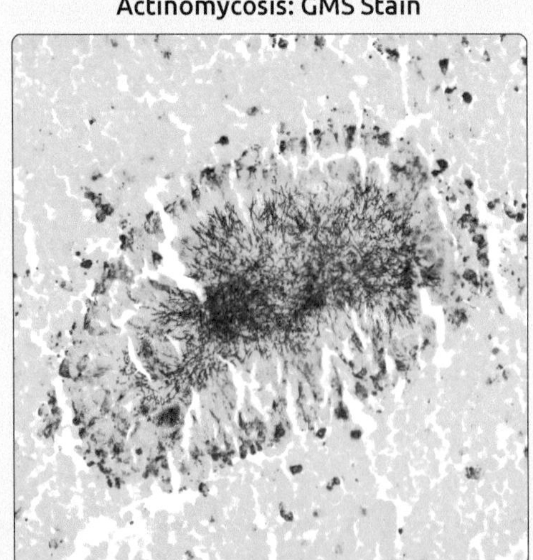

Actinomycosis: Gram Stain

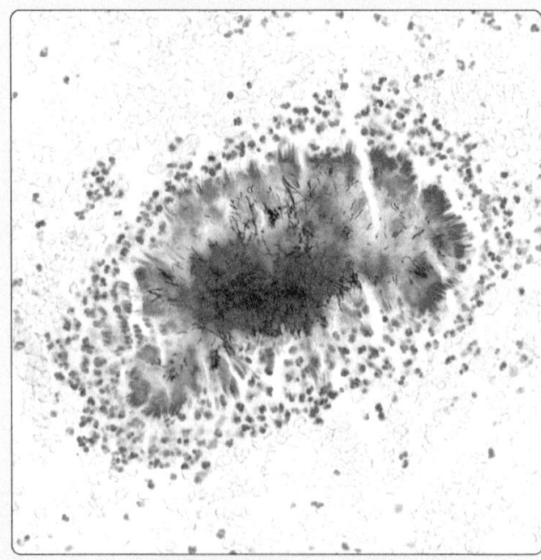

TERMINOLOGY

Synonyms

- Lumpy jaw

ETIOLOGY/PATHOGENESIS

Infectious Agents

- Infection with *Actinomyces* spp., anaerobic, gram-positive, filamentous bacteria that are part of normal flora at different anatomical sites and cause disease following breach of mucosal lining
- > 25 spp. isolated from human samples; *Actinomyces israelii* most frequent pathogenic spp.; others include *A. meyeri*, *A. viscosus*, *A. neuii*, *A. turicensis*, *A. odontolyticus*, *A. georgiae*, *A. gerencseriae*, *A. naeslundii*, and *A. oris*

CLINICAL ISSUES

Epidemiology

- Risk factors include poor oral hygiene, smoking, alcohol abuse, antiinflammatory drugs (e.g., chronic steroid use), leukemia, HIV, organ transplantation, diabetes mellitus, and bisphosphonate or radiation-associated osteonecrosis

Presentation

- Orocervicofacial (most common site of infection): Fever, pain, and localized swelling that may be mistaken for neoplastic process; ± sinus tract formation; disease may involve adjacent bone and skeletal muscle
- Thoracic (2nd most common site of infection): Pneumonia, low-grade fever, cough, and shortness of breath, sometimes with notable weight loss and hemoptysis
- Abdominopelvic: Ruptured appendix or prolonged intrauterine device (IUD) use with fever, vaginal discharge, pain, or weight loss
- Central nervous system (rare): Direct extension from orocervicofacial disease or by hematogenous spread; typically abscess
- Musculoskeletal (rare): Trauma, prostheses, or direct infiltration from soft tissue infection

Treatment

- Surgical debridement (with extensive necrosis) or sinus tract excision (chronic)
- Penicillin is 1st-line antibiotic therapy
- Removal of IUD

Prognosis

- Varies by site, extent of disease, and time to therapy

MICROBIOLOGY

Culture

- Growth on enriched media (serum or blood) in anaerobic conditions produces colonies in 2-4 days but may require extended period of time; colony morphology of some spp. has characteristic molar tooth appearance
- Bacterial identification by MALDI-TOF or PCR
- 50% negative culture rate due to previous antibiotic therapy, inhibition of growth in polymicrobial infections, exposure to oxygen during transportation and culture, or insufficient incubation time

MACROSCOPIC

General Features

- Mass-forming lesions with tissue necrosis, abscess formation, ± sinus tract formation with sulfur granules (firm yellow granular material)

MICROSCOPIC

Histologic Features

- Basophilic filamentous branching bacterial forms (1-2 µm in diameter); frequently associated with other bacteria, including staphylococci, streptococci, fusobacteria, and colonizing microbiota
- Sulfur granules (up to 2 mm in size) composed of clumped colonies of bacteria in center with eosinophilic periphery with club-like projections due to Splendore-Hoeppli phenomenon
- Tissue necrosis, abscess formation, acute and chronic inflammation, granulomatous inflammation, ± sinus tract formation

ANCILLARY TESTS

Special Stains

- Gram and methenamine silver stains highlight filamentous *Actinomyces* spp. and other associated bacteria
- Modified acid-fast stains are negative

DIFFERENTIAL DIAGNOSIS

Nocardiosis

- Gram-positive, partially acid-fast filamentous bacteria that may also form granules

Eumycetoma

- Fungal mycetomas may appear similar with sulfur granules; distinguished by presence of fungal hyphae

Botryomycosis

- May similarly form colonies mimicking sulfur granules
- Composed of clumps of nonfilamentous bacteria highlighted by Gram or Warthin-Starry stains

Pseudoactinomycotic Radiate Granules in Intrauterine Device Use

- May be found in endometrial biopsies and curettings
- Refractile without dense core and negative for organisms on Gram and GMS stains

SELECTED REFERENCES

1. Boot M et al: The diagnosis and management of pulmonary actinomycosis. J Infect Public Health. 16(4):490-500, 2023
2. McHugh KE et al: The cytopathology of Actinomyces, Nocardia, and their mimickers. Diagn Cytopathol. 45(12):1105-15, 2017
3. Könönen E et al: Actinomyces and related organisms in human infections. Clin Microbiol Rev. 28(2):419-42, 2015
4. Garner O et al: Multi-centre evaluation of mass spectrometric identification of anaerobic bacteria using the VITEK® MS system. Clin Microbiol Infect. 20(4):335-9, 2014
5. Valour F et al: Actinomycosis: etiology, clinical features, diagnosis, treatment, and management. Infect Drug Resist. 7:183-97, 2014
6. Haggerty CJ et al: Actinomycotic brain abscess and subdural empyema of odontogenic origin: case report and review of the literature. J Oral Maxillofac Surg. 70(3):e210-3, 2012
7. Pritt B et al: Pseudoactinomycotic radiate granules of the gynaecological tract: review of a diagnostic pitfall. J Clin Pathol. 59(1):17-20, 2006

Bacillus Species Infections

KEY FACTS

ETIOLOGY/PATHOGENESIS

- Infection with *Bacillus* spp., gram-positive bacilli widely present in environment; spores are extremely resistant and have been found in virtually every habitat

CLINICAL ISSUES

- *B. anthracis* (anthrax) has 3 clinical types: Cutaneous (95%), pulmonary (5%), and gastrointestinal (1%)
- *B. cereus*: Opportunistic pathogen and causative agent of food-borne illness and occasional nosocomial outbreaks
- *B. thuringiensis*: Predominantly insect pathogen, uncommon cause of gastroenteritis and wound and burn infections

MICROBIOLOGY

- Culture is gold standard for diagnosis; medium, gray, flat, irregular (Medusa head), nonhemolytic colonies

MICROSCOPIC

- Gram-positive bacilli (1.2 μm wide) highlighted by Gram, Silver, and IHC stains
- Pulmonary anthrax: Pleural effusions, pulmonary edema, and hyaline membrane formation
- Lymphatics anthrax: Hemorrhagic mediastinitis
- Cutaneous anthrax: Epidermal necrosis, hemorrhage, acantholysis, and ulceration; dermal edema, coagulation necrosis, hemorrhage, and vasculitis
- CNS anthrax: Low- and high-pressure hemorrhages along with vasculitis composed of fibrinoid necrosis and neutrophils in meninges and parenchyma

TOP DIFFERENTIAL DIAGNOSES

- Skin lesions mimicking cutaneous anthrax: Brown recluse spider bite, ulceroglandular tularemia, plague, ecthyma gangrenosum, spotted fever rickettsial infection, scrub typhus (differentiated by culture and IHC)
- Gastrointestinal Infections: *Clostridioides difficile* infection, inflammatory bowel disease, ischemia
- Respiratory Infections: Pneumonia, transfusion-associated acute lung injury

Anthrax Hemorrhagic Meningoencephalitis

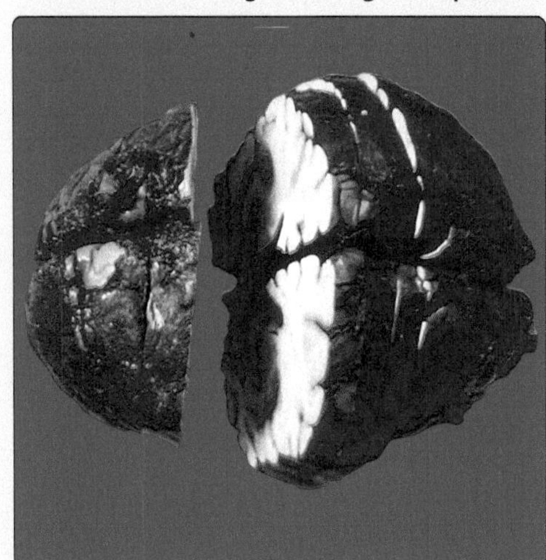

***Bacillus anthracis* Gram Stain**

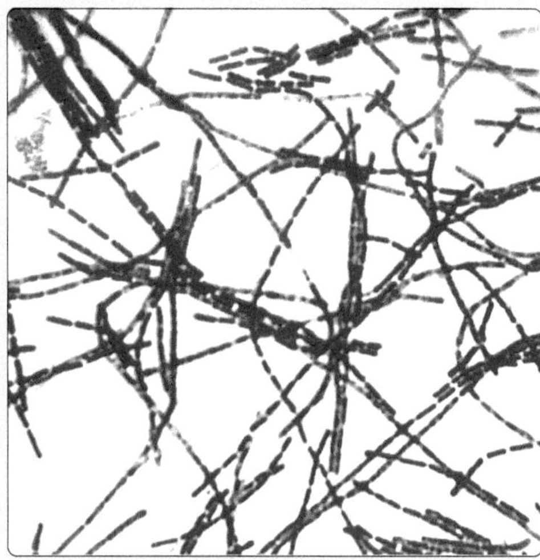

(Left) *A brain from a patient with disseminated Bacillus anthracis infection demonstrates diffuse hemorrhagic meningoencephalitis, which is pathognomonic for the disease. (Courtesy CDC/PHIL.)* **(Right)** *Bacillus anthracis appears on Gram stain as long chains of rod-shaped bacilli. Infections with Bacillus species warrant careful clinical investigation. (Courtesy CDC/PHIL.)*

Cutaneous Anthrax

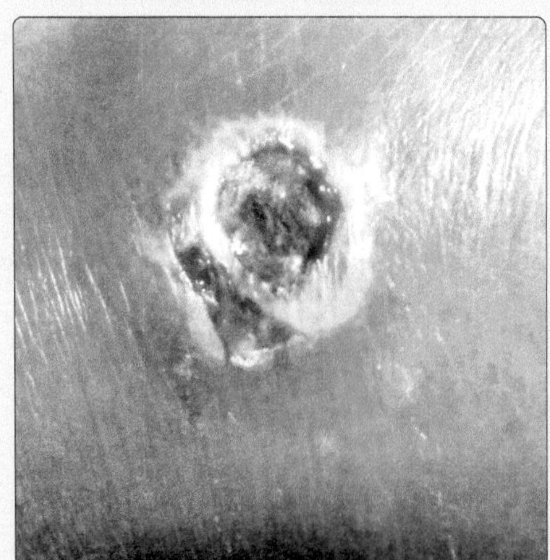

***Bacillus anthracis* Culture**

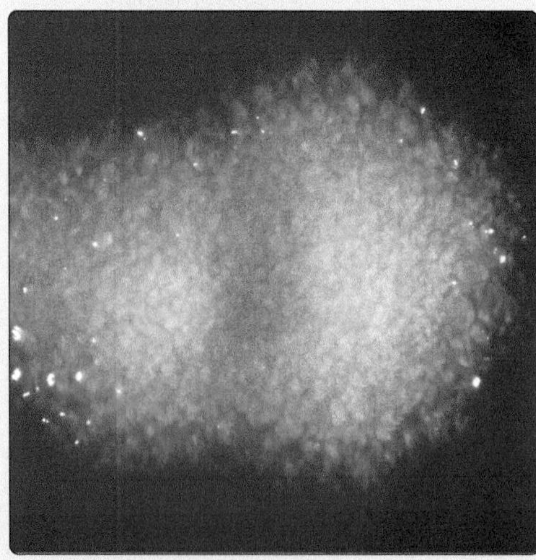

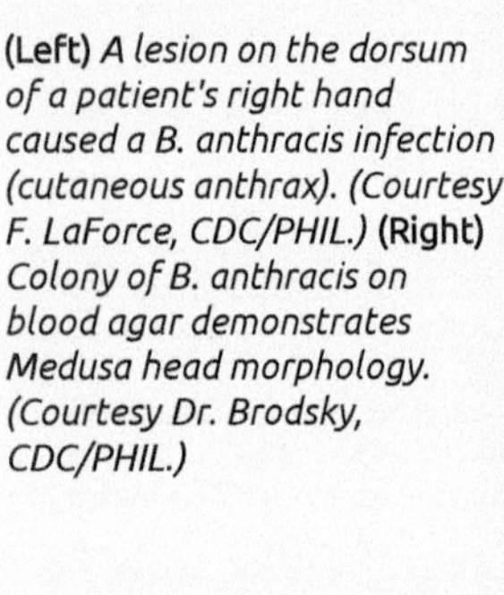

(Left) *A lesion on the dorsum of a patient's right hand caused a B. anthracis infection (cutaneous anthrax). (Courtesy F. LaForce, CDC/PHIL.)* **(Right)** *Colony of B. anthracis on blood agar demonstrates Medusa head morphology. (Courtesy Dr. Brodsky, CDC/PHIL.)*

TERMINOLOGY

Synonyms

- Charbon, Siberian plague, splenic fever, Cumberland disease, malignant edema, woolsorter's disease, la maladie de Bradford

Definitions

- *Bacillus anthracis* derived from Latin "bacillum" (walking stick due to rod-shaped organism) and Greek "anthrakos" (coal, referring to black eschars from cutaneous Anthrax)

ETIOLOGY/PATHOGENESIS

Infectious Agents

- Infection with *Bacillus* species, gram-positive bacilli widely present in environment; spores are extremely resistant and have been found in virtually every habitat
- Spore contamination can underlie both true outbreaks and pseudooutbreaks (i.e., contaminated blood culture bottles)
- *Bacillus anthracis*, *Bacillus cereus*, and *Bacillus thuringiensis* are most clinically relevant species, collectively as "*B. cereus* group"
- *B. anthracis* infection occurs naturally by contact with infected animals and animal products (e.g., hides) as well as through laboratory accidents, biological warfare, and contaminated heroin; contains 2 large plasmids (pXO1 and pXO2) that encode virulence factors (lethal toxin, edema toxin) and polyglutamate capsule
- *B. cereus* associated with food-borne illness and transmitted by contaminated laundry and disinfectant wipes can occur within hospital environment; produces plasmid-encoded emetic toxin and enterotoxin; virulent strains may carry plasmids similar to *B. anthracis*
- *B. thuringiensis* used as biopesticides, which can result in occupational exposure; produces insecticidal toxins (Cry and Cyt) that form parasporal crystals
- Species less commonly associated with clinical syndrome include *Bacillus circulans*, *Bacillus licheniformis*, *Bacillus megaterium*, *Bacillus pumilus*, *Bacillus sphaericus*, and *Bacillus subtilis*; may represent blood culture contaminants

CLINICAL ISSUES

Presentation

- *B. anthracis* (anthrax) has 3 clinical types: Cutaneous (95%), pulmonary (5%), and gastrointestinal (1%)
  - Cutaneous anthrax is most common cause of naturally acquired anthrax
    - Characteristic lesion is ulceration with blackened eschar, unaccompanied by fever, pus, or pain
    - Eschars may be surrounded by substantial edema
  - Pulmonary anthrax occurs with breathing of spores
    - Active infection occurs in lymph nodes
    - Presents with fever, dyspnea, and cyanosis
    - Can rapidly progress to circulatory collapse and death
  - Gastrointestinal anthrax can develop after eating raw or undercooked meat of infected animals
    - Ulcerations can be confined to oral cavity or develop throughout gastrointestinal tract
    - Can present with significant edema of throat
- *B. cereus* is opportunistic pathogen and causative agent of food-borne illness and occasional nosocomial outbreaks
  - Foodborne illness can be associated with wide variety of foods and be of emetic (commonly associated with rice) and diarrheal types
  - Illness in immunocompromised individuals can be severe and includes bacteremia/sepsis, pneumoniae, abscess, osteomyelitis, meningitis, ocular infections, and brain hemorrhage; endophthalmitis from ocular penetrating injury
- *B. thuringiensis* is predominantly insect pathogen and uncommon cause of human gastroenteritis and wound and burn infections
- *B. circulans*, *B. licheniformis*, *B. megaterium*, *B. pumilus*, *B. sphaericus*, and *B. subtilis* may have variety of clinical presentations ranging from meningitis to bacteremia to food poisoning

Laboratory Tests

- PCR (fresh and FFPE samples)
  - Laboratory Response Network (LRN) real-time assay for *B. anthracis* (detects plasmid and chromosomal components)
  - 16S rRNA sequencing has limited ability to differentiate members of *B. cereus* group; whole-genome sequencing may be required
  - PCR assays are available for detection of *B. cereus* enterotoxin and emetic toxin, but their reliability has not been established
- Serology: Antibodies to anthrax toxin proteins, protective antigen (PA) lethal factor (LF), and edema factor (EF) are commercially available and have been used for ELISA testing of patient serum and direct fluorescent-antibody (DFA) assays

Treatment

- *B. anthracis*: Usually susceptible to penicillin (other useful drugs include tetracyclines, fluoroquinolones, and chloramphenicol)
- *B. cereus* and *B. thuringiensis*
  - Produce β-lactamases, resistant to all β-lactams except carbapenems
  - Options include vancomycin, clindamycin, fluoroquinolones, aminoglycosides, and carbapenems
  - Susceptibilities should be performed on *Bacillus* spp. (nonanthracis) isolated from sterile body sites or in serious infection; not performed when thought to be contaminant

Prognosis

- *B. anthracis* mortality
  - Cutaneous: 10-20% with no treatment, 1% with treatment
  - Inhalation: 65-89% with treatment
- *B. cereus* mortality varies widely with immunocompetency of patient

MICROBIOLOGY

Characteristics

- **Phylum**: Firmicutes; **class**: Bacilli; **order**: Bacillales; **family**: *Bacillaceae*; **genus**: *Bacillus*
- Gram-positive (though some may appear gram variable or even gram negative), large rod-shaped organism (~ 1.2 μm wide), frequently present in chains

- Aerobic (or facultatively anaerobic) growth
- Forms endospores (usually elliptical and subterminal, not associated with swollen sporangium in *B. anthracis*, *B. cereus*, or *B. thuringiensis*); highlighted by spore stains (e.g., malachite green)
- Capsule (not produced by majority of *B. cereus* and *B. thuringiensis* isolates) identified by India ink exclusion, McFadyean reaction (polychrome methylene blue), and DFA stains with antibodies specific for polyglutamate capsule
- *B. thuringiensis* also characteristically produces parasporal crystals
- Catalase positive, often motile (except *B. anthracis* and *B. mycoides*); any nonmotile, nonhemolytic, catalase-positive, gram-positive rods presumed *B. anthracis* until ruled out

Culture

- Culture identification is gold standard for diagnosis
- *Bacillus* spp. grow on routine blood and chocolate agar
- Spores can be generated by heat treatment
- *B. anthracis*
  - Forms medium, gray, flat, irregular (Medusa head), nonhemolytic colonies on blood agar that are susceptible to gamma phage
  - May be incorrectly or not identified by matrix-assisted laser desorption/ionization (MALDI)
  - Categorized as tier 1 select agent: Once identified, must be transferred to laboratory registered by CDC or Animal and Plant Health Inspection Service (APHIS); remaining material must be destroyed within 7 days
  - PLET agar can be used for selective media (not routinely available in diagnostic laboratories)
- *B. cereus* and *B. thuringiensis*
  - Form variety of colony morphologies on blood agar, generally motile
  - Often demonstrate some β-hemolysis (differentiates from *B. anthracis*)
  - MALDI may identify to species level if validated (varies by institution)

MACROSCOPIC

Gross Features

- Diffuse hemorrhagic meninges is pathognomic of anthrax
- Disseminated *B. cereus* shows small to large focal hemorrhages
- Pleural effusions (most characteristic feature of anthrax) and pulmonary edema
- Lymphatogenous spread from lungs results in hemorrhagic mediastinitis in anthrax ("shotgun thorax")
- Endophthalmitis (*B. cereus*)

MICROSCOPIC

Histologic Features

- Cutaneous anthrax: Epidermal necrosis, hemorrhage, acantholysis, and ulceration with polymorphonuclear infiltrates; dermis shows edema, coagulation necrosis, hemorrhage, and vasculitis with marked perivascular inflammatory infiltrate
- Pulmonary anthrax has hyaline membrane formation more so than true pneumonia with limited neutrophilic reaction
- Gastrointestinal anthrax has 2 main forms: Hemorrhagic ulcers confined to oropharyngeal region and concentrated in terminal ileum and cecum with mesenteric hemorrhagic lymphadenitis and peritonitis
- *B. cereus* infection shows liver abscesses, pancolitis, typhlitis
- Central nervous system anthrax with low- and high-pressure hemorrhages along with vasculitis composed of fibrinoid necrosis and neutrophils in meninges and parenchyma
- Central nervous system *B. cereus* infection in immunosuppressed patients (usually in setting of malignancy) with meningitis, meningoencephalitis, subarachnoid hemorrhage, and brain abscesses

ANCILLARY TESTS

Special Stains

- Gram stain highlights bacilli (may appear gram negative after antibiotic treatment)
- Silver stains (Warthin-Starry, Steiner), GMS, and PAS with diastase may better highlight organisms in tissue

Immunohistochemistry

- Antibodies for *B. anthracis* cell wall antigen and capsule highlight bacilli, bacillary fragments, and granular antigen staining

DIFFERENTIAL DIAGNOSIS

Skin Lesions Mimicking Cutaneous Anthrax

- Brown recluse spider bite, ulceroglandular tularemia, plague, ecthyma gangrenosum, spotted fever rickettsial infection, scrub typhus (differentiated by culture and IHC)

Gastrointestinal Infections

- *Clostridioides difficile* infection, inflammatory bowel disease, ischemia

Respiratory Infections

- Pneumonia, transfusion-associated acute lung injury

SELECTED REFERENCES

1. Lotte R et al: Bacillus cereus invasive infections in preterm neonates: an up-to-date review of the literature. Clin Microbiol Rev. 35(2):e0008821, 2022
2. Dietrich R et al: The food poisoning toxins of Bacillus cereus. Toxins (Basel). 13(2), 2021
3. Ehling-Schulz M et al: The Bacillus cereus group: Bacillus species with pathogenic potential. Microbiol Spectr. 7(3), 2019
4. Zasada AA: Injectional anthrax in human: a new face of the old disease. Adv Clin Exp Med. 27(4):553-8, 2018
5. Rudrik JT et al: Safety and accuracy of matrix-assisted laser desorption ionization-time of flight mass spectrometry for identification of highly pathogenic organisms. J Clin Microbiol. 55(12):3513-29, 2017
6. Vodopivec I et al: A cluster of cns infections due to B. cereus in the setting of acute myeloid leukemia: neuropathology in 5 patients. J Neuropathol Exp Neurol. 74(10):1000-11, 2015
7. Kolstø AB et al: What sets Bacillus anthracis apart from other Bacillus species? Annu Rev Microbiol. 63:451-76, 2009
8. Guarner J et al: Histopathology and immunohistochemistry in the diagnosis of bioterrorism agents. J Histochem Cytochem. 54(1):3-11, 2006
9. Guarner J et al: Pathology and pathogenesis of bioterrorism-related inhalational anthrax. Am J Pathol. 163(2):701-9, 2003
10. Shieh WJ et al: The critical role of pathology in the investigation of bioterrorism-related cutaneous anthrax. Am J Pathol. 163(5):1901-10, 2003

***Bacillus cereus* Cerebral Hemorrhages**

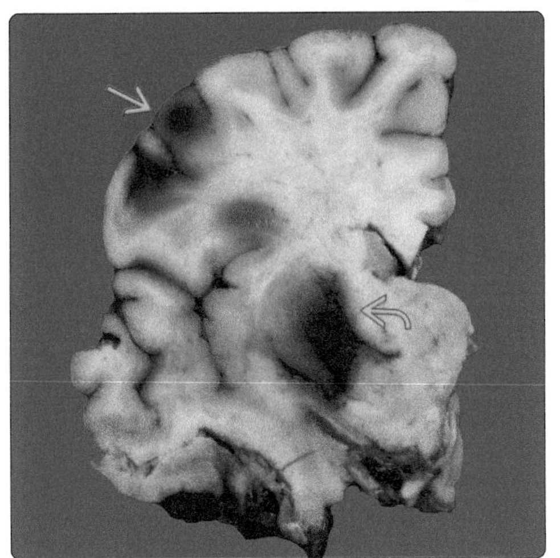

***Bacillus cereus* Cerebral Hemorrhage**

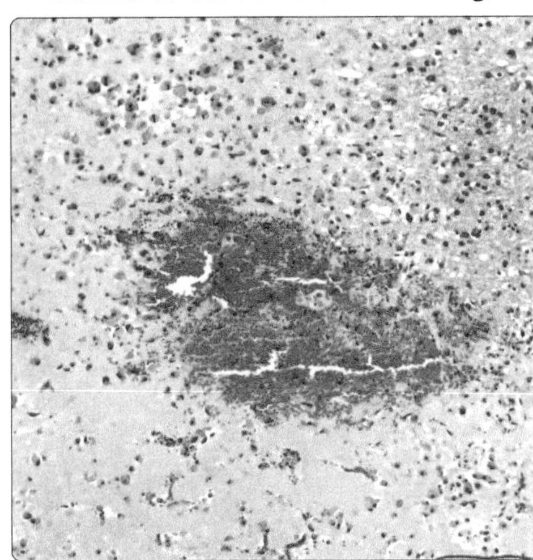

(Left) *Large parenchymal hemorrhages involving the cerebral cortex and subcortical white matter ➙, as well as the basal ganglia ➙, were identified in this patient with acute myeloid leukemia and disseminated Bacillus cereus infection.* **(Right)** *A small cerebral hemorrhage is seen within the brain of a patient with disseminated B. cereus infection.*

***Bacillus cereus* Fibrin Thrombi**

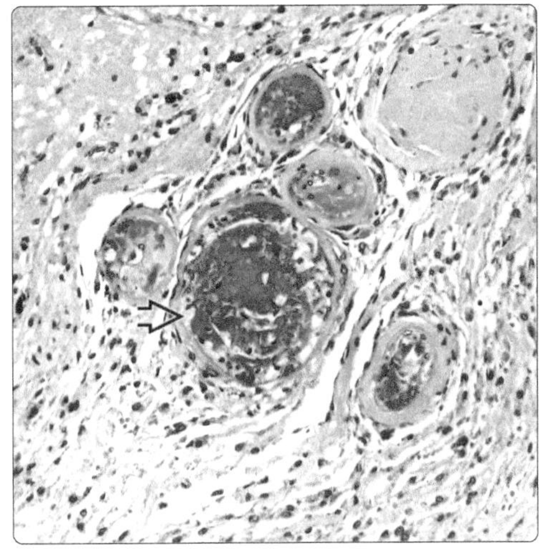

***Bacillus cereus* Cerebral Abscess**

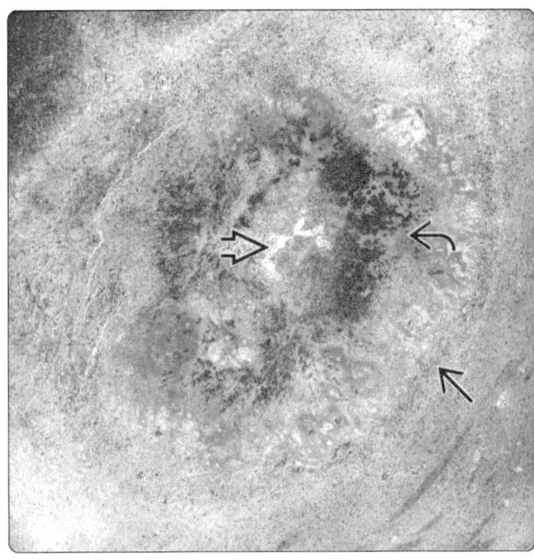

(Left) *Meningeal vessels from a case of disseminated B. cereus infection show fibrin thrombi ➙.* **(Right)** *A large cerebral abscess is present in this brain tissue from a patient with disseminated B. cereus infection. Note the central necrosis ➙, rim of inflammation ➙, and scattered fibrin ➙, consistent with hematogenous spread.*

***Bacillus cereus* Gram Stain**

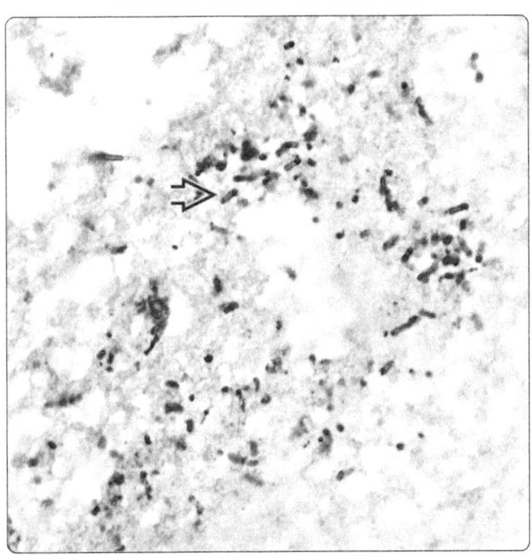

***Bacillus cereus* GMS Stain**

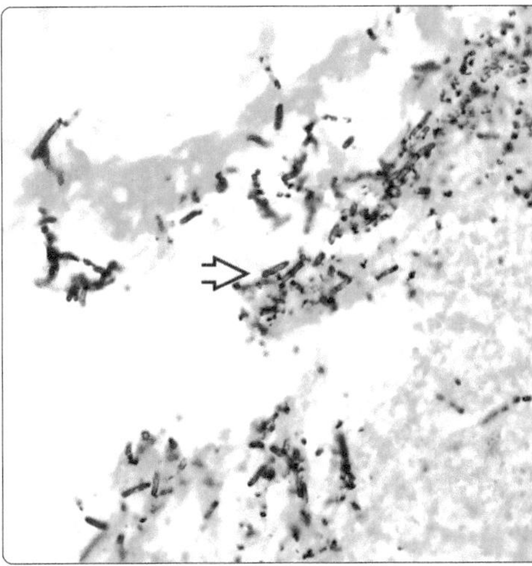

(Left) *A brain abscess from a patient with acute myelogenous leukemia and disseminated B. cereus infection is shown with large rods ➙ seen on Gram staining. Note that the normally gram-positive bacteria are only partially picking up the tissue on Gram stain.* **(Right)** *A brain abscess from a patient with acute myelogenous leukemia and disseminated B. cereus infection is shown with large rods ➙ on methenamine silver staining.*

Clostridioides and Other Gram-Positive Anaerobes

KEY FACTS

ETIOLOGY/PATHOGENESIS

- Infection with clostridia, resilient sporulating bacteria found in wide variety of natural habitats (e.g., soil, sewage, water), which produce number of protein toxins

CLINICAL ISSUES

- Range of infections, including soft tissue infections (gas gangrene) (*Clostridium perfringens* and *Clostridium septicum*) and antibiotic-associated pseudomembranous colitis (*Clostridioides difficile*)
- *Clostridium difficile* commonly diagnosed by 2-step algorithm (i.e., immunoassay followed by PCR)

MICROBIOLOGY

- Most species are obligate anaerobes; variety of selective and differential agars are available
- RapID ANA assay strips and MALDI for identification

MICROSCOPIC

- Gram stain shows large, club-shaped, gram-positive rods
- *C. difficile* colitis: Mild disease with inflamed colonic mucosa and luminal mucus, severe disease with characteristic pseudomembranes
- *C. perfringens* (type C): Enteritis necroticans lesions in proximal jejunum are characterized by mucosal ulceration, submucosal edema, mixed inflammatory infiltrate, and necrosis
- Clostridial myonecrosis (*C. perfringens, C. septicum, Clostridium histolyticum, C. novyi*): Necrosis of skin, soft tissue, and muscle

TOP DIFFERENTIAL DIAGNOSES

- Colitis: Inflammatory bowel disease (IBD), diverticulitis, other infectious colitis; differentiated by positive stool toxin assay for *C. difficile*
- Necrotizing enterocolitis: Bowel ischemia, Crohn disease; no associated bacteria present
- Necrotizing Fasciitis: Differentiated by lack of gas in tissue, gram-positive cocci or other organisms present on tissue Gram stain

***Clostridium* spp. Gram Stain**

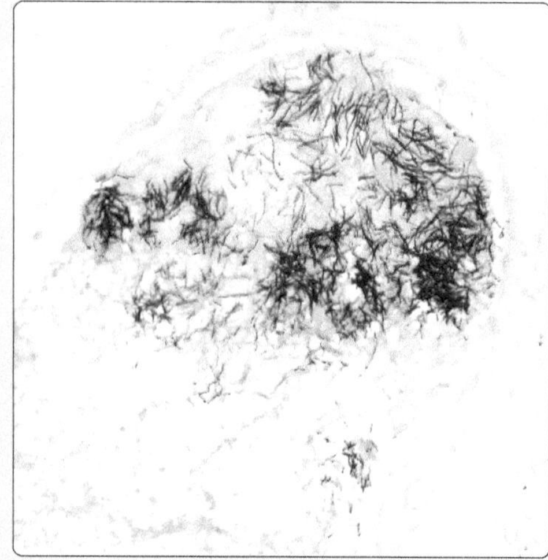

Clostridial Myonecrosis

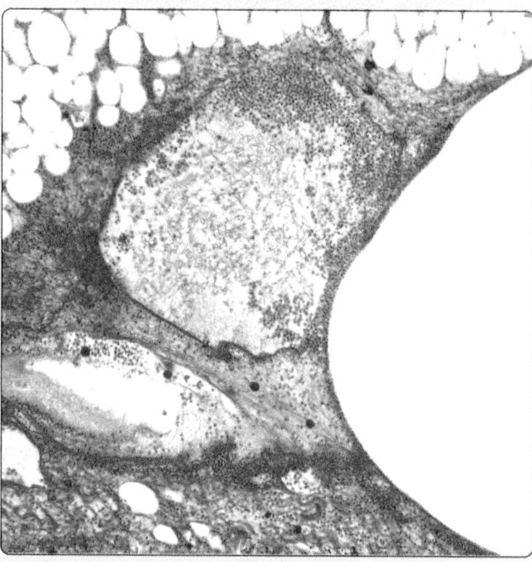

(Left) *Gram stain from an autopsy of a patient who died of myonecrosis shows dense growth of Clostridium septicum gram-positive rods.* **(Right)** *Clostridial myonecrosis is characterized by abundant coagulative necrosis of the soft tissues, often tracking along fascial planes. Inflammation may be sparse in neutropenia.*

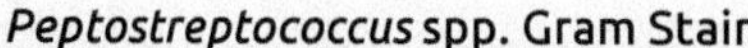

***Peptostreptococcus* spp. Gram Stain**

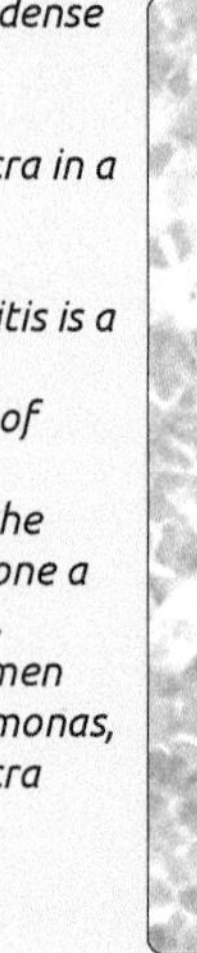

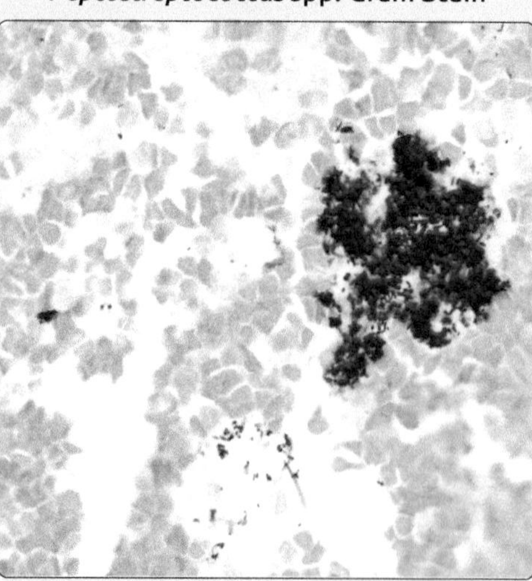

***Peptostreptococcus* spp. Osteomyelitis**

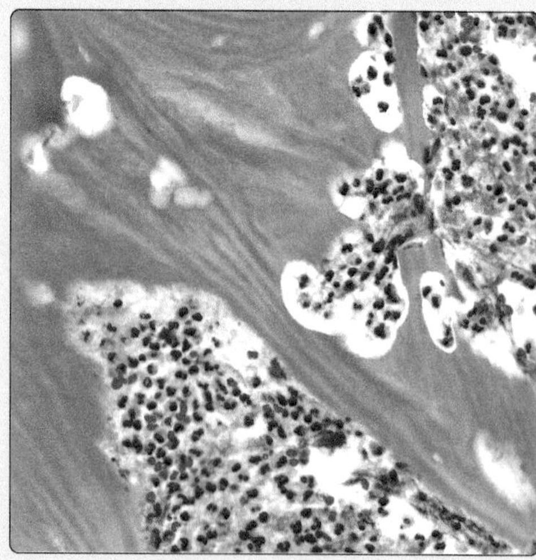

(Left) *Gram stain shows dense colonies of Parvimonas (formerly Micromonas, Peptostreptococcus) micra in a patient who developed anaerobic osteomyelitis.* **(Right)** *Acute osteomyelitis is a diagnosis that is strictly defined by the presence of neutrophils in close association with pits in the bone, often giving the bone a moth-eaten appearance. Cultures from this specimen grew P. (formerly Micromonas, Peptostreptococcus) micra and Fusobacterium nucleatum.*

TERMINOLOGY

Definitions

- Greek: "Kloster" (spindle)

ETIOLOGY/PATHOGENESIS

Infectious Agents

- Infection with clostridia, resilient sporulating bacteria found in wide variety of natural habitats (e.g., soil, sewage, water), which produce number of protein toxins
- *Clostridioides difficile* (formerly *Clostridium difficile*) produces TcdA (enterotoxin) and TcdB (cytotoxin)
- *Clostridium botulinum* produces BoNT, one of most potent toxins described for any organism
- *Clostridium perfringens* produces many different toxins, including alpha and theta toxins implicated in gas gangrene
- *Clostridium septicum* produces 4 major toxins (alpha, beta, gamma, delta) with hemolytic, DNAse, and hyaluronidase activities
- *Clostridium sordellii* produces up to 7 toxins
- *Clostridium tetani* produces tetanospasmin (TeNT), neurotoxin produced at site of infection
- *Clostridium tertium* is aerotolerant clostridial species that does not produce toxins (often mistaken for *Bacillus* or *Lactobacillus* spp.)
- Gram-positive anaerobic cocci include *Finegoldia* (formerly *Peptostreptococcus*) *magna*, *Parvimonas* (formerly *Micromonas*, *Peptostreptococcus*) *micra*, *Peptoniphilus asaccharolyticus*, *Peptostreptococcus anaerobius*
- Gram-positive nonsporulating bacilli include *Propionibacterium acnes*, *Lactobacillus* spp., *Bifidobacterium* spp.

CLINICAL ISSUES

Epidemiology

- *C. difficile*: Part of intestinal flora of 3-5% of healthy adults; disease associated with age, hospital or long-term care facility, bowel surgery, antibiotic use, inflammatory bowel disease (IBD), use of proton pump inhibitors
- *C. botulinum*: Infant botulism associated with soil, dust, and honey; ingestion of preformed toxin in food or production of toxin by organisms in wound
- *C. perfringens*: Skin and soft tissue infections associated with crush-type injury, artery laceration, soil-contaminated open long-bone fractures, penetrating injuries involving bowel leakage into abdominal cavity; enteric infections associated with improperly cooked meat or meat products (due to survival of spores)
- *C. septicum*: Associated with occult colon cancer, diverticulitis, bowel surgery, hematologic malignancy, diabetes, AIDS, radiation and chemotherapy, neutropenia
- *C. sordellii*: Associated with induced or spontaneous abortion as well as childbirth
- *C. tetani*: Associated with puncture wounds and injection drugs (also *Clostridium novyi*)
- Other gram-positive anaerobes are colonizers of oral/gut/genital sites; disease often associated with barrier breach of colonized sites (frequently polymicrobial)

Presentation

- Clostridial disease
  - *C. difficile*: Diarrhea (± blood and mucus), pseudomembranous colitis, toxic megacolon
  - *C. botulinum*: Food-borne disease (acute flaccid paralysis) can be preceded by general GI upset
  - *C. perfringens*: Soft tissue infections (gas gangrene, clostridial myonecrosis)
  - *C. perfringens* enteric infections: Mild diarrhea unless in context of compromised immune system (usually *C. perfringens* enterotoxin-producing type A)
    - Necrotizing enterocolitis is also associated with *C. perfringens* type A and predominately affects low-birth-weight infants
  - *C. septicum*: Spontaneous gas gangrene
  - *C. sordellii*: Gas gangrene of uterus
  - *C. tetani*: Paralysis and muscle spasms
- Other gram-positive anaerobes
  - Infections are generally proximal to colonization sites (pelvis, abdomen, etc.) and often mixed as reflection of breach of colonization site
  - *Peptostreptococcus* spp.: Implicated in wide variety of infections, particularly obstetric, postsurgical, intraoral
  - *Finegoldia* spp.: Associated with skin, soft tissue, and joint infections, among others (sometimes in pure culture)
  - *Parvimonas* spp.: Common member of oral flora, implicated in variety of oral infections (some pelvic as well)
  - *Peptoniphilus* spp.: Commonly associated with venous leg and decubitus ulcers (among others)
  - *P. acnes*: Common skin commensal (and occasional specimen contaminant), implicated in endocarditis (30% complicated by intracardiac abscess) and prosthetic joint infections (particularly shoulders) as well as acne lesions and others
  - *Lactobacillus* spp.: *L. rhamnosus*, *L. casei*, *L. fermentum*, *L. gasseri*, *L. plantarum*, *L. acidophilus*, and *L. ultunensis* most commonly associated with infection
    - *L. crispatus*, *L. gasseri*, *L. jensenii*, *L. iners* associated with vaginal health and prevention of vaginosis
    - Highly associated with caries and oral pathology
    - Some concern that probiotic strains may be pathogenic in vulnerable individuals

Laboratory Tests

- Direct examination (smear and Gram stain)
  - Gram stain of wound smear (showing gram-positive rods, ± spores) is critical for diagnosis of clostridial gas gangrene
  - Some species/strains may appear Gram variable
- *C. botulinum* toxin may be detected by mouse bioassay with neutralization or PCR (only done in select public health laboratories)
- *C. difficile* (commonly 2-step algorithm, i.e., immunoassay followed by PCR)
  - Immunoassays: Targets include glutamate dehydrogenase (GDH) (general target for all *C. difficile*) along with TcdA and TcdB (sensitivity 45-58%)
  - PCR: Highly sensitive (94-99%) for detection directly in stool (usually *tcdB*); concern that PCR-only testing strategies may not differentiate colonizing from disease-causing strains

- Cell culture/animal cytotoxicity assay: Traditional gold standard for detection of toxogenic *C. difficile* (sensitivity: 94-100%; specificity: 99%), though now infrequently done outside of reference labs/research studies

Treatment

- Surgical approaches
  - Radical amputation remains best treatment for gas gangrene or necrotizing fasciitis
  - Fulminant *C. difficile* colitis may result in toxic megacolon and possibly require colostomy
  - Anaerobic abscess may require surgical drainage
- Drugs
  - *C. difficile*
    - Fidaxomicin, oral or rectal vancomycin, metronidazole
    - Fecal transplant for recurrent disease
  - For anaerobic infections caused by other organisms, drug choice is guided by typical (community) resistance patterns of organism in question
  - Typical choices include β-lactam/inhibitor combinations, carbapenems, clindamycin, tigecycline, and metronidazole
  - Antitoxin for some clostridial disease

Prognosis

- Varies widely depending on organism and immune status of patient

IMAGING

CT Findings

- Tissue gas present in gas gangrene may be apparent by CT
- *C. difficile* colitis: Toxic megacolon characterized by colonic dilation, "thumbprinting," and pericolic fat stranding from mucosal edema; signs of pneumoperitoneum if dilatation has progressed to perforation

MICROBIOLOGY

Biochemical Characteristics and Morphology

- Clostridia are gram-positive (though may appear gram variable or even gram negative), rod-shaped organisms with round or pointed ends, arranged in short chains or pairs
- Endospores (if present) are often wider than cell, conferring swollen end or spindle-shaped appearance
- Most clostridia are catalase, oxidase, and superoxide dismutase negative

Culture and Identification

- Most species are obligate anaerobes, though some species can grow (though not sporulate) in low-oxygen environments; variety of selective and differential agars are available
- *C. difficile* culture is not routinely offered in clinical laboratories, though selective and differential media is available, including cycloserine, cefoxitin, fructose agar (CCFA), and CHROMID *C. difficile* (chromogenic agar for isolation directly from stool)
- RapID ANA assay strips (Remel) are commonly used in clinical labs to identify dozens of medically important anaerobes
- Matrix-assisted laser desorption/ionization (MALDI) is becoming standard for anaerobic identification

MICROSCOPIC

Histologic Features

- No histopathologic findings present in botulism or tetanus
- *C. difficile* colitis
  - Mild disease associated with mildly inflamed colonic mucosa with luminal mucus
  - Advanced disease with inflammatory erosion of lamina propria and development of fibrinopurulent cap that can extend to form pseudomembrane in severe disease
- *C. perfringens*
  - Enteritis necroticans lesions occur in proximal jejunum and are characterized by mucosal ulceration, submucosal edema, mixed inflammatory infiltrate, and necrosis
  - Involved vasculature may show congestion, thrombi, fibrinoid necrosis, and arteritis
  - Pneumatosis intestinalis and pseudomembranes may be observed
  - May cause massive hemolysis presenting as "ghost cells" on blood smear
- Clostridial myonecrosis (*C. perfringens, C. septicum, Clostridium histolyticum, C. novyi*)
  - Necrosis of skin, soft tissue, and muscle
  - Characteristic pauciinflammatory response

ANCILLARY TESTS

Special Stains

- Gram stain of clostridia shows large, club-shaped, gram-positive rods; may also be highlighted by silver stains and PAS

DIFFERENTIAL DIAGNOSIS

Colitis

- IBD, diverticulitis, other infectious colitis
- Differentiated by positive stool toxin assay for *C. difficile*

Necrotizing Enterocolitis

- Bowel ischemia, Crohn disease
- No associated bacteria present

Necrotizing Fasciitis

- Differentiated by lack of gas in tissue, gram-positive cocci or other organisms present on tissue Gram stain

SELECTED REFERENCES

1. Johnson S et al: Clinical practice guideline by the Infectious Diseases Society of America (IDSA) and Society for Healthcare Epidemiology of America (SHEA): 2021 focused update guidelines on management of Clostridioides difficile infection in adults. Clin Infect Dis. 73(5):e1029-44, 2021
2. Rao AK et al: Clinical guidelines for diagnosis and treatment of botulism, 2021. MMWR Recomm Rep. 70(2):1-30, 2021
3. Kraft CS et al: A laboratory medicine best practices systematic review and meta-analysis of nucleic acid amplification tests (NAATs) and algorithms including NAATs for the diagnosis of clostridioides (Clostridium) difficile in adults. Clin Microbiol Rev. 32(3), 2019
4. Lawson PA et al: Reclassification of Clostridium difficile as Clostridioides difficile (Hall and O'Toole 1935) Prévot 1938. Anaerobe. 40:95-9, 2016
5. Onderdonk AB et al: Gas gangrene and other Clostridium-associated diseases. In Mandell et al: Mandell, Douglas, and Bennett's Principles and Practice of Infectious Diseases. 8th Edition. Philadelphia: Elsevier/Saunders. 2768-72, 2015

Clostridioides spp. Colonic Necrosis

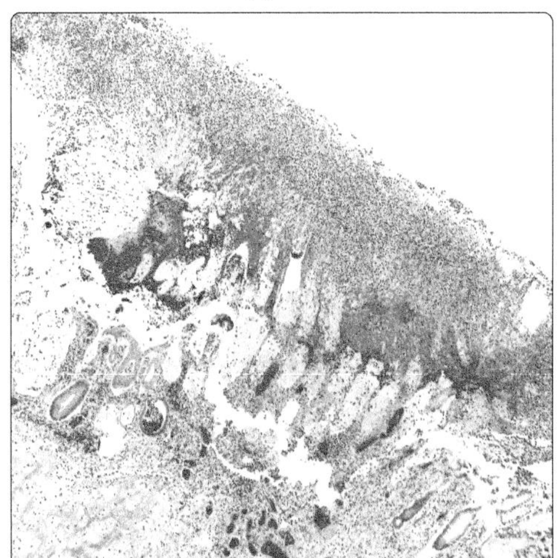

Clostridial Myonecrosis

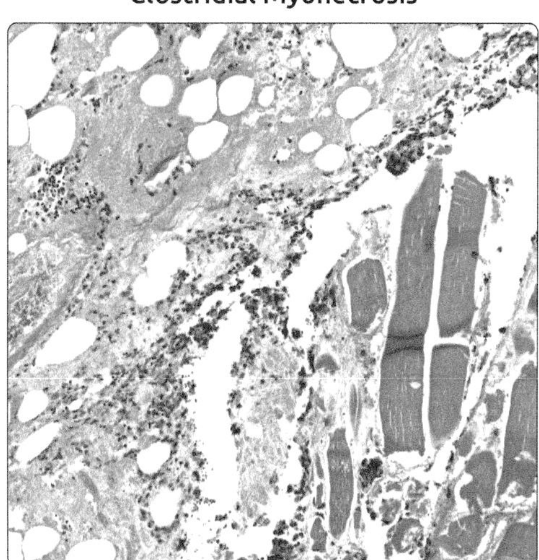

(Left) *H&E section demonstrates colon with necrosis of the epithelium and pseudomembrane formation in fulminant Clostridioides difficile colitis.* **(Right)** *This acute clostridial myonecrosis is characterized by abundant necrotic debris, including skeletal muscle fibers with coagulative necrosis and large spaces within the tissue, the histologic correlate of gas gangrene.*

Peptostreptococcus spp. Gram Stain

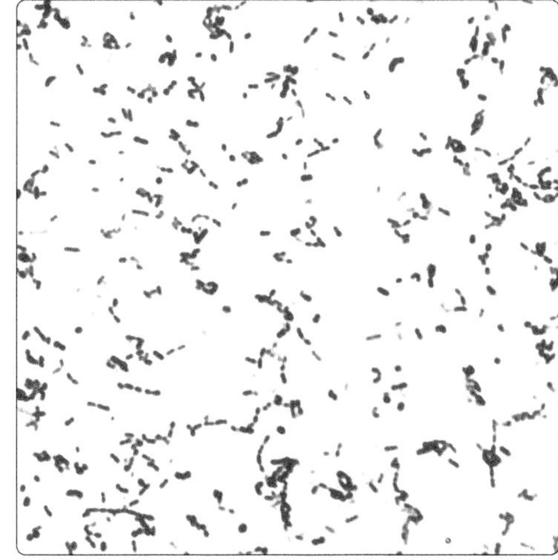

Propionibacterium acnes Gram Stain

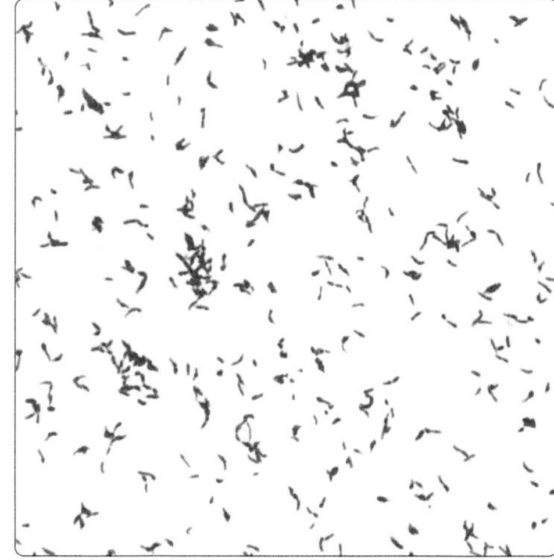

(Left) *Gram stain of Peptostreptococcus spp. demonstrates gram-positive cocci in pairs and chains (100x magnification).* **(Right)** *Gram stain of Cutibacterium acnes (formerly Propionibacterium acnes) from cultured isolate demonstrates pleomorphic gram-positive rods (100x magnification).*

Clostridium novyi Gram Stain

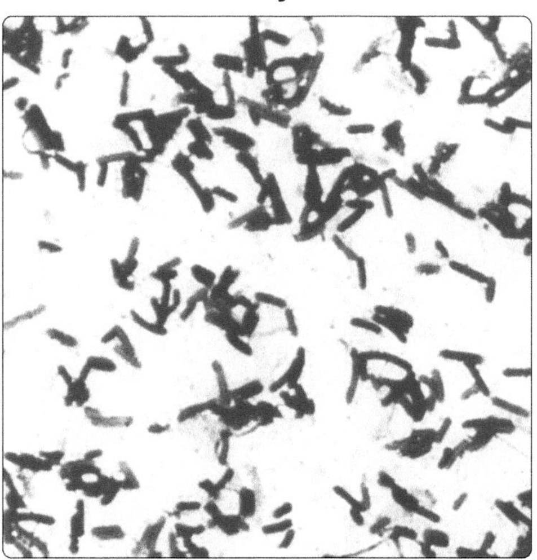

Clostridioides difficile Gram Stain

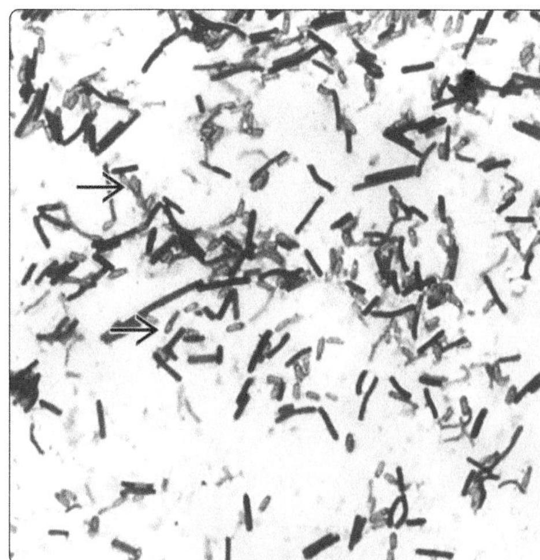

(Left) *Gram stain of Clostridium novyi demonstrates large, gram-positive rods.* **(Right)** *Gram stain of C. difficile demonstrates large, gram-positive rods with visible spores (100x magnification) ⮕.*

Corynebacterium Species Infections

KEY FACTS

ETIOLOGY/PATHOGENESIS

- Corynebacteria are practically split between *Corynebacterium diphtheriae* and all other species, collectively known as diphtheroids
- *C. diphtheriae*: Respiratory disease, cardiac involvement, muscle paralysis, and ulcerative skin lesions; caused by toxin encoded by *TOX* gene
- Diphtheroids: Pharyngitis, endocarditis, genitourinary tract infections, prostatitis, periodontal infections, and line-associated, device-related, and surgical site infections

MICROBIOLOGY

- Grow on 5% sheep blood agar; speciated by API CORYNE system (bioMérieux), MALDI-TOF MS, and 16S rRNA sequencing
- Since (nondiphtheria group) corynebacteria are prevalent as skin commensals, it is important to differentiate pathogens from contaminants

MICROSCOPIC

- Diphtheria (*C. diphtheriae*): Respiratory pseudomembrane on tonsils and pharynx; cutaneous ulcer with dense cap
- Erythrasma (*C. minutissimum*): Organisms often visible in stratum corneum; minimal host response
- Cystic granulomatous neutrophilic mastitis with diphtheroids demonstrable in cystic spaces
- Gram stain demonstrates gram-positive rods with slight curve and club shape

TOP DIFFERENTIAL DIAGNOSES

- Anthrax and noninfectious ulcers: Epidermal necrosis, hemorrhage, acantholysis, and ulceration with polymorphonuclear infiltrates; cutaneous diphtheria differentiated by identification of corynebacteria
- Yeast and fungal infections: Dermal inflammation with fungal elements in stratum corneum highlighted by PAS or GMS stains; erythrasma differentiated by identification of corynebacteria

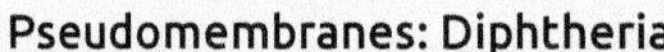

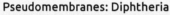

Pseudomembranes: Diphtheria

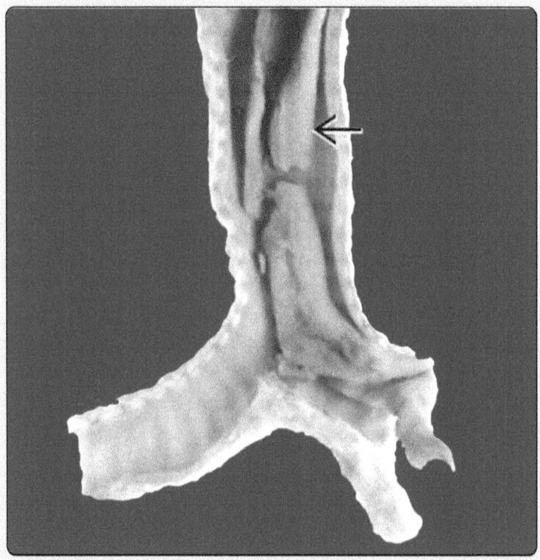

Diphtheria: Inflammatory Exudate

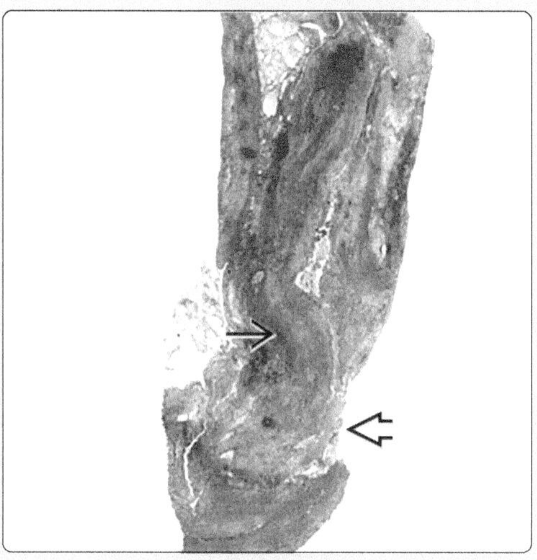

(Left) *Gross photograph of the trachea from a patient who died of diphtheria shows classic pseudomembranes →. (Courtesy R. Cooke, MD.)* **(Right)** *Histologic examination of the pseudomembranes associated with diphtheria reveals sheets of sloughed, largely necrotic epithelium ⇨ admixed with fibrin and an inflammatory exudate →. (Courtesy R. Cooke, MD.)*

Erythrasma

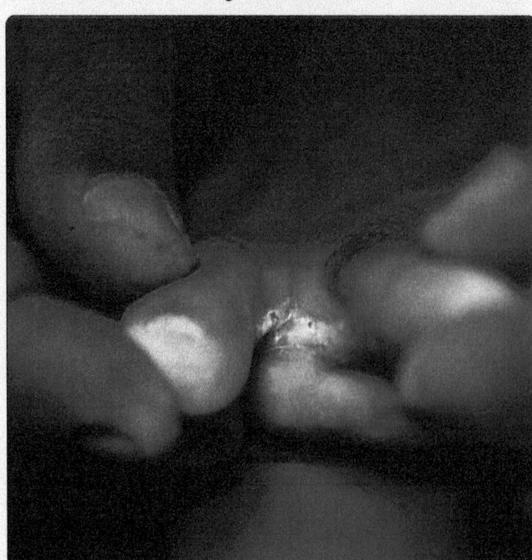

***Corynebacterium ulcerans*: Gram Stain**

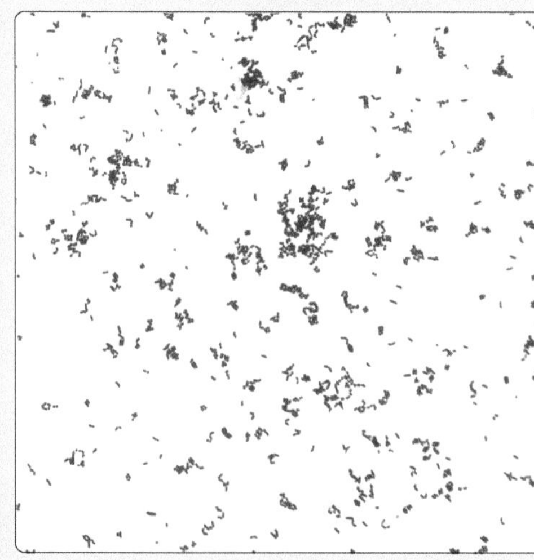

(Left) *Erythrasma is demonstrated by fluorescence under Wood lamp illumination. (Courtesy L. Georg, PhD, CDC/PHIL.)* **(Right)** *Gram stain shows Corynebacterium ulcerans, which was cultured from a foot ulcer, demonstrating pleomorphic, gram-positive rods arranged like match sticks (10x).*

TERMINOLOGY

Definitions

- Greek: "Korune" (club, club-shaped morphology)
- Greek: "Diphthera" (pair of leather scrolls, for pseudomembrane appearance)

ETIOLOGY/PATHOGENESIS

Infectious Agents

- Infection with corynebacteria, gram-positive bacilli split into *Corynebacterium diphtheriae* group and diphtheroids (all other species), via respiratory droplets or contact with skin lesions
- *C. diphtheriae*
  - 3 subtypes: *C. d. gravis*, *C. d. intermedius*, and *C. d. mitis*, in decreasing order of pathogenicity
  - Manifestations of disease are caused by toxin, encoded by *TOX* gene, encoded by lysogenic phage
  - Widespread toxin-mediated necrosis leads to characteristic thick, adherent, leathery "membrane" of diphtheria, composed of bacteria, necrotic epithelium, fibrin, and inflammatory cells
  - Other systemic aspects of disease (e.g., myocarditis) result from dissemination of toxin rather than hematogenous spread of bacteria
  - Strains of *C. diphtheriae* that do not produce toxin (but may encode it) are increasingly associated with disease; mechanisms of their pathogenicity are poorly understood
  - *C. ulcerans* and *C. pseudotuberculosis* are part of *C. diphtheriae* group (zoonotic, possibly toxigenic)
- Diphtheroids: Many species colonize skin; clinically relevant species include *C. jeikeium*, *C. glucuronolyticum*, *C. minutissimum*, *C. pseudodiphtheriticum*, *C. striatum*, and *C. urealyticum*

CLINICAL ISSUES

Epidemiology

- *C. diphtheriae* is extremely uncommon in USA
  - Increasing use of matrix-assisted laser desorption/ionization (MALDI) in diagnostic laboratories may identify *C. diphtheria* and other potentially toxigenic species, which would not have been speciated/identified using traditional methods and algorithms
  - Risk factors include extremes of age, nonvaccinated status, migrant from endemic area (e.g., India)
  - Route of infection is by airborne respiratory droplets or contact with respiratory excretions or skin lesions (humans are sole reservoir)
- Diphtheroids: Risk factors include extremes of age, compromised immune system, residence in hospital; growing recognition as agents of device-associated infection

Presentation

- *C. diphtheriae* (causative agent of diphtheria)
  - Respiratory disease often occurs 2-4 days after exposure (cough, hoarseness, sore throat, dyspnea, odynophagia); tonsils may be enlarged and associated with grayish-white membranes
  - Cardiac involvement (due to toxin) manifests 1-2 weeks after infection with arrhythmias and symptoms of congestive heart failure
  - Neurologic involvement can occur at any time and typically begins with bulbar symptoms; may progress to proximal then distal muscle paralysis
  - Cutaneous infections present as vesicles that progress to nonhealing ulcers (mm to cm in size)
- Diphtheroids
  - Community-acquired infections include pharyngitis, native valve endocarditis, genitourinary tract infections, acute and chronic prostatitis, mastitis, and periodontal infections
  - Nosocomial infections include line-associated infections, native and prosthetic valve endocarditis, device-related infections, and surgical site infections
  - *C. striatum*: Emerging multidrug-resistant organism implicated in pneumonia, sepsis, etc.; usually in immunocompromised patients
  - *C. minutissimum*: Associated with erythrasma and, rarely, septicemia and endocarditis in vulnerable patients
  - *C. amycolatum*: Historically confused with several other species; rarely associated with wide variety of infections in vulnerable patients
  - *C. glucuronolyticum*: Normal genitourinary flora; associated with chronic prostatitis
  - *C. pseudodiphtheriticum*: Normal upper respiratory flora; associated with endocarditis, respiratory infections, and others
  - *C. jeikeium*: Associated with nosocomial infections (can be severe), such as septicemia, endocarditis, CSF shunt infections, meningitis, skin and soft tissue infections, prosthetic joint infections, etc.
  - *C. urealyticum*: Chronic and recurrent urinary tract infections in vulnerable populations
  - *C. kroppenstedtii*: Granulomatous mastitis associated with recurrent abscesses

Laboratory Tests

- Direct examination of swabs or blood smear
  - Swabs should be taken from involved area of nasopharynx and, if present, underneath membranes
  - Neisser or Loeffler methylene blue staining demonstrates metachromatic granules (limited sensitivity)
- Toxin detection
  - Toxin genes now commonly detected by PCR at public health and reference laboratories
  - Elek test: Traditional toxin assay that uses strips embedded with antitoxin, detects *TOX* gene-producing strains on agar plates

Treatment

- *C. diphtheriae*
  - Vaccine often included with DTaP; recommendations vary by age
  - Antitoxin antibodies levels of 0.1 to 0.01 IU are considered protective; boosters are recommended every 10 years
  - Postexposure: Booster and antibiotics (penicillin and erythromycin are preferred drugs)

- Treatment of infections with antibiotics as above, antisera [diphtheria antitoxin (DAT) produced in horses], and vaccine when convalescent (formalin-inactivated toxin)
- Diphtheroids: Preferred antibiotics differ by species; some are highly resistant to multiple classes

Prognosis

- *C. diphtheriae*: Mortality ranges from 3.5-12.0%; highest at extremes of age and in unvaccinated individuals

MICROBIOLOGY

Morphologic and Biochemical Characteristics

- Cells are aerobic, nonspore forming, catalase positive, and nonmotile
- With 50 medically relevant species, there is great deal of diversity in biochemical profile of corynebacteria
- Cell wall is distinct, containing mesodiaminopimelic acid and short-chain mycolic acids 22-36 carbons in length in many, but not all, species
- Gram stain demonstrates gram-positive rods with slight curve and club shape
- Arrangement is in "V"s or palisades with what has been termed pile of matchsticks appearance

Culture

- Grow on 5% sheep blood agar
- Selective media: Cysteine-tellurite blood agar (CTBA) and Tinsdale media (differentiates diphtheria group from diphtheroids by formation of brown-black halos from tellurite reduction)

Microbiological Identification

- API CORYNE system (bioMérieux)
- MALDI (may not be present in standard libraries)
- Gas chromatography of medium-length fatty acids with Sherlock system (MIDI) can assist with genus and possible species-level identifications
- Sequencing of 16S rRNA gene can differentiate most species

Interpretation Guidelines

- Since (nondiphtheria group) corynebacteria are prevalent as skin commensals, it is important to differentiate pathogens from contaminants
- Guidelines have been proposed to indicate true disease association: Isolation from normally sterile sites (if blood, from > 1 bottle of multiple bottles), predominant organism from adequately collected clinical material, or from urine if > 10^4/mL and only organism isolated or predominant organism and > 10^5/mL
- Clinical significance is strengthened by isolate recovered from > 1 specimen, organisms seen in direct Gram stains of tissue with inflammatory response, and no other pathogenic organisms observed in lesion

MACROSCOPIC

General Features

- Diphtheria
  - Pharynx, larynx, trachea, and main bronchi may be covered by grayish pseudomembranes
  - In severe cases, lungs are hemorrhagic and moderately solid
  - With cardiac involvement, heart appears dilated and pale
- Diphtheroids: Erythrasma appears as brownish discoloration in axilla, groin, and inframammary regions

MICROSCOPIC

Histologic Features

- *C. diphtheriae*
  - Respiratory: Forms characteristic pseudomembrane on tonsils and pharynx, which can descend further down respiratory tree; satellite infections may be found in lower airway or upper GI tract; *C. diphtheriae* proliferates on surface of pseudomembrane
  - Cutaneous lesions have diverse appearances due to superinfection of preexisting lesions; primary infection begins as vesicle and progresses to ulcer with punched-out appearance and dense "cap" or membrane; lesions commonly occur on lower legs, feet, or hands
- Diphtheroids
  - Erythrasma (*C. minutissimum*): Organisms often visible in stratum corneum; minimal host response
  - Pitted keratolysis (multiple species): Infection of stratum corneum of soles of feet, which develop small pits
  - Cystic granulomatous neutrophilic mastitis with diphtheroids demonstrable in cystic spaces

ANCILLARY TESTS

Special Stains

- Bacilli are highlighted (positive) on Gram stains

DIFFERENTIAL DIAGNOSIS

Anthrax and Noninfectious Ulcers

- Epidermal necrosis, hemorrhage, acantholysis, and ulceration with polymorphonuclear infiltrates; cutaneous diphtheria differentiated by identification of corynebacteria

Yeast and Fungal Infections

- Dermal inflammation with fungal elements in stratum corneum highlighted by PAS or GMS stains; erythrasma differentiated by identification of corynebacteria

Darier Disease

- Greasy hyperkeratotic papules in seborrheic regions with acantholysis and dyskeratosis; not associated with bacteria

SELECTED REFERENCES

1. Tariq H et al: Detection of Corynebacterium kroppenstedtii in granulomatous lobular mastitis using real-time polymerase chain reaction and sanger sequencing on formalin-fixed, paraffin-embedded tissues. Arch Pathol Lab Med. 146(6):749-54, 2022
2. Williams MM et al: Detection and characterization of diphtheria toxin gene-bearing Corynebacterium species through a new real-time PCR assay. J Clin Microbiol. 58(10), 2020
3. Wu JM et al: Cystic neutrophilic granulomatous mastitis: an update. J Clin Pathol. 73(8):445-53, 2020
4. Sharma NC et al: Diphtheria. Nat Rev Dis Primers. 5(1):81, 2019
5. Oliveira A et al: Insight of genus Corynebacterium: ascertaining the role of pathogenic and non-pathogenic species. Front Microbiol. 8:1937, 2017
6. Hacker E et al: Corynebacterium ulcerans, an emerging human pathogen. Future Microbiol. 11:1191-208, 2016

Pseudomembranes: Diphtheria

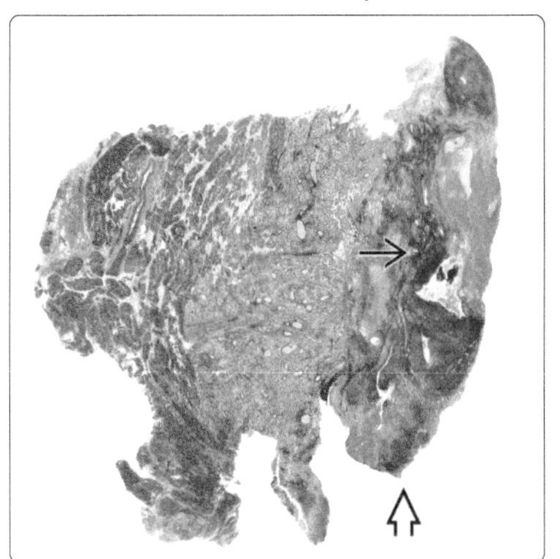

Pseudomembranes and Inflammation

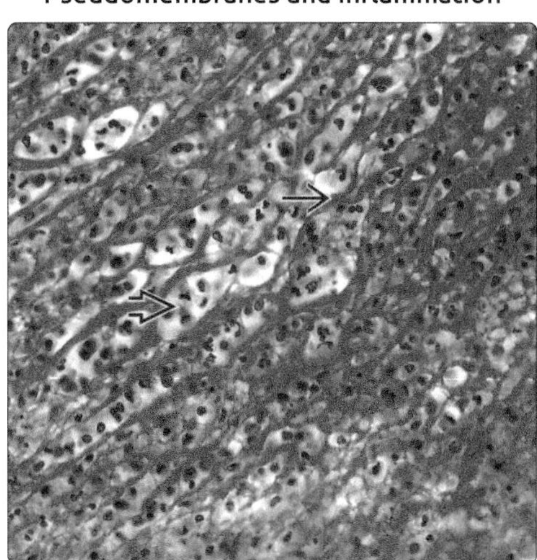

(Left) *Low magnification of the pseudomembranes associated with diphtheria reveals sheets of sloughed, largely necrotic epithelium* ⇨ *admixed with fibrin and an inflammatory exudate* →*. (Courtesy R. Cooke, MD.)* **(Right)** *High-power image of pseudomembranes from a patient with diphtheria reveals sheets of sloughed epithelium admixed with acute inflammation* ⇨ *and entrapped in fibrin* →*.*

Coagulative Necrosis: Diphtheria

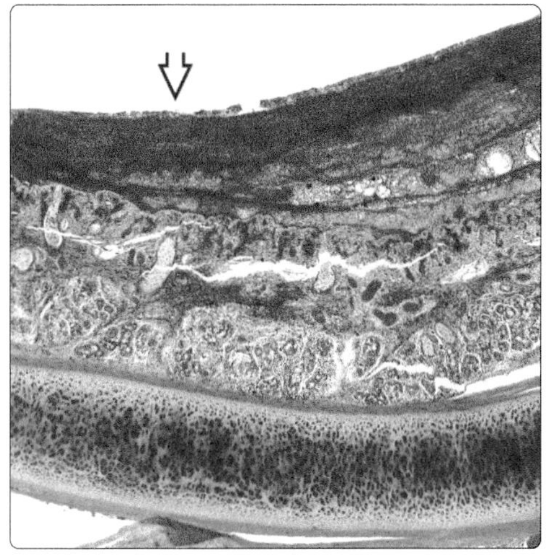

Diphtheria: Spleen

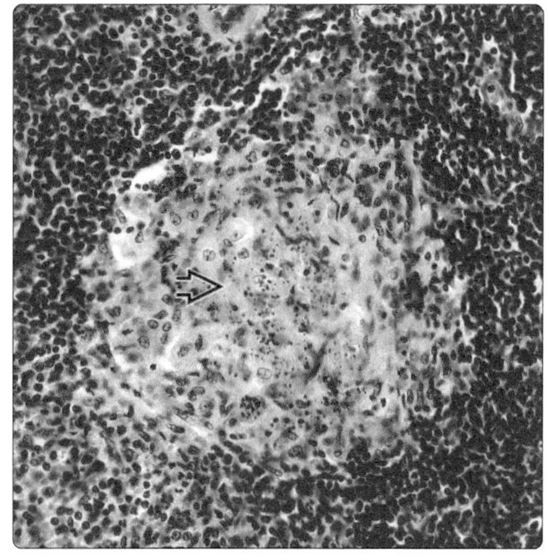

(Left) *Diphtheria trachea with coagulative necrosis of the mucosa* ⇨ *is shown earlier in progression than pseudomembrane formation.* **(Right)** *Diphtheria infection in the spleen is characterized by tight granulomas of epithelioid histiocytes* ⇨ *with the relatively unusual finding of pyknotic debris.*

Cystic Neutrophilic Granulomatous Mastitis

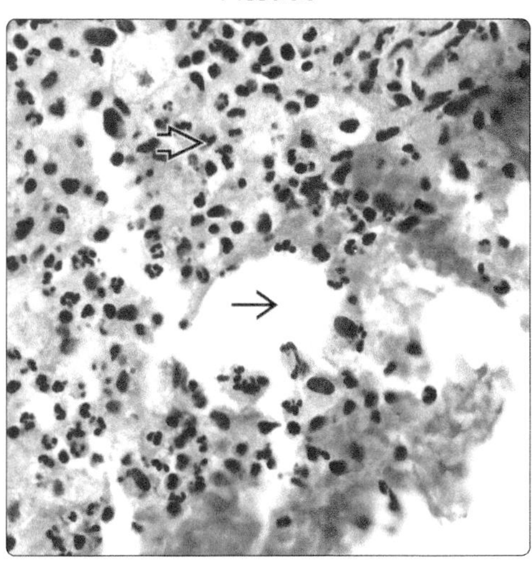

Diphtheroids: Gram Stain

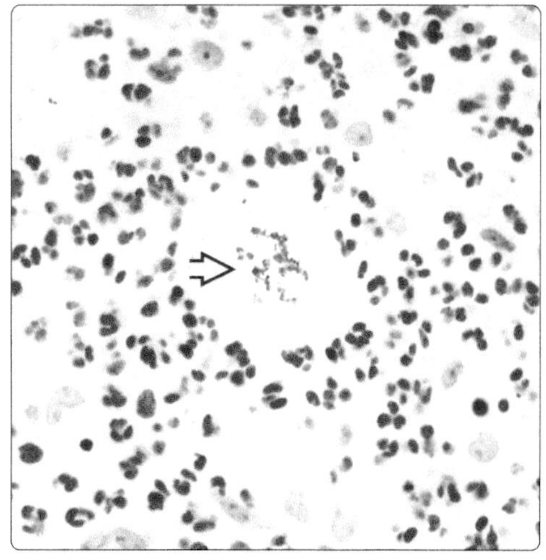

(Left) *Cystic neutrophilic granulomatous mastitis is a form of breast abscess characterized by sheets of neutrophils* ⇨ *with the unusual circumscribed spaces* → *surrounded by neutrophils.* **(Right)** *The morphology of diphtheroids* ⇨ *is best visualized on Gram stain showing gram-positive, club-shaped organisms, which form clumps reminiscent of a pile of matchsticks.*

Listeria Species Infection

KEY FACTS

ETIOLOGY/PATHOGENESIS

- Infection with *Listeria monocytogenes* and *Listeria ivanovii*, gram-positive bacilli widely present in environment as saprophytic organisms
- Most infections are foodborne, associated with fruits and vegetables, deli meats, smoked meats, and unpasteurized milk and cheese; can multiply at refrigeration temperatures

CLINICAL ISSUES

- Disease is most severe at extremes of age, in immunosuppressed patients, and in pregnant women
- Febrile gastroenteritis, maternal-fetal/neonatal listeriosis, or bacteremia ± CNS involvement
- Causes 1,600 illnesses and 260 deaths annually in USA; 83 outbreaks reported to CDC from 2012-2021

MICROBIOLOGY

- Gram-positive, non-spore-forming, facultative anaerobe shaped as short rods arranged as singles or short chains
- Nonfastidious organisms that grow in wide temperature range (0-50 °C), typically isolated on blood agar, with small zone of β-hemolysis
- Classified to species level by automated platforms, MALDI TOF MS, and 16S rRNA sequencing

MICROSCOPIC

- Gram-positive bacilli highlighted by Gram and silver stains
- CNS: Meningitis, encephalitis, and abscess
- Liver: Granulomas and abscesses
- Placenta: Acute villitis, abscesses and granulomas, and necrotizing acute chorioamnionitis

TOP DIFFERENTIAL DIAGNOSES

- Other causes of bacterial abscess and meningitis (e.g., *Streptococcus pneumoniae* and *Escherichia coli*): Differentiate by morphology on special stains, cultures, or molecular diagnosis

(Left) *Section of the skin from a fetal autopsy of maternal-fetal listeriosis shows mixed chronic inflammation involving the superficial dermis with focal erosion of the overlying epidermis.* **(Right)** *This section shows Listeria chorioamnionitis with focal villitis ⇨. (Courtesy Franz von Lichtenberg Collection of Infectious Disease Pathology, BWH.)*

Fetal Listeriosis

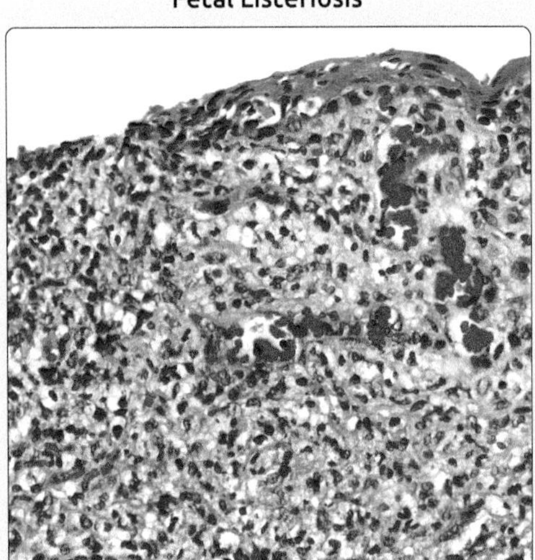

***Listeria* spp. Chorioamnionitis**

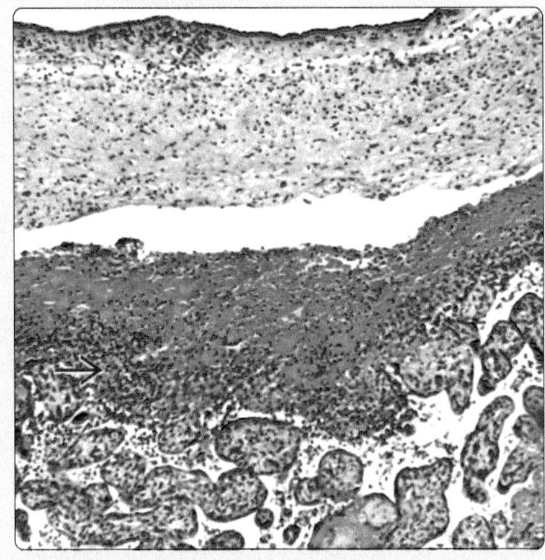

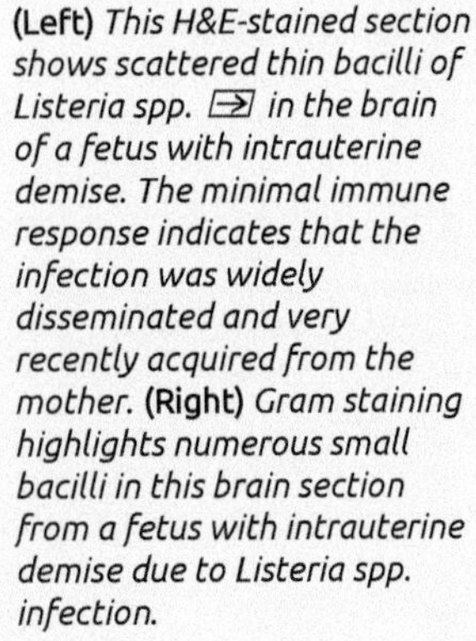

(Left) *This H&E-stained section shows scattered thin bacilli of Listeria spp. ⇨ in the brain of a fetus with intrauterine demise. The minimal immune response indicates that the infection was widely disseminated and very recently acquired from the mother.* **(Right)** *Gram staining highlights numerous small bacilli in this brain section from a fetus with intrauterine demise due to Listeria spp. infection.*

***Listeria* spp. Brain Involvement**

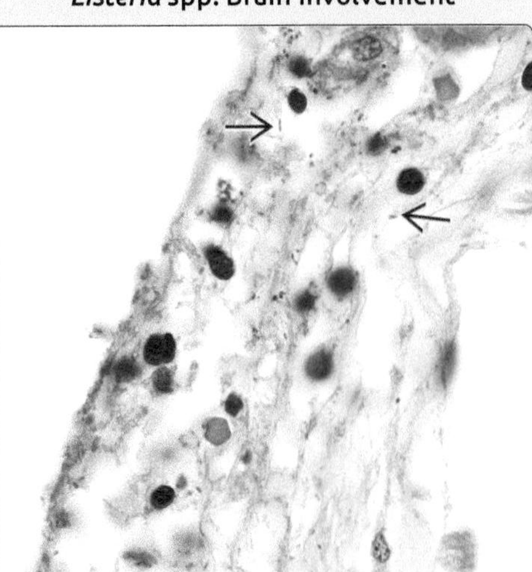

***Listeria* spp. Gram Stain**

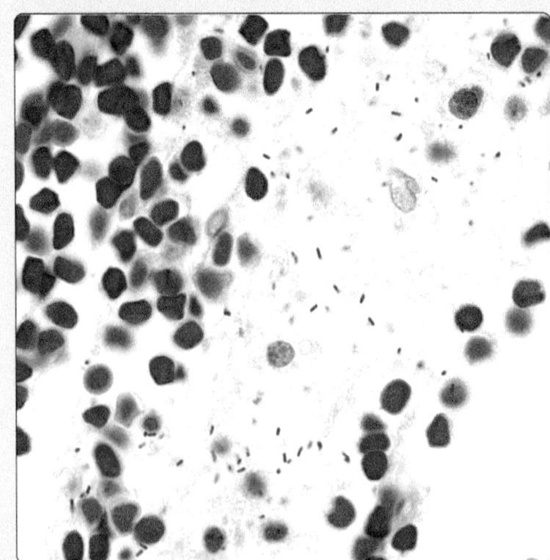

TERMINOLOGY

Definitions

- Named after English surgeon Joseph Lister (1827-1912)

ETIOLOGY/PATHOGENESIS

Infectious Agents

- Infection with *Listeria monocytogenes* and *Listeria ivanovii*, gram-positive bacilli widely present in environment as saprophytic organisms
- Most infections are foodborne, associated with fruits and vegetables, deli meats, smoked meats, and unpasteurized milk and cheese; can multiply at refrigeration temperatures
- Invades CNS by transport across blood brain barrier within host immune cells, direct invasion of endothelial cells, and retrograde movement up axons of involved nerves

CLINICAL ISSUES

Epidemiology

- Disease is most severe at extremes of age, in immunosuppressed patients, and in pregnant women
- Causes 1,600 illnesses and 260 deaths annually in USA
- 83 outbreaks reported in National Outbreak Reporting System (NORS) from 2012-2021

Presentation

- Febrile gastroenteritis typically occurs in immunocompetent patients after 5-49 hour incubation
- Maternal-fetal/neonatal listeriosis generally presents as bacteremia in mother, and may result in stillbirth or abortion in ~ 20% of pregnancies, preterm delivery
  - Early disease (before delivery) disseminated microabscesses (granulomatosis infantiseptica) is typically fatal; pneumonia, meningitis, or bacteremia
  - Late disease (at time of delivery from uncomplicated pregnancy) manifests as meningitis
- Bacteremia ± CNS involvement in ~ 50% of patients: Meningitis, meningoencephalitis, rhomboencephalitis, and brain abscess
- Cutaneous listeriosis may result from contact with infected animals (generally occupational) or, rarely, from hematogenous spread

Laboratory Tests

- CSF analysis: With meningitis/meningoencephalitis, Gram stain is positive in < 30% of cases, but cultures are positive in 80%; with abscess, culture is positive in < 50%
- Cervix, amniotic fluid, and placental cultures may reveal organism in maternal listeriosis
- Multiplex PCR: CSF and positive blood culture bottles

Treatment

- Gastroenteritis is self-limited and should subside in 3-4 days
- For invasive disease, ampicillin or penicillin plus trimethoprim-sulfamethoxazole or gentamicin
- Imipenem, meropenem, and linezolid are also active

Prognosis

- Mortality averages 36% with CNS involvement

IMAGING

MR Findings

- Rhomboencephalitis involving dorsal brainstem and cerebellum

MICROBIOLOGY

Morphologic and Biochemical Characteristics

- Gram-positive, non-spore-forming, facultative anaerobe shaped as short rods arranged as singles or short chains; characteristic tumbling motility, particularly at 20-28 °C due to temperature-regulated flagella
- Positive assays include catalase, Voges-Proskauer (acetoin production), methyl red (acidic fermentation products), and esculin hydrolysis

Culture and Identification

- Nonfastidious organisms that grow in wide temperature range (0-50 °C), typically isolated on blood agar, with small zone of β-hemolysis (due to hemolysin production)
- Classified to species level by automated platforms and MALDI TOF MS
- Selective and differential agars include LPM (colonies are blue), Oxford and PALCAM (colonies are black), and several chromogenic agars (i.e., Oxoid Brilliance, can differentiate between *L. monocytogenes* and *L. ivanovii*)

MACROSCOPIC

General Features

- Placental infection can be indicated by yellowish membranes with fruity odor and large abscesses

MICROSCOPIC

Histologic Features

- CNS: Meningitis, encephalitis, and abscess
- Liver: Granulomas and abscesses
- Placenta: Acute villitis, abscesses and granulomas, and necrotizing acute chorioamnionitis

ANCILLARY TESTS

Special Stains

- Short bacilli highlighted by Gram and silver stains

DIFFERENTIAL DIAGNOSIS

Bacterial Abscess and Meningitis

- Differentiate from other infectious causes (e.g., *Streptococcus pneumoniae* and *Escherichia coli*) by special stains, culture, or molecular diagnosis

SELECTED REFERENCES

1. Khsim IEF et al: Listeriosis in pregnancy: an umbrella review of maternal exposure, treatment and neonatal complications. BJOG. 129(9):1427-33, 2022
2. Koopmans MM et al: Human listeriosis. Clin Microbiol Rev. e0006019, 2022
3. Pogreba-Brown K et al: Complications associated with foodborne listeriosis: a scoping review. Foodborne Pathog Dis. 19(11):725-43, 2022
4. Engelen-Lee JY et al: Histopathology of Listeria meningitis. J Neuropathol Exp Neurol. 77(10):950-7, 2018

Rhodococcus Species Infection

KEY FACTS

ETIOLOGY/PATHOGENESIS

- Rhodococci are bacteria widely present in environment that cause infection via inhalation of contaminated dirt and dust or by direct inoculation

CLINICAL ISSUES

- 85-90% of human cases immunocompromised patients
- Pulmonary disease (cavitary upper lobe pneumonia) is most common manifestation; may be complicated by pleural effusions &/or severe hemoptysis
- Dissemination may occur in rare instances
- Mortality ranges up to 50% in HIV patients

MICROBIOLOGY

- Gram-positive coccobacilli or pleomorphic rods; may be partially acid-fast
- Obligate aerobes, which can tolerate wide temperature range (optimum 30 °C) and grow on most nonspecific laboratory media, including blood agar

MICROSCOPIC

- Typically appears in necrotizing, granulomatous pattern dominated by macrophages; also associated with malakoplakia
- Coccobacillary organisms can be visualized by Gram, silver, and acid-fast stains

TOP DIFFERENTIAL DIAGNOSES

- Necrotizing granulomas associated with other members of aerobic actinomyces, *Corynebacterium* and *Mycobacterium* spp., and fungi
- Histiocytic aggregates with *Mycobacterium avium* complex (MAC), *M. genavense*, *H. capsulatum*, and *C. neoformans*
- Malakoplakia is most commonly associated with gram-negative infections of genitourinary tract
- Cavitary lung lesions also associated with *Mycobacterium tuberculosis*, nontuberculous mycobacteria, *Blastomyces* spp., *Histoplasma* spp., *Coccidioides* spp., *Aspergillus* spp., *Burkholderia pseudomallei*

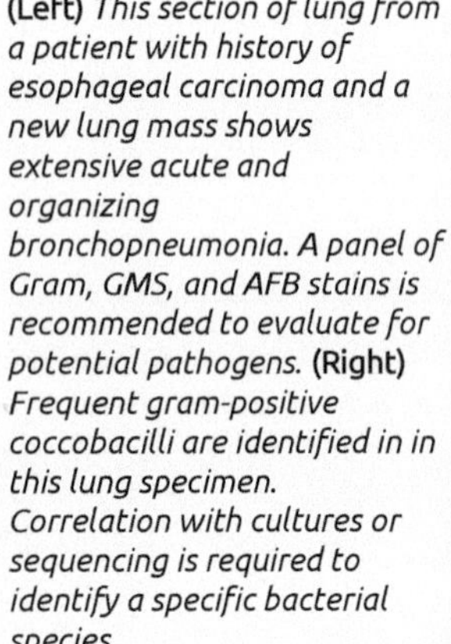
(Left) *This section of lung from a patient with history of esophageal carcinoma and a new lung mass shows extensive acute and organizing bronchopneumonia. A panel of Gram, GMS, and AFB stains is recommended to evaluate for potential pathogens.* **(Right)** *Frequent gram-positive coccobacilli are identified in in this lung specimen. Correlation with cultures or sequencing is required to identify a specific bacterial species.*

Rhodoccus **Suppurative Lung Abscess**

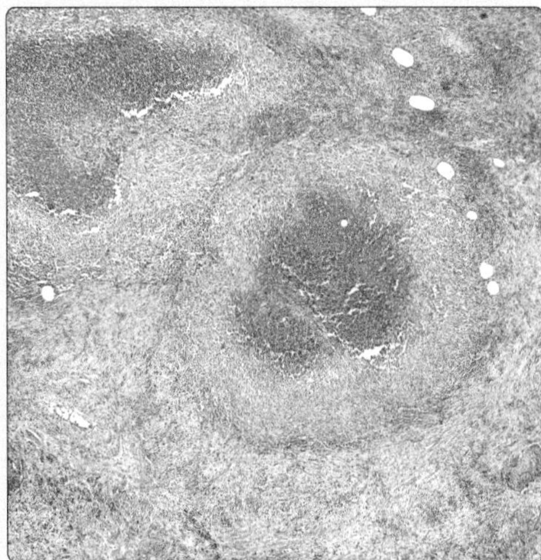

Rhodoccus **spp.: Gram Stain**

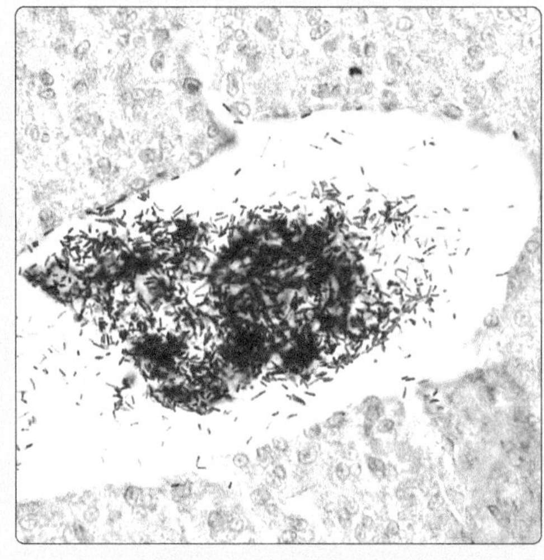

(Left) *Rhodoccus species can exhibit acid-fast staining due to the presence of mycolic acids in the cell wall, which may cause misidentification as mycobacteria. This case was confirmed to be Rhodoccus rhodochrous from concurrent lung and BAL cultures.* **(Right)** *Rhodococcus spp. colonies can appear as rough, smooth, or mucoid and buff cream, yellow, orange, or red colorless, and may become increasingly pigmented and rough with age. [Courtesy E. Crowe, MLS(ASCP)CM.]*

Rhodoccus **spp.: Acid-Fast Stain**

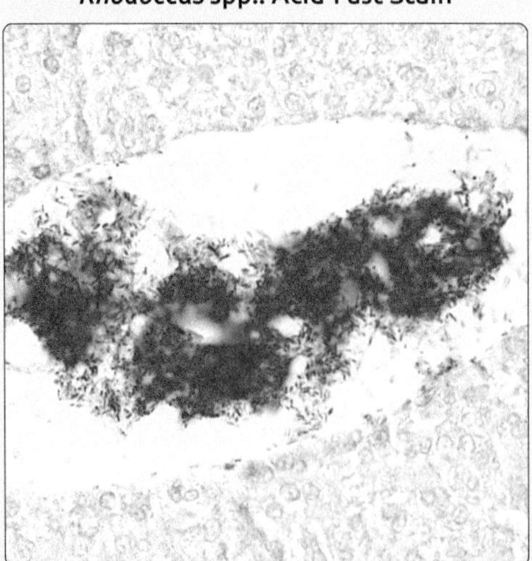

Rhodococcus ruber **Isolated in Culture**

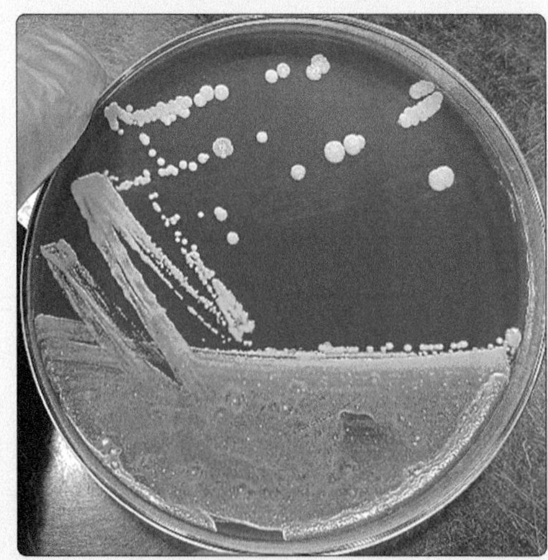

TERMINOLOGY

Definitions

- Greek: "Rhodon" (rose) + "kokkos" (berry, grain)

ETIOLOGY/PATHOGENESIS

Infectious Agents

- Rhodococci are bacteria widely present in environment that cause infection via inhalation of contaminated dirt and dust or by direct inoculation
- *R. equi* is important veterinary pathogen and is also associated with disease in humans; rare reports of nosocomial infections (ventriculoperitoneal shunts and dialysis tubing) and person-to-person spread
- Rhodococcus bacteremias in cancer patients are often associated with biofilm formations on central lines
- Other uncommon pathogens include *R. rhodochrous*, *R. erythropolis*, *R. ruber*, *R. gordoniae*, and *R. fascians*

CLINICAL ISSUES

Epidemiology

- Exposure to livestock, farming, or gardening increases risk
- 85-90% of human cases occur in immunocompromised patients, e.g., HIV, transplant recipients, corticosteroid use

Presentation

- Pulmonary disease (cavitary upper lobe pneumonia) is most common manifestation of rhodococcal infection (80% of cases); cavitation, pleural effusions, and life-threatening hemoptysis are potential complications
- Disseminated disease in immunocompromised patients
- Less commonly, endophthalmitis, wound infection, osteomyelitis, peritonitis, chronic corneal ulcer, brain abscess, and purulent meningitis

Treatment

- Drugs: Combination of 2-3 drugs during induction phase (e.g., vancomycin, imipenem, or ciprofloxacin, with erythromycin or rifampin); maintenance therapy (weeks to months) with ciprofloxacin or erythromycin
- Surgical debulking of extensive disease, particularly in immunocompromised patients (not usually required)

Prognosis

- Mortality ranges from ~ 11% in immunocompetent to 50% in HIV patients

IMAGING

Radiographic Findings

- Imaging generally reveals upper lung lesions, which can expand to cavitary lesions (> 50% of pulmonary cases) &/or pleural effusion (~ 20%)

MICROBIOLOGY

Morphologic/Biochemical

- Gram-positive coccobacilli (from solid media or tissue) or pleomorphic rods (from liquid culture); may be partially acid-fast
- Organisms are generally catalase, urease, lipase, and phosphatase positive; sugars and alcohols are not fermented or oxidized

Culture

- Obligate aerobes that grow on most nonspecific laboratory media, including blood agar
- Mucoid, smooth, irregular colonies within 48 hours that may turn salmon-pink color after ~ 4 days
- Selective media for enrichment include: CNA agar, PEA agar, and ceftazidime-novobiocin agar

Microbiologic Identification

- Laboratory platforms that can be used to identify rhodococci include API Coryne strip (bioMérieux), MALDI-TOF, 16s rRNA sequencing, and medium-chain fatty acid analysis (Sherlock System, MIDI Inc.)

MICROSCOPIC

Histologic Features

- Typically appears in necrotizing, granulomatous pattern dominated by macrophages, which may contain coccobacillary organisms, visualized by Gram and silver stains
- Organisms are partially acid-fast and must be differentiated from *Mycobacterium* spp.
- Can demonstrate malakoplakia inflammatory pattern consisting of histiocytes and von Kossa-positive Michaelis-Gutmann bodies (mineralized remnants of incompletely digested bacteria)
- Endophthalmitis and keratitis in ocular tissue

Cytologic Features

- Preparations of fine-needle aspirations (FNAs) and bronchoalveolar lavages may demonstrate malakoplakia

DIFFERENTIAL DIAGNOSIS

Other Bacterial and Fungal Infections

- Necrotizing granulomas are associated with other members of aerobic actinomyces, *Corynebacterium* and *Mycobacterium* spp., and fungi
- Histiocytic aggregates may also be caused by *Mycobacterium avium* complex (MAC), *Mycobacterium genavense*, *Histoplasma capsulatum*, and *Cryptococcus neoformans*
- Malakoplakia is most commonly associated with gram-negative infections of genitourinary tract
- Cavitary lung lesions also associated with *Mycobacterium tuberculosis*, nontuberculous mycobacteria, *Blastomyces* spp., *Histoplasma* spp., *Coccidioides* spp., *Aspergillus* spp., *Burkholderia pseudomallei*

SELECTED REFERENCES

1. Sanz MG: Rhodococcus equi-what is new this decade? Vet Clin North Am Equine Pract. 39(1):1-14, 2023
2. Val-Calvo J et al: International spread of multidrug-resistant Rhodococcus equi. Emerg Infect Dis. 28(9):1899-903, 2022
3. Lin WV et al: Diagnosis and management of pulmonary infection due to Rhodococcus equi. Clin Microbiol Infect. 25(3):310-5, 2019
4. Majidzadeh M et al: Current taxonomy of Rhodococcus species and their role in infections. Eur J Clin Microbiol Infect Dis. 37(11):2045-62, 2018

KEY FACTS

ETIOLOGY/PATHOGENESIS

- *Staphylococcus* species found widely on skin and mucous membranes of humans and animals; divided into coagulase-positive (*S. aureus*) and coagulase-negative (major species: *S. epidermidis*)
- *S. aureus:* Skin and soft tissue infections, bloodstream infection, endocarditis, pneumonia, osteomyelitis, toxin-mediated diseases include TSS, SSSS, and food poisoning
- Coagulase-negative *Staphylococcus* (CoNS): Intravascular catheter and device-/material-related infections and endocarditis
- With routine use of MALDI in diagnostic laboratories, many species will be diagnosed, which were formerly called CoNS

MICROSCOPIC

- Gram and silver stains highlight gram-positive cocci
- SSSS: Sloughed stratum corneum, regular, smooth keratinocytes, absence of inflammation
- TSS: Spongiotic reaction with neutrophils, scattered necrotic keratinocytes, edematous dermis
- Impetigo: Subcorneal pustules with neutrophils and acantholytic cells
- Endocarditis: Defective/mechanical and native valves; large (> 1-cm) vegetations; septic emboli and mycotic aneurysms
- Pneumonia: Necrotic lesions with abscess formation
- Osteomyelitis: Neutrophils adjacent to bony trabeculae with erosive changes

TOP DIFFERENTIAL DIAGNOSES

- Toxic epidermal necrolysis: Effects entire epidermis vs. SSSS, which only involves stratum corneum
- Pemphigus foliaceus: Lacks organisms, which differentiates from impetigo
- Endocarditis, pneumonia, osteomyelitis, cellulitis, and necrotizing fasciitis can be caused by organisms other than *S. aureus* (or as copathogens); specific organisms identified by Gram and silver stains, culture, PCR

Bacterial Folliculitis

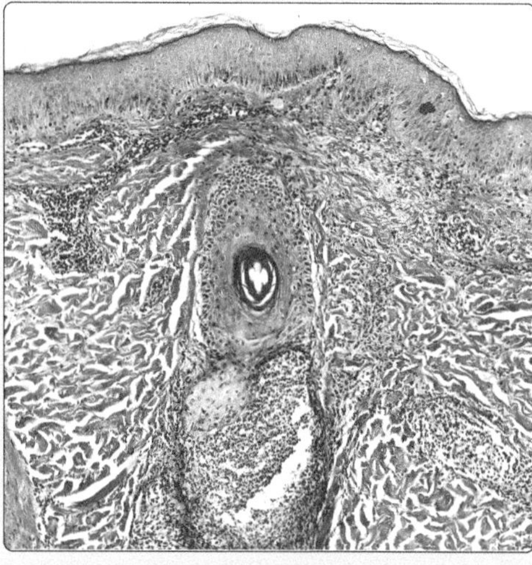

Bullous Impetigo

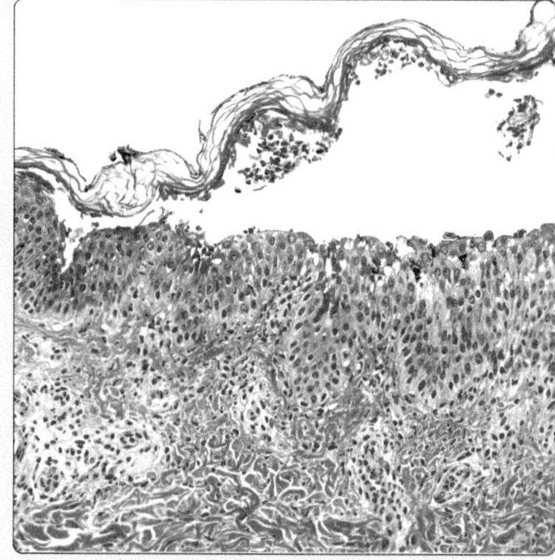

(Left) *Folliculitis is characterized by sheets of neutrophilic inflammation centered on hair follicles and adnexal structures, most often caused by Staphylococcus aureus. (Courtesy B. Smoller, MD.)* **(Right)** *Bullous impetigo is shown with subcorneal clefting and neutrophilic exudate within the resultant blister. (Courtesy B. Smoller, MD.)*

Gross Photograph: Staphylococcal Pneumonia

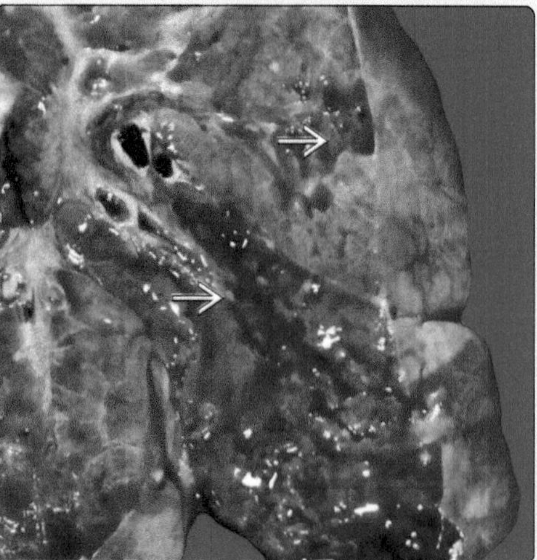

Staphylococcal Pneumonia With Necrosis

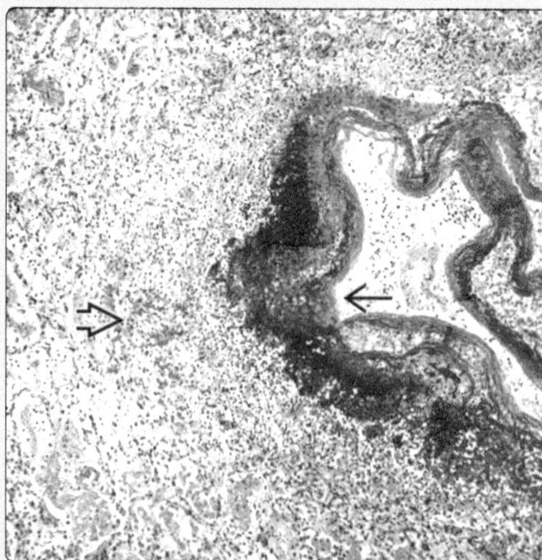

(Left) *Gross photograph of hemorrhagic, necrotizing staphylococcal pneumonia shows bronchial erosion and empyema ➡. (Courtesy Franz von Lichtenberg Collection of Infectious Disease Pathology, BWH.)* **(Right)** *Staphylococcal pneumonia demonstrates bronchial wall necrosis ➡ and diffuse consolidation ➡ of adjacent alveoli. (Courtesy Franz von Lichtenberg Collection of Infectious Disease Pathology, BWH.)*

TERMINOLOGY

Abbreviations

- Methicillin-sensitive *Staphylococcus aureus* (MSSA)
- Methicillin-resistant *S. aureus* (MRSA)
- Vancomycin-intermediate *S. aureus* (VISA)
- Coagulase-negative *Staphylococcus* (CoNS)

Definitions

- Greek: "Staphyle" (grape) + "kokkus" (grain, seed)

ETIOLOGY/PATHOGENESIS

Infectious Agents

- *Staphylococcus* species found widely on skin and mucous membranes of humans and animals; hardy in multiple environments and can survive on surfaces for months
- Split into coagulase-positive and coagulase-negative species
- Coagulase-positive staphylococci
  - *S. aureus* is major pathogen; often colonizes nares
  - Virulence factors: Coagulase, hyaluronidase, lipase, enterotoxin type B, TSST-1, exfoliative toxins, alpha toxin, beta toxin, delta toxin, Panton-Valentine leukocidin
- Coagulase-negative staphylococci; recent move to change CoNS to "SOSA" or Staph species other than *S. aureus*
  - Trophism for distinct regions of host (i.e., axillae, head, etc.); commonly isolated from human skin
  - *Staphylococcus epidermidis* is major pathogen; others include *S. lugdunensis, S. saprophyticus, S. hemolyticus, S. capitis, S. hominis, S. saccharolyticus*, and *S. warneri*
- Majority of methicillin resistance mediated by PBP2a, penicillin-binding protein with reduced affinity for most β-lactam antibiotics; PBP2a is encoded by gene mecA (rarely, MecC)

CLINICAL ISSUES

Epidemiology

- *S. aureus* is one of most common pathogens in both nosocomial and community-acquired infections
  - Risk factors include male sex, extremes of age, dialysis, diabetes, cancer, rheumatoid arthritis, HIV infection, IV drug use and alcohol abuse, defects in phagocytosis and chemotaxis
  - Highly clonal (particularly MRSA) with most pandemic strains linking back to 3 clonal complexes (CC5, CC8, and CC30)
  - MRSA is common in both hospital and community (59% in ICU patients, 55% in non-ICU patients, 48% in outpatients)
  - Carriage is most important predisposing factor for infection; large percentage of population (> 50%) either persistently or intermittently
  - Community-acquired (CA-MRSA) and healthcare-acquired (HCA-MRSA) *S. aureus* strains are responsible for distinct clinical syndromes
- CoNS
  - *S. epidermidis*: 9 clonal types prevalent worldwide (CC2 is major one)
  - Strongly associated with intravascular catheters and other devices

Presentation

- *S. aureus* causes wide spectrum of disease
  - Toxin-mediated diseases
    - Toxic shock syndrome (TSS) associated with children, tampon use, postoperative wound, or soft tissue infections; high fever, hypotension, and diffuse rash that eventually desquamates (involvement of ≥ 3 organ systems)
    - Staphylococcal scalded skin syndrome (SSSS) in infants or young children: Bullous exfoliative dermatitis with diffuse (Ritter disease) and localized (pemphigus neonatorum) forms; bright red skin on head, which then spreads downward toward extremities (with constitutional symptoms)
    - Gastroenteritis: Improperly stored prepared food, particularly dairy; toxin can remain active under conditions that kill organism; nausea, vomiting, diarrhea, and abdominal pain, generally 2-6 hours after ingestion
  - Skin and soft tissue infections (SSTI); account for 1/3 of SSTI
    - Can be relatively superficial (folliculitis, furuncles, carbuncles, and impetigo in epidermis and dermis) or deep (cellulitis, fasciitis, and pyomyositis in dermis and subcutaneous tissues)
    - Folliculitis: Nodule centered on hair follicle, which may have apparent pus, may evolve into large furuncles
    - Carbuncles: Collections of furuncles and may demonstrate several openings to discharge pus
    - Impetigo: Pustules or bullae with honey-colored crusting and negative Nikolsky sign; often occurs as complication of other dermatoses, typically on face
    - Cellulitis: Painful, bright red macules or plaques, which can demonstrate scaling and ulceration over time
    - Necrotizing fasciitis: Typically presents subsequent to trauma with pain out of proportion to clinical findings; fever, malaise, and myalgias follow, and pain can eventually progress to anesthesia, considered surgical emergency
  - Bloodstream infection (BSI); 2nd most common cause of bacteremia
    - Community-associated BSI generally occurs in patients without other major risk factors and often can be traced to distinct focus of infection (i.e., endocarditis)
    - Healthcare-associated or nosocomial BSI is often related to intravascular catheters or other instrumentation and surgical site infections
    - Carries risk of metastatic foci, particularly endocarditis (10%)
  - Endocarditis
    - Usually presents acutely with fever, dyspnea, tachycardia, pleuritic chest pain, hypotension
    - Clinical signs include murmur, petechiae, and Janeway lesions (from septic emboli), possibly CNS findings
  - Pneumonia; < 5% of community-acquired and 25-47% of healthcare-associated pneumonia
    - Can be initiated by airway exposure or hematogenous seeding and often follows severe course
    - Community-acquired pneumonia can often be preceded by influenza-like illness

- Signs and symptoms include marked dyspnea, hemoptysis, fever, leukopenia, hypotension, and elevated C-reactive protein
- Chest x-ray demonstrates multilobar cavitating alveolar infiltrates
- Sequelae can include abscess and empyema

- Osteomyelitis: Responsible for 50-70% of cases
  - Infection can be result of hematogenous or contiguous spread
  - Hematogenous spread usually results in acute picture with chills, fever, malaise, pain, and swelling
  - Contiguous spread (usually from complications of diabetes, vascular disease, or prosthesis) often follows chronic, subacute course with low-grade inflammation, necrosis, and fistulas
  - May be painless due to neuritis
- *S. aureus* may also cause meningitis, pericarditis, prosthetic joint infections (usually stage I, occurring within 3 months of surgery), septic arthritis, and pyomyositis

- CoNS infections generally more indolent than those caused by *S. aureus*
  - Intravascular catheter and device/material-related infections
    - Most common cause of BSIs (associated with intravascular catheters)
    - Infection of vascular grafts are also most commonly caused by CoNS
    - CoNS accounts for ~ 25% of pacemaker-associated infections
    - Stage II prosthetic joint infections (occurring between 3 months and 2 years after surgery) are often caused by CoNS and follow indolent course (pain without fever or drainage)
  - Endocarditis
    - Usually occurs on prosthetic valves and occurs at time of placement (manifests within 12 months)
    - Heart failure occurs in 54% of cases with abscess and valve dysfunction occurring frequently
  - Neonatal infections
    - CoNS is responsible for 31% of all nosocomial infections and 73% of bacteremias in USA NICUs
    - Neonates are more likely to develop wider range of disease (wound abscess, pneumonia, urinary tract infection, meningitis, enterocolitis, omphalitis)
    - Infections are usually nosocomial (not acquired from mother)
  - *S. saprophyticus* frequently (2nd to *Escherichia coli*) causes urinary tract infections in young, sexually active women
  - *S. lugdunensis* is distinguished by causing similar spectrum and severity of infections to *S. aureus*
    - Endocarditis caused by *S. lugdunensis* follows more virulent course than that of other CoNS and often results in valve dysfunction and abscess formation (mortality: 50-70%)
    - Also frequent cause of SSTIs below waist (where it resides among skin flora)
    - Emerging cause of prosthetic joint infections
  - *S. hemolyticus* is common cause of bacteremia and is increasingly multidrug resistant

Laboratory Tests

- Serologic testing for antistaphylococcal antibodies does not play role in diagnosis due to lack of specificity
- PCR/sequencing of 16S rRNA and *rpoB* genes for speciation of culture isolates and frozen or formalin-fixed paraffin-embedded tissue

Treatment

- Necrotizing fasciitis requires emergent drainage and debridement
- Removal of infected hardware &/or devices
- MRSA can account for 50-60% of staphylococci in USA hospitals; vancomycin and linezolid are often used to treat infections in these settings
- CA-MRSA tends to carry fewer resistance determinants to other drugs than HCA-MRSA does
- CoNS antibiotic susceptibility varies by species (many are resistant to multiple drugs)

Prognosis

- Variable by species and site of infection
- *S. aureus:* Toxin-mediated disease mortality ranges from very low in food poisoning to quite high in adult SSSS (> 50%) or CA-MRSA necrotizing pneumonia (60%)
- CoNS: Mortality is highest with *S. lugdunensis* endocarditis (50-70%) and is generally low with most other manifestations

MICROBIOLOGY

Morphologic/Biochemical

- Catalase-positive, gram-positive cocci arranged in clusters
- All are facultative anaerobes, except for anaerobic species *S. saccharolyticus* and *S. aureus* subspecies *anaerobius*
- Grows in temperature range from 18-40 °C; tolerates 10% NaCl

Culture

- Staphylococci are usually isolated on blood agar plates
  - *S. aureus* appears as smooth, creamy, yellowish to orange colonies, while CoNS are often nonpigmented
  - *S. aureus* usually demonstrates β-hemolysis, while CoNS are generally nonhemolytic (except for *S. hemolyticus* and *S. lugdunensis*)
- Selective agars for *S. aureus* include mannitol salt agar, egg yolk-tellurite pyruvate containing Baird-Parker medium, Columbia colistin-nalidixic acid agar, lipase-salt-mannitol agar, and phenylethyl alcohol agar
- Also several chromogenic agars available (including those that can differentiate MRSA)

Microbiological Identification

- Organisms presumptively identified as staphylococci if catalase-positive, gram-positive cocci
- Coagulase production differentiates *S. aureus* from most CoNS (except *S. lugdunensis*: Coagulase positive, clumping factor negative)
- Within CoNS, pathogenic *S. saprophyticus* is differentiated by resistance to novobiocin
- With routine use of MALDI-TOF MS in diagnostic laboratories, many species will be diagnosed, which were formerly called "CoNS"

- Rapid molecular platforms are available to detect presence of *S. aureus* and CoNS directly from primary specimens and positive blood bottles (as well as to identify MRSA)
- *S. aureus*, as well as many species of CoNS, can be identified by gram-positive card on Vitek 2 (BioMérieux) automated platform
- API Staph strip (BioMérieux), consisting of 19 reactions, is also used within clinical laboratories to differentiate staphylococcal species (can distinguish 20)

MICROSCOPIC

Histologic Features

- *S. aureus*
  - SSSS: Sloughed stratum corneum, keratinocytes regular and smooth with occasional acantholytic cells, inflammation is not present; mediated by toxin, thus, organisms are not present
  - TSS: Spongiotic reaction with neutrophils and scattered necrotic keratinocytes over edematous dermis, superficial perivascular and mixed cell infiltrate with neutrophils and possibly eosinophils; pustular or necrotic vasculitis and neutrophilic abscesses may be present; mediated by toxin, thus, no organisms present
  - Impetigo: Subcorneal pustules with variable numbers of neutrophils and acantholytic cells; cocci may be present
  - Folliculitis, furuncles, and carbuncles: Inflammatory cells, predominantly neutrophils, centered on 1 or several hair follicles
  - Cellulitis: Edema in dermis and subcuticular regions and dilated blood vessels and lymphatics, diffuse infiltrate of neutrophils; organisms are very rarely observed
  - Chronic cellulitis: Spongiosis of epidermis with vesicles, pustules, ulceration, and necrosis ± fibrosis
  - Necrotizing fasciitis: Fascia and deep soft tissue necrosis, hemorrhage, thrombosis, and secondary vasculitis
  - Endocarditis: *S. aureus* can colonize both defective/mechanical and native valves (often damaging them); relatively large (> 1-cm) vegetations; often results in septic emboli and mycotic aneurysms
  - Pneumonia: Primary pneumonia or as sequelae of influenza; necrotic lesions with abscess formation, which may metastasize to distant organs or rupture into pleural space, causing empyema; clusters of organisms may be seen
  - Osteomyelitis: Neutrophils adjacent to bony trabeculae with erosive changes; organisms may be seen
- CoNS
  - Lesser degree of pus and necrosis compares to *S. aureus* infections
  - Colonized devices and catheters usually appear to be coated with tan, fibrinous material and microscopically demonstrate clusters of cocci with acute inflammatory infiltrates

ANCILLARY TESTS

Immunohistochemistry

- Not widely used due to cross reactivity between species; may be available at reference laboratories

Special Stains

- Tissue Gram stain highlights gram-positive cocci in pairs or clusters; gram positivity may be weak or absent due to staining quality or antibiotic treatment effects
- Methenamine silver stains can highlight cocci with negative Gram staining; may be difficult to interpret if high background is present

DIFFERENTIAL DIAGNOSIS

Other Causes of Endocarditis

- Streptococcal and enterococcal endocarditis: Less severe course, less suppurative reaction; causative organism identified by culture or PCR
- Noninfectious endocarditis: Lack of inflammatory reaction, no visible organisms, and negative cultures

Toxic Epidermal Necrolysis

- Effects entire epidermis vs. SSSS, which only involves stratum corneum

Pemphigus Foliaceus

- Lacks organisms, which differentiates from impetigo

Other Bacterial Skin and Soft Tissue Infections

- Cellulitis and necrotizing fasciitis can be caused by organisms other than *S. aureus* (or as copathogens); specific organisms identified by Gram and silver stains, culture, PCR

SELECTED REFERENCES

1. Howden BP et al: Staphylococcus aureus host interactions and adaptation. Nat Rev Microbiol. 21(6):380-95, 2023
2. Severn MM et al: Staphylococcus epidermidis and its dual lifestyle in skin health and infection. Nat Rev Microbiol. 21(2):97-111, 2023
3. Duan R et al: Rapid and simple approaches for diagnosis of Staphylococcus aureus in bloodstream infections. Pol J Microbiol. 71(4):481-9, 2022
4. Cheung GYC et al: Pathogenicity and virulence of Staphylococcus aureus. Virulence. 12(1):547-69, 2021
5. Heilbronner S et al: Staphylococcus lugdunensis: a skin commensal with invasive pathogenic potential. Clin Microbiol Rev. 34(2), 2021
6. Kavanagh N et al: Staphylococcal osteomyelitis: disease progression, treatment challenges, and future directions. Clin Microbiol Rev. 31(2), 2018
7. Lakhundi S et al: Methicillin-resistant Staphylococcus aureus: molecular characterization, evolution, and epidemiology. Clin Microbiol Rev. 31(4), 2018
8. Natsis NE et al: Coagulase-negative Staphylococcus skin and soft tissue infections. Am J Clin Dermatol. 19(5):671-7, 2018
9. Becker K et al: Coagulase-negative staphylococci. Clin Microbiol Rev. 27(4):870-926, 2014
10. Stach CS et al: Staphylococcal superantigens interact with multiple host receptors to cause serious diseases. Immunol Res. 59(1-3):177-81, 2014
11. Guarner J et al: Immunohistochemical evidence of Clostridium sp, Staphylococcus aureus, and group A Streptococcus in severe soft tissue infections related to injection drug use. Hum Pathol. 37(11):1482-8, 2006
12. Lichtenberg, F: Pathology of Infectious Diseases. Raven Press, 1991

(Left) *Gross photograph of lethal staphylococcal pneumonia demonstrates a bronchopleural fistula →. (Courtesy Franz von Lichtenberg Collection of Infectious Disease Pathology, BWH.)* **(Right)** *Staphylococcal bronchopneumonia demonstrates fibrinopurulent exudate → lining the partially necrotic alveolar walls. (Courtesy Franz von Lichtenberg Collection of Infectious Disease Pathology, BWH.)*

Gross Photograph Pleural Pneumonia

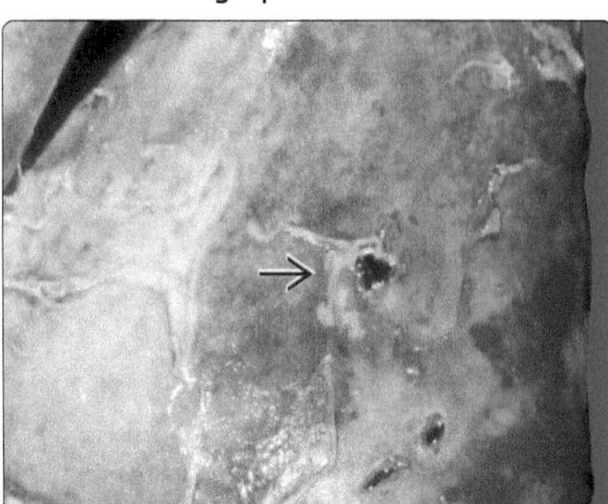

Staphylococcal Bronchopneumonia Exudate

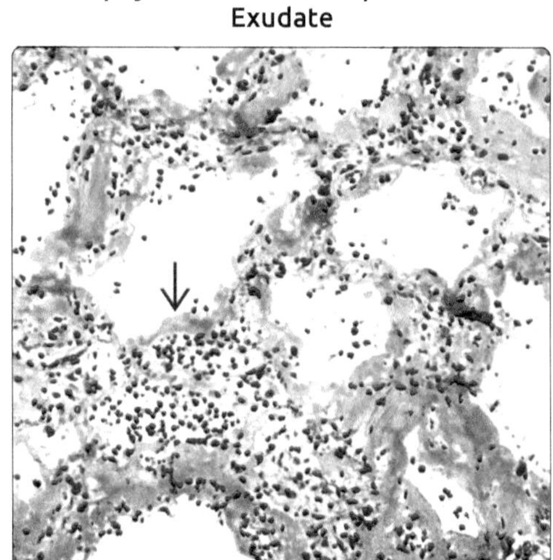

(Left) *Staphylococcal colonies → are easily visualized by Gram stain in bronchopneumonia and can also be seen as basophilic clusters on H&E. (Courtesy Franz von Lichtenberg Collection of Infectious Disease Pathology, BWH.)* **(Right)** *S. aureus appears as gram-positive cocci in clusters → in a positive blood culture on this Gram stain.*

Bronchopneumonia: Gram Stain

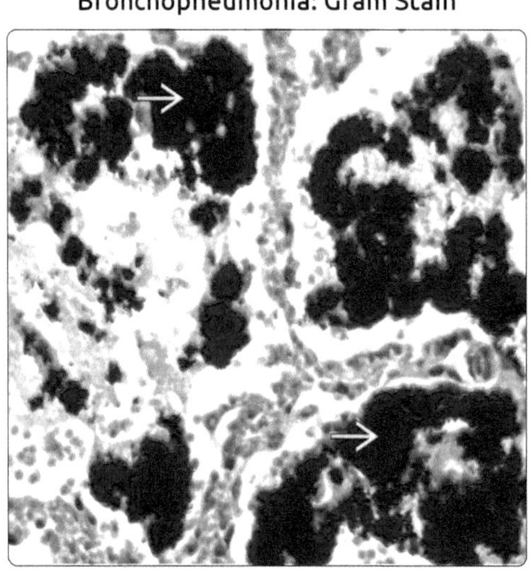

Staphylococcus aureus Gram Stain

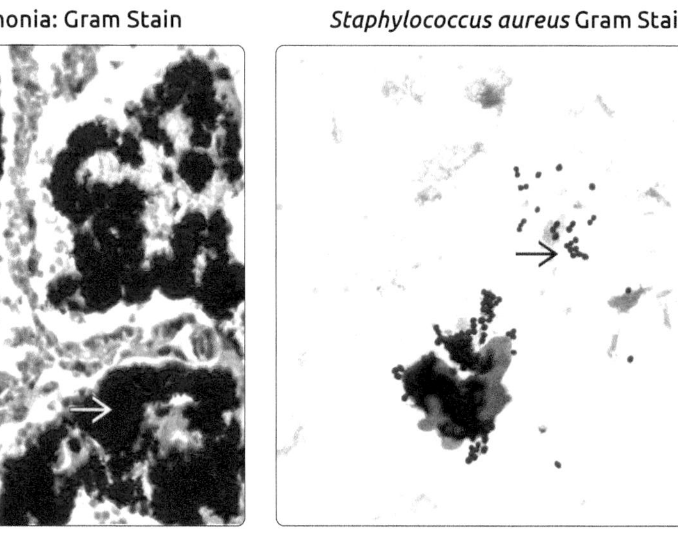

(Left) *S. aureus osteomyelitis shows sheets of neutrophils and mononuclear cells intimately admixed with devitalized bone and necrotic debris.* **(Right)** *Brown and Brenn stain of S. aureus osteomyelitis is shown, which reveals gram-positive cocci in clusters →.*

Staphylococcus aureus Osteomyelitis

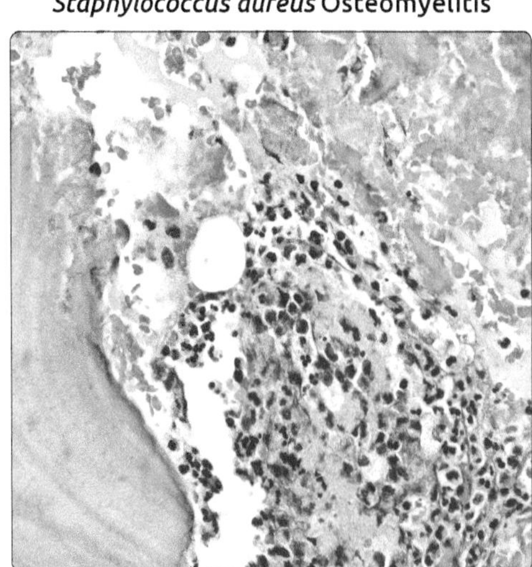

Osteomyelitis Gram Stain

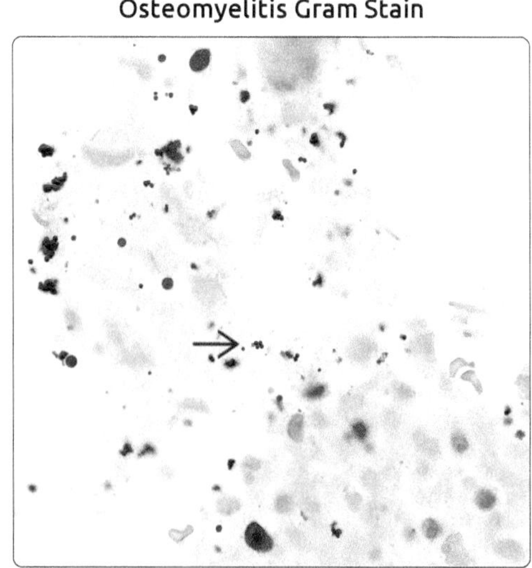

Staphylococcus aureus Miliary Abscess

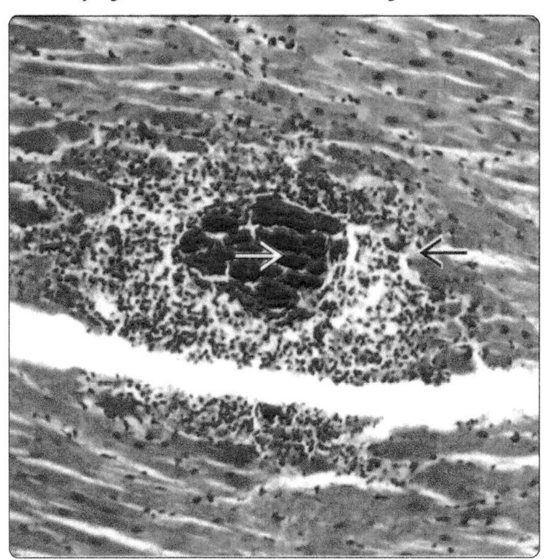

Staphylococcus Endocarditis

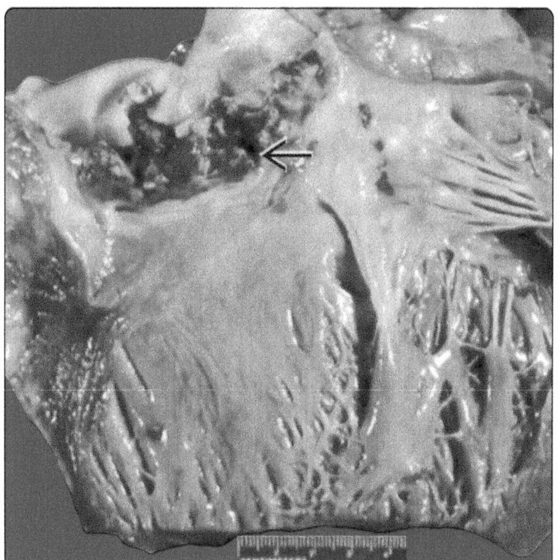

(Left) *S. aureus sepsis can also cause miliary abscesses (here in the myocardium). Note the colony of bacteria ➡ surrounded by abscess formation ➡. (Courtesy Franz von Lichtenberg Collection of Infectious Disease Pathology, BWH.)* **(Right)** *Gross photograph depicts large vegetations ➡ in staphylococcal endocarditis. (Courtesy Franz von Lichtenberg Collection of Infectious Disease Pathology, BWH.)*

Staphylococcus Endocarditis Aortic Valve Vegetations

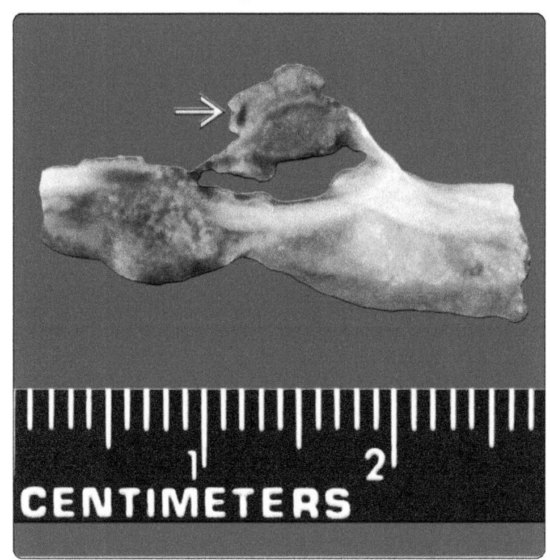

Septic Embolus to Hepatic Artery

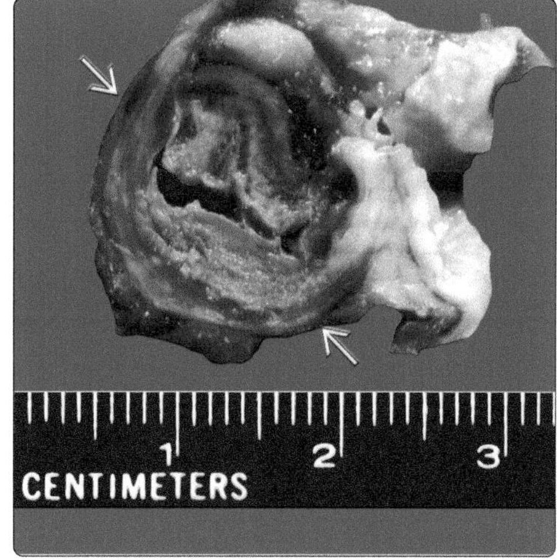

(Left) *Gross photograph illustrates large, "shaggy" aortic valve vegetations ➡ in staphylococcal endocarditis. (Courtesy Franz von Lichtenberg Collection of Infectious Disease Pathology, BWH.)* **(Right)** *Septic emboli from staphylococcal endocarditis can cause mycotic aneurysms ➡ of distant vessels (here, the hepatic artery). (Courtesy Franz von Lichtenberg Collection of Infectious Disease Pathology, BWH.)*

Septic Emboli With Brain Infarction

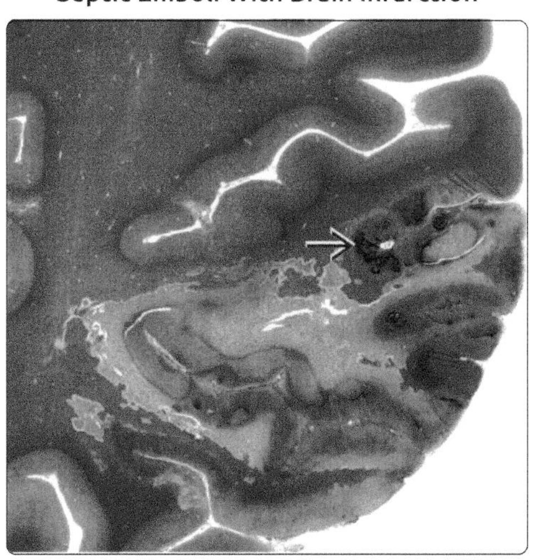

Septic Emboli With Lung Infarction

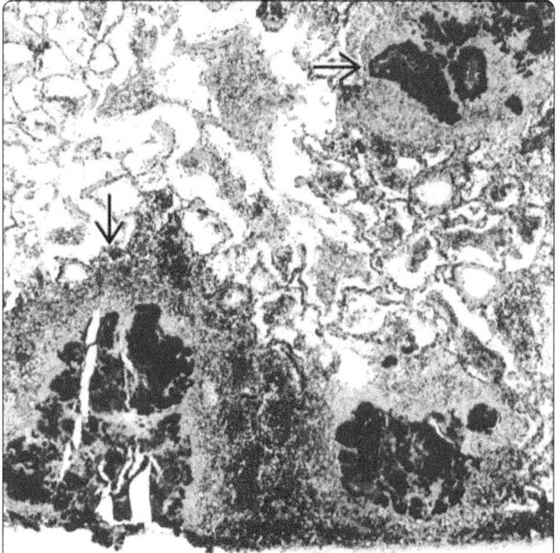

(Left) *Septic emboli from staphylococcal endocarditis can cause infected infarcts of distant organs ➡ (here, the brain). (Courtesy Franz von Lichtenberg Collection of Infectious Disease Pathology, BWH.)* **(Right)** *Septic emboli from staphylococcal endocarditis can cause infected infarcts of distant organs ➡ (here, the lung). (Courtesy Franz von Lichtenberg Collection of Infectious Disease Pathology, BWH.)*

KEY FACTS

ETIOLOGY/PATHOGENESIS

- *Streptococcus* spp. reside upon human or animal oropharyngeal, urogenital, and GI mucous membranes
- *Enterococcus* spp. reside within human or animal GI tract but able to persist in harsh environmental conditions
- Clinically relevant spp. include *S. pyogenes* (group A), *S. agalactiae* (group B), *S. dysgalactiae*, *S. pneumoniae*, *S. mitis* group, *S. anginosus* group, *S. salivarius* group, *S. mutans* group, *S. bovis* (*gallolyticus*) group, *E. faecium*, and *E. faecalis*

CLINICAL ISSUES

- *S. pyogenes*: Acute pharyngitis, skin/soft tissue infections
- *S. pneumoniae*: Pneumonia, bacteremia, meningitis, sinusitis, otitis media
- Viridans streptococci: Bacteremia, infective endocarditis, abscess, dental caries
- *S. agalactiae*: Infection of endometrium, placenta, cesarean section wounds, neonatal sepsis, meningitis
- *Enterococcus spp.*: Bacteremia, endocarditis, urinary tract infection, soft tissue infections

MICROSCOPIC

- Gram-positive cocci highlighted by Gram and silver stains
- *S. pyogenes* pneumonia: Marked edema, hemorrhage, abscess, and empyema; necrotic macrophages
- *S. pneumoniae* pneumonia: Nonnecrotizing; early-phase "red hepatization," marked by extensive edema, hemorrhage, and acute inflammation; late-phase "gray hepatization," marked by macrophage infiltrate
- Chorioamnionitis: Necrotizing, organisms often present

TOP DIFFERENTIAL DIAGNOSES

- Other bacterial infections: Gram-positive cocci (typically *Staphylococcus* spp.) and gram-positive or gram-negative bacilli; culture/PCR required for definitive diagnosis
- Viral pneumonia: Lack of gram staining for bacteria ± viral cytopathic effect; confirm by PCR

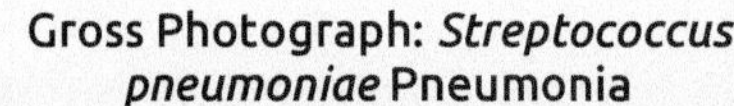

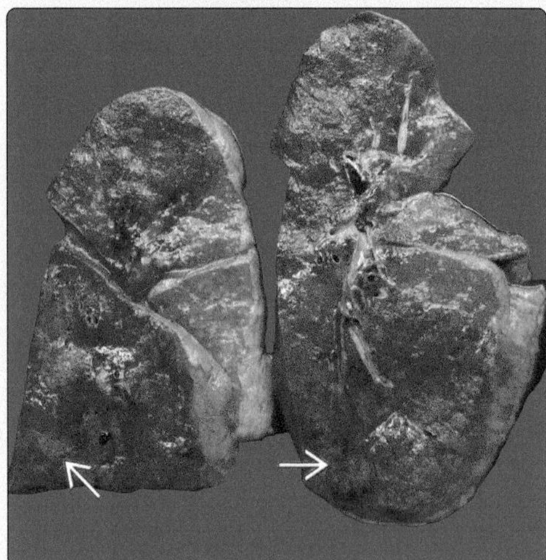

Streptococcus pneumoniae Gram Stain

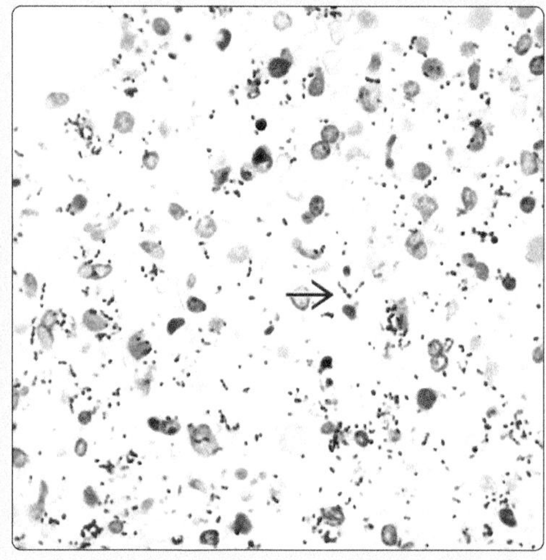

(Left) *These lungs from a patient who died of Streptococcus pneumoniae pneumonia demonstrate the heavy, mixed inflammatory exudates of red hepatization* ➡. **(Right)** *Numerous gram-positive cocci in pairs and chains* ➡ *are visible in the lungs of this patient who died from S. pneumoniae pneumonia.*

Acute Pneumonia With Hemorrhage

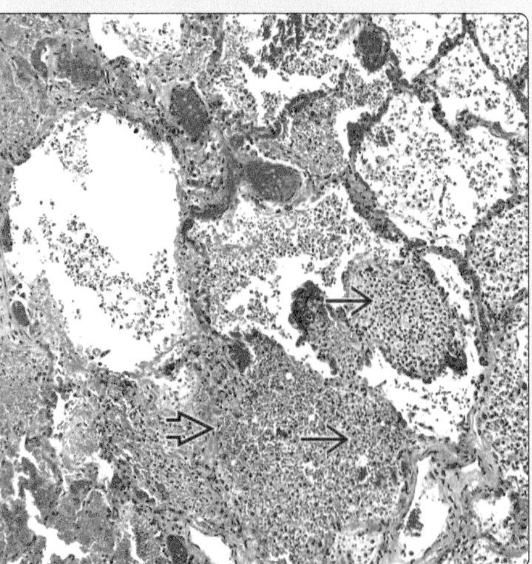

Bacteria on Tissue Section

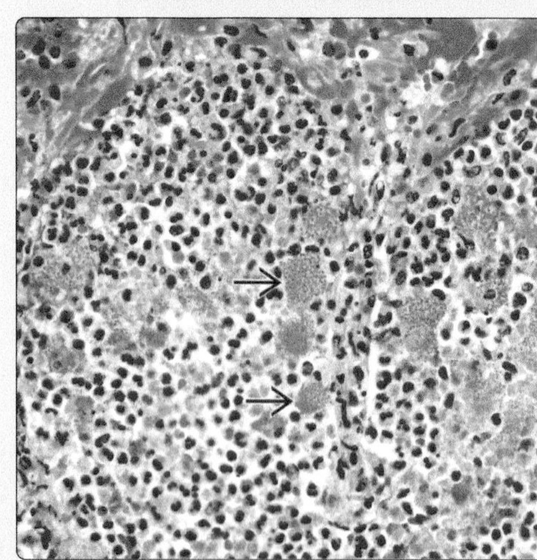

(Left) *Medium-power H&E shows acute pneumonia with patchy hemorrhage* ➡ *and dense, acute inflammation* ➡, *which is the histologic correlate of "red hepatization" noted on gross examination.* **(Right)** *This section is from the lung of a 20-year-old woman who died of sepsis. Blood cultures grew group C streptococci. Numerous clusters of cocci* ➡ *are seen.*

TERMINOLOGY

Definitions

- Greek: "Streptos" (twisted chain) + "kokkus" (grain)
- Greek: "Entero" (intestine) + "kokkus" (grain)

ETIOLOGY/PATHOGENESIS

Infectious Agents

- Streptococci reside upon human or animal oropharyngeal, urogenital, and GI mucous membranes, spread through direct contact or droplet exposure; clinically relevant species divided by hemolysis patterns
  - α-hemolytic groups: *S. pneumoniae*, *S. mitis* group, *S. salivarius* group, *S. mutans* group
  - β-hemolytic groups: *S. pyogenes* (group A), *S. agalactiae* (group B, a.k.a. GBS), and *S. dysgalactiae* (group C or G)
  - Nonhemolytic groups: *S. bovis* (*gallolyticus*) group
- Enterococci reside within human or animal GI tract; clinically relevant species (formerly known as group D streptococci) include nonhemolytic *E. faecium* and *E. faecalis*

CLINICAL ISSUES

Epidemiology

- *S. pyogenes* acute pharyngitis in 5-15 year olds
- *S. agalactiae* (GBS) neonatal disease from colonized mothers (10-30% of healthy adults); infections in patients with diabetes, alcoholism, and cancer
- *S. mutans* is primary colonizer of tooth surface
- *S. pneumoniae* colonizes nasopharynges of 30-70% of young children and 5% of adults
- *S. mitis*, *S. anginosus*, *S. salivarius*, and *S. mutans* groups (collectively called viridans streptococci) are most heavily concentrated in oral cavity but also found as commensals in GI tract, on skin, and in female genital tract
- *S. bovis* group found in alimentary tracts of ruminants
- *Enterococcus* spp. colonize large intestine, which is thought to be prerequisite for invasive disease

Presentation

- *S. pyogenes*, group A streptococci
  - Streptococcal pharyngitis ("strep throat"): Sore throat, malaise, high fever, headache, and GI symptoms; complicated by Scarlet fever, abscess, meningitis, pneumonia, rheumatic fever, poststreptococcal glomerulonephritis (PSGN)
  - Erysipelas: Infection of dermis (face or lower extremities) with lymphatic involvement; raised lesions, clear border between involved and uninvolved skin, strong red color
  - Streptococcal cellulitis: Infection involving skin (compromised by trauma or wounds) and subcutaneous tissues; lesions neither raised nor well demarcated
  - Necrotizing fasciitis: Infection of subcutaneous tissue and fascia, which results in rapidly spreading tissue necrosis (can evolve into myonecrosis); generally begins from site of minor trauma or surgery
  - Impetigo (pyoderma): Papule that evolves into vesicle and then into pustule (eventually crusts over and heals)
  - Also can present as bacteremia, pneumonia, and streptococcal toxic shock syndrome
- *S. pneumoniae*
  - Pneumonia (~ 25% of community-acquired pneumonia in USA); acute-onset cough, fatigue, shortness of breath, dyspnea, fever/sweats/chills, purulent sputum, and pleuritic chest pain; complicated by pleural effusion, empyema, endocarditis, meningitis
  - Common cause of otitis media and sinusitis
  - Meningitis: Caused by hematogenous or, less commonly, contiguous spread from sinuses or middle ear; headache, fever, neck stiffness
- *S. agalactiae* (GBS)
  - Bacteremia: Fever, chills, and change in mental status
  - Endometrium, placenta, infection of cesarean section wounds; endometritis low-grade fever, malaise, uterine tenderness; complicated by pelvic abscess, septic shock, or septic thrombophlebitis
  - Newborns infection include bacteremia, meningitis, and pneumonia
- Viridans streptococci
  - Transient bacteremia due to routine oral manipulations (e.g., tooth brushing) or contamination from skin; clinically significant in context of chemotherapy-induced neutropenia
  - Infective endocarditis (20% of cases): Background of preexisting heart disease, organisms from oral cavity; subacute progression with B symptoms, splenomegaly, Osler nodes, splinter hemorrhages, murmur
  - Meningitis, pneumonia, and endophthalmitis (particularly with injections for macular degeneration)
  - Anginosus group (*S. anginosus*, *S. intermedius*, and *S. constellatus*): Abscess formation of head and neck, CNS, abdominal cavity
  - *S. bovis* group (*S. gallolyticus*, *S. pasteurianus*, and *S. infantarius*): 11-17% of infective endocarditis cases; affects aortic valve; associated with colorectal malignancy and hepatobiliary disease
  - *S. mutans*: Dental caries
- *Enterococcus* spp.
  - Bacteremia: Source can be patient's own GI/GU tracts, wounds, or synthetic surfaces of urinary or intravascular catheters
  - Endocarditis (particularly *E. faecalis*): In context of damaged heart, procedures that perturb GI/GU tracts; typically subacute with B symptoms, fevers, murmurs
  - Also urinary tract infections (usually in catheterized patients), meningitis (uncommon), skin and soft tissue infections, and abdominal and pelvic infections (often as part of polymicrobial infection)
  - Common agent of wide spectrum of neonatal disease (due to presence in vagina)
  - Asymptomatic colonization: Hospitals may perform rectal screening for vancomycin-resistant enterococci (VRE) to guide isolation practices

Laboratory Tests

- Rapid antigen tests are useful for *S. pyogenes*: sensitivity (~ 80%) and specificity (~ 95%)
- Rapid assay BinaxNOW can detect C polysaccharide antigen of *S. pneumoniae* in urine and is 58-93% sensitive but not useful in children
- Detection of antibodies to streptolysin O and DNase B can be useful when evaluating for sequelae of streptococcal infection (e.g., rheumatic fever and PSGN)

- Several nucleic acid amplification technique (NAAT)-based platforms can diagnose streptococcal and enterococcal spp. directly from clinical specimens, including positive blood bottles and respiratory and CSF specimens
- NAAT detection of GBS directly from vaginorectal swabs (without broth enrichment) is not standard of care due to concerns for lower sensitivity
- Gram stains of clinical specimens (e.g., CSF, abscess, peritoneal fluid) can identify infections directly

Treatment

- Necrotizing fasciitis requires surgical debridement
- Endocarditis may require surgical repair of damaged valves
- *S. pyogenes* and *S. agalactiae:* Penicillin for treatment and prophylaxis of colonized pregnant women
- *S. pneumoniae*: Penicillin/amoxicillin, fluoroquinolones, doxycycline
- Enterococci: Vancomycin resistance is serious issue for *E. faecium* (VRE), ampicillin if susceptible

Prognosis

- Mortality ranges from 20-70% in streptococcal necrotizing fasciitis up to 80% in streptococcal myonecrosis

MICROBIOLOGY

Morphologic/Biochemical

- Facultatively anaerobic, catalase-negative, gram-positive cocci arranged in pairs and chains

Culture

- Cultured on 5% sheep's blood agar; colonies are usually white or gray (particularly enterococci) and glistening
- Small (< 0.5-mm) β-hemolytic colonies: Typical of *S. anginosus* group (along with strong "butterscotch" or "movie theater popcorn" smell)
- Large (0.5-mm) β-hemolytic colonies: *S. pyogenes, S. dysgalactiae, S. agalactiae*
- α-hemolytic colonies: Often formed by viridans streptococci as well as *S. pneumoniae*, which also can have characteristic depression in colony center
- γ-hemolytic (nonhemolytic) colonies: Enterococci

Microbiological Identification

- Streptococci divided into Lancefield groupings based on antibody reactivity to cell wall-associated carbohydrates (e.g., group B streptococci refers to Lancefield grouping)
  - Most medically significant groups are A, B, C, D, F, and G
  - Rapid assays to determine Lancefield group (e.g., Thermo Scientific/Remel PathoDextra and Streptex grouping kits) are widely available in clinical laboratories
- Both MALDI and VITEK platforms are widely used
- Several smaller scale identification strips can differentiate among streptococci, e.g., API strep strip (bioMérieux) and RapID strep strip (Remel)
- 16S rRNA sequencing can reliably distinguish genus but not always species-level identification

MACROSCOPIC

General Features

- Endocarditis: Vegetation may be seen on heart valves, size may range from thin veneer to bulky and obstructing
- Meningitis: Exudate may be seen coating surfaces of leptomeninges

MICROSCOPIC

Histologic Features

- Endocarditis: Subacute with few leukocytes; vegetations composed of fibrin, platelets, cellular debris, organisms, leukocytes
- Tonsillitis and peritonsillar abscess: Reactive lymphoid hyperplasia and fibrosis, may be complicated by abscess underneath capsule of palatine tonsil
- *S. pyogenes* pneumonia: Marked edema, hemorrhage, abscess, and empyema; necrotic macrophages and numerous bacteria may be seen
- *S. pneumoniae* pneumonia: Less acute, nonnecrotizing; early-phase "red hepatization," marked by extensive edema, hemorrhage, and acute inflammation; late-phase "gray hepatization," marked by macrophage infiltrate
- Erysipelas: Acute inflammation, edema, and, occasionally, subepidermal bullae
- Cellulitis: Inflammation in dermis and subcutaneous tissue, fat necrosis
- Necrotizing fasciitis: Acute inflammation and necrosis along fascial planes, more extensive than apparent from clinical exam
- Meningitis: Meningeal and parenchymal hemorrhage, neutrophilic infiltrate, arteritis obliterans, infarct, thrombosis, vasculitis, abscess
- CNS abscess: Core of necrotic debris, organisms, and neutrophils; rim of granulation tissue that matures into fibrous capsule
- Chorioamnionitis: Necrotizing, organisms often present

ANCILLARY TESTS

Special Stains

- Organisms typically highlighted by tissue Gram stain (may appear partially gram positive due to staining quality)
- Cocci may appear gram negative with slightly increased size due to antibiotic treatment effects

DIFFERENTIAL DIAGNOSIS

Other Bacterial Infections

- Gram-positive cocci: Most commonly *Staphylococcus* spp.
- Gram-positive or -negative rods: Culture required for definitive diagnosis

Viral Pneumonia

- Lack of gram staining for bacteria ± viral cytopathic effect

SELECTED REFERENCES

1. Brouwer S et al: Pathogenesis, epidemiology and control of Group A Streptococcus infection. Nat Rev Microbiol. 21(7):431-47, 2023
2. Dotters-Katz SK et al: Group B Streptococcus and pregnancy: critical concepts and management nuances. Obstet Gynecol Surv. 77(12):753-62, 2022
3. Pilarczyk-Zurek M et al: The clinical view on Streptococcus anginosus group - opportunistic pathogens coming out of hiding. Front Microbiol. 13:956677, 2022
4. Weiser JN et al: Streptococcus pneumoniae: transmission, colonization and invasion. Nat Rev Microbiol. 16(6):355-67, 2018
5. Arias CA et al: The rise of the Enterococcus: beyond vancomycin resistance. Nat Rev Microbiol. 10(4):266-78, 2012

Acute Rheumatic Fever

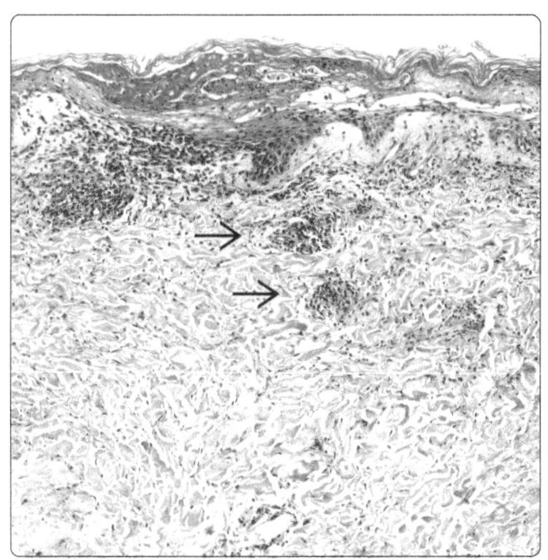

Rheumatic Fever Endocarditis

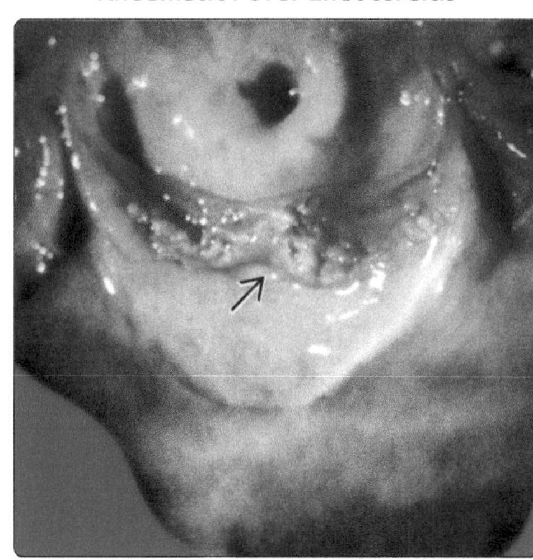

(Left) *Erythema marginatum is an uncommon manifestation of acute rheumatic fever (and a major Jones criterion). This specimen demonstrates perivascular infiltration of lymphocytes and neutrophils in the dermis* ➙*. (Courtesy B. Smoller, MD.)* **(Right)** *Gross photograph of poststreptococcal rheumatic fever demonstrates verrucae on the aortic valve cusp* ➙*. (Courtesy Franz von Lichtenberg Collection of Infectious Disease Pathology, BWH.)*

MR: Brain Abscess

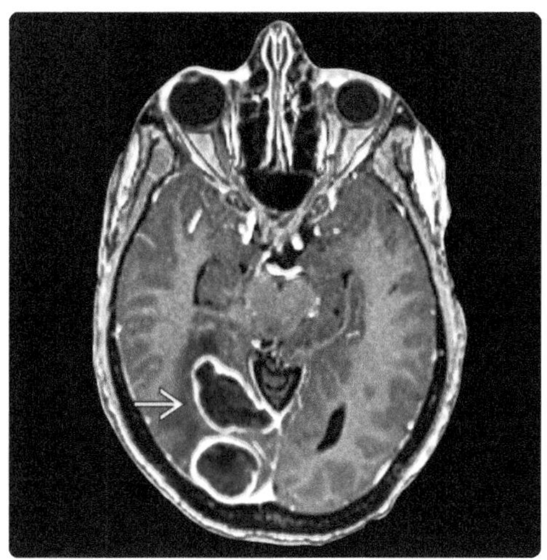

Brain Abscess

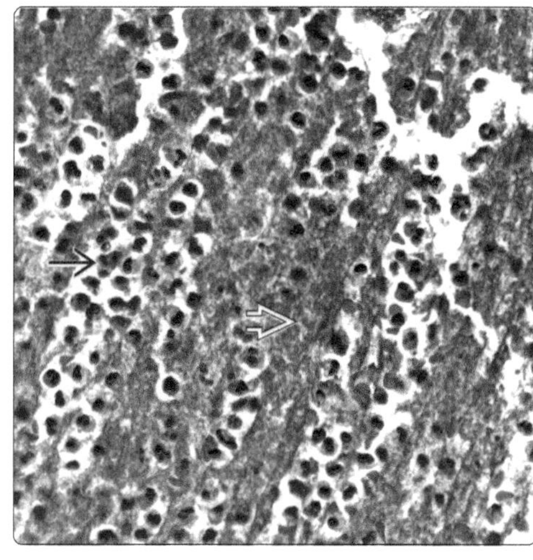

(Left) *This MR from a patient with a streptococcal brain abscess demonstrates ring-enhancing lesions* ➙*.* **(Right)** *High-power H&E from a streptococcal brain abscess shows sheets of neutrophils* ➙ *among a background of necrotic brain matter and necroinflammatory debris* ➙*.*

Staphylococcus intermedius Gram Stain

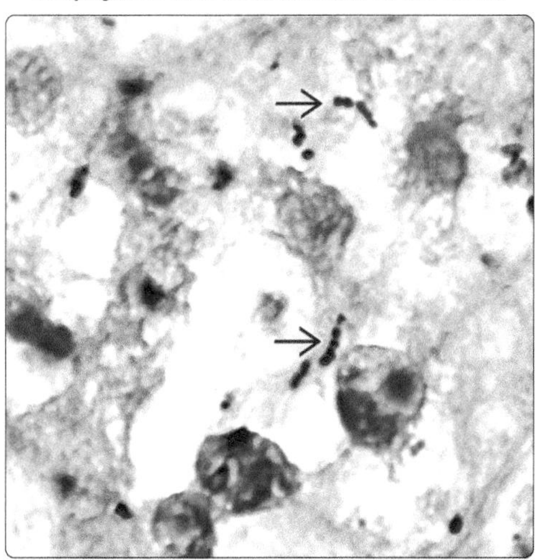

Erysipelas

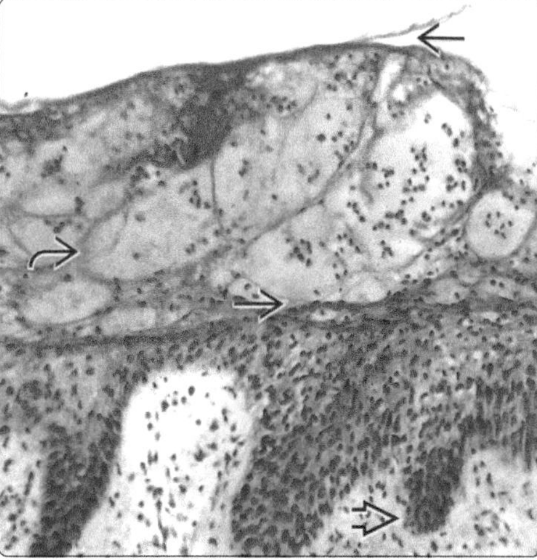

(Left) *This brain biopsy from a patient with streptococcal brain abscess demonstrates numerous gram-positive cocci in pairs and chains* ➙*. Cultures grew S. intermedius, a member of the anginosus group of streptococci known for its ability to cause invasive disease.* **(Right)** *In streptococcal erysipelas, there is intense, acute, exudative inflammation of all skin layers with edema* ➙*, blunting the dermal papillae* ➙*, and lifting the corneal layer* ➙*. (Courtesy Franz von Lichtenberg Collection of Infectious Disease Pathology, BWH.)*

Whipple Disease

KEY FACTS

ETIOLOGY/PATHOGENESIS

- Infection with *Tropheryma whipplei* (gram-positive bacilli)
- Extremely rare condition (1 case per million annually) with likely genetic predisposition
- Affects gastrointestinal tract, heart valves, central nervous system, and joints
- Asymptomatic carriage common

CLINICAL ISSUES

- Multisystem chronic infection in middle-aged adults (M > F)
- Considered great mimicker, diagnosis difficult
- Cardinal symptoms: Arthralgia, diarrhea, abdominal discomfort, and weight loss

MICROSCOPIC

- Dense collections of foamy macrophages within mucosa of small bowel is classic
- Loss of microvilli, lymphatic obstruction, and deposits of lipid in tissues
- In sites outside of gastrointestinal tract, macrophages containing organisms are found in variable numbers
- Organisms strongly PAS positive (diastase resistant); highlighted by GMS, Warthin-Starry, anti-*T. whipplei* IHC, *T. whipplei* RNA ISH; negative for AFB and tissue Gram stains
- PCR: Confirms presence of DNA in tissue sections

TOP DIFFERENTIAL DIAGNOSES

- *Mycobacterium avium* complex infection: AFB positive intracellular organisms
- *Rhodococcus* species infection: Gram-positive, AFB-positive coccobacilli associated with necrotizing granulomata or malakoplakia
- Histoplasmosis: Small oval yeast (2-4 μm) with narrow-based budding, associated with granulomatous inflammation; clustered within macrophages
- Sarcoidosis: Epithelioid granulomatous inflammation with multinucleated giant cells; PAS negative

Duodenal Mucosal Plaques

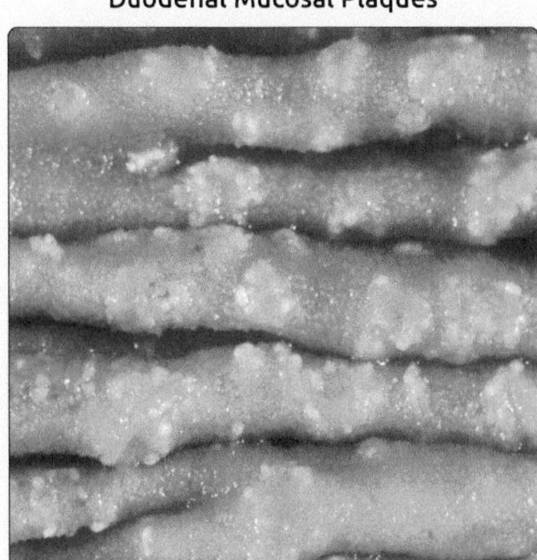

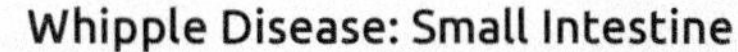

Whipple Disease: Small Intestine

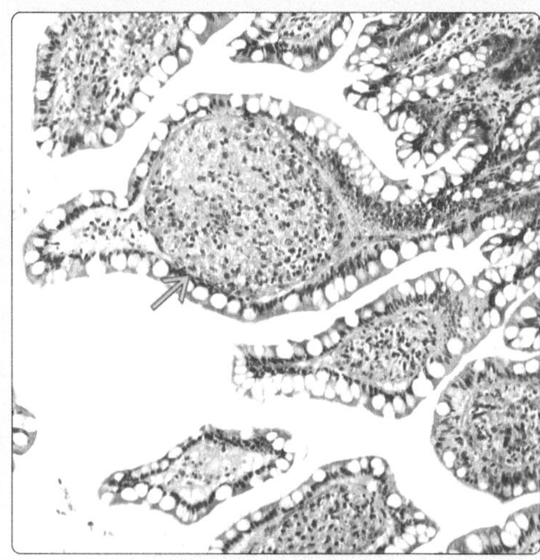

(Left) *Innumerable nodular, white-yellow plaques are present on the duodenal mucosal surface in this patient with Whipple disease. (Courtesy F. Mitros, MD, A. Bellizzi, MD.)* **(Right)** *This H&E-stained section shows distended small intestinal villi ⇒ filled with foamy histiocytes.*

***Tropheryma whipplei*: PAS-D Stain**

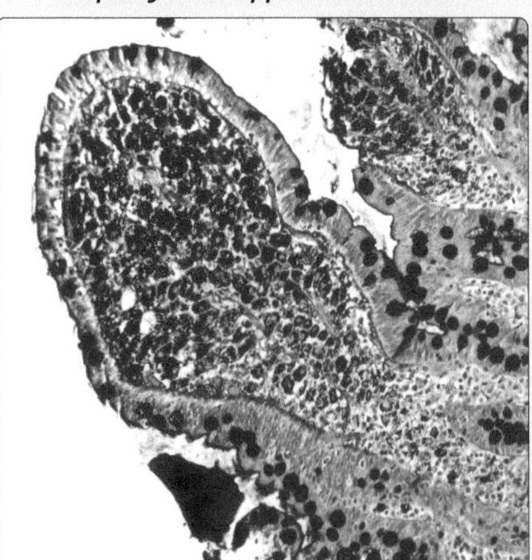

Negative AFB Staining

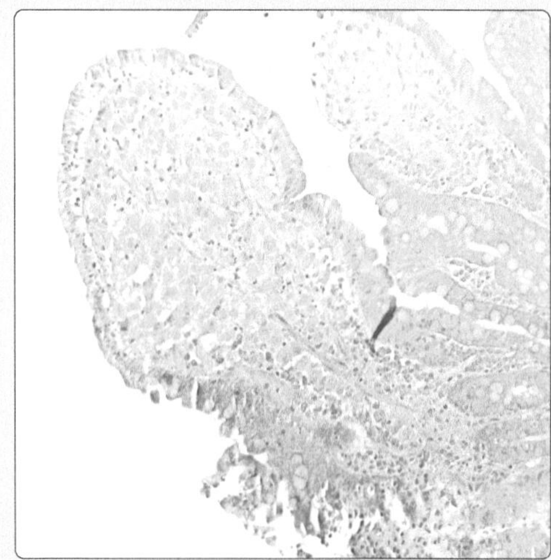

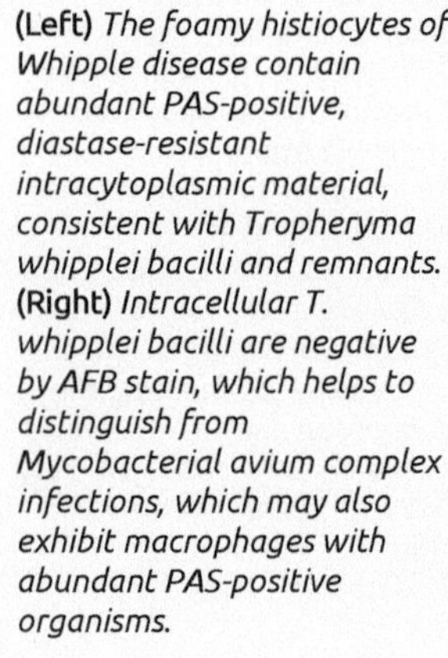

(Left) *The foamy histiocytes of Whipple disease contain abundant PAS-positive, diastase-resistant intracytoplasmic material, consistent with Tropheryma whipplei bacilli and remnants.* **(Right)** *Intracellular T. whipplei bacilli are negative by AFB stain, which helps to distinguish from Mycobacterial avium complex infections, which may also exhibit macrophages with abundant PAS-positive organisms.*

TERMINOLOGY

Synonyms

- Intestinal lipodystrophy, *Tropheryma whipplei* infection

Definitions

- Greek: "Trophe" (food) + "eruma" (barrier)
- From George Hoyt Whipple (first described)

ETIOLOGY/PATHOGENESIS

Infectious Agents

- Infection with *T. whipplei* (gram-positive bacilli) via fecal-oral transmission; bacteria infect and replicate in macrophages
- Commonly found in soil, sewage, and gastrointestinal tract and oral cavity of healthy persons

CLINICAL ISSUES

Epidemiology

- Extremely rare condition (1 case per million annually); most cases reported in Europe and USA
- Male predominance (> 85%)
- Genetic predispositions (e.g., HLA DRB1*13 and DQB1*06)

Presentation

- Chronic systemic infection affecting gastrointestinal tract, joints, and central nervous system, usually middle aged (~ 55 years)
- Weight loss, hypoalbuminemia, diarrhea (steatorrhea), arthralgias, migratory arthritis, and anemia in > 80%
- Lymphadenopathy, abdominal pain, skin pigmentation, fever, and neurologic signs (headaches, cognitive changes) in < 50% of patients
- Culture-negative endocarditis (native or implants): Slowly progressive, signs of heart failure without fever
- CNS involvement: Mass lesion, dementia, ataxia, diplopia; oculomasticatory myorhythmia is pathognomonic
- Other presentations: Fever and cough, pneumonia, isolated gastroenteritis (children)
- Asymptomatic carriage varies by geographic region and age (2-75%), highest in children and in regions with poor sanitary conditions
- May be associated with immunosuppression and immune reconstitution syndrome

Laboratory Tests

- PCR (16S rRNA or targeted PCR) may be performed on CSF, joint fluid, urine, saliva, or stool
  - High rates of asymptomatic carriage may make result interpretation difficult; confirmed by 2nd test (biopsy, PCR from sterile site, etc.)
  - Can be used to gauge treatment response
- Role of serology uncertain due to high rates of exposure and reduced/abnormal immune responses in diseased

Treatment

- Regimens vary, most recommendations include parental course for 2-4 weeks (ceftriaxone, penicillin, trimethoprim-sulfamethoxazole), followed by 1+ year(s) of oral therapy
- For CNS treatment, intravenous drugs are required
- For immune reconstitution inflammatory syndrome (IRIS), supportive therapy (corticosteroids, cytokines) is required in addition to antibiotics

Prognosis

- CNS involvement: Mortality 100% without antibiotic therapy, relapse common
- Endocarditis: Mortality 10-25%

IMAGING

Radiographic Findings

- Chest x-ray: Pleural effusions and pulmonary infiltrates
- Abdominal CT: Duodenum may show thickening and lymphadenopathy

MICROBIOLOGY

Bacterial Characteristics and Culture

- Small (0.25-0.30 μm by 0.80-1.7 μm) nonmotile gram-positive bacilli (actinobacteria)
- Potentially obligate intracellular pathogen due to its reduced genome size (depleted of several crucial pathways) and proteome similar to other intracellular pathogens
- Unable to culture by routine methods (slow growth rate, requires cell cocultivation)

MACROSCOPIC

General Features

- Small intestine: Endoscopy may show villous flattening, mucosal edema, with yellow speckled appearance
- Heart: Infected valves contain small, yellow vegetations

MICROSCOPIC

Histologic Features

- Small intestine: Dense collections of mucosal foamy macrophages with vacuolated, pale blue-gray cytoplasm
- Liver, esophagus, stomach, colon, heart, brain, and other tissues show variable numbers of macrophages in sheets, cords, or nests; loss of microvilli, lymphatic obstruction, and deposits of lipid in tissues
- Lymph nodes: Macrophage infiltrates with nonnecrotizing granulomatous inflammation
- In minimal disease, macrophages may be scattered, and special stains difficult to interpret

ANCILLARY TESTS

Histochemistry

- Bacilli within macrophages appear as PAS-positive, diastase-resistant granular material
- Positive on Warthin-Starry, Steiner, and GMS stains
- Weak to negative staining with tissue Gram stains
- Negative acid-fast bacilli stains

Immunohistochemistry

- Anti-*T. whipplei* antibodies confirm presence of bacteria in tissue

In Situ Hybridization

- Confirms infection (vs. contamination) in tissue sections using RNA targets

Electron Microscopy

- Bacteria with trilaminar cell wall structure

DIFFERENTIAL DIAGNOSIS

Mycobacterium avium Complex Infection

- Dense collections of AFB-positive macrophages in gastrointestinal tract (usually small bowel)

Rhodococcus Species Infection

- Coccobacillary organisms highlighted by Gram, GMS, and AFB stains, associated with necrotizing granulomatous inflammation or malakoplakia

Histoplasmosis

- Small oval yeast (2-4 μm) with narrow-based budding, frequently clustered within macrophages, and associated with granulomatous inflammation

Sarcoidosis

- Epithelioid granulomatous inflammation with multinucleated giant cells; negative for PAS

SELECTED REFERENCES

1. Ioannou P et al: Whipple's disease-associated infective endocarditis: a systematic review. Infect Dis (Lond). 55(7):447-57, 2023
2. Meyer S et al: Contribution of PCR to differential diagnosis between patients with Whipple disease and Tropheryma whipplei carriers. J Clin Microbiol. 61(2):e0145722, 2023
3. Makka S et al: Tropheryma whipplei intestinal colonization in migrant children, Greece. Emerg Infect Dis. 28(9):1926-8, 2022
4. Duss FR et al: Whipple disease: a 15-year retrospective study on 36 patients with positive polymerase chain reaction for Tropheryma whipplei. Clin Microbiol Infect. 27(6):910.e9-13, 2021
5. Feurle GE et al: Tropheryma whipplei in feces of patients with diarrhea in 3 locations on different continents. Emerg Infect Dis. 27(3):932-5, 2021
6. Moter A et al: Potential role for urine polymerase chain reaction in the diagnosis of Whipple's disease. Clin Infect Dis. 68(7):1089-97, 2019
7. Loiodice A et al: Transmission electron microscopy helpfulness in Whipple's disease masked by immunosuppressant therapy for arthritis. APMIS. 126(1):92-6, 2018
8. Saito H et al: Whipple's disease with long-term endoscopic follow-up. Intern Med. 57(12):1707-13, 2018
9. Boban M et al: Cytology of cerebrospinal fluid in CNS Whipple disease. Acta Neurol Belg. 117(4):935-6, 2017
10. Dolmans RA et al: Clinical manifestations, treatment, and diagnosis of Tropheryma whipplei infections. Clin Microbiol Rev. 30(2):529-55, 2017

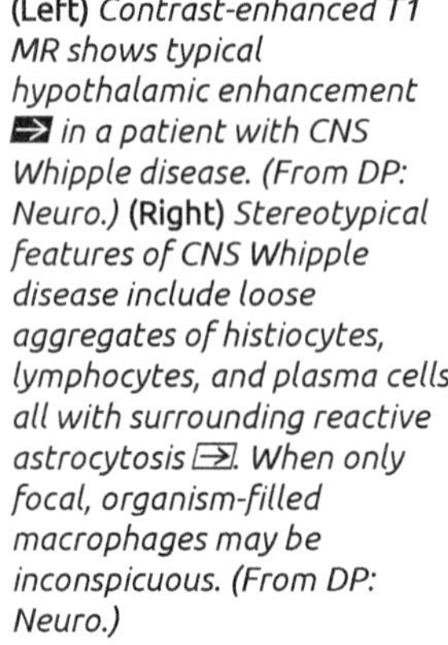

(Left) *Contrast-enhanced T1 MR shows typical hypothalamic enhancement ➡ in a patient with CNS Whipple disease. (From DP: Neuro.)* **(Right)** *Stereotypical features of CNS Whipple disease include loose aggregates of histiocytes, lymphocytes, and plasma cells, all with surrounding reactive astrocytosis ➡. When only focal, organism-filled macrophages may be inconspicuous. (From DP: Neuro.)*

CNS Whipple Disease: MR Features

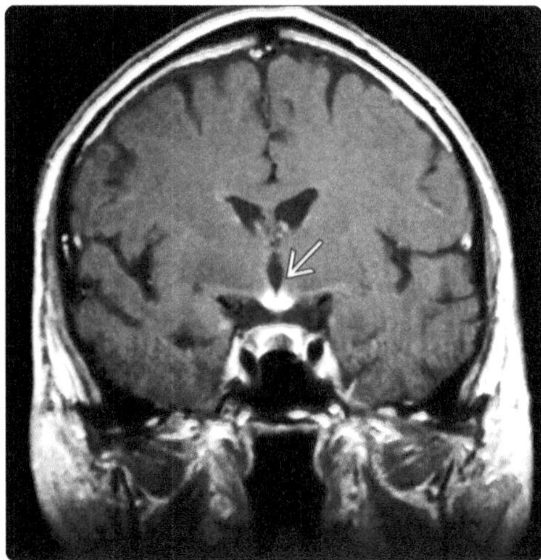

CNS Whipple Disease: Inflammation and Reactive Astrocytes

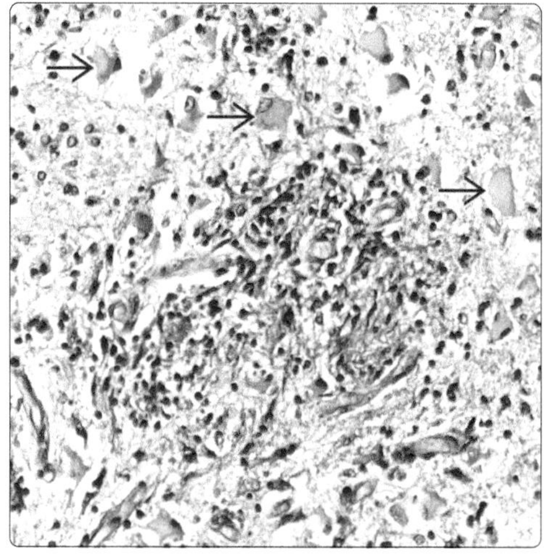

(Left) *A grayish tinge is helpful when suspecting that the cytoplasm of macrophages is filled with organisms rather than generic, phagocytized debris. Organisms are so numerous that they cannot be individually resolved. (From DP: Neuro.)* **(Right)** *Immunostaining for the bacteria T. whipplei is a definitive diagnostic test, although not widely available outside of reference laboratories. (From DP: Neuro.)*

CNS Whipple Disease: Infected Macrophages

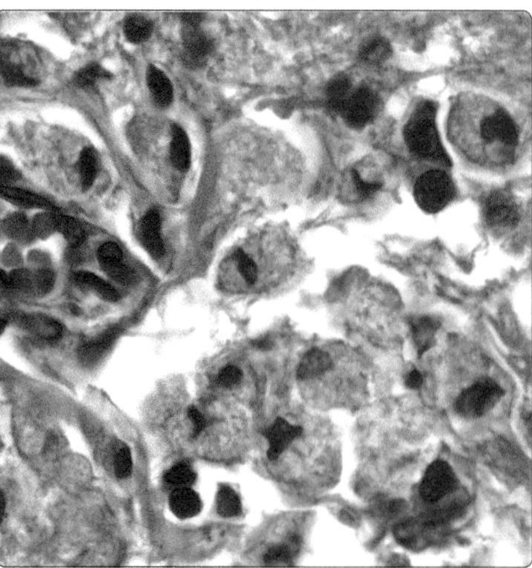

CNS Whipple Disease: *Tropheryma whipplei* IHC

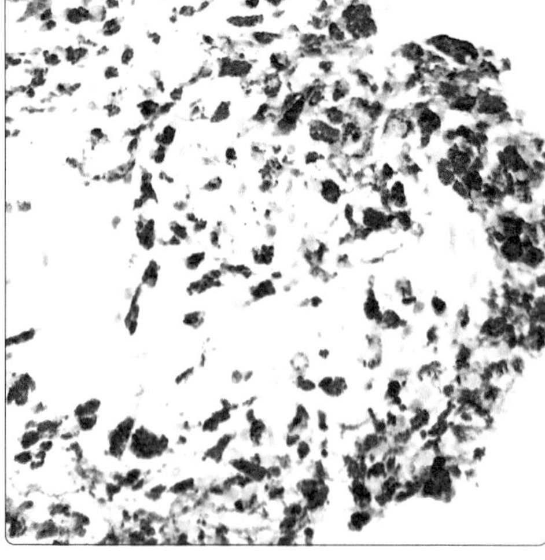

Cardiac Involvement of Whipple Disease

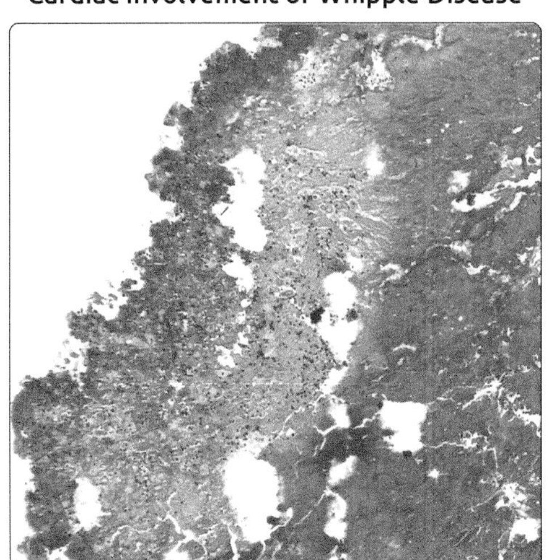

Cardiac Vegetation: Foamy Histiocytes

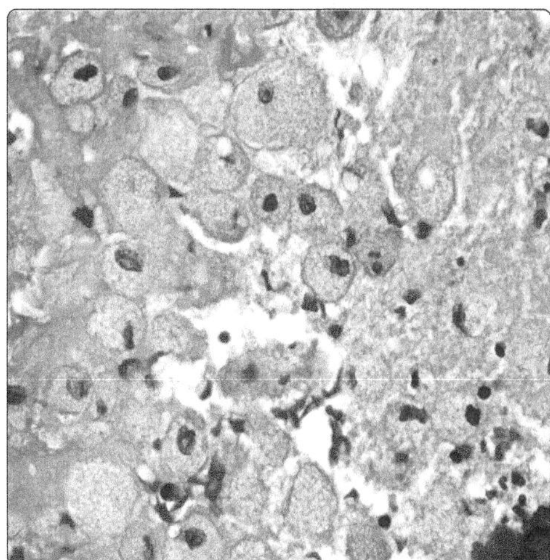

(Left) *H&E sections of heart valve vegetation from a case of culture-negative endocarditis shows foci of foamy histiocytes.* **(Right)** *High magnification images reveal numerous histiocytes with abundant, intracytoplasmic, amphophilic material with a bluish hue.*

Cardiac Vegetation: PAS-D Stain

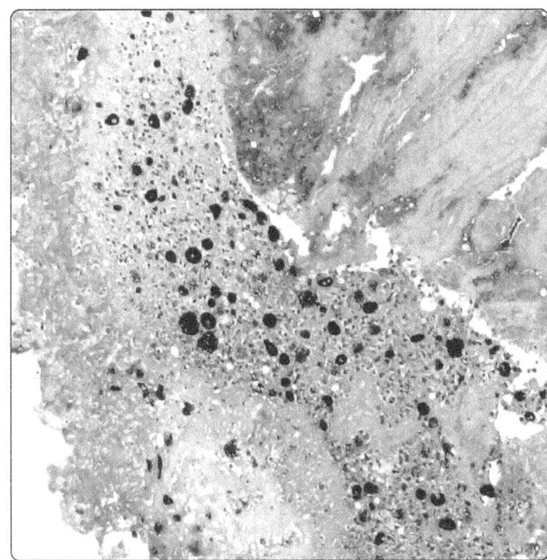

Cardiac Involvement of Whipple Disease: PAS-D Stain

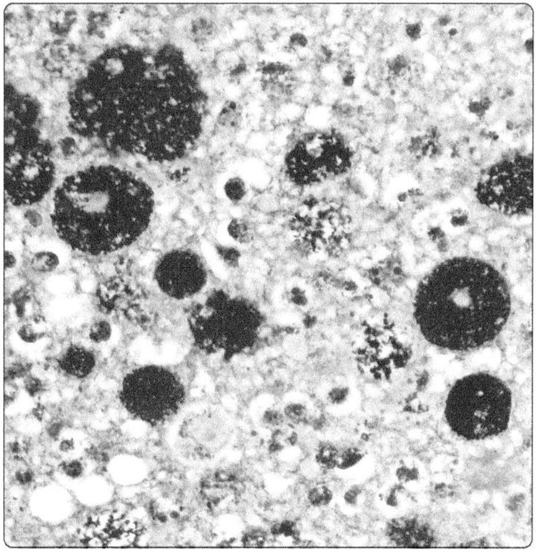

(Left) *Scattered foamy macrophages in this heart valve vegetation specimen are strongly PAS positive, consistent with cardiac involvement of Whipple disease.* **(Right)** *The foamy histiocytes contain abundant PAS-positive, diastase-resistant intracytoplasmic material, consistent with T. whipplei bacilli and remnants.*

Methenamine Silver Stain

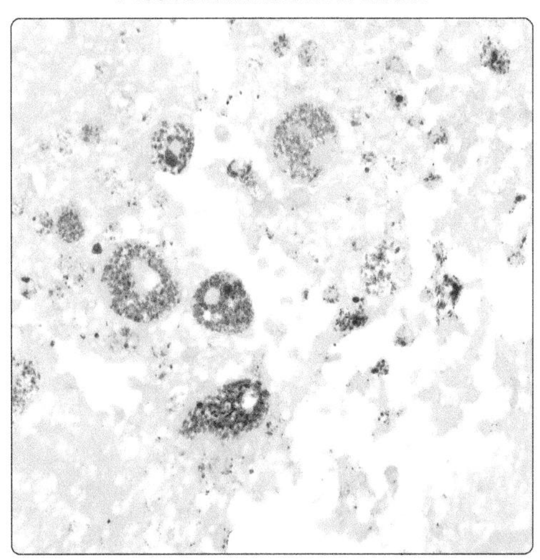

Tissue Gram Stain

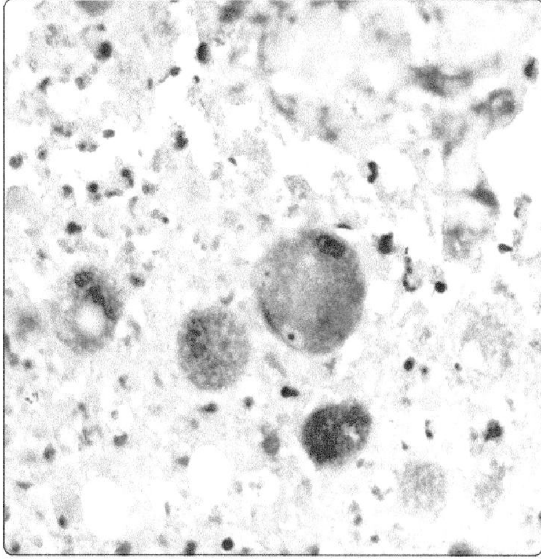

(Left) *T. whipplei bacilli can be highlighted by Gomori methenamine silver stain (as shown here) as well as by Warthin-Starry and Steiner silver stains.* **(Right)** *While T. whipplei is a gram-positive bacillus, tissue Gram staining of the bacterium within macrophages is typically negative due to the abundance of PAS-positive material coating the bacterial surface.*

Pathologically Important Enterobacterales: *Escherichia, Shigella, Salmonella, Klebsiella*, and *Yersinia* Species Infections

KEY FACTS

ETIOLOGY/PATHOGENESIS AND CLINICAL ISSUES

- Enterobacterales are facultatively anaerobic, gram-negative bacilli, residing both within gut and widely in nature
- Intestinal *Escherichia coli* include enterotoxigenic *E. coli* (ETEC), enteropathogenic *E. coli* (EPEC), enteroaggregative *E. coli* (EAEC), enterohemorrhagic *E. coli* (EHEC), and enteroinvasive *E. coli* (EIEC)
- Shiga toxin-producing *E. coli* (STEC) and EHEC associated with hemorrhagic colitis and hemolytic-uremic syndrome
- Extraintestinal *E. coli* (ExPEC): UTIs, sepsis, etc.
- *Shigella* species: Enteritis and bacillary dysentery
- *Salmonella* species: Typhoid and enteritis
- *Enterobacter, Serratia, Citrobacter, Proteus, Providencia, Morganella* species: Wide spectrum of disease (UTI, bacteremia, pneumonia, liver abscess)
- *Klebsiella* species: Pneumonia, UTIs, liver abscess; rhinoscleroma (*K. rhinoscleromatis),* granuloma inguinale (*K. granulomatis*)
- *Y. enterocolitica*: Enterocolitis, mesenteric adenitis, terminal ileitis, exudative pharyngitis
- *Y. pestis*: Plague (3 forms): Primary bubonic (majority of cases), septicemic, pneumonic

MICROBIOLOGY

- Most species grow on standard laboratory media (1-2 days); identified by automated typing systems (including MALDI)
- Molecular detection directly from stool, blood, or respiratory samples; usually part of syndromic panels

DIFFERENTIAL DIAGNOSIS

- Gastroenteritis caused by other bacteria (e.g., *Clostridioides difficile, Campylobacter jejuni*) and viruses (rotavirus, norovirus); confirm by culture, PCR
- Pneumonia caused by other bacteria (e.g., pneumococcus, *Mycoplasma pneumoniae*); confirm by culture, PCR
- Other infectious causes of granulomatous nasal swellings: tuberculosis, leprosy, leishmaniasis, sarcoidosis; lack Mikulicz cells of rhinoscleroma

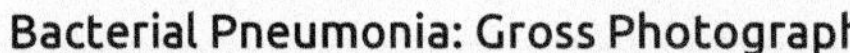

Bacterial Pneumonia: Gross Photograph

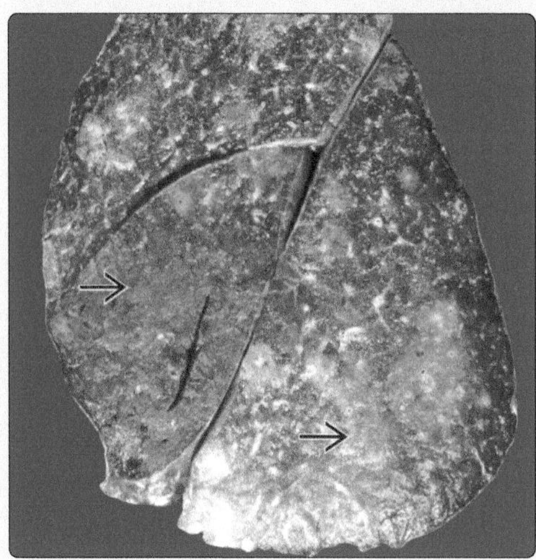

Air Space Inflammation

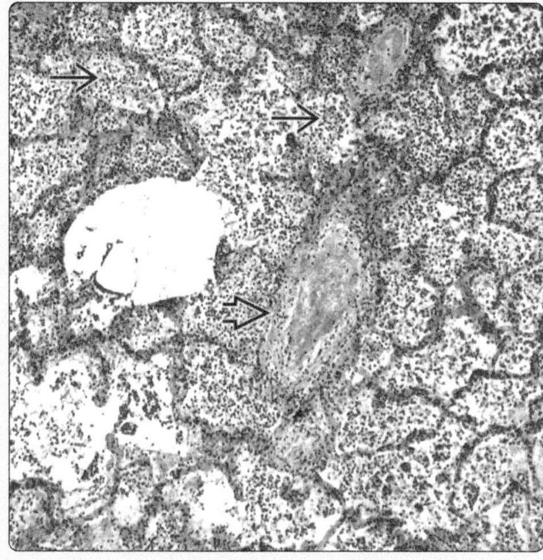

(Left) *This gross photograph demonstrates confluent pneumonia ⇨ caused by Escherichia coli and Enterobacter cloacae. (Courtesy Franz von Lichtenberg Collection of Infectious Disease Pathology, BWH.)* **(Right)** *A lung with enteric pneumonia shows inflammation filling air spaces ⇨ and involving bronchioles and vessels ⇨. (Courtesy Franz von Lichtenberg Collection of Infectious Disease Pathology, BWH.)*

Bronchopneumonia: Gross Photograph

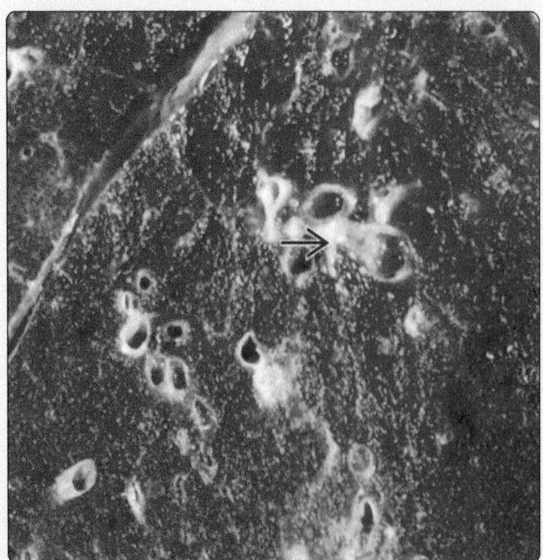

Alveolar Wall Necrosis

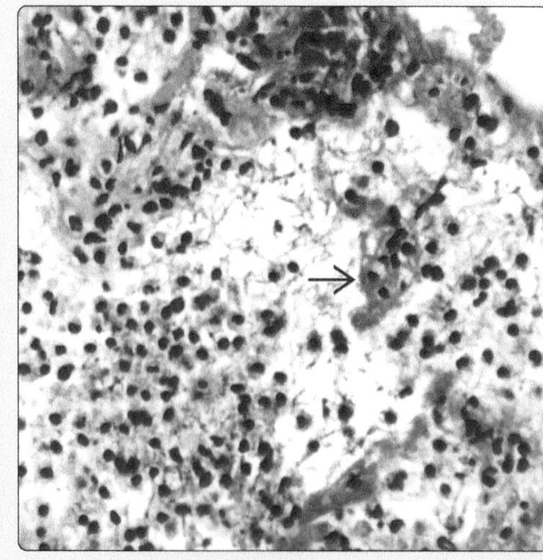

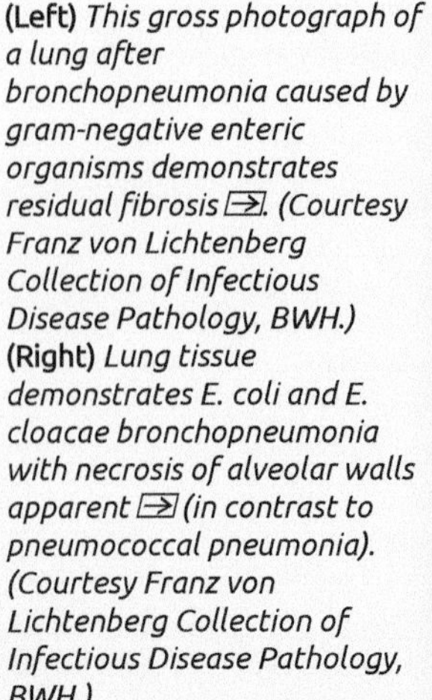

(Left) *This gross photograph of a lung after bronchopneumonia caused by gram-negative enteric organisms demonstrates residual fibrosis ⇨. (Courtesy Franz von Lichtenberg Collection of Infectious Disease Pathology, BWH.)* **(Right)** *Lung tissue demonstrates E. coli and E. cloacae bronchopneumonia with necrosis of alveolar walls apparent ⇨ (in contrast to pneumococcal pneumonia). (Courtesy Franz von Lichtenberg Collection of Infectious Disease Pathology, BWH.)*

TERMINOLOGY

Synonyms

- *Yersinia* infection: Plague, pneumonic or bubonic plague
- *Salmonella enterica* serotype typhi: Typhoid fever, enteric fever

Definitions

- "*Escherichia*" named after German-Austrian pediatrician Theodor Escherich who found organism in stool "coli"
- "*Klebsiella*" named after microbiologist Edwin Klebs; also referred to as Friedlander bacillus after Carl Friedlander
- "Shigellosis" named after Kiyoshi Shiga
- "Salmonellosis" named after Daniel Elmer Salmon (veterinary surgeon and pathologist)
- "*Yersinia*" named after Alexandre Yersin (1863-1943), who discovered that *Yersinia pestis* was causative agent of plague

INFECTIOUS AGENTS: EPIDEMIOLOGY, CLINICAL PRESENTATION, AND PATHOGENESIS

General Characteristics

- Enterobacterales are facultatively anaerobic, gram-negative bacilli consisting of many members, residing both within gut and widely in nature

Escherichia coli

- Enterotoxigenic *E. coli* (ETEC)
  - Associated with "traveler's diarrhea" and is spread via contaminated food and water
  - Causes watery diarrhea, nausea, and cramps (no fecal blood, mucus, or leukocytes)
- Enteropathogenic *E. coli* (EPEC)
  - In developed world, mainly associated with nosocomial diarrhea
  - Spread person to person
  - Disease may be more severe than that caused by ETEC, and symptoms may include fever, vomiting, weight loss, and malnutrition
- Shiga toxin-producing and enterohemorrhagic *E. coli* (STEC and EHEC)
  - Causes mostly food-borne illness, bloody or watery diarrhea (± fever); associated with undercooked beef and produce
  - Hemorrhagic colitis and hemolytic-uremic syndrome (HUS) are serious complications
  - Pathogenesis of STEC strains is mediated by Shiga toxins, STX1, and STX2 (Shiga-like toxins) and encoded on temperate bacteriophage, which is toxic to host cell ribosome
  - Stressors to bacterial cell (such as antibiotics) cause induction of toxin and are therefore contraindicated
  - Once released, toxin can disseminate throughout body
  - Targeting of endothelial cells is linked with creation of microvascular thrombi and development of HUS
- Enteroaggregative *E. coli* (EAEC)
  - Growing cause of diarrhea among many groups, including children, travelers, and immunocompromised
  - May be associated with both acute and chronic diarrhea
  - Clinical course is marked by abdominal cramping, hematochezia, and passage of mucus
- Enteroinvasive *E. coli* (EIEC)
  - Very similar to strains of *Shigella*
  - Ranges clinically from watery diarrhea to dysentery
  - Once taken up by phagocytic cell, EIEC can escape from phagosome, replicate in cytoplasm, and employ host actin to spread from cell to cell
- Extraintestinal pathogenic *E. coli* (ExPEC)
  - Grouping of strains that cause infection outside gut
  - UTIs and sepsis most common
  - Particular virulence factors tend to be associated with these strains as opposed to intestinal *E. coli*

Shigella Species

- Clinically important species include *Shigella sonnei* (most common), *Shigella dysenteriae*, and *Shigella flexneri*
- Spread from person to person and is considered most infectious bacterial diarrhea (requires very small inoculum)
- *Shigella* (along with EIEC) is causative agent of bacillary dysentery; fever, abdominal cramping, and watery diarrhea followed by frequent, smaller volume bowel movements containing mucus &/or blood
- Some strains express Shiga toxin (usually *S. dysenteriae*)

Enterobacter, Serratia, Citrobacter, Proteus, Providencia, Morganella Species

- Usually implicated as agents of wide spectrum of disease (UTI, bacteremia, pneumonia) in hospital patients
- Virulence factors include inducible, chromosomal β-lactamase in *Enterobacter*, *Serratia*, *Citrobacter*, and *Morganella* species
- *Proteus* species, particularly *Proteus mirabilis*, are noteworthy cause of UTIs, particularly in catheterized patients
- *Proteus* species UTI more severe than *E. coli* with higher proportion developing into pyelonephritis and causing bacteremia

Salmonella Species

- Clinically relevant strains are serotypes of *Salmonella enterica* subspecies *enterica*
  - Within these, there is basic division between *Salmonella* ser. Typhi and nontyphoidal *Salmonella*, including serotypes Typhimurium, Enteritidis, and Newport
- *Salmonella* ser. Typhi
  - Humans are only known reservoir; bacteria can be shed in stools of convalescent patients
  - Typhoid (enteric fever) is characteristically bimodal with initial period (1-2 weeks) of fever and constipation with positive blood cultures followed by diarrheic phase with positive stool cultures
  - Complications include intestinal hemorrhage and perforation, encephalitis, neuropsychiatric symptoms
- Most other nontyphoidal *Salmonella* serotypes cause food-borne illness and are associated with animals (poultry, beef, and dairy products) as well as fresh produce
  - Also associated with certain pets, e.g., lizards, turtles, frogs, and snakes
  - Most common clinical manifestation of *Salmonella* infection is gastroenteritis

- Usually presents 1-2 days after eating contaminated food; watery, nonbloody diarrhea, fever, nausea, vomiting, and abdominal cramping
- Symptoms generally last 3-7 days with fecal carriage of organisms continuing for 4-5 weeks
- Bacteremia occurs in up to 8% of patients
- *Salmonella* may infect vascular sites or disseminate to extraintestinal sites, such as blood, bone, and joints, meninges
- Patients with sickle cell disease, HIV, acute or recent malaria are particularly vulnerable

Klebsiella Species

- Clinically relevant species are *Klebsiella pneumoniae*, *Klebsiella oxytoca*, and *Klebsiella granulomatis*
  - *K. pneumoniae*
    - Implicated in pneumonia, UTIs, and liver abscess in immunocompetent patients
    - Among hospital patients, *K. pneumoniae* is isolated as frequent cause of wound infection, sepsis, and other manifestations
    - Pneumonia caused by *K. pneumoniae* is termed Friedlander disease due to characteristic severity, tendency to include abscess, location in upper lobes, association with currant-jelly-sputum appearance and bulging-fissure sign on radiographs, and propensity for alcoholic patients
  - *K. pneumoniae* subspecies *rhinoscleromatis* is agent of rhinoscleroma
    - Chronic granulomatous infection of respiratory tract (particularly nasal passages)
    - Most common in developing countries
  - *K. oxytoca*
    - Less frequently isolated than *K. pneumoniae* but responsible for similar spectrum of disease in hospitalized patients
  - *K. granulomatis*
    - Responsible for chronic genital ulcerative disease (granuloma inguinale)
    - Spreads through contact with open sores

Yersinia Species

- Clinically relevant species: *Yersinia enterocolitica*, *Y. pseudotuberculosis*, and *Y. pestis*
  - *Y. enterocolitica*
    - Food-borne pathogen with reports of diverse sources (often pigs and pork products)
    - Clinical manifestations of *Y. enterocolitica* infection include enterocolitis (fever, diarrhea ± blood/mucous, abdominal pain), mesenteric adenitis, terminal ileitis, and exudative pharyngitis
    - May be mistaken for acute appendicitis
    - Extraintestinal manifestations
      - Septicemia is uncommon but severe manifestation in immunocompromised, older adults, and patients with iron overload and can be associated with contaminated blood products
      - Reactive polyarthritis in 15% of patients, erythema nodosum reported
  - *Y. pseudotuberculosis*
    - Mesenteric adenitis (fever and right lower quadrant pain)
  - *Y. pestis*
    - Associated with exposure to rodents and their fleas
    - Exposure can be cutaneous or inhalational
    - Within USA, most common in western states
    - Causative agent of plague; 3 distinct forms: Primary bubonic (majority of cases), septicemic, and pneumonic
    - Primary bubonic plague presents with headache, chills, high fever, and buboes (swollen lymph nodes) developing in neck, groin, or axilla
    - Septicemic plague is rapidly progressive disease leading to organ failure; buboes are not apparent
    - Pneumonic plague (primary from inhalation or secondary via hematogenous spread) is also rapidly progressive, moving from fever, malaise, headache, and cough to hypoxia, hemoptysis, chest pain, and dyspnea within 1-2 days

LABORATORY TESTING, TREATMENT, AND PROGNOSIS

Laboratory Tests

- Gram stain and culture
- Detection of Shiga toxin from primary samples (PCR, immunoassay)
- Molecular detection directly from stool, blood, or respiratory samples; usually part of larger (syndromic) panels

Treatment

- Certain cases of gastrointestinal tract-origin, gram-negative infections require surgical interventions, such as infective endocarditis (valve replacement)
- Antibiotic treatment typically based on isolate susceptibility and source of infection
- Acquired resistance to multiple classes of antibiotics is major problem among Enterobacterales

Prognosis

- Varies widely with host status and organism

MICROBIOLOGY

Morphologic and Biochemical Characteristics

- Gram-negative bacilli
- Ability to ferment lactose is major branchpoint in identification of enteric gram-negative rods
  - Species of *Salmonella*, *Shigella*, *Proteus*, and *Yersinia* do not ferment lactose

Culture

- Organisms with specific culture requirements/characteristics
  - *E. coli* O157:H7, prominent EHEC organism, is identified by culture on sorbitol-MacConkey agar
  - Cefsulodin-irgasan-novobiocin (CIN) agar is used for selection and differentiation of *Yersinia* species

Microbiologic Identification

- Several tests for biochemical reactions are available as rapid, bench-top assays that make most routine identifications, e.g., oxidase and indole production

- Automated typing systems [including matrix-assisted laser desorption/ionization (MALDI)] and manual strips are widely used in clinical laboratories to identify enteric organisms
- *Yersinia* species
  - *Y. pestis* may be cultured and identified in normal clinical laboratory, though lab may not store or continue to work on strain for > 7 days after identification
  - Automated typing systems are notoriously poor at identifying *Yersinia* species
  - MALDI can detect several species but may not diagnose *Y. pestis* unless appropriate library is used
- Intestinal *E. coli* strains are not differentiated in routine clinical laboratories (i.e., ETEC) with exception of detection of Shiga toxin
  - Several assays are available for specific detection of Shiga toxin (PCR, immunoassay, etc.)

HISTOPATHOLOGY BY ORGAN SYSTEM

Central Nervous System

- Meningitis
  - Gram-negative meningitis is associated with sepsis, trauma, neurosurgical procedures, and disseminated strongyloidiasis in hyperinfection syndrome
  - Cytospin preparations demonstrate sheets of neutrophils in CSF
  - Gram-negative bacilli likely present on Gram stain (extracellular and within phagocytic cells)
- Brain abscess
  - Organisms: Any organism causing gram-negative sepsis, especially in setting of thrombosis
  - Associated with neurosurgical procedures
  - *Citrobacter* species has propensity to form abscess as complication of meningitis in neonates

Pulmonic

- Aspiration pneumonia
  - Organisms: All members of Enterobacterales (pneumonia caused by *K. pneumoniae* can be particularly severe and sometimes chronic)
  - Patchy distribution of acute inflammation with admixed macrophages alternating with areas of nodular, fibroblastic foci (organizing)
  - Often associated with hemorrhage and abscess formation
  - Clusters of gram-negative rods often visible
- Pneumonic plague (*Y. pestis* infection)
  - Suppurative, hemorrhagic, necrotizing pneumonia
  - Primary pneumonic plague may demonstrate organisms in intraalveolar space, while secondary pneumonic plague from hematogenous spread may be more likely to demonstrate organisms in interstitium

Cardiac

- Endocarditis
  - Organisms: *E. coli* and *Salmonella* are most common causes of gram-negative endocarditis (2% of all endocarditis)
  - *Salmonella* has proclivity for damaged heart valves (particularly on left side)
  - Acute inflammatory infiltrates, atrial thrombus, and valve perforation or destruction may be seen
  - Organisms often visible with Gram or silver stains
- Infected aortic aneurysm
  - Organisms: *E. coli* and *Salmonella*
  - Acute inflammation is commonly, but not always, superimposed on atherosclerosis
  - Gram stain often does not reveal organisms, and culture or other methods are required for identification

Hepatic

- Abscess
  - Organisms: *E. coli* and *K. pneumoniae* are most common gastrointestinal-source bacteria associated with liver abscess, but other Enterobacterales may also be seen
  - Often necrotic center, neutrophilic infiltrates

Reticuloendothelial/Lymphatic

- Splenic abscess
  - Organisms: Any of Enterobacterales family, predominantly *E. coli* and *Klebsiella*
  - Diagnosis is by imaging
- Primary bubonic plague (*Y. pestis*)
  - Primary bubonic plague in draining lymph nodes can demonstrate edema, hemorrhage, and necrosis
  - Masses of organisms may be seen

Gastrointestinal

- Hemorrhagic diarrheal diseases
  - Organisms: *E. coli* (STEC or EHEC, EAEC, EIEC), *Shigella*, *Salmonella*, *Y. enterocolitica*
  - Nontyphoidal *Salmonella* infection tends to produce acute, self-limited colitis picture with polymorphonuclear infiltrate in lamina propria, cryptitis, and occasional crypt abscess
    - In general, crypt architecture is preserved (except in severe disease)
    - Neutrophils may be less prominent in *Salmonella* infection than other pathogens
  - *Shigella* infection may also produce acute, self-limited picture but can also cause pseudomembrane and ulcer formation
    - Crypt architecture may be markedly distorted with heavy, neutrophilic infiltrate in lamina propria
    - Generally affects left colon and can be very difficult to distinguish from inflammatory bowel disease
  - EHEC may present similarly to *Shigella* infection with addition of bowel edema (can be very prominent), necrosis, crypt withering, and microthrombi in small vessels; preferentially affects right colon
  - Enteritis caused by *Yersinia* infection can be differentiated from that caused by other pathogens by its propensity to promote granulomatous inflammation with lymphoid cuffing, but pattern can be mixed with diffuse, neutrophilic infiltrate
    - Other features include lymphoid hyperplasia, transmural lymphoid aggregates, giant cells, and ulceration
- Nonhemorrhagic diarrheal diseases
  - Organisms: *E. coli* (ETEC, EPEC, and others), *Salmonella* (generally nontyphoidal)
  - Minimal or no inflammatory change

Genitourinary

- HUS/renal microangiopathy
  - Organisms: *E. coli*
  - Schistocytes in peripheral blood
  - Microangiopathic changes with fibrin thrombi in kidneys (glomeruli) and other organs (systemic)
  - Cortical necrosis may be present
- Pyelonephritis
  - Organisms: Any uropathogen (e.g., *E. coli, P. mirabilis, Klebsiella*, and *Enterobacter*)
  - Neutrophilic infiltrates may be observed in tubules and collecting ducts
  - Abscesses may be present, but if they are small and concentrated in cortex, this may indicate hematogenous spread rather than ascending infection from lower urinary tract
  - Glomeruli are generally spared except in severe cases
  - Emphysematous pyelonephritis may be complication when gas collects in necrotic areas, usually in organ with preexisting diabetic glomerulosclerosis
- Cystitis
  - Organisms: Any uropathogen (e.g., *E. coli, P. mirabilis, Klebsiella*, and *Enterobacter*)
  - May display acute or chronic inflammation
  - Emphysematous cystitis may arise in background of chronic UTI, neurogenic bladder, trauma, urinary stasis, or instrumentation
    - Characterized by empty cavities in lamina propria
    - Foreign body giant cells may be present
- Prostatitis/epididymitis
  - Uropathogens are typical cause of prostatitis and epididymitis with *E. coli* being most frequently isolated
- Granuloma inguinale (donovanosis)
  - Organisms: *K. granulomatis*
  - Ulcerating disease of genital areas
  - PAP smear or ulcer biopsy may demonstrate nonnecrotizing granulomatous inflammation with epithelioid histiocytes, giant cells, and lymphocytes
  - Intracellular organisms may be seen within histiocytes (Donovan bodies)
  - Ulcerations can be quite severe and engulf entire genital region if left untreated

Bone

- Osteomyelitis
  - Hematogenous spread
    - Organisms: Generally monomicrobial
    - Commonly isolated gram-negative organisms include *Salmonella* (especially in sickle cell disease), *E. coli*, and *Klebsiella*
    - Gram-negative organisms are most common in children or adults with some pathology (IV drug abuse, diabetes, sickle cell disease, etc.)
    - Typically manifests as suppurative lesion with edema, hemorrhage, and necrosis
    - Salmonella may produce granulomatous inflammation
    - Bacteria may be visible on Gram or silver stain
  - Contiguous spread or direct inoculation
    - Organisms: Generally polymicrobial as consequence of spread from open, infected ulcer or wound (e.g., periodontal abscess, decubitus ulcer, or open fracture)
      - *E. coli, Proteus, Klebsiella* are all commonly isolated
    - In addition to features of osteomyelitis by hematogenous spread, disease by contiguous spread may demonstrate chronic inflammation (especially in case of spread from ulcer)

Skin

- Cellulitis
  - Enterobacterales are uncommon causes of cellulitis except in diabetic patients, particularly as complication of decubitus ulcers

Soft Tissue

- Myositis: Very rarely caused by Enterobacterales
- Rhinoscleroma
  - Organisms: *K. pneumoniae* subspecies *rhinoscleromatis*
  - Disease occurs in 3 phases: Rhinitic, proliferative (granulomatous), and cicatricial (sclerotic)
  - Proliferative stage: Epithelial hyperplasia with mixed inflammatory infiltrate of plasma cells, foamy histiocytes (Mikulicz cells), lymphocytes, and neutrophils in underlying stroma; usually arranged in sheets, but microabscesses may also be present
  - Sclerotic stage is defined by fibrosis and scant cellularity (mostly lymphocytes and plasma cells)
  - Organisms can often by seen with H&E or silver stain

DIFFERENTIAL DIAGNOSIS

Other Infectious Causes of Gastroenteritis

- Bacterial (e.g., *Clostridioides difficile, Campylobacter jejuni*) and viral (e.g., rotavirus, norovirus)
- Confirm by Gram stain, IHC, culture, PCR

Other Infectious Causes of Pneumonia

- Bacterial (e.g., pneumococcus, *Mycoplasma pneumoniae*) and viral (e.g., influenza, respiratory syncytial virus)
- Confirm by VCPE, Gram stain, IHC, culture, PCR

Other Infectious Causes of Granulomatous Nasal Swellings

- e.g., tuberculosis, leprosy, leishmaniasis, sarcoidosis
- Confirm by acid-fast stains, Giemsa, IHC, culture, PCR
- Lack Mikulicz cells of rhinoscleroma

SELECTED REFERENCES

1. Janda JM et al: The changing face of the family Enterobacteriaceae (Order: "Enterobacterales"): new members, taxonomic issues, geographic expansion, and new diseases and disease syndromes. Clin Microbiol Rev. 34(2), 2021
2. Baker S et al: Recent insights into Shigella. Curr Opin Infect Dis. 31(5):449-54, 2018
3. Umphress B et al: Rhinoscleroma. Arch Pathol Lab Med. 142(12):1533-6, 2018
4. Lamps LW: Update on infectious enterocolitides and the diseases that they mimic. Histopathology. 66(1):3-14, 2015
5. Wain J et al: Typhoid fever. Lancet. 385(9973):1136-45, 2015
6. Melton-Celsa AR: Shiga toxin (Stx) classification, structure, and function. Microbiol Spectr. 2(4):EHEC-0024-2013, 2014
7. Guarner J et al: Immunohistochemical detection of Yersinia pestis in formalin-fixed, paraffin-embedded tissue. Am J Clin Pathol. 117(2):205-9, 2002

Acute Necrotizing Pneumonia

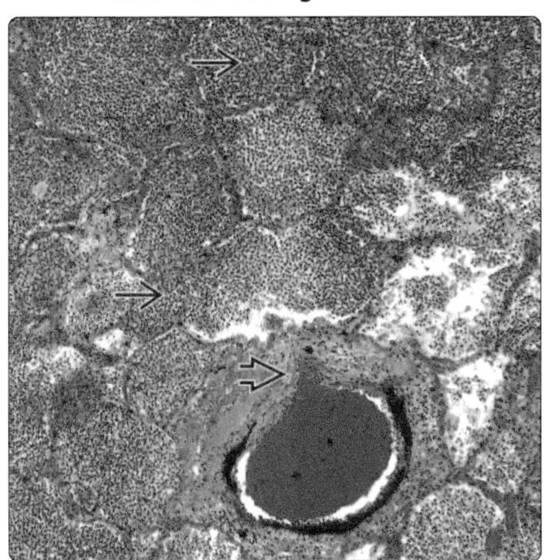

Pyelonephritis: Gross Photograph

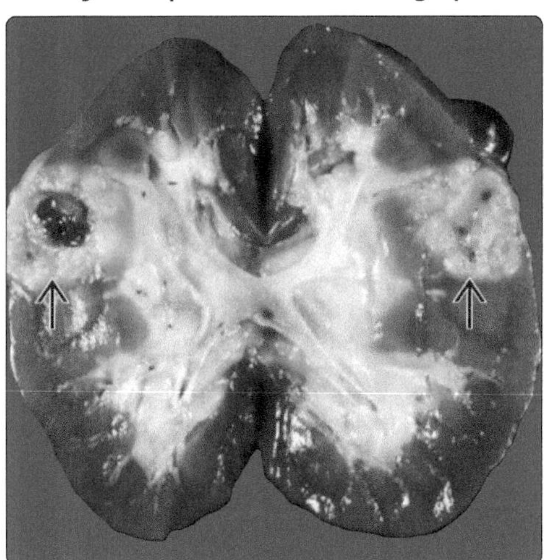

(Left) *Friedlander disease (Klebsiella pneumoniae) is an acute, necrotizing pneumonia. The alveoli are filled with neutrophils ➡, and necrosis ⇨ is present.* **(Right)** *This gross photograph depicts xanthogranulomatous pyelonephritis with an expanding local mass mimicking tumor ➡. Proteus mirabilis and E. coli are most frequently isolated from this lesion. (Courtesy Franz von Lichtenberg Collection of Infectious Disease Pathology, BWH.)*

Liver Abscess: Gross Photograph

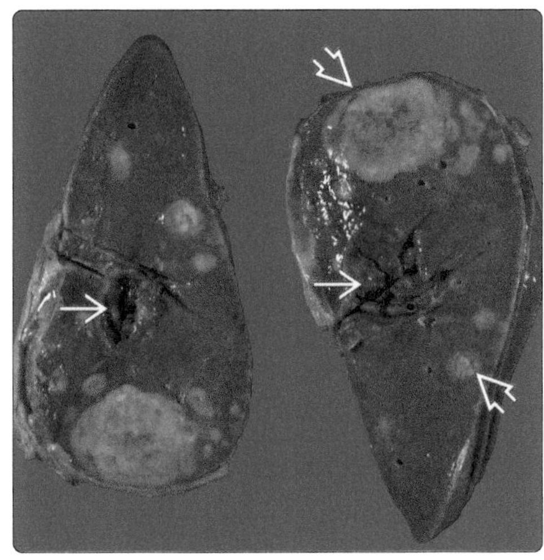

Hepatic Abscess

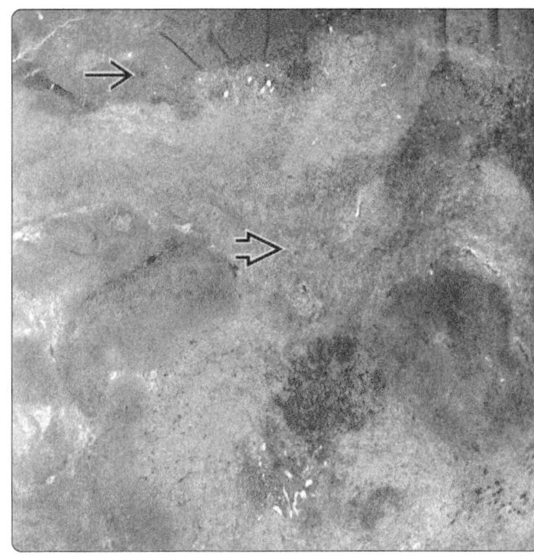

(Left) *Gross photograph of a liver from a patient who died of metastatic carcinoid tumor ⇨ shows a drained abscess ➡, which grew K. pneumoniae, Enterococcus faecium, and E. cloacae.* **(Right)** *The histology of a hepatic abscess shows necrotic tissue ➡ and abundant, acute inflammation ⇨. As this is an early, acute lesion, there is no reactive capsule. The abscess cavity is filled with necrotic debris mixed with bile. Cultures grew Klebsiella species.*

Bacillary Dysentery

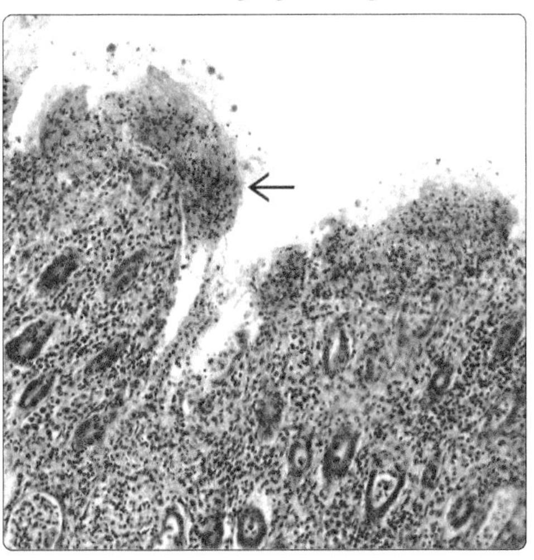

Salmonella Enteritis in Ulcerative Colitis

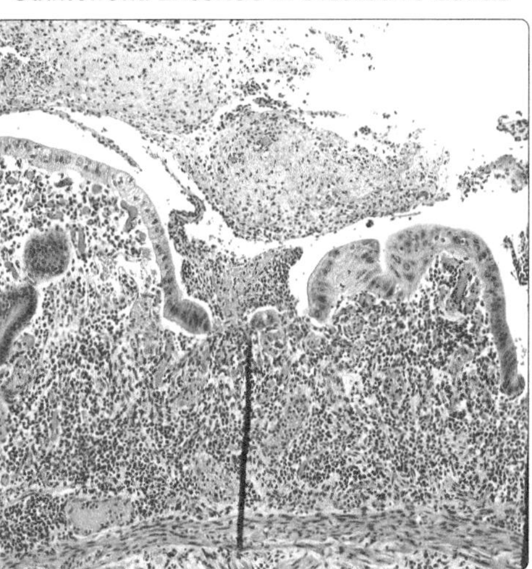

(Left) *In a case of bacillary dysentery, this medium-power image shows an earlier phase of acute necrosis with loss of the surface epithelium and replacement by a tenacious clot of fibrin ➡ with admixed necroinflammatory debris.* **(Right)** *Total abdominal colectomy shows an area of ileum with neutrophilic exudate forming pseudomembranes. This patient had ulcerative colitis complicated by Salmonella enteritis. (Courtesy M. Drage, MD, PhD.)*

Ulcers in *Salmonella*

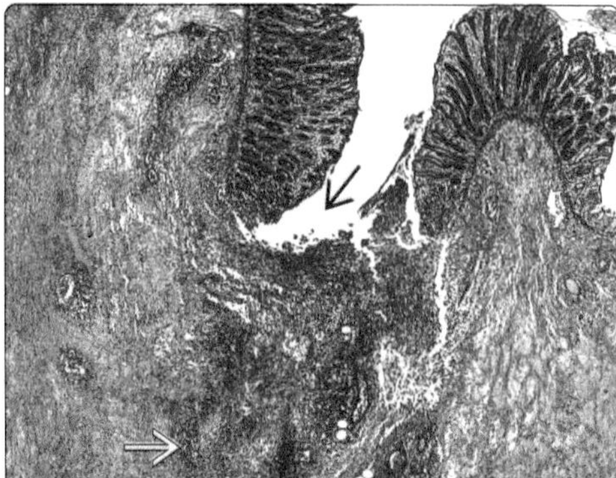

***Shigella* Colitis**

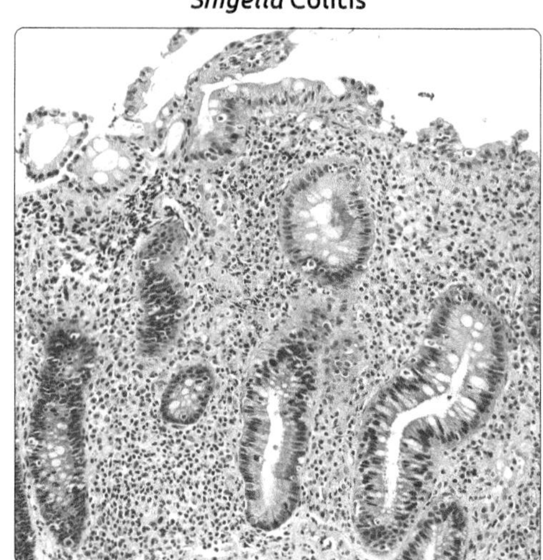

(Left) *This patient underwent right colectomy for severe bleeding due to Salmonella infection. Scattered, sharply demarcated ulcers ⇨ extend into the submucosa and are associated with dense inflammation with fibrosis ➡. (From DP: Endoscopy.)* **(Right)** *Shigella flexneri colon biopsy shows diffuse, mixed lamina propria inflammation with some distortion of crypt architecture. The endoscopic and histologic impressions may be mistaken for inflammatory bowel disease. (Courtesy M. Drage, MD, PhD.)*

***Shigella* Colitis**

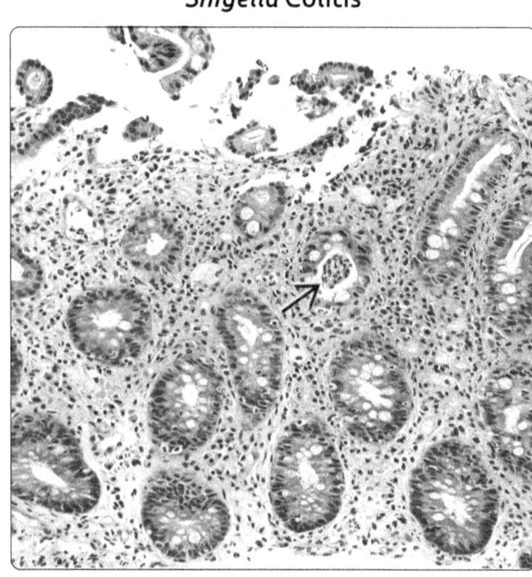

Typhoid

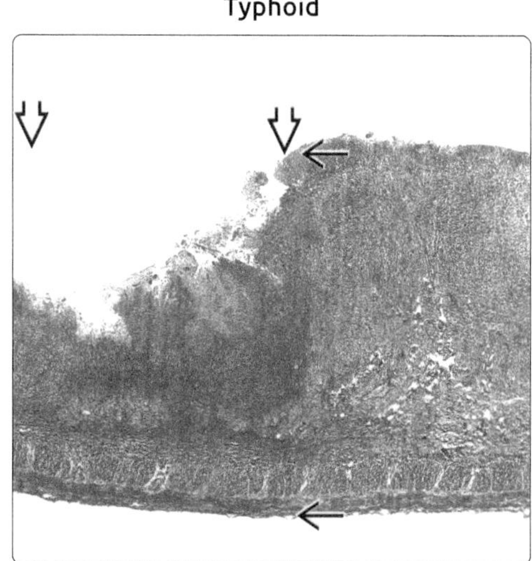

(Left) *This biopsy in a case of S. flexneri colitis shows epithelial injury, lamina propria edema, and neutrophilic crypt abscess ⇨ in the absence of histologic features of chronic injury. (Courtesy M. Drage, MD, PhD.)* **(Right)** *Low-power image shows intestinal typhoid with transmural coagulative necrosis (between ⇨), loss of epithelium (between ⇩), edema, and inflammation.*

Renal Typhoid

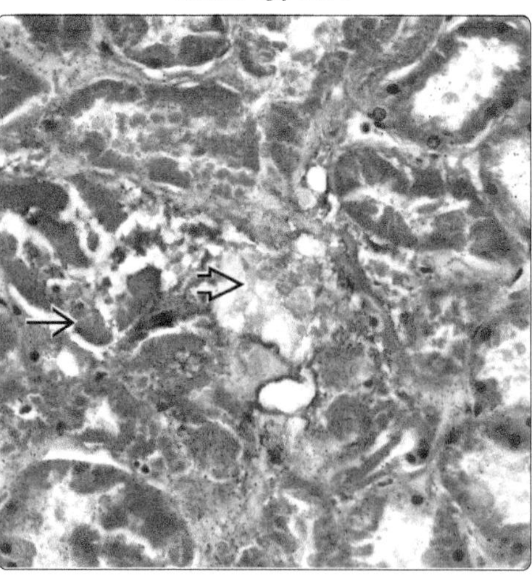

Granuloma Inguinale

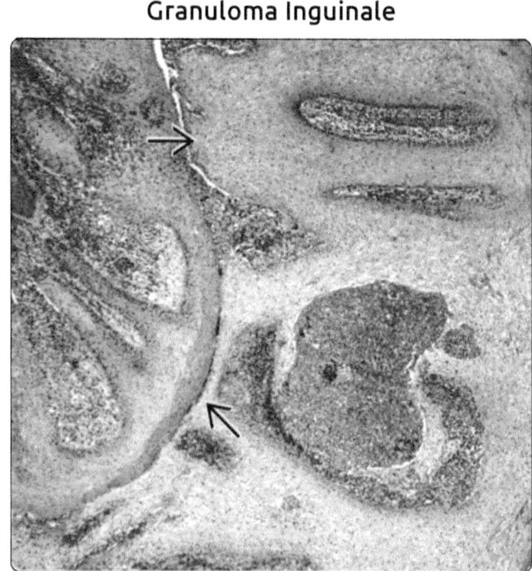

(Left) *Renal typhoid is an acute nephritis with marked coagulative necrosis. This high-power image shows coagulative necrosis of the proximal tubules ⇨ and clouds of bacteria in the center ⇨.* **(Right)** *H&E section demonstrates the pseudoepitheliomatous proliferation ⇨ in granuloma inguinale (donovanosis). (Courtesy Franz von Lichtenberg Collection of Infectious Disease Pathology, BWH.)*

Leishman-Donovan Bodies

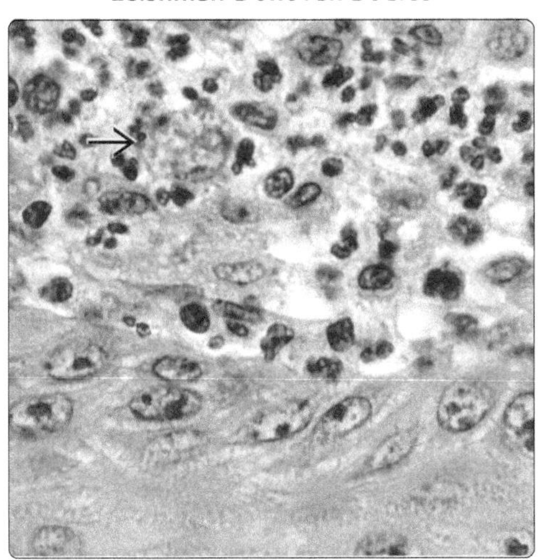

Leishman-Donovan Bodies: Silver Stain

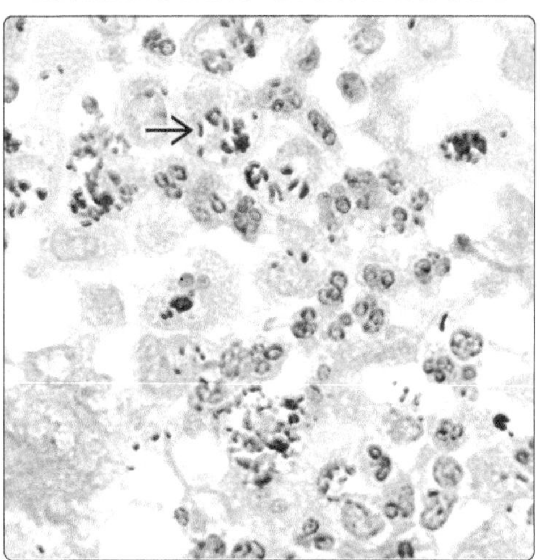

(Left) *High-power view of granuloma inguinale demonstrates weakly basophilic corpuscles in cytoplasmic vacuoles (Leishman-Donovan bodies* ⇒*). (Courtesy Franz von Lichtenberg Collection of Infectious Disease Pathology, BWH.)* **(Right)** *Silver stain reveals that Leishman-Donovan bodies contain short rods* ⇒ *corresponding to K. pneumoniae subspecies granulomatis. (Courtesy Franz von Lichtenberg Collection of Infectious Disease Pathology, BWH.)*

Rhinoscleroma

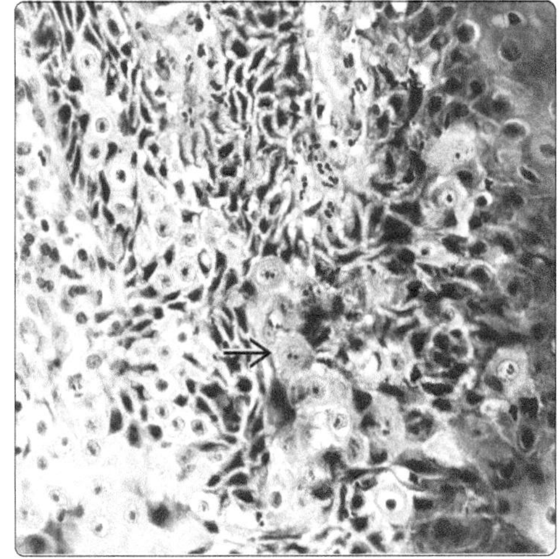

Bubonic Plague: Lymph Node

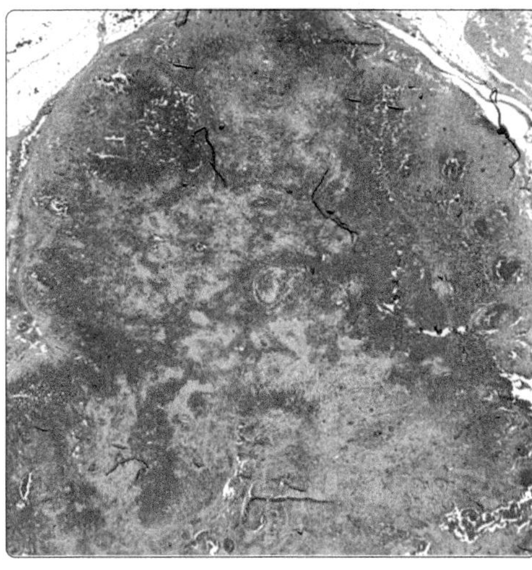

(Left) *This specimen of rhinoscleroma demonstrates numerous foamy histiocytes (Mikulicz cells)* ⇒. **(Right)** *H&E section of an inguinal lymph node from a bubonic plague victim shows widespread hemorrhagic necrosis causing swelling and effacement of normal architecture. (Courtesy Franz von Lichtenberg Collection of Infectious Disease Pathology, BWH.)*

Bubonic Plague: Gram Stain

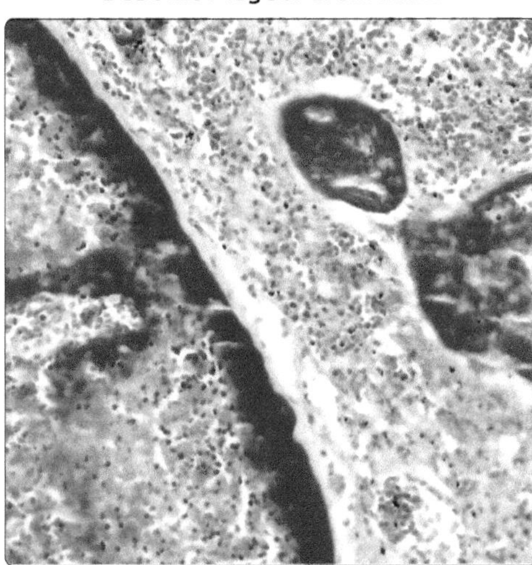

Colonic Ulcers: *Yersinia* Infection

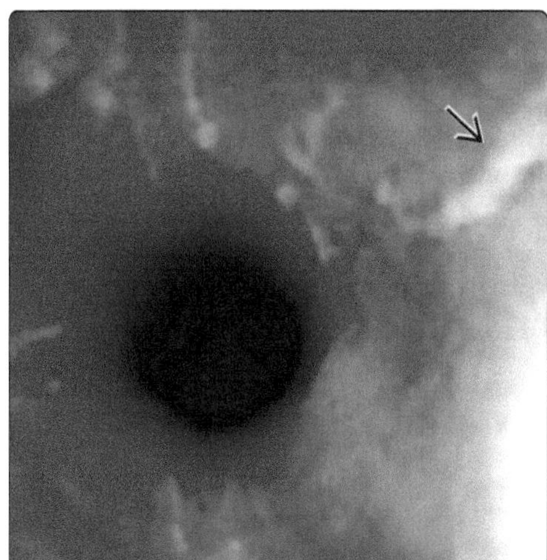

(Left) *Gram stain of a Yersinia pestis-infected inguinal lymph node shows massive proliferation of organisms, particularly at the sinus margins. (Courtesy Franz von Lichtenberg Collection of Infectious Disease Pathology, BWH.)* **(Right)** *Yersinia infection caused diffuse erythema and linear ulcers* ⇒ *in this patient with acute-onset diarrhea. (From DP: Endoscopic.)*

Fastidious Organisms: *Brucella*, *Francisella*, *Haemophilus*, and *Legionella* Species Infections

KEY FACTS

ETIOLOGY/PATHOGENESIS AND CLINICAL ISSUES

- *Brucella* spp.: Meat packing and unpasteurized dairy products; nonspecific symptoms (fever, osteoarticular, constitutional) affecting all organs
- *Francisella* spp.: Transmitted via arthropod vector; ulceroglandular and pneumonic forms
- *Haemophilus influenzae* and *Haemophilus parainfluenzae*: Normal flora in oropharynx and nasopharynx; wide range of infections with mucosal invasion
- *Haemophilus ducreyi* (chancroid): Painful genital ulceration with associated inguinal lymphadenopathy
- *Legionella pneumophila*: Consolidating pneumonia, myalgia, diarrhea, elevated LFTs, electrolyte imbalances

MICROSCOPIC

- *Brucella* spp.: Granulomas and mixed inflammatory infiltrate (commonly liver but can affect any site); endocarditis
- *Francisella* spp.: Necrosis, abscess, and granuloma in lymph nodes as well as necrotizing pneumonia
- *H. influenzae* type b: Meningitis, pneumonia, cellulitis
- Untypeable *H. influenzae*: Pneumonia, sinusitis, conjunctivitis
- *H. ducreyi* chancroid: Mononuclear infiltrates extending deep into dermis
- *Legionella* spp.: Acute fibrinopurulent bronchopneumonia
- Small rods visible with silver stains; not well detected by tissue Gram stains

TOP DIFFERENTIAL DIAGNOSIS

- Mycobacteria, *Bartonella*, *Burkholderia pseudomallei*, *Nocardia*, *Listeria*, and *Actinomycetes* infections also associated with granulomatous inflammation
- Anthrax, plague, pneumococcus, *Staphylococcus aureus* also associated with necrotizing pneumonia
- Plague, anthrax, mycobacteria, *Bartonella* also associated with skin lesions and lymphadenopathy
- Syphilis and herpes also associated with ulceration
- Differentiate by special stains, IHC, PCR, serology, culture

Epidemiology of *Brucella* spp. Infections

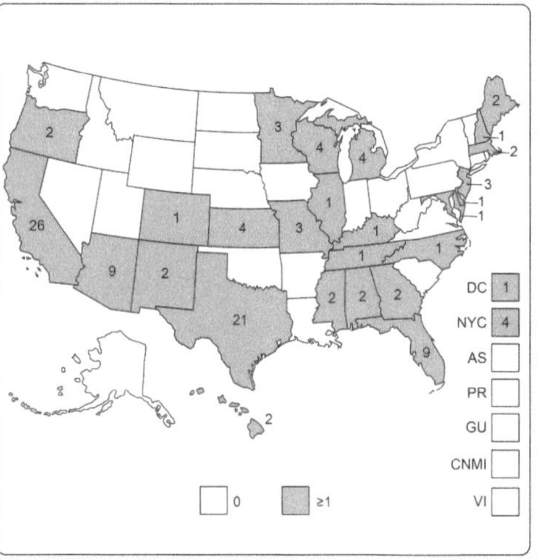

Brucella spp. Psoas Abscesses

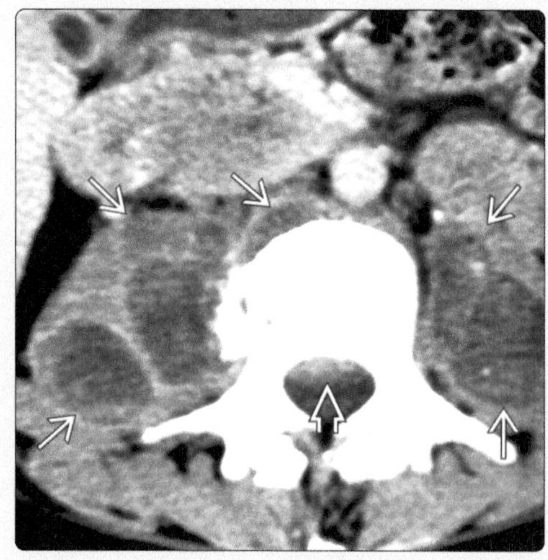

(Left) *The number of reported cases of brucellosis in the USA and its territories (2010 n=115) is shown. The highest number (56.5%) of brucellosis cases were reported by California, Texas, Arizona, and Florida. (Courtesy CDC.)* **(Right)** *Bilateral psoas abscesses ➡ (with calcification) and narrowed canal ⇨ would be typical of tuberculosis. This patient worked in a meat-packing plant, and titers were positive for brucellosis. (From DI: MSK Non-Trauma.)*

Liver With Brucellosis

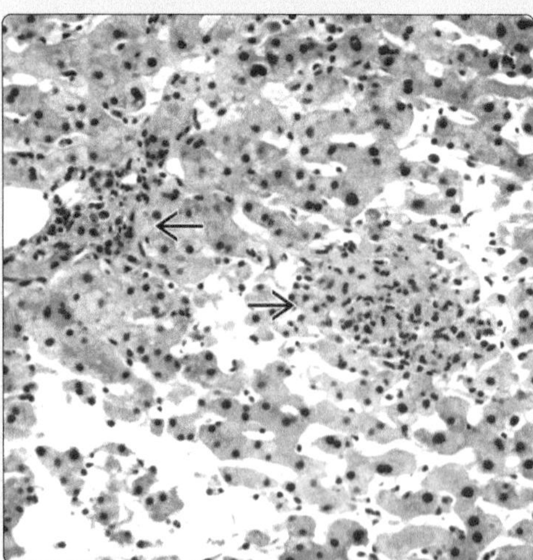

Liver With Brucellosis

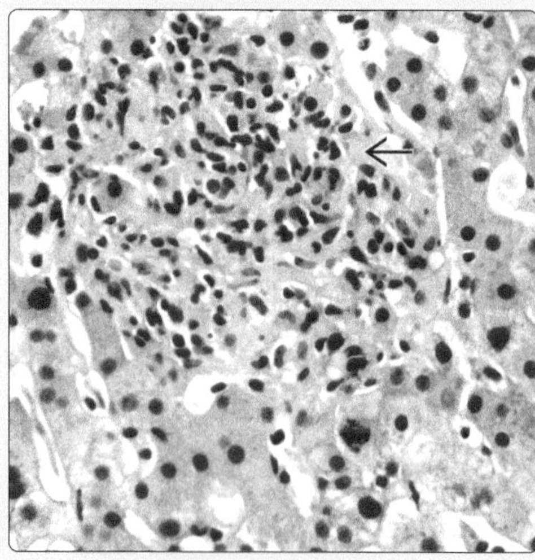

(Left) *Liver biopsy from a patient with brucellosis demonstrates granulomata ⇨ in the liver parenchyma, which are loosely organized and not restricted to the portal triads.* **(Right)** *Liver biopsy from a patient with brucellosis demonstrates granulomata ⇨ in the liver parenchyma with hepatocyte necrosis. Clinically, patients present with elevated transaminases due to multifocal granulomatous diseases.*

TERMINOLOGY

Definitions

- *Brucella* infection: Undulant fever, Gibraltar fever, Mediterranean fever, and Malta fever; named after British physician David Bruce (1855-1931)
- *Francisella* infection: Tularemia, rabbit fever, deer fly fever, and market men's disease; named after American bacteriologist Edward Francis (1872-1957)
- *Haemophilus* infection: a.k.a. Pfeiffer bacillus, bacterial influenza, chancroid; named for Richard Pfeiffer, who proposed it was causative agent of influenza
- *Legionella* infection: Legionnaire disease, Pontiac fever; named for 1st documented outbreak at hotel among members of American Legion in 1976

INFECTIOUS AGENTS: EPIDEMIOLOGY, CLINICAL PRESENTATION, AND PATHOGENESIS

Brucella spp.

- Infection with *B. melitensis*, *B. suis*, and *B. abortus* via occupational exposure (e.g., meat packing, dairy) or consumption of unpasteurized milk products (cows or goats); considered potential agent of bioterrorism
- Entry via cuts or abrasions on skin or through mucous membranes of respiratory and digestive tracts
- Taken up by macrophages and dendritic cells and disseminated widely via lymphatics
- Most commonly presents with fever, osteoarticular involvement, sweating, and constitutional symptoms
  - Hepatosplenomegaly (30%), lymphadenopathy (10%)
  - Osteoarticular involvement (50%): Sacroiliitis, spondylitis, arthritis, osteomyelitis
  - Hepatobiliary manifestations: Reactive hepatitis with granulomas, liver abscess
  - Genitourinary findings (10%): Orchiepididymitis, glomerulonephritis, renal abscess
  - Neurological manifestations (6-7%): Peripheral neuropathy, chorea, meningoencephalitis, cranial nerve damage (i.e., VI, VIII); psychiatric disturbances
  - Pulmonary features (1%): Pleural effusions, pneumonia, granulomas, abscesses
  - Skin involvement: Erythematous papular lesions, purpura, dermal cysts, Stevens-Johnson syndrome
  - Hematologic: Leukocytosis, leukopenia, thrombocytopenia, anemia
  - Endocarditis (1%; aortic valve most common): Myocarditis, pericarditis, endarteritis, thrombophlebitis, and mycotic aneurysms also reported
  - Ocular lesions: Anterior uveitis, chorioretinitis, optic neuritis, papilledema, keratitis
  - Pregnancy: Intrauterine infection, fetal death, spontaneous abortion, prematurity, low birth weight

Francisella spp.

- Infection with *Francisella tularensis* via arthropod vector, usually tick or biting fly, airborne exposure to contaminated dusts and aerosols, ingestion of contaminated food and water, or cutaneous exposure to infected animals
- *F. tularensis* subspecies *tularensis* (type A) is most virulent and common cause of infections in North America; considered potential agent of bioterrorism
- Other subspecies that may infect humans are *F. holarctica* (type B), *F. novicida* (sometimes considered separate species), and *F. mediasiatica*
- *F. hispaniensis* and *F. philomiragia* rarely cause human disease
- Few cases in USA (Arkansas, Missouri, Kansas, South Dakota, California, Oklahoma, and Massachusetts); incidence peaks in summer (tick exposure) and winter (hunting); most common in children and older men
- Organisms spread via lymphohematogenous route, both as free organisms and within diverse array of host cells
- Clinical presentation: Fever, chills, headache, malaise, fatigue, cough, vomiting, sore throat, abdominal pain, and diarrhea (incubation period: 1-20 days)
- 6 classic forms of tularemia: Ulceroglandular, pneumonic, glandular, oculoglandular, pharyngeal, and typhoidal
- Ulceroglandular tularemia: Painful, isolated lymphadenopathy; skin lesion evolves from red, painful papules, sometimes with vesicles, to necrotic lesion, to painful ulcer with raised border
- Pneumonic tularemia: Primary from inhalation or secondary from hematogenous seeding of lung; fever, cough, minimal sputum production, pleuritic chest pain; exudative, lymphocytic-predominant pleural fluid

Haemophilus spp.

- Infection with *Haemophilus* spp., many of which are normal flora but may cause disease following mucosal invasion
- Member of HACEK group of organisms (*Haemophilus* spp., *Aggregatibacter* spp., *Cardiobacterium hominis*, *Eikenella corrodens*, and *Kingella* spp.), infrequent cause of infective endocarditis
- *H. influenzae:* Normal flora in oropharynx and nasopharynx, spread by airborne droplets or contact with secretions; disease with invasion of oropharyngeal mucosa and subsequent dissemination
  - 6 different capsular types (serotypes a-f): Virulence factor for evasion of phagocytosis; may be unencapsulated/untypeable
  - *H. influenzae* type b (Hib) vaccine based on capsular antigen; in postvaccine era, most colonizing strains are untypeable
  - *H. influenzae* type b: Meningitis, epiglottitis, empyema, pneumonia, cellulitis, bacteremia, septic arthritis
  - Untypeable *H. influenzae*: Otitis media, chronic obstructive pulmonary disease exacerbation, pneumonia, sinusitis, conjunctivitis, sepsis
- *H. parainfluenzae:* Predominant *Haemophilus* spp. in upper respiratory tract; less frequently associated with otitis media, sinusitis, and, rarely, infective endocarditis
- *H. ducreyi:* Sexually transmitted infection (chancroid), most common in developing countries; painful genital ulceration with associated inguinal lymphadenopathy
- *H. aegyptius:* Unencapsulated species resembling biotype III of *H. influenzae;* acute purulent conjunctivitis
- *H. hemolyticus:* Commensal strain

Legionella spp.

- Infection most commonly with *Legionella pneumophila* serogroup 1 via inhalation in contaminated air droplets from man-made water source (e.g., air conditioning)
- Widespread in warm aqueous environments, growth fostered by replication within free-living amebas
- Legionnaire disease: Consolidating pneumonia with pulse-temperature dissociation (Faget sign), myalgia, diarrhea, elevated LFTs, electrolyte imbalances; headache and confusion; metastatic infection in immunocompromised; pulmonary symptoms not prominent
- Pontiac fever: Self-limited syndrome marked by fever, headache, and myalgias

LABORATORY TESTING, TREATMENT, AND PROGNOSIS

Laboratory Tests

- *Brucella* spp.
  - Blood culture is gold standard (70-90% sensitive with lysis centrifugation method); cultures of bone marrow and other potentially involved tissues and fluids cultures may be useful
  - Commercially available ELISA assays (based on antibodies to smooth LPS); highly sensitive, though cross reactivity with other gram-negative bacteria can be issue
  - PCR assays using primers to 16S rRNA or BCP31 genes as well as IS711 insertion sequence may be employed on clinical samples (sensitivity may be superior to blood culture)
- *Francisella* spp.
  - Gram stains of tissues and fluids are generally negative
  - Cultures are generally negative unless plated on supportive (cysteine-containing) media
  - Rapid diagnostic tests can be run directly on clinical samples, including direct fluorescent antibody (DFA) and immunohistochemistry
  - Serology: IgM and IgG appear together within 2 weeks of infection and peak at 4-5 weeks
- *Legionella* spp.
  - Urinary antigen is rapid test for Legionnaire disease (limited to serogroup 1); sensitivity 70-100%, specificity 95-100%
  - PCR is highly sensitive but not commonly offered in clinical laboratories
  - Serologies not generally used for diagnosis or monitoring

Treatment

- *Brucella* spp.
  - Surgical intervention for some cases of abscess formation
  - Multiple drugs for extended periods of time
    - Daily doxycycline and streptomycin for 6 weeks
    - Doxycycline/streptomycin for extended periods of time for severe disease
    - Ceftriaxone/doxycycline/rifampin for neurobrucellosis
- *Francisella* spp.
  - Surgical drainage occasionally for suppurative nodes
  - Streptomycin and gentamicin for all forms of tularemia except meningitis (require additional drugs with superior penetration into CSF)
  - Fluoroquinolones or doxycycline for less severe disease
- *Haemophilus* spp.
  - Treatment of *H. ducreyi* must also cover syphilis due to 10% coinfection (preferred azithromycin/ceftriaxone)
  - Treatment of *H. influenza* often amoxicillin (alternatives are ceftriaxone or fluoroquinolone)
- *Legionella* spp.
  - Levofloxacin and azithromycin are 1st line, though other fluoroquinolones, macrolides, and tetracyclines may be considered

Prognosis

- Brucellosis relapse is common (5-25%), due to organism persistence in protected niches; fatalities rare, most often consequence of endocarditis
- Fatalities are also low (~ 4%) in tularemia (with treatment) and are often associated with pulmonic disease

MICROBIOLOGY

Culture and Microbiological Identification

- Biosafety considerations
  - Due to high risk of infection of laboratory personnel, any cultures from patients suspected of being infected by *Brucella* or *Francisella* should be handled in biological safety cabinet
  - Work-up within typical microbiology lab will stop as soon as presumed identification is made, usually via serum agglutination test; further testing is generally done in reference laboratory within Laboratory Response Network (LRN)
- *Brucella* spp.
  - Small, aerobic, non-spore-forming, gram-negative rods or coccobacilli
  - All are catalase positive, most are oxidase and urease positive, with variable hydrogen sulfide production
  - Growth on blood and Mueller-Hinton agars; small, smooth, and glistening colonies after 24-48 hours
  - Some strains can grow on MacConkey agar; *B. abortus* and *B. suis* require 5-10% CO2; Thayer-Martin medium may be used to isolate *Brucella* from contaminated specimens
  - Best method from clinical specimens is inoculation into bottles for monitoring by continuously monitored automatic alert systems, such as BACTEC or BacT/ALERT (usually positive in 1 week)
  - In specialized laboratories, *Brucella* may be identified and typed down to species &/or biovar level
- *Francisella* spp.
  - Small, aerobic, non-spore-forming, gram-negative coccobacilli
  - All are hydrogen sulfide and (weakly) catalase positive, and both oxidase and urease negative
  - Common media that can support growth include chocolate agar, buffered charcoal-yeast extract agar, and Thayer-Martin agar; growth is slow, and colonies may take 48 hours to appear
  - Cysteine heart agar media that has been supplemented with 9% chocolatized sheep's blood (CHAB) can be used for diagnostic purposes, as *Francisella* displays distinct colony morphology on this media
- *Haemophilus* spp.

- Small, facultatively anaerobic, non-spore-forming, gram-negative rods or coccobacilli
- Depending on species, may require X (protoporphyrin IX) &/or V (nicotinamide) factors; X and V factors are in chocolate agar, or can be provided separately on quad plates for diagnostics
- HACEK agents of endocarditis are readily grown in modern blood culture bottles and do not require extended incubation times
- Biochemical systems include smaller panels as well as cards for Vitek 2 (some incorporate *Neisseria* spp. as well as other HACEK organisms)

- *Legionella* spp.
  - Small, aerobic, pleomorphic gram-negative rod (coccobacillary in clinical specimens, slender rods on laboratory media)
  - Cannot be grown on standard laboratory media due to its requirement for cysteine and soluble iron; BCYE-α is commonly used; colonies have speckled, blue-green appearance that matures into opalescence
  - Standard identification is based on culture characteristics along with serotyping to distinguish serogroup 1 strains
- MALDI-TOF MS and 16S rRNA sequencing may be used for identification

MICROSCOPIC

Histologic Features

- *Brucella* spp.
  - Liver: Granulomas, mixed inflammatory cell infiltrate in sinusoids, focal and centrilobular necrosis, abscess
  - Brucelloma: Liver mass with central calcification, manifestation of chronic or reactivated granulomatous disease
  - Heart: Valve vegetations (most commonly) on aortic and mitral valves; granulomatous lesions of myocardium also reported
  - Spleen: Giant cells and increased numbers of macrophages, along with granulomas
  - Testes and epididymides: Widespread inflammation, predominantly lymphocytic by some reports
- *Francisella* spp.
  - Lymph nodes: Mixed cellular inflammatory infiltrate and necrosis [focal (outer cortex) or widespread], occasional granulomas, and inflammation extending beyond lymph node capsule
    - Fine-needle aspirations of affected lymph nodes may demonstrate suppuration, necrosis, granulomas, and abscess formation
    - Macrophages are often present, and phagocytosed bacteria may rarely be observed
  - Lung: Necrotizing pneumonia with abundant fibrin and neutrophils within alveolar walls and spaces, edema, and widespread necrosis
  - Liver and spleen: Microabscesses
  - Other: Suppurative leptomeningitis and ulcerations of small and large bowels
- *Haemophilus* spp.
  - *H. ducreyi* chancroid lesions characterized by perivascular and interstitial mononuclear cell infiltrates extending deep into dermis
  - Infectious endocarditis caused by HACEK organisms may result in larger and more numerous vegetations that are caused by viridans group *Streptococci*
- *Legionella* spp.
  - Acute fibrinopurulent bronchopneumonia, alveoli with numerous neutrophils, macrophages and abundant fibrin, focal necrosis of bronchiolar epithelium, relatively well-preserved pulmonary architecture

Special Stains

- Organisms stain poorly (if at all) with Gram stain
- Small rods visible with silver stains (e.g., Steiner, Warthin-Starry, Dieterle)

Immunohistochemistry

- Not widely used but may be available at reference laboratories

DIFFERENTIAL DIAGNOSIS

Other Causes of Granulomatous Inflammation

- Other infectious etiologies
  - Bacteria (e.g., mycobacteria, *Bartonella, Burkholderia pseudomallei, Nocardia, Listeria, Actinomycetes),* fungi (e.g., *Histoplasma, Sporothrix, Candida, Cryptococcus, Aspergillus*), and parasites (e.g., *Schistosoma, Leishmania, Toxoplasma*)
  - Differentiate by morphology if organisms are visualized in tissue sections, culture, or molecular and serological testing
- Noninfectious etiologies (e.g., sarcoidosis and Crohn disease): Differentiate by chronicity and lack of infectious agent

Other Causes of Necrotizing Pneumonia

- Other pathogens (e.g., anthrax) may cause similar abrupt-onset, fulminant pneumonia
- Differentiate by clinical findings, serology, and culture

Other Causes of Skin Lesions and Lymphadenopathy

- e.g., pasteurellosis, plague, anthrax, mycobacteriosis, bartonellosis
- Other causes of ulcerated lesions, e.g., syphilis and herpes
- Differentiate by clinical findings, culture, and serology

SELECTED REFERENCES

1. Moffa MA et al: Legionellosis on the rise: a scoping review of sporadic, community-acquired incidence in the United States. Epidemiol Infect. 151:e133, 2023
2. Soares CN et al: Neurobrucellosis. Curr Opin Infect Dis. 36(3):192-7, 2023
3. Kurmanov B et al: Assays for identification and differentiation of Brucella species: a review. Microorganisms. 10(8), 2022
4. Slack MPE et al: Invasive Haemophilus influenzae infections after 3 decades of hib protein conjugate vaccine use. Clin Microbiol Rev. 34(3):e0002821, 2021
5. Brothwell JA et al: Interactions of the skin pathogen Haemophilus ducreyi with the human host. Front Immunol. 11:615402, 2020
6. Vaidya T et al: Cutaneous Legionella infections in allogeneic hematopoietic cell transplantation recipients. Dermatol Online J. 26(6), 2020
7. Ambrosioni J et al: HACEK infective endocarditis: epidemiology, clinical features, and outcome: a case-control study. Int J Infect Dis. 76:120-5, 2018
8. Tuncer E et al: Tularemia: potential role of cytopathology in differential diagnosis of cervical lymphadenitis: multicenter experience in 53 cases and literature review. APMIS. 122(3):236-42, 2014
9. Guarner J et al: Histopathology and immunohistochemistry in the diagnosis of bioterrorism agents. J Histochem Cytochem. 54(1):3-11, 2006

Epidemiology of Tularemia

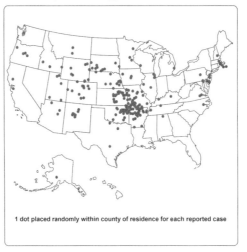

1 dot placed randomly within county of residence for each reported case

Francisella tularensis Pneumonia

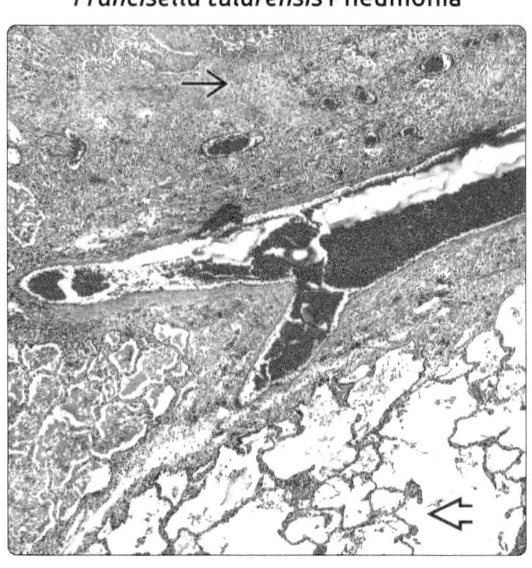

(Left) *Map of tularemia cases (2016) is shown. Although uncommon (100-300 cases per year), tularemia has been reported across most of the USA. It most frequently found in the south central and the Pacific Northwest regions and parts of Massachusetts, including Martha's Vineyard. (Courtesy CDC.)* **(Right)** *Lung section shows focal necrotizing pneumonia ⇨ caused by Francisella tularensis adjacent to relatively normal lung with emphysematous change ⇨. Special stains for organisms may be negative.*

Francisella tularensis Necrotizing Pneumonia

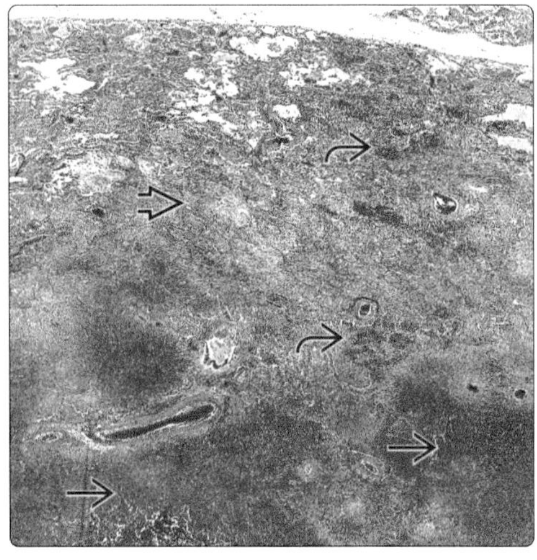

Francisella tularensis Pneumonia

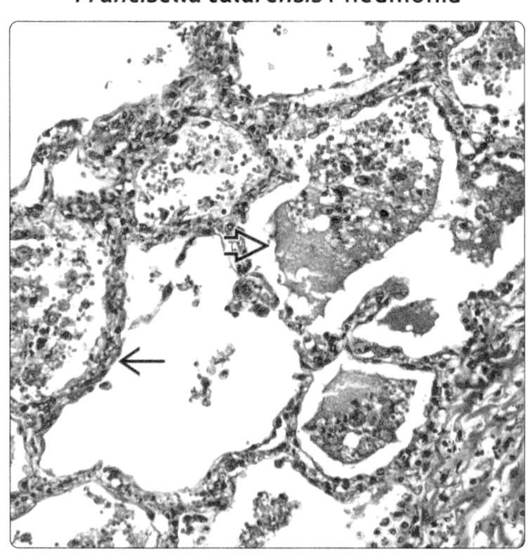

(Left) *Lung section shows focal necrotizing pneumonia ⇨ caused by F. tularensis adjacent to areas of active cellular pneumonia ⇨ with congestion and focal hemorrhage ⇨.* **(Right)** *Lung section shows pneumonia filling alveolar spaces caused by F. tularensis with proteinaceous debris ⇨ and thickened alveolar septa ⇨.*

Francisella tularensis Silver Stain

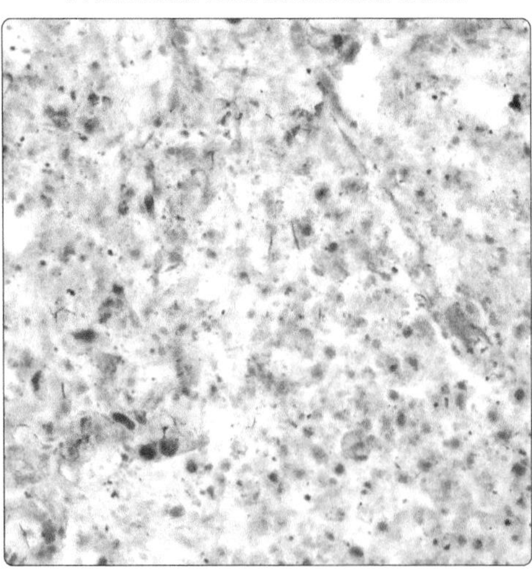

Panniculitis: Tularemia

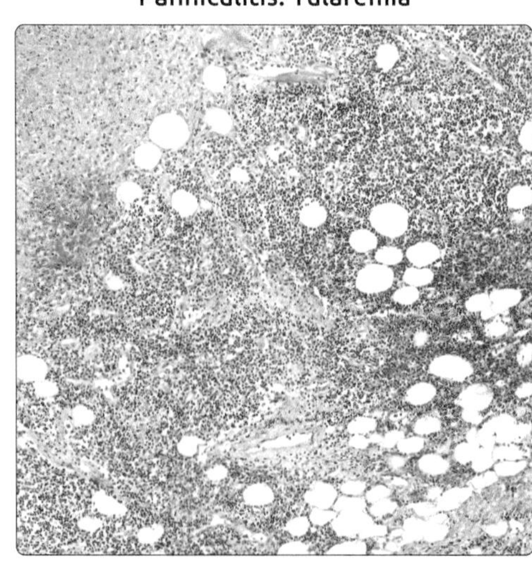

(Left) *Lung section demonstrates numerous rods within the tissue, consistent with Francisella on silver stain. Because the organism is highly infectious, caution is required for culture conditions.* **(Right)** *Tularemia panniculitis can be limited to lymph nodes (glandular) or nodal and extranodal compartments (ulceroglandular) and can be associated with Erythema nodosum. (Courtesy B. Smoller, MD.)*

Haemophilus ducreyi Chancroid

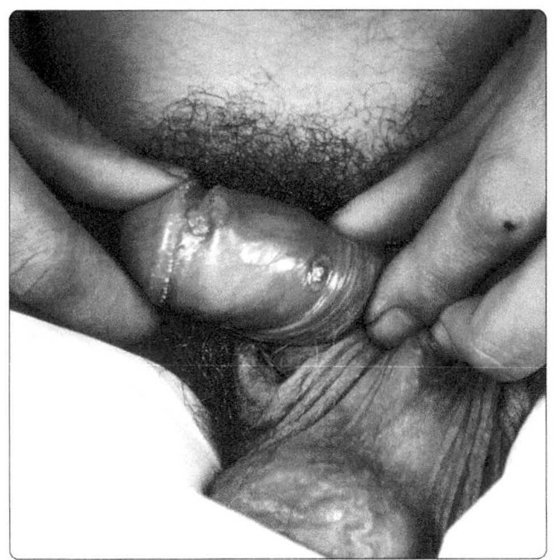

Chancroid

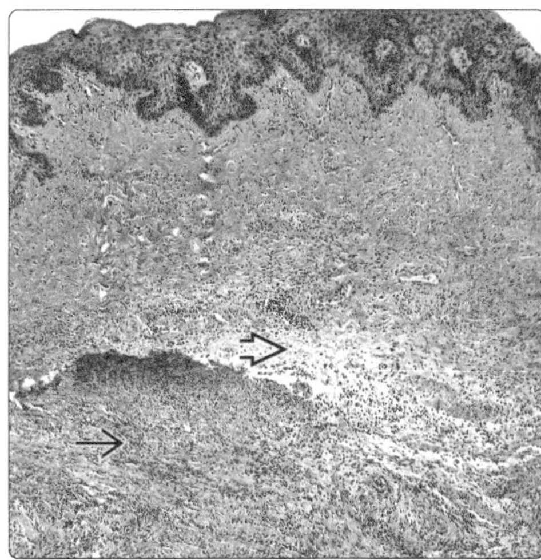

(Left) *Chancroid, caused by Haemophilus ducreyi, must be distinguished from syphilis chancre. (Courtesy D. Pirozzi, MD, CDC/PHIL.)* **(Right)** *Skin biopsy from a patient with chancroid (H. ducreyi infection) demonstrates a nonulcerated lesion with edema ⊡ and deep lymphoplasmacytic inflammation ⊡. Classic lesions are ulcerated with 3 layers, including an upper layer of neutrophils, fibrin, and debris (not seen here) overlying central granulation tissue with chronic inflammation below.*

Legionella spp. Culture Isolate

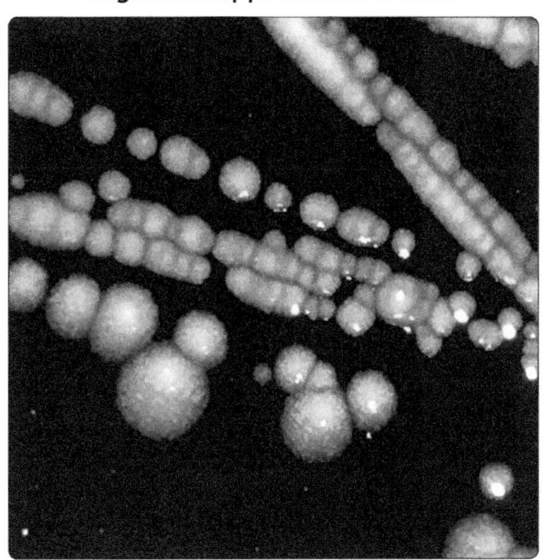

Legionellosis Gross Lung Pathology

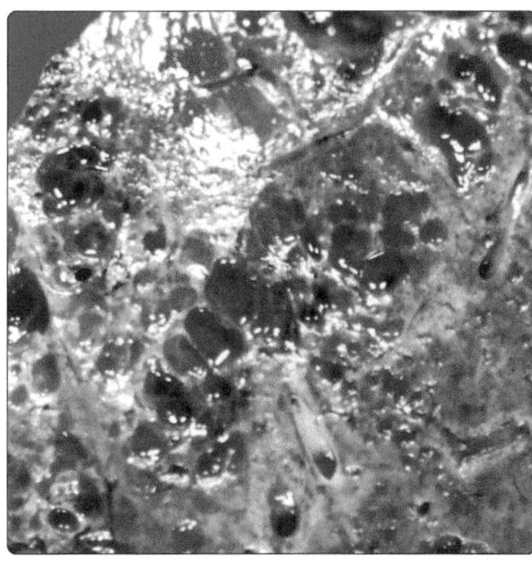

(Left) *Legionella pneumophila forms characteristic bluish, speckled colonies on BCYE-a agar.* **(Right)** *Section of lung tissue from a fatal case of legionellosis demonstrates large amounts of a clear alveolar infiltrate. (Courtesy J. Blackmon, MD, CDC/PHIL.)*

Legionnaire Disease

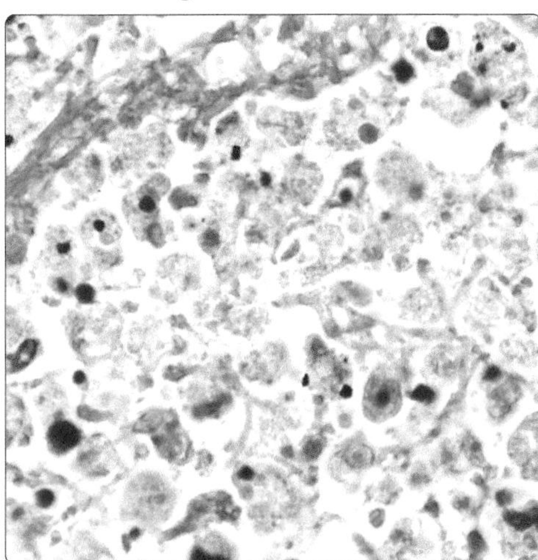

Legionella pneumophila Silver Stain

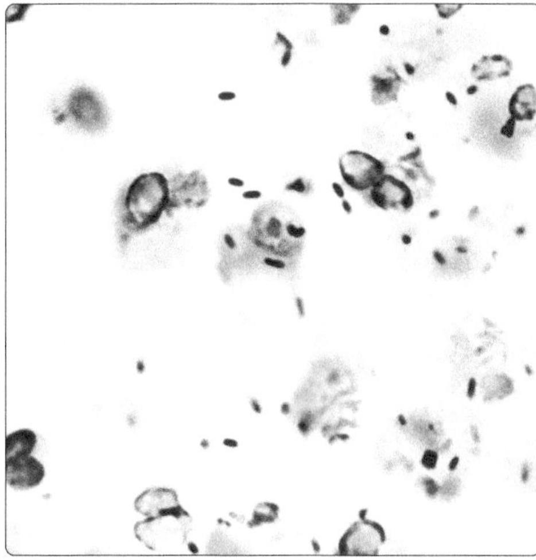

(Left) *Inflammatory congestion of alveolar spaces is shown in this case of fatal pneumonia due to Legionnaire disease. (Courtesy W. Cherry PhD, CDC/PHIL.)* **(Right)** *Biopsied lung tissue specimen, stained with modified Dieterle silver impregnation procedure, reveals small, blunt, pleomorphic intracellular, and extracellular bacilli, which stain brown to black against a pale yellow background. (Courtesy W. Cherry PhD, CDC/PHIL.)*

KEY FACTS

ETIOLOGY/PATHOGENESIS AND CLINICAL ISSUES

- *Acinetobacter baumannii* complex: Pneumonia, line-associated bloodstream infection, postsurgical meningitis and wound infection, trauma-associated skin and soft tissue infection
- *Burkholderia cepacia* complex: Pneumonia, catheter-associated infections, abscesses, bone and joint infections, varied skin and soft tissue involvement, endocarditis, genitourinary infections
- *Burkholderia mallei*: Glanders disease
- *Burkholderia pseudomallei*: Melioidosis (Whitmore disease): Skin and soft tissue infections, pulmonary involvement, disseminated disease involving abscesses of spleen, kidney, prostate, and liver, and encephalomyelitis
- *Pseudomonas aeruginosa:* Hospital-/healthcare-associated and community-acquired pneumonia, chronic colonization in patients with respiratory tract diseases, bloodstream and urinary tract infections, infective endocarditis, ecthyma gangrenosum, osteomyelitis, and septic arthritis

MICROBIOLOGY

- Most *Acinetobacter*, *Burkholderia*, and *Pseudomonas* organisms will grow on standard laboratory media
- Culture characteristics, automated platforms, and identification strips (MALDI, Vitek, API strips, etc.) are used to identify most spp.

DIFFERENTIAL DIAGNOSIS

- Other causes of pneumonia: Bacterial (e.g., *Klebsiella pneumoniae, Mycoplasma pneumoniae*) and viral (e.g., influenza, RSV)
- Other causes of hepatosplenic abscesses: Bacterial (e.g., *Escherichia coli, Bacteroides* spp.) and parasitic (e.g., *Entamoeba histolytica*)
- Other infectious causes of keratitis: Bacterial (e.g., *Staphylococcus aureus*, Enterobacteriaceae) and parasitic (e.g., *Acanthamoeba* spp.)
- Confirm by presence of trophozoites/cysts, Gram- or silver-stained bacteria, IHC, culture, PCR

(Left) *Coronal section gross photograph demonstrates Pseudomonas aeruginosa necrotizing hemorrhagic pneumonia ➡. (Courtesy Franz von Lichtenberg Infectious Disease Collection, BWH.)* **(Right)** *Gross photograph demonstrates necrosis of terminal airways ➡ in a patient with P. aeruginosa pneumonia. (Courtesy Franz von Lichtenberg Infectious Disease Collection, BWH.)*

***Pseudomonas aeruginosa* Pneumonia**

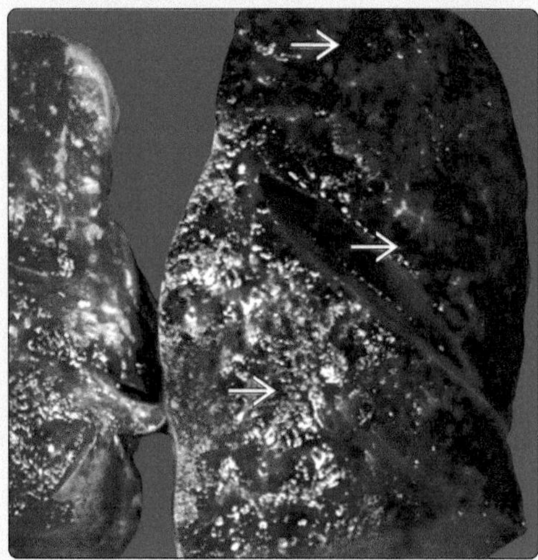

***Pseudomonas aeruginosa* Pneumonia**

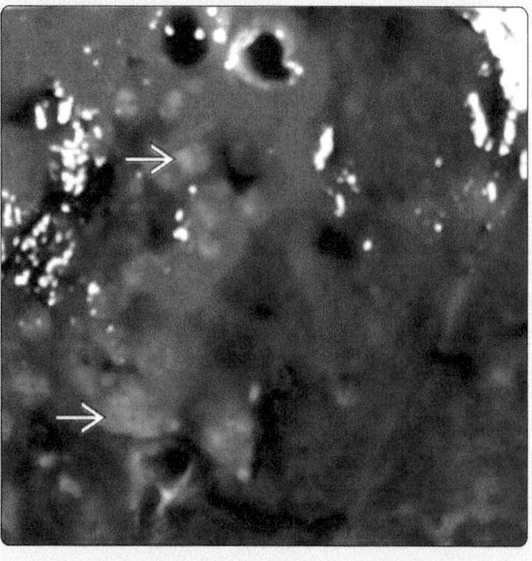

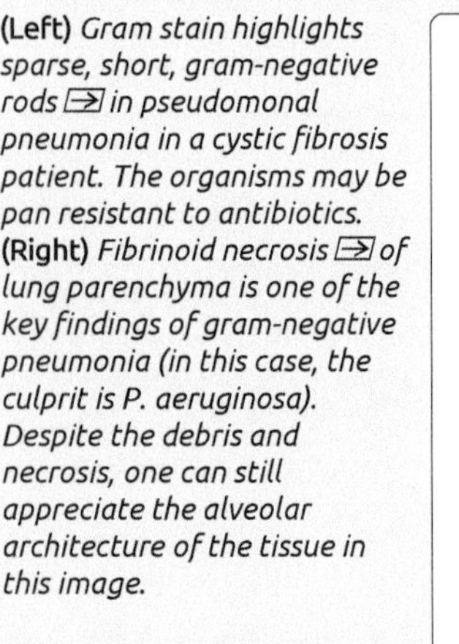

(Left) *Gram stain highlights sparse, short, gram-negative rods ➡ in pseudomonal pneumonia in a cystic fibrosis patient. The organisms may be pan resistant to antibiotics.* **(Right)** *Fibrinoid necrosis ➡ of lung parenchyma is one of the key findings of gram-negative pneumonia (in this case, the culprit is P. aeruginosa). Despite the debris and necrosis, one can still appreciate the alveolar architecture of the tissue in this image.*

***Pseudomonas aeruginosa* Gram Stain**

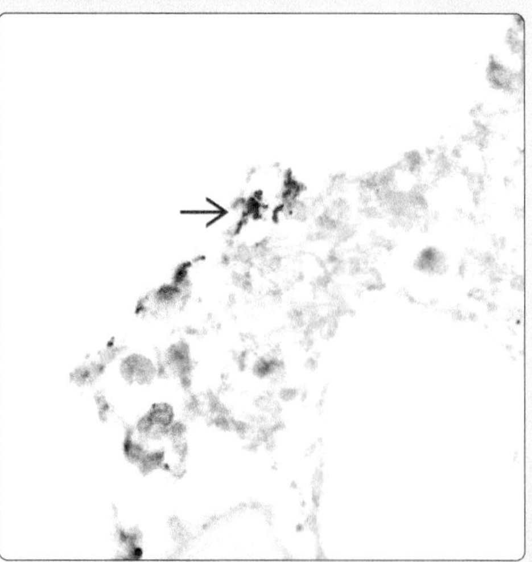

***Pseudomonas aeruginosa* Fibrinoid Necrosis**

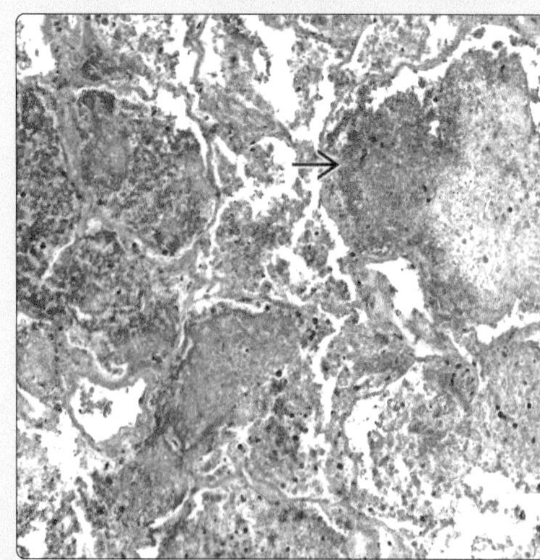

TERMINOLOGY

Definitions

- *Acinetobacter*: Derived from Greek "a kineto" (nonmotile) + "bacter" (rod)
- *Burkholderia*: Walter H. Burkholder (plant pathologist at Cornell University)
- *Pseudomonas*: Derived from Greek "pseudes" (false) + "monas" (nonflagellated protist)

INFECTIOUS AGENTS: EPIDEMIOLOGY, CLINICAL PRESENTATION, AND PATHOGENESIS

Acinetobacter spp.

- *Acinetobacter baumannii* complex; can be colonizer or cause of infection; difficult to differentiate from *Acinetobacter calcoaceticus* (often reported as complex)
  - Healthcare-associated infections, environmental (nicknamed "Iraqibacter" due to emergence as prominent pathogen in military facilities during Iraq War)
  - Frequent resistance to multiple classes of antibiotics, "carbapenem-resistant *A. baumannii* spp. (CRAB)" considered high-risk pathogen
  - Healthcare-associated presentations include pneumonia, bloodstream infection (line associated), postsurgical meningitis, and wound infection
  - Community-associated pneumonia may be severe
  - Trauma-associated skin and soft tissue infections
- *Acinetobacter johnsonii*, *A. lwoffii*, and *A. radioresistens* are skin flora rarely associated with nosocomial infections

Burkholderia spp.

- *B. cepacia* complex is composed of many distinct spp., designated genomovars
  - Widely distributed environmental saprophyte in soil and water; some spp. used in agriculture as components of pesticides or herbicide; can be difficult to discern between colonizer vs. pathogen
  - Have been described as contaminants of disinfectants, such as chlorhexidine, IV solutions, medical devices used in urologic and obstetric procedures, and cosmetics
  - Transmission likely from environment, nosocomially via exposure to contaminated medicines and devices and person-to-person contact
  - Predisposed include patients with cystic fibrosis (impaired mucociliary clearance and reduced antimicrobial production), chronic granulomatous disease (defective oxidative killing), burns, sickle cell anemia, and immunocompromised
  - *B. cepacia* complex spp. have been isolated in ~ 3% of positive respiratory cultures isolated from cystic fibrosis patients; contraindication to lung transplantation in cystic fibrosis (poor postoperative prognosis)
  - Pneumonia, catheter-associated infections, abscesses, bone and joint infections, varied skin and soft tissue involvement (ulcers to ecthyma gangrenosum), endocarditis, genitourinary infections
  - Pathogenesis: Proteases, lipases, siderophores, and pili help to establish invasive disease
- *B. mallei* is causative agent of Glanders disease
  - Tier 1 biological select agent: Potential to pose severe threat to public health and safety; laboratory infections reported
  - Endemic in Africa, Asia, Middle East, Central and South America
  - Transmission mainly through broken skin via direct contact with horses, donkeys, mules, and other animals but also may be inhaled
  - Dependent on route of exposure, e.g., with skin ulcerations or abscesses, increased mucus production in eyes, nose, and respiratory tract or signs and symptoms of pneumonia
  - If untreated, dissemination can occur within 1-4 weeks of initial infection, leading to abscesses in liver and spleen
- *B. pseudomallei* is causative agent of melioidosis, a.k.a. Whitmore disease
  - Tier 1 biological select agent: Potential to pose severe threat to public health and safety
  - Endemic in tropical climates, particularly Southeast Asia and Australia but also in Middle East, India, China, and Central and South America
  - In endemic geographic regions, annual incidence of melioidosis up to 50 cases per 100,000
  - Transmission via percutaneous inoculation and inhalation in wet seasons; rarely, mother-infant transmission (in setting of mastitis), laboratory acquired, and iatrogenic infections
  - Most infections are subclinical
  - Usually presents in patients in 5th-6th decades with underlying conditions (diabetes, alcoholism, renal insufficiency, chronic lung disease, immunosuppression, thalassemia, and kava consumption); incubation is usually 1-21 days but can be up to months or years
  - Acute form defined as < 2 months of symptoms: Skin and soft tissue infections, pulmonary involvement, disseminated disease involving abscesses of spleen, kidney, prostate, and liver, and encephalomyelitis
  - Parenchymal abscesses and suppurative parotitis and, more rarely, mycotic aneurysms, mediastinal masses, pericardial collections, and adrenal abscesses have also been described
  - Chronic form defined as > 2 months of symptoms: Usually involves skin and soft tissue as well as pulmonary infections mimicking tuberculosis (a.k.a. Vietnamese tuberculosis)
  - Reactivation can occur many years after primary infection with latency lasting as long as 62 years; relapse is reported in up to 20% of cases

Pseudomonas spp.

- *P. aeruginosa* is most significant cause of human disease, but other spp. (e.g., *P. putida*) may be isolated; widely present in environment
  - Most common in immunocompromised, those at extremes of life, with cystic fibrosis (accounts for 60-70% of respiratory infections in this group), on ventilators, or with burns or other wounds
  - Many diverse antibiotic-resistance mechanisms, including efflux pumps, drug-modifying enzymes, and mutations in porins (alter permeability)

- If cultured from normally sterile site, likely true infection vs. possible colonization in respiratory tract cultures; cultures from colonized patients may demonstrate numerous strains/subpopulations
- Hospital-/healthcare-associated pneumonia (ventilated and nonventilated patients), community-acquired pneumonia, and chronic colonization in patients with respiratory tract diseases
- Bloodstream and urinary tract infections
- Infective endocarditis
- Ecthyma gangrenosum: In gluteal region or extremities that progress from macules to vesicles and bullous lesions: Dark, central eschar, in setting of bacteremia in immunocompromised patients but can be caused by other organisms
- Osteomyelitis and septic arthritis: Particularly sternoclavicular septic arthritis, vertebral osteomyelitis, temporal bone and skull base osteomyelitis, septic arthritis and osteomyelitis of pubic symphysis, and osteomyelitis caused by nail puncture or combat wounds
- Immunocompetent hosts: Skin and soft tissue infections (folliculitis, paronychia) and otitis externa (swimmer's ear): Keratitis with malignant otitis externa and endophthalmitis are 2 severe, aggressive manifestations
- Establishment in cystic fibrosis patients is long-term and associated changes in phenotype include mucoid appearance, lack of pigmentation, and loss of motility (poor prognosis)
- Pathogenesis: Pili and fimbriae (adhesion and mobility), toxins (alkaline phosphatase, exotoxin A, phospholipase C, protease IV, elastase, pyocyanin, etc.), intercellular communication systems (quorum sensing), pyoverdine (access to iron), lipopolysaccharide, and alginate (modify host immune response)

LABORATORY TESTING, TREATMENT, AND PROGNOSIS

Laboratory Tests

- Culture and Gram stain of affected site (sputum, wound, blood, etc.)
- Serology may be useful to diagnose *B. pseudomallei* infection in nonendemic areas, i.e., to assess for laboratory exposure
- For *B. pseudomallei* encephalomyelitis, CSF may show elevated white blood cell counts (mononuclear predominance), normal or slightly decreased glucose, and intermittently elevated protein

Treatment

- *Acinetobacter* spp.
  - Several agents available for susceptible organisms, including ampicillin-sulbactam, cefepime, and meropenem
  - For extensively resistant organisms, options may include polymyxins, cefiderocol
- *Burkholderia* spp.
  - *B. cepacia* complex
    - Guided by isolate susceptibility, trimethoprim-sulfamethoxazole, levofloxacin, carbapenems, minocycline may be options; combination therapy often required
  - *B. mallei* and *B. pseudomallei* diseases
    - Induction IV therapy (ceftazidime, meropenem, or imipenem) followed by oral eradication therapy for several months (trimethoprim-sulfamethoxazole is preferred)
    - Lab exposure: Trimethoprim-sulfamethoxazole or amoxicillin-clavulanate (21 days)
- *P. aeruginosa* infection
  - Guided by isolate susceptibility
  - Options include piperacillin-tazobactam, cefepime, meropenem, and aminoglycosides, among others

Prognosis

- Morbidity and mortality range widely depending on organism and host

MICROBIOLOGY

Morphologic and Biochemical Characteristics

- Aerobic, gram-negative, non-spore-forming rods
  - *Acinetobacter* organisms may appear as coccobacilli, diplococci, or cocci; may be difficult to destain and can sometimes be incorrectly identified as gram positive
  - *B. pseudomallei* may demonstrate bipolar staining resembling safety pins (neither sensitive nor specific)
  - *P. aeruginosa* may have apparent mucoid material or be present within polymorphonuclear cells (both clinically significant)
- "Nonfermenter" refers to organisms that do not ferment glucose
  - In addition to *Pseudomonas*, *Burkholderia*, and *Acinetobacter* spp., also includes *Stenotrophomonas*, *Ralstonia*, and *Achromobacter* spp., among others

Culture

- *Acinetobacter* organisms grow on standard laboratory media
- Most *Burkholderia* spp. will grow on standard laboratory media, including 5% sheep blood and MacConkey
  - *B. pseudomallei* is selected by Ashdown agar (containing gentamicin) or liquid transport broth (containing colistin) when used to culture samples from nonsterile sites
    - Culture propagation can be associated with laboratory-acquired infections (laboratory staff should take precautions when working with potential or suspect samples)
    - Colonies appear smooth and creamy at first, then often mature to dry, wrinkled colonies after few days
- *Pseudomonas* organisms grow on most laboratory media
  - Mueller-Hinton agar often used to highlight production of blue-green pigments (pyocyanin and pyoverdine) associated with *P. aeruginosa*
  - *P. aeruginosa* can grow at 42 °C and have characteristic grape-like odor
  - *P. fluorescens* can grow at 4 °C

Microbiologic Identification

- Large part of laboratory identification of these organisms is by culture characteristics
- Automated platforms and identification strips (MALDI, Vitek, API strips, etc.) are used in clinical laboratory to identify most of these spp.
  - *Pseudomonas* isolates from cystic fibrosis patients may be more difficult to identify due to altered phenotype

- *Burkholderia* spp. may be misidentified as other nonfermentative spp. on automated platforms
- *B. pseudomallei* and *B. mallei* require enhanced biosafety environment and will not be worked up in standard clinical laboratory
- *B. cepacia* complex requires sequencing of multiple targets to be identified past "complex" level

HISTOPATHOLOGY BY ORGAN SYSTEM

Central Nervous System

- *P. aeruginosa*: Less common cause of meningitis; often associated with neurosurgical procedures
- *B. pseudomallei*: Abscess and encephalitis

Ocular

- *P. aeruginosa*: Contact lens-associated keratitis and endophthalmitis (associated with penetrating injuries and surgical procedures)

Pulmonic

- Pneumonia
  - *Acinetobacter* spp. in pulmonary specimens may be due to colonization or infection; increasingly reported as cause of hospital-acquired pneumonia (particularly in ventilated patients)
  - Pneumonia is common manifestation of *B. pseudomallei* infection (melioidosis): Presentation can range from septic shock to mild disease; severe cases often associated with caseous necrosis and metastatic abscesses throughout both lungs
  - *P. aeruginosa* is most common cause of gram-negative, hospital-acquired, and ventilator-associated pneumonia; virulent pneumonia characterized by hemorrhage and necrosis (high mortality); can involve microvasculature, resulting in bacteremia and sepsis
- Chronic lung disease associated with cystic fibrosis
  - *P. aeruginosa* is predominant pathogen, though presence of *B. cepacia* complex, nontuberculous mycobacteria, and MRSA are common and carry poor prognosis
  - Progressive course punctuated by acute pulmonary exacerbations (APEs) with increased sputum volume, change in sputum color, hemoptysis, cough, and fatigue, among others; clinical spectrum includes chronic airway and parenchymal infection, bronchopneumonia, and necrotizing pneumonia

Cardiac

- *P. aeruginosa* is rare (3%) cause of suppurative gram-negative endocarditis; associated with IV drug use (right-sided endocarditis)

Hepatic

- *B. mallei* or *B. pseudomallei*: Liver abscess

Reticuloendothelial

- *B. mallei* or *B. pseudomallei*: Splenic abscess

Bone

- *P. aeruginosa*
  - Osteomyelitis via hematogenous spread or direct inoculation
  - Associated with sternoclavicular and symphysis pubis septic arthritis, vertebral and skull base osteomyelitis, osteomyelitis associated with nail puncture, osteomyelitis associated with combat
  - Contiguous spread is often from chronic, decubitus, or diabetic foot ulcers; will likely be polymicrobial and demonstrate chronic infection
  - Poor prognosis (higher recurrence and need for amputation)

Skin

- *Acinetobacter* spp. is associated with trauma-induced skin and soft tissue infections
- *B. pseudomallei*: Reported to cause nodules and ulcers with microabscesses, though range of reported findings varies widely
- *P. aeruginosa*
  - Ecthyma gangrenosum: Characterized by epidermal and dermal necrosis, necrotizing vasculitis, and mixed inflammatory infiltrate; bacteria can be isolated from lesion
  - Malakoplakia (nodules characterized by von Hansemann cells, macrophages with eosinophilic granules, and, occasionally, basophilic Michaelis-Gutmann bodies)
  - Botryomycosis (purulent abscess filled with basophilic granules of varying size, corresponding to colonies of bacteria, embedded in hyaline matrix)

Urogenital

- *P. aeruginosa* is common cause of nosocomial- and healthcare-associated urinary tract infections

DIFFERENTIAL DIAGNOSIS

Other Infectious Causes of Pneumonia

- Bacterial (e.g., *Klebsiella pneumoniae*, *Mycoplasma pneumoniae*) and viral (e.g., influenza, RSV)
- Confirm by Gram or silver stains, IHC, culture, PCR

Other Infectious Causes of Hepatosplenic Abscesses

- Bacterial (e.g., *Escherichia coli*, *Bacteroides* spp.) and parasitic (e.g., *Entamoeba histolytica*)
- Confirm by presence of trophozoites/cysts, Gram- or silver-stained bacteria, IHC, culture, PCR

Other Infectious Causes of Keratitis

- Bacterial (e.g., *Staphylococcus aureus*, Enterobacteriaceae) and parasitic (e.g., *Acanthamoeba* spp.)
- Confirm by presence of trophozoites/cysts, Gram- or silver-stained bacteria, IHC, culture, PCR

SELECTED REFERENCES

1. Bzdyl NM et al: Pathogenicity and virulence of Burkholderia pseudomallei. Virulence. 13(1):1945-65, 2022
2. Gee JE et al: Multistate outbreak of melioidosis associated with imported aromatherapy spray. N Engl J Med. 386(9):861-8, 2022
3. Tamma PD et al: Infectious Diseases Society of America guidance on the treatment of AmpC β-lactamase-producing enterobacterales, carbapenem-resistant Acinetobacter baumannii, and Stenotrophomonas maltophilia Infections. Clin Infect Dis. 74(12):2089-114, 2022
4. Rossi E et al: Pseudomonas aeruginosa adaptation and evolution in patients with cystic fibrosis. Nat Rev Microbiol. 19(5):331-42, 2021
5. Harding CM et al: Uncovering the mechanisms of Acinetobacter baumannii virulence. Nat Rev Microbiol. 16(2):91-102, 2018
6. Prasad SC et al: Osteomyelitis of the temporal bone: terminology, diagnosis, and management. J Neurol Surg B Skull Base. 75(5):324-31, 2014

(Left) *Acute inflammatory exudate rims expansile hemorrhage in a necrotic lung in this case of P. aeruginosa. In severe cases, such as this, both necrotizing pneumonia and eventually diffuse alveolar damage result in high mortality.* **(Right)** *This image shows acute P. aeruginosa pneumonia associated with ectatic bronchiole in a 35-year-old patient with advanced cystic fibrosis. The chronic inflammation is a consistent feature of cystic fibrosis regardless of colonization.*

Pseudomonas aeruginosa **Necrotizing Pneumonia**

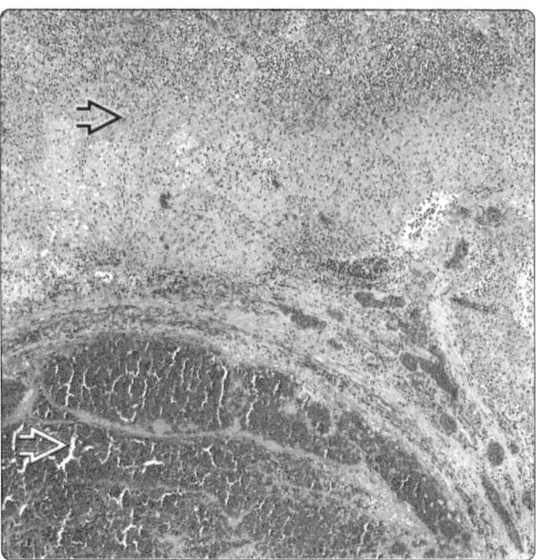

Pseudomonas aeruginosa **in Cystic Fibrosis**

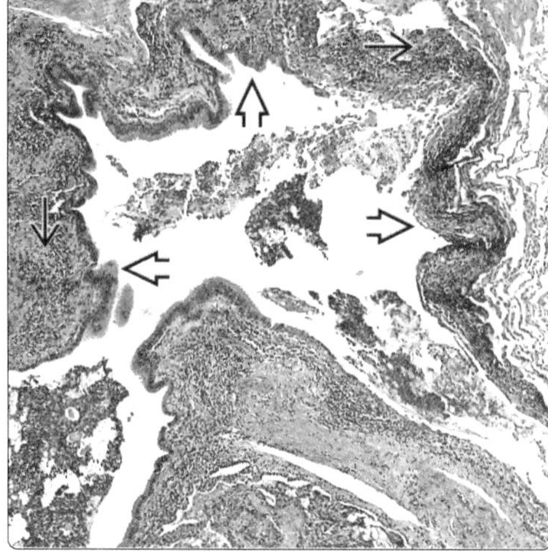

(Left) *Section shows acute P. aeruginosa pneumonia centered on airways with sparing of the adjacent pulmonary parenchyma in a patient with cystic fibrosis. As the disease progresses, the organisms may break through bronchial walls and cause spillover pneumonia in the alveoli.* **(Right)** *Gross photograph demonstrates P. aeruginosa vegetative endocarditis. (Courtesy Franz von Lichtenberg Infectious Disease Collection, BWH.)*

Pseudomonas aeruginosa **Pneumonia Progression**

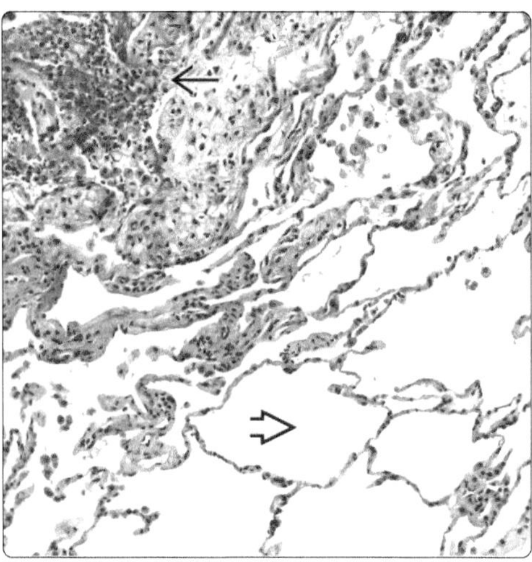

Pseudomonas aeruginosa **Endocarditis**

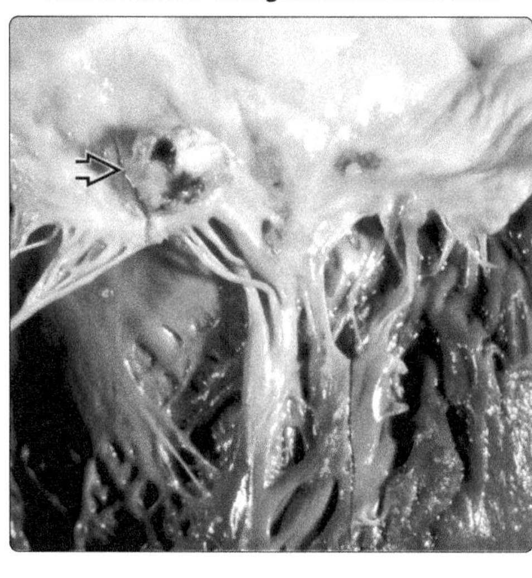

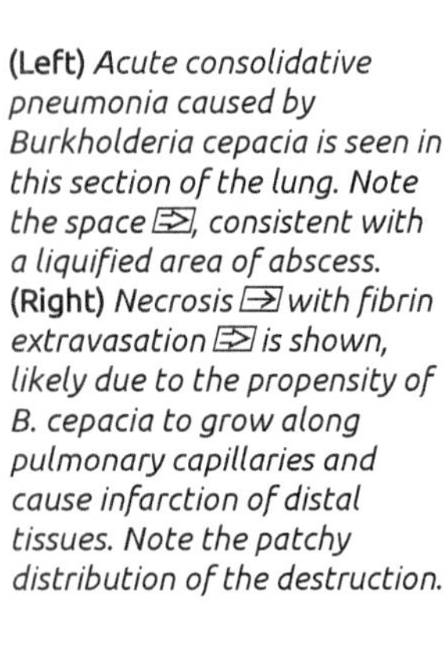

(Left) *Acute consolidative pneumonia caused by Burkholderia cepacia is seen in this section of the lung. Note the space, consistent with a liquified area of abscess.* **(Right)** *Necrosis with fibrin extravasation is shown, likely due to the propensity of B. cepacia to grow along pulmonary capillaries and cause infarction of distal tissues. Note the patchy distribution of the destruction.*

Burkholderia cepacia **Acute Pneumonia**

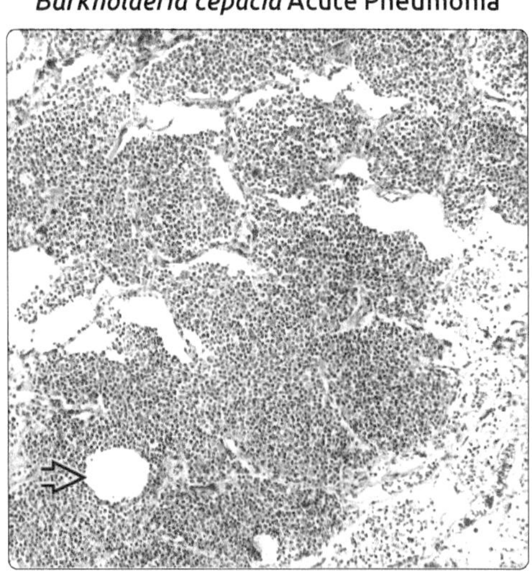

Burkholderia cepacia **Pulmonary Necrosis**

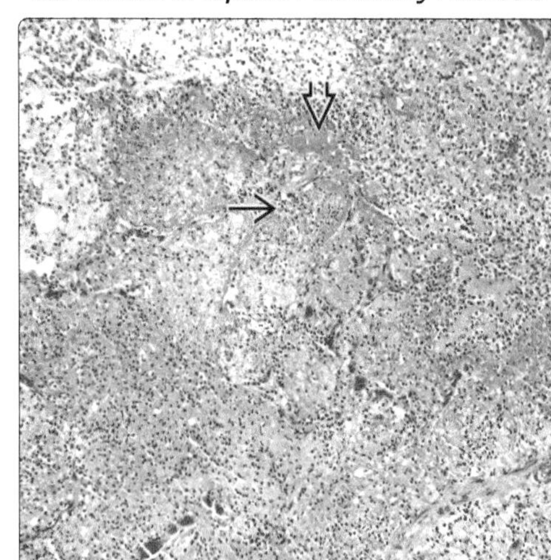

Reactive Pathology

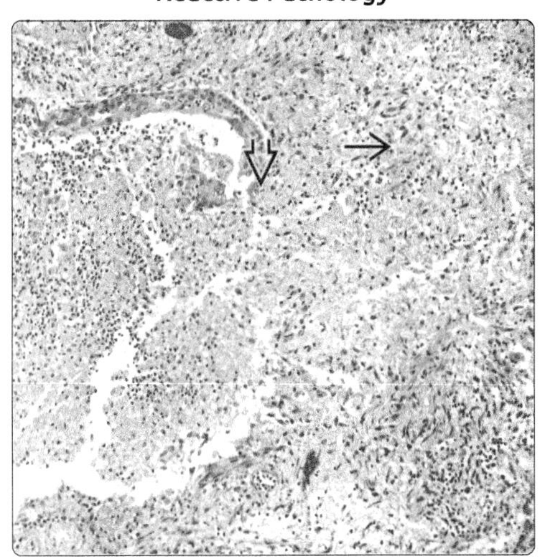

Burkholderia pseudomallei (Melioidosis)

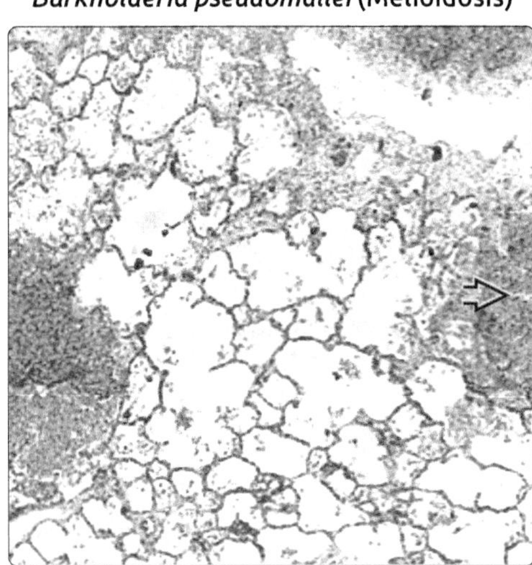

(Left) *Bronchiolar rupture ⇒ with reactive fibroblastic proliferation ⇒, which might have formed an abscess cavity, is shown. This patient's cultures grew B. cepacia but could have also been of a Pseudomonas species.* **(Right)** *Miliary lung lesions rich in macrophages ⇒ are demonstrated in this patient with melioidosis sepsis caused by Burkholderia pseudomallei.*

Burkholderia pseudomallei Gram Stain

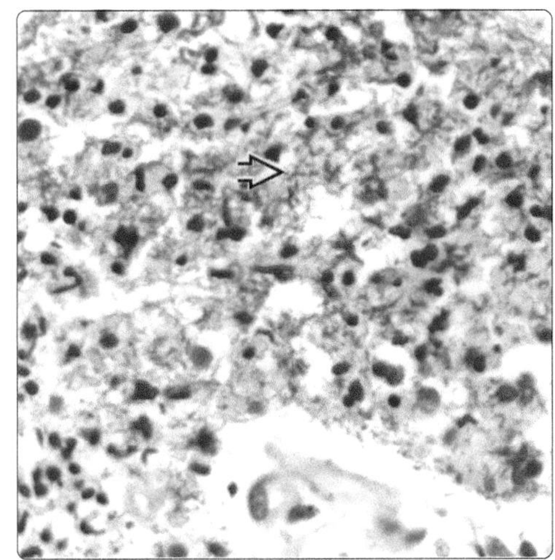

Acinetobacter baumannii Gram Stain

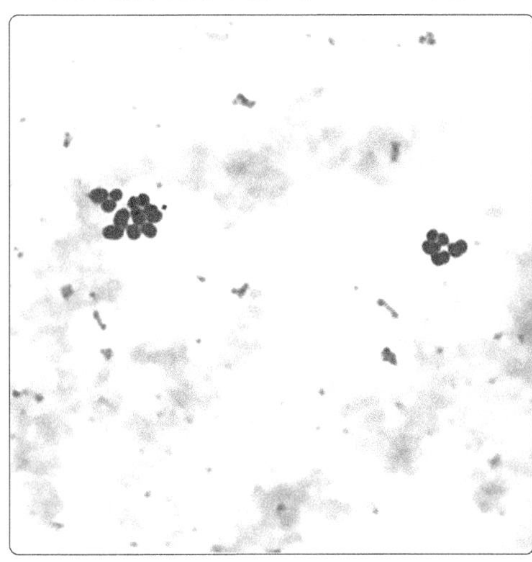

(Left) *Gram stain elucidates dense growth of B. pseudomallei ⇒ in lung lesions in a patient with melioidosis.* **(Right)** *Gram stain of a positive blood culture bottle demonstrates the appearance of Acinetobacter baumannii complex as plump, gram-negative diplococci.*

Necrotizing Vasculitis

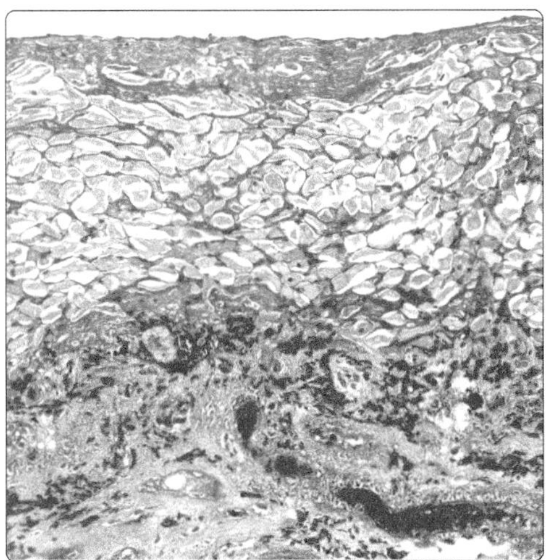

Coagulative Necrosis

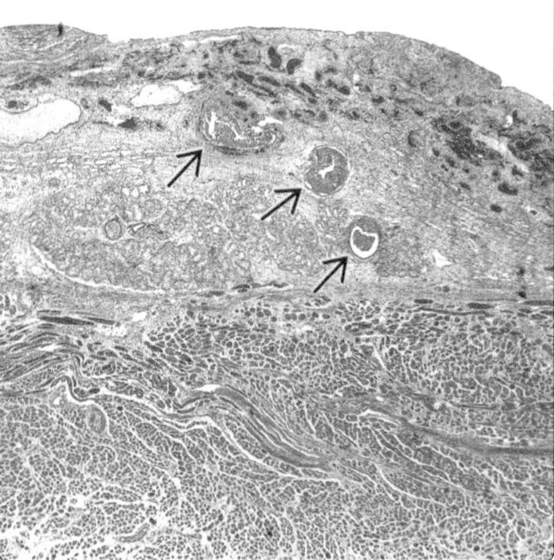

(Left) *Ecthyma gangrenosum (often associated with P. aeruginosa bacteremia) is characterized by necrotizing vasculitis with coagulative necrosis of the superficial skin. Often, these specimens are remarkably pauciinflammatory, as these patients are often profoundly immunosuppressed. (Courtesy B. Smoller, MD.)* **(Right)** *Skin sample shows the characteristic features of euthymic gangrenosum: Superficial coagulative necrosis in a pauciinflammatory context ⇒. (Courtesy B. Smoller, MD.)*

KEY FACTS

ETIOLOGY/PATHOGENESIS

- Much of normal human intestinal, vaginal, and oral microbiota is composed of anaerobes, which can cause invasive infections

CLINICAL ISSUES

- *Bacteroides* spp.: Polymicrobial anaerobic infections, propensity for abscess formation
- *Fusobacterium nucleatum:* Periodontal disease, obstetric infections, multiorgan disseminated disease
- *Fusobacterium necrophorum*: Lemierre syndrome, joint infections, peritonsillar abscess
- *Leptotrichia* spp.: Bacteremia, infective endocarditis
- *Porphyromonas* spp.: Chronic periodontitis, necrotizing ulcerative gingivitis, intraabdominal infections
- *Prevotella* spp.: Empyema, lung abscess, periodontal disease, bacterial vaginosis, PID, tuboovarian abscess
- *Veillonella* spp.: Bacteremia, endocarditis, osteomyelitis, meningitis, pleuropulmonary and joint infections

MICROSCOPIC

- Gram-negative anaerobes often members of polymicrobial infections; highlighted by Gram and silver stains
- Histopathologic findings are nonspecific compared to other bacteria associated with periodontitis and peritonsillar abscess, osteomyelitis, septic arthritis, and intraabdominal, brain, or liver abscess

TOP DIFFERENTIAL DIAGNOSES

- Actinomycosis: Gram-positive filamentous bacilli, frequently with Splendore-Hoeppli phenomenon; other bacteria may be intermixed
- Other bacterial causes of abscess: Gram-positive (e.g., *Staphylococcus* spp., *Streptococcus* spp.) and gram-negative aerobes (e.g., *Escherichia coli*)
- Other causes of chorioamnionitis: Bacteria (e.g., *Escherichia coli,* group B strep, *Mycoplasma pneumoniae*) and fungi (e.g., *Candida* spp.)
- Confirm with Gram and silver stains, IHC, PCR, culture

(Left) *Lung with severe diffuse alveolar damage and superimposed peribronchial necrosis from a previously healthy 20-year-old woman who succumbed to Fusobacterium necrophorum infection is shown.* **(Right)** *Lung with a sharply circumscribed area of necrotic inflammatory cells is shown. The periphery is densely packed with mixed mononuclear and neutrophilic inflammation.*

***Fusobacterium* Infection in Lung**

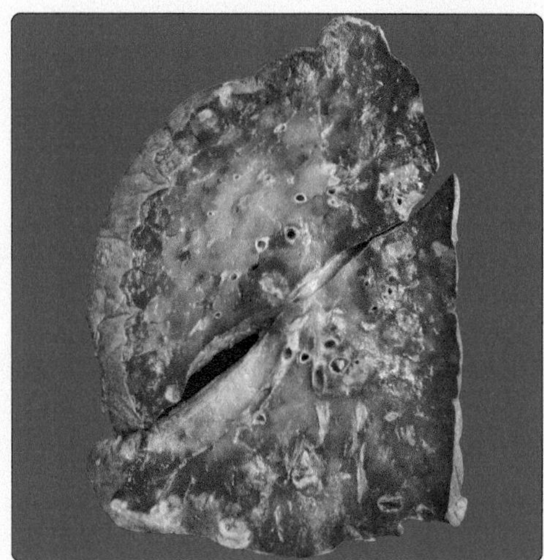

***Fusobacterium necrophorum* Necrotizing Pneumonia**

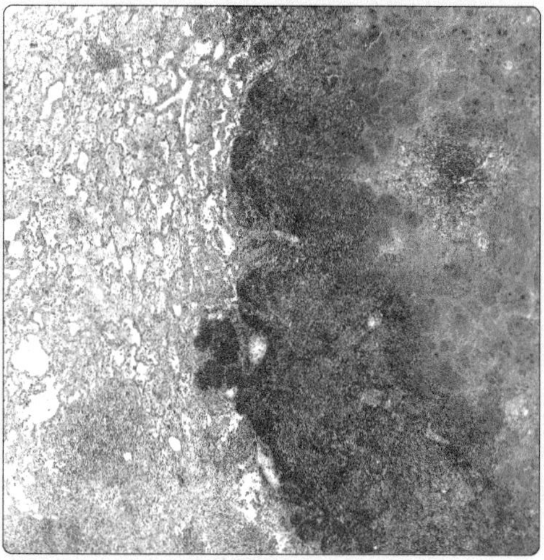

(Left) *High-power image from the same autopsied lung reveals numerous gram-negative, short rods/coccobacilli at the interface between viable and necrotic inflammatory cells.* **(Right)** *This section shows monochorionic, diamniotic twin-dividing membranes with a Fusobacterium infection in twin A ⇒ but not in twin B ⇨. Because twin A is usually located closer to the cervix, its amniotic sac is more susceptible to ascending infection than that of twin B. (From DP: Placenta.)*

***Fusobacterium necrophorum* Gram Stain**

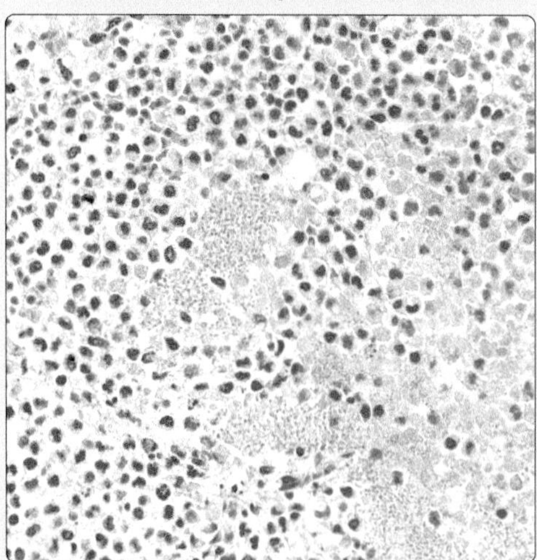

***Fusobacterium* Infection in Placenta**

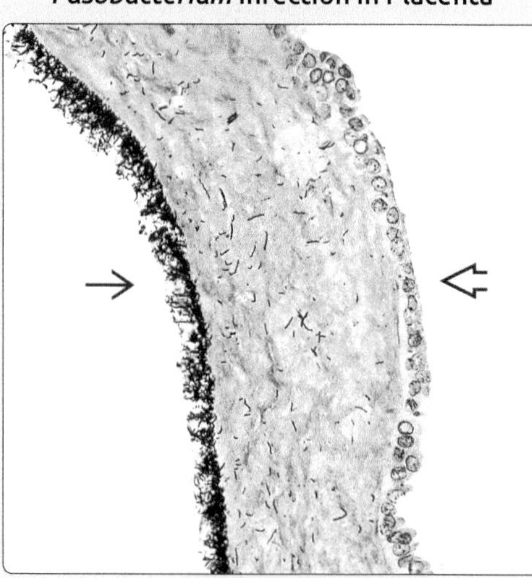

TERMINOLOGY

Synonyms

- Necrobacillosis, postanginal sepsis, or Lemierre syndrome all refer to infection with *Fusobacterium necrophorum*

Definitions

- *Fusobacterium*: Latin: fūs(us) (spindle)
- *Prevotella*: André R. Prévot (French bacteriologist)
- *Porphyromonas*: Greek: Porphyreos (purple), monas (unit)
- *Veillonella*: Adrien Veillon (French bacteriologist)
- *Leptotrichia:* Leptos (fine) thricos (hair)

ETIOLOGY/PATHOGENESIS

Infectious Agents

- Much of normal human intestinal, vaginal, and oral microbiota is composed of anaerobes
- *Bacteroides* spp.
  - Composes 30% of total gut bacteria (most of which are benign commensals); *B. tectus* also associated with dog and cat bites
  - *B. fragilis* group organisms are most prominent pathogens among gram-negative anaerobes (and are most likely species to cause monomicrobial infection)
  - Other clinically relevant species include *B. thetaiotaomicron*, *B. vulgatus, B. distasonis, B. ovatus, B. uniformis, B. caccae*
  - Pathogenicity associated with distinctive capsular component (polysaccharide A)
- *Fusobacterium* spp.
  - Invasive *Fusobacterium* spp. have been shown to be rich in adhesions and other surface-associated proteins, as compared to noninvasive strains
  - Clinically relevant species include *F. nucleatum* and *F. necrophorum*
  - *F. nucleatum* is major component of dental plaque, associated with mature biofilms in periodontitis, and some suggestion of linkage with colorectal cancer
- *Leptotrichia* spp.
  - Part of normal oral and intestinal human flora
  - Invasive infections in immunosuppressed patients
- *Porphyromonas* spp.
  - Major constituents of dental plaque
  - Clinically significant species include *P. gingivalis* and *P. endodontalis*
  - Able to invade periodontal tissue and is potent biofilm producer
- *Prevotella* spp.
  - Prevalent in oral, vaginal, and gut microbiota; enriched among gut flora in association with plant-rich diet
  - Inverse association with prevalence of *Bacteroides* spp. within gut
  - Possible association with inflammatory conditions, such as rheumatoid arthritis
- *Veillonella* spp.
  - Inhabitants of normal human oral flora (and gastrointestinal tract and vagina to lesser degree)
  - Often not speciated, though *V. parvula* is most often associated with significant infection

CLINICAL ISSUES

Epidemiology

- Poor dental hygiene may predispose patients to invasive infection by oral anaerobes
- Infections associated with gastrointestinal and gynecological malignancies, infection, &/or procedures

Presentation

- *Bacteroides* spp.
  - Major component of polymicrobial anaerobic infections and most common cause of anaerobic bacteremia
  - Associated with intraabdominal and gynecological infection, trauma, and malignancy
  - Isolated from joints, heart valves, abdominal abscesses, ulcers, bronchial secretions, bones, and brain
- *F. nucleatum*
  - Periodontal disease
  - Obstetric and perinatal infections causing preterm birth, term stillbirth, and fetal demise
  - Brain abscess complicating periodontal disease, joint infection, pleuropulmonary infections, and, rarely, bacteremia
- *F. necrophorum*
  - Lemierre syndrome: Pharyngitis, high fever, cervical lymphadenopathy, thrombophlebitis of internal jugular vein, intensely painful metastatic abscess (commonly lungs, joints, and long bones)
  - Peritonsillar abscess
  - Anaerobic joint infections, polymicrobial intraabdominal infections
- *Leptotrichia* spp.
  - Infrequent cause of bacteremia and infective endocarditis, associated with neutropenia
- *Porphyromonas* spp.
  - Strongly correlated with chronic periodontitis
  - Necrotizing ulcerative gingivitis, infected root canals, intraabdominal infections
  - *P. uenonis* specifically associated with (polymicrobial) infections below waistline (appendicitis, pilonidal abscess, etc.)
  - Induces high levels of proinflammatory cytokines, associated with development of cerebrovascular disease
  - *P. gingivalis* expresses citrullinating peptidylarginine deiminase enzyme that converts arginine residues in proteins to citrulline and is associated with autoimmune conditions, such as rheumatoid arthritis
- *Prevotella* spp.
  - Typically part of polymicrobial infection
  - Cariogenic organism and other oral infections
  - Rare reports of brain abscess following dental procedures
  - Associated with empyema, lung abscess, periodontal disease, bacterial vaginosis, pelvic inflammatory disease (PID), and tuboovarian abscess
  - Presence may correlate localized and systemic inflammatory conditions; direct infections are uncommonly reported
- *Veillonella* spp.
  - Most significant pathogen among anaerobic gram-negative cocci

- Rarely isolated as causative agent of serious infection, reports include bacteremia, osteomyelitis, meningitis, prosthetic joint infection, pleuropulmonary infection, and endocarditis

Laboratory Tests

- Monomicrobial infections may be identified with 16S rRNA Sanger sequencing, while next-generation sequencing required for polymicrobial infections

Treatment

- Due to common presence in polymicrobial infections, treatment regimens are often directed toward broad coverage (including coinfecting enteric organisms)
- Metronidazole, β-lactam/β-lactamase inhibitors, carbapenems, etc. all have role in treatment
- *B. fragilis* group is penicillin resistant
- Surgery for abscess, debridement of necrotic tissue

Prognosis

- *Bacteroides* spp. high mortality (27% for bacteremias)

MICROBIOLOGY

Morphology

- *Bacteroides* spp.: Gram-negative rods (may be pleomorphic, can appear as coccobacilli); when grown in liquid medium, cells develop bipolar vacuoles ("safety pins")
- *Fusobacterium nucleatum*: Filamentous gram-negative rods with slender, pointed ends (needle shape)
- *Fusobacterium necrophorum*: Pleomorphic, from coccoid to long rods with rounded ends
- *Leptotrichia* spp.: Distinct pencil-shaped, fusiform, gram-negative rods
- *Prevotella* and *Porphyromonas* spp.: Pleomorphic, gram-negative rods; often pigmented colonies (brown/black)
- *Veillonella* spp.: Gram-negative diplococci

Biochemical Characteristics

- *Bacteroides* spp.: Bile tolerant, non-spore-forming; resistant to kanamycin, vancomycin, and colistin; production of short-chain fatty acids may be used to speciate
- *Fusobacterium* spp.: Bile sensitive, indole positive; resistant to vancomycin, sensitive to kanamycin and colistin; produces butyrate during glucose fermentation

Culture and Identification

- Care must be taken to maintain anaerobic environment when transporting specimens to laboratory for anaerobic culture (e.g., anaerobic swabs or ESwabs); laboratory growth requires use of anaerobic chamber or anaerobic jars to avoid toxic effects of oxygen
- Many specialized anaerobic agars are available, i.e.,
  - *Bacteroides* bile esculin agar: Selective growth of *Bacteroides* spp.
  - Egg yolk agar: Assessment of lecithinase and lipase production by *Fusobacterium* spp.
  - Laked Kanamycin-vancomycin blood agar (LKV): Selective growth of *Prevotella* and *Bacteroides* spp.
- Due to colonization of mucosal surfaces with anaerobic flora, aspirates and biopsies are preferred over swabs for detection of clinically relevant organisms
- Identification has traditionally been by biochemical/susceptibility profiles; MALDI-TOF MS currently plays major role in identification
- Identification of *F. necrophorum* as cause of pharyngotonsillitis may be missed, as most diagnostics for that syndrome are geared toward detection of group A *Streptococcus* (*S. pyogenes*)
- Susceptibility testing rarely performed

MICROSCOPIC

Histologic Features

- Gram-negative anaerobes often members of polymicrobial infections
- Histopathologic findings are nonspecific compared to other bacteria associated with periodontitis and peritonsillar abscess, osteomyelitis, septic arthritis, and intraabdominal, brain, or liver abscess
- *F. necrophorum* associated with Lemierre syndrome: Suppurative thrombophlebitis of internal jugular vein, metastatic abscesses of lungs, joints, and long bones
- *F. nucleatum* associated with chorioamnionitis

ANCILLARY TESTS

Special Stains

- Gram and silver stains (e.g., Warthin-Starry) highlight organisms

DIFFERENTIAL DIAGNOSIS

Actinomycosis

- Gram-positive filamentous bacilli, frequently with Splendore-Hoeppli phenomenon; other bacteria may be intermixed
- Confirm with Gram and silver stains, PCR, culture

Other Bacterial Causes of Abscess

- Includes gram-positive (e.g., *Staphylococcus* spp., *Streptococcus* spp.) and gram-negative aerobes (e.g., *Escherichia coli*)
- Confirm with Gram and silver stains, PCR, culture

Other Causes of Chorioamnionitis

- Includes diverse bacteria (e.g., *Escherichia coli,* group B strep, *Mycoplasma pneumoniae*) and fungi (e.g., *Candida* spp.)
- Confirm with Gram and silver stains, IHC, PCR, culture

SELECTED REFERENCES

1. Kajihara T et al: Distribution, trends, and antimicrobial susceptibility of Bacteroides, Clostridium, Fusobacterium, and Prevotella Species causing bacteremia in Japan During 2011-2020: a retrospective observational study based on national surveillance data. Open Forum Infect Dis. 10(7):ofad334, 2023
2. Ranganath N et al: Leptotrichia bacteremia: 10-year retrospective clinical analysis and antimicrobial susceptibility profiles. J Clin Microbiol. 61(2):e0173322, 2023
3. Tett A et al: Prevotella diversity, niches and interactions with the human host. Nat Rev Microbiol. 19(9):585-99, 2021
4. Bullman S et al: Analysis of Fusobacterium persistence and antibiotic response in colorectal cancer. Science. 358(6369):1443-8, 2017
5. Riordan T: Human infection with Fusobacterium necrophorum (Necrobacillosis), with a focus on Lemierre's syndrome. Clin Microbiol Rev. 20(4):622-59, 2007

Fusobacterium spp. Gram Stain

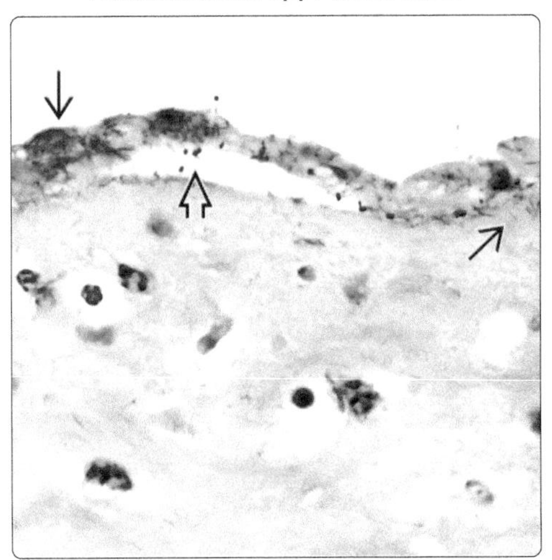

Fusobacterium spp. Warthin-Starry Stain

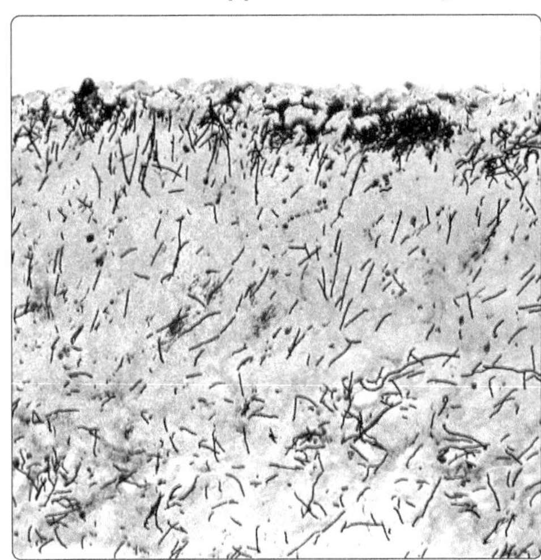

(Left) *Gram stain shows mixed infection with gram-negative filamentous Fusobacterium spp.* ➔ *and gram-positive cocci* ➔. *Fusobacterium spp. are a frequent component of polymicrobial infections. (From DP: Placenta.)* **(Right)** *Warthin-Starry stain is very useful in highlighting the organisms within the amnion and subamniotic connective tissue. (From DP: Placenta.)*

Fusobacterium Chorioamnionitis

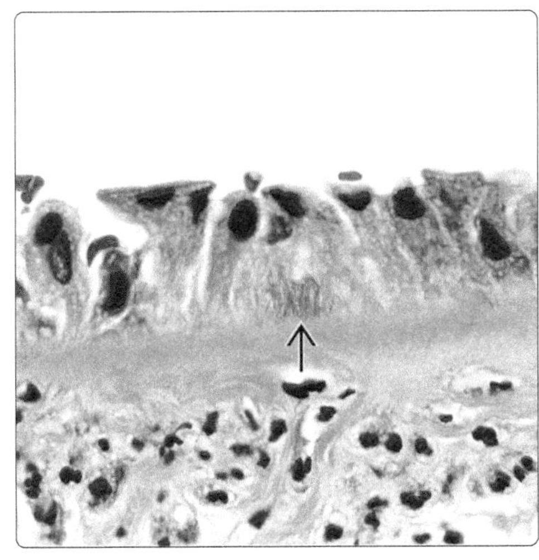

Veillonella spp. Gram Stain

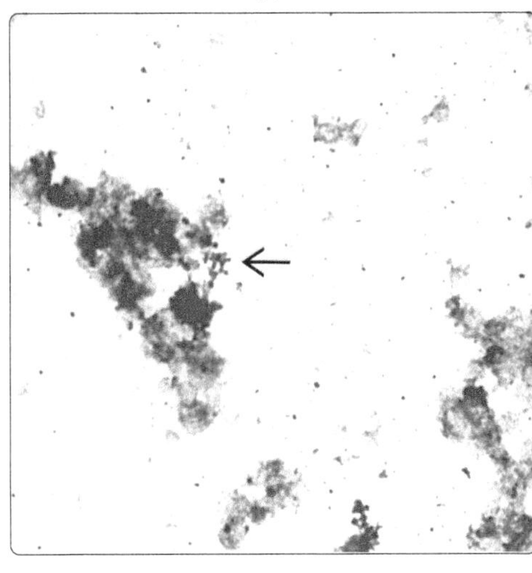

(Left) *Fusobacterium spp. are very long, thin, filamentous bacterium* ➔ *usually found vertically oriented in the amnion. They are associated with severe chorioamnionitis. (From DP: Placenta.)* **(Right)** *Gram stain of Veillonella spp. from a blood bottle demonstrates small, gram-negative cocci* ➔.

Bacteroides spp. Gram Stain

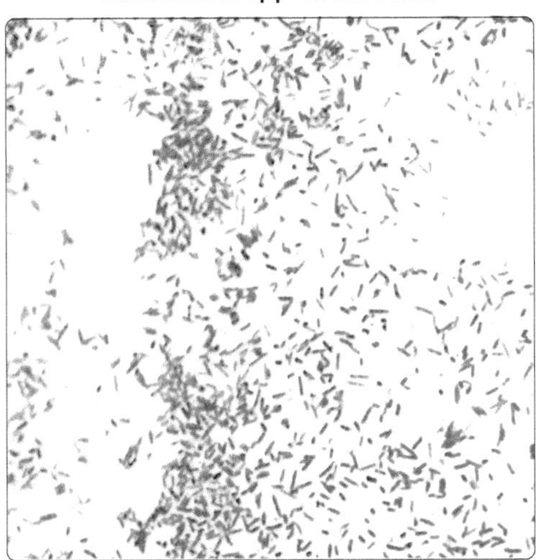

Prevotella spp. Gram Stain

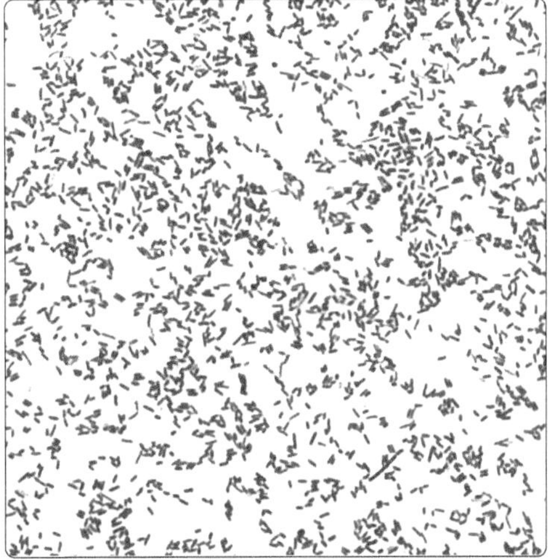

(Left) *Gram stain of Bacteroides fragilis demonstrates medium-sized, gram-negative rods.* **(Right)** *Gram stain of Prevotella spp. demonstrates short, gram-negative rods.*

Bartonella Species Infections

KEY FACTS

ETIOLOGY/PATHOGENESIS

- Infection with *Bartonella* spp. facultative intracellular, pleomorphic, gram-negative bacilli that invade RBCs; transmitted by arthropods via blood meals, scratch or saliva of infected animal, or blood transfusion

CLINICAL ISSUES

- Carrion disease (*Bartonella bacilliformis*): Oroya fever with acute hemolytic anemia, verruga peruana cutaneous lesions
- Cat-scratch disease (*Bartonella henselae*): Papule or pustule at scratch site; lymphadenopathy; typically self-limited
- Trench fever (*Bartonella quintana*): 5-day cycles of fever
- Bacillary angiomatosis (*B. quintana, B. henselae*): Vasoproliferative lesions in skin/bones of immunosuppressed

MICROSCOPIC

- Cat-scratch disease: Lymph nodes with coalescent stellate granulomas; necrotic center, palisaded histiocytes, and rare multinucleated giant cells
- Bacillary angiomatosis and verruga peruana: Capillary proliferation, plump endothelial cells, vascular stroma with neutrophilic infiltrate
- Bacilli (1-3 μm) highlighted with silver stains (e.g., Warthin-Starry, Dieterle) or IHC, often clustered around vessels or in areas of necrosis

TOP DIFFERENTIAL DIAGNOSES

- Mycobacterial and fungal lymphadenitis: Necrotizing granulomatous inflammation; organisms identified by special stain, culture, or molecular testing
- Sarcoidosis: Nonnecrotizing granulomas without distinct layers; no associated microorganisms; rarely in children
- Culture-negative endocarditis (*Coxiella burnetii, Tropheryma whipplei*): Confirmed by serology, IHC, molecular testing
- Other vascular skin lesions: Kaposi sarcoma, angiosarcoma, pyogenic granuloma

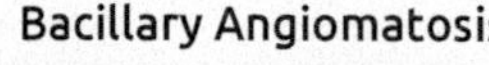

Bacillary Angiomatosis

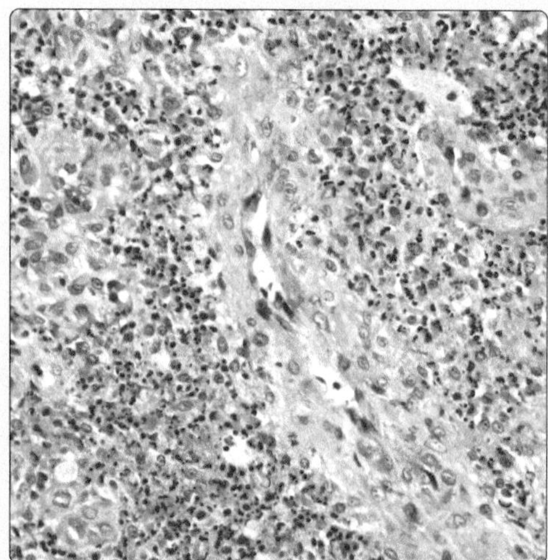

Cat-Scratch Disease

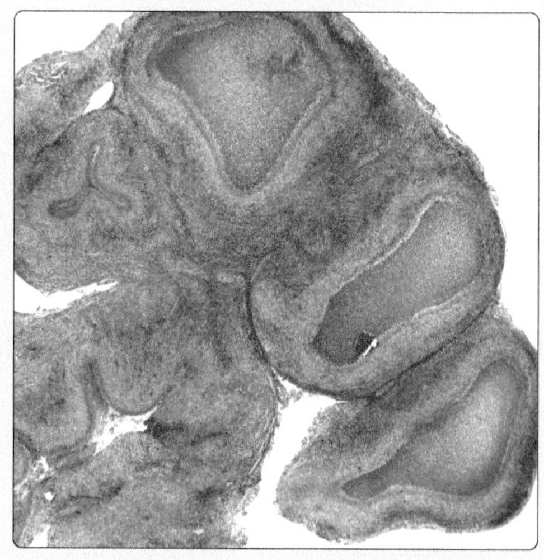

(Left) *This skin biopsy from a patient with HIV shows plump endothelial cells and neutrophilic inflammation, characteristic of bacillary angiomatosis due to Bartonella quintana or Bartonella henselae.* **(Right)** *This axillary lymph node in a patient with cat-scratch disease shows characteristic stellate granulomas with necrotic centers.*

Verruga Peruana

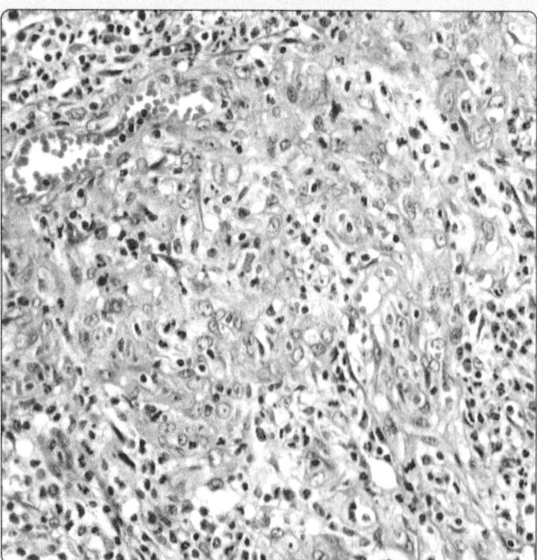

***Bartonella* spp. Silver Stain**

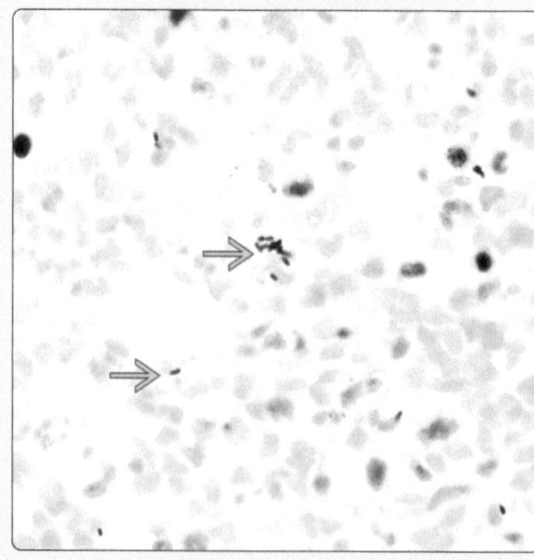

(Left) *Skin biopsy of a verruga peruana due to B. bacilliformis infection shows capillary proliferation, plump endothelial cells, and fibrotic vascular stroma with a neutrophilic infiltrate.* **(Right)** *Silver nitrate impregnation methods, including Dieterle stain, can highlight Bartonella spp. bacilli* ⇒*, which may appear singly or in clusters around blood vessels.*

TERMINOLOGY

Definitions

- *Bartonella* genus named for microbiologist Alberto Barton (discovered cause of Carrion disease)

ETIOLOGY/PATHOGENESIS

Infectious Agents

- Infection with *Bartonella* spp. facultative intracellular, pleomorphic, gram-negative bacilli that invade RBCs; transmitted by arthropods via blood meals, scratch or saliva of infected animal, or blood transfusion

CLINICAL ISSUES

Epidemiology

- *Bartonella bacilliformis*: Andes region; human reservoir, transmitted by sand fly (*Lutzomyia verrucarum*); can infect up to 100% of host's RBCs, resulting in hemolytic anemia
- *Bartonella henselae*: Worldwide distribution; domesticated cat reservoir, transmitted predominately by cat fleas (*Ctenocephalides felis*); most infections in children
- *Bartonella quintana*: Worldwide distribution; human reservoir, transmitted predominantly by human body louse (*Pediculus humanus*)

Presentation

- Carrion disease (*B. bacilliformis*): Oroya fever (early phase) with acute hemolytic anemia; can be complicated by cardiopulmonary or meningeal disease and secondary bacterial infections; verruga peruana (Peruvian warts; chronic phase) with cutaneous lesions
- Cat-scratch disease (mostly *B. henselae*): Inflammation at site of scratch with papule or pustule; fever, malaise, lymphadenopathy 1-3 weeks after exposure, eye involvement (Parinaud oculoglandular syndrome); heart and neurologic complications rarely occur
- Trench fever (*B. quintana*): 5-day cycles of fever, retroorbital headache, myalgia, skin rash, bone pain; cardiac involvement in chronic infections; bacillary angiomatosis (also with *B. henselae*) papulonodular vasoproliferative lesions in skin or bones of immunosuppressed individuals

Laboratory Tests

- Serology (IgM, IgG): Does not reliably differentiate among *Bartonella* spp.; positive results may persist for years
- PCR (e.g., 16S rRNA) performed on blood, fresh/FFPE tissue
- Bacilli may be observed in peripheral blood smears during Oroya fever (acute infection)

Treatment

- Cat-scratch disease is self-limited and does not require treatment; range of antibiotics used for other infections

Prognosis

- Carrion disease has mortality rate of 90%

MICROBIOLOGY

Culture Conditions

- Slow growth (~ 3 weeks) that may require direct inoculation into chocolate agar plates or cocultivation in cell culture

MICROSCOPIC

Histologic Features

- Cat-scratch disease
  - Skin papule with mixed inflammatory infiltrate effacing dermoepidermal interface, swollen endothelial cells; epidermis with acanthosis, parakeratosis, orthohyperkeratosis, focal necrosis
  - Lymph nodes with follicular hyperplasia, microabscesses, and foci of cortical necrosis, followed by coalescent stellate granulomas with necrotic center, palisaded histiocytes, and rare multinucleated giant cells
- Bacillary angiomatosis and verruga peruana: Capillary proliferation with lobular arrangement; plump endothelial cells, fibrotic or myxoid vascular stroma with neutrophilic infiltrate; epidermal acanthosis and hyperkeratosis
- Granular basophilic clumps of bacteria may be visualized
- Rocha-Lima inclusions: Endothelial cell cytoplasmic inclusions from bacteria-containing phagosomes

ANCILLARY TESTS

Special Stains and Immunohistochemistry

- Bacilli (1-3 μm) highlighted with silver stains (e.g., Warthin-Starry, Dieterle), often clustered around vessels or in areas of necrosis
- Bacilli highlighted by anti-*Bartonella* spp. antibodies

DIFFERENTIAL DIAGNOSIS

Mycobacterial and Fungal Lymphadenitis

- Necrotizing granulomatous inflammation associated with *Mycobacterium tuberculosis*, *Coccidioides* spp., etc.; organisms identified by special stain, culture, or molecular testing

Sarcoidosis

- Nonnecrotizing granulomas without distinct layers; no associated microorganisms; rarely in children

Other Causes of Culture-Negative Endocarditis

- e.g., *Coxiella burnetii* and *Tropheryma whipplei*, confirmed by serology, IHC, molecular testing

Other Vascular Skin Lesions

- Kaposi Sarcoma: HHV8-positive spindled cells with interconnecting vascular channels, extravasated RBCs, hyaline globules
- Angiosarcoma: Mitotically active atypical endothelial cells; interconnecting, ramifying vascular channels with tufting
- Pyogenic granuloma: Polypoid lesion of capillary-type vessels with overlying ulceration

SELECTED REFERENCES

1. McCormick DW et al: Bartonella spp. Infections identified by molecular methods, United States. Emerg Infect Dis. 29(3):467-76, 2023
2. Garcia-Quintanilla M et al: Carrion's disease: more than a neglected disease. Parasit Vectors. 12(1):141, 2019
3. Lins KA et al: Cutaneous manifestations of bartonellosis. An Bras Dermatol. 94(5):594-602, 2019
4. Okaro U et al: Bartonella species, an emerging cause of blood-culture-negative endocarditis. Clin Microbiol Rev. 30(3):709-46, 2017
5. Caponetti GC et al: Evaluation of immunohistochemistry in identifying Bartonella henselae in cat-scratch disease. Am J Clin Pathol. 131(2):250-6, 2009

Campylobacter and *Vibrio* Species Infections

KEY FACTS

ETIOLOGY/PATHOGENESIS

- *Campylobacter* spp. (*Campylobacter jejuni* and *Campylobacter fetus* most common)
    - Infection through contaminated food and water (particularly undercooked chicken)
- *Vibrio* spp. (*Vibrio cholerae, Vibrio parahaemolyticus,* and *Vibrio vulnificus* are clinically relevant)
    - Present in brackish water (*V. parahaemolyticus* and *V. vulnificus* associated with oysters and other shellfish)

CLINICAL ISSUES

- *C. jejuni* often presents as acute enteritis (abdominal pain, watery or bloody diarrhea, malaise, fever)
    - Tends to produce acute, self-limited colitis picture with polymorphonuclear infiltrate in lamina propria, cryptitis, and occasional crypt abscess
    - Reactive arthritis, Guillain-Barré syndrome may occur
- *C. fetus* associated with systemic disease (bacteremia, meningitis, vascular infection, abscess, etc.)
- *V. cholerae*: Severe, noninflammatory, watery diarrhea (can be 1 L/hour)
- *V. parahaemolyticus*: Major cause of acute diarrheal disease (particularly in Asia) but generally acute self-limited colitis
- *V. vulnificus*: Severe soft tissue infections with bullous lesions separating epidermis from dermis

TOP DIFFERENTIAL DIAGNOSES

- *C. jejuni* enteritis: Other causes of "bloody diarrhea," inflammatory bowel disease, ischemic colitis
- *C. fetus* sepsis: Other causes of "severe sepsis," requiring blood cultures for diagnosis
- *V. parahaemolyticus* gastroenteritis: Manifests in similar but usually more mild, manner to shigellosis
- *V. vulnificus* soft tissue infection: Necrotizing fasciitis caused by other organisms (i.e., *Streptococcus pyogenes)*

Persistent *Campylobacter* Infection

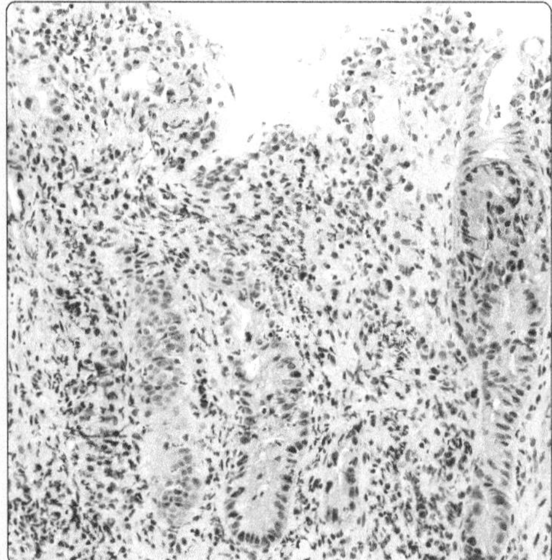

Persistent *Campylobacter* Infection

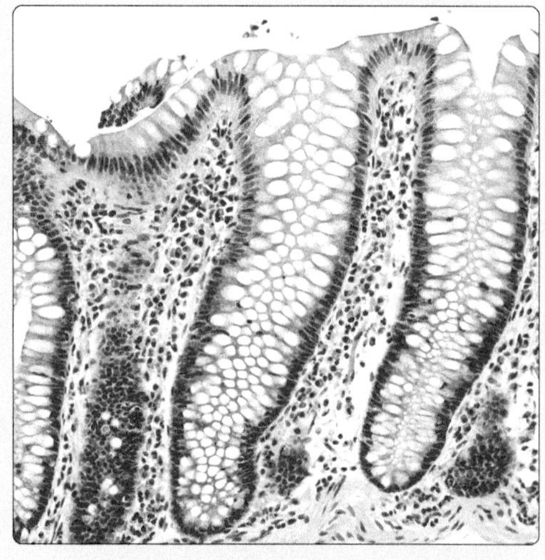

(Left) *Persistent Campylobacter infection with preserved architecture is shown. Histologic and endoscopic differential includes inflammatory bowel disease. (Courtesy M. Drage, MD, PhD.)* **(Right)** *Follow-up colonoscopy at 3 months post antibiotic treatment confirms complete recovery (normal colonic mucosa). (Courtesy M. Drage, MD, PhD.)*

Persistent *Campylobacter* Infection

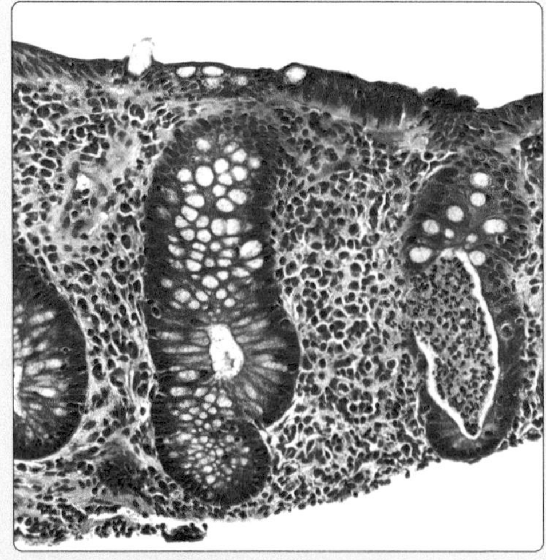

Acute *Campylobacter* Infection

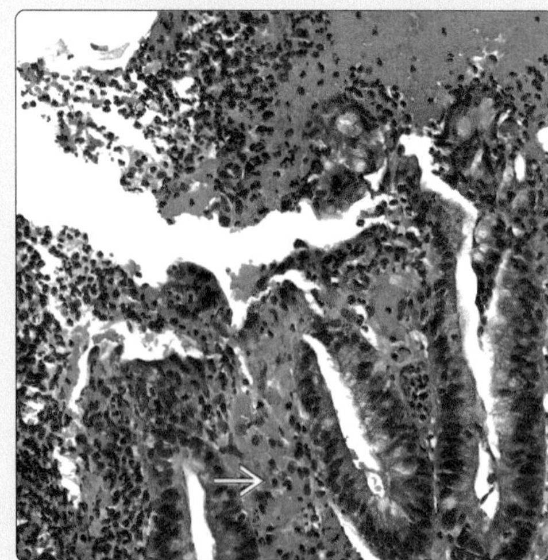

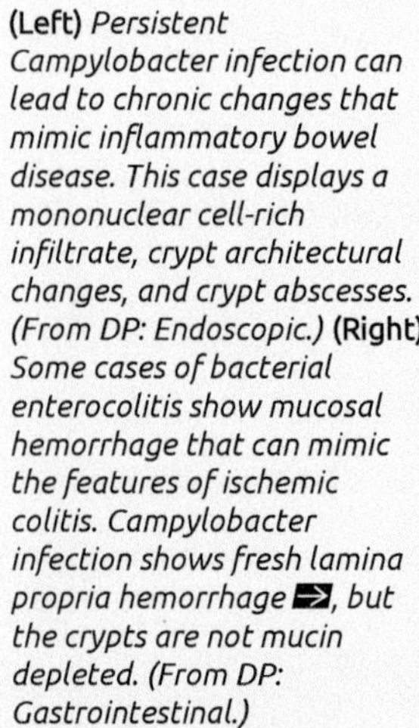

(Left) *Persistent Campylobacter infection can lead to chronic changes that mimic inflammatory bowel disease. This case displays a mononuclear cell-rich infiltrate, crypt architectural changes, and crypt abscesses. (From DP: Endoscopic.)* **(Right)** *Some cases of bacterial enterocolitis show mucosal hemorrhage that can mimic the features of ischemic colitis. Campylobacter infection shows fresh lamina propria hemorrhage ➔, but the crypts are not mucin depleted. (From DP: Gastrointestinal.)*

TERMINOLOGY

Definitions

- Greek: "Campylos" (curved) + "baktron" (rod)
- Latin: "Vibrio" (to quiver) + Greek: "Khole" (bile)
  - "Vibrion": Coined by Filipo Pacini who 1st characterized *Vibrio cholerae* during pandemic

ETIOLOGY/PATHOGENESIS

Environmental Exposure

- *Campylobacter* spp.
  - Diverse animal reservoirs (worldwide)
  - Infection through contaminated food and water (particularly undercooked chicken), animal contact
- *Vibrio* spp.
  - Present in brackish water, bacterial levels increased in warm months
  - *Vibrio parahaemolyticus* and *Vibrio vulnificus* associated with oysters and other shellfish
    - *V. vulnificus* can be transmitted either through contaminated food or directly from contaminated water into cutaneous lesion

Infectious Agents

- *Campylobacter jejuni* and *Campylobacter fetus* most commonly isolated species from humans
  - Virulence factors not extensively characterized
  - *C. jejuni* can multiply in bile, aiding infection in small intestine
  - Susceptible to hairy cell leukemia; disease more common in those who take proton pump inhibitors
  - Able to invade gut mucosa by inducing uptake by nonphagocytic cells
  - *C. ureolyticus* is emerging cause of gastroenteritis
- *V. cholerae*, *V. parahaemolyticus*, and *V. vulnificus* are most clinically relevant species
  - *V. cholerae*
    - Strains divided into > 200 serogroups based on O polysaccharide cell wall antigens
    - Not invasive; epidemic strains of *V. cholerae* include O1 and O139 subtypes
      - Virulence factors include **toxin-coregulated pili (TCP)**, which allows colonization and adherence to small intestine, and **cholera toxin (CT)**, which causes increased cAMP/chloride secretion in intestinal epithelial cells
    - Can colonize small intestine
  - *V. parahaemolyticus*
    - Virulence mainly mediated by enterotoxic hemolysins [thermostable direct hemolysin (TDH) and TDH-related hemolysin (TRH)]
    - Infection primary in distal small intestine
  - *V. vulnificus*
    - Virulence factors not well characterized, include polysaccharide capsule
- *Aeromonas* and *Plesiomonas* spp. are related, curved, gram-negative bacilli
  - *Aeromonas* may be associated with gastroenteritis and wound infection
  - *Plesiomonas* is occasionally isolated as cause of acute infectious gastroenteritis
- *Helicobacter* spp. are curved, gram-negative rods, which are also related to *Campylobacter* and *Vibrio*

CLINICAL ISSUES

Presentation

- *Campylobacter* spp.
  - *C. jejuni* often presents as acute enteritis (abdominal pain, watery or bloody diarrhea, malaise, fever)
    - Symptoms appear 2-4 days after infection (range: 1-7 days) and typically last for 1 week
    - Persistent disease occurs in minority (notable in children and those with immunoglobulin deficiencies)
    - Systemic disease in small minority of patients (bacteremia, meningitis, endocarditis), often immunocompromised
    - Infection may be followed by reactive arthritis
    - Guillain-Barré syndrome may follow small minority of infections by 2-3 weeks
      - Accounts for 20-50% of Guillain-Barré cases
  - *C. fetus* associated with systemic disease (bacteremia, meningitis, vascular infection, abscess, etc.)
    - More likely to be isolated from bloodstream than feces
    - Also associated with *C. jejuni*-like diarrheal illness
    - Vascular involvement may manifest as mycotic aneurysm, endocarditis, vasculitis, thrombophlebitis, or pericarditis
    - May cause spontaneous abortion in pregnant women or sepsis &/or meningitis in live-born infants
- *Vibrio* spp.
  - *V. cholerae*
    - Severe, noninflammatory, watery diarrhea (can be 1 L/hour), sometimes called "rice water stools"
    - Vomiting, abdominal cramps
    - Acute tubular necrosis, stroke, and aspiration pneumonia may also be present
    - Death from dehydration
  - *V. parahaemolyticus*
    - Major cause of acute diarrheal disease (particularly in Asia)
    - Diarrhea may be watery or bloody (less fluid loss than in cholera)
    - Intestinal damage is less severe than in shigellosis
  - *V. vulnificus*
    - Severe soft tissue wound infections
      - Manifest as erythematous lesions that evolve into bullae and necrotic ulcers
    - Septicemia
    - Disease is particularly severe in individuals with liver disease and iron overload syndromes

Treatment

- *Campylobacter* spp.
  - Usually supportive except for serious &/or extraintestinal disease
    - Preferred agents include erythromycin for intestinal and aminoglycosides for extraintestinal
    - Growing resistance to macrolides and fluoroquinolones
- *V. cholerae*

- Focus is on rehydration
- Antibiotics in patients with severe disease or immunocompromised
- Antibiotics may decrease diarrhea/fluid loss (macrolides or fluoroquinolones)

- *V. parahaemolyticus*
  - Gastroenteritis is usually not treated
    - Doxycycline or fluoroquinolone for severe cases
- *V. vulnificus*
  - Surgical debridement plays major role
  - Antibiotics include fluoroquinolones, doxycycline, and 3rd-generation cephalosporins

Prognosis

- Varies greatly; mortality can be very high with *V. vulnificus* septicemia and systemic disease (> 50%)

MICROBIOLOGY

Morphologic and Biochemical Characteristics

- *Campylobacter* spp.
  - Motile, non-spore-forming, curved or spiral-shaped, gram-negative rods
  - Some spp. (e.g., *Campylobacter urealyticus*) may not appear curved
  - *C. jejuni* is typically able to hydrolyze hippurate
- *Vibrio* spp.
  - Motile, non-spore-forming, curved or straight, gram-negative rods
  - Oxidase positive fermenter (common with *Aeromonas*, *Plesiomonas*, and *Chromobacterium*)

Culture

- *Campylobacter* spp.
  - Requires microaerophilic environment
  - 1-3 days to produce colonies
  - Selective media is often used to prevent overgrowth of other spp.
  - *C. jejuni* grows at 42 °C (other spp. grow at 37 °C)
  - Blood cultures useful for extraintestinal *C. jejuni* and *C. fetus* infections
- *Vibrio* spp.
  - Facultative anaerobe; requires salt for growth
  - Selective agars include taurocholate tellurite gelatin agar (TTGA) and thiosulfate citrate bile sucrose agar (TCBS)
    - *V. cholerae* colonies are yellowish, whereas *V. parahaemolyticus* and *V. vulnificus* may appear blue-green
  - Grows easily on standard laboratory medium

Microbiologic Identification

- *Campylobacter* spp.
  - Specialized growth requirements, oxidase, and hippurate are key elements of identification
  - Rapid antigen tests are available for *Campylobacter* diagnosis directly from stool
  - MALDI is becoming more routine
  - *Campylobacter* targets may be included in commercially available multiplex PCR panels for stool
- *Vibrio* spp.
  - Appearance on selective agars
  - All are oxidase positive; *V. cholerae* and *V. vulnificus* are lactose positive; *V. parahaemolyticus* is lactose negative
  - Commercial identification systems can confuse *Vibrio* spp. with *Aeromonas* spp.
  - MALDI can identify many *Vibrio* spp. to species level
  - Polyvalent antisera for *V. cholerae* serotyping performed in endemic areas; otherwise, may be available in specialized reference labs
  - *Vibrio* targets may be included in commercially available multiplex PCR panels for stool

MICROSCOPIC

Histologic Features

- *C. jejuni*
  - Affects jejunum, ileum, and colon
  - Tends to produce acute, self-limited colitis picture with polymorphonuclear infiltrate in lamina propria, cryptitis, and occasional crypt abscess
- *V. cholerae*
  - Despite severity of diarrhea, little to no inflammatory picture
- *V. parahaemolyticus*
  - Rarely biopsied
  - Generally acute self-limited colitis
- *V. vulnificus*
  - Rarely biopsied
  - Bullous lesions with separation of epidermis from dermis
  - Clusters of bacteria may be visible in dermal vasculature

DIFFERENTIAL DIAGNOSIS

Campylobacter jejuni Enteritis

- Other causes of "bloody diarrhea" (*Escherichia coli*, *Salmonella*, *Shigella*, *Yersinia*), inflammatory bowel disease, ischemic colitis
- Other infectious causes of pseudoappendicitis (*Yersinia*)

Campylobacter fetus Systemic Infection

- Other causes of "severe sepsis," requiring blood cultures for diagnosis

Vibrio parahaemolyticus Gastroenteritis

- Manifests in similar but usually more mild, manner to shigellosis

Vibrio vulnificus Skin and Soft Tissue Infections

- Necrotizing fasciitis caused by other organisms (i.e., *Streptococcus pyogenes*)

SELECTED REFERENCES

1. Epping L et al: Population biology and comparative genomics of Campylobacter species. Curr Top Microbiol Immunol. 431:59-78, 2021
2. Baker-Austin C et al: Vibrio vulnificus: new insights into a deadly opportunistic pathogen. Environ Microbiol. 20(2):423-30, 2018
3. Baker-Austin C et al: Vibrio spp. infections. Nat Rev Dis Primers. 4(1):8, 2018
4. Weil AA et al: Cholera: recent updates. Curr Opin Infect Dis. 31(5):455-61, 2018
5. Fitzgerald C: Campylobacter. Clin Lab Med. 35(2):289-98, 2015
6. Lamps LW: Update on infectious enterocolitides and the diseases that they mimic. Histopathology. 66(1):3-14, 2015

Campylobacter fetus

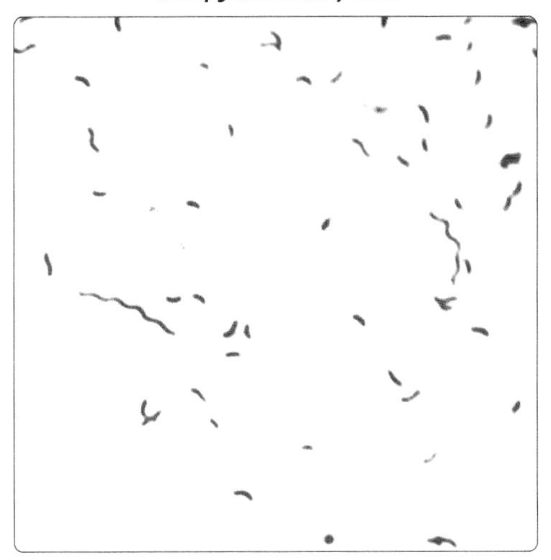

Vibrio cholerae Infection

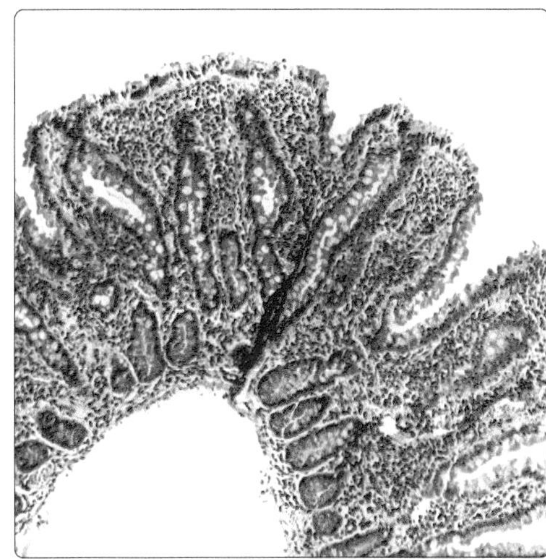

(Left) *Gram stain of cultured Campylobacter fetus demonstrates its pleomorphic appearance with occasional spiral forms. (Courtesy CDC/PHIL.)* **(Right)** *Small intestine from a patient with an acute case of cholera shows intact mucosa with villous blunting and only mild active inflammation. (Courtesy E. Gangarosa, MD, CDC/PHIL.)*

Vibrio vulnificus Infection

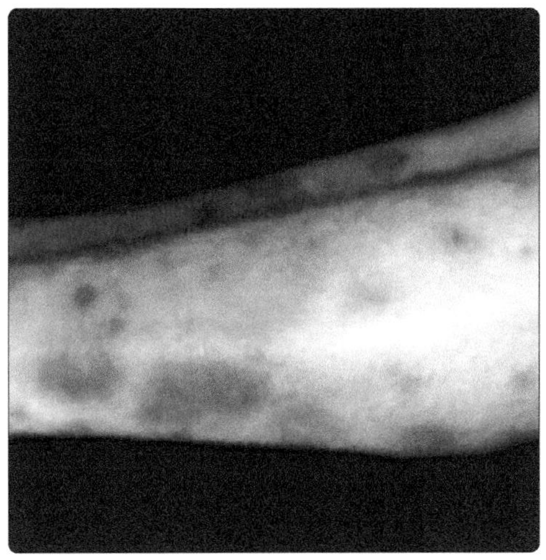

Vibrio vulnificus Infection

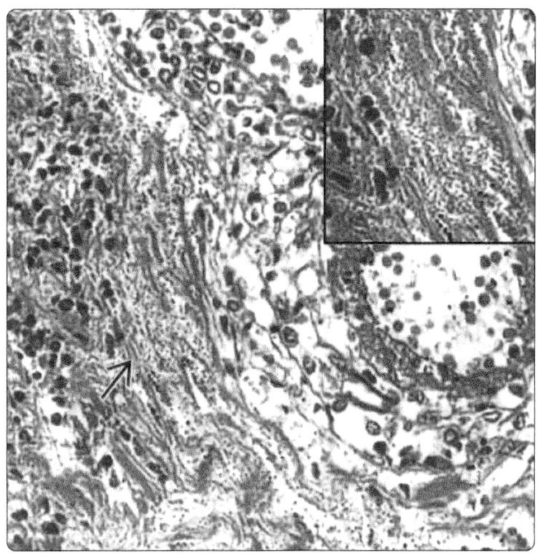

(Left) *Cutaneous lesions are shown on a patient who succumbed to Vibrio vulnificus infection with urticarial rash, petechial hemorrhage, purpura, and swelling. (Courtesy Chen et al, 2002.)* **(Right)** *Microscopically, dermal tissue from a patient who succumbed to V. vulnificus shows inflammation surrounding blood vessels with abundant bacteria ⇒. Inset shows higher magnification of the bacteria. (Courtesy Chen et al, 2002.)*

Vibrio parahaemolyticus Gastroenteritis (Acute)

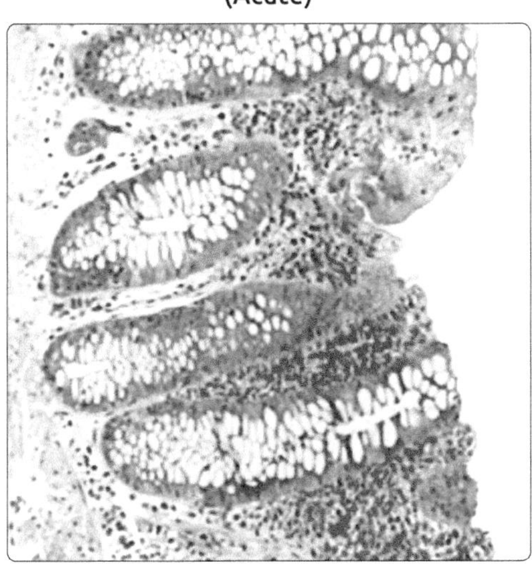

Vibrio parahaemolyticus Gastroenteritis (Convalescent)

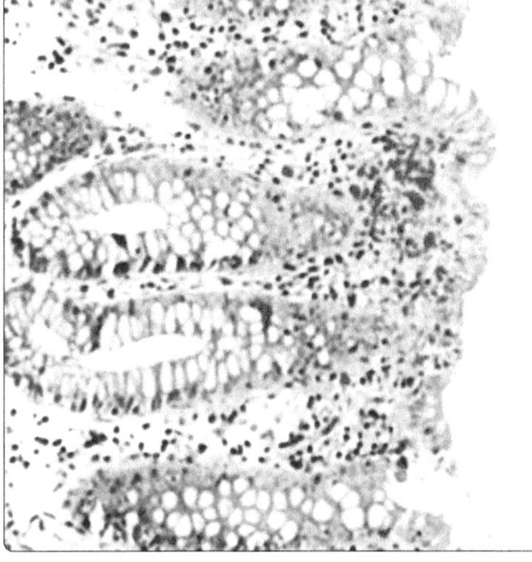

(Left) *Rectal biopsy 2 days after onset of diarrhea in a patient infected with Vibrio parahaemolyticus demonstrates lamina propria hemorrhage and surface epithelial degenerative change. (Courtesy Qadri et al, 2003.)* **(Right)** *Rectal mucosa at convalescence (day 30) in a patient infected with V. parahaemolyticus infection shows recovery of epithelium. (Courtesy Qadri et al, 2003.)*

Helicobacteriosis

KEY FACTS

ETIOLOGY/PATHOGENESIS

- Gram-negative microaerophilic, spiral-shaped, flagellated bacteria transmitted by fecal-oral or oral-oral routes
- *Helicobacter pylori* accounts for 99% of infections; 1% of infections due to *Helicobacter heilmannii*

CLINICAL ISSUES

- Worldwide distribution
- 20% risk of ulcer; < 5% risk of cancer
- Breath urease/urea test is highly sensitive and specific
- Serum antibody test detects exposure, but not presence, of bacteria
- Stool antigen test can determine eradication

MICROSCOPIC

- *H. pylori*: Long, faint, curved rods present adhered to foveolar epithelial cells or present in lumen; may appear coccoid after PPI treatment
- *H. heilmannii*: Longer and thicker than *H. pylori*
- Chronic gastritis with increased plasma cells and lymphoid aggregates; active infection with neutrophils
- Mild chronic inflammation can persist after treatment

ANCILLARY TESTS

- Organisms seen on Gram stain (negative), Giemsa (faint), Warthin-Starry (black), Alcian yellow (blue-green), Wright-Giemsa (blue), and toluidine blue (dark blue)
- Anti-*H. pylori* antibodies are more sensitive and specific than histochemistry; both curved rod forms and coccoid forms (after therapy) are detected

TOP DIFFERENTIAL DIAGNOSES

- Autoimmune gastritis: Corpus-restricted atrophy of oxyntic glands, hyperplasia of enterochromaffin-like cells; negative *Helicobacter* spp. IHC
- Focally enhanced gastritis: Focally prominent infiltrate of lymphocytes, histiocytes, &/or neutrophils

Lymphoid Aggregates

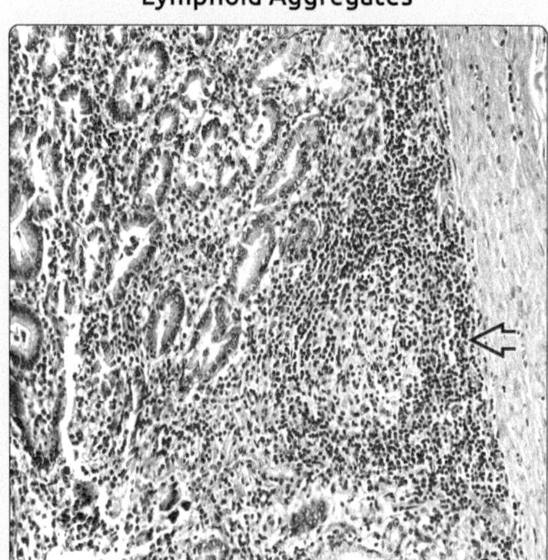

Helicobacter pylori

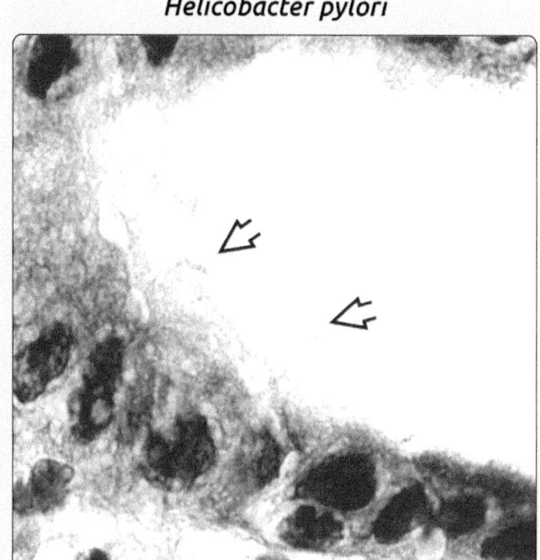

(Left) *Stomach biopsy with a lymphoid aggregate ⇨ (strongly suggestive of Helicobacter pylori infections in Western populations) is shown. Lymphoid aggregates are more common in developing countries.* **(Right)** *High-power view of a crypt containing H. pylori is shown with several, faintly staining organisms ⇨ all along the epithelial border. Special stains or IHC can confirm the diagnosis, although histology of tissue and organisms on routine staining is usually sufficient.*

Helicobacter heilmannii

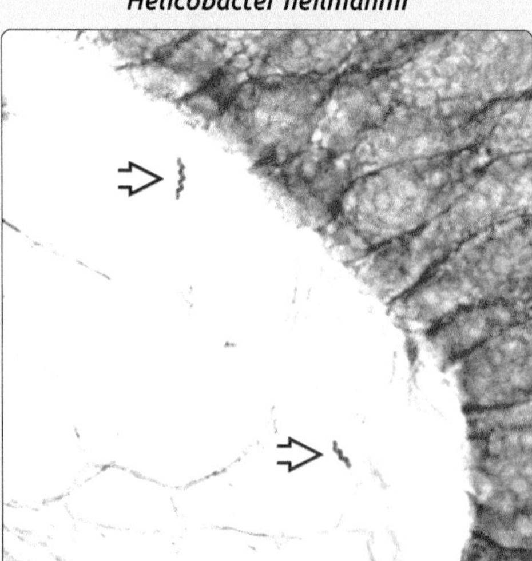

***Helicobacter* spp. Immunohistochemistry**

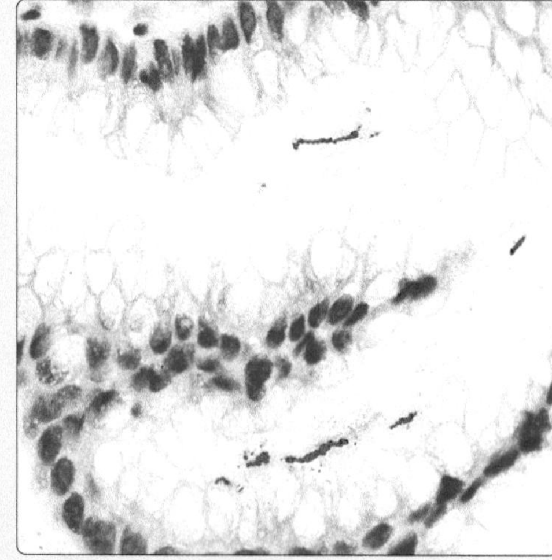

(Left) *Compared to H. pylori, Helicobacter heilmannii are longer, thicker, and more easily identifiable on H&E-stained sections ⇨.* **(Right)** *Immunohistochemical stain for Helicobacter spp. demonstrates organisms (red) lining the epithelium of an infected patient.*

TERMINOLOGY

Definitions

- Greek: "Hélix" (twisted or spiral) + "bakterion" (small staff)
- *heilmannii* named for German pathologist Konrad Heilmann

ETIOLOGY/PATHOGENESIS

Infectious Agents

- Infection with gram-negative microaerophilic, spiral-shaped, flagellated *Helicobacter* spp. bacteria; transmitted by fecal-oral or oral-oral routes and produces urease for protection from stomach acid
- *Helicobacter pylori* (formerly *Campylobacter pylori*) accounts for 99% of infections; 1% of infections due to *Helicobacter heilmannii;* other species have been isolated from human patients
- Risk of gastric adenocarcinoma (< 5%) with chronic untreated infection with ulceration and mucosa-associated lymphoid tissue (MALT)-type lymphoma due to chronic inflammation

CLINICAL ISSUES

Epidemiology

- Upper gastrointestinal tract colonization/infection in 50% of world population

Presentation

- 80% of infections are asymptomatic
- Symptoms include nausea, vomiting, abdominal pain, heartburn, halitosis, morning hunger, diarrhea
- Gastric ulcers worsen with food due to increased acid production, while duodenal ulcers (associated with antral gastritis) improve with food due to closing of pylorus

Laboratory Tests

- Serum antibody test detects exposure, but not presence, of bacteria; sensitivity and specificity > 90% (new infection)
- Stool antigen test detects presence of bacteria, does not indicate degree of disease, can determine eradication; sensitivity 98% and specificity 94% (initial stage of disease)
- Breath urease/urea test detects active production of urease enzyme; highly sensitive and specific
- PCR/sequencing (fresh, FFPE tissue): Used for diagnosis and detection of antibiotic resistance mutations in 23S rRNA, gyrA, rdxA, pbp1, 16S rRNA, and rpoB genes

Treatment

- Triple-drug therapy with antibiotics and antacid medications to heal ulcer and eradicate organism

Prognosis

- In patients where infection is eradicated, risk of cancer is reduced; reinfection may occur

MICROBIOLOGY

Culture

- Homogenized stomach biopsies are plated onto trypticase soy sheep blood agar and incubated at 5-7% oxygen/5% carbon dioxide at 35 °C (growth within 2-4 days)
- Indicated if patient fails basic triple-regimen therapy for eradication of organism
- Battery of antibiotics tested to determine resistance and select additional treatment

MACROSCOPIC

Endoscopy

- Ulceration of mucosa (active infection); puckered ulcers with fixed borders (carcinoma); large, fixed masses (lymphoma)

MICROSCOPIC

Histologic Features

- *H. pylori* seen as small, faint collections of long, curved rods at epithelia cell border adherent to foveolar epithelial cells or collections in lumen; may appear coccoid after PPI treatment
- *H. heilmannii* are longer and thicker than *H. pylori* with spiral/corkscrew shape in lumen; milder inflammatory changes
- Chronic gastritis with increased plasma cells in lamina propria and lymphoid aggregates in mucosa; active infection with neutrophils
- Mild chronic inflammation can persist after treatment
- Superficial microerosions, intestinal metaplasia, and regenerative foveolar hyperplasia may be present
- Gastric adenocarcinoma and MALT lymphoma

ANCILLARY TESTS

Histochemistry

- Organisms seen on Gram stain (negative), Giemsa (faint), Warthin-Starry (black), Alcian yellow (blue-green), Wright-Giemsa (blue), and toluidine blue (dark blue)

Immunohistochemistry

- Anti-*H. pylori* antibodies are more sensitive and specific than histochemistry; both curved rod forms and coccoid forms (after therapy) are detected

DIFFERENTIAL DIAGNOSIS

Autoimmune Gastritis

- Corpus-restricted atrophy of oxyntic glands, hyperplasia of enterochromaffin-like cells; negative *Helicobacter* spp. IHC

Focally Enhanced Gastritis

- Focally prominent infiltrate of lymphocytes, histiocytes, &/or neutrophils; resembles partially treated *H. pylori* gastritis

SELECTED REFERENCES

1. Malfertheiner P et al: Helicobacter pylori infection. Nat Rev Dis Primers. 9(1):19, 2023
2. Mannion A et al: Helicobacter pylori antimicrobial resistance and gene variants in high- and low-gastric-cancer-risk populations. J Clin Microbiol. 59(5), 2021
3. Robinson K et al: The spectrum of helicobacter-mediated diseases. Annu Rev Pathol. 16:123-44, 2021
4. Bento-Miranda M et al: Helicobacter heilmannii sensu lato: an overview of the infection in humans. World J Gastroenterol. 20(47):17779-87, 2014
5. Batts KP et al: Appropriate use of special stains for identifying Helicobacter pylori: recommendations from the Rodger C. Haggitt Gastrointestinal Pathology Society. Am J Surg Pathol. 37(11):e12-22, 2013

Neisseria and *Moraxella* Species Infections

KEY FACTS

ETIOLOGY/PATHOGENESIS

- Infection with *Neisseria meningitidis*, *Neisseria gonorrhoeae*, and *Moraxella catarrhalis*; humans are only known host

CLINICAL ISSUES

- *N. meningitidis* (meningococcus): Bacteremia ± shock and meningitis
- *N. gonorrhoeae* (gonococcus): Acute urethritis, epididymitis, rectal involvement, prostatitis (males); endocervicitis, urethritis, anal involvement, pelvic inflammatory disease (females); pharyngitis, conjunctivitis, disseminated gonococcal infection with arthritis-dermatitis syndrome
- *M. catarrhalis:* Otitis media, sinusitis, chronic obstructive pulmonary disease (COPD) exacerbation
- Meningococcal conjugate (MenACWY) and serogroup B meningococcal (MenB) vaccines available

MICROSCOPIC

- Gram and silver stains highlight clumps of gram-negative cocci (including within neutrophils)
- *N. meningitidis*: Dense neutrophilic leptomeningitis; dermal vessel microthrombi, suppurative or sterile arthritis
- *N. gonorrhoeae*: Suppurative epididymitis, chronic endometritis, purulent cervicitis, acute salpingitis, tuboovarian abscess
- Arthritis-dermatitis syndrome: Suppurative or sterile arthritis; skin pustule surrounded by erythema, pustular vasculitis with abscesses
- *M. catarrhalis*: Acute sinusitis, otitis media, and COPD exacerbations rarely biopsied

TOP DIFFERENTIAL DIAGNOSES

- Other causes of bacterial meningitis: e.g., *Group B Streptococcus, S. pneumoniae, Escherichia coli*
- Other causes of infectious arthritis: e.g., *Staphylococcus aureus, Pseudomonas aeruginosa*, polymicrobial
- Other causes of pelvic inflammatory disease: e.g., *Chlamydia trachomatis*
- Differentiate by Gram stain, culture, PCR

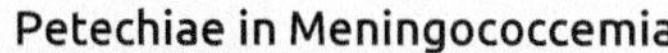

Petechiae in Meningococcemia

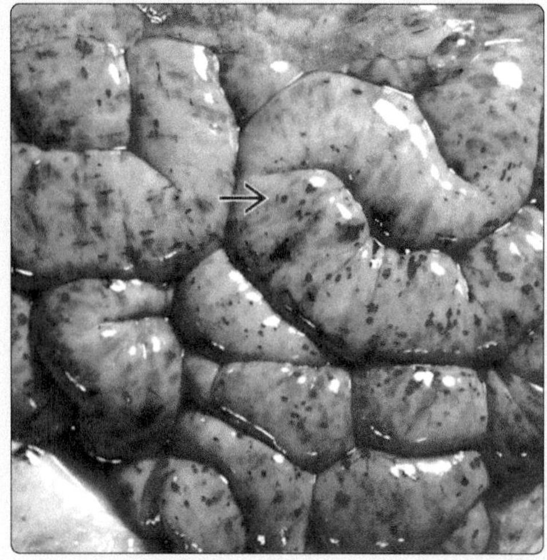

Purpura Fulminans

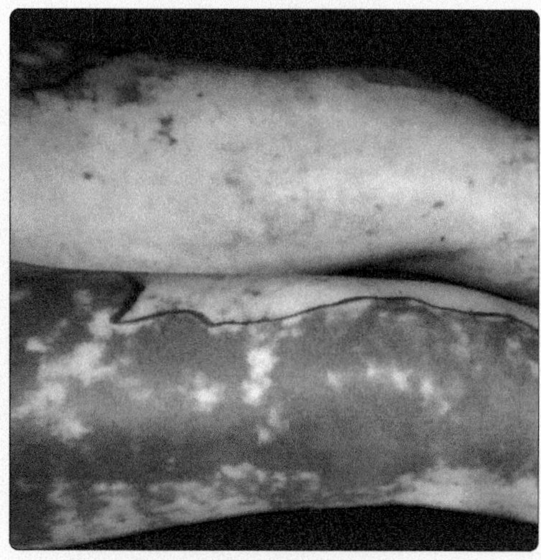

(Left) *Fulminant meningococcemia with disseminated intravascular coagulation (DIC) shows ecchymoses and petechiae throughout the visceral peritoneum →. (Courtesy Franz von Lichtenberg Collection of Infectious Disease Pathology, BWH.)* **(Right)** *This patient demonstrated fulminant meningococcemia with purpuric hemorrhage. (Courtesy Franz von Lichtenberg Collection of Infectious Disease Pathology, BWH.)*

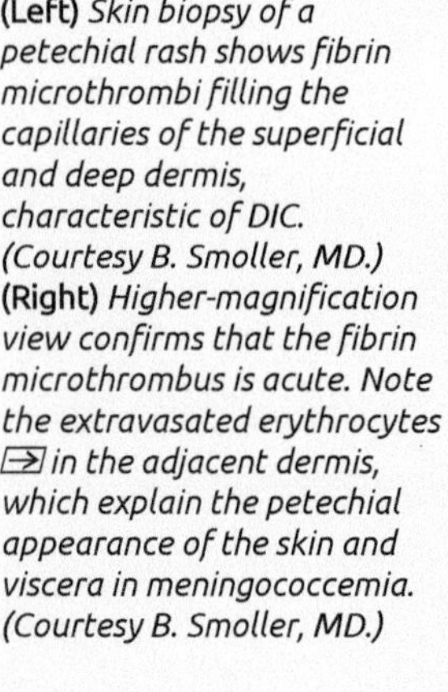

Fibrin Microthrombi

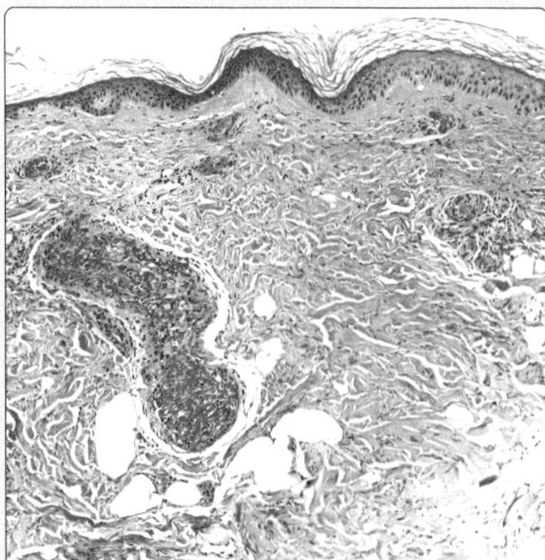

Fibrin Microthrombus and Extravasated Erythrocytes

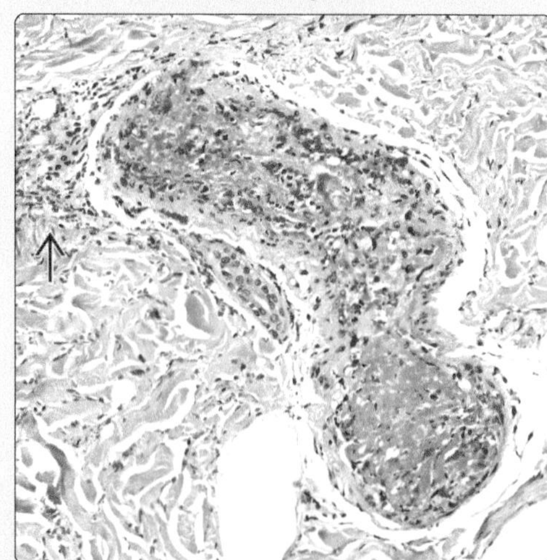

(Left) *Skin biopsy of a petechial rash shows fibrin microthrombi filling the capillaries of the superficial and deep dermis, characteristic of DIC. (Courtesy B. Smoller, MD.)* **(Right)** *Higher-magnification view confirms that the fibrin microthrombus is acute. Note the extravasated erythrocytes → in the adjacent dermis, which explain the petechial appearance of the skin and viscera in meningococcemia. (Courtesy B. Smoller, MD.)*

TERMINOLOGY

Definitions

- *Neisseria*: From Albert Neisser, who discovered etiologic agent of gonorrhea
- Greek: "Gonorrhoeae" (seminal flux)

ETIOLOGY/PATHOGENESIS

Infectious Agents

- Infection with *Neisseria meningitidis*, *Neisseria gonorrhoeae*, and *Moraxella catarrhalis*; humans are only known host
- *N. meningitidis* (meningococcus)
  - Major site of colonization is nasopharynx; invasive disease typically caused by encapsulated strains
  - In bloodstream, attach to and invade vascular endothelium (forming aggregates or microcolonies)
  - In brain, tight junctions are dissociated, opening access to subarachnoid space
  - Transmitted by inhalation of infected droplets, contact with respiratory secretions, or through sexual contact
- *N. gonorrhoeae* (gonococcus)
  - Always pathogenic, never colonizer
  - Primarily infects urogenital epithelia, though disseminated disease is possible
  - Spread is by sexual contact in both sexes or maternal-fetal transmission at time of birth
- *M. catarrhalis*
  - Historically described as commensal organism of nasopharynx, now considered pathogen
  - Spread by inhalation of droplets or other contact with respiratory secretions
  - Disease often caused by spread of colonizing organisms to other sites (e.g., middle ear, lower respiratory tract)

CLINICAL ISSUES

Epidemiology

- *N. meningitidis* is carried asymptomatically in nasopharynx in 5-25% of population (highest in adolescents and those in crowded living conditions)
  - Hosts with particular immune deficiencies (e.g., defects in terminal complement pathway) are susceptible
  - Large burden of disease in sub-Saharan Africa with high attack rate (ranging from 100 per 100,000 to 1 per 100)
  - Increasing cause of sexually transmitted urethritis
- *N. gonorrhoeae* is far more common in USA than in other industrialized countries
  - Highest attack rates in 15- to 19-year-old Black female patients
  - MSM are also at increased risk
- *M. catarrhalis* colonizes large percentage of infants and 1-5% of healthy adults

Presentation

- *N. meningitidis*
  - Invasive disease usually consists of bacteremia ± shock and meningitis
  - Less common manifestations: Pneumonia, septic arthritis, purulent pericarditis, conjunctivitis, epiglottitis, sinusitis, otitis, urethritis, and proctitis
  - Onset is usually abrupt, and signs and symptoms progress rapidly [fever, weakness, cold and pallor of extremities, organ failure, and disseminated intravascular coagulation (DIC)]
  - Often characteristic purpuric or petechial rash
  - Complications can include Waterhouse-Friderichsen syndrome (adrenal hemorrhage) and myocarditis (seen in < 1/2 of patients at autopsy)
- *N. gonorrhoeae*
  - Male patients: Acute urethritis with purulent discharge and dysuria; epididymitis and rectal involvement ± prostatitis may be present
  - Female patients: Predominant site is endocervix, but urethra and anus may also be involved
    - Vaginal discharge, dysuria, and vaginal bleeding
    - ~ 10-20% of women develop infection of upper genital tract [pelvic inflammatory disease (PID)]
    - Signs and symptoms of PID include abdominal tenderness, fever, nausea, and vomiting; exam findings include adnexal tenderness and pain with cervical movement
    - Complications of PID include infertility, ovarian abscess, and perihepatitis (Fitz-Hugh-Curtis syndrome)
  - Other manifestations in both men and women include pharyngitis, conjunctivitis, and disseminated gonococcal infection (DGI) presenting as arthritis-dermatitis syndrome
    - Arthritis is usually asymmetric polyarthritis and can progress to septic arthritis
    - Dermatitis is usually confined to extremities and consists of multiple papules and pustules, some with evidence of hemorrhage or necrosis
  - Infection in pregnancy can result in spontaneous abortion or premature labor with increased infant mortality
- *M. catarrhalis*
  - Otitis media in children and sinusitis in children and adults
  - Very common cause of COPD exacerbations
  - Can cause pneumonia in older adults, particularly if there are underlying conditions

Laboratory Tests

- *N. meningitidis*
  - Blood and CSF Gram stain and culture can reveal organisms
  - Large number of neutrophils in CSF
  - Direct PCR (e.g., *ctrA* gene) or multiplex panels (e.g., FilmArray ME Panel) may be useful
- *N. gonorrhoeae*
  - Urethral/rectal/endocervical specimens can be tested by culture or (more commonly) nucleic acid amplification tests (NAATs)
  - Direct Gram staining of specimens is most useful in male urethritis
  - In disseminated infection, blood culture often positive, and synovial culture often negative
  - Skin biopsies can demonstrate bacteria with immunohistochemistry but are usually culture negative
- *M. catarrhalis*
  - Most often diagnosed in context of COPD exacerbation by sputum culture

- Cultures of middle ear and sinus aspirates can grow organisms but are rarely done

Treatment

- Meningococcal conjugate (MenACWY) vaccination recommended for 11-12 year olds with booster at age 16 as well as other individuals with increased risk for disease
- Serogroup B meningococcal (MenB) vaccination may be given to 16-23 year olds as well as > 10 year olds with increased risk for disease
- Antibiotics
  - *N. meningitidis*: Preferred treatment is 3rd-generation cephalosporin
  - *N. gonorrhoeae*: Ceftriaxone is mainstay of treatment
  - *M. catarrhalis*: Several drugs are routinely used (cephalosporins, tetracycline, trimethoprim-sulfamethoxazole, etc.); most strains are resistant to penicillin, ampicillin, vancomycin, and clindamycin
- Surgical treatment may be required for survivors of fulminant meningococcemia (e.g., limb and digit amputations)

Prognosis

- Meningococcal meningitis has mortality of 5-18%; long-term complications include loss of digits or limbs, neurologic impairment, and disruption/asymmetry of growth
- Mortality is rare with gonococcal infection; long-term complications vary from blindness in neonates to infertility in women with PID
- Mortality and long-term complications are rare with *Moraxella* infection

MICROBIOLOGY

Culture and Identification

- Gram-negative diplococci ("coffee beans")
- *N. meningitidis* and *N. gonorrhoeae* commonly isolated on modified Thayer-Martin media; *Moraxella* spp. grow on wide variety of agar types
- Colonies can be differentiated from commensal *Neisseria* spp. by their appearance (larger and pinker) and hockey-puck sign (can be easily pushed along agar surface)
- Carbohydrate utilization patterns for differentiation: *N. meningitidis* utilizes both glucose and maltose, and *N. gonorrhoeae* utilizes only glucose
- Platforms for identification include MALDI-TOF MS, *Neisseria-Haemophilus* (NH) ID card for VITEK 2 and API-NH or CarbFerm strips

MICROSCOPIC

Histologic Features

- *N. meningitidis*
  - Meningitis: Sheets of neutrophils in leptomeninges; bacteria are often observable (usually within neutrophils); death associated with cerebral edema and impingement of midbrain
  - Meningococcemia: Skin with microthrombi in dermal vessels, necrotizing vasculitis
  - Interstitial pneumonitis (mononuclear inflammation mainly confined to alveolar septa), adrenal hemorrhage and necrosis, myocarditis, and glomerular fibrin thrombi
  - Meningococcal arthritis: Joints with sterile arthritis; suppurative inflammation or mixed inflammatory cell infiltrate
- *N. gonorrhoeae*
  - Infection in male patients may produce epididymitis with suppurative inflammation
  - Common cause of purulent cervicitis but rarely biopsied
  - PID
    - Gonococcal endometritis: Chronic with numerous plasma cells in mixed inflammatory cell infiltrate
    - Acute salpingitis: Edematous fallopian tubes; plicae may be adherent and are edematous and inflamed
    - Can progress to tuboovarian abscess with purulent inflammation and adhesions
    - Can form cystic structures upon healing
  - DGI: Arthritis-dermatitis syndrome
    - Suppurative, septic arthritis or "sterile" arthritis
    - Characteristic skin lesion is pustule surrounded by erythema: Pustular vasculitis with intra- or subepidermal abscesses
- *M. catarrhalis*: Specimens from acute sinusitis, otitis media, and COPD exacerbations rarely evaluated by pathologists

ANCILLARY TESTS

Immunohistochemistry

- IHC not widely used due to cross reactivity between species but may be available at reference laboratories

Special Stains

- Gram and silver stains highlight clumps of gram-negative cocci (including within neutrophils)

DIFFERENTIAL DIAGNOSIS

Other Causes of Bacterial Meningitis

- e.g., *Group B Streptococcus, S. pneumoniae, Escherichia coli*
- Differentiate by Gram stain, culture, PCR

Other Causes of Infectious Arthritis

- e.g., *Staphylococcus aureus, Pseudomonas aeruginosa*, polymicrobial
- Differentiate by Gram stain, culture, PCR

Other Causes of Pelvic Inflammatory Disease

- e.g., *Chlamydia trachomatis*
- Differentiate by Gram stain, culture, PCR

SELECTED REFERENCES

1. Cox BK et al: The histopathology of anorectal Neisseria gonorrhoeae Infection. Am J Clin Pathol. 158(5):559-63, 2022
2. Adamson PC et al: Point-of-care testing for sexually transmitted infections: a review of recent developments. Arch Pathol Lab Med. 144(11):1344-51, 2020
3. Caugant DA et al: Neisseria meningitidis: using genomics to understand diversity, evolution and pathogenesis. Nat Rev Microbiol. 18(2):84-96, 2020
4. Unemo M et al: Gonorrhoea. Nat Rev Dis Primers. 5(1):79, 2019
5. Ridpath AD et al: Postmortem diagnosis of invasive meningococcal disease. Emerg Infect Dis. 20(3):453-5, 2014
6. Guarner J et al: Neutrophilic bacterial meningitis: pathology and etiologic diagnosis of fatal cases. Mod Pathol. 26(8):1076-85, 2013
7. Guarner J et al: Pathogenesis and diagnosis of human meningococcal disease using immunohistochemical and PCR assays. Am J Clin Pathol. 122(5):754-64, 2004

Fulminant Meningococcemia

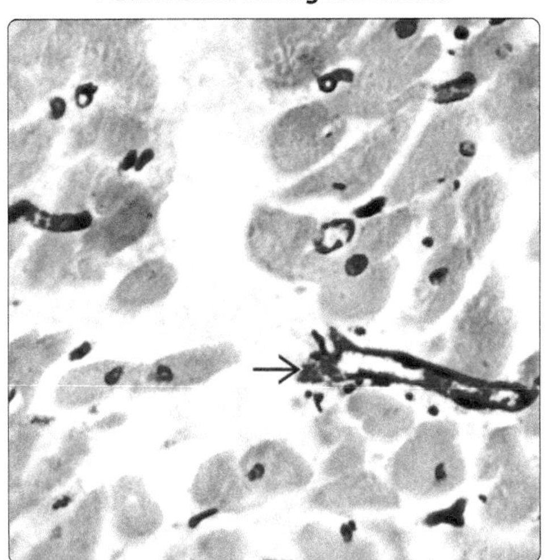

Neisseria meningitidis Gram Stain

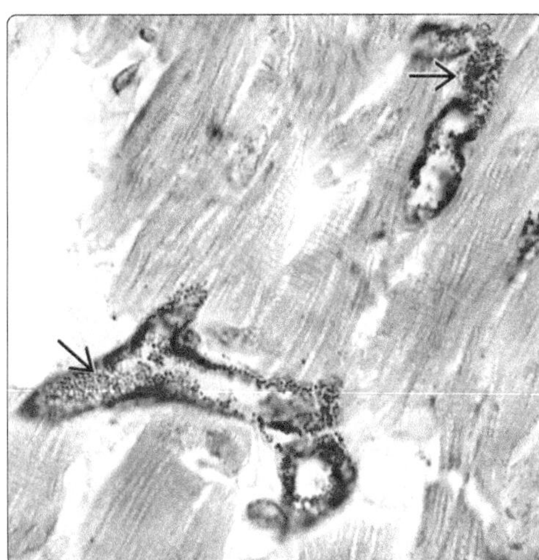

(Left) *H&E section of heart tissue from a patient with fulminant meningococcemia demonstrates widespread intravascular meningococcal colony growth ➞. Note the absence of a cellular reaction.* **(Right)** *Gram stain of heart tissue from a patient with fulminant meningococcemia demonstrates thick colonies ➞ in the intravascular space. (Courtesy Franz von Lichtenberg Collection of Infectious Disease Pathology, BWH.)*

Neutrophilic Leptomeningitis

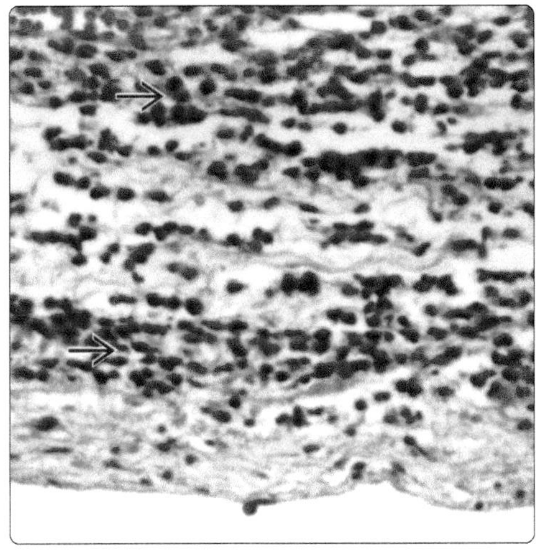

Neisseria meningitidis Diplococci

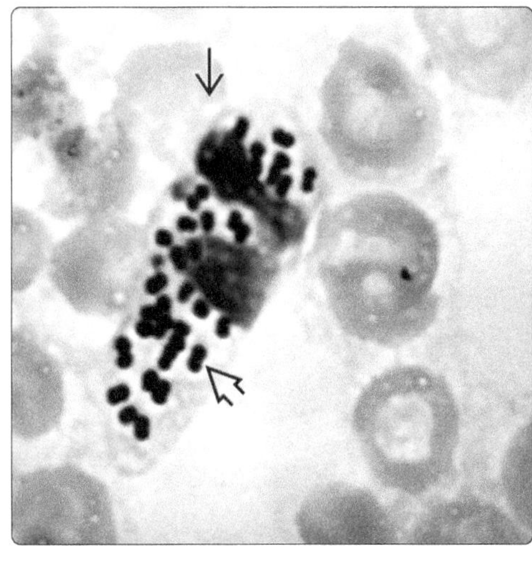

(Left) *In meningococcal meningitis, a diffuse polymorphonuclear infiltrate ➞ of the leptomeninges can be seen. In the absence of neutrophils, petechial hemorrhages may be seen due to fibrin thrombi in meningococcemia.* **(Right)** *This image demonstrates a neutrophil ➞ from the cerebrospinal fluid of an infected patient packed with Neisseria meningitidis diplococci ➞. (Courtesy Franz von Lichtenberg Collection of Infectious Disease Pathology, BWH.)*

Fibrin Microthrombi

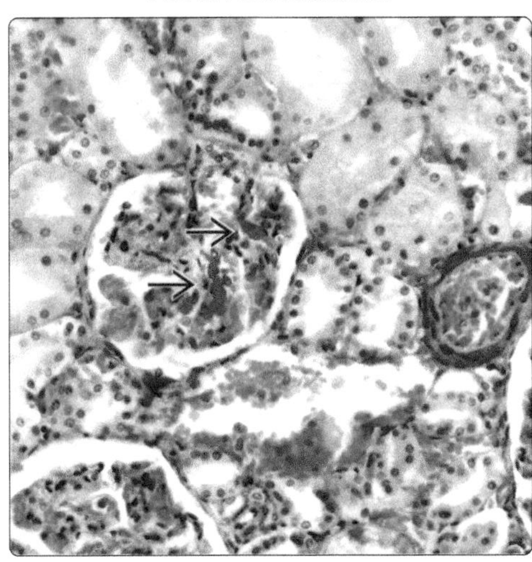

Neisseria gonorrhoeae Gram Stain

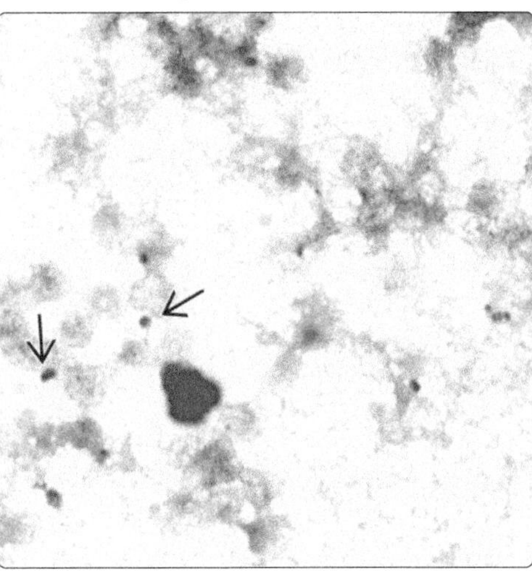

(Left) *In meningococcemia with DIC, fibrin microthrombi ➞ can be seen plugging glomerular capillaries. These same thrombi are responsible for skin petechiae.* **(Right)** *Neisseria gonorrhoeae from a disseminated infection is apparent on this gram-stained blood culture as Gram-negative diplococci ➞.*

Pertussis

KEY FACTS

ETIOLOGY/PATHOGENESIS

- Infection with *Bordetella pertussis*, gram-negative, encapsulated, nonmotile, aerobic bacillus, spread by respiratory droplets

CLINICAL ISSUES

- Affects ~ 40 million people worldwide with ~ 300,000 deaths annually
- Progresses to violent coughing with inspiratory "whoop"
- Diagnosis primarily by culture from nasopharyngeal or oropharyngeal swab; PCR and serology can be performed but are less reliable
- Vaccines (DTap, Tdap) for disease prevention
- Antibiotics shorten duration of illness and decrease transmissibility

MICROSCOPIC

- Necrotizing bronchiolitis, intraalveolar hemorrhage, and fibrinous edema
- Respiratory epithelium is coated with bacteria; may be denuded with secondary infection, neutrophils within walls of trachea/bronchi are seen
- Bronchopneumonia with extension into alveolar spaces with secondary infection
- Interstitial pneumonia or bronchiolitis obliterans organizing pneumonia as complications of progressive disease; diffuse alveolar damage in some fatal infections
- Gram-negative bacilli seen with silver and Giemsa stains

TOP DIFFERENTIAL DIAGNOSES

- Adenovirus and other viral infections: Viral cytopathic effect present; special stains negative for bacteria
- Diphtheria: Respiratory tract pseudomembranes with Gram positive bacilli on surface
- *Mycoplasma pneumonia*: Nonspecific lymphocytic/neutrophilic bronchiolitis; special stains negative for bacteria

Pertussis in Epithelium

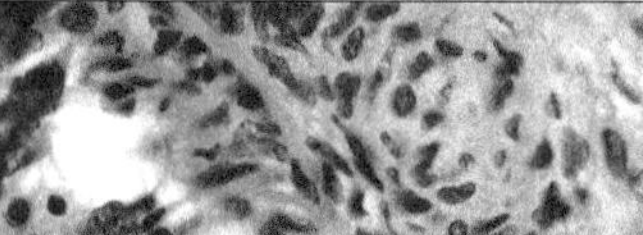

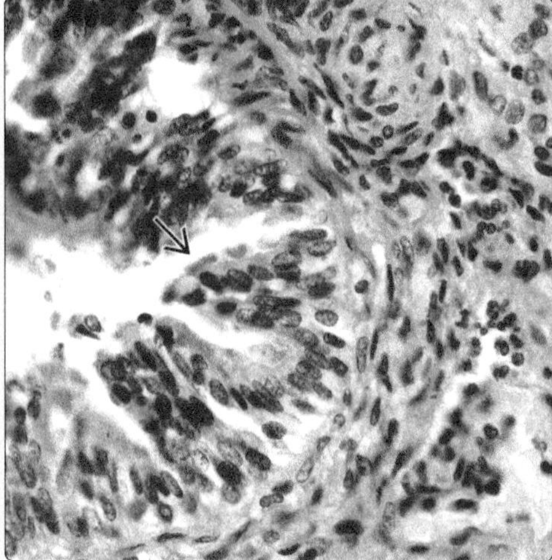

Pertussis in Epithelium: Giemsa

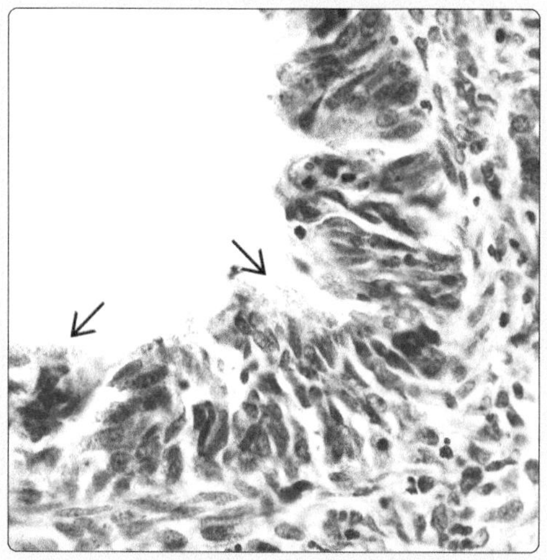

(Left) *A small airway from an infant who died of pertussis shows clumps of bacteria ⇨ lining the ciliated respiratory epithelium at autopsy.* **(Right)** *Bordetella pertussis is a gram-negative coccobacillus, which can be highlighted with Giemsa ⇨ and silver stains to demonstrate the adherence to epithelium.*

Pertussis in Epithelium and Alveoli

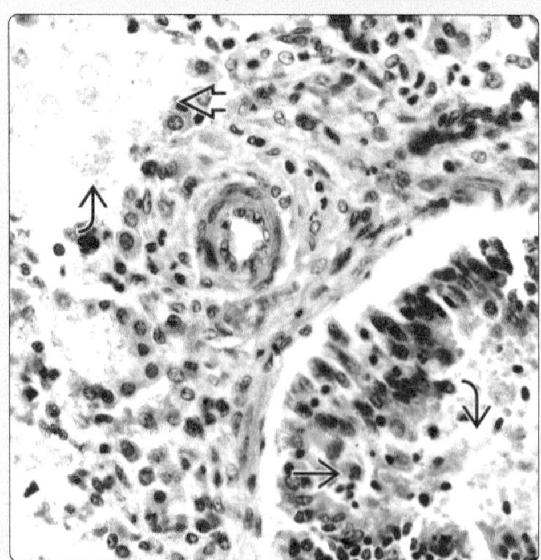

Pertussis in Epithelium

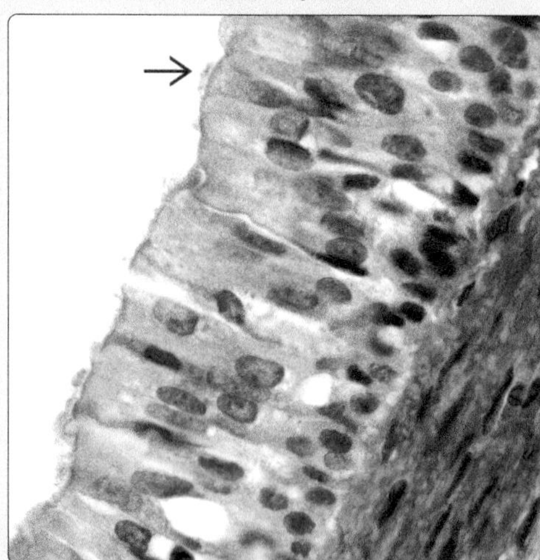

(Left) *A small airway ⇨ and the adjacent alveolar spaces ⇨ demonstrate innumerable bacteria ⇨ in clouds as part of a secondary bacterial infection in fatal pertussis.* **(Right)** *In this section of trachea from a fatal pertussis infection, the normal ciliated epithelium is interrupted by blue/gray clumps ⇨ of bacteria on the surface.*

TERMINOLOGY

Synonyms

- Whooping cough, 100 days cough

Definitions

- From Jules Bordet (Belgian bacteriologist)
- Latin: "Per" (away, extreme) + "tussis" (cough)

ETIOLOGY/PATHOGENESIS

Infectious Agents

- Infection with *Bordetella pertussis*, gram-negative, encapsulated, nonmotile, aerobic bacillus, which is spread by respiratory droplets (1- to 2-week incubation period); humans are only known host
- Upon entry into respiratory tract, bacteria bind to cilia via filamentous hemagglutinin adhesin; tracheal cytotoxins inhibit movement of cilia, decreasing clearance of mucus, which leads to extreme cough
- Bacteria further inhibit phagocytosis through pertussis toxin (PT) that disrupts phagocyte adenylate cyclase production of cyclic AMP
- *Bordetella parapertussis* and *Bordetella holmesii* may cause pertussis-like illness as well as other nonpertussis illness symptoms

CLINICAL ISSUES

Epidemiology

- Affects 15-40 million people worldwide with 200,000-300,000 deaths annually
- USA: Markedly decreased after introduction of vaccines in 1940s; 1,609-48,277 cases/year (2010-2022)

Presentation

- Initial fever, rhinorrhea, cough
- Progresses to violent coughing with inspiratory "whoop"; may be followed by with emesis or cyanosis
- Complications include insomnia, weight loss, rib fracture, urinary incontinence, respiratory failure, and death

Laboratory Tests

- Lymphocytosis (> 4,000 cells/μL (adults) or 8,000 cells/μL (pediatric)
- Diagnosis primarily by culture from nasopharyngeal or oropharyngeal swab
- PCR for species specific insertional sequences (e.g., *B. pertussis* IS*481; B. parapertussis* IS *1001*)
- ELISA test for antibodies (IgG, IgA, or IgM) to filamentous hemagglutinin adhesin (FHA) or PT

Treatment

- Vaccines for disease prevention (e.g., DTP, DTap, Tdap)
- Antibiotics (erythromycin, clarithromycin, azithromycin, trimethoprim-sulfamethoxazole) may shorten duration of illness (if given early) and decrease transmissibility
- Postexposure prophylaxis recommended for infants, women in 3rd trimester of pregnancy, immunocompromised, and people with asthma

Prognosis

- Mortality is 1.2% (primarily occurs in unvaccinated children)

MICROBIOLOGY

Culture

- Growth on Bordet-Gengou agar or buffered charcoal yeast extract (BCYE) agar with selective antibiotic (cephalosporin)
- Nonmotile organism that is positive for oxidase but negative for urease, citrate, and nitrate reductase

MACROSCOPIC

Patterns of Infection Found in Fatal Cases

- Otitis media, laryngitis, tracheitis, bronchitis, pneumonia

MICROSCOPIC

Histologic Features

- Necrotizing bronchiolitis, intraalveolar hemorrhage, and fibrinous edema
- Respiratory epithelium is coated with bacteria; may be denuded with secondary infection, neutrophils within walls of trachea/bronchi
- Bronchopneumonia with extension into alveolar spaces with secondary infection
- Interstitial pneumonia or bronchiolitis obliterans organizing pneumonia as complications of progressive disease
- Diffuse alveolar damage in some fatal infections

ANCILLARY TESTS

Histochemistry

- Gram-negative bacilli seen with silver and Giemsa stains

Immunohistochemistry

- Available in reference labs for confirming diagnosis
- May show intracellular bacteria and bacteria antigens within phagocytic cells and respiratory epithelium

DIFFERENTIAL DIAGNOSIS

Adenovirus and Other Viral Infections

- Similar appearance but with viral cytopathic effect, negative special stains for bacteria

Diphtheria

- Nonvaccinated patient with trachea pseudomembrane, mostly upper airway but may have secondary pneumonia

Mycoplasma pneumonia

- Similar appearance with nonspecific lymphocytic or neutrophilic bronchiolitis; organisms not identified by Gram or silver stains

SELECTED REFERENCES

1. Bridel S et al: A comprehensive resource for Bordetella genomic epidemiology and biodiversity studies. Nat Commun. 13(1):3807, 2022
2. Lefrancq N et al: Global spatial dynamics and vaccine-induced fitness changes of Bordetella pertussis. Sci Transl Med. 14(642):eabn3253, 2022
3. Palvo F et al: Severe pertussis infection: a clinicopathological study. Medicine (Baltimore). 96(48):e8823, 2017
4. Arbefeville S et al: Development of a multiplex real-time PCR assay for the detection of Bordetella pertussis and Bordetella parapertussis in a single tube reaction. J Microbiol Methods. 97:15-9, 2014
5. Paddock CD et al: Pathology and pathogenesis of fatal Bordetella pertussis infection in infants. Clin Infect Dis. 47(3):328-38, 2008

Intestinal Spirochetosis

KEY FACTS

ETIOLOGY/PATHOGENESIS

- Infection/colonization of with noninvasive spirochetes *Brachyspira aalborgi* and *Brachyspira pilosicoli*

CLINICAL ISSUES

- Highest prevalence in HIV patients, men who have sex with men, and in developing countries
- Associated with chronic diarrhea and abdominal pain
- Most healthy adult carriers are asymptomatic
- May affect any region of colon, including rectum and appendix
- Endoscopy: Usually normal colonic mucosa
- Treatment with antidiarrheals and antibiotics

MICROSCOPIC

- Basophilic, fringed layer of organisms (3-6 μm thick) present at surface of epithelium
- Organisms have corkscrew or spirillar appearance and do not invade mucosa
- Usually no associated inflammatory infiltrate
- Organisms highlighted by Warthin-Starry, Dieterle, Steiner, Alcian blue (pH 2.5), PAS, and antispirochetal IHC

TOP DIFFERENTIAL DIAGNOSES

- Syphilis: Spirochetes highlighted by Warthin-Starry and spirochete IHC; organisms are invasive and associated with plasma cell-rich inflammation; confirm with serology
- Helicobacteriosis: Spiral-shaped bacteria highlighted by Warthin-Starry but negative for spirochete IHC; organisms luminal but associated with plasma cell-rich inflammation; confirm with anti-*Helicobacter* spp. IHC
- Enteroadherent *Escherichia coli* infection: Gram-negative, Warthin-Starry-positive, noncurvy (straight) rods
- Prominent luminal glycocalyx: Warthin-Starry stain negative

Intestinal Spirochetosis

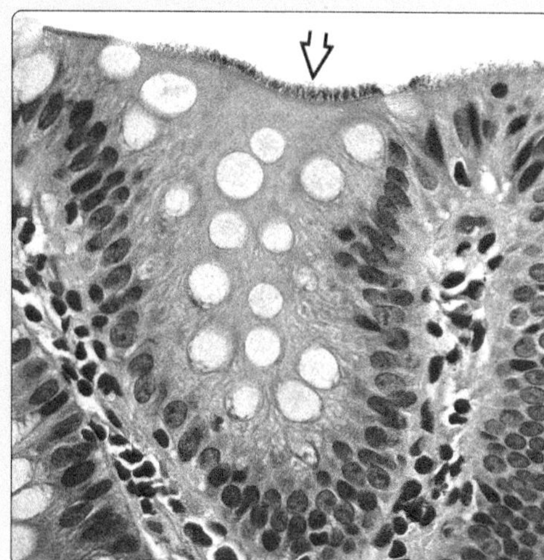

Patchy Involvement of Spirochetosis

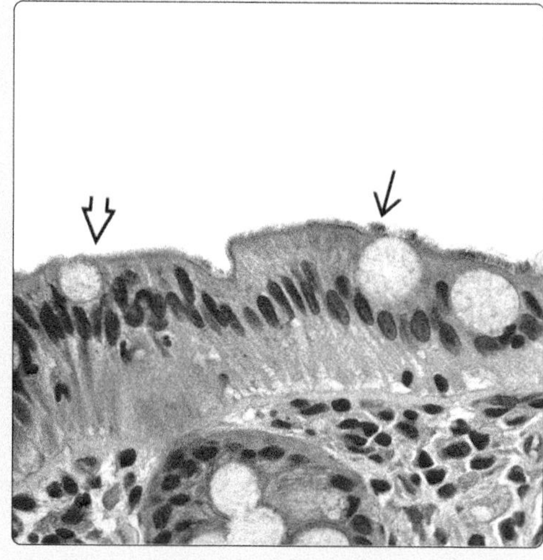

(Left) *Intestinal biopsy demonstrates purple adherent spirochetes ⇨ to the brush border, consistent with spirochetosis, most commonly due to Brachyspira aalborgi or Brachyspira pilosicoli.* **(Right)** *High-power view of an intestinal biopsy is shown in a patient with spirochetosis where organisms ⇨ are adherent to the brush border. Note the unaffected area ⇨.*

Spirochete IHC

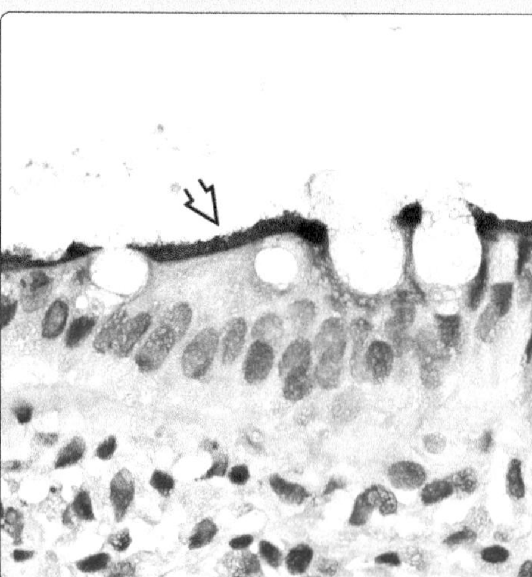

Spirochete Morphology: IHC

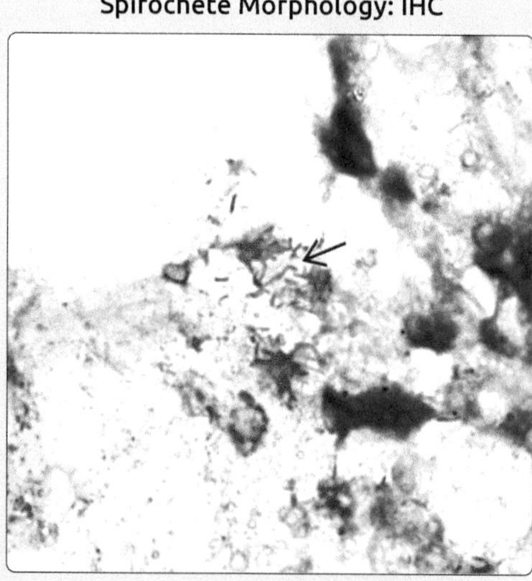

(Left) *Immunohistochemical stain for spirochetes (cross reacts with Treponema spp., Borrelia spp., and Brachyspira spp.) highlights the organisms ⇨ at the brush border in spirochetosis, which may appear as a solid strip of staining due to high density of organisms.* **(Right)** *Corkscrew appearance can be easier to visualize in organisms detached from the epithelial surface, as shown by this spirochete immunostain ⇨.*

TERMINOLOGY

Definitions

- Greek: "Spira" (spiral) + "khaite" (long hair)
- Greek: "Brachys" (short) + "spira" (spiral)

ETIOLOGY/PATHOGENESIS

Infectious Agents

- Infection/colonization of with noninvasive spirochetes *Brachyspira aalborgi* and *Brachyspira pilosicoli* (*Brachyspiraceae* family) via fecal-oral route or oral-anal contact
- Highly debated whether *Brachyspira* are human pathogens or commensals
- *B. pilosicoli* cause diarrheal illness in animals

CLINICAL ISSUES

Epidemiology

- Histologic prevalence of 2-16% in western countries
- Higher prevalence of 20-62% in HIV patients and men who have sex with men (MSM)
  - No correlation between prevalence and immune status/CD4 count
  - Some hypothesize intestinal spirochetosis could be sexually transmitted disease
- Higher but variable prevalence in developing countries

Site

- May affect any region of colon, including rectum and appendix

Presentation

- Most healthy adults with histologic evidence of colonization are asymptomatic
- Vague abdominal pain and chronic diarrhea
- In children: Nausea, weight loss, failure to thrive

Treatment

- Antibiotics: Penicillin benzathine, metronidazole
- Antidiarrheals

Prognosis

- Varies from complete resolution to continued chronic diarrhea
- Some reports suggest outcome after therapy is independent of histologic resolution

MICROBIOLOGY

Bacterial Features

- Fastidious anaerobic spirochetes with slender tapered ends
  - *B. aalborgi*: 2-6 μm in length, 0.2 μm in diameter
  - *B. pilosicoli*: 4-20 μm in length, 0.2-0.5 μm in diameter

Culture

- Although organisms can be cultured, not part of routine diagnosis

MACROSCOPIC

Endoscopic Findings

- Typically normal colonic mucosa
- Rare reports of mucosal erosion, edema, erythema, polypoid appearance
- Biopsies should be taken in at-risk populations, even if colonic mucosa is normal

MICROSCOPIC

Histologic Features

- Basophilic, fringed layer of organisms (3-6 μm thick) present at surface of epithelium (may be focal or patchy)
- Organisms have corkscrew or spirillar appearance and do not invade the mucosa
- Usually no associated inflammatory infiltrate

ANCILLARY TESTS

Special Stains

- Organisms highlighted by Warthin-Starry, Dieterle, Steiner, Alcian blue (pH 2.5), and PAS stains
- Negative for tissue Gram stain

Immunohistochemistry

- Antispirochetal antibodies (also stain *Treponema* and *Borrelia*) will be strongly positive

DIFFERENTIAL DIAGNOSIS

Syphilis

- *Treponema pallidum* spirochetes morphologically similar to *Brachyspira* spp. and also highlighted by Warthin-Starry stain and spirochete IHC
- Organisms invade into mucosa and are associated with dense plasma cell-rich inflammation; confirm with serology

Helicobacteriosis

- *Helicobacter pylori* and *Helicobacter heilmannii* are also spiral-shaped bacteria highlighted by Warthin-Starry stain but negative by spirochete IHC
- Organisms located in lumen and can be highlighted by anti-*Helicobacter* spp. IHC; associated with plasma cell-rich inflammation

Enteroadherent *Escherichia coli* Infection

- Gram-negative, silver-positive, noncurvy (straight) rods
- Bacilli (not spirillar in form)

Prominent Luminal Glycocalyx

- Negative for silver impregnation stains

SELECTED REFERENCES

1. Eslick GD et al: Clinical and pathologic factors associated with colonic spirochete (Brachyspira pilosicoli and Brachyspira aalborgi) infection: a comprehensive systematic review and pooled analysis. Am J Clin Pathol. 160(4):335-40, 2023
2. Pérez-Tanoira R et al: Increased prevalence of symptomatic human intestinal spirochetosis in MSM with high-risk sexual behavior in a cohort of 165 individuals. Trop Med Infect Dis. 8(5), 2023
3. Graham RP et al: Treponema pallidum Immunohistochemistry is positive in human intestinal Spirochetosis. Diagn Pathol. 13(1):7, 2018
4. Hampson DJ: The spirochete Brachyspira pilosicoli, enteric pathogen of animals and humans. Clin Microbiol Rev. 31(1), 2018
5. Ena J et al: Intestinal spirochetosis as a cause of chronic diarrhoea in patients with HIV infection: case report and review of the literature. Int J STD AIDS. 20(11):803-5, 2009
6. Calderaro A et al: Infective colitis associated with human intestinal spirochetosis. J Gastroenterol Hepatol. 22(11):1772-9, 2007. Erratum in: J Gastroenterol Hepatol. 22(11):2049, 2007

Borrelia Species Infections

KEY FACTS

ETIOLOGY/PATHOGENESIS

- Infection with *Borellia* spp., helical gram-negative bacteria transmitted by arthropods
- Lyme: *B. burgdorferi* group, transmitted by *Ixodes* spp. ticks
- Tick-borne relapsing fever: *B. hermsii* and other spp., transmitted by *Ornithodoros hermsi*
- Louse-borne relapsing fever: *B. recurrentis*
- Hard tick relapsing fever: *B. miyamotoi*

CLINICAL ISSUES

- Serology: ELISA screen followed by Western blot confirmation
- PCR: CSF, synovial joint fluid, blood, tissue
- Oral doxycycline is mainstay of treatment

MICROSCOPIC

- Erythema migrans: Superficial and deep perivascular infiltrate; central eosinophils and peripheral plasma cells
- Lymphocytoma: Diffuse lymphocytic infiltrate
- Acrodermatitis chronica atrophicans: Superficial and deep lymphoplasmacytic infiltrate, fibrous bands, and pseudosclerodermatous changes
- Synovium: Marked edema and neutrophilic infiltrate
- Cardiac: Diffuse, focal, or perivascular inflammation
- Spirochetes highlighted by IHC and Warthin-Starry stain

TOP DIFFERENTIAL DIAGNOSES

- Syphilis: Spirochetes and plasma cell-rich inflammation; distinguish with serology, PCR
- Leptospirosis: Spirochetes, can involve many organs; distinguish with serology, PCR
- *Rickettsia* infections: Endothelial injury and vasculitis affecting any organ; confirm with PCR, IHC
- Babesiosis: Also transmitted by *Ixodes* spp.; pear-shaped and cross forms in RBCs
- Anaplasmosis/ehrlichiosis: Also transmitted by *Ixodes* spp.; morulae in monocytes and granulocytes

(Left) *Erythema migrans, with its bull's-eye appearance, is pathognomonic for Lyme disease. (Courtesy J. Gathany, CDC/PHIL.)* **(Right)** *Spirochetes ⇨ are extracellular organisms that vary from 8-30 µm in length and have 3-10 helical coils, as would be seen in Borrelia recurrentis or Borrelia hermsii. (From DP: Blood & Bone Marrow.)*

Erythema Migrans

Tick-Borne Relapsing Fever

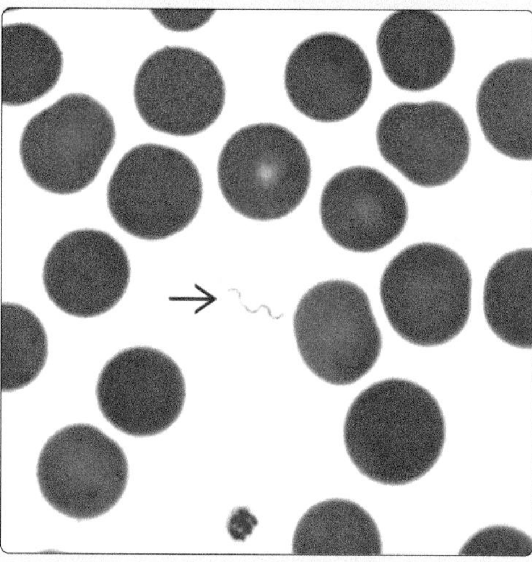

(Left) *Warthin-Starry silver staining highlights scattered spirochetes in heart tissue, consistent with Lyme carditis. (Courtesy S. Zaki, MD, PhD, CDC/PHIL.)* **(Right)** *Scattered spirochetes are highlighted by immunohistochemistry (red) in the midgut of an Ixodes spp. tick, consistent with Borrelia spp. Antibodies may show cross reactivity between Treponema, Borrellia, and Leptospira spp., necessitating correlation with clinical history and other laboratory findings.*

***Borrelia burgdorferi*: Warthin-Starry Stain**

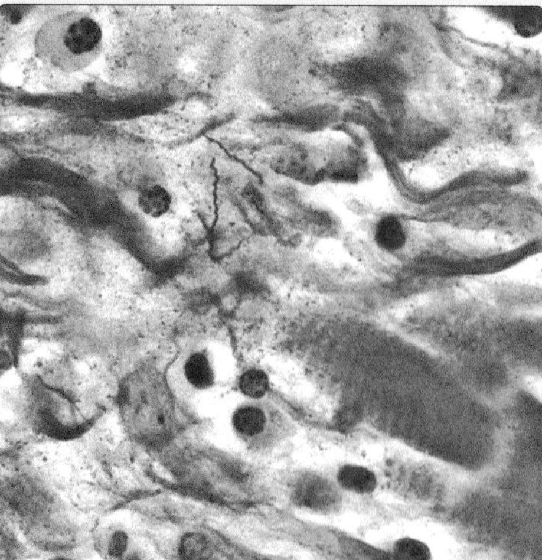

Spirochete Immunohistochemistry

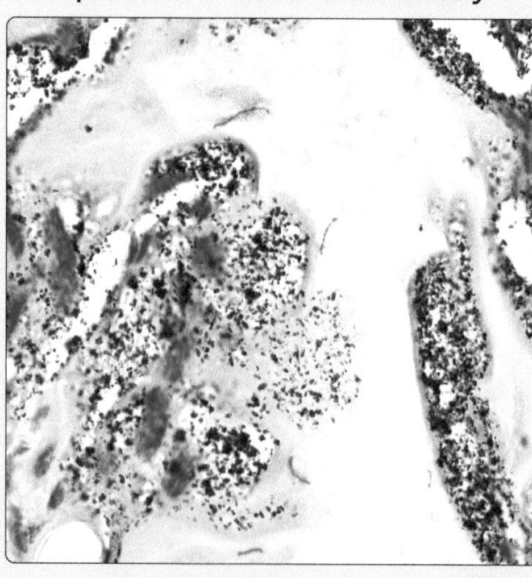

TERMINOLOGY

Definitions

- *Borrelia* named in honor of Amédée Borrel
- "Lyme" from Lyme, Connecticut (1st disease description)

ETIOLOGY/PATHOGENESIS

Infectious Agents

- Infection with *Borellia* spp., helical gram-negative bacteria transmitted by arthropods
- Lyme disease
  - Caused by *B. burgdorferi* or *B. mayonii* in USA and *B. afzelii* or *B. garinii* in Europe
  - Transmitted by *Ixodes scapularis* (deer tick) in Northeastern and midwestern USA, *I. pacificus* (western black-legged tick) in Western USA, *I. ricinus* (sheep tick) in Europe, and *I. persulcatus* (taiga tick) in Asia
  - *Borellia* spp. in tick midgut are transferred to mammalian host during blood meal; local replication occurs, resulting in inflammatory response creating target-shaped rash (erythema migrans); wide dissemination after days to weeks
- Tick-borne relapsing fever (TBRF) caused by *B. hermsii*, *B. parkerii*, *B. turicatae*, transmitted by *Ornithodoros hermsi* (soft-bodied tick)
- Louse-borne relapsing fever (LBRF) caused by *B. recurrentis*; spread by *Pediculus humanus*
- Hard tick relapsing fever (HTRF) caused by *B. miyamotoi* in Japan, Russia, Europe, North America; spread primarily by *Ixodes* spp.
- TBRF-like illness caused by *B. crocidurae* in West Africa, *B. hispanica* in Spain and Morocco, *B. duttoni* in Africa, and *B. turicatae* in New World
- Antigenic variation is responsible for relapsing pattern (febrile episodes during time of high replication)

CLINICAL ISSUES

Epidemiology

- Lyme disease most common vector-borne infection in USA; 35,000 cases reported/year to CDC with total cases estimated up to 476,000/year; associated with outdoor activities from spring until early autumn
- Highest incidence of Lyme is in Northeast (particularly Connecticut); also found in Midwest (Wisconsin, Minnesota, Michigan) and West (northern California)
- TBRF: USA patient exposure to rodent-infested cabin or woodpile in Rocky Mountain region; globally, variable exposure to ticks and, rarely, vertical transmission
- LBRF: Associated with refugee settings in developing or displaced nations

Presentation

- Lyme disease
  - Initial presentation is most commonly erythema migrans at site of tick bite but may be absent or not have classic target appearance with central clearing; systemic symptoms may include fatigue, headache, fever and chills, and lymphadenopathy
  - After days to weeks, additional cutaneous lesions may develop (indicating cutaneous spread)
  - After weeks to months, additional complications may include Lyme arthritis, neuroborreliosis, cardiac Lyme borreliosis, and, rarely, *Borrelia* lymphocytoma and conjunctivitis
  - Chronic manifestations may include acrodermatitis chronica atrophicans (red/bluish lesions on extensor surfaces of extremities), chronic arthritis, and neurological symptoms
- TBRF and LBRF
  - After ~ 7-day incubation, patient experiences cycles consisting of 3 days of fever followed by 7 afebrile days, which can repeat up to 30x without treatment
  - Associated symptoms include myalgias, arthralgias, headache, dizziness, and vomiting; less commonly lymphadenopathy, hepatosplenomegaly, rash, and myocarditis

Laboratory Tests

- Lyme disease
  - Serology
    - ELISA assays are available for whole-cell lysates, groups of antigens, or single targets (i.e., C6 peptide)
    - Standard recommendation is for 2-tiered approach (ELISA screen followed by Western blot confirmation), though 2-tiered ELISA approaches have been proposed as alternative
    - IgM and IgG testing useful to determine acute vs. chronic infection, though IgM can persist for months to years; acute vs. convalescent serum needed to demonstrate seroconversion
  - PCR: CSF, synovial joint fluid, blood, tissue
  - Lumbar puncture: Lymphocytic pleocytosis, elevated protein, normal glucose, and anti-*Borrelia* antibodies (in cases of Lyme meningitis)
- TBRF and LBRF
  - Peripheral blood smear will often demonstrate organisms during febrile periods
  - Serologic testing and direct PCR can also aid diagnosis

Treatment

- Oral doxycycline is mainstay of treatment
- IV ceftriaxone is standard treatment for neuroborreliosis

Prognosis

- Mortality in Lyme disease is rare and usually due to cardiac involvement; ~ 60% of untreated patients develop persistent infection, which generally clears after several years
- Mortality in untreated TBRF is ~ 10%
- Jarisch-Herxheimer reactions in 10-20% of LBRF patients (Africa) with < 5% overall mortality with antibiotics

MICROBIOLOGY

Morphologic and Biochemical Characteristics

- Microaerophilic, helical-shaped (8-30 μm long x 0.2-0.5 μm wide), multiple endoflagella, motile

Culture and Microbiologic Identification

- Difficult to culture; may take up to 12 weeks; highest sensitivity early in infection, before antibiotics

- Highly enriched media is required; high lot-to-lot variability in efficacy; formulations include Barbour-Stoenner-Kelly II medium (BSK II), BSH-H medium, and Kelly medium Preac-Mursic (MKP)
- Most identification is done via PCR (16S rRNA, OspA, etc.)

MICROSCOPIC

Histologic Features of Lyme Disease

- Cutaneous
  - Erythema migrans: Typical features include superficial and deep perivascular infiltrate with central eosinophils and peripheral plasma cells
  - Lymphocytoma involving ear lobe, nipple, or scrotum: Diffuse lymphocytic infiltrate; may have follicular structures resembling germinal centers; interfollicular areas demonstrate lymphocytic infiltrate, plasma cells, eosinophils, mast cells, macrophages
  - Acrodermatitis chronica atrophicans: Dermal changes in absence of epidermal changes; superficial and deep lymphoplasmacytic infiltrate, fibrous bands, and pseudosclerodermatous changes sometimes with prominent telangiectasia of lymphatics
- Synovium: Marked edema and neutrophilic infiltrate in acute stages, followed by nonspecific chronic mixed inflammation and fibrin deposition with neovascularization in persistent stage
- Cardiac: Diffuse, focal, or perivascular infiltrates composed of either lymphocytes or mixed inflammation (highly variable); myocyte necrosis may be observed
- CNS: Mild fibrosis of meninges and lymphocytic infiltrates, intimal hyperplasia of meningeal arteries, spongiform changes, diffuse astrocytosis, microglial activation with microglial nodules, and diffuse demyelination of cerebral and cerebellar white matter
- Peripheral nerves: Mixed inflammatory infiltrate of epineurial vasa nervorum and endoneurial capillaries, and axonal degeneration

Histologic Features of Relapsing Fevers

- Autopsy findings may include hepatitis, miliary splenic abscess, central nervous system hemorrhage with perivascular infiltrate, and gastrointestinal and renal hemorrhagic lesions

ANCILLARY TESTS

Immunohistochemistry

- Spirochete antibodies highlight organisms in skin lesions more commonly than deep tissue sites (brain, heart)

Special Stains

- Organisms may be visualized by Warthin-Starry and other bacterial silver stains

DIFFERENTIAL DIAGNOSIS

Syphilis (*Treponema pallidum*)

- Spirochetes morphologically similar; also highlighted by Warthin-Starry stain and spirochete IHC
- Plasma cell-rich inflammation, can affect any organ in secondary or tertiary syphilis; confirm with serology, PCR

Leptospirosis (*Leptospira* spp.)

- Spirochetes morphologically similar; also highlighted by Warthin-Starry stain and spirochete IHC
- Pulmonary, renal, hepatic, and cardiac manifestations; confirm with PCR, serology

Rickettsia spp. Infections

- Many spp. transmitted by ticks (including *Amblyomma* and *Dermacentor* spp.)
- Endothelial injury and vasculitis can affect any organ system; confirm with PCR, IHC

Babesiosis (*Babesia* spp.)

- Mixed infections can occur due to shared vectors (*Ixodes* spp. ticks)
- *Babesia* spp. infect red blood cells with diagnostic pear-shaped and cross forms

Anaplasmosis and Ehrlichiosis

- Mixed infections can occur due to shared vectors (*Ixodes* spp. ticks)
- Morulae present in peripheral blood monocytes and granulocytes; confirm with PCR, serology

RNA Viral Infection (Noncytopathic)

- Clinical history and inflammatory pattern similar to viral myocarditis and viral encephalitis
- Powassan virus also spread by *Ixodes* spp. ticks
- Serology, PCR, and IHC to distinguish from arbovirus infections

SELECTED REFERENCES

1. Pratt GW et al: Utility of whole blood real-time PCR testing for the diagnosis of early Lyme disease. Am J Clin Pathol. 158(3):327-30, 2022
2. Rodino KG et al: When to think about other Borreliae:: hard tick relapsing fever (Borrelia miyamotoi), Borrelia mayonii, and beyond. Infect Dis Clin North Am. 36(3):689-701, 2022
3. Branda JA et al: Laboratory diagnosis of Lyme borreliosis. Clin Microbiol Rev. 34(2), 2021
4. Lochhead RB et al: Lyme arthritis: linking infection, inflammation and autoimmunity. Nat Rev Rheumatol. 17(8):449-61, 2021
5. Galan A et al: Detection of Borrelia in Ixodes scapularis ticks by silver stain, immunohistochemical and direct immunofluorescent methods. J Cutan Pathol. 45(7):473-7, 2018
6. Rudolf J et al: Laboratory testing for tick-borne infections in a large northeastern academic medical center: an 11-year experience. Am J Clin Pathol. 150(5):415-20, 2018
7. Talagrand-Reboul E et al: Relapsing fevers: neglected tick-borne diseases. Front Cell Infect Microbiol. 8:98, 2018
8. Knudtzen FC et al: Characteristics and clinical outcome of Lyme neuroborreliosis in a high endemic area, 1995-2014: a retrospective cohort study in Denmark. Clin Infect Dis. 65(9):1489-95, 2017
9. Koedel U et al: Lyme neuroborreliosis. Curr Opin Infect Dis. 30(1):101-7, 2017
10. Muehlenbachs A et al: Cardiac tropism of Borrelia burgdorferi: an autopsy study of sudden cardiac death associated with Lyme carditis. Am J Pathol. 186(5):1195-205, 2016
11. Tee SI et al: Acrodermatitis chronica atrophicans with pseudolymphomatous infiltrates. Am J Dermatopathol. 35(3):338-42, 2013
12. Wilson TC et al: Erythema migrans: a spectrum of histopathologic changes. Am J Dermatopathol. 34(8):834-7, 2012

Lyme Disease Incidence in USA

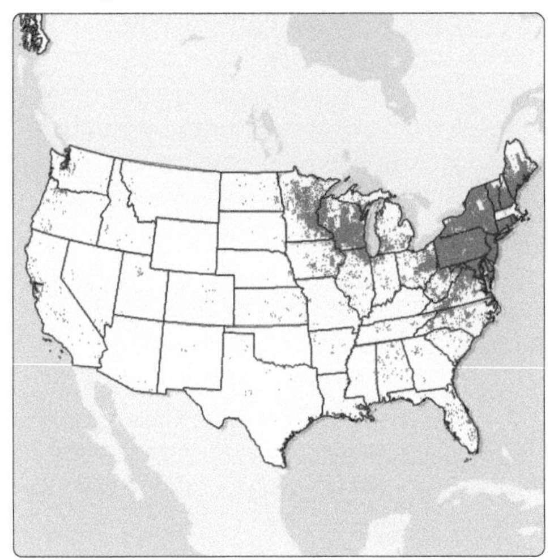

Ixodes scapularis (Deer Tick)

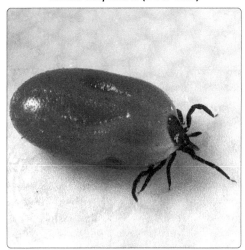

(Left) *Data from the CDC demonstrates the geographic incidence of Lyme disease in the USA in 2019. Dots displayed randomly throughout a county based on the number of reported cases. (Courtesy CDC.)* **(Right)** *This female Ixodes scapularis shows an engorged abdomen following a host blood meal. (Courtesy G. Alpert, CDC/PHIL.) In addition to Borrelia spp., I. scapularis serves as a vector for Anaplasma phagocytophilum, Ehrlichia muris eauclairensis, Babesia microti, and Powassan virus.*

Erythema Migrans

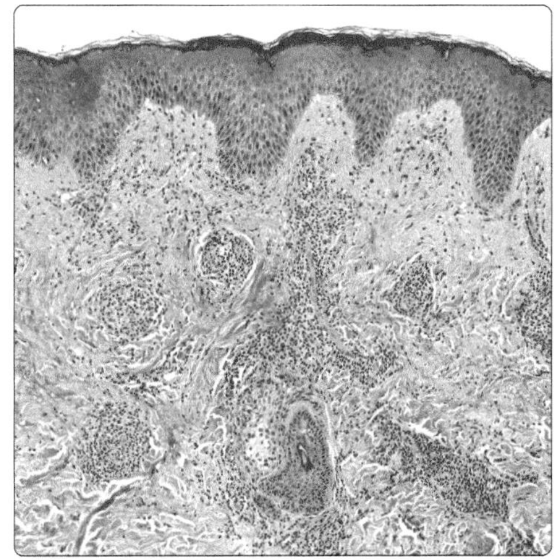

Acrodermatitis Chronica Atrophicans

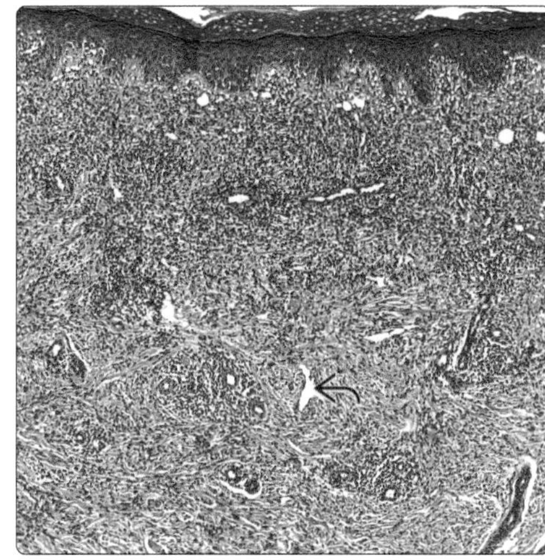

(Left) *Erythema migrans is characterized by a superficial and deep dermal perivascular lymphoplasmacytic infiltrate. (Courtesy B. Smoller, MD.)* **(Right)** *Acrodermatitis chronica atrophicans (3rd stage of Lyme disease) shows slight acanthosis with a dense, patchy, superficial, and deep infiltrate with dilated and ectatic vessels ➙. (From DP: Nonneoplastic Derm.)*

Lymphocytoma Cutis

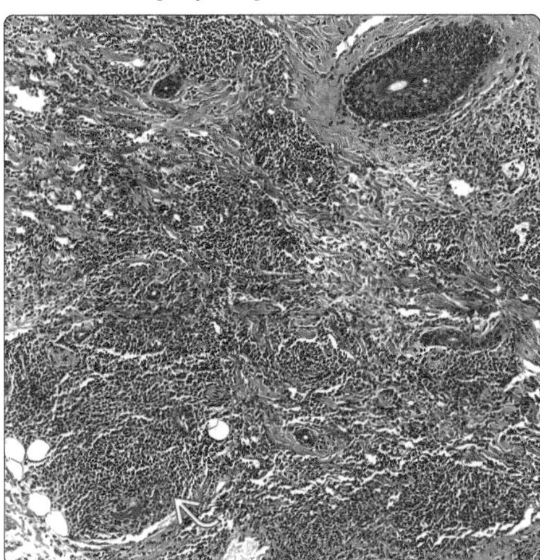

Lyme Myocarditis

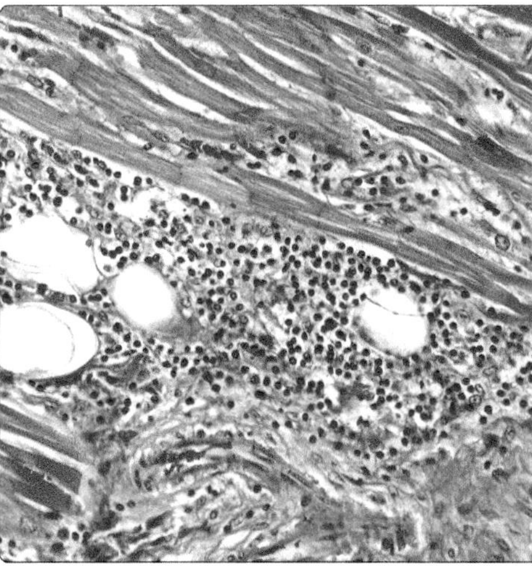

(Left) *Lymphocytoma cutis, a nonspecific skin inflammatory pattern that may be seen in Lyme disease, shows a much more dense, superficial, and deep inflammatory infiltrate ➙ that can simulate lymphoma. (From DP: Nonneoplastic Derm.)* **(Right)** *Lyme myocarditis, shown here, includes a wide range of histologic findings, including locally destructive, predominantly lymphocytic myocarditis. This patient was untreated and died of myocardial complications.*

Leptospira Species Infection

KEY FACTS

ETIOLOGY/PATHOGENESIS

- Infection with *Leptospira* spp. spirochetes via exposure to water contaminated with urine from infected animals

CLINICAL ISSUES

- Global disease but most common in warmer climates
- Septicemic phase (after 2-30 day incubation): Week-long febrile illness
- Immune phase: Severe, late-stage presentation can occur in 5-15% of patients
- Serology is most common means of diagnosis
- Organisms can be detected directly via dark-field microscopy, PCR, or culture
- Treated with oral doxycycline or IV penicillin/ceftriaxone

MICROSCOPIC

- Liver: Disorganization of liver cell plates, spotty necrosis, Kupffer cell hyperplasia, cholestasis, and portal infiltrates
- Lungs: Intraalveolar hemorrhage, vasculitis, diffuse alveolar damage
- Kidneys: Acute interstitial nephritis/acute tubular necrosis
- Liver: Disorganization of liver cell plates, spotty necrosis, Kupffer cell hyperplasia, cholestasis, and portal infiltrates
- Heart: Interstitial myocarditis with hemorrhage
- Organisms highlighted by silver stains and spirochete IHC

TOP DIFFERENTIAL DIAGNOSES

- Borreliosis: Spirochetes highlighted by Warthin-Starry stain and spirochete IHC; cutaneous, synovial, cardiac, and CNS manifestations with Lyme disease; confirm with PCR, serology
- Syphilis: Spirochetes highlighted by Warthin-Starry stain and spirochete IHC; plasma cell-rich inflammation, can affect any organ in secondary or tertiary syphilis; confirm with serology

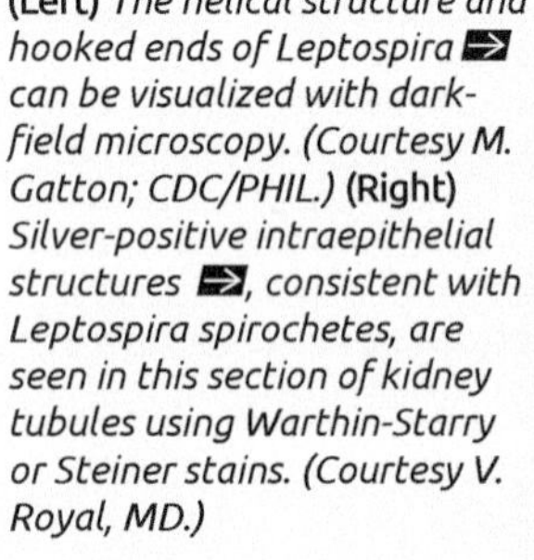

(Left) *The helical structure and hooked ends of Leptospira ➡ can be visualized with dark-field microscopy. (Courtesy M. Gatton; CDC/PHIL.)* **(Right)** *Silver-positive intraepithelial structures ➡, consistent with Leptospira spirochetes, are seen in this section of kidney tubules using Warthin-Starry or Steiner stains. (Courtesy V. Royal, MD.)*

Leptospira **Morphology: Dark Field**

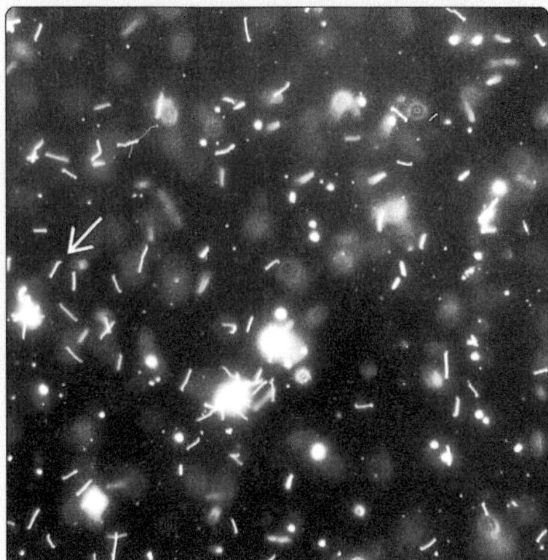

Leptospira **spp.: Silver Stain**

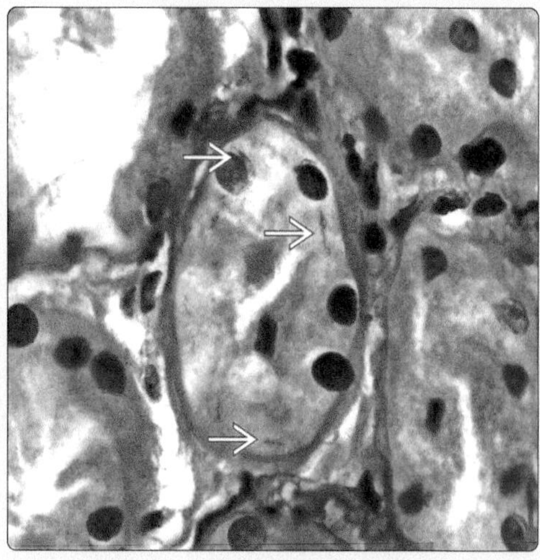

(Left) *Silver staining has made numerous Leptospira visible ➡ in this liver section taken at autopsy. (Courtesy M. Hicklin, CDC/PHIL.)* **(Right)** *Mononuclear inflammation, tubulitis ➡, casts, and focal cast extrusion ➡ can be seen in leptospirosis. (Courtesy V. Royal, MD.)*

Leptospira **spp. in Liver**

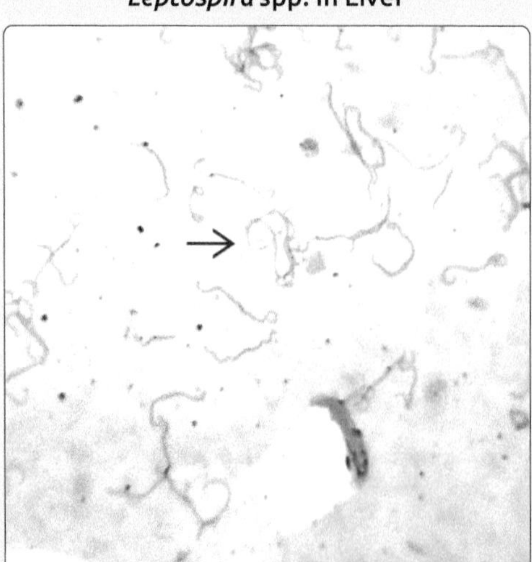

Leptospirosis in Kidney

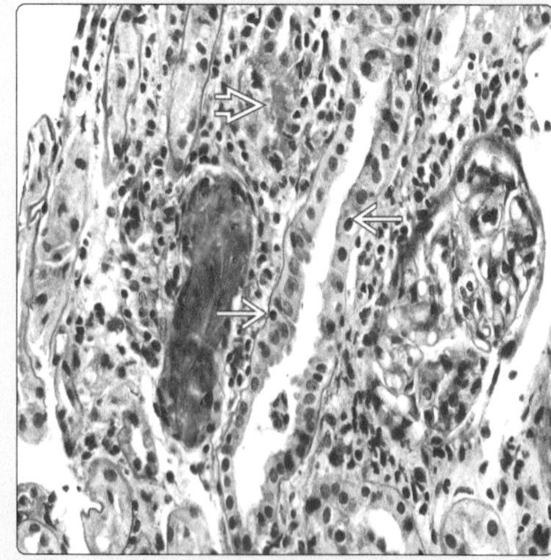

TERMINOLOGY

Definitions

- Greek: Leptos (thin) + Latin: Spira (coiled)

ETIOLOGY/PATHOGENESIS

Infectious Agents

- Infection with *Leptospira* spp. spirochetes via exposure of mucous membranes and cuts and scrapes in skin to contaminated water; rapidly enter bloodstream and spread hematogenously throughout body
- Large, zoonotic reservoir as chronic renal infections in many animals (e.g., rodents, livestock, and companion animals), which shed organisms in urine
- Organisms may be present in untreated water and damp soil; outbreaks can be linked to heavy rainfall and flooding
- *Leptospira interrogans* is most clinically relevant spp.; many pathogenic serotypes (serovars)
- Humans experience acute infection but are not carriers

CLINICAL ISSUES

Epidemiology

- Global disease but most common in warmer climates; estimated 1 million cases/year (60,000 deaths)
- USA: 100-200 cases/year (highest in Puerto Rico, Hawaii)

Presentation

- Septicemic phase (after 2-30 day incubation): Week-long febrile illness with high fever, headache, chills, rigors, myalgias (particularly in calf and lumbar region), conjunctival suffusion, abdominal pain, nausea, vomiting, cough, and pharyngitis
- Immune phase: Severe, late-stage presentation can occur in 5-15% of patients with jaundice, renal failure, arrhythmias, pulmonary symptoms, aseptic meningitis, photophobia, eye pain, adenopathy, hepatosplenomegaly, petechial rash, and disseminated intravascular coagulation
- Weil disease: Severe manifestation marked by liver and kidney failure, hemorrhagic pneumonitis, arrhythmias, and circulatory collapse

Laboratory Tests

- Serology is most common means of diagnosis
- Organisms can be detected directly via dark-field microscopy, PCR, or culture
- *Leptospira* detected in blood, CSF, and urine during initial septicemic phase
- During immune phase, organisms detected in tissue and urine but not blood or CSF

Treatment

- No FDA-approved vaccine
- Oral doxycycline for most cases
- IV penicillin or ceftriaxone for more severe infections

Prognosis

- Most patients experience subclinical or mild disease; mortality with severe disease approaches 40%

MICROBIOLOGY

Morphologic and Biochemical Characteristics

- *Leptospira* spp. are obligately aerobic, thin, tightly coiled spirochetes with pointed ends that may be bent into hook
- Catalase and oxidase positive

Culture and Microbiologic Identification

- After 2-4 weeks, it will grow on media supplemented with B vitamins, long-chain fatty acids, and ammonium salts [e.g., Ellinghausen-McCullough-Johnson-Harris media (EMJH)]
- Dark-field microscopy to identify colonies

MICROSCOPIC

Histologic Features

- Lungs: Intraalveolar hemorrhage, interstitial inflammation, vasculitis, pulmonary edema; occasionally diffuse alveolar damage with hyaline membranes
- Kidneys: Acute interstitial nephritis/acute tubular necrosis with mixed but predominantly mononuclear inflammatory infiltrate
- Liver: Disorganization of liver cell plates, spotty necrosis, Kupffer cell hyperplasia, cholestasis, and portal infiltrates; submassive centrilobular hepatocellular necrosis with intense hemorrhage in Weil disease
- Interstitial myocarditis accompanied by hemorrhage; can involve epicardium, valves, coronary arteries, and aorta

ANCILLARY TESTS

Special Stains

- Silver stains may reveal helical to filamentous or granular aggregates of organisms

Immunohistochemistry

- Antispirochete antibodies highlight organisms but frequently cross react with *Borrelia* and *Treponema* spp.

DIFFERENTIAL DIAGNOSIS

Borreliosis

- *Borrelia burgdorferi* and other spp. highlighted by Warthin-Starry stain and spirochete IHC
- Cutaneous, synovial, cardiac, and CNS manifestations with Lyme disease; confirm with PCR, serology

Syphilis

- *Treponema pallidum* spirochetes morphologically similar to *Leptospira* spp. and also highlighted by Warthin-Starry stain and spirochete IHC
- Plasma cell-rich inflammation, can affect any organ in secondary or tertiary syphilis; confirm with serology

SELECTED REFERENCES

1. Stone NE et al: Diverse lineages of pathogenic Leptospira species are widespread in the environment in Puerto Rico, USA. PLoS Negl Trop Dis. 16(5):e0009959, 2022
2. Sykes JE et al: Role of diagnostics in epidemiology, management, surveillance, and control of leptospirosis. Pathogens. 11(4), 2022
3. Picardeau M: Virulence of the zoonotic agent of leptospirosis: still terra incognita? Nat Rev Microbiol. 15(5):297-307, 2017
4. Waggoner JJ et al: Molecular diagnostics for human leptospirosis. Curr Opin Infect Dis. 29(5):440-5, 2016
5. Salkade HP et al: A study of autopsy findings in 62 cases of leptospirosis in a metropolitan city in India. J Postgrad Med. 51(3):169-73, 2005

Syphilis and Other Treponematoses

KEY FACTS

ETIOLOGY/PATHOGENESIS

- Infections with *Treponema* spp., gram-negative spirochetes, including syphilis (*Treponema pallidum* subspecies *pallidum*), yaws (*T. pallidum* subspecies *pertenue*), Bejel (*T. pallidum* subspecies *endemicum*), pinta (*T. pallidum* subspecies *carateum*)

CLINICAL ISSUES

- Presentation/symptoms vary with primary, secondary, and tertiary phases and congenital infections

MICROSCOPIC

- Warthin-Starry stain and anti-*T. pallidum* IHC highlight spirochetes
- Primary: Acanthotic epidermis, ulceration, endothelial swelling, and dense lymphoplasmacytic infiltrate
- Secondary: Lymphoplasma histiocytic infiltrate with some neutrophils, epithelioid cells, and occasional giant cells
- Tertiary: Necrotizing granulomatous inflammation
- Congenital: Placenta with enlarged hypercellular villi, proliferative fetal vascular changes, acute/chronic villitis
- Yaws: Dermal and perivascular infiltrate of lymphocytes and plasma cells; limited endothelial proliferation/swelling
- Bejel: Perivascular lymphoplasmacytic infiltrate, granulomas
- Pinta: Endothelial swelling and perivascular lymphoplasmacytic infiltrate; hyperchromic lesions

TOP DIFFERENTIAL DIAGNOSES

- Other ulcerated lesions (e.g., chancroid, granuloma inguinale, herpes simplex, lymphogranuloma venereum)
- Other skin rashes: Psoriasiform hyperplasia with stratum corneum neutrophils (psoriasis); eosinophils and plasma cells (drug and lichenoid hypersensitivity reactions)
- Other causes of granulomatous inflammation: Nonnecrotizing granulomatous inflammation with (*Brucella* spp.) or without (sarcoid) infectious etiology
- Negative serology, no spirochetes, and negative PCR

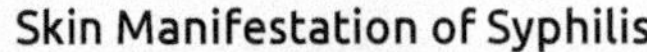

Skin Manifestation of Syphilis

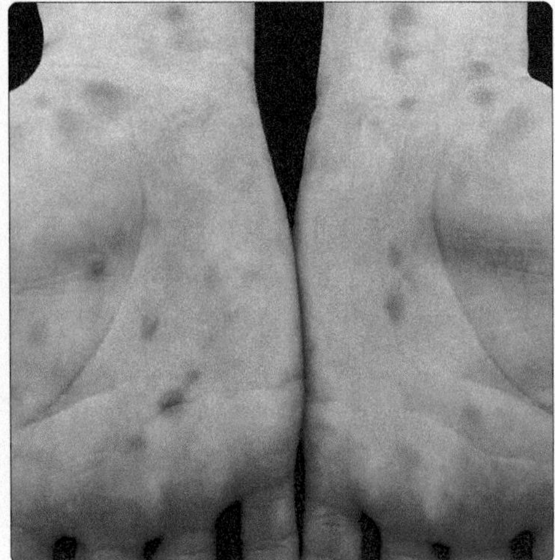

Secondary Syphilis

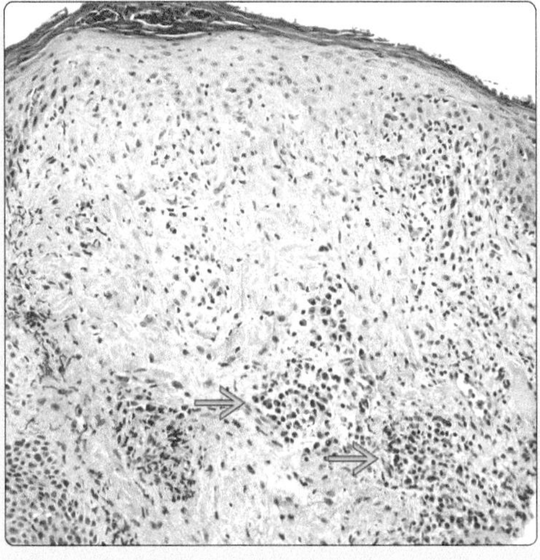

(Left) *Very few diseases cause an erythematous maculopapular eruption involving the palms and soles, and clinical history and laboratory testing are useful for confirming syphilis. (Courtesy G. Strauch, MD.)* **(Right)** *A subtle lichenoid dermatitis with superficial perivascular aggregates of plasma cells ➡ is characteristic of secondary syphilis.*

***Treponema pallidum* Warthin-Starry Stain**

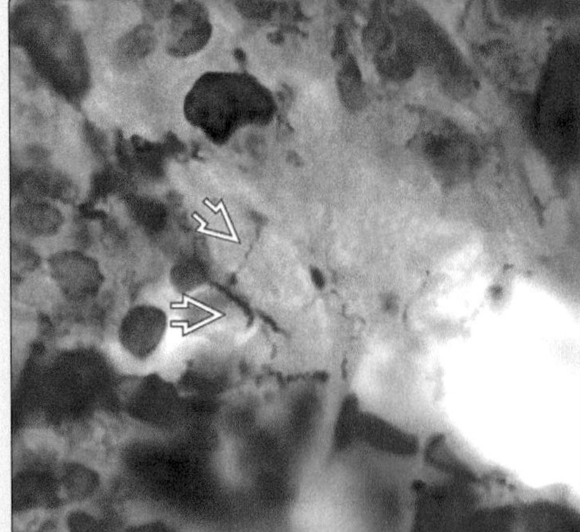

***Treponema pallidum* Immunohistochemistry**

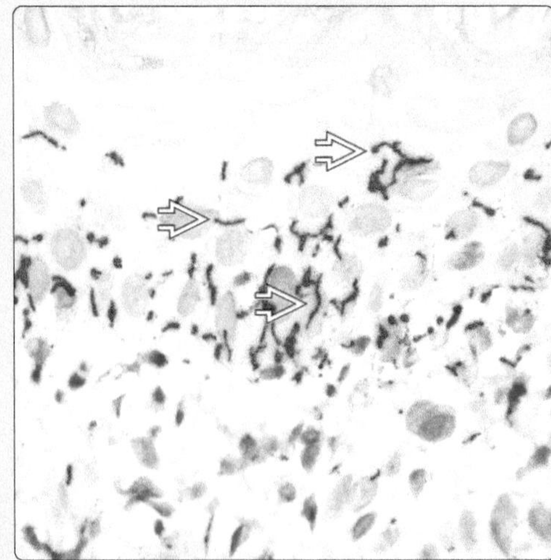

(Left) *Spirochetes ➡ seen on this Warthin-Starry stain are 5- to 20-µm long, < 0.5-µm-wide spirals, typical of Treponema pallidum infection.* **(Right)** *Numerous spirochetes ➡ are frequently detected in secondary syphilis using a polyclonal antibody. Notice the clean signal and preserved corkscrew morphology, highly valuable in distinguishing true signal from artifact.*

TERMINOLOGY

Synonyms

- Venereal syphilis: Lues, great pox, French disease, Italian disease
- Yaws: Pian, parangi, frambesia, paru, patek, buba, coko, tona
- Bejel: Endemic syphilis, dichuchwa, frenga, njovera, siti, belesh, bishel, nonvenereal syphilis
- Pinta: Mal del pinto, carate, azul, empeines, lota, tina

Definitions

- Greek: "Trepein" (to turn) + "nema" (thread)

ETIOLOGY/PATHOGENESIS

Infectious Agents

- All human treponematoses are similar in pathogenesis and clinical manifestations; differences in ages affected, mode of acquisition and capacity for CNS, and transplacental invasion are debatable
- Syphilis is sexually transmitted infection caused by gram-negative bacterium *Treponema pallidum* subspecies *pallidum*, in *Spirochaetaceae* family
- Yaws is tropical disease acquired by direct skin contact with infectious lesions and facilitated by skin breaks caused by *T. pallidum* subspecies *pertenue*
- Bejel is caused by *T. pallidum* subspecies *endemicum* and believed to be transmitted through mucosal and skin contact and sharing of eating and drinking utensils
- Pinta is caused by *Treponema carateum*, and it is regarded as mildest of treponematoses and believed to be transmitted by repeated skin-to-skin contact

CLINICAL ISSUES

Epidemiology

- Any sexually active person can get venereal syphilis through unprotected vaginal, anal, oral sex
- Estimated incidence of 12 million new cases each year
- North America and Western Europe: Men who have sex with men (MSM), coinfection with HIV, and heterosexual couples
- Although several low-income countries have achieved WHO targets for elimination of congenital syphilis, alarming increase in prevalence of syphilis has resulted in recent resurgence of congenital infections
- CDC reported 918 babies born with syphilis in USA in 2017 and 1,870 in 2019, and number is still increasing
- Other treponematoses often affect skin and present with skin lesions following contact with infected person
  - Almost 75% of people affected are children < 15 years
  - Overcrowding and poor personal hygiene and sanitation facilitate spread of disease in warm communities

Presentation

- Primary syphilis
  - Single small, red, painless papule with ulceration (chancre) lasts 3-6 weeks and heals without treatment
  - Without treatment, progresses to secondary stage
- Secondary syphilis
  - 3 weeks to 3 months after primary stage
  - Widespread skin rash mainly affects soles and palms but can spread to whole body
  - Raised patches (condyloma lata)
  - Fever, muscle and joint pains, headache, and swollen lymph glands; can affect any organ (e.g., CNS, liver, kidneys, skeletal muscles)
- Latent syphilis
  - Begins when all clinical symptoms disappear
  - With no treatment, may resolve or remain latent for years; most people do not develop tertiary stage syphilis
- Tertiary syphilis
  - May develop 3-10 or more years later
  - Solitary lesion (gummas)
  - Brain involvement (neurosyphilis), spinal cord disease
  - Can affect heart, eyes, or any other organs
    - Panuveitis is typical presenting sign in ocular syphilis
    - Optic nerve involvement is common
    - Syphilitic aortic aneurysm occurs most commonly in ascending aorta in either saccular or fusiform shape
  - Symptoms of late stage can include difficulty coordinating muscle movements, paralysis, numbness, gradual blindness, and dementia
- Congenital syphilis
  - One of TORCH infections (O = others)
  - Cause of spontaneous abortion and stillbirth
  - Live-born neonates may present with secondary syphilis and progress to latent stages
  - Remains major public health problem worldwide
  - Screening for syphilis infection in pregnant women is associated with reduced incidence of congenital syphilis
- Yaws
  - Primary lesion ("mother yaw") is erythematous papule often on lower extremities that may grow into typically painless papilloma (up to 5 cm in diameter)
  - Secondary papules are smaller scaly irregular macules; may grow and ulcerate, releasing highly infectious fluid
- Bejel
  - Primary lesion is painless papule or ulcer in oral or nasopharyngeal mucosa, often unobserved
  - Secondary lesions are very similar to secondary syphilis, including condylomata lata and split papules
- Pinta
  - Primary lesion is erythematosquamous plaque on areas of exposed skin
  - Disseminated secondary lesions (called pintids) present as scaly papules that coalesce into psoriasiform plaques, which may become hyper- or hypopigmented

Laboratory Tests

- Serology
  - Screening: Venereal disease research laboratory (VDRL), rapid plasma reagin (RPR), enzyme immunoassay (EIA) tests
  - Diagnosis: Fluorescent treponemal antibody absorption (FTA-ABS) test, *T. pallidum* particle agglutination assay (TPA), microhemagglutination assay (MA-PT)
- PCR
  - Nested PCR is sensitive method for detecting blood TP-DNA and is especially useful for detecting early syphilis
  - In late stages, sensitivity of PCR is lower than IHC techniques

- *T. pallidum* cannot be cultured

Treatment

- High-dose penicillin for syphilis and endemic treponematoses
- Jarisch-Herxheimer reaction: Febrile inflammatory reaction that may occur in patients after treatment of syphilis
- Oral single-dose azithromycin effective in patients with latent yaws

Prognosis

- Syphilis is easily cured in early stages
- Congenital and tertiary disease associated with significant morbidity and may be fatal

MICROSCOPIC

Histologic Features

- While venereal syphilis is common, other treponematoses are rare, except in endemic areas, and biopsies are extremely infrequent
- Spirochetes not visible on routine H&E but may be visualized with darkfield microscopy (mainly used in early stages)
- Primary syphilis: Acanthotic epidermis, ulceration, endothelial swelling, dense lymphoplasmacytic inflammation
- Secondary syphilis: Lichenoid inflammatory infiltrate composed of lymphocytes, plasma cells, some neutrophils, epithelioid histiocytes, and occasional giant cells or poorly formed granulomas; psoriasiform hyperplasia commonly seen in condyloma lata
- Tertiary syphilis: Necrotizing granulomatous inflammation
- Congenital syphilis: Placental histologic features include triad of enlarged hypercellular villi, proliferative fetal vascular changes, and acute or chronic villitis
- Yaws: Dermal and perivascular infiltrate of lymphocytes and plasma cells; limited or no endothelial proliferation and swelling (in contrast with venereal syphilis)
- Bejel: Early lesions show perivascular lymphoplasmacytic infiltrate and granulomas, very similar to primary syphilis
- Pinta: Primary and secondary pinta lesions show endothelial swelling and perivascular lymphocytes, plasma cells, and neutrophils; hyperchromic lesions show dermal melanin deposition; hypochromic (late) lesions show epidermal atrophy and absence of melanin

ANCILLARY TESTS

Special Stains

- Warthin-Starry (WS) stain highlights corkscrew-shaped spirochetes
  - Primary, secondary, and congenital syphilis: Numerous spirochetes present around vessels
  - Secondary syphilis, yaws: Numerous spirochetes within epidermis, between keratinocytes, on inflamed surface, and within dermis
  - Tertiary syphilis: Spirochetes occasionally in gummas
  - Pinta: Spirochetes in melanophages of hyperchromic lesions (absent in hypochromic lesions)

Immunohistochemistry

- Anti-*T. pallidum* IHC typically easier to perform and faster to interpret than WS stain
- Cross reactivity with other spirochetes (e.g., *Borrelia* spp., *Leptospira* spp., *Brachyspira* spp.)

DIFFERENTIAL DIAGNOSIS

Other Infectious Causes of Ulcerated Lesions

- e.g., candidiasis, chancroid, granuloma inguinale, herpes simplex, herpes zoster, lymphogranuloma venereum
- Lack of spirochetes by IHC or WS stain; specific etiology identified by special stains, IHC, culture, PCR

Other Infectious and Noninfectious Skin Rashes

- Broad differential, including Rocky Mountain spotted fever, graft-vs.-host disease, erythema migrans, and meningococcemia, amongst many others; syphilis has been dubbed "great mimic"
- Psoriasis: Psoriasiform hyperplasia with neutrophils in stratum corneum
- Drug reaction: Eosinophils and plasma cell infiltrate
- Lichenoid hypersensitivity reaction: Eosinophils and plasma cell infiltrate
- Negative serology, no spirochetes, and negative PCR for syphilis

Other Causes of Granulomatous Inflammation

- Sarcoidosis: Nonnecrotizing granulomatous inflammation without identified infectious etiology
- Brucellosis: Nonnecrotizing granulomatous inflammation due to gram-negative *Brucella* spp.

SELECTED REFERENCES

1. Peeling RW et al: Syphilis. Lancet. 402(10398):336-46, 2023
2. Suñer C et al: Rapid serologic test for diagnosis of yaws in patients with suspicious skin ulcers. Emerg Infect Dis. 29(8):1682-4, 2023
3. Ghanem KG et al: The modern epidemic of syphilis. N Engl J Med. 382(9):845-54, 2020
4. Ozturk-Engin D et al: Predictors of unfavorable outcome in neurosyphilis: multicenter ID-IRI Study. Eur J Clin Microbiol Infect Dis. 38(1):125-34, 2019
5. Sonmez C et al: Performance evaluation of nine different syphilis serological tests in comparison with the FTA-abs test. J Immunol Methods. 464:9-14, 2019
6. Arando M et al: The Jarisch-Herxheimer reaction in syphilis: could molecular typing help to understand it better? J Eur Acad Dermatol Venereol. 32(10):1791-5, 2018
7. Cooper JM et al: Congenital syphilis. Semin Perinatol. 42(3):176-84, 2018
8. Graham RP et al: Treponema pallidum immunohistochemistry is positive in human intestinal spirochetosis. Diagn Pathol. 13(1):7, 2018
9. Heston S et al: Syphilis in children. Infect Dis Clin North Am. 32(1):129-44, 2018
10. Klein A et al: The great imitator on the rise: ocular and optic nerve manifestations in patients with newly diagnosed syphilis. Acta Ophthalmol. 97(4):e641-7, 2018
11. Wang C et al: Sensitive detection of Treponema pallidum DNA from the whole blood of patients with syphilis by the nested PCR assay. Emerg Microbes Infect. 7(1):83, 2018
12. Yuan SM: Syphilitic aortic aneurysm. Z Rheumatol. 77(8):741-8, 2018
13. Chen B et al: The tradition algorithm approach underestimates the prevalence of serodiagnosis of syphilis in HIV-infected individuals. PLoS Negl Trop Dis. 11(7):e0005758, 2017
14. Stamm LV: Pinta: Latin America's forgotten disease? Am J Trop Med Hyg. 93(5):901-3, 2015
15. Giacani L et al: The endemic treponematoses. Clin Microbiol Rev. 27(1):89-115, 2014

Primary Syphilis: Chancre

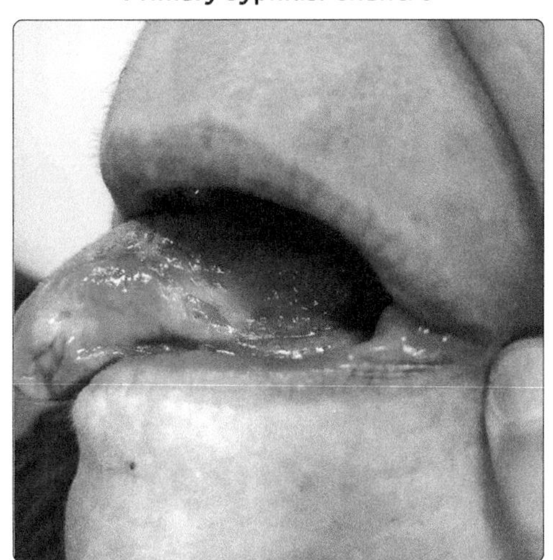

Primary Syphilis: Chancre

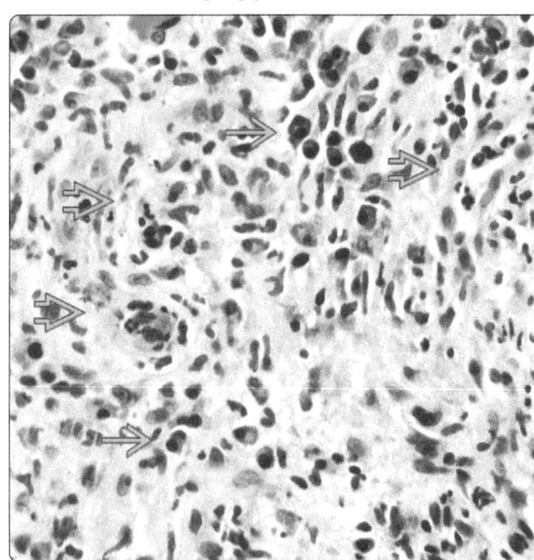

(Left) *A painless ulcer in the mucosae is characteristic of primary syphilis.* **(Right)** *Marked endothelial swelling ➲ and a plasma cell-rich ➲ inflammatory infiltrate are characteristic of the primary lesion of syphilis, termed endarteritis obliterans.*

Primary Syphilis Immunohistochemistry

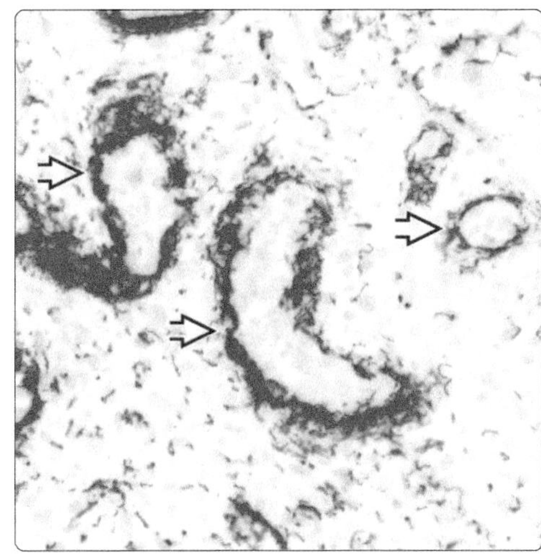

Syphilitic Alopecia

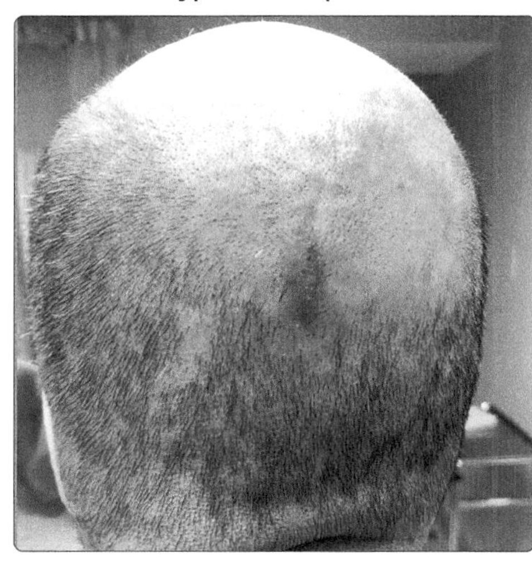

(Left) *Numerous spirochetes decorating the wall of vessels ➲ (mimicking an immunohistochemical vascular marker) are noted in primary syphilis.* **(Right)** *Alopecia is an uncommon manifestation of syphilis and characteristically presents with irregular alopecic patches imparting a characteristic moth-eaten pattern.*

Secondary Syphilis: Condyloma Latum

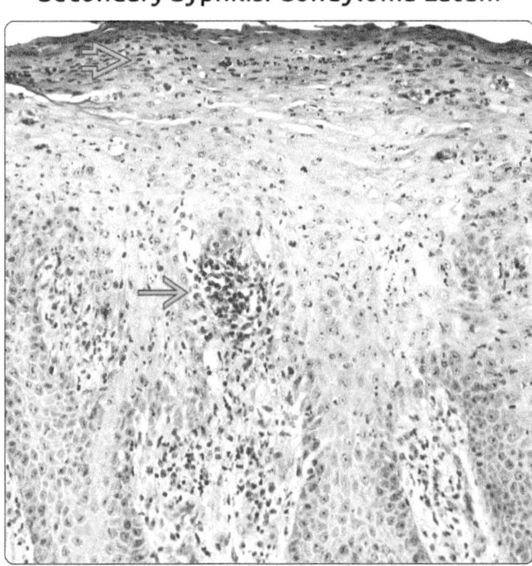

Condyloma Lata Immunohistochemistry

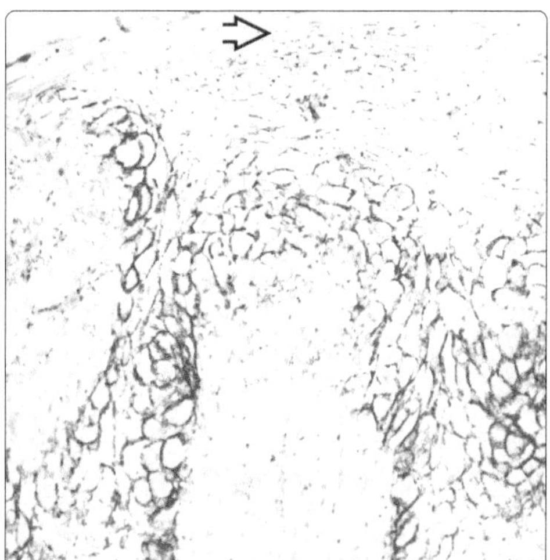

(Left) *Psoriasiform epidermal hyperplasia with parakeratotic scale infiltrated by neutrophils ➲ and plasma cell aggregates at the dermal papilla ➲ are typical of condyloma lata.* **(Right)** *Numerous spirochetes at all epidermal levels are easily noted on immunohistochemistry in condyloma lata. Notice treponema are abundant, including in the scale ➲, correlative with it being highly contagious.*

(**Left**) *This HIV-positive patient shows a widespread maculopapular eruption indicative of secondary syphilis. (Courtesy G. Strauch, MD.)* (**Right**) *This photograph depicts chronic progressive interstitial keratitis of the corneal stroma due to a congenital syphilitic infection, which often results in blindness. (Courtesy R. Sumpter, CDC/PHIL.)*

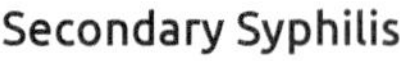

Secondary Syphilis

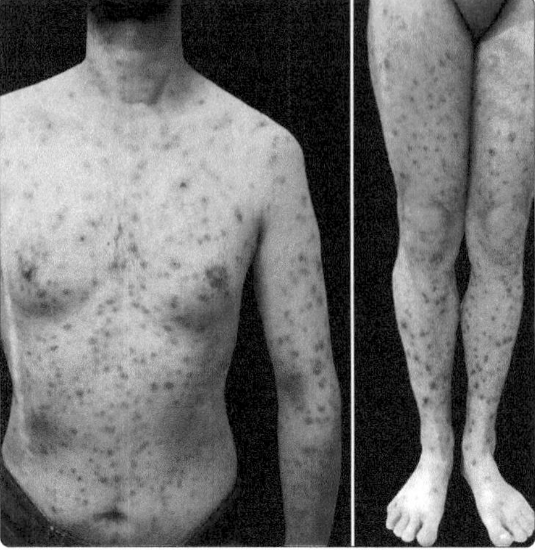

Congenital Syphilis: Interstitial Corneal Keratitis

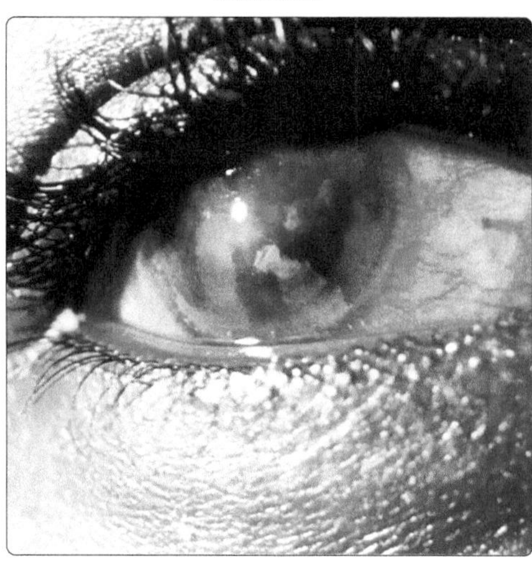

(**Left**) *This photograph from a patient with congenital syphilis shows mulberry molars, or Moon molars, a condition where the bite surface of the permanent, 1st lower molar teeth, develop rounded surfaces to their cusps, resembling the surface of a mulberry. (Courtesy R. Sumpter, CDC/PHIL.)* (**Right**) *This photograph of a patient with congenital syphilis infection shows a perforation in the midline of the palate's midline. (Courtesy S. Lindsley, CDC/PHIL.)*

Congenital Syphilis: Mulberry Molars

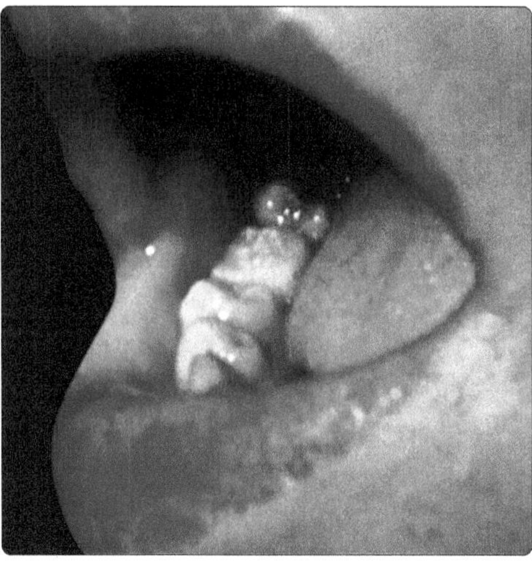

Congenital Syphilis: Perforation of Palate

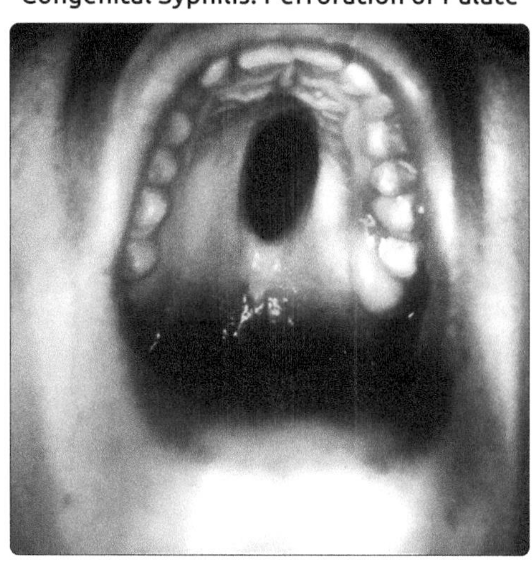

(**Left**) *This patient presented with an intraoral gummatous lesion of the soft palate due to a longstanding tertiary, syphilitic infection. (Courtesy CDC/PHIL.)* (**Right**) *This cardiac muscle image shows a microgumma lesion, consisting of a central zone of necrosis, surrounded by large numbers of plasma cells and lymphocytes, while vascular proliferation is present on the periphery. (Courtesy S. Lindsley, CDC/PHIL.)*

Tertiary Syphilis: Gumma

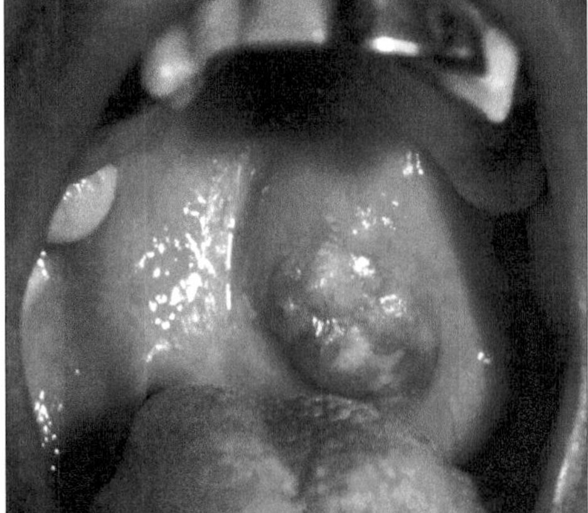

Gumma Histology

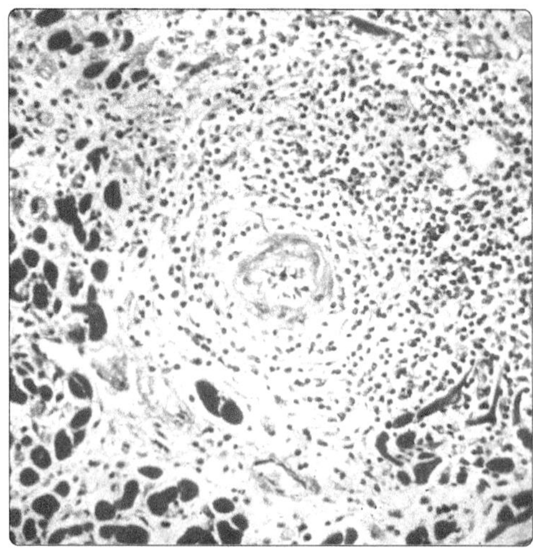

Tertiary Syphilis: Gumma

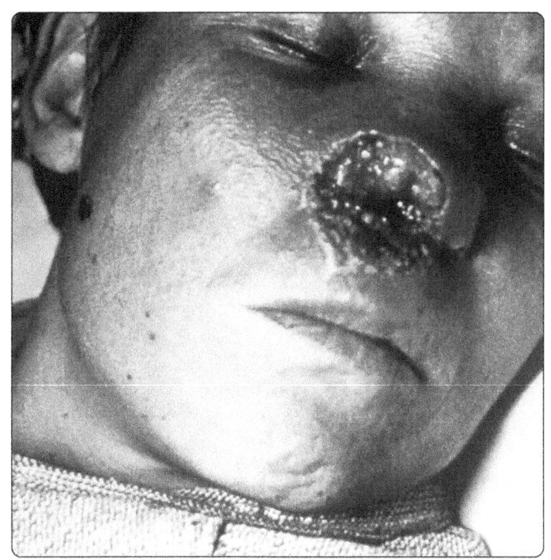

Yaws Skin Lesions

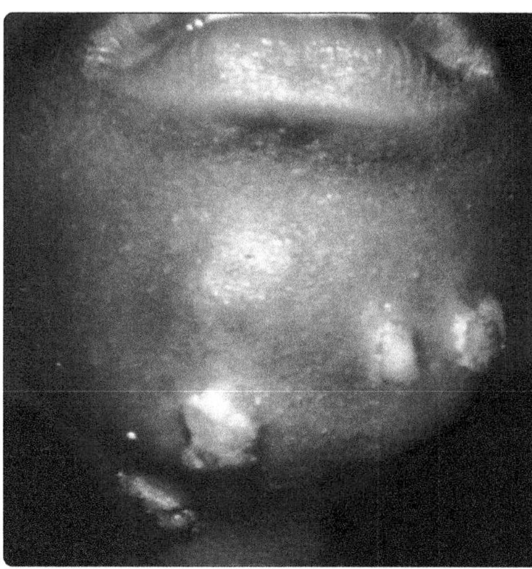

(Left) *This photograph of a patient's face shows an erosive lesion of the nose, known as a gumma, associated with tertiary syphilis. (Courtesy CDC/PHIL.)* **(Right)** *This photograph of a patient's chin shows papillomatous lesions diagnosed as yaws with a positive VDRL test (1:8) and positive/reactive microhemagglutination assay (MHA-TP) test. (Courtesy P. Perine, MD, CDC/PHIL.)*

Crab Yaws

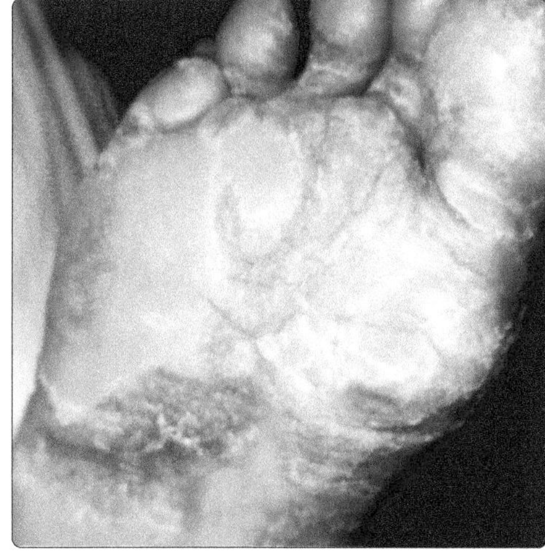

Tertiary Yaws

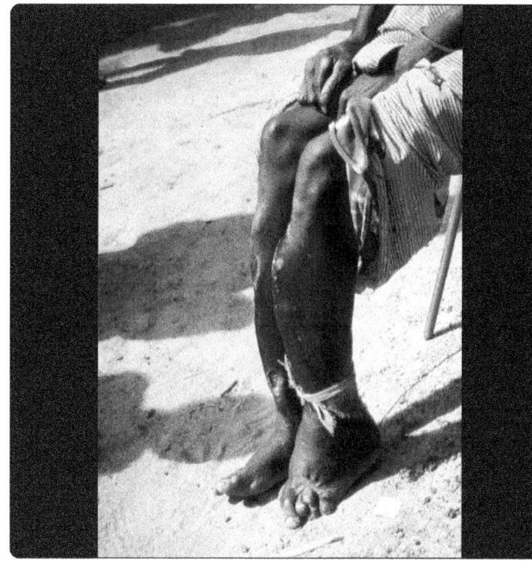

(Left) *This photograph shows tumor-like masses, which can cause individuals to walk in an odd and characteristic fashion, on the sides of a foot, leading to the nickname crab yaws. (Courtesy S. Lindsley, CDC/PHIL.)* **(Right)** *This photograph shows a tibial sabre deformity, characterized by marked anterior bowing of the lower leg, due to a late tertiary yaws infection. VDRL testing was positive (1:16) with positive/reactive microhemagglutination assay (MHA-TP) test. (Courtesy P. Perine, MD, CDC/PHIL.)*

***Treponema carateum* Dark Field Visualization**

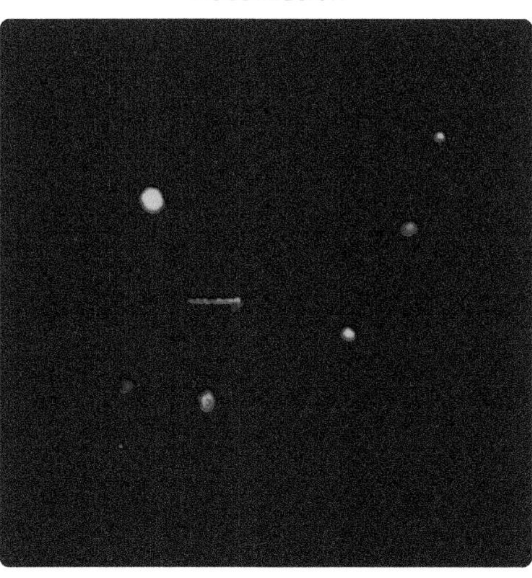

Pinta Histology

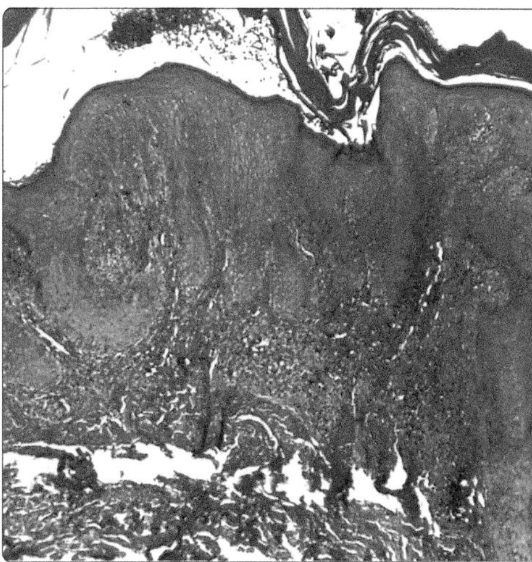

(Left) *This dark-field image shows corkscrew-shaped Treponema carateum spirochetes, which cause pinta. (Courtesy G. Keever, CDC/PHIL.)* **(Right)** *This image of a 20-month-old pinta lesion, caused by Treponema carateum, shows hyperkeratosis, parakeratosis, acanthosis, elongation of rete pegs, and a dermal inflammatory infiltrate. (Courtesy CDC/PHIL.)*

KEY FACTS

ETIOLOGY/PATHOGENESIS

- Infection with *Anaplasma phagocytophilum, Ehrlichia chaffeensis, Ehrlichia ewingii,* and *Ehrlichia muris eauclairensis,* small obligate gram-negative intracellular bacteria transmitted by tick bites, blood transfusions, and organ transplantation

CLINICAL ISSUES

- Symptoms (1-2 weeks after tick bite) include fever, headache, muscle pain, malaise, GI symptoms, cough, confusion; maculopapular petechiae rash (< 30%)
- PCR (blood): Highest sensitivity within 1 week of illness; decreased by doxycycline
- Indirect immunofluorescence assay: 4x rise in IgG between acute and convalescent stages is > 90% sensitive

MICROSCOPIC

- Morulae (intracytoplasmic microcolonies) can be seen in peripheral blood cells, but presence in particular cell type is not sufficiently specific to differentiate between spp.
- *A. phagocytophilum* and *E. ewingii* morulae most commonly identified in granulocytes; *E. chaffeensis* in monocytes; no target cell identified for *E. muris eauclairensis*
- Morulae seen in bone marrow aspirates/biopsies and in autopsy tissue sections from most organs, highlighted by IHC and ISH

TOP DIFFERENTIAL DIAGNOSES

- Other tick-borne infections/coinfections in differential
- Rocky Mountain spotted fever (*Rickettsia rickettsii*): Rash more common; confirm with PCR, IHC, serology
- Babesiosis (*Babesia* spp.): RBC infected with pear-shaped and cross forms
- Lyme (*Borrelia burgdorferi*): Erythema migrans (bull's-eye rash): Confirm with PCR, IHC, Warthin-Starry stain, serology
- Heartland virus infection: Similar symptoms to ehrlichiosis in tick-exposed patient from affected area, nonresponsive to doxycycline

(Left) *Wright stain of a peripheral blood smear shows an intramonocytic morula (Latin for mulberry) ⇒ associated with Ehrlichia chaffeensis infection. [From Biggs et al. MMWR Recomm Rep 2016;65(No. RR-2):1-44.]* **(Right)** *Giemsa-stained peripheral blood shows intragranulocytic morulae ➡, consistent with Ehrlichia ewingii or Anaplasma phagocytophilum, which require geography, serology, and PCR to distinguish. (Courtesy S. Kroft, MD.)*

Ehrlichia chaffeensis Morula in Monocyte

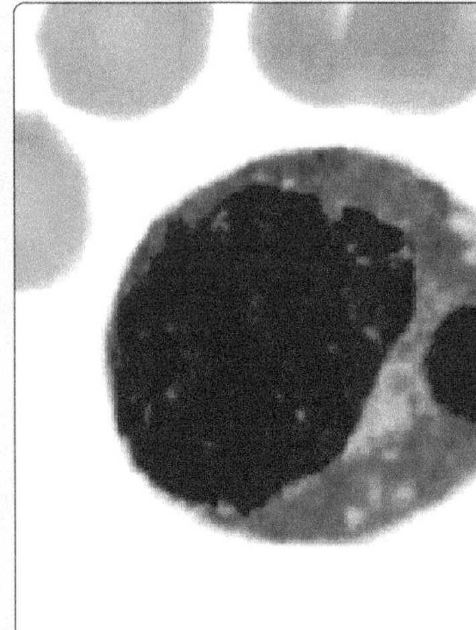

Anaplasma phagocytophilum or Ehrlichia _ewingii_ Morulae in Granulocyte

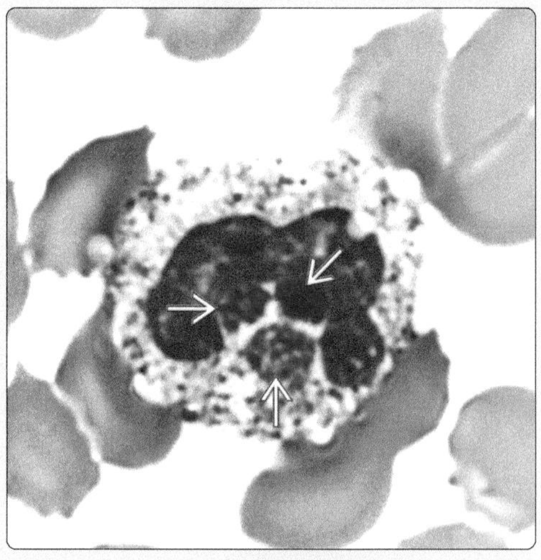

(Left) *E. chaffeensis immunohistochemistry highlights morulae (red) within monocytes in the kidney of a patient with ehrlichiosis. [From Biggs et al. MMWR Recomm Rep 2016;65(No. RR-2):1-44.]* **(Right)** *A. phagocytophilum immunohistochemistry highlights morulae (red) in the spleen of a patient with splenic rupture associated with anaplasmosis. [From Biggs et al. MMWR Recomm Rep 2016;65(No. RR-2):1-44.]*

Ehrlichia chaffeensis Immunohistochemistry

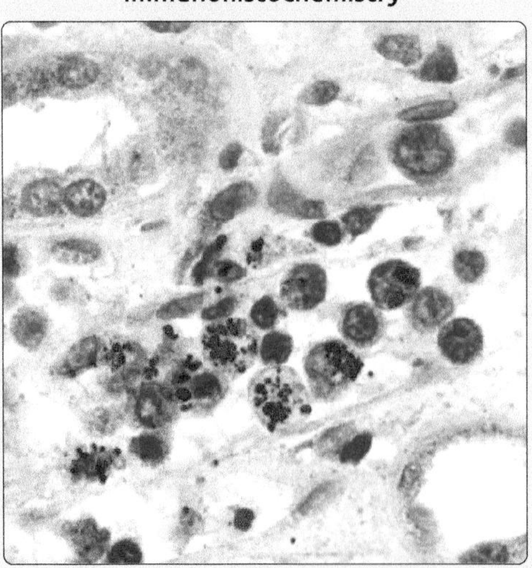

Anaplasma phagocytophilum Immunohistochemistry

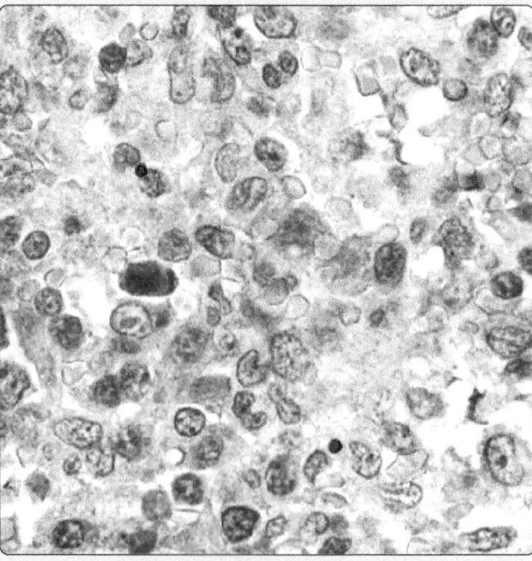

TERMINOLOGY

Definitions

- *Anaplasma phagocytophilum* derived from Greek (without plasma + loving phagocytes)
- *Ehrlichia* (after Paul Ehrlich) *chaffeensis* [after Fort Chaffee (1st patient identified)]; *ewingii* [after Sidney A. Ewing (pioneer of agent)]

ETIOLOGY/PATHOGENESIS

Infectious Agents

- Infection with *Anaplasma* spp. and *Ehrlichia* spp., small obligate gram-negative intracellular bacteria transmitted by tick bites, blood transfusions, and organ transplantation
- Organisms reside in hematopoietic or endothelial cells and multiply in cytoplasmic membrane-bound vacuoles as microcolonies called morulae
- *A. phagocytophilum* (human granulocytic anaplasmosis) transmitted by *Ixodes scapularis* in Northeast and upper Midwest and *I. pacificus* in Northern California; also reported in Central Europe and Scandinavia
- *E. chaffeensis* ehrlichiosis (human monocytic ehrlichiosis): Transmitted by *Amblyomma americanum*; endemic in Southeast, South Central, and mid-Atlantic USA; also in Mexico, Central and South America, East Asia, Europe, and central Africa
- *E. ewingii* ehrlichiosis: Transmitted by *A. americanum* in South Central and Southeast USA
- *E. muris eauclairensis* ehrlichiosis (formerly *E. muris*-like agent) transmitted by *I. scapularis* in Minnesota/Wisconsin

CLINICAL ISSUES

Epidemiology

- *A. phagocytophilum*: 1,764-5,762 cases/year reported in USA (2010-2019); 5-10% of healthy people in high-prevalence areas have serologic evidence of prior exposure
- *E. chaffeensis*: 946-2,093 cases/year reported in USA (2010-2019)
- *E. ewingii*: Total of 261 cases reported in USA (2008-2019)
- *E. muris eauclairensis:* 115 cases reported (2009-2019)
- Highest in summer months with most nymphal ticks

Presentation

- Acute symptoms 1-2 weeks after painless tick bite
- Anaplasmosis: Fever, headache, muscle pain, malaise, chills, nausea, abdominal pain, cough, confusion; maculopapular ± petechiae rash (10% of patients)
- Ehrlichiosis: Malaise, headache, chills/fever, GI symptoms, mental status changes, stiff neck, clonus; maculopapular petechial rash in 1/3 of cases (predominantly *E. chaffeensis)*

Laboratory Tests

- Mild anemia, thrombocytopenia, leukopenia, transaminitis
- PCR (blood): 60-70% sensitive for *Anaplasma* spp., and 52-87% sensitive for *Ehrlichia* spp. within 1 week of illness; decreased by doxycycline treatment
- Serology: Indirect immunofluorescence assay (IFA) on paired serum samples to demonstrate 4x rise in IgG titers in first 4 weeks (> 90% sensitive); antibody titers are frequently negative in 1st week of illness
- IgM titers can remain elevated for years and are not reliable for acute infection

Treatment

- Doxycycline is 1st-line treatment

Prognosis

- Anaplasmosis rarely fatal (< 1%); complications, including renal failure, acute respiratory distress syndrome, toxic shock-like syndrome, hemophagocytosis, rhabdomyolysis, pancreatitis, and opportunistic infections
- Ehrlichiosis rarely fatal (3%; no fatalities reported with *E. ewingii* or *E. muris eauclairensis*); complications include renal failure, acute respiratory distress syndrome, coagulopathy, myocarditis, encephalopathy
- Severity increased in immunosuppression, HIV infection

MICROBIOLOGY

Bacterial Features

- Small obligate intracellular bacteria (0.2-2.0 μm)
- Cultures require specialized systems involving human promyelocytic leukemia cells and are not routinely performed for diagnosis

MICROSCOPIC

Peripheral Blood Smear (Direct Exam Stained With Eosin-Azure-Type Dyes)

- *A. phagocytophilum* morulae (intracytoplasmic microcolonies) present most commonly in granulocytes (20-80% of patients within 1st week of illness)
- *E. chaffeensis* morulae present most commonly in monocytes (1-20% of patients)
- *E. ewingii* morulae more commonly present in granulocytes
- *E. muris eauclairensis* morulae have not yet been observed in peripheral blood cells
- Presence of morulae in particular cell type is not sufficiently specific to differentiate between *Anaplasma* and *Ehrlichia* spp.
- Ehrlichiosis may also show atypical lymphocytes with large, hyperchromatic nuclei, abundant basophilic cytoplasm, and prominent cytoplasmic granules
- Evidence of mixed infections may be identified, e.g., intraerythrocytic rings and "Maltese cross," suggestive of Babesiosis

Histopathology

- Bone marrow aspirate/biopsy: Normocellular or hypercellular marrow with rare morulae in monocytes or granulocytes
- Fatal cases of *E. chaffeensis* ehrlichiosis show systemic, multiorgan involvement; bacteria most abundant in spleen, lymph nodes, and bone marrow, less frequently in liver and lung, and occasionally in other organs; direct vasculitis and endothelial injury are rare

ANCILLARY TESTS

Immunohistochemistry/In Situ Hybridization

- Morulae may be highlighted by IHC and ISH in granulocytes or monocytes within spleen, lymph nodes, and bone marrow

DIFFERENTIAL DIAGNOSIS

Rocky Mountain Spotted Fever (*Rickettsia rickettsii*)

- Also transmitted by tick bites (*Amblyomma* and *Dermacentor* spp.)
- Rash more common (~ 90% of patients)
- Endothelial injury and vasculitis can affect any organ system; confirm with PCR, IHC

Babesiosis (*Babesia* spp.)

- Mixed infections can occur due to shared vectors (*Ixodes* spp. ticks)
- *Babesia* spp. infect RBCs with diagnostic pear-shaped and cross forms

Lyme (*Borrelia burgdorferi*)

- Mixed infections can occur due to shared vectors (*Ixodes* spp. ticks)
- Erythema migrans (bull's-eye rash) should warrant investigation for Lyme
- Lymphoplasmacytic to mixed inflammation; confirm with PCR, IHC, Warthin-Starry stain, serology

Heartland Virus Infection

- Clinical signs/symptoms similar to ehrlichiosis with tick exposure (Missouri and Tennessee)
- Patients fail to respond to doxycycline, but there is no current clinical test or therapy available

SELECTED REFERENCES

1. Dixon DM et al: Ehrlichiosis and anaplasmosis subcommittee report to the tick-borne disease working group. Ticks Tick Borne Dis. 12(6):101823, 2021
2. Biggs HM et al: Diagnosis and management of tickborne rickettsial diseases: Rocky Mountain spotted fever and other spotted fever group Rickettsioses, Ehrlichioses, and Anaplasmosis - United States. MMWR Recomm Rep. 65(2):1-44, 2016
3. Allen MB et al: First reported case of Ehrlichia ewingii involving human bone marrow. J Clin Microbiol. 52(11):4102-4, 2014
4. Rand JV et al: Intracytoplasmic granulocytic morulae counts on confirmed cases of ehrlichiosis/anaplasmosis in the Northeast. Am J Clin Pathol. 141(5):683-6, 2014
5. Hamilton KS et al: Characteristic peripheral blood findings in human ehrlichiosis. Mod Pathol. 17(5):512-7, 2004
6. Dawson JE et al: Tissue diagnosis of Ehrlichia chaffeensis in patients with fatal ehrlichiosis by use of immunohistochemistry, in situ hybridization, and polymerase chain reaction. Am J Trop Med Hyg. 65(5):603-9, 2001

Epidemiology: Ehrlichia *chaffeensis*

0 ●0 to < 0.31 ●0.31 to < 3.69 ●3.69 to < 11.07 ●11.07+ Not Notifiable

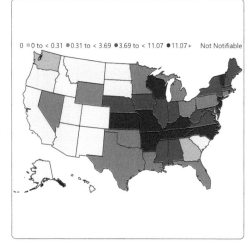

Epidemiology: *Anaplasma phagocytophilum*

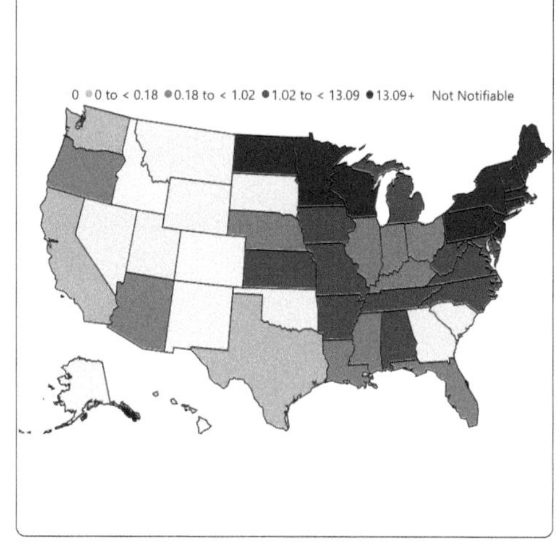

(Left) *Incidence of E. chaffeensis ehrlichiosis by state in 2019 per 1 million persons is illustrated. E. chaffeensis is spread by Amblyomma americanum ticks. (Courtesy CDC.)* **(Right)** *Incidence of anaplasmosis by state in 2019 per 1 million persons is illustrated. A. phagocytophilum is spread by Ixodes scapularis and Ixodes pacificus in the eastern and western parts of the USA, respectively. (Courtesy CDC.)*

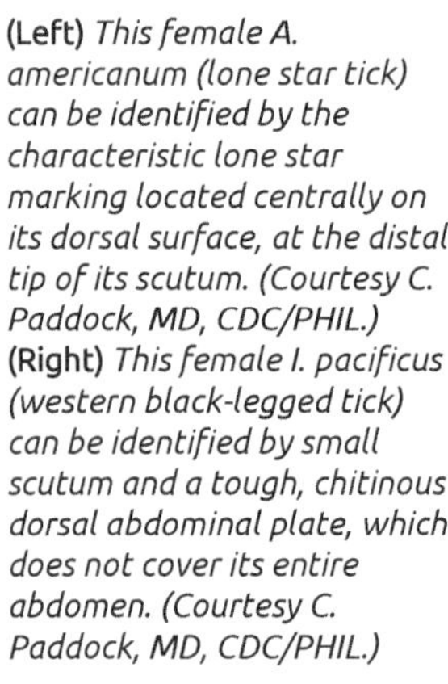

(Left) *This female A. americanum (lone star tick) can be identified by the characteristic lone star marking located centrally on its dorsal surface, at the distal tip of its scutum. (Courtesy C. Paddock, MD, CDC/PHIL.)* **(Right)** *This female I. pacificus (western black-legged tick) can be identified by small scutum and a tough, chitinous dorsal abdominal plate, which does not cover its entire abdomen. (Courtesy C. Paddock, MD, CDC/PHIL.)*

***Amblyomma americanum* (Lone Star Tick)**

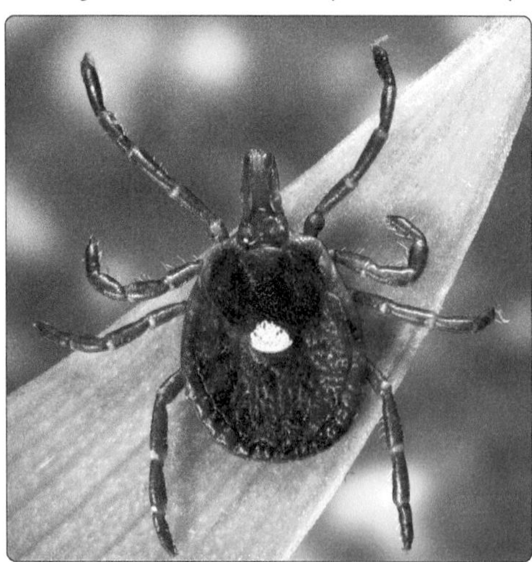

***Ixodes pacificus* (Western Black-Legged Tick)**

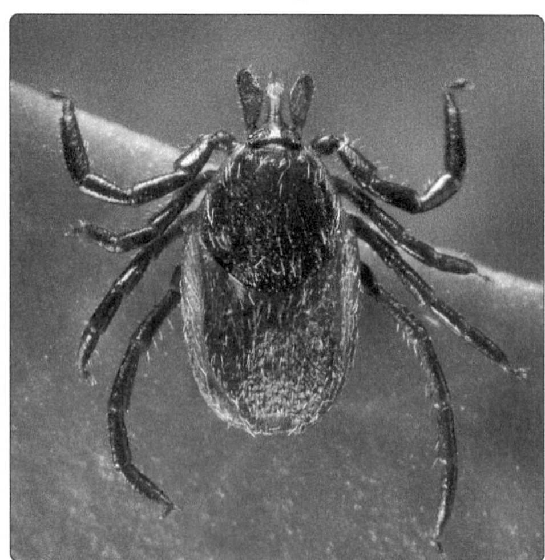

Intracellular *Anaplasma* Bacteria

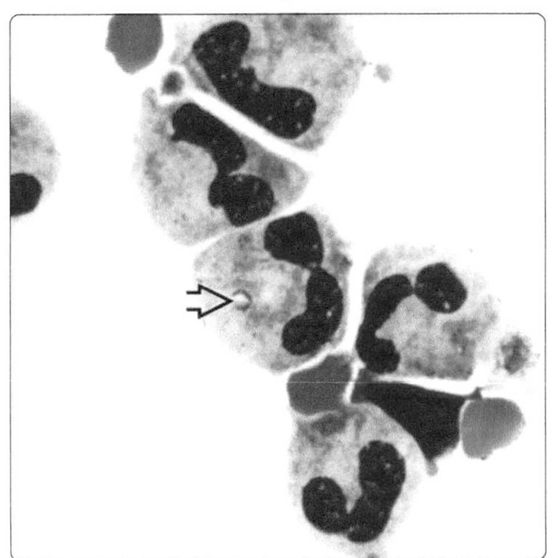

***Anaplasma* Bacteria vs. Toxic Granulations**

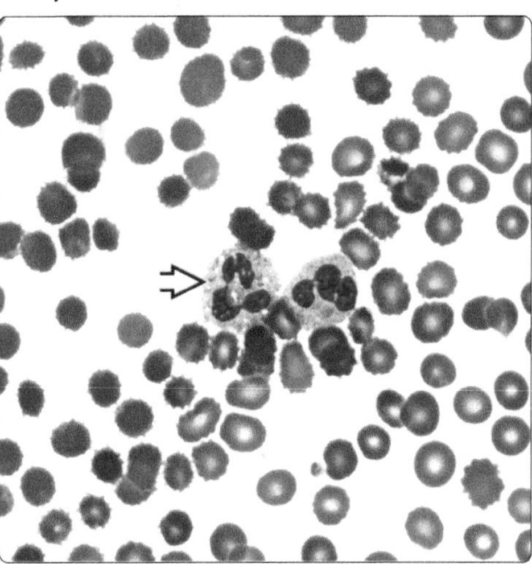

(Left) *A smaller inclusion consistent with the intracellular bacteria, Anaplasma, is shown ⇨. Note the hyposegmented and band-form neutrophils without toxic granulations. (Courtesy T. Wieczorek, MD, PhD.)* **(Right)** *Inclusions ⇨ consistent with the intracellular bacteria, Anaplasma, are shown. Note the 3- to 4-lobed neutrophils and toxic granulations. Large numbers of toxic granulations (as in sepsis) may be confused with the bacteria. (Courtesy T. Wieczorek, MD, PhD.)*

***Ehrlichia* Inclusion**

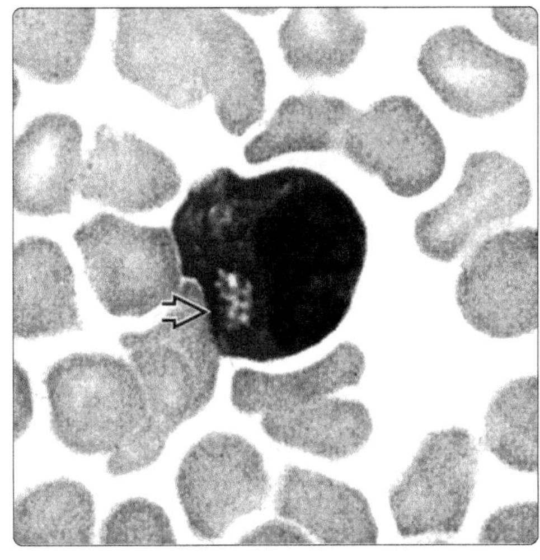

***Anaplasma* Inclusions**

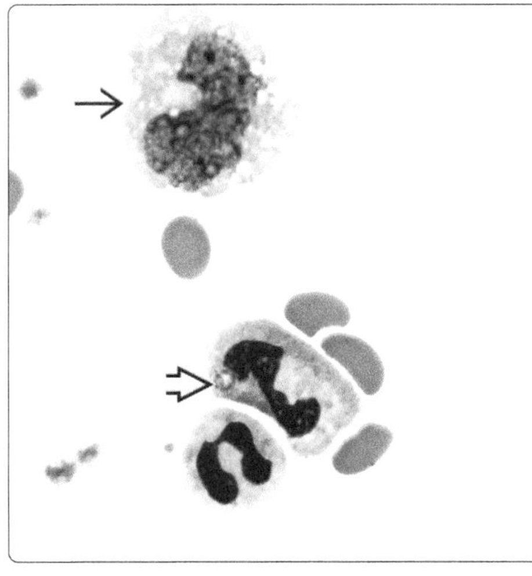

(Left) *A large inclusion ⇨ consistent with the intracellular bacteria, Ehrlichia, is shown. Note the monocyte containing the organism, which is typical of human monocytic ehrlichiosis.* **(Right)** *An inclusion ⇨ consistent with Anaplasma is shown. Note the hyposegmented neutrophils and lack of toxic granulations. A monocyte → is shown for comparison. Although mixed infections with other agents are common, Anaplasma and Ehrlichia do not commonly coexist. (Courtesy T. Wieczorek, MD, PhD.)*

***Anaplasma* Inclusions**

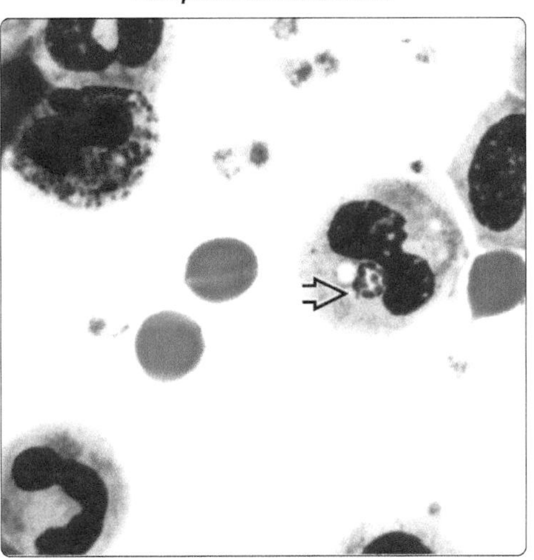

***Anaplasma* Inclusion vs. Platelets**

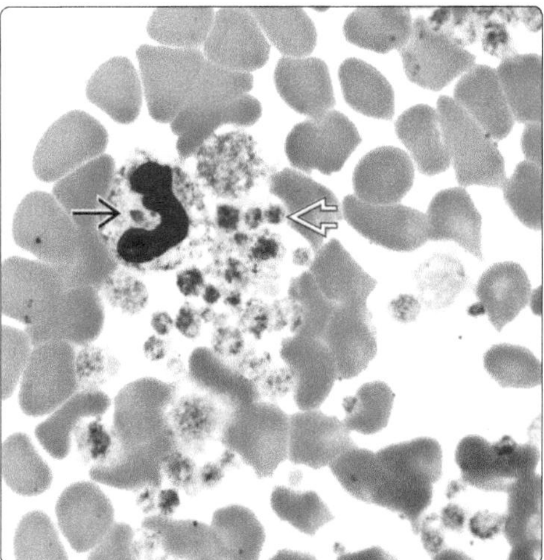

(Left) *A large inclusion ⇨ consistent with intracellular bacteria, Anaplasma, is shown in the cytoplasm of this neutrophil. (Courtesy T. Wieczorek, MD, PhD.)* **(Right)** *An inclusion → consistent with Anaplasma is shown. Note hyposegmented neutrophil with toxic granulations. Large aggregates of giant platelets ⇦ can be seen, and overlapping platelets on leukocytes can be confusing. (Courtesy T. Wieczorek, MD, PhD.)*

KEY FACTS

ETIOLOGY/PATHOGENESIS

- Infection with *Chlamydiaceae*, obligate intracellular organisms with biphasic lifestyle (elementary and reticulate bodies)

CLINICAL ISSUES

- *Chlamydia trachomatis*: Trachoma, genital infections, conjunctivitis, lymphogranuloma venereum, proctocolitis
- *Chlamydia pneumoniae*: Common cause of atypical pneumonia
- *Chlamydia psittaci*: Multiple presentations (e.g., fever, pharyngitis, hepatosplenomegaly, adenopathy) with wide range in severity
- Nucleic acid amplification tests (NAATs) are preferred method for detection in clinical specimens

MICROSCOPIC

- General: Organisms observable in intracellular vacuoles (optimally visualized with silver stains and IHC)
- Trachoma: Chronic follicular conjunctivitis with papillary hypertrophy; intracellular (bacterial) inclusions on Giemsa-stained conjunctiva smears
- Genital disease: Endometritis, salpingitis, and tuboovarian abscess; epididymitis
- Lymphogranuloma venereum (LGV): Cutaneous lesions and proctitis demonstrate chronic inflammation; lymph nodes with suppurative inflammation and necrosis, "stellate abscess"

TOP DIFFERENTIAL DIAGNOSES

- Bacteria conjunctivitis (e.g., *Staphylococcus aureus*, *Streptococcus pneumoniae*, and *Haemophilus influenzae*); differentiate by special stains, IHC, positive culture, PCR
- Viral conjunctivitis (e.g., adenoviruses): Negative bacterial culture, concurrent upper respiratory infection
- Chancroid (*Haemophilus ducreyi*): Larger, more painful ulcers

(Left) *Chlamydia trachomatis in tissue culture is shown with elementary bodies →. Standard microbiology culture techniques do not detect Chlamydia organisms. Confirmatory diagnosis is made with PCR or serology.* **(Right)** *C. trachomatis infection in tissue culture demonstrates reticulate bodies →. Reticulate bodies indicate replication of the bacteria, while elementary bodies are infectious and transmit disease.*

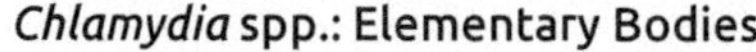

Chlamydia spp.: Elementary Bodies

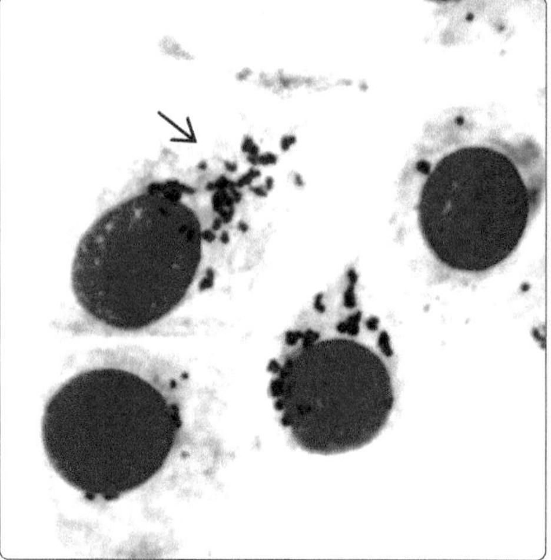

Chlamydia spp.: Reticulate Bodies

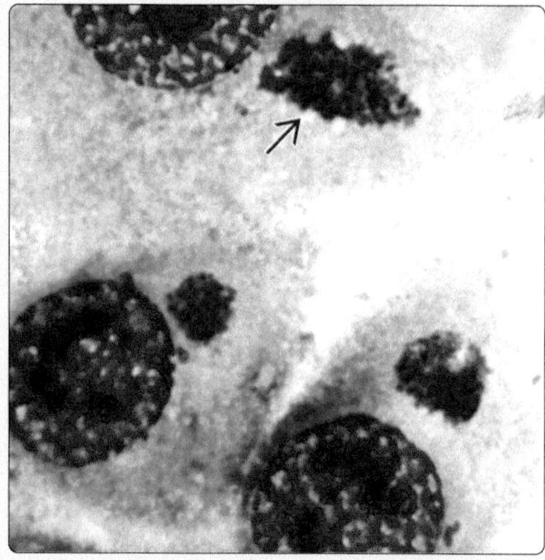

(Left) *The histologic signature of early stage lymphogranuloma venereum (LGV) is a "stellate abscess" or granuloma →. In later stages, histologic findings are nonspecific, and granulomas are rare.* **(Right)** *Image shows sheets of necrotic debris and mixed inflammation from a lesion in LGV. The histologic findings are not specific. Knowledge of the clinical scenario (and cultures) is key to the diagnosis.*

Lymphogranuloma Venereum: "Stellate Abscess"

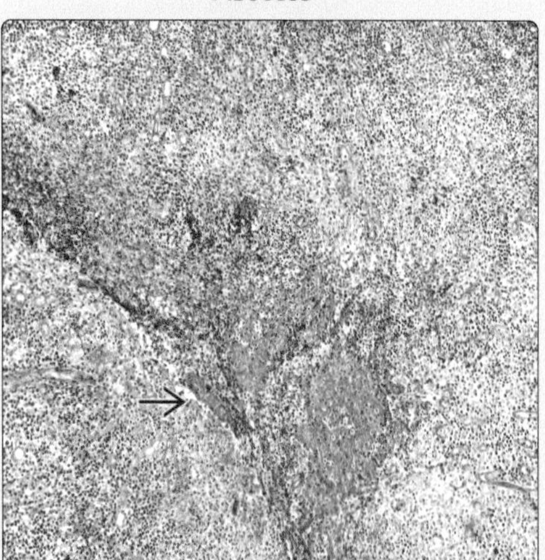

Lymphogranuloma Venereum: Necrosis

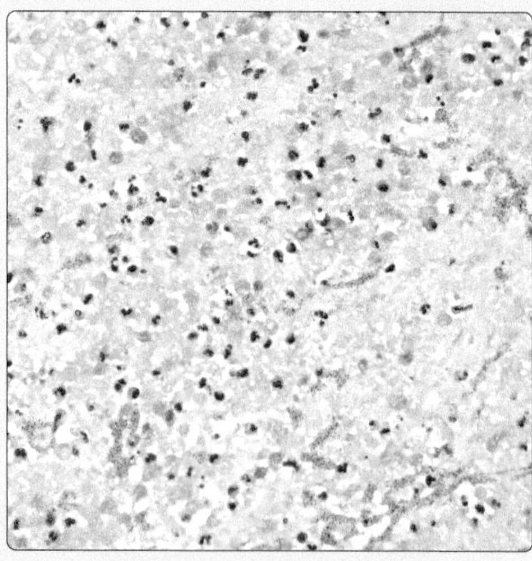

TERMINOLOGY

Synonyms

- Trachoma
- Lymphogranuloma venereum (LGV)
- Psittacosis, parrot fever

Definitions

- Greek: "Chlamys/khlamus" (cloak)

ETIOLOGY/PATHOGENESIS

Infectious Agents

- Infection with *Chlamydiaceae* (*Chlamydia* spp. and *Chlamydophila* spp.), ancient group of obligate intracellular organisms with tiny genomes; pleomorphic organisms with basic components of gram-negative envelope, though they do not express peptidoglycan
- In 1999, molecular analysis reassigned *Chlamydia* species into 2 groups, *Chlamydia* (including *C. trachomatis*) and *Chlamydophila* (including *C. pneumoniae* and *C. psittaci*); more recent data suggest these organisms should be reunited, and controversy has not been settled
- All species share biphasic lifestyle with 2 different developmental forms
  - Elementary bodies (EB) are metabolically slowed down, spore-like forms that are specialized for environmental survival and host cell attachment
  - Upon uptake (clathrin-mediated endocytosis) by epithelial cell, EBs differentiate into reticulate bodies (RB) within host cell vacuoles
  - RBs are germinal forms, which actively divide 8-10x before differentiating back into EBs, which exit cell by slow extrusion or cell lysis and reinfect new cells
- *C. trachomatis* divided into 15 serovars [based on OmpA (MOMP) antigenicity]
  - Group 1 causes trachoma, genital tract disease, and conjunctivitis (trachoma biovar)
    - Serovars Ab, B, Ba, and C are causes of trachoma leading to blindness
    - Serovars D, E, F, G, H, I, J, and K have been reported in diseases of genitourinary tract [urethritis, pelvic inflammatory disease (PID)] and complications of pregnancy (ectopic pregnancy, conjunctivitis &/or pneumonia in neonates)
    - Bind to squamocolumnar cells or conjunctiva, urethra, and rectum in women and men, endocervix and upper genital tract in women, and respiratory tract in infants
  - Group 2 causes LGV and proctocolitis (LGV biovar)
    - Serovars L1, L2, and L3 are responsible for LGV; not all serologic tests for LGV cover all 3 serovars
    - Invade beyond mucosal epithelium and enter lymphatics, where they multiply inside monocytes and macrophages
  - Plasticity zone encodes perforin and phospholipase D proteins; contact with host cells induces IL-8 and neutrophilic response
  - Spread is by sexual contact, childbirth, or hand-to-eye contact (trachoma); exclusively infects humans
- *C. pneumoniae*
  - Virulence factors poorly characterized
  - Transmission poorly described; evidence for person-to-person spread as well as zoonoses (infects horses, marsupials, and frogs)
- *C. psittaci*
  - Pathogenesis is less well characterized, but genomic analysis of plasticity zone indicates that toxin gene may be partially responsible for more virulent strains
  - Developed as agent of biological warfare by both USA and former Soviet Union in early 20th century
  - Spread is by contact with birds (even casual) or other domestic animals (infects numerous mammalian species)

CLINICAL ISSUES

Epidemiology

- Trachoma: Most common among young children in developing countries
- Genital infection: Most common in young, sexually active men and women (most common bacterial sexually transmitted disease)
  - LGV is most common in developing countries, though epidemiology has begun to change with increasing prevalence in western Europe and USA, particularly among men who have sex with men
- *C. pneumoniae* has been demonstrated by serology to have infected sizable percentages of adult populations in several countries (e.g., 9% of 6 week to 19 year olds in USA)

Presentation

- *C. trachomatis*
  - Trachoma
    - Chronic keratoconjunctivitis
    - Sequelae from scarring can cause trichiasis with ulceration, scarring, and eventual blindness
  - Genital infection in male patients
    - Major cause of nongonococcal urethritis: Whitish/clear discharge, may be scant; 1% develop reactive arthritis
    - Epididymitis, prostatitis, and proctitis
  - Genital infection in women
    - Often asymptomatic, sometimes mucopurulent cervicitis/urethritis
    - Endometritis/salpingitis/peritonitis (PID)
    - Sequelae can include infertility and ectopic pregnancy
  - LGV (3 stages)
    - Formation of small genital papule
    - Adenitis (buboes) and development of systemic symptoms (fever, headache, myalgia) and lymphadenopathy (may be severe)
    - Chronic disease that can include fistulas, fibrosis, scarring, and elephantiasis of genitalia due to lymphatic obstruction
    - Alternatively, may present as severe proctitis, generally in men who have sex with men
- *C. pneumoniae*
  - Typically mild respiratory infections
  - Common cause of atypical pneumonia
- *C. psittaci*
  - Several described presentations with wide range in severity (subclinical to rapidly fatal)
    - Subclinical or mild, nonspecific, viral-like symptoms
    - Fever, pharyngitis, hepatosplenomegaly, adenopathy
    - Fever, bradycardia, malaise, and splenomegaly

- Atypical pneumonia (more severe than that caused by *C. pneumoniae*)
- Common symptoms and signs are diverse and wide ranging
  - Fever, headache, myalgias, reactive arthritis
  - Pharyngeal erythema, cough, rales
  - Peri-/myocarditis, endocarditis
  - Hepatomegaly, hepatitis, jaundice
  - Hemolytic anemia, disseminated intravascular coagulation (DIC)
  - Glomerulonephritis, acute tubulointerstitial nephritis, and acute tubular necrosis
  - Multiple neurologic and dermatologic manifestations (e.g., Horder spots)
- Gestational psittacosis
  - Severe, progressive febrile illness
  - Headache, DIC, hepatitis, renal failure
  - Significant fetomaternal morbidity and mortality

Laboratory Tests

- Nucleic acid amplification tests (NAATs) are preferred method for detecting *Chlamydia* in clinical specimens
- 16S rRNA PCR may also be used
- As intracellular pathogen, *Chlamydia* species has to be cultured in cells, which is rarely done for diagnostic purposes
- Serologies may be used to diagnose some types of chlamydial disease (e.g., *C. psittaci* infection)

Treatment

- Macrolides, tetracycline, and quinolones are mainstays of treatment

Prognosis

- Mortality is generally low (up to 1% with treated *C. psittaci* infection, 20% untreated), though several manifestations have significant long-term morbidity

MICROBIOLOGY

Culture

- Obligate intracellular pathogens and must be cultured within eukaryotic cells, which is not routinely done in most clinical laboratories

MACROSCOPIC

Trachoma

- Initial infection may present with "pink eye" or mild irritation
- Lymphoid hyperplasia may produce large, white nodules on mucosa surface of eyelid in early stages
- Advanced stages (repeated infection) lead to scarring with eyelash inversion and corneal ulceration (blindness)

MICROSCOPIC

Histologic Features

- Trachoma: Chronic follicular conjunctivitis with papillary hypertrophy
- Genital disease: Urethritis and cervicitis specimens rarely sent for surgical pathology
  - Upper genital tract infection in women may demonstrate endometritis, salpingitis, and tuboovarian abscess
  - Epididymitis in men is usually characterized by suppurative inflammation with fibrin covering
- LGV
  - Cutaneous lesions and proctitis demonstrate chronic inflammation, giant cells, plasma cells, lymphocytes, necrosis, and granulation tissue
    - Granulomas with epithelioid histiocytes
    - Fibrosis and scarring with chronicity
  - Lymph nodes with suppurative inflammation and necrosis followed by plasma cell infiltration and lymphocytic hyperplasia
    - Histologic hallmark is "stellate abscess"
    - Suppurative lesions surrounded by epithelioid and multinucleated giant cells
- Psittacosis: Histopathologic features are not well described; may include myocarditis
- Pneumonia: Standard features of atypical bacterial pneumonia

Cytologic Features

- Trachoma: Giemsa-stained smear from conjunctiva should demonstrate large intracellular (bacterial) inclusions in cytoplasm of histiocytes

ANCILLARY TESTS

Special Stains and Immunohistochemistry

- Organisms may be observable in intracellular vacuoles
- Silver staining and IHC are optimal means to visualization (especially in genital disease)

DIFFERENTIAL DIAGNOSIS

Bacterial Conjunctivitis

- Cause by numerous organisms (e.g., *Staphylococcus aureus*, *Streptococcus pneumoniae*, and *Haemophilus influenzae*); differentiate by special stains, IHC, positive culture, PCR

Viral Conjunctivitis

- Most commonly due to adenoviruses; negative bacterial culture, concurrent upper respiratory infection

Chancroid

- *Haemophilus ducreyi*; larger, more painful ulcers

SELECTED REFERENCES

1. Stelzner K et al: Intracellular lifestyle of Chlamydia trachomatis and host-pathogen interactions. Nat Rev Microbiol. 21(7):448-62, 2023
2. Wolff BJ et al: Multiplex real-time PCR assay for the detection of all Chlamydia species and simultaneous differentiation of C. psittaci and C. pneumoniae in human clinical specimens. Ann Lab Med. 43(4):375-80, 2023
3. de Vries HJC et al: Call for consensus in Chlamydia trachomatis nomenclature: moving from biovars, serovars, and serotypes to genovariants and genotypes. Clin Microbiol Infect. 28(6):761-3, 2022
4. Solomon AW et al: Trachoma. Nat Rev Dis Primers. 8(1):32, 2022
5. Paul L et al: Gestational psittacosis resulting in neonatal death identified by next-generation RNA sequencing of postmortem, formalin-fixed lung tissue. Open Forum Infect Dis. 5(8):ofy172, 2018
6. Elwell C et al: Chlamydia cell biology and pathogenesis. Nat Rev Microbiol. 14(6):385-400, 2016

Early Trachoma

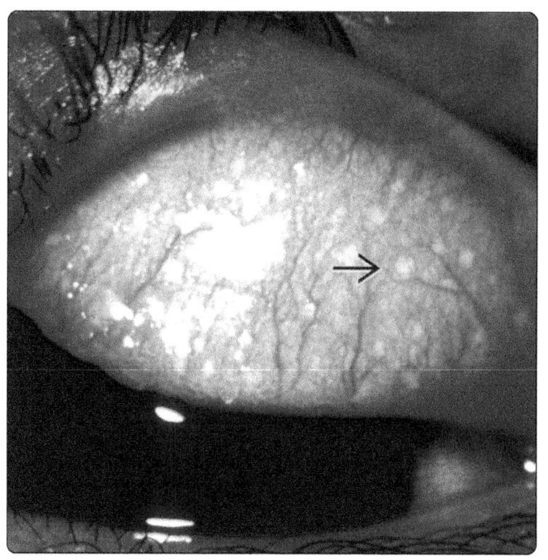

Advanced Trachoma

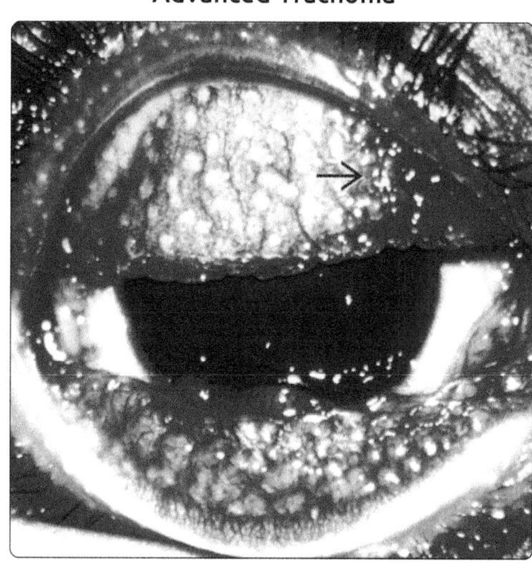

(Left) *This patient has stage I trachoma demonstrating multiple small lymphoid follicles ⇒. At this stage, the eye may only appear slightly red and swollen ± discharge. (Courtesy D. M. Albert, MD.)* **(Right)** *This patient has trachoma stage IIa, demonstrating advanced follicular inflammation ⇒ with a grossly swollen, red eye. As the disease advances, scarring and increased inflammation lead to corneal ulcers. (Courtesy D. M. Albert, MD.)*

Trachoma: Inflammation

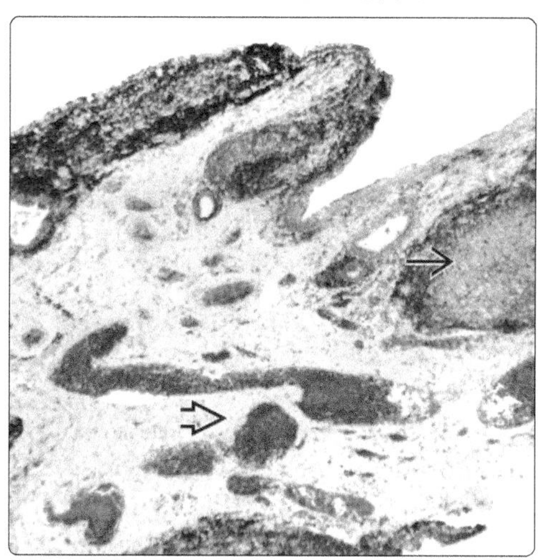

Trachoma: Fibrosis

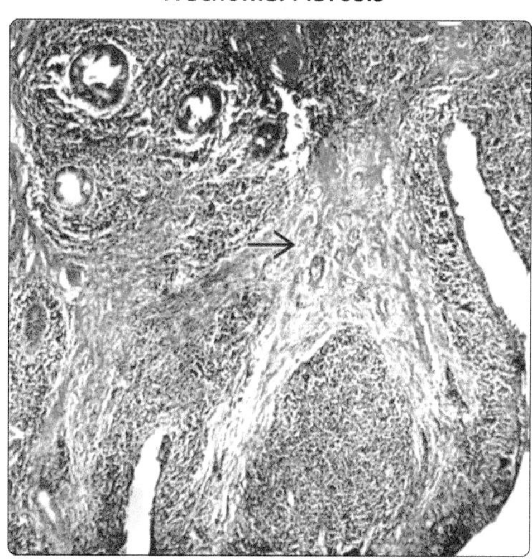

(Left) *Conjunctiva in a patient with trachoma demonstrates follicular inflammation ⇒ and neovascularization ⇒.* **(Right)** *In later stages of trachoma, increased fibrosis ⇒ and scarring is seen in the cicatricial stages. Scarring disrupts eye lashes with inversion, which aggravates corneal ulcerations. (Courtesy Franz von Lichtenberg Infectious Disease Collection, BWH.)*

End-Stage Trachoma

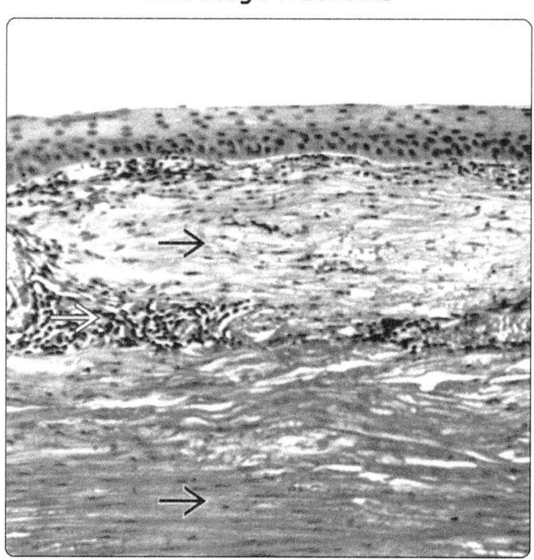

Life Cycle of *Chlamydia* spp.

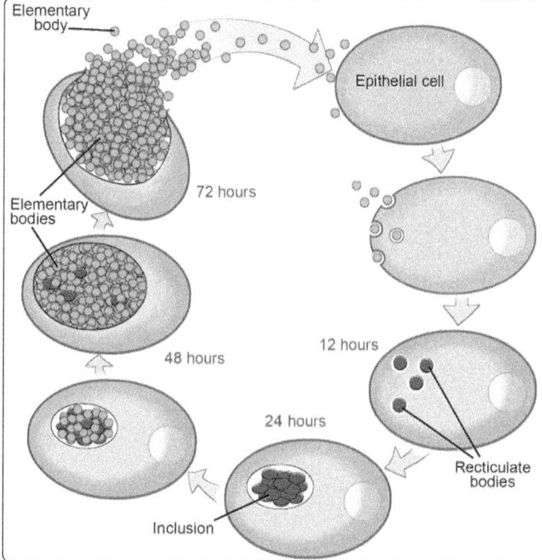

(Left) *In end-stage trachoma, there is dense fibrosis ⇒ and reduced inflammation ➡.* **(Right)** *Illustration shows the life cycle of Chlamydia spp., including the intracellular, noninfectious form (reticulate bodies) and the extracellular, infectious form (elementary bodies). (Courtesy CDC.)*

Coxiella Species Infection

KEY FACTS

ETIOLOGY/PATHOGENESIS

- Zoonotic infection (Q fever) with *Coxiella burnetii*, Gram-negative intracellular bacteria, spread primarily through inhalation of aerosols

CLINICAL ISSUES

- Acute Q fever: Febrile syndrome/flu-like illness, pneumonia, hepatitis, cardiac and neurologic manifestations
- Persistent infection: Endocarditis, vascular involvement, liver involvement, osteoarticular infection
- Pregnancy: May result in miscarriage, fetal death, malformations, growth retardation, or premature delivery
- Serology is mainstay of diagnosis; PCR from blood or tissue

MICROSCOPIC

- Endocarditis: Fibrosis and calcifications, limited inflammation, small or absent vegetations; bacteria present as coarse granular material within macrophages
- Liver: Mononuclear inflammation, fibrin ring granulomas, Kupffer cells, fatty change, eosinophilia, cirrhosis
- Pulmonary: Interstitial edema, mixed inflammation, intraalveolar histiocytes and focal necrosis, hemorrhage
- Skeletal: Osteomyelitis (often multifocal), spondylodiscitis, prosthetic joint infection

TOP DIFFERENTIAL DIAGNOSES

- Whipple disease: Culture-negative endocarditis with foamy macrophages filled with PAS-positive, acid fast-negative bacilli; confirm with PCR, IHC/ISH
- *Bartonella* spp. infection: Culture-negative endocarditis associated with gram-negative coccobacilli highlighted by Warthin-Starry stain; confirm with IHC, PCR, serology
- Other causes of fibrin-ring granuloma: CMV, EBV, allopurinol toxicity, leishmaniasis, boutonneuse fever, salmonella, and toxoplasmosis

Fibrin Ring Granuloma

Q Fever Endocarditis

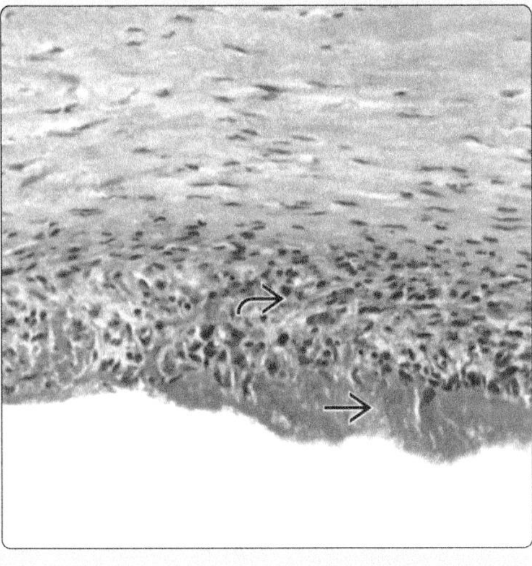

(Left) *Fibrin ring granuloma from a patient with Q fever is characterized by a central fat vacuole surrounded by macrophages and a thin network of fibrin. Other etiologies include CMV, EBV, Hodgkin lymphoma, drug (ipilimumab), and lupus. (Courtesy M. Drage, MD, PhD.)* **(Right)** *Mitral valve from a patient with Q fever endocarditis shows a small vegetation on the valve and a mononuclear inflammatory cell infiltrate. [J Infect Dis. 187(7):1097-106, 2003.]*

***Coxiella burnetii* Ultrastructural Features**

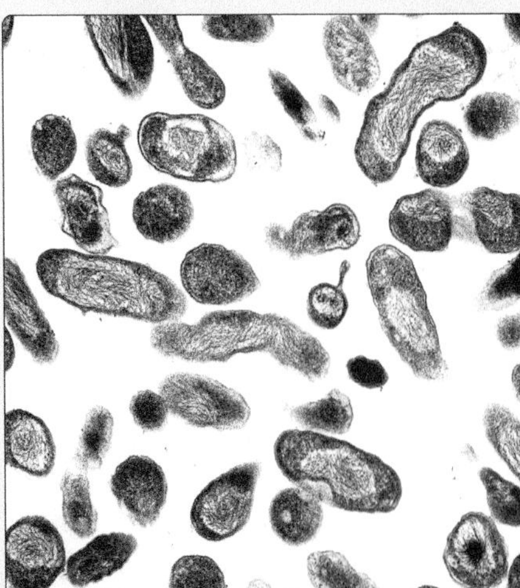

Gram-Negative *Coxiella* Species

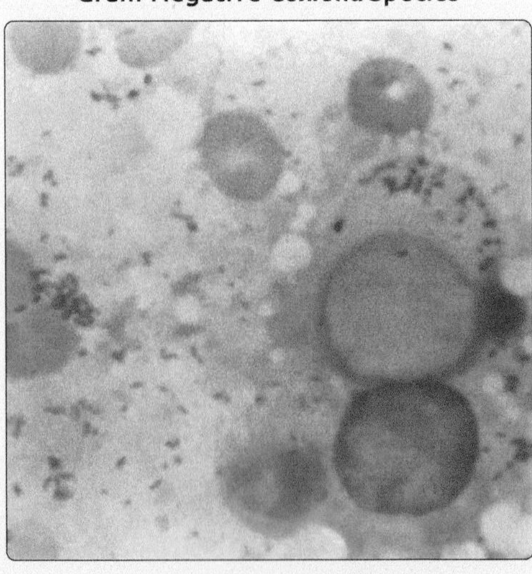

(Left) *Transmission electron micrograph shows multiple bacilli of Coxiella burnetii bacilli, gram-negative intracellular bacteria that cause Q fever. (Courtesy National Institute of Allergy and Infectious Diseases, Rocky Mountain Laboratories, CDC/PHIL.)* **(Right)** *Photomicrograph of an unknown tissue sample shows numerous gram-negative C. burnetii, the pathogen responsible for causing Q fever. (Courtesy CDC/PHIL.)*

TERMINOLOGY

Definitions

- Q fever; so-called "Query fever" in 1935, when syndrome was suspected to be new disease
- *Coxiella burnetii* after Herald Rea Cox (American bacteriologist) and McFarlane Burnet (Australian virologist)

ETIOLOGY/PATHOGENESIS

Infectious Agents

- Zoonotic infection with *Coxiella burnetii*, gram-negative intracellular bacteria, spread via inhalation of aerosols as well as through tick bites, ingestion of unpasteurized dairy products, blood transfusion, transplacentally, or sexual contact
- Associated with exposure to sheep, goats, and cattle; highest concentration of organism in birth products but also present in urine, feces, and milk
- Classified as potential agent of bioterrorism due to combination of virulence with environmental stability

CLINICAL ISSUES

Epidemiology

- Worldwide distribution; seroprevalence up to 30% in Africa
- Pooled estimate of seroprevalence is > 20% among slaughterhouse workers and veterinarians
- USA: 109-179 cases/year of acute and 23-40 cases/year of chronic Q fever (2010-2019); ~ 24% of soil samples PCR positive for *C. burnetii*

Presentation

- Acute Q fever (50% of infections; 2-3 week incubation): Febrile syndrome/flu-like illness, pneumonia, hepatitis; cardiac and neurologic manifestations rare
- Persistent infection (< 5%; weeks to years after acute infection) causes ~ 10% of culture-negative endocarditis; vascular involvement with aortoduodenal fistula, spondylodiscitis with psoas abscess, graft or aneurysm rupture; osteoarticular infections and lymphadenitis rare
- In utero infection may result in miscarriage, fetal death, malformations, growth restriction, premature delivery

Laboratory Tests

- PCR detection from blood/serum, fresh or FFPE tissue
- Serology is mainstay of diagnosis
  - Acute infection: Phase II antibodies directed against common protein antigens are present 7-15 days after symptom onset and decrease after 3-6 months; > 200 IgG or 4x rise over 3-6-weeks or > 50 IgM
  - Persistent infection: Phase I antibodies directed against full-length LPS; > 800 IgG
- Cultures: Not cultured on clinical media; require biosafety level 3 containment

Treatment

- Depends on manifestation, i.e., tetracycline for pneumonia, doxycycline with ciprofloxacin, or rifampin for endocarditis

Prognosis

- Endocarditis: 5-9% mortality
- Vascular involvement: 18-26% mortality

MICROSCOPIC

Histologic Features

- Endocarditis: Extensive fibrosis and calcifications, limited lymphohistiocytic inflammation, vascularization, small or absent vegetations, absence of microabscesses or granulomata; bacteria present as coarse granular material within macrophages
- Liver: Mononuclear cell infiltration of portal tracts, granulomas (fibrin ring or "doughnut"), prominent sinusoidal Kupffer cells, fatty change, sinusoidal wall eosinophilia, cirrhosis
- Pulmonary: Interstitial edema, mixed inflammatory infiltrate, intraalveolar histiocytes and focal necrosis, hemorrhage; microorganisms rarely apparent
- Skeletal: Osteomyelitis (often multifocal), spondylodiscitis, prosthetic joint infection

ANCILLARY TESTS

Histochemistry

- Gimenez stain to detect organisms; does not stain with Gram

Immunohistochemistry

- Antibodies for detection of *C. burnetii* are available though not widely used clinically

DIFFERENTIAL DIAGNOSIS

Whipple Disease (*Tropheryma whipplei*)

- Culture-negative endocarditis associated with abundant foamy macrophages filled with PAS-positive, acid fast-negative bacilli; confirm with PCR, IHC/ISH

Bartonella spp. Infection

- Culture-negative endocarditis associated with gram-negative coccobacilli highlighted by Warthin-Starry stains; confirm with IHC, PCR, serology

Other Causes of Fibrin-Ring Granulomas

- CMV, EBV, allopurinol toxicity, leishmaniasis, boutonneuse fever, salmonella, and toxoplasmosis

SELECTED REFERENCES

1. Cherry CC et al: Acute and chronic Q fever national surveillance - United States, 2008-2017. Zoonoses Public Health. 69(2):73-82, 2022
2. Yessinou RE et al: Prevalence of Coxiella-infections in ticks - review and meta-analysis. Ticks Tick Borne Dis. 13(3):101926, 2022
3. de Lange MMA et al: High Coxiella burnetii seroconversion rate in veterinary students, the Netherlands, 2006-2010. Emerg Infect Dis. 26(12):3086-8, 2020
4. Sahu R et al: Current approaches for the detection of Coxiella burnetii infection in humans and animals. J Microbiol Methods. 179:106087, 2020
5. Faucon AL et al: Coxiella burnetii endocarditis on bioprosthetic aortic valve, with peripheral arterial embolism. Cardiovasc Pathol. 34:38-9, 2018
6. Meriglier E et al: Osteoarticular manifestations of Q fever: a case series and literature review. Clin Microbiol Infect. 24(8):912-3, 2018
7. Miller HK et al: Trends in Q fever serologic testing by immunofluorescence from four large reference laboratories in the United States, 2012-2016. Sci Rep. 8(1):16670, 2018
8. Woldeyohannes SM et al: Seroprevlance of Coxiella burnetii among abattoir and slaughterhouse workers: A meta-analysis. One Health. 6:23-8, 2018
9. Jang YR et al: Molecular detection of Coxiella burnetii from the formalin-fixed tissues of Q fever patients with acute hepatitis. PLoS One. 12(7):e0180237, 2017
10. Million M et al: Antiphospholipid antibody syndrome with valvular vegetations in acute Q fever. Clin Infect Dis. 62(5):537-44, 2016

Rickettsia and *Orientia* Species Infections

KEY FACTS

ETIOLOGY/PATHOGENESIS

- Infection with obligate intracellular gram-negative bacteria in *Rickettsiaceae* family, spread via arthropod bites
- Spotted fever group includes *Rickettsia rickettsii* (Rocky Mountain spotted fever), transmitted by ticks
- Typus group includes louse-borne *R. prowazekii* (epidemic typhus) and flea-borne *R. typhi* (Murine typhus)
- Scrub typus group consists of *Orientia tsutsugamushi* transmitted by mites/chiggers

CLINICAL ISSUES

- Diagnosis is mainly clinical &/or serologic
- RMSF: 7-day incubation followed by fever, myalgias, gastrointestinal distress, and headache; characteristic petechial maculopapular rash (90% of patients)
- PCR can be done on primary specimens (targets: 17-kDa lipoprotein, OmpA, etc.)
- Culture is rarely performed by clinical laboratories
- Doxycycline is mainstay of treatment

MICROSCOPIC

- Endothelial injury with increased permeability/edema, hemorrhage, thrombi, perivascular inflammation (usually lymphohistiocytic), and vasculitis in any organ system
- Organisms are best visualized in tissue using immunohistochemistry in infected endothelial cells

TOP DIFFERENTIAL DIAGNOSES

- Other tick-borne infections in differential
- Lyme (*Borrelia burgdorferi*): Erythema migrans (bull's-eye rash): Confirm with PCR, IHC, Warthin-Starry stain, serology
- Anaplasmosis and ehrlichiosis: Rash less common; morulae present in peripheral blood monocytes and granulocytes; confirm with PCR, serology
- Babesiosis (*Babesia* spp.): RBCs infected with pear-shaped and cross forms
- Heartland virus infection: Similar symptoms to ehrlichiosis in tick-exposed patient from affected area, nonresponsive to doxycycline

Rash in RMSF

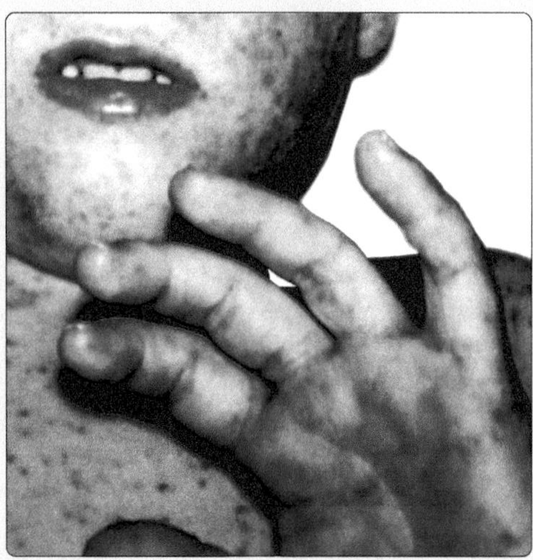

***Rickettsia* Within Macrophages**

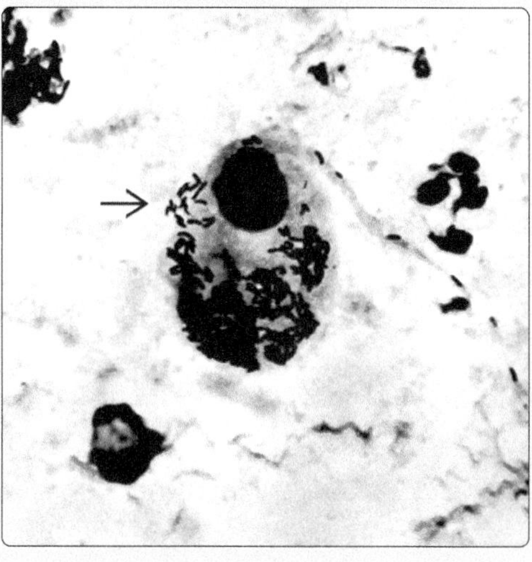

(Left) *This child with Rocky Mountain spotted fever (RMSF) demonstrates the characteristic petechial maculopapular rash involving the palms.* **(Right)** *Rickettsia* → *are able to proliferate inside of macrophages, as seen on this Macchiavello stain, oil immersion.*

Acute Vasculitis in RMSF

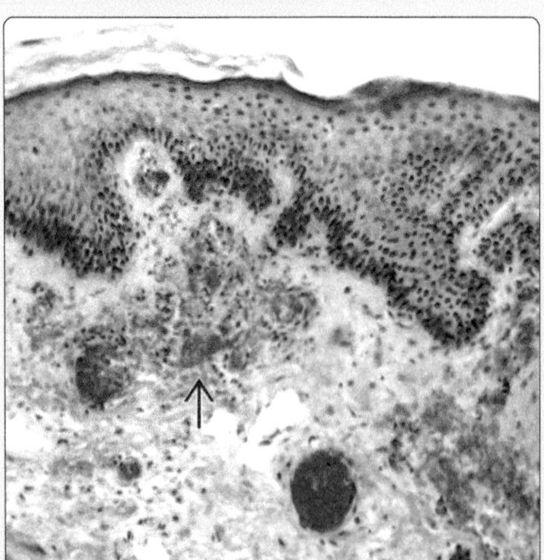

Arteritis: *Rickettsia* spp. IHC

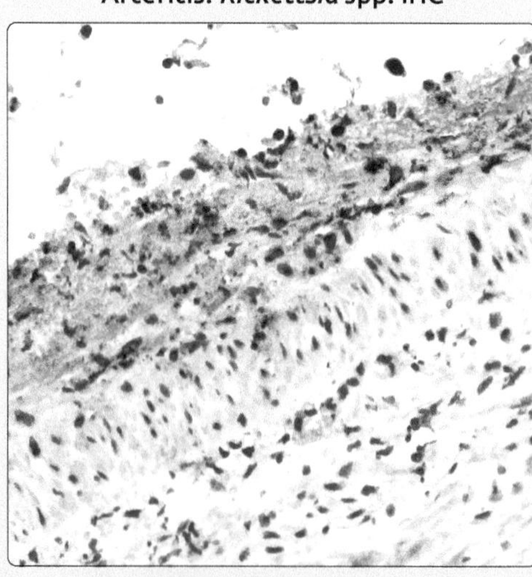

(Left) *This skin biopsy from a patient with RMSF demonstrates acute vasculitis causing endothelial damage and focal hemorrhage* →. **(Right)** *Immunohistochemistry using an antirickettsial antibody highlights rickettsial antigen in a thickened arterial intima. H&E staining of another section revealed intimal fibrinoid change and leukocytoclasis. (Courtesy J. Olano, MD.)*

TERMINOLOGY

Definitions

- *Rickettsia* from Howard Taylor Ricketts: Studied rickettsial disease and died from typhus
- Greek: "Typhos" (smoky or hazy for mental status of patients)

ETIOLOGY/PATHOGENESIS

Infectious Agents

- Infection with *Rickettsia* spp. or *Orientia* spp., obligate intracellular gram-negative bacteria in *Rickettsiaceae* family, spread via arthropod bites
- After introduction into skin, organisms spread rapidly, targeting vascular endothelium; endothelial cell injury results in increased permeability, edema, hypovolemia, hypotension, and hypoalbuminemia

Spotted Fever Group

- Transmitted predominantly by ticks, including *Dermacentor* spp. (e.g., *D. variabilis, D. similis, D. andersoni*), *Amblyomma* spp., and *Rhipicephalus* spp.
- *R. rickettsii* (Rocky Mountain spotted fever; RMSF): North, Central, and South America
- *R. aeschlimannii* (Rickettsiosis): South Africa, Morocco, Mediterranean
- *R. africae* (African tick-bite fever): Sub-Saharan Africa, West Indies
- *R. akari* (Rickettsialpox): South Africa, North and South America, Korea, southern and eastern Europe; transmitted by *Liponyssoides sanguineus* (mouse mite)
- *R. australis* (Queensland tick typhus): Australia, Tasmania
- *R. conorii* subsp. *caspiae* (Astrakhan spotted fever): North Caspian region of Russia
- *R. conorii* subsp. *conorii* (Mediterranean spotted fever/Boutonneuse fever): Africa, southern Europe, southern and western Asia (India)
- *R. conorii* subsp. *indica* (Indian tick typhus): South Asia
- *R. conorii* subsp. *israelensis* (Israeli tick typhus): Southern Europe, Middle East
- *R. felis* (Cat flea rickettsiosis): Africa, North and South America, Asia, Europe; transmitted by fleas
- *R. heilongjiangensis* (Far eastern spotted fever): East Asia, northern China, far east Russia
- *R. helvetica* (aneruptive fever): Asia, central and northern Europe
- *R. honei* including strain "marmionii" (Flinders Island spotted fever/Thai tick typhus): Australia, Thailand
- *R. japonica* (Japanese spotted fever): Japan
- *R. massiliae* (Mediterranean spotted fever-like illness): Central Africa, North America, Europe
- *R. monacensis* (Mediterranean spotted fever-like illness): North Africa, Europe
- *R. parkeri* (Maculatum infection): North and South America
- *R. raoultii* (Tick-borne lymphadenopathy): Asia, Europe
- *R. sibirica* (North Asian tick typhus/Siberian tick typhus): China, Mongolia, Russia
- *R. sibirica mongolotimonae* (Lymphangitis-associated rickettsiosis): Africa, Asia, Europe
- *R. slovaca* (Tick-borne lymphadenopathy): Asia, southern and eastern Europe

Typhus Group

- Transmitted by louse and fleas
- *R. prowazekii* (Epidemic typhus; Sylvatic typhus): Central Africa, North, Central, and South America, Asia
- *R. typhi* (Murine typhus): Temperate, tropical, and subtropical areas, worldwide

Scrub Typus Group

- Transmitted by Trombiculid mites and chiggers
- *Orientia tsutsugamushi* (Scrub typhus): Asia-Pacific region, Middle East
- *O. chuto* (Scrub typhus): United Arab Emirates
- *O. chiloensis* (Scrub typhus): Southern Chile

CLINICAL ISSUES

Epidemiology

- RMSF is most prevalent in late spring/summer in children, adults > 60 years, and with increased exposure to ticks
- Epidemic typhus is most often diagnosed in developing countries in crowded conditions, which favor spread of lice
- Scrub typhus is most prevalent in Tsutsugamushi Triangle connecting Japan, NW Australia, and central Russia; most common in autumn

Presentation

- RMSF: 7-day incubation followed by fever, myalgias, gastrointestinal distress, and headache; petechial maculopapular rash (90% of patients) starting on wrists and ankles; meningeal symptoms, abnormal EEG, ocular pathology, renal failure, and pulmonary compromise
- Epidemic typhus: 11-day incubation followed by rigors, malaise, mental status changes, and headache; petechial/maculopapular rash sparing palms, soles, and face; can reactivate later in life with milder clinical course (Brill-Zinsser disease)
- Murine typhus (more mild disease than epidemic typhus): 1- to 2-week incubation period followed by acute onset of fever, headache, nausea and vomiting, headache, and rash that is predominantly maculopapular sparing palms and soles; progression of disease can include worsening gastrointestinal distress, pulmonary involvement, hepatosplenomegaly, and neurologic manifestations
- Scrub typhus: Fever, headaches, and myalgia ~ 10 days after bite (indicated by erythematous papule/eschar); pulmonary involvement is common and can progress to acute respiratory distress syndrome

Laboratory Tests

- Serology is used for retrospective confirmation (look for 4x rise in titer over course of disease); cross reactivity across rickettsial spp.
- PCR assays are available for blood and tissue (offered by national reference/public health laboratories); targets include 17-kDa lipoprotein, OmpA, etc.

Treatment

- Doxycycline is mainstay of treatment for both RMSF and typhus

Prognosis

- Untreated RMSF and typhus can be rapidly fatal, but with treatment, mortality is usually < 5% in healthy individuals

MICROBIOLOGY

Morphologic and Biochemical Characteristics

- Small, gram-negative, pleomorphic, obligate intracellular organisms
- Stained by Gimenez method or acridine orange

Culture and Microbiologic Identification

- Must be cultured in eukaryotic cell lines, guinea pigs, or embryonated hen's eggs
- Rarely done in clinical laboratory; culture is generally followed by molecular methods for identification

MICROSCOPIC

Histologic Features

- Overall pathology is connected with endothelial injury and subsequent increased permeability/edema, hemorrhage, thrombi, perivascular inflammation (usually lymphohistiocytic), and vasculitis (present in any organ system)
- RMSF
  - Cutaneous: Lymphohistiocytic capillaritis and venulitis with extravasation of erythrocytes, edema, and perivascular and interstitial infiltrates; leukocytoclastic vasculitis with neutrophilic infiltrate, basal layer vacuolar degeneration, and dermoepidermal interface lymphocytic exocytosis
  - Pulmonary: Diffuse interstitial mononuclear (including numerous lymphoblasts) inflammatory infiltrate, pulmonary edema and intraalveolar hemorrhage, vasculitis of arterioles and venules
  - Liver: Marked portal mixed inflammation, spotty lobular necrosis
  - Kidney: Mixed inflammatory infiltrate of vessels and interstitium, acute tubular necrosis, focal segmental tuft necrosis (less common)
  - Brain: Parenchymal lesions often restricted to white matter and consist of microinfarcts
- Epidemic typhus and murine typhus have similar histopathologic presentation to RMSF
- Scrub typhus
  - Cutaneous: Eschars characterized by leukocytoclastic vasculitis and neutrophil infiltration; perieschar region has epidermal exocytosis of mononuclear cells and basal vacuolar changesand dermal perivascular, interstitial, and perineural mononuclear cell infiltration, thrombosis, atypical lymphocyte infiltration, and mitotic figures in dermis
  - Cardiac: Myocarditis, mixed inflammatory infiltrate
  - Pulmonary: Interstitial pneumonitis (more pronounced/common than in RMSF), bacterial bronchopneumonia
  - Liver: Spotty lobular necrosis, typically associated with less of granulocytic infiltrate than in RMSF; periportal steatosis, erythrophagocytosis, sinusoidal infiltrate with activated Kupffer cells and lymphocytes
  - Lymph nodes: Hyperplasia and necrosis (more so than with RMSF)
  - Kidney: Glomerulonephritis, foci of interstitial nephritis
  - Brain: Mononuclear cell meningitis, typhus nodules (predominantly oligodendroglial cells), perivascular cuffing of arteries, focal hemorrhages in parenchyma and meninges, degeneration of ganglion cells

ANCILLARY TESTS

Immunohistochemistry/Immunofluorescence

- Rickettsial antigens present in endothelial cells

Electron Microscopy

- Membrane-bound bacilli (1-2 μm) in cytoplasm and nucleus

DIFFERENTIAL DIAGNOSIS

Lyme (*Borrelia burgdorferi*)

- Also transmitted by tick bites (*Ixodes* spp.)
- Erythema migrans (bull's-eye rash) should warrant investigation for Lyme
- Lymphoplasmacytic inflammation with spirochetes; confirm with PCR, IHC, Warthin-Starry stain, serology

Anaplasmosis and Ehrlichiosis

- Also transmitted by tick bites (*Ixodes* and *Amblyomma* spp.)
- Rash less common in anaplasmosis (10%) and ehrlichiosis (< 40%)
- Morulae present in peripheral blood monocytes and granulocytes; confirm with PCR, serology

Babesiosis (*Babesia* spp.)

- Also transmitted by tick bites (*Ixodes* spp.)
- *Babesia* spp. infect RBCs with diagnostic pear-shaped and cross forms

Heartland Virus Infection

- Clinical signs/symptoms similar to ehrlichiosis with tick exposure (Missouri and Tennessee)
- Patients fail to respond to doxycycline, but there is no current clinical test or therapy available

SELECTED REFERENCES

1. CDC Yellow Book 2024: Rickettsial diseases. Updated May 01, 2023. Accessed June 25, 2023. https://wwwnc.cdc.gov/travel/yellowbook/2024/infections-diseases/rickettsial-diseases
2. Gillespie JJ et al: Orientia and Rickettsia: different flowers from the same garden. Curr Opin Microbiol. 74:102318, 2023
3. Walker DH et al: Rickettsiosis subcommittee report to the tick-borne disease working group. Ticks Tick Borne Dis. 13(1):101855, 2022
4. Salje J: Cells within cells: Rickettsiales and the obligate intracellular bacterial lifestyle. Nat Rev Microbiol. 19(6):375-90, 2021
5. Bradshaw MJ et al: Meningoencephalitis due to spotted fever rickettsioses, including Rocky Mountain spotted fever. Clin Infect Dis. 71(1):188-95, 2020
6. Doppler JF et al: A systematic review of the untreated mortality of murine typhus. PLoS Negl Trop Dis. 14(9):e0008641, 2020
7. Jay R et al: Clinical characteristics of Rocky Mountain spotted fever in the United States: a literature review. J Vector Borne Dis. 57(2):114-20, 2020
8. Vyas NS et al: Investigating the histopathological findings and immunolocalization of rickettsialpox infection in skin biopsies: a case series and review of the literature. J Cutan Pathol. 47(5):451-8, 2020
9. Sekeyová Z et al: Rickettsial infections of the central nervous system. PLoS Negl Trop Dis. 13(8):e0007469, 2019
10. Jang MS et al: Histopathologic finding of perieschar lesions in Tsutsugamushi disease shows lymphocytic vasculitis mimicking angiocentric lymphoma. Ann Dermatol. 30(1):29-35, 2018

Spotted Fever Rickettsiosis in USA, 2019

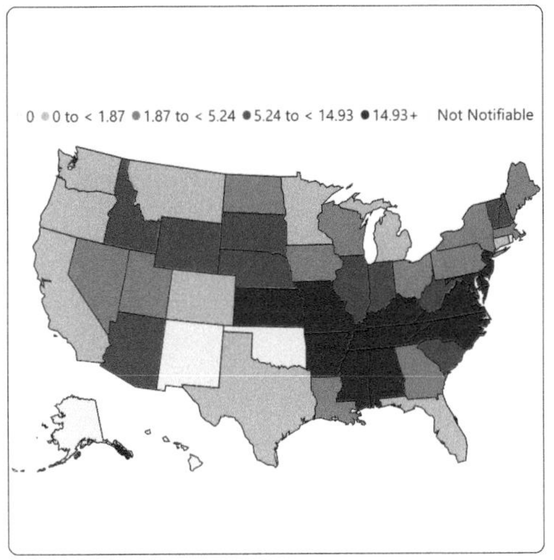

Dermacentor andersoni (Rocky Mountain Wood Tick)

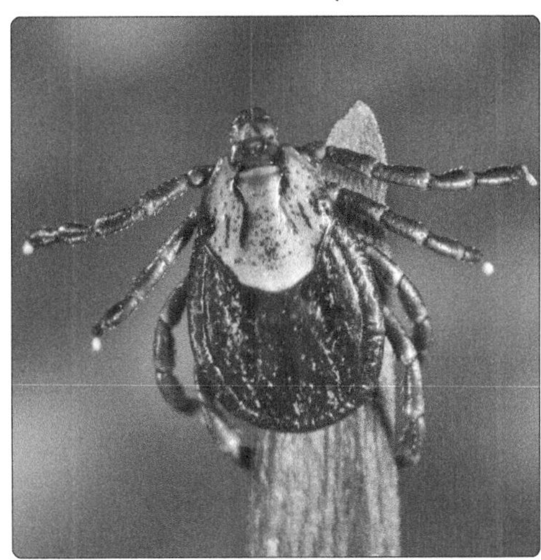

(Left) *Map shows annual incidence (per million persons) for spotted fever rickettsiosis in the USA in 2019. Several ticks with characteristic geographic distributions serve as vectors for Rickettsia spp. infections, including D. variabilis, D. similis, D. andersoni, A. maculatum, and R. sanguineus. (Courtesy CDC.)* **(Right)** *A female D. andersoni is pictured here, identifiable by a bright red, tear drop-shaped body and white-colored shield. (Courtesy, C. Paddock, MD, CDC/PHIL.)*

Orientia tsutsugamushi: Ultrastructural Features

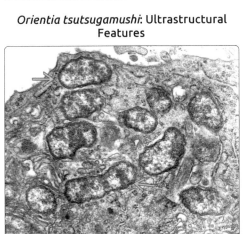

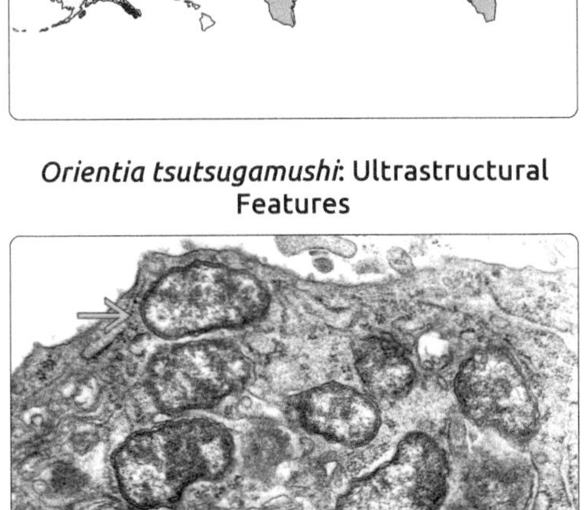

Rickettsial Tubulointerstitial Nephritis

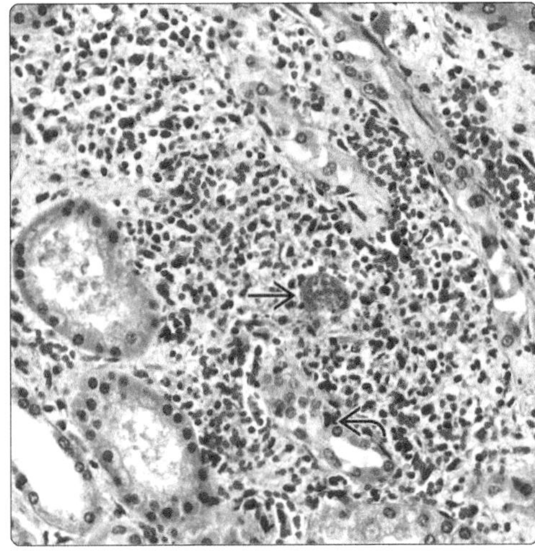

(Left) *This electron micrograph of a hypertrophic peritoneal mesothelial cell of a mouse that experimentally infected with Orientia tsutsugamushi shows several organisms ⇒ visible free within the cell cytoplasm. (Courtesy, E. Ewing, CDC/PHIL.)* **(Right)** *Peritubular capillary thrombosis ⇒ with interstitial hemorrhage and a predominantly mononuclear inflammatory infiltrate are characteristic of rickettsial tubulointerstitial nephritis (TIN). Focal tubulitis is also evident ⇗. (Courtesy J. Olano, MD.)*

Fibrinoid Necrosis in RMSF

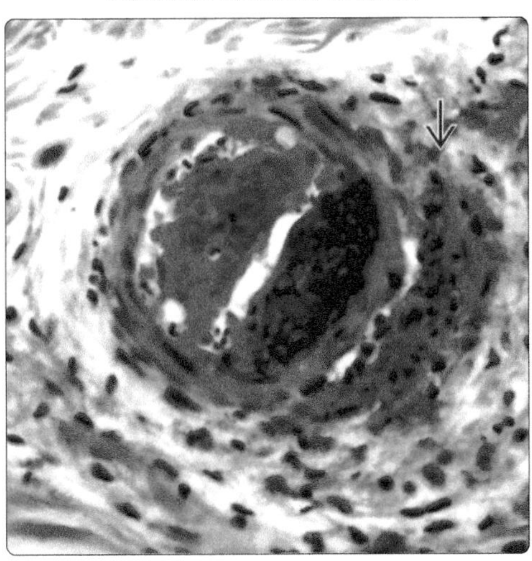

CNS Vasculitis in Epidemic Typhus

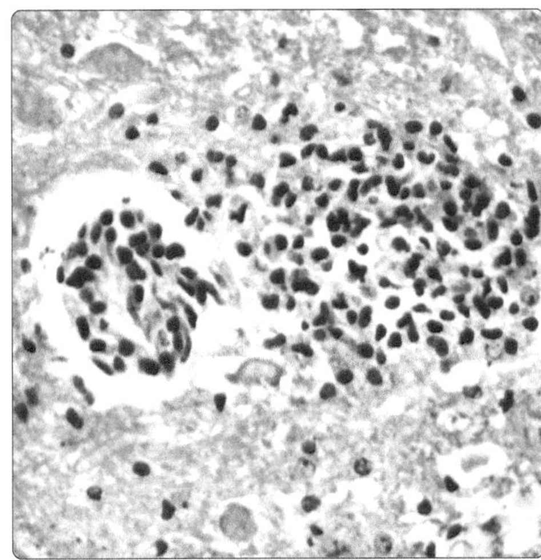

(Left) *In this lethal case of RMSF, fibrinoid necrosis of small arteries with mural thrombi ⇒ are seen.* **(Right)** *Spotty CNS vasculitis in a pontine arteriole with adjacent mononuclear "typhus nodule" is seen in this case of Brill-Zinsser disease (epidemic typhus).*

Mycoplasma and *Ureaplasma* Species Infections

KEY FACTS

ETIOLOGY/PATHOGENESIS

- Infections with *Mycoplasma* and *Ureaplasma* spp., bacteria in class Mollicutes, smallest free-living organisms (0.2-0.3 μm in diameter), which lack cell wall

CLINICAL ISSUES

- *M. pneumoniae*: "Walking" pneumonia, tracheobronchitis, pharyngitis; disseminated disease, hemolytic anemia, skin rash, myocarditis, encephalitis
- *M. hominis, M. genitalium*: Bacterial vaginitis, pelvic inflammatory disease, pyelonephritis, neonatal infection; disseminated disease (immunocompromised)
- *Ureaplasma* spp.: Urogenital infections, urethritis, renal calculi; preterm birth with pulmonary/CNS disease; hyperammonemia syndrome
- Laboratory: PCR testing (including multiplex panels) is preferred method of detection; may reflect colonization
- Culture and susceptibility testing requires specialized media (typically performed at reference labs)
- Treatment: Fluoroquinolones, tetracyclines, macrolides

MICROSCOPIC

- Organisms not visualized by Gram stain, but antigen can be highlighted by targeted IHC
- *M. pneumoniae*: Nonspecific lymphocytic/neutrophilic bronchiolitis, epithelial injury, sloughing, intraalveolar mucus/proteinaceous material; DAD in severe cases
- *M. hominis*-associated chorioamnionitis, vaginal abscess

TOP DIFFERENTIAL DIAGNOSES

- Other atypical pneumonias (e.g., *Legionella* spp., *Chlamydia* spp., *Coxiella burnetii, Bordetella* spp.) confirmed by IHC, molecular, or serology testing
- Pulmonary viral infections (e.g., RSV, adenovirus, and influenzas A and B) confirmed by viral inclusions, IHC, PCR, antigen testing, or culture
- Other urogenital bacterial infections (e.g., *Chlamydia trachomatis, Neisseria gonorrhea, Gardnerella vaginalis*) confirmed by IHC, molecular testing or culture

Mycoplasma pneumoniae **Colony Morphology**

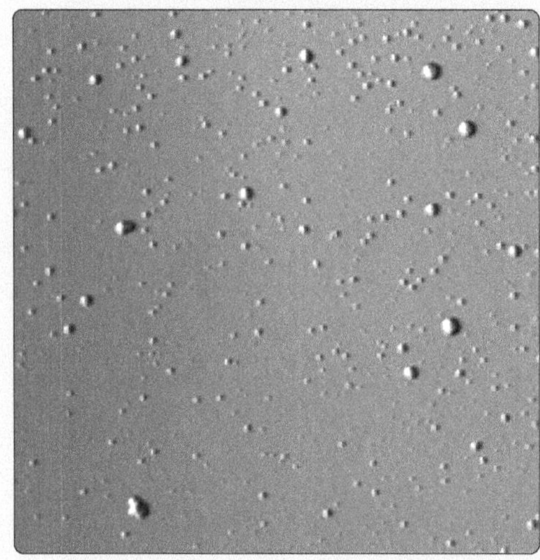

Mycoplasma pneumoniae **Chest Radiograph**

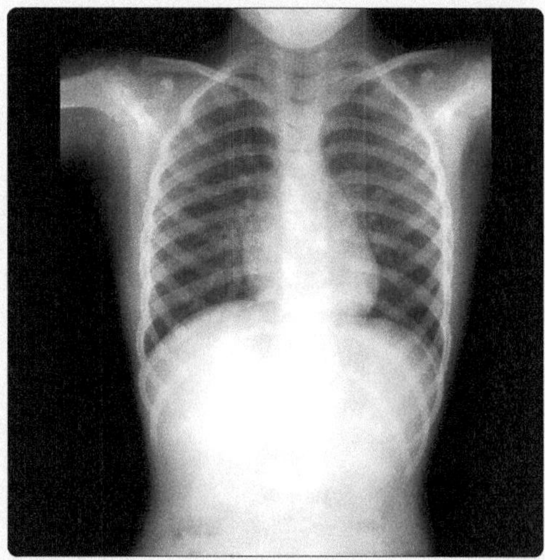

(Left) *Small, colorless, punctate colonies (dissection scope needed) grow on SP4 agar within 5-14 days when cultured aerobically at 37 °C. (Courtesy S.M. Leal Jr., MD, PhD.)* **(Right)** *Mycoplasma pneumoniae pulmonary infection demonstrates diffuse hazy infiltrates and bilateral hilar lymphadenopathy. (Courtesy H. B. Dull, MD, CDC/PHIL.)*

Bartholin Cyst Abscess

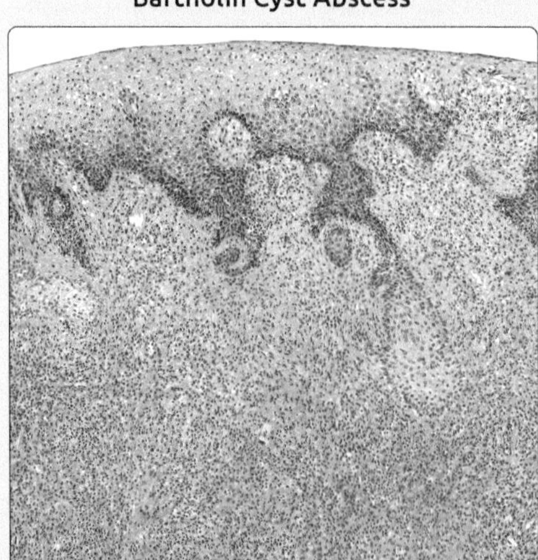

Mycoplasma pneumoniae **IHC**

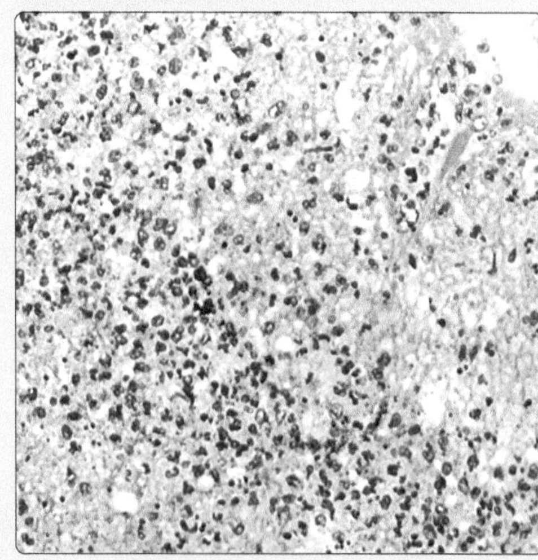

(Left) *This section shows reactive epithelial change and severe acute inflammation and necrosis, consistent with abscess. 16S rRNA gene sequencing was positive for Mycoplasma hominis.* **(Right)** *M. pneumoniae antigen is identified by IHC in perivascular histiocytes in necrotic brain tissue in a patient with fatal acute disseminated encephalomyelitis following M. pneumoniae pneumonia. (Courtesy Stamm et al. Emerg Infect Dis. 14(4):641-3, 2008.)*

TERMINOLOGY

Synonyms

- Walking pneumonia, nongonococcal urethritis

Definitions

- Greek: "Mykes" (fungus), "plasma" (formed)

ETIOLOGY/PATHOGENESIS

Infectious Agents

- Infections with bacteria in *Mycoplasma* and *Ureaplasma* genera, members of class Mollicutes, which are smallest free-living organisms (0.2-0.3 μm in diameter), known for lacking cell wall around their cell membrane
- *Mycoplasma* spp. demonstrate high variation in cell surface proteins allowing for evasion of host immune system
- *M. pneumoniae* P1 adhesion protein interacts with sialylated glycoprotein receptors on epithelial cells, destroying cilia, resulting in respiratory illness
- *Ureaplasma* spp. produce IgA protease to degrade immunoglobulins, release urea, and form urinary calculi

CLINICAL ISSUES

Epidemiology

- *M. pneumoniae* spreads in crowded environments
- Colonization with genital *M. hominis, M. genitalium, U. urealyticum*, or *U. parvum* is common and increases with number of sexual partners
- Neonates exposed in utero/intrapartum
- Higher burden of disease in patients with HIV or other immune defects (especially hypogammaglobulinemia)

Presentation

- *M. pneumoniae* infection can present with "walking" (nonsevere) pneumonia, tracheobronchitis, pharyngitis; extrapulmonary manifestations include disseminated disease, immune-mediated hemolytic anemia, skin rash (e.g., erythema multiforme), myocarditis, encephalitis
- *M. hominis, M. genitalium* can cause bacterial vaginitis and pelvic inflammatory disease (typically bacterial copathogen), pyelonephritis, neonatal infection; disseminated infection occurs rarely in immunocompromised patients
- *Ureaplasma* spp. cause urogenital infections, nongonococcal urethritis, renal calculi; preterm birth, postpartum fever, pulmonary, CNS infection in neonates; hyperammonemia syndrome after lung transplantation

Laboratory Tests

- PCR testing (including multiplex panels) is preferred method of detection, although may reflect colonization
- EIA antibodies lack sensitivity and specificity
- Complement fixation titers peak in 4 weeks and persists 6-12 months

Treatment

- Fluoroquinolones, tetracyclines, macrolides (*Ureaplasma* spp. only)

Prognosis

- Intraamniotic infection with *M. hominis* and *Ureaplasma* spp. associated with poorer fetal outcomes
- Atypical "walking" pneumonia generally nonsevere

IMAGING

Radiographic Findings

- *M. pneumoniae* pulmonary infection with bilateral diffuse patchy, reticulonodular opacities, severity out of proportion to clinical status

MICROBIOLOGY

Culture, Morphology, and Biochemical Features

- Organisms not visualized by Gram stain
- Slow-growing (2-6 weeks), facultative anaerobes (*M. pneumoniae* is strict aerobe)
- Requires complex lipid cholesterol in growth media; specialized agar required (SP4 or A8) at 37 °C (culture and susceptibility testing generally performed in reference labs)
- *M. pneumoniae, Ureaplasma* spp. form small punctate colonies that require dissection scope for visualization
- *M. hominis*: Colonies show typical "fried egg" within 2-4 days; occasionally will grow on blood on or chocolate agar
- *Mycoplasma* spp. typically utilize glucose and or arginine, *Ureaplasma* spp. are urease positive

MICROSCOPIC

Histologic Features

- *M. pneumoniae*: Nonspecific lymphocytic or neutrophilic bronchiolitis, epithelial injury with sloughing, intraalveolar mucus or proteinaceous material; diffuse alveolar damage in severe cases
- *M. hominis* associated chorioamnionitis, vaginal abscess

ANCILLARY TESTS

PCR

- 16S rRNA sequencing can be performed on FFPE tissue

Immunohistochemistry

- Bacterial antigens highlighted by IHC in affected tissues (available at some reference laboratories)

DIFFERENTIAL DIAGNOSIS

Pulmonary Infections

- Other atypical pneumonias (e.g., *Legionella* spp., *Chlamydia* spp., *Coxiella burnetii, Bordetella* spp.) confirmed by IHC, molecular, or serology testing
- Viral infections (e.g., RSV, adenovirus, and influenzas A and B) confirmed by viral inclusions, IHC, PCR, antigen testing, or culture

Urogenital Infections

- Other bacterial infections (e.g., *Chlamydia trachomatis, Neisseria gonorrhea, Gardnerella vaginalis*) confirmed by IHC, molecular testing or culture

SELECTED REFERENCES

1. Hu J et al: Insight into the pathogenic mechanism of Mycoplasma pneumoniae. Curr Microbiol. 80(1):14, 2022
2. Ahmed J et al: Mycoplasma hominis: an under recognized pathogen. Indian J Med Microbiol. 39(1):88-97, 2021
3. Stamm B et al: Neuroinvasion by Mycoplasma pneumoniae in acute disseminated encephalomyelitis. Emerg Infect Dis. 14(4):641-3, 2008

Mycobacterium tuberculosis Complex Infections

KEY FACTS

ETIOLOGY/PATHOGENESIS

- *Mycobacterium tuberculosis* (MTB) complex: Rod-shaped, acid-fast, aerobic, slow-growing intracellular pathogens that subvert phagosomal cells in order to persist and evade immune system
- Drug resistance is serious problem, and some infections are virtually untreatable
- Transmission mainly by inhalation of contaminated droplets; *Mycobacterium bovis* transmitted from cattle via undercooked meat or unpasteurized milk
- May establish itself in subclinical, latent state or immediately progress to active disease (~ 10%)

CLINICAL ISSUES

- Pulmonary tuberculosis: Usually presents with nonspecific, constitutional symptoms and productive cough
- Extrapulmonary tuberculosis results from contiguous or lymphohematogenous spread and can affect any organ
- Diagnosis: Tuberculin skin testing, interferon release assays, sputum analysis; acid-fast staining, culture, and direct detection of organisms by PCR

MICROSCOPIC

- Histopathologic hallmark is necrotizing granuloma with giant cells and epithelioid histiocytes
- Bacilli highlighted by acid-fast stains and by IHC

TOP DIFFERENTIAL DIAGNOSES

- Nontuberculous mycobacterial infections: Granulomatous inflammation (± necrosis) with positive AFB stains; distinguish by culture, PCR
- Fungal infections (e.g., cryptococcosis, histoplasmosis): Necrotizing granulomatous inflammation with fungal elements highlighted by GMS, PAS-D stains
- Sarcoidosis: Granulomatous inflammation (± focal necrosis) without identified infectious etiology
- Crohn disease: Small, nonnecrotizing granulomas confined to GI tract; AFB stain negative

(Left) *This image of a Ziehl-Neelsen-stained sputum smear shows an AFB. While morphologically compatible with Mycobacterium tuberculosis (MTB), species identification must be confirmed by cultures or molecular testing. (Courtesy R. Smithwick, MS, CDC/PHIL.)* **(Right)** *H&E shows 4 examples of the hallmark lesion of MTB infection: Granuloma with centrally located Langerhans giant cells → surrounded by layers of inflammatory cells.*

MTB: Ziehl-Neelsen Stain

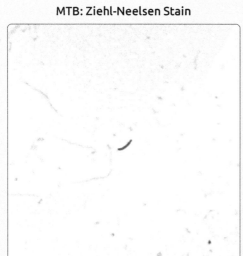

Hallmark Lesions of Tuberculosis

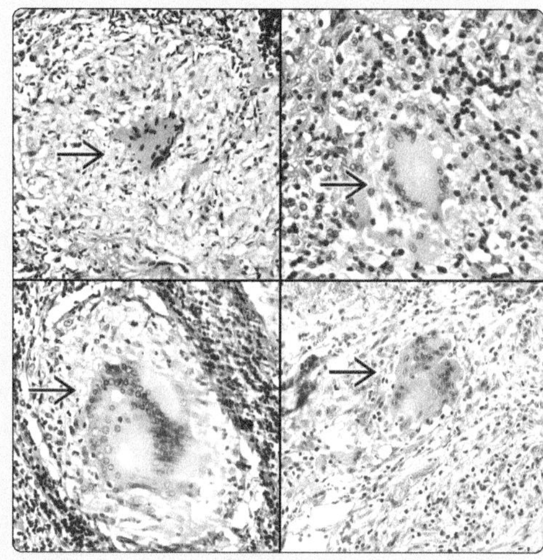

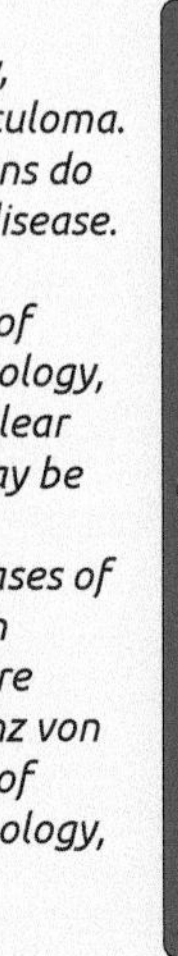

(Left) *This specimen demonstrates a solitary, caseous, primary tuberculoma. The majority of infections do not progress to active disease. (Courtesy Franz von Lichtenberg Collection of Infectious Disease Pathology, BWH.)* **(Right)** *Despite clear granulomas, AFB → may be scarce and require a painstaking search in cases of tuberculosis. Cases with innumerable bacteria are possible. (Courtesy Franz von Lichtenberg Collection of Infectious Disease Pathology, BWH.)*

MTB: Caseous Necrosis

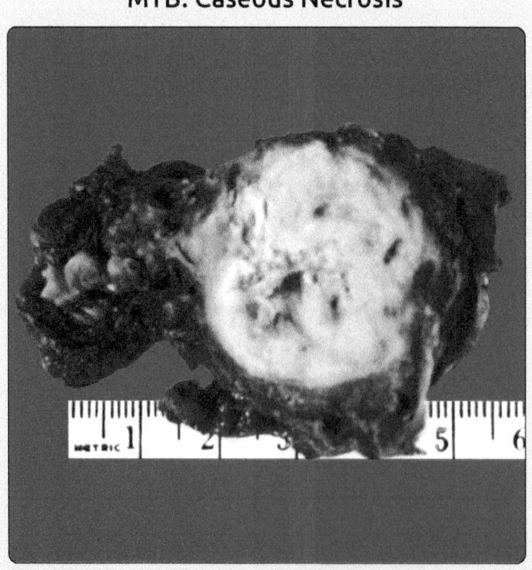

MTB: Acid-Fast Stain in Tissue

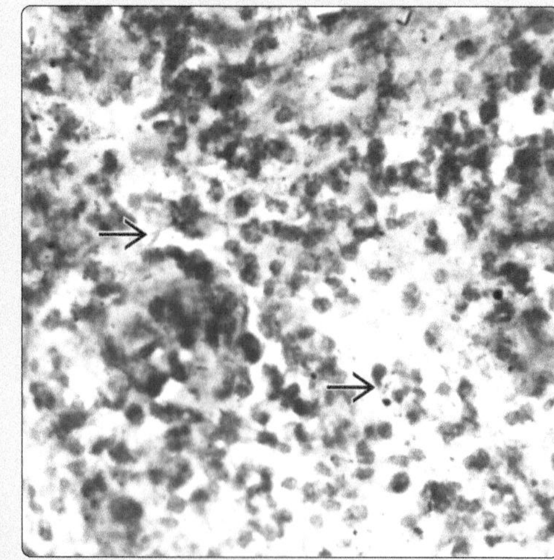

TERMINOLOGY

Synonyms

- Tuberculosis, phthisis, consumption, tubercle bacillus, Koch bacillus

Definitions

- Greek "myco" (fungi, for similarity to fungal growth on liquid media surfaces) and Latin "tuber" (lump or swelling)

ETIOLOGY/PATHOGENESIS

Infectious Agents

- *Mycobacterium tuberculosis* (MTB) complex composes several species with > 99.9% identity, including *M. tuberculosis, M. africanum, M. canettii, M. bovis, M. caprae,* and *M. pinnipedii*
- Transmission mainly by inhalation of contaminated droplets; *M. bovis* can be transmitted from cattle via undercooked meat or unpasteurized milk
- Intracellular pathogens subvert phagosomal compartment in order to persist and evade immune system
- Cell wall contains lipomannan, lipoarabinomannan, and mycolic acids, responsible for acid-fast properties
- Humans are only natural reservoir for *M. tuberculosis, M. africanum,* and *M. canettii*; cattle are reservoirs for *M. bovis* and *M. caprae,* and seals are reservoir for *M. pinnipedii*

CLINICAL ISSUES

Presentation

- Initial infection can lead to subclinical, latent state or progress immediately to active disease (~ 10%)
- Latent disease may reactivate in older age, periods of stress or nutrient deprivation, or due to immunosuppression (e.g., HIV infection)
- Pulmonary tuberculosis (TB): Frequently asymptomatic early in disease (may be detected radiologically); progresses to nonspecific, constitutional symptoms, productive cough; hemoptysis may indicate endobronchial erosion
- Extrapulmonary TB can result from contiguous or lymphohematogenous spread
  - Miliary TB: Progressive, widely disseminated disease (foci resemble millet seeds)
  - CNS TB: Common complication of childhood disease; headache, vomiting, mental status changes, meningismus, focal neurologic signs, and coma
  - Pleurisy: Most common in young children
  - Pericarditis: Most common in HIV-positive patients
  - Skeletal TB (Pott disease) occurs in 1/3 of cases: Typically begins on anterior aspect of vertebral body, spreads to discs and other vertebra; paraspinal abscess common
  - Lymphadenitis (scrofula): Most common form of extrapulmonary TB
    - HIV negative: Usually unilateral and cervical; no systemic symptoms
    - HIV positive and AIDS: Often multifocal and marked systemic symptoms
    - Commonly complicated by suppuration, sinus formation, and enlargement of surrounding nodes (may represent immune activation rather than spread)
  - Renal: Asymptomatic lesions common; sterile pyuria; advanced disease with papillary necrosis, uretal stricture, hydronephrosis, cavitation, and autonephrectomy
  - Genitourinary
    - Male patients: Often tender, scrotal mass with draining sinus; may have calcified foci in prostate
    - Female patients: Hematogenous spread commonly involves endometrium and ovaries; may mimic carcinoma in cervix or peritoneal carcinomatosis
  - GI: Can affect any part of GI tract (also hepatic and pancreatic inflammation and masses)
  - Cutaneous: May result from exogenous infection, spread from underlying focus, or hematogenous spread
    - Primary MTB: Exogenous infection in unsensitized individual; affects any mucocutaneous surface; may remain localized or involve underlying lymph nodes (similar to Ghon complex)
    - TB verrucosa cutis (prosector's wart): Exogenous infection in sensitized individual; no underlying adenopathy, rarely ulcerates
    - Scrofuloderma: Contiguous spread from underlying lesion, lymph nodes, bones, etc.; may present as chronic draining sinus tract or cutaneous abscess
    - Lupus vulgaris: Chronic cutaneous process resulting from hematogenous spread in highly sensitized individual; typically solitary plaques or nodules (often face or neck) with central ulceration; malignancy (i.e., squamous cell carcinoma) in longstanding cases
- Other MTB complex organisms cause clinically and histologically equivalent TB-like disease
  - *M. africanum*: Predominantly in west Africa; symptomatic patients usually immunocompromised; lacks "region of difference 9," likely related to differences in pathogenesis
  - *M. canettii*: Predominantly in Horn of Africa; symptomatic patients may be immunocompetent or immunocompromised; species has novel phenolic glycolipid and lipooligosaccharide
  - *M. bovis*: Associated with animal exposure; control primarily through culling of affected animals; inherently resistant to pyrazinamide
  - *M. caprae*: Associated with animal exposure in Eastern Europe; control primarily through culling of affected animals; distinguished by molecular testing
  - *M. pinnipedii*: Associated with exposure to seals, guinea pigs, rabbits, or tapirs; distinguished by molecular testing

Laboratory Tests

- Tuberculin skin testing: Screen to detect exposure by reaction to intradermal dose of purified protein derivative (PPD)
- Interferon-γ release assays: ELISA-based assay to determine response to multiple, purified MTB products; does not cross react with bacille Calmette-Guerin (BCG) but may with other mycobacterial species (e.g., *M. kansasii, M. szulgai, M. marinum*)
- Sputum: Acid-fast staining, culture, and direct detection of organisms by PCR; 2-3 sputa are required to rule out/rule in infection in suspected patient
- CSF: High protein, low glucose, lymphocytic predominance with detection of organisms (by culture or AFB stain) in meningitis

- Fine-needle aspiration: May show organisms in lymphadenitis; often smear positive in HIV-positive patients but may need biopsy and culture for detection in HIV-negative patients
- PCR/sequencing of 16S rRNA, *rpoB*, etc. or detection of IS*6110* of primary specimens, culture isolates, or formalin-fixed paraffin-embedded tissue

Treatment

- Lymphadenitis may require surgical excision; large lesions of any organ may be resected to prevent catastrophic erosions (e.g., aorta)
- Active disease treated with months-long, multidrug regimens; usually some combination of isoniazid, rifampin, pyrazinamide, and ethambutol
- Drug resistance is serious problem in MTB therapy, and some or all commonly used agents may be ineffective
- Standard treatment for latent MTB infection consists of 9 months of daily isoniazid or alternative regimen
- BCG vaccine used in high-prevalence regions to prevent childhood TB meningitis and miliary disease; not recommended for regions with low risk of infection due to variable effectiveness against adult pulmonary TB and potential for false-positive tuberculin skin tests
- BCG vaccine also used as immunotherapy for bladder cancer, which may cause cystitis, prostatitis, or systemic infection

Prognosis

- Excellent in immunocompetent individuals with drug-susceptible infections
- Outcomes can be quite poor in ill/immunocompromised patients, particularly if infected with resistant strains

IMAGING

Radiographic Findings

- Classically, upper lobe involvement with apical scarring
- Miliary TB, pleural effusions, lobar pneumonias, and hilar masses also possible
- Pulmonary sites may show cavitation
- Nonpulmonary sites may show small (miliary) nodules or large, solid or cavitary lesions with variable calcification

MICROBIOLOGY

Culture and Microbiologic Identification

- Acid-fast, aerobic rods (3 x 0.5 μm); weakly gram-positive
- Detected on smears by acid-fast (e.g., Ziehl-Neelsen, Kinyoun) and fluorescent stains (e.g., auramine O)
- Slow growing: Doubling time may be > 20 hours; time to detection is 2-8 weeks; colonies can be beige to yellowish and have piled-up or crinkled appearance
- Commonly cultured in liquid media as part of automated BACTEC mycobacterial growth indicator tube (MGIT) system: Time to detection is 1-3 weeks
- Traditionally identified by biochemical tests on cultured isolates, now increasingly identified by MALDI-TOF MS or nucleic acid amplification test (NAAT)
- Growing role for whole-genome sequencing from cultured isolates for fine-tuned speciation, epidemiology, and prediction of antibiotic resistance

MACROSCOPIC

General Features

- Lungs: Cavities, caseating (necrotic) zones, and old calcified foci; commonly involves hilar and mediastinal lymph nodes; may heal and calcify (Ghon foci)
- Extrapulmonary: Widespread, caseating granulomas
- Intestinal ulcers may be transversal, granular, and punched out against smooth, hyperemic mucosa (tubercles may proliferate along edges)

MICROSCOPIC

Histologic Features

- Pulmonary TB can involve airways, parenchyma, and pleura
  - Langerhans giant cells with nuclei in horseshoe arrangement and epithelioid macrophages
  - As granulomas progress, center becomes necrotic (caseous necrosis, coagulative necrosis speckled with basophilic particles of hydroxyapatite)
- Extrapulmonary
  - Intestinal: Clubbing of villi, inflammatory infiltrates, necrosis of lamina propria and submucosa
  - Hepatitis: Caseating granulomas or diffuse, inflammatory, and fibrous lesions (usually in context of miliary TB)
  - Lymphadenitis: Usually demonstrates well-formed granulomas with scarce bacilli
  - CNS: Caseating granulomas of brain parenchyma, leptomeningitis, pachymeningitis
  - Primary cutaneous: Chronic inflammation, granulomatous inflammation
  - Verrucosa cutis: Hyperkeratosis
  - Scrofuloderma: Ulcerative lesions arising from contiguous spread of underlying affected lymph nodes
  - Lupus vulgaris: Focal, chronic, granulomatous dermatitis
  - Erythema induratum: Granulomatous panniculitis with necrosis and vasculitis on posterior aspect of legs
  - Skeletal: Granulomatous lesions with degeneration of bone and discs; commonly spreads into contiguous soft tissue with abscess formation

ANCILLARY TESTS

Special Stains

- Carbol fuchsin-based AFB (e.g., Ziehl-Neelsen, Kinyoun) detect AFB but cannot distinguish between MTB and nontuberculous mycobacteria
- Modified AFB stains (e.g., Fite-Faraco) increase sensitivity but decrease specificity (i.e., also highlight *Nocardia* spp.)
- May be visualized by other stains (e.g., Gram, GMS) with high organism concentration

Immunohistochemistry

- Antimycobacterial antibodies increase sensitivity compared to AFB stains, as bacilli may appear larger depending on IHC detection method
- Specificity may be lower depending on antibody (e.g., polyclonal antibodies stain all *Mycobacterium* spp., including *M. leprae*, and *Nocardia* spp.)

DIFFERENTIAL DIAGNOSIS

Nontuberculous Mycobacterial Infections

- Other mycobacteria may exhibit necrotizing granulomatous inflammation with positive AFB stains
- Distinguish with molecular or culture methods

Fungal Infections

- *Cryptococcus* spp., *Histoplasma* spp., *Coccidioides* spp. may be associated with necrotizing granulomatous inflammation
- Fungal elements (e.g., yeast, spherules, endospores) identified by GMS or PAS-D stains; AFB stain negative

Sarcoidosis

- Generally small, tightly circumscribed granulomas, which may show limited necrosis
- May contain asteroid bodies or small calcifications
- Negative AFB stains, cultures, molecular testing

Crohn Disease

- Granulomas tend to be small and nonnecrotizing, confined to GI tract
- Other features of chronic injury should be present; AFB stain negative

SELECTED REFERENCES

1. Kaul S et al: Cutaneous tuberculosis. Part II: complications, diagnostic workup, histopathological features, and treatment. J Am Acad Dermatol. 89(6):1107-19, 2023
2. Lange C et al: 100 years of Mycobacterium bovis bacille Calmette-Guérin. Lancet Infect Dis. 22(1):e2-12, 2022
3. Crothers JW et al: Clinical performance of mycobacterial immunohistochemistry in anatomic pathology specimens. Am J Clin Pathol. 155(1):97-105, 2021
4. Eraksoy H: Gastrointestinal and abdominal tuberculosis. Gastroenterol Clin North Am. 50(2):341-60, 2021
5. Pantanowitz L et al: Artificial intelligence-based screening for mycobacteria in whole-slide images of tissue samples. Am J Clin Pathol. 156(1):117-28, 2021
6. Furin J et al: Tuberculosis. Lancet. 393(10181):1642-56, 2019
7. Meehan CJ et al: Whole genome sequencing of Mycobacterium tuberculosis: current standards and open issues. Nat Rev Microbiol. 17(9):533-45, 2019

MTB: Culture Isolate

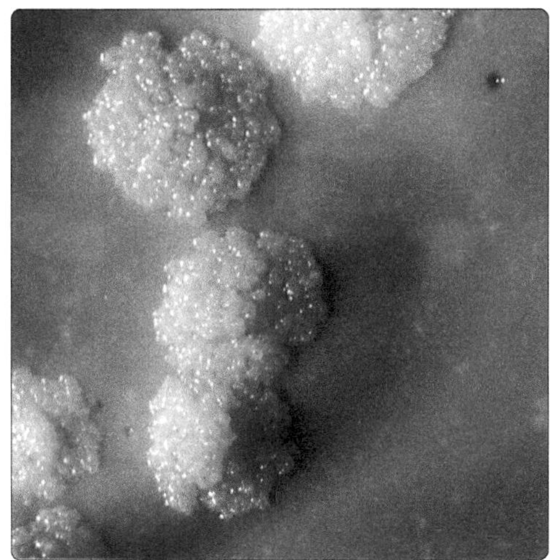

MTB: Ultrastructural Features

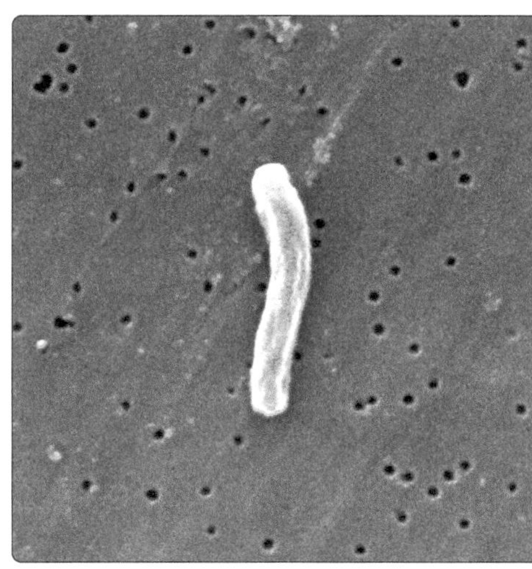

(Left) *This culture plate shows colonies of MTB, characterized by a colorless, rough surface. Speciation is increasingly achieved by MALDI-TOF MS. (Courtesy G. Kubica, PhD, CDC/PHIL.)* **(Right)** *This scanning electron microscopic image depicts a single MTB bacterium, which can range 2.0-4.0 µm in length and 0.2-0.5 µm in width. (Courtesy R. Butler, MS, CDC/PHIL.)*

MTB: Auramine-Rhodamine Stain

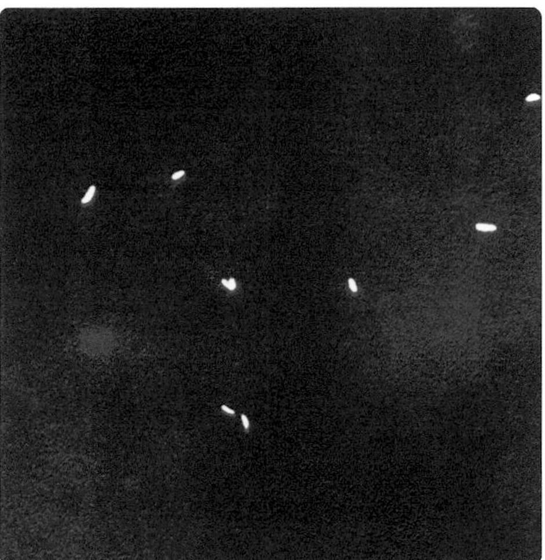

MTB Cording

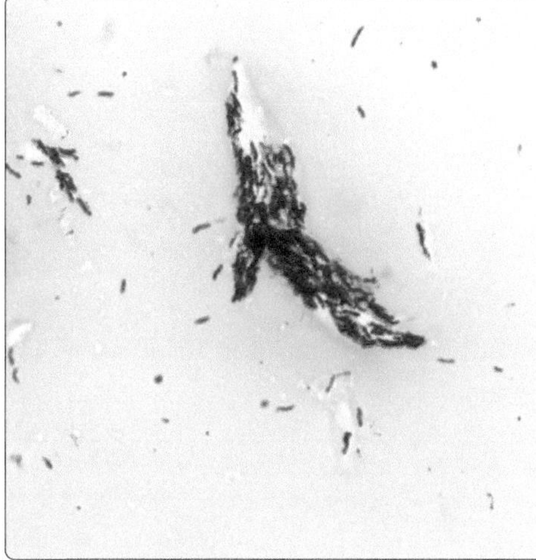

(Left) *Auramine-rhodamine staining of this BAL smear highlights scattered MTB bacteria. (Courtesy W. Jones, Jr., PhD, CDC/PHIL.)* **(Right)** *Ziehl-Neelsen staining highlights aggregates of bacilli forming microscopic structures that resemble cords, referred to as cord formation or cording, and is considered a virulence factor. (Courtesy J. Crothers, MD.)*

(Left) *In tuberculosis, necrotizing granulomas* ➡ *are the histologic correlate of caseous necrosis (a term used only for the gross appearance). (Courtesy Franz von Lichtenberg Collection of Infectious Disease Pathology, BWH.)* **(Right)** *The lungs from a patient with advanced pulmonary tuberculosis demonstrate both caseous necrosis* → *and cavitation* ⇨*. (Courtesy Franz von Lichtenberg Collection of Infectious Disease Pathology, BWH.)*

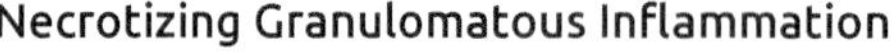

Necrotizing Granulomatous Inflammation

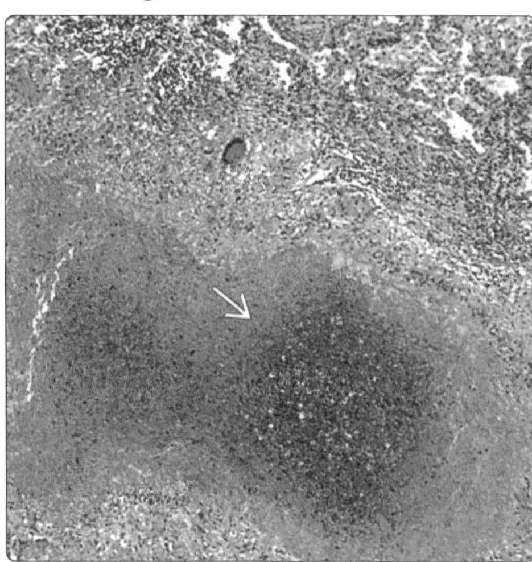

Caseous Necrosis in Lung

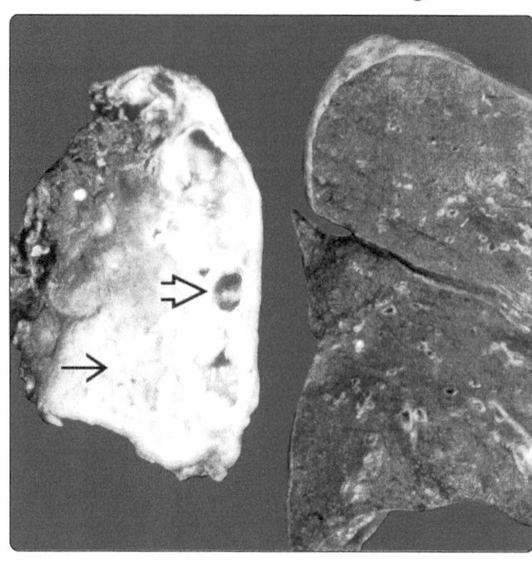

(Left) *In reactivation tuberculosis, lesions tend to be subapical, such as the caseating mass* ➡ *seen in this gross photograph. (Courtesy Franz von Lichtenberg Collection of Infectious Disease Pathology, BWH.)* **(Right)** *In active pulmonary tuberculosis, granulomas are mixed with exudative lesions, including purulent bronchial content* →*. (Courtesy Franz von Lichtenberg Collection of Infectious Disease Pathology, BWH.)*

Large Tuberculosis Mass

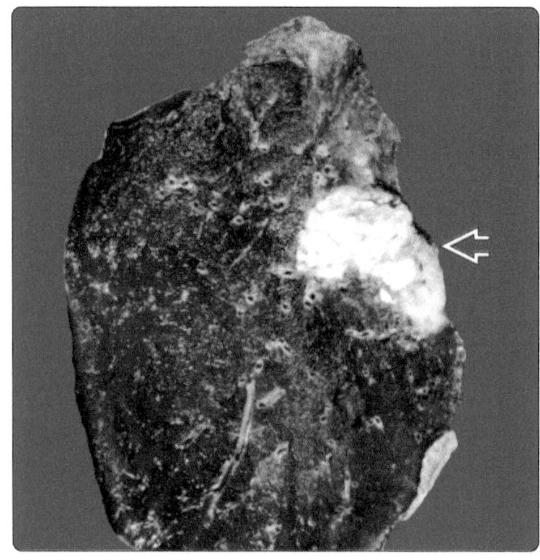

Tuberculosis Exudative Lesions

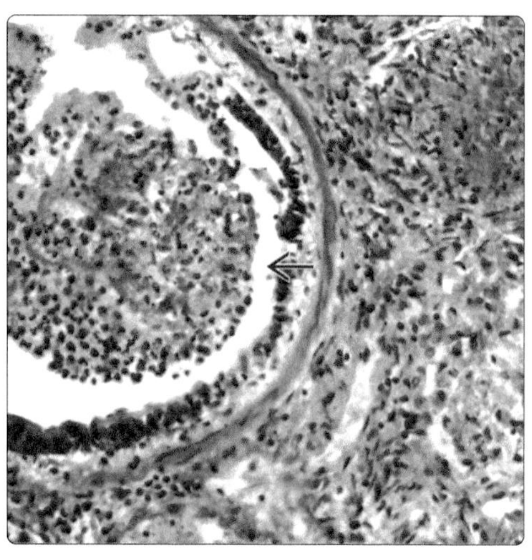

(Left) *H&E shows that hematogenous spread has caused miliary tubercles* ⇨ *to form in the omental fat. Note the rim of lymphocytes* →*. (Courtesy Franz von Lichtenberg Collection of Infectious Disease Pathology, BWH.)* **(Right)** *Both bronchioles and alveoli are targets of necrotizing granulomatous inflammation* → *in tuberculous bronchopneumonia. Note the areas of necrosis* ⇨*. (Courtesy Franz von Lichtenberg Collection of Infectious Disease Pathology, BWH.)*

Miliary Tuberculosis

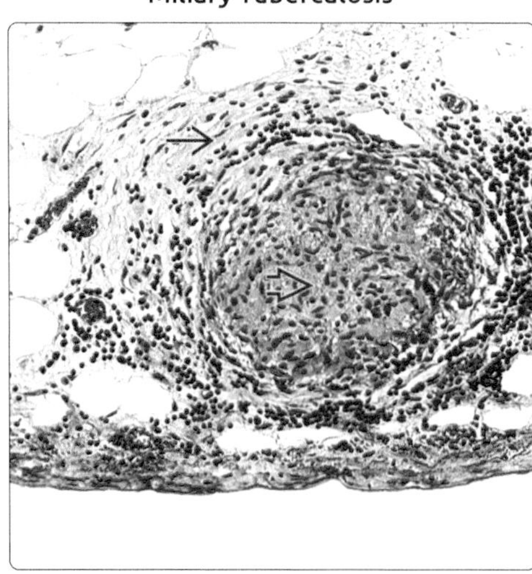

Necrotizing Pneumonia

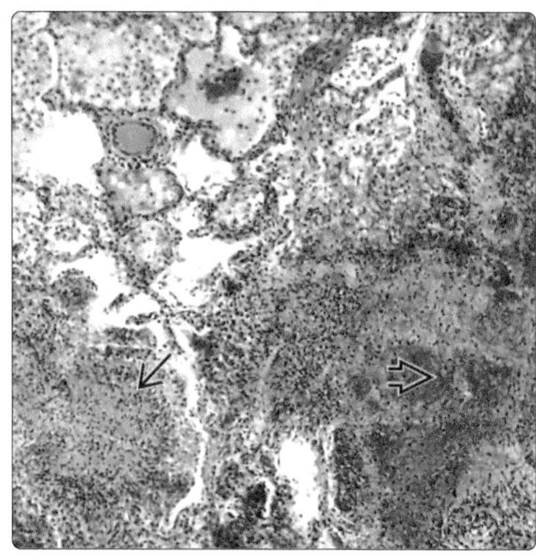

Tuberculous Lymphadenitis

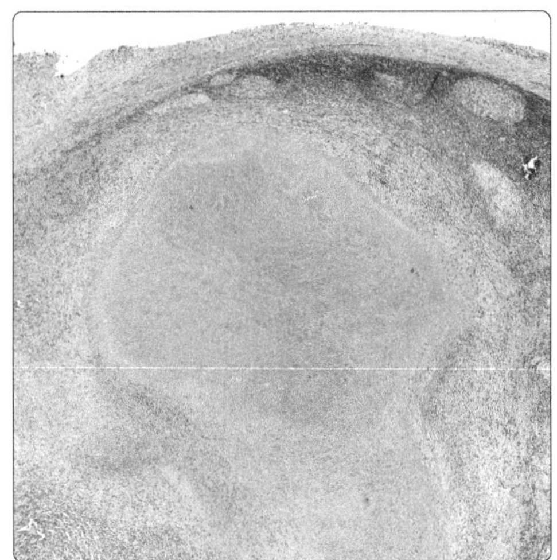

***Mycobacterium* spp. IHC**

(Left) *This cervical lymph node biopsy from a patient who previously lived in Africa shows necrotizing granulomatous inflammation. While highly suspicious for MTB, confirmation with AFB stains, culture, or PCR is recommended to exclude other infectious etiologies.* **(Right)** *IHC may serve as an efficient screening tool for detection of mycobacteria due to the wider size of bacilli compared to histochemical stains.*

Tuberculous Meningitis

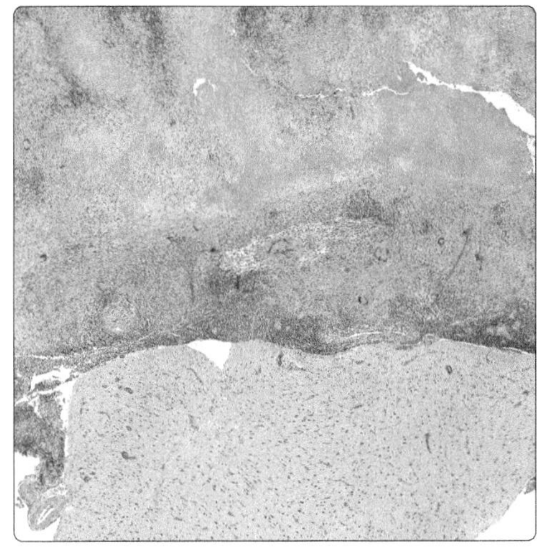

Intestinal Ulcers: Tuberculosis

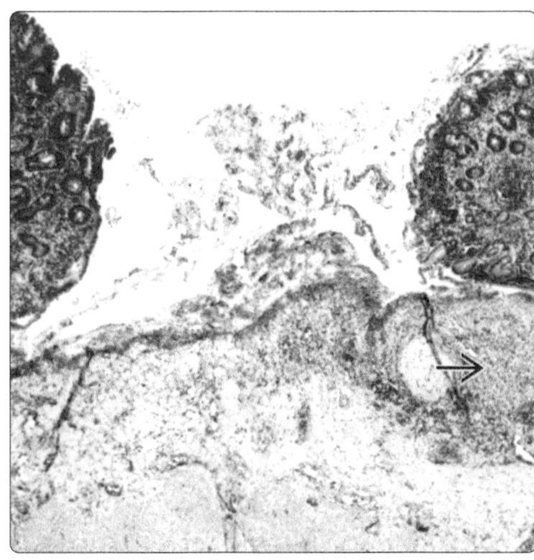

(Left) *Tuberculous meningitis is associated with necrotizing granulomatous inflammation and giant cells, which can be patchy in distribution, involving the leptomeninges &/or dura.* **(Right)** *Intestinal ulcers in tuberculosis are transversal, granular, and punched out against smooth, hyperemic mucosa. They undermine the mucosa with tubercles proliferating along the edge ➔. (Courtesy Franz von Lichtenberg Collection of Infectious Disease Pathology, BWH.)*

Tuberculosis Verrucosa Cutis

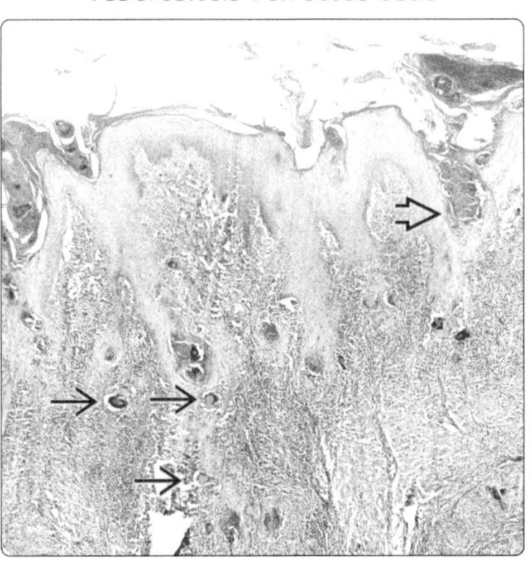

Lupus Vulgaris

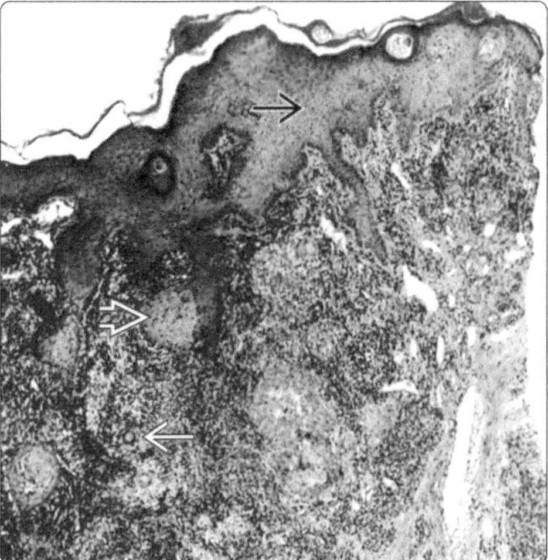

(Left) *Tuberculosis verrucosa cutis is characterized by verrucous hyperkeratosis ➔ with parakeratosis, hypergranulosis, and pseudoepitheliomatous hyperplasia. Nonnecrotizing granulomas are often present. This example has numerous Langhans cells ➔. (Courtesy B. Smoller, MD.)* **(Right)** *Lupus vulgaris demonstrates epidermal acanthosis ➔, and numerous tubercles ➔ are seen with giant cells ➔. (Courtesy Franz von Lichtenberg Collection of Infectious Disease Pathology, BWH.)*

Leprosy

KEY FACTS

ETIOLOGY/PATHOGENESIS

- Infection with *Mycobacterium leprae* or *Mycobacterium lepromatosis*, gram-positive, acid-fast, obligatory intracellular, rod-shaped bacilli

CLINICAL ISSUES

- Affects millions of people worldwide; endemic mainly in sub-Saharan Africa, Brazil, Indian subcontinent, and Southeast Asia
- Multidrug therapy is primarily used; curable with initiation and completion of therapy
- Skin involvement ranges from single hypopigmented macule to erythematous plaques and alopecia
- Peripheral nerve involvement includes thickened nerve (inflammation) with loss of sensation

MICROSCOPIC

- AFB best highlighted by Fite-Faraco stain (modified Ziehl-Neelsen)
- Lepromatous leprosy: Sheets of macrophages filled with numerous intracellular organisms
- Tuberculoid leprosy: "Tuberculoid" granulomatous reaction and extensive infiltration to nerves throughout dermis
- Intracellular and extracellular masses (globi): Clumps of bacilli (erythema nodosum leprosum)
- Positive skin smears but can be negative in tuberculoid or borderline forms

TOP DIFFERENTIAL DIAGNOSES

- MTB and NTM infections: Bacilli appear similar but positive by unmodified AFB stains; confirm with cultures or PCR
- Syphilis: *Treponema pallidum* spirochetes identified by Warthin-Starry stain or immunohistochemistry
- Leishmaniasis: Parasitized macrophages with amastigotes
- Sarcoidosis: Nonnecrotizing granulomata, negative for organisms
- Lymphoma: May have histiocytic component; negative for organisms

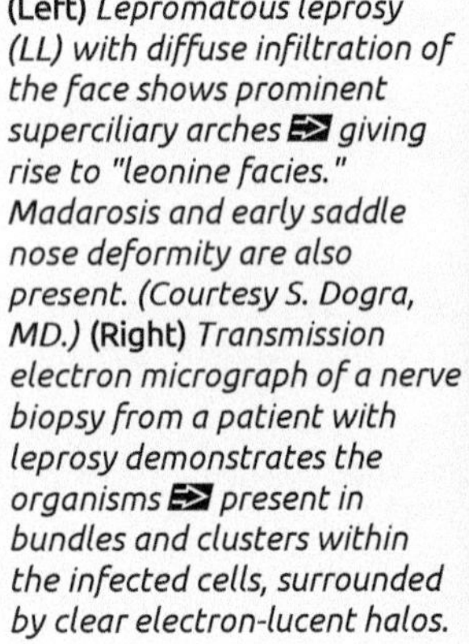

(Left) *Lepromatous leprosy (LL) with diffuse infiltration of the face shows prominent superciliary arches ➡ giving rise to "leonine facies." Madarosis and early saddle nose deformity are also present. (Courtesy S. Dogra, MD.)* **(Right)** *Transmission electron micrograph of a nerve biopsy from a patient with leprosy demonstrates the organisms ➡ present in bundles and clusters within the infected cells, surrounded by clear electron-lucent halos.*

Leonine Facies of Leprosy

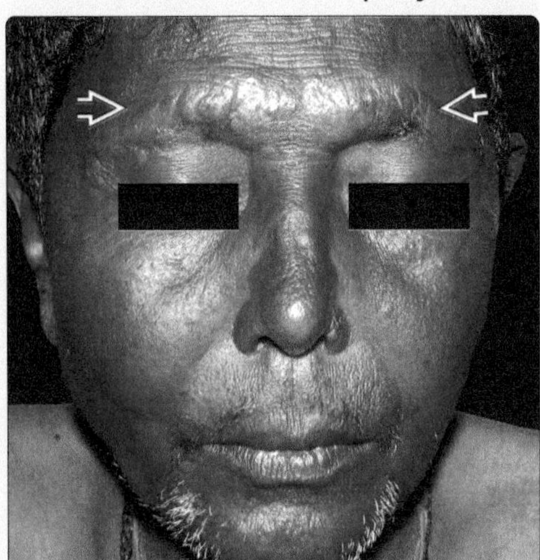

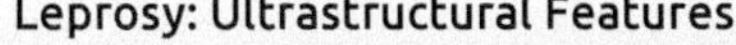

Leprosy: Ultrastructural Features

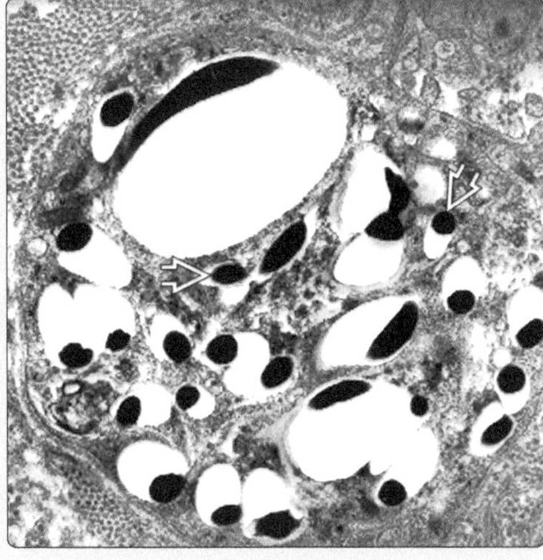

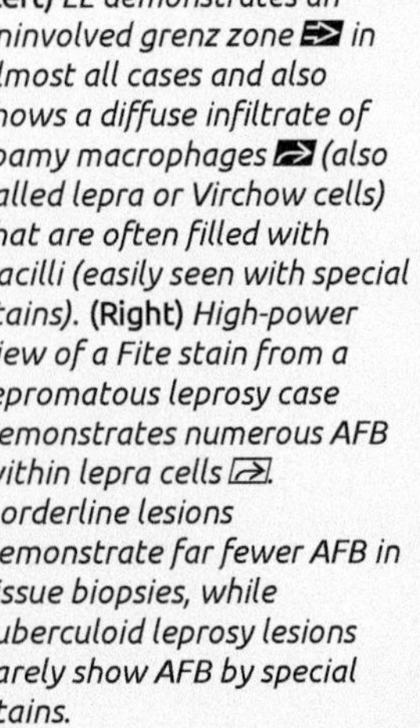

(Left) *LL demonstrates an uninvolved grenz zone ➡ in almost all cases and also shows a diffuse infiltrate of foamy macrophages ➡ (also called lepra or Virchow cells) that are often filled with bacilli (easily seen with special stains).* **(Right)** *High-power view of a Fite stain from a lepromatous leprosy case demonstrates numerous AFB within lepra cells ➡. Borderline lesions demonstrate far fewer AFB in tissue biopsies, while tuberculoid leprosy lesions rarely show AFB by special stains.*

Leprosy in Skin

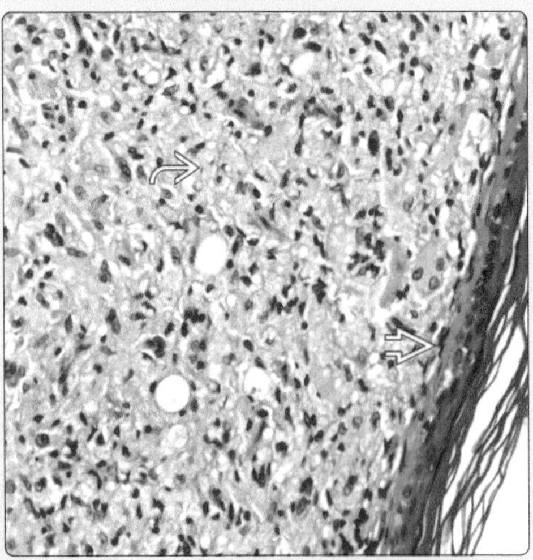

Acid-Fast Bacilli Morphology

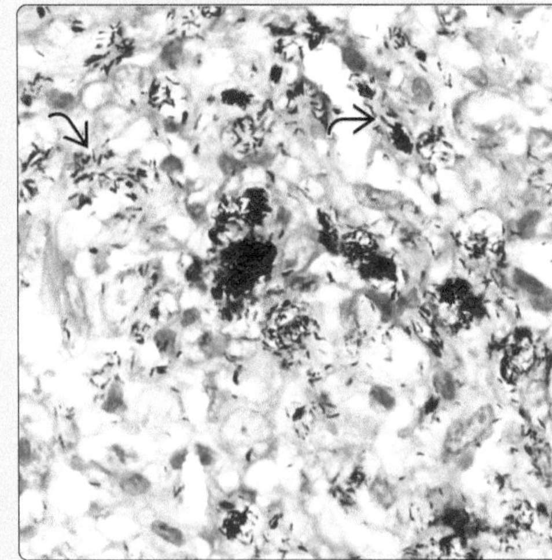

TERMINOLOGY

Synonyms

- Hansen disease

Definitions

- Middle English: "Lepry" (covered with scales, scaly)

ETIOLOGY/PATHOGENESIS

Infectious Agents

- Infection with *Mycobacterium leprae* or *Mycobacterium lepromatosis*, gram-positive, acid-fast, obligatory intracellular, rod-shaped bacilli
- Exact mechanism of transmission is unclear; possibly via droplets; no evidence of skin-skin contact producing infection (estimated 3- to 5-year incubation)
- Organisms spread to different organs (mainly skin and nerves), infect macrophages, endothelial cells and Schwann cells, and induce immune reaction

CLINICAL ISSUES

Epidemiology

- Affects millions of people; ~ 200,000 new cases/year
- Endemic mainly in sub-Saharan Africa, Brazil, Indian subcontinent, and Southeast Asia
- *M. lepromatosis* mainly in Mexico and Central America
- Armadillos may be source of infection in USA

Presentation

- May be entirely asymptomatic
- Skin involvement ranges from single hypopigmented macule to erythematous plaques and alopecia
- Peripheral nerve involvement includes thickened nerve (inflammation) with loss of sensation
- **WHO Classification**
  - Paucibacillary: No bacilli on skin smear test; < 5 lesions
  - Multibacillary: Bacilli on skin smear test; ≥ 6 lesions
- **Ridley-Jopling Classification**
  - Tuberculoid leprosy (TL): Strong immunity; few hypopigmented asymmetric lesions; minimal loss of sensation or nerve thickening
  - Borderline leprosy (BL): Most common form, intermediate severity; numerous macules, papules, plaques; loss of sensation, swollen lymph nodes
  - Lepromatous leprosy (LL): Limited immunity; symmetric widespread lesions, lepromas, alopecia, madarosis, sensation loss, bone and cartilage destruction, and systemic involvement
  - Indeterminate: Hypopigmented macules and slight loss of sensation; may resolve or progress
- **Types of Leprosy Reactions**
  - Type 1 reaction: Reversal reaction, occurs in TL or BL; edema and erythema of preexisting lesions and neuritis
  - Type 2 reaction (erythema nodosum leprosum): Occurs in LL; painful erythematous nodules and fever; inflammation of other tissues
  - Lucio leprosy (*M. lepromatosis*): Multiple bizarre-patterned skin ulcers

Laboratory Tests

- Serology not used for diagnosis
- PCR (fresh, FFPE samples) can confirm diagnosis
  - Multiple targets, including 16S rRNA, *rpoB*, *folP*, and *gyrA*
  - RLPM: Unique repetitive element present in *M. lepromatosis*

Treatment

- Antibiotics include dapsone, rifampicin, and clofazimine
- Steroids and other antiinflammatory medications to relieve nerve swelling and prevent long-term deformity
- Surgery to drain abscesses or correct deformities

Prognosis

- Curable with initiation and completion of therapy

MICROBIOLOGY

Culture

- Has not been cultured on artificial media
- Foot pads of mice or armadillos (impractical for routine diagnosis)

MICROSCOPIC

Histologic Features

- TL: Lymphocytes, epithelioid histiocytes, and multinucleated giant cells with necrosis, predominantly around nerves and cutaneous adnexa; rare organisms
- BL: Foamy macrophages and circumscribed granulomatous reaction with lymphocytic response involving perineural and periadnexal regions; numerous organisms
- LL: Sheets of foamy macrophages (Virchow cells) with abundant pink to pale cytoplasm filled with numerous intracellular organisms (globi) diffusely involving dermis
- Lucio phenomenon: Leukocytoclastic vasculitis and epidermal infarction

Cytologic Features

- Positive skin smears but can be negative in TL or BL forms

ANCILLARY TESTS

Special Stains and Immunohistochemistry

- Acid-fast, rod-shaped bacilli (1-8 μm long x 0.2-0.5 μm in diameter), best highlighted with modified Ziehl-Neelsen stains, such as Fite-Faraco or Wade-Fite
- When organisms are abundant, they may also be identified standard Ziehl-Neelsen or Kinyoun AFB stains, GMS, Gram, and H&E
- Positive with antimycobacterial antibodies (but may cross react with other species)

DIFFERENTIAL DIAGNOSIS

Tuberculosis and Nontuberculous Mycobacteria Infections

- Inflammatory patterns range from necrotizing granulomatous to diffuse histiocytic infiltrate
- Organisms strongly positive on Fite and unmodified AFB stains; however, morphology alone cannot be used to distinguish, and confirmation with cultures or PCR is required

Syphilis

- Lymphoplasmacytic inflammatory infiltrate with epithelioid cells and occasional giant cells
- *Treponema pallidum* spirochetes identified by Warthin-Starry stain or immunohistochemistry

Leishmaniasis

- Ulcerated epidermis, lymphoplasmacytic infiltrate, parasitized macrophages containing *Leishmania* spp. amastigotes

Sarcoidosis

- Predominantly nonnecrotizing granulomatous inflammation
- Negative for organisms by stains, PCR, and cultures

Lymphoma

- May include histocytic infiltrate mimicking leprosy
- Negative for organisms by stains, PCR, and cultures

SELECTED REFERENCES

1. HRSA: National Hansen's disease (leprosy) program. Updated May 2023. Accessed June 4, 2023. https://www.hrsa.gov/hansens-disease
2. Chen KH et al: Leprosy: a review of epidemiology, clinical diagnosis, and management. J Trop Med. 2022:8652062, 2022
3. Romero-Navarrete M et al: Leprosy caused by Mycobacterium lepromatosis. Am J Clin Pathol. 158(6):678-86, 2022
4. Hockings KJ et al: Leprosy in wild chimpanzees. Nature. 598(7882):652-6, 2021
5. Carlock S et al: Hansen disease (leprosy) and armadillo exposure in arkansas: a case series. Am J Dermatopathol. 42(10):769-73, 2020
6. Sharma R et al: Isolation of Mycobacterium lepromatosis and development of molecular diagnostic assays to distinguish Mycobacterium leprae and M. lepromatosis. Clin Infect Dis. 71(8):e262-9, 2020
7. Wroblewski KJ et al: The AFIP history of ocular leprosy. Saudi J Ophthalmol. 33(3):255-9, 2019
8. Pinheiro RO et al: Innate immune responses in leprosy. Front Immunol. 9:518, 2018
9. Singh A et al: Histopathological features in leprosy, post-kala-azar dermal leishmaniasis, and cutaneous leishmaniasis. Indian J Dermatol Venereol Leprol. 79(3):360-6, 2013
10. Grimaud J: [Peripheral nerve damage in patients with leprosy.] Rev Neurol (Paris). 168(12):967-74, 2012

(Left) *LL demonstrates diffuse infiltration with nodules involving the ear lobules and face. Leprosy prefers cooler areas of the body (ears, nose, and peripheral nerves). (Courtesy S. Dogra, MD.)* **(Right)** *Medium-power view of a case of LL demonstrates a diffuse infiltration of the arrector pili muscle by the histocytic cells and lymphocytes.*

Nodular Lepromatous Leprosy

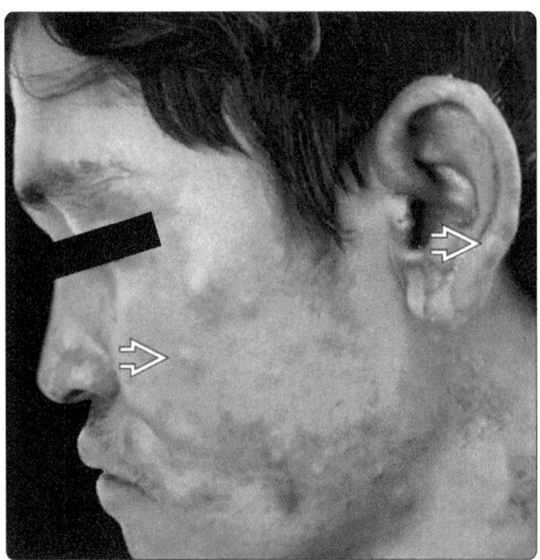

Lepromatous Infiltrates

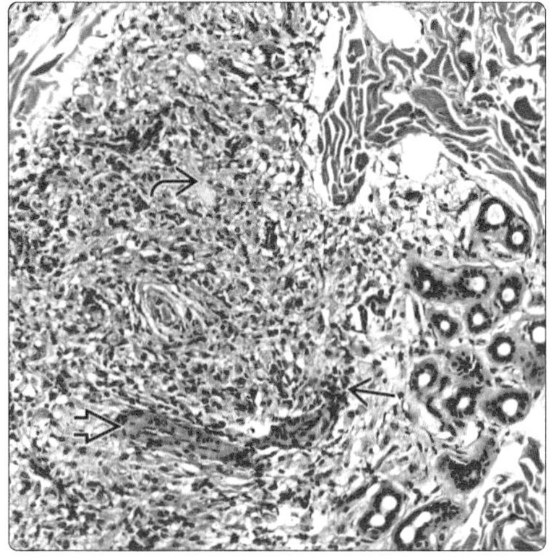

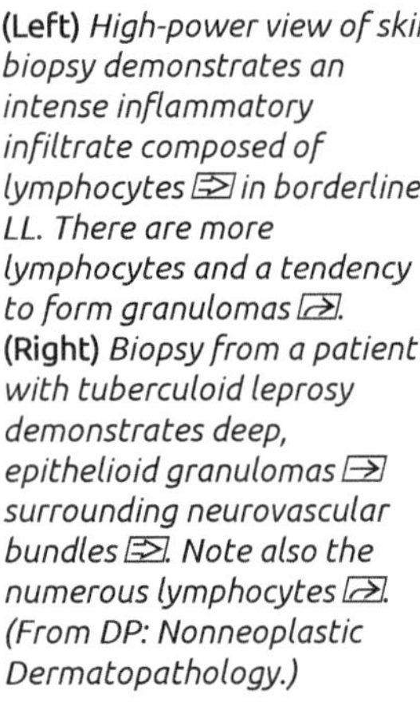

(Left) *High-power view of skin biopsy demonstrates an intense inflammatory infiltrate composed of lymphocytes in borderline LL. There are more lymphocytes and a tendency to form granulomas.* **(Right)** *Biopsy from a patient with tuberculoid leprosy demonstrates deep, epithelioid granulomas surrounding neurovascular bundles. Note also the numerous lymphocytes. (From DP: Nonneoplastic Dermatopathology.)*

Lymphocytes and Granulomata

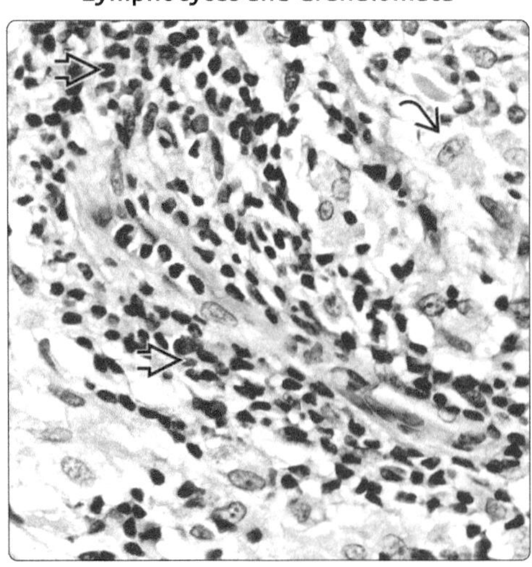

Tuberculoid Leprosy

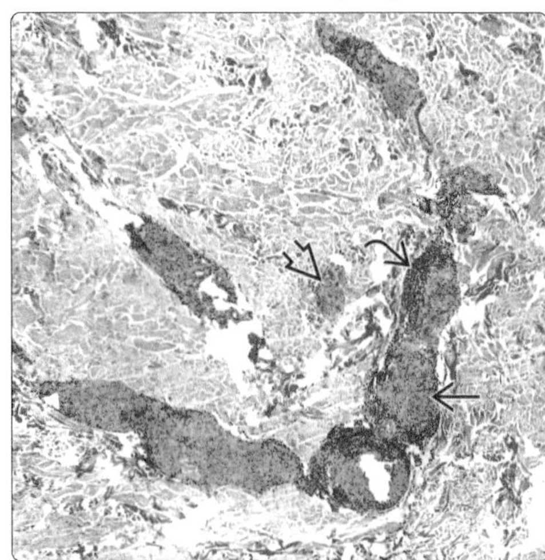

Skin Biopsy: Fite Stain

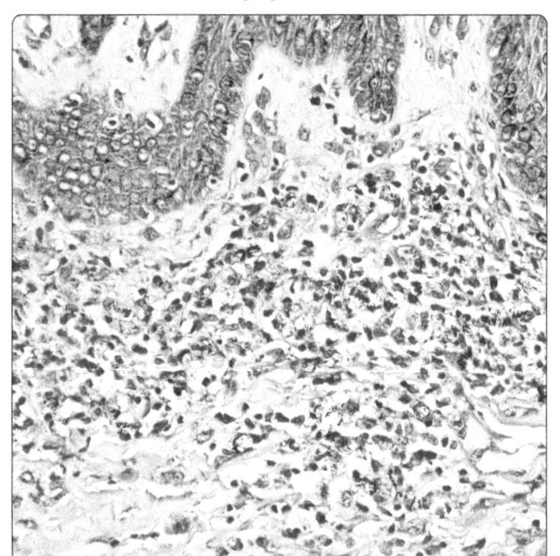

Skin Biopsy: Immunohistochemistry

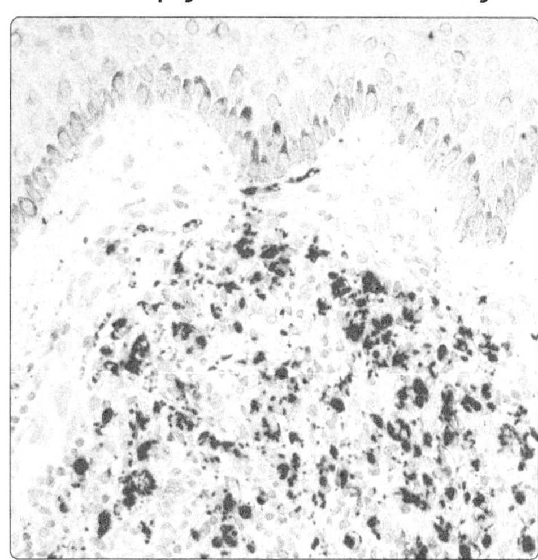

(Left) *Fite staining of this skin biopsy highlights numerous AFB within foamy macrophages (lepra cells; Virchow cells).* **(Right)** *Immunohistochemistry using a polyclonal antimycobacterial antibody highlights numerous individual and clumps of AFB within foamy macrophages. Bacilli appear wider than with Fite staining due to the alkaline phosphatase red chromogen, which can be helpful in identifying rare organisms in tuberculous leprosy.*

Lucio Phenomenon

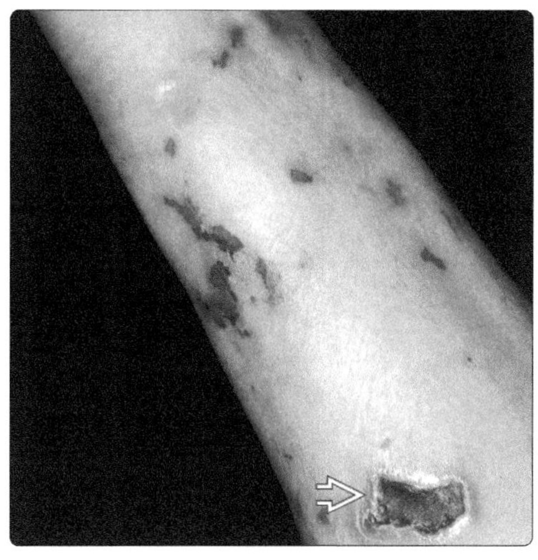

Thrombotic Vasculopathy

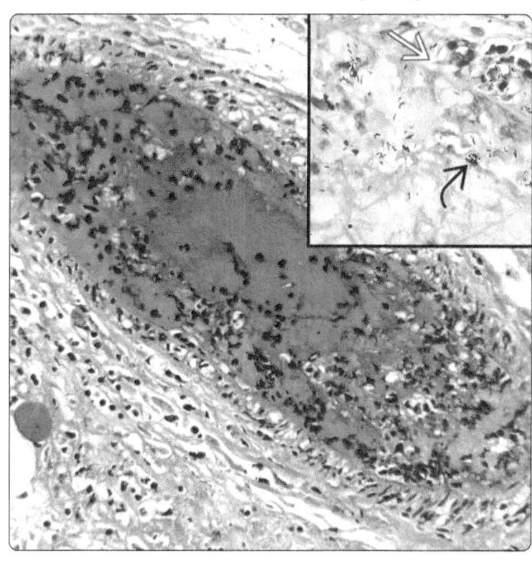

(Left) *A case of Lucio phenomenon (due to Mycobacterium lepromatosis infection) shows ulcerated skin nodules ➡. (Courtesy E. Kraus, MD.)* **(Right)** *This biopsy of Lucio phenomenon shows a thrombotic vasculopathy pattern with a large thrombus in a vessel, surrounding mononuclear inflammation, and a mild endothelial proliferation that can be quite marked at times. A Fite stain demonstrates positive-staining AFB within the thrombus ➡ and vessel wall ➡. (Courtesy D. Scollard, MD, PhD.)*

Nerve Biopsy

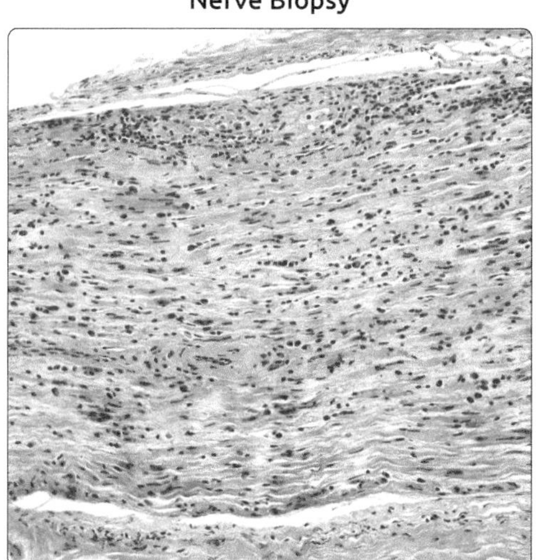

Nerve Biopsy: Fite Stain

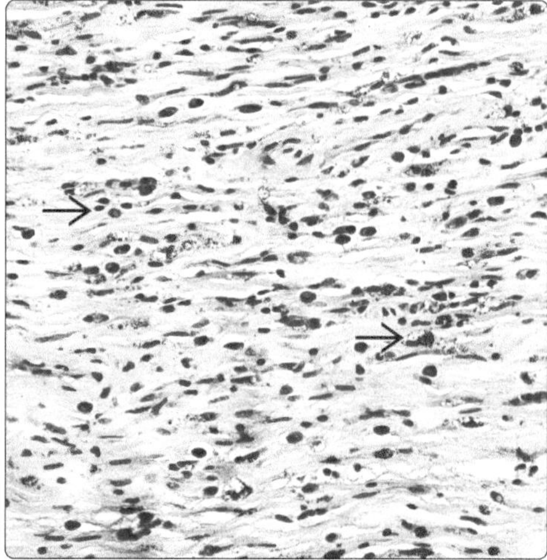

(Left) *Biopsy of a sural nerve from a patient with lepromatous leprosy shows moderate lymphocytic inflammation and numerous foamy-appearing macrophages.* **(Right)** *Fite staining of a sural nerve biopsy from a patient with lepromatous leprosy highlights abundant red-staining bacilli within foamy macrophages ➡ and Schwann cells.*

Buruli Ulcer

KEY FACTS

ETIOLOGY/PATHOGENESIS

- Chronic necrotizing skin and soft tissue infection, caused by *Mycobacterium ulcerans*, predominantly observed in West Africa and South Australia
- Mode of transmission poorly understood; presumably acquired from stagnant water in ponds, swamps, backwaters, dams

CLINICAL ISSUES

- May begins with papule, nodule, or edematous plaque that progresses to necrotizing ulcer
- Ulcer is typically painless or mildly painful, despite extensive tissue destruction
- Ulcers may take months to years to heal and leave contracting scars, even with appropriate antibiotic treatment but inadequate would management

MICROBIOLOGY

- Bacilli may be observed on smears stained with Ziehl-Neelsen, Kinyoun, or auramine-rhodamine methods
- Yellowish colonies grow in 6-12 weeks at 29-33 °C; species confirmed by MALDI-TOF or PCR

MICROSCOPIC

- Extensive cutaneous necrosis extending into subcutis
- Edema with few inflammatory cells in absence of secondary infection (by pyogenic bacteria)
- Vasculitis and thrombosis present around areas of necrosis with bluish globular clumps of extracellular bacilli
- AFB stains highlight numerous bacilli during necrotic, nonulcerative and ulcerative stages

TOP DIFFERENTIAL DIAGNOSES

- Arterial and venous ulcers: Older adult patients, localized to legs and feet; no AFBs
- Diabetic ulcer: Diabetic patients with neuropathy and peripheral vascular disease; no AFBs
- Leishmaniasis: Mixed acute and chronic inflammation with poorly formed granulomas and amastigotes

Buruli Ulcer

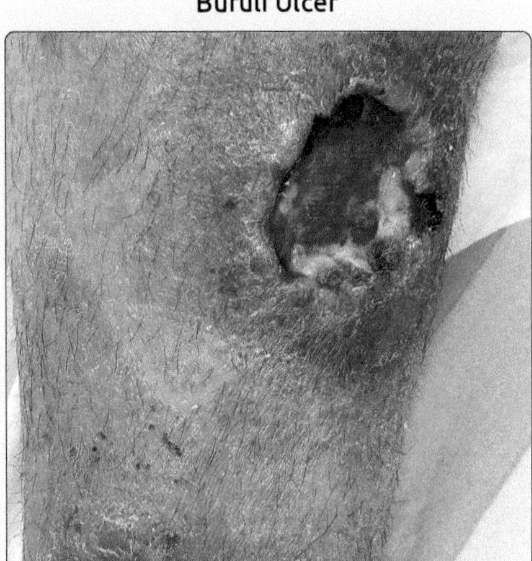

Buruli Ulcer

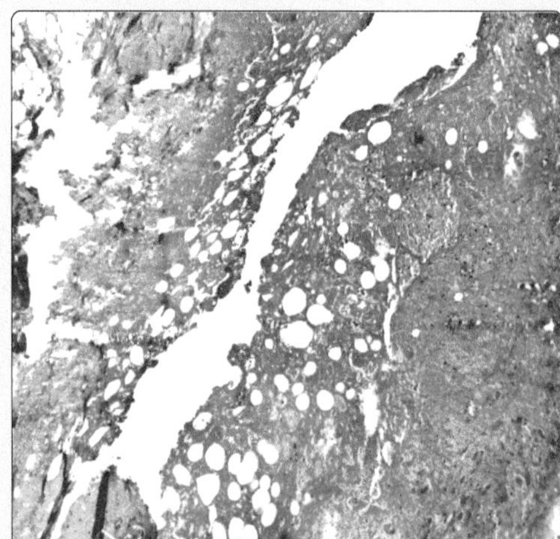

(Left) *A deep ulcer with undermined borders develops from an edematous papule or plaque characteristically. Of note, these are frequently asymptomatic. (Courtesy D. Diaz, MD.)* **(Right)** *Extensive necrosis of the dermis and subcutaneous tissue is observed in this H&E-stained section, findings characteristic of Buruli ulcer. (Courtesy D. Diaz, MD.)*

Buruli Ulcer Acid-Fast Stain

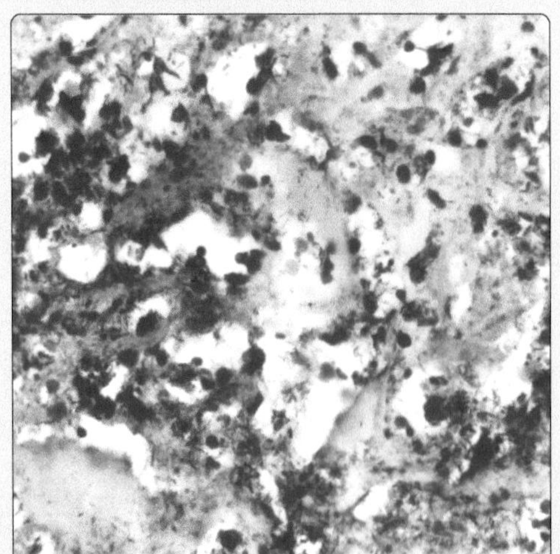

Buruli Ulcer: Clumps of Acid-Fast Bacilli

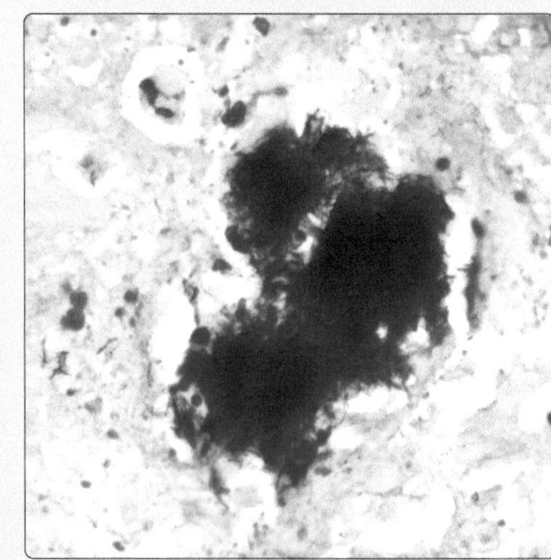

(Left) *The presence of abundant acid-fast bacilli within necrotic tissue is typical of Mycobacterium ulcerans infection. (Courtesy D. Diaz, MD.)* **(Right)** *Large "clumps" of acid-fast, alcohol-resistant bacilli within necrotic tissue from an ulcer are virtually pathognomonic of a Buruli ulcer. (Courtesy D. Diaz, MD.)*

TERMINOLOGY

Synonyms

- Buruli ulcer (BU), Bairnsdale ulcer, Searles ulcer, Daintree ulcer, Mossman ulcer, Kumasi ulcer, Sik-belonga-sepik

ETIOLOGY/PATHOGENESIS

Infectious Agents

- Chronic necrotizing skin and soft tissue infection, caused by *Mycobacterium ulcerans*, 1st described in Australia in 1948; considered neglected tropical disease
- Pathology due to lipid-like, diffusible exotoxin mycolactone and not mycobacterium itself
- Mode of transmission poorly understood; human-to-human transmission has not been documented
- Presumably acquired from stagnant water in ponds, swamps, backwaters, dams; mosquitoes may be vector in certain regions, including Australia

CLINICAL ISSUES

Epidemiology

- BU is 3rd most commonly reported mycobacterial infection after tuberculosis and leprosy; estimated as high as 5,000-6,000 cases annually, equal distribution between males and females
- Predominantly observed in Central and West Africa and South Australia but has also been reported in other countries with temperate and subtropical climates (e.g., Central and South America)
- Recent increased incidence in urban settings in Australia (Victoria) likely associated with increased rainfall and exposure to possums and koalas (who also have disease)
- In Africa, ~ 50% cases occur in children < 15 years old; in Australia and Japan, mostly in adults

Presentation

- May begin with papule, nodule, or edematous plaque that progresses to expansive necrotizing ulcer
- Ulcer is typically painless or mildly painful, despite extensive tissue destruction
- Mostly affects exposed body areas, such as arms and legs
- Not all infected individuals manifest disease, and spontaneous healing has been documented

Laboratory Tests

- PCR targeting IS*2404* insertion sequence of *M. ulcerans* can be performed on tissue biopsies (~ 98% sensitivity) and fine-needle aspirates (~ 86% sensitivity)

Treatment

- 1st-line treatment is 8 weeks of rifampicin/streptomycin
- Paradoxical worsening of symptoms is characteristic during effective antibiotic therapy
- Wound management is essential and frequently neglected

Prognosis

- Dependent on extent of disease; favorable with complete healing with antibiotic therapy and wound management
- Ulcers may take months to years to heal and leave contracting scars, even with appropriate antibiotic treatment but inadequate would management

MICROBIOLOGY

Culture and Identification

- Sample center of nonulcerated lesion or beneath undermined edge of ulcerative lesion, down to fascia
- Bacilli may be observed on smears stained with Ziehl-Neelsen (ZN), Kinyoun, or auramine-rhodamine methods
- Grows in 6-12 weeks at 29-33 °C on Löwenstein-Jensen medium or Middlebrook 7H12B (BACTEC system)
- Cultures appear yellowish and rough with well-demarcated edges; species confirmed by MALDI-TOF or PCR

MACROSCOPIC

General Features

- Ulcer has deep undermining edges with extensive cutaneous and soft tissue destruction and exposure of underlying structures (e.g., tendons)

MICROSCOPIC

Histologic Features

- Extensive cutaneous necrosis extending into subcutis; adipose ghost cells
- Edema with few inflammatory cells in absence of secondary infection (by pyogenic bacteria)
- Vasculitis and thrombosis present around areas of necrosis with bluish globular clumps of extracellular bacilli
- Granulomatous inflammation with early healing, followed by granulation tissue, fibrosis, and scar

Cytologic Features

- Pus or extensive necrotic tissue, depending on stage

ANCILLARY TESTS

Special Stains

- AFBs (ZN, Fite-Faraco) highlight numerous bacilli during necrotic, nonulcerative, and ulcerative stages

DIFFERENTIAL DIAGNOSIS

Arterial and Venous Ulcers

- Older adult patients, localized to legs and feet; no AFBs

Diabetic Ulcer

- Diabetic patients with neuropathy and peripheral vascular disease; no AFBs

Leishmaniasis

- Mixed acute and chronic inflammation with poorly formed granulomas and amastigotes

SELECTED REFERENCES

1. Muleta AJ et al: Understanding the transmission of Mycobacterium ulcerans: a step towards controlling Buruli ulcer. PLoS Negl Trop Dis. 15(8):e0009678, 2021
2. Guarner J: Buruli ulcer: review of a neglected skin mycobacterial disease. J Clin Microbiol. 56(4), 2018
3. Yotsu RR et al: Buruli ulcer: a review of the current knowledge. Curr Trop Med Rep. 5(4):247-56, 2018
4. Phillips RO et al: Sensitivity of PCR targeting Mycobacterium ulcerans by use of fine-needle aspirates for diagnosis of Buruli ulcer. J Clin Microbiol. 47(4):924-6, 2009
5. Guarner J et al: Histopathologic features of Mycobacterium ulcerans infection. Emerg Infect Dis. 9(6):651-6, 2003

Mycobacterium avium Complex and Other Nontuberculous Mycobacterial Infections

KEY FACTS

ETIOLOGY/PATHOGENESIS

- Infection with nontuberculous mycobacteria (NTM), aerobic, rod-shaped non-spore-forming, acid-fast organisms
- *Mycobacterium avium* complex (MAC)
- Slow-growing NTM (colonies > 7 days): *M. kansasii, M. xenopi, M. ulcerans, M. marinum, M. haemophilum*
- Rapidly growing mycobacteria (RGM): *M. fortuitum, M. chelonae, M. abscessus, M. smegmatis, M. goodii, M. flavescens, M. vaccae*
- MALDI-TOF MS or sequencing (16S rRNA, *hsp65*) for speciation

MICROSCOPIC

- MAC: Lungs/lymph nodes with necrotizing granulomas or histiocyte infiltrate with many intracellular AFB
- *M. kansasii*: Necrotizing granulomas, suppurative abscess, spindle cell proliferations, granular eosinophilic necrosis
- *M. marinum*: Epidermal changes, prominent necrosis, subcutaneous infiltrates, abscess, and granulomas
- *M. chelonae*: Necrotizing folliculitis
- Scrofula: Granulomas with necrotic centers; overlying dermis with inflammatory infiltrate
- Osteomyelitis: Granulomatous inflammation, necrosis
- Bacilli highlighted by acid-fast stains (e.g., Ziehl-Neelsen, Kinyoun, Fite-Faraco) and IHC

TOP DIFFERENTIAL DIAGNOSES

- Tuberculosis: Necrotizing granulomatous inflammation; positive AFB stain; culture/PCR to distinguish
- Leprosy: Skin and peripheral nerve involvement; rare to abundant AFB (highlighted by Fite-Faraco); confirm by PCR
- Fungal infections (e.g., *Cryptococcus* spp., *Histoplasma* spp.): Fungal elements highlighted by GMS or PAS-D stains
- Bartonellosis: Gram-negative bacilli highlighted by silver stains; confirm by PCR
- Bacterial abscess (e.g., *Staphylococcus* spp., *Streptococcus* spp.): Positive Gram or silver stain; speciation by culture/PCR

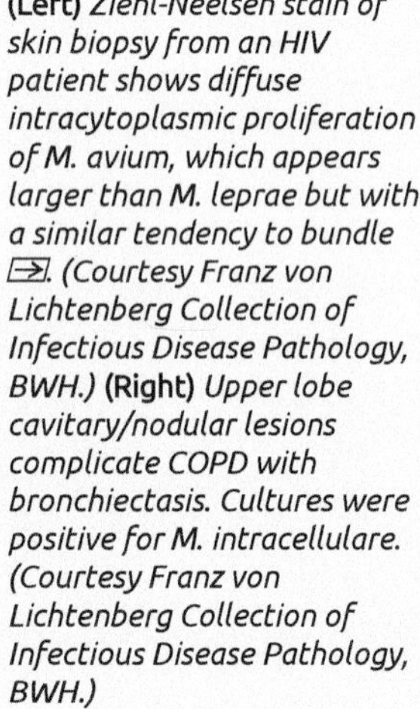

(Left) *Ziehl-Neelsen stain of skin biopsy from an HIV patient shows diffuse intracytoplasmic proliferation of M. avium, which appears larger than M. leprae but with a similar tendency to bundle →. (Courtesy Franz von Lichtenberg Collection of Infectious Disease Pathology, BWH.)* **(Right)** *Upper lobe cavitary/nodular lesions complicate COPD with bronchiectasis. Cultures were positive for M. intracellulare. (Courtesy Franz von Lichtenberg Collection of Infectious Disease Pathology, BWH.)*

Mycobacterium avium Acid-Fast Stain

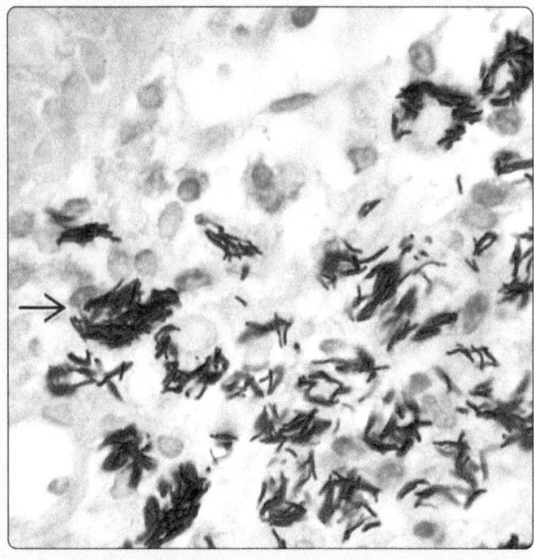

Mycobacterium intracellulare Lung Pathology

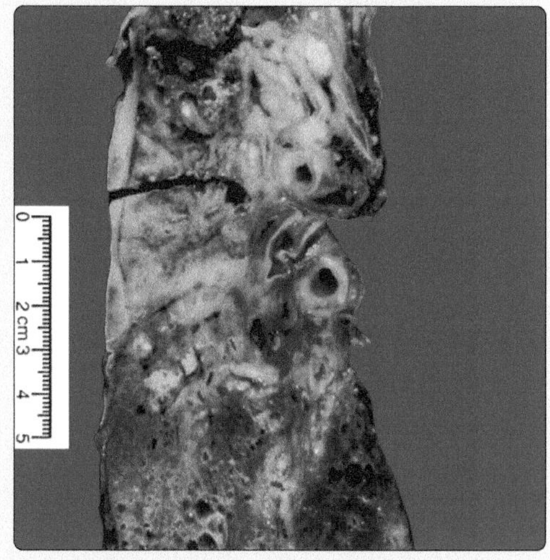

(Left) *A skin punch biopsy from a patient who presented with several weeks of acid-fast bacillus (+) nodules is shown with areas of superficial abscess formation ➡ and deep organized chronic inflammation →.* **(Right)** *High magnification of a tissue section from a patient with atypical Mycobacterium spp. infection demonstrates giant cells → of various morphologies admixed with epithelioid histiocytes ⇨.*

Skin With Necrotizing Abscess

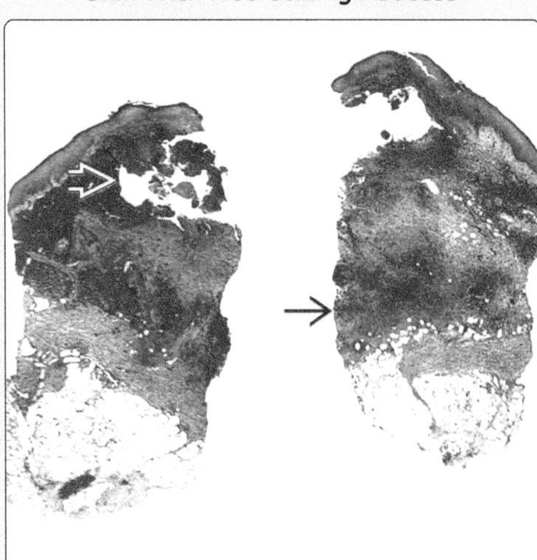

Giant Cells

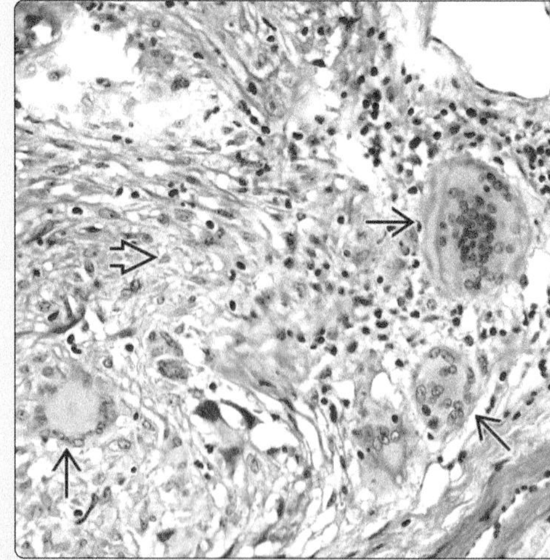

ETIOLOGY/PATHOGENESIS

Infectious Agents

- > 200 *Mycobacterium* spp. identified, many of which cause disease in humans
- *M. avium* complex (MAC): *M. avium, M. intracellulare, M. chimera, M. colombiense*; widely present in environment; transmission by inhalation or ingestion of contaminated food or water
- Slow-growing nontuberculous mycobacteria (NTM): *M. kansasii, M. xenopi, M. simiae, M. ulcerans, M. marinum, M. haemophilum*, and *M. gordonae*
- Rapidly growing mycobacteria (RGM): Nonpigmented (*M. fortuitum, M. chelonae/M. abscessus*), late pigmenting (*M. smegmatis, M. goodii*), early pigmenting (*M. flavescens, M. vaccae*)
- Whole-genome sequencing analyses have led to proposals for splitting *Mycobacterium* genus into 5 genera

CLINICAL ISSUES

Presentation

- MAC
  - Sputum cultures can be positive in patients without disease (need to be accompanied by clinical symptoms, positive imaging, etc.)
  - Pulmonary disease in HIV(+): Upper lobe fibronodular and cavitary disease
  - Older, thin women (Lady Windermere disease): Lung nodules associated with bronchiectasis, and tree-in-bud opacities on imaging
  - Chronic obstructive pulmonary disease (COPD) associated: Fibrocavitary lung disease
  - Pigeon or hot tub exposure: Hypersensitivity pneumonitis vs. direct infection; subacute/chronic course
  - Lymphadenitis: Children < 5 years old; nontender, firm, unilateral, enlarged cervical nodes often associated with ulceration and fistula formation
  - Disseminated disease in HIV(+), hairy cell leukemia, and primary immunodeficiencies: Fever, weight loss, anemia, abdominal pain, diarrhea, hepatosplenomegaly
- Slow-growing NTM
  - *M. kansasii*: Upper lobe, fibronodular cavitary disease similar to MAC
  - *M. xenopi*: Osteomyelitis
  - *M. ulcerans*: Buruli ulcers
  - *M. marinum*: Papules and ulcerations on hands and arms associated with cleaning fish tank
  - *M. haemophilum*: Skin nodules, sometimes associated with soft tissue abscess, fistulas, and osteomyelitis
  - *M. gordonae*: Rarely, if ever, cause of clinical disease
- RGM
  - Community-acquired infections of skin and soft tissue; can be associated with tattoos, nail salon furunculosis, plastic surgery
  - Also implicated in bone and joint infections, catheter-associated infections, and disseminated infections; more commonly in immunocompromised
  - *M. abscessus*: Chronic lung infection, especially in patients with cystic fibrosis

Laboratory Tests

- PCR/sequencing (e.g.,16S rRNA, *hsp65*, and *rpoB* genes) from primary specimens; formalin-fixed, paraffin-embedded tissue; or culture isolates

Treatment

- MAC: Difficult to treat, requires multiple-drug regimen given over many months; agents include clarithromycin, ethambutol, rifampin, amikacin, and streptomycin
- Isolated lymphadenitis often treated with surgical excision alone
- NTMs can be difficult to treat with antimicrobials; standard treatment varies by species

Prognosis

- MAC: Excellent prognosis in childhood lymphadenitis; extremely poor in disseminated disease in AIDS patients

MICROBIOLOGY

Culture and Microbiologic Identification

- Mycobacteria are aerobic, rod-shaped (0.2-0.6 µm wide x 1.0-10 µm long), non-spore-forming, acid-fast organisms
- Some rods can appear bent or beaded; some demonstrate cording (e.g., *M. gordonae, M. chelonae, M. marinum*)
- Commonly used media include Löwenstein-Jensen- and Middlebrook-based formulations; RGM produce colonies within 7 days while slow growers take longer
  - *M. haemophilum* requires hemoglobin, hemin (factor X), or ferric ammonium citrate
  - *M. marinum, M. ulcerans*, and *M. haemophilum* grow best at lower temperatures (28-30 °C)
- MAC and *M. kansasii* can be identified by nucleic acid hybridization assays (Gen-Probe)
- MALDI-TOF MS is becoming standard for identification; sequencing may also be used for speciation

MACROSCOPIC

Gross Features

- RGM: Small to large abscess with purulent centers
- Slow-growing NTM: Granulomatous inflammation with caseous (yellow, cheese-like) appearance; may include dense fibrous capsule and calcifications in older lesions
- Spindle cell nodules of MAC may appear white and solid similar to tumors

MICROSCOPIC

Histologic Features

- Lungs
  - MAC in immunocompromised: Cavitating lesions with necrotizing granulomas (similar to MTB); loose histiocytic infiltrate with many intracellular bacilli may be present (with increasing immunosuppression)
  - MAC in immunocompetent (older women): Often in right middle lobe, extensive swaths of nonnecrotizing epithelioid histiocytes ± well-organized necrotizing granulomas; extensive underlying pulmonary pathology is frequently present
  - MAC hypersensitivity pneumonitis ("hot tub lung"): Well-formed granulomas, often peribronchial; organisms rarely detected

- *M. kansasii*: Necrotizing granulomas, suppurative abscess, spindle cell proliferations, and foci of granular eosinophilic necrosis; organisms described as coarsely beaded, folded, or cross-linked curved ends
- Skin
  - Manifestations range widely by species and host immune status; most characteristic pattern is granulomas with necrotic, neutrophilic centers surrounded by histiocytes and peripheral lymphocytic infiltrate; granulomas less tightly formed than with MTB
  - *M. marinum*: Acanthosis, pseudoepitheliomatous hyperplasia, and exocytosis; necrosis may be prominent; immunosuppressed associated with deeper (subcutaneous), more diffuse infiltrates, abscess, and more prominent granulomas
  - *M. chelonae:* Necrotizing folliculitis
  - *M. ulcerans* (Buruli ulcer): Extensive necrosis of subcutaneous tissue with minimal inflammatory reaction
- Lymph nodes
  - Lymphadenitis requires excisional biopsy (needle aspirations are generally avoided due to complications, such as fistulas)
  - Scrofula: Involved lymph nodes have multiple granulomas with necrotic centers; overlying dermis can be involved by extensive inflammatory infiltrate; organisms rarely observed (culture needed for definitive diagnosis)
  - MAC lymphadenitis in HIV(+) patients may be more marked by histiocytic infiltrate containing large numbers of intracellular bacilli
- Other
  - Osteomyelitis: Granulomatous inflammation in immunocompetent patients; mixed inflammatory infiltrate, necrosis
  - Virtually any organ may be affected in disseminated disease; general histopathologic feature is necrotizing granuloma but varies widely with organism and immune status of patient
  - MAC is most common agent associated with immune reconstitution syndrome in HIV infection
  - Mycobacterial spindle cell pseudotumor may be found in lymph nodes, lung, skin, brain, etc.: Spindle cells are foamy histiocytes containing many mycobacteria but may be mistaken for neoplasm

ANCILLARY TESTS

Special Stains

- Number of acid-fast bacilli (AFB) seen on Ziehl-Neelsen (standard AFB stain) or Kinyoun (modified AFB) may be few/scattered to large numbers
- Fite (modified by addition of vegetable oil) for organisms, such as *M. leprae*, also stains other *Mycobacterium* spp.
- Gram and silver stains may be weakly positive when large numbers or organisms are present

Immunohistochemistry

- Anti-*Mycobacterium* spp. IHC may have increased sensitivity but decreased specificity compared to histochemical stains (varies with antibody)

PCR

- Molecular testing can distinguish between *Mycobacterium* spp.; most useful to detect slow-growing species (i.e., cultures negative at 1 week); low yield in absence of histologically identified AFBs

DIFFERENTIAL DIAGNOSIS

Tuberculosis

- *M. tuberculosis* complex infection with necrotizing granulomatous inflammation
- Positive AFB stain; requires culture/PCR to distinguish

Leprosy

- *M. leprae* infection involving skin and peripheral nerves
- Abundant (lepromatous) or rare (tuberculous) numbers of AFB; best highlighted by Fite-Faraco stain
- Does not grow in culture; confirm by PCR

Fungal Infections

- e.g., *Cryptococcus* spp., *Histoplasma* spp. *Coccidioides* spp. infections; may be associated with necrotizing granulomatous inflammation
- Fungal elements (e.g., yeast, spherules, endospores) identified by GMS or PAS-D stains; AFB stain negative

Bartonellosis

- *Bartonella* spp. infections with necrotizing granulomatous inflammation
- Negative AFB stain; gram-negative bacilli highlighted by silver stains; confirm by PCR

Bacterial Abscess

- e.g., *Staphylococcus* spp., *Streptococcus* spp., polymicrobial infections; abundant neutrophils and necrotic debris
- Negative AFB stain; positive Gram or silver stain (depending on organism); culture/PCR to confirm

SELECTED REFERENCES

1. Bekina-Sreenivasan D et al: Mycobacterium xenopi native vertebral osteomyelitis and discitis: case & review of published cases. IDCases. 33:e01835, 2023
2. El Zein S et al: Clinical manifestations, treatment and outcomes of patients infected with Mycobacterium haemophilum with a focus on immune reconstitution inflammatory syndrome: a retrospective multi-site study. Infect Dis (Lond). 55(7):467-79, 2023
3. Varley CD et al: Nontuberculous mycobacteria: diagnosis and therapy. Clin Chest Med. 43(1):89-98, 2022
4. Johansen MD et al: Non-tuberculous mycobacteria and the rise of Mycobacterium abscessus. Nat Rev Microbiol. 18(7):392-407, 2020
5. Hogan JI et al: Mycobacterial musculoskeletal infections. Thorac Surg Clin. 29(1):85-94, 2019
6. Martiniano SL et al: Nontuberculous mycobacterial infections in cystic fibrosis. Thorac Surg Clin. 29(1):95-108, 2019
7. Cenci E et al: Evaluation of IVD 3.0 Vitek MS matrix-assisted laser desorption ionization-time of flight mass spectrometry for identification of Mycobacterium tuberculosis and nontuberculous mycobacteria and its use in routine diagnostics. Eur J Clin Microbiol Infect Dis. 37(10):2027-9, 2018
8. Franco-Paredes C et al: Cutaneous mycobacterial infections. Clin Microbiol Rev. 32(1), 2018
9. Griffin I et al: Outbreak of tattoo-associated nontuberculous mycobacterial skin infections. Clin Infect Dis. 69(6):949-55, 2018
10. Gupta RS et al: Phylogenomics and comparative genomic studies robustly support division of the genus Mycobacterium into an emended genus Mycobacterium and four novel genera. Front Microbiol. 9:67, 2018
11. Sia TY et al: Clinical and pathological evaluation of Mycobacterium marinum group skin infections associated with fish markets in New York City. Clin Infect Dis. 62(5):590-5, 2016

Neutrophilic Abscess

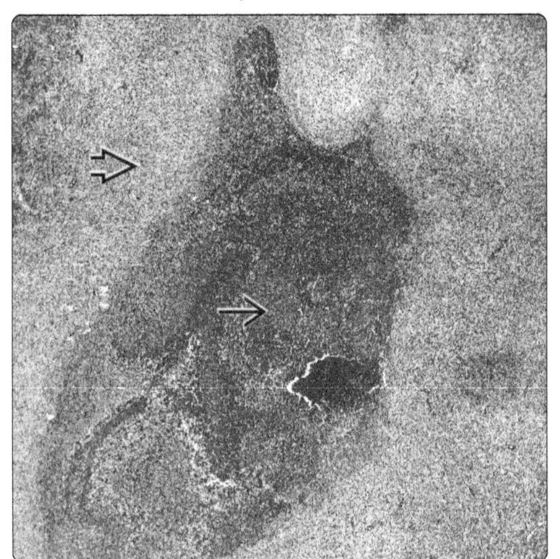

Epithelioid Histiocytes

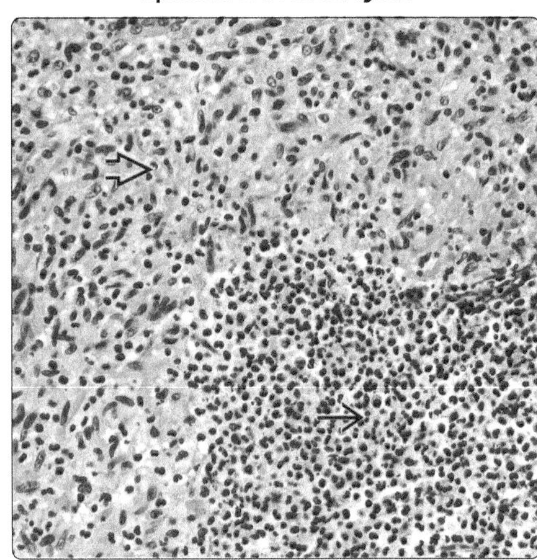

(Left) *Low-power view shows a large granulomatous mass with central neutrophilic abscess ⇨ formation surrounded by dense granulomatous inflammation ⇨ in a lymph node of a patient with an atypical Mycobacterium infection.* **(Right)** *High magnification shows epithelioid granulomatous inflammation ⇨ with central neutrophilic abscess ⇨ formation in a lymph node of a patient with an atypical Mycobacterium infection.*

Abscess Formation

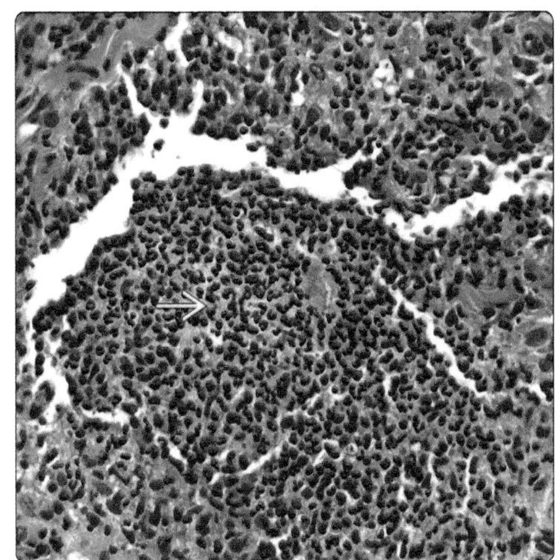

Mycobacterium kansasii Acid-Fast Stain

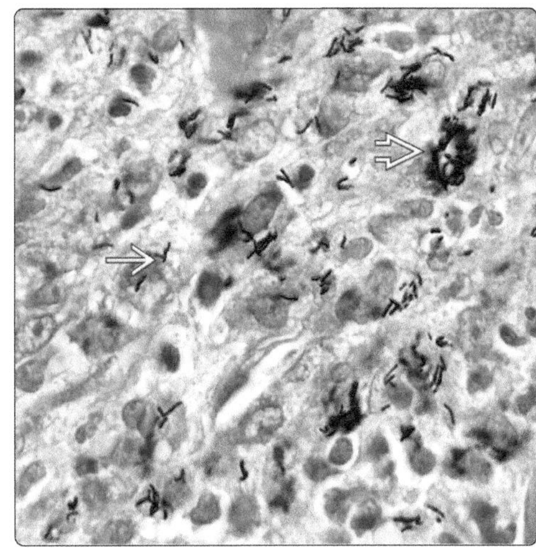

(Left) *A section from a well-developed skin abscess in a patient with a chronic history of lesions for several weeks demonstrates large collections of neutrophils ➡ in a case of atypical mycobacterial infection.* **(Right)** *An acid-fast stain from a patient with Mycobacterium kansasii infection of the skin demonstrates individual ➡ and aggregates ➡ of the organisms both free in tissue and within macrophages.*

Abscess Formation

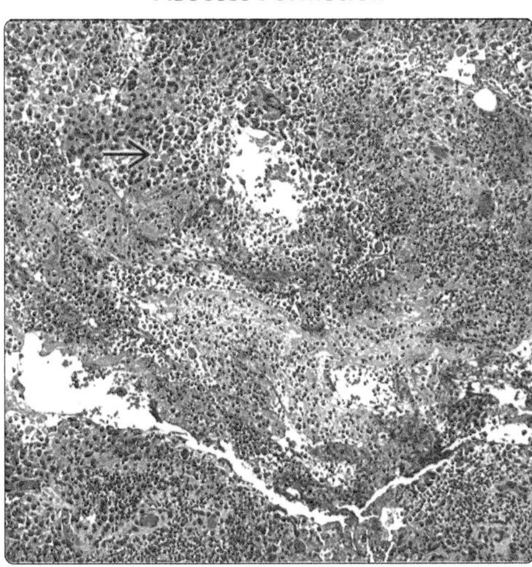

Mycobacterium fortuitum Acid-Fast Stain

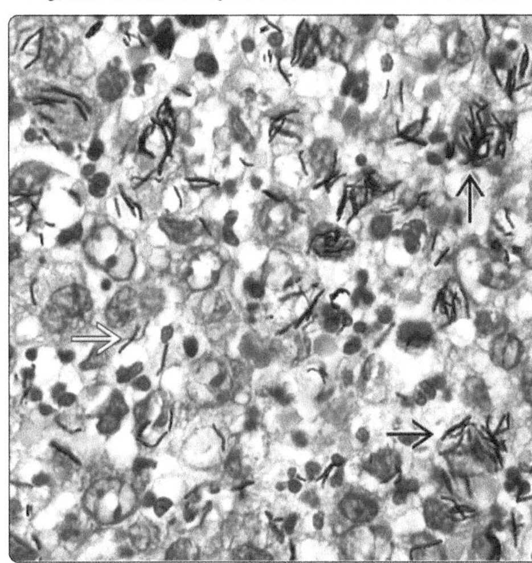

(Left) *A section from a skin abscess in a patient with a fulminant history demonstrates large collections of neutrophils ⇨ admixed with necrosis and edema in a case of rapidly growing mycobacteria.* **(Right)** *An acid-fast stain from a patient with rapidly growing Mycobacterium fortuitum infection of the skin demonstrates individual ➡ and clumps ⇨ of the organisms free in tissue.*

KEY FACTS

ETIOLOGY/PATHOGENESIS

- Infection with *Nocardia* species, gram-variable, weakly acid-fast bacteria present in soil, standing water, and decaying plants, transmitted by dust inhalation or skin/wound inoculation

CLINICAL ISSUES

- Pulmonary, skin (primary or secondary), disseminated, and neurologic disease
- Majority of cases are in immunosuppressed hosts
- High mortality with neurologic involvement

IMAGING

- Lungs with infiltrates with central necrosis (cavitation)
- Brain with abscesses or subtle meningitis

MICROBIOLOGY

- Grow as strict aerobes on wide range of media and temperatures (3 days to several weeks)
- MALDI-TOF and 16S rRNA sequencing faster and more reliable than phenotypic testing for speciation

MICROSCOPIC

- Necrotic abscess with neutrophils, neutrophil debris, and liquefactive necrosis
- Organisms subtle on H&E; lesions may be paucibacillary
- GMS: Thin, branching filamentous bacilli (~ 1-µm diameter and up to 20 µm long)
- Gram variable, mAFB positive with beaded staining pattern
- Negative on routine AFB stains

TOP DIFFERENTIAL DIAGNOSES

- Actinomycosis: Filamentous bacilli negative on mAFB stains
- Mycobacteria infections: Shorter bacilli strongly positive on routine and modified AFB stains
- Candidiasis: Thin hyphal forms of wider than *Nocardia* and mAFB negative

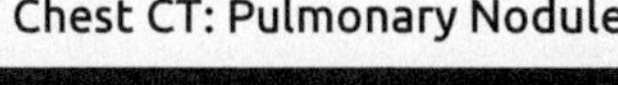
Chest CT: Pulmonary Nodule

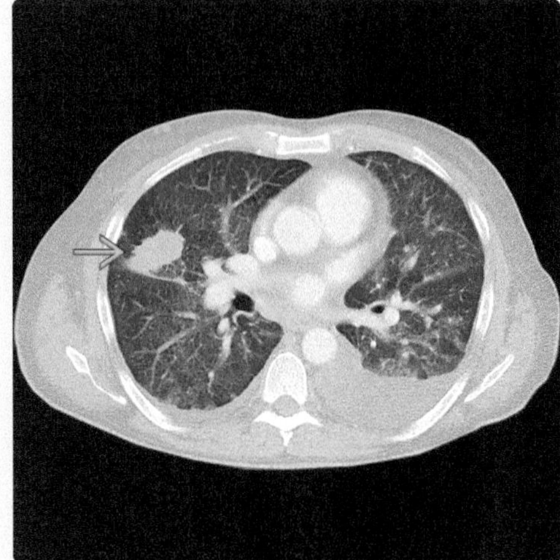

Pulmonary Abscess Cavities

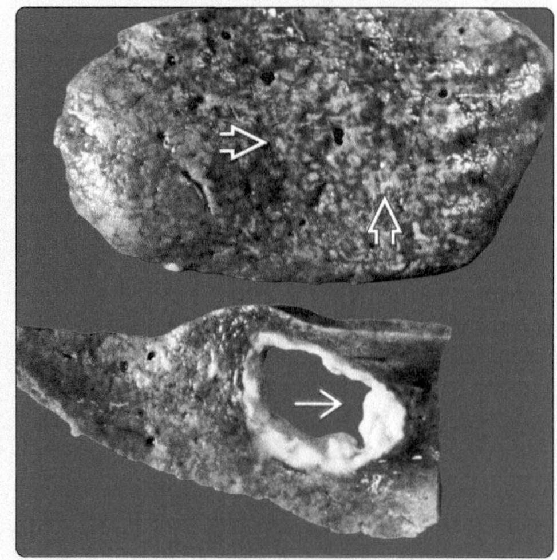

(Left) *This chest CT (lung window settings) shows a large right middle lobe nodule with irregular margins ⇨, typical findings for pulmonary nocardiosis.* **(Right)** *A large cavitary abscess ➡ is shown from pulmonary nocardiosis with satellite areas of small abscesses formed in adjacent lung tissue ➡.*

Nocardia Pulmonary Abscess

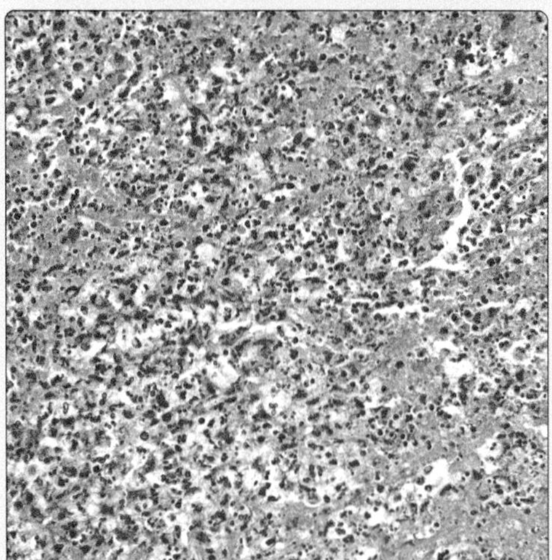

Nocardia spp. Modified AFB Stain

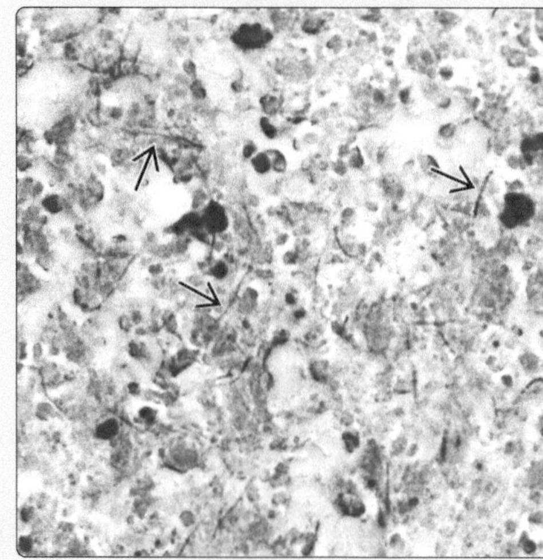

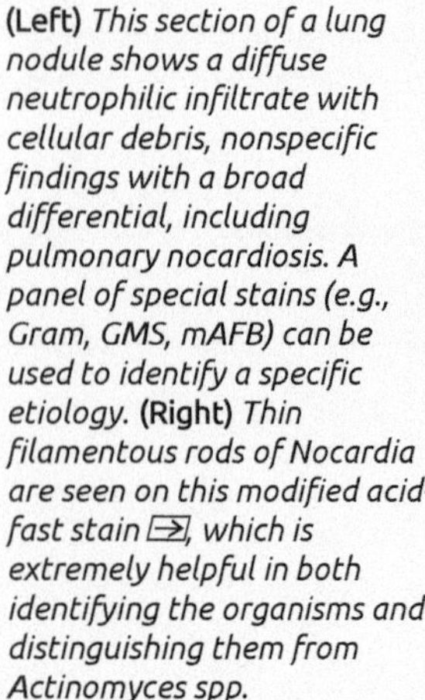
(Left) *This section of a lung nodule shows a diffuse neutrophilic infiltrate with cellular debris, nonspecific findings with a broad differential, including pulmonary nocardiosis. A panel of special stains (e.g., Gram, GMS, mAFB) can be used to identify a specific etiology.* **(Right)** *Thin filamentous rods of Nocardia are seen on this modified acid-fast stain ⇨, which is extremely helpful in both identifying the organisms and distinguishing them from Actinomyces spp.*

TERMINOLOGY

Definitions

- *Nocardia* from Edmond Nocard (French veterinarian)

ETIOLOGY/PATHOGENESIS

Infectious Agents

- Infection with *Nocardia* species, gram-variable, weakly acid-fast bacteria present in soil, standing water, and decaying plants, transmitted by dust inhalation or skin/wound inoculation
- > 100 species with < 1/2 infecting humans; *N. abscessus*, *N. asteroides*, *N. brasiliensis*, *N. cyriacigeorgica*, *N. farcinica*, and *N. nova* are most common isolates
- Most species contain virulence factor, cord factor (trehalose-6-6'-dimycolate)

CLINICAL ISSUES

Epidemiology

- USA: Estimated 500-1,000 new cases/year
- Majority of cases are in immunosuppressed hosts

Presentation

- Pulmonary disease: Fever, cough, night sweats, chest pain
- Disseminated nocardiosis: Fever with multiple organ involvement (brain most common site)
- Neurologic disease: Focal neurologic deficits, headache, seizures, behavioral changes
- Rare presentations: Endocarditis, keratitis, endophthalmitis, sporotrichosis-like lymphangitis, cellulitis, mycetoma

Laboratory Tests

- 16S rRNA, hsp65 sequencing of primary specimen or isolate for species identification

Treatment

- Surgical drainage may speed treatment and recovery
- Prolonged antibiotic therapy (up to 6 months) with sulfonamides or trimethoprim/sulfamethoxazole

Prognosis

- Neurologic involvement: 80% mortality
- Other sites: 50% mortality

IMAGING

Radiographic Findings

- Lungs with infiltrates with central necrosis (cavitation)
- Brain with abscesses or subtle meningitis

MICROBIOLOGY

Culture

- Grow as strict aerobes on wide range of media and temperatures (3 days to several weeks for growth)
- Identification by determining antibiotic resistance to gentamicin, tobramycin, amikacin, and erythromycin, then reaction to acetamide, adonitol, inositol, citrate, and colony pigment on Mueller-Hinton agar
- MALDI-TOF and 16S rRNA sequencing faster and more reliable for speciation

MACROSCOPIC

General Features

- Large abscesses may be found in affected organs containing necrotic, liquefactive material

MICROSCOPIC

Histologic Features

- Necrotic abscess with neutrophils, neutrophil debris, and liquefactive necrosis found in any affected site
- Organisms subtle on H&E; lesions may be paucibacillary
- Skin lesions may have larger clumps ("sulfur granules") associated with Splendore-Hoeppli phenomenon

ANCILLARY TESTS

Histochemistry

- GMS: Organisms are easily visualized as thin, branching filamentous bacilli (~ 1-μm diameter and up to 20 μm long); may appear as shorter bacilli or cocci due to fragmentation
- Bacilli are gram variable with beaded staining pattern
- Modified acid-fast stain (Kinyoun or Fite-Faraco) positive with beaded pattern
- Negative on routine AFB stains

DIFFERENTIAL DIAGNOSIS

Actinomycosis

- Similar appearance of filamentous bacilli on Gram and GMS stains; larger "sulfur granules," negative on mAFB stains, and much less common cause of disseminated disease

Mycobacteria Infections

- Shorter bacilli that are strongly positive on routine and modified AFB stains; *Nocardia* species may be isolated on mycobacteria cultures (Löwenstein-Jensen media)

Rhodococcus, *Tsukamurella*, and *Gordonia* Infections

- Bacteria that are also weakly mAFB positive but have shorter coryneform morphology

Candidiasis

- Very thin hyphal forms of *Candida* may be confused with *Nocardia* but will not be acid-fast and should have yeast forms present

SELECTED REFERENCES

1. Traxler RM et al: Updated review on Nocardia species: 2006-2021. Clin Microbiol Rev. 35(4):e0002721, 2022
2. Restrepo A et al: Nocardia infections in solid organ transplantation: guidelines from the Infectious Diseases Community of Practice of the American Society of Transplantation. Clin Transplant. 33(9):e13509, 2019
3. Sood R et al: Role of FNA and special stains in rapid cytopathological diagnosis of pulmonary nocardiosis. Acta Cytol. 62(3):178-82, 2018
4. McHugh KE et al: The cytopathology of Actinomyces, Nocardia, and their mimickers. Diagn Cytopathol. 45(12):1105-15, 2017
5. Yarbrough ML et al: Identification of Nocardia, Streptomyces, and Tsukamurella using MALDI-TOF MS with the Bruker Biotyper. Diagn Microbiol Infect Dis. 89(2):92-7, 2017
6. Wang HL et al: Nocardiosis in 132 patients with cancer: microbiological and clinical analyses. Am J Clin Pathol. 142(4):513-23, 2014
7. Yu X et al: Nocardia infection in kidney transplant recipients: case report and analysis of 66 published cases. Transpl Infect Dis. 13(4):385-91, 2011

(Left) *N. farcinica is shown growing on a blood agar plate. Colonial morphology of Nocardia varies between spp. and isolates and may appear chalky, matte or velvety, powdery, and either irregular, wrinkled, and heaped or smooth on the surface, may be brown, tan, pink, orange, red, purple, gray, yellow, peach, or white. [Courtesy E. Crowe, MLS(ASCP)CM.]* **(Right)** *Kinyoun staining of a N. farcinica isolate demonstrates weak modified AFB positivity, which is most prominent in coccal forms. [Courtesy E. Crowe, MLS(ASCP)CM.]*

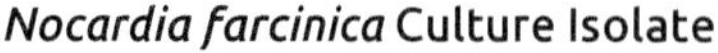

Nocardia farcinica **Culture Isolate**

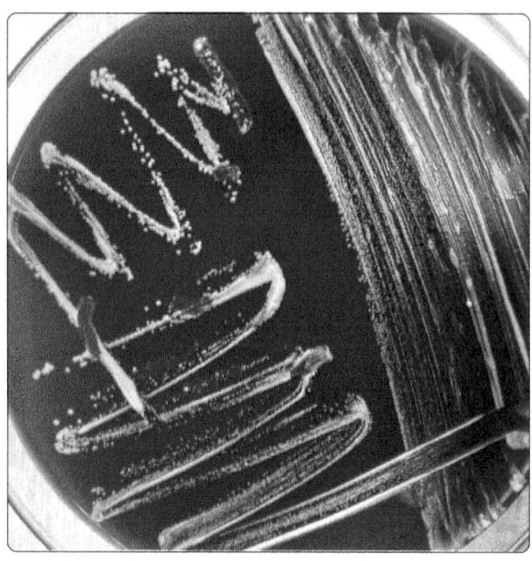

Nocardia farcinica **Kinyoun Stain**

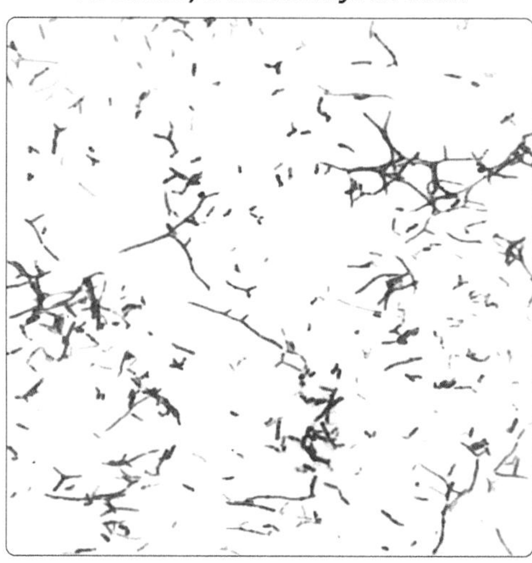

(Left) *Nocardia appear as thin, filamentous gram-positive bacilli with a beaded pattern →. While morphologically similar to Actinomyces, Nocardia can be distinguished by acid-fast stains.* **(Right)** *Nocardia stains very well with methenamine silver staining, making this an ideal stain to screen for bacteria in tissue samples. Nocardia filamentous bacilli are easily distinguished from fungal hyphae due to their significantly smaller size (~ 1-µm diameter).*

Nocardia **spp. Gram Stain**

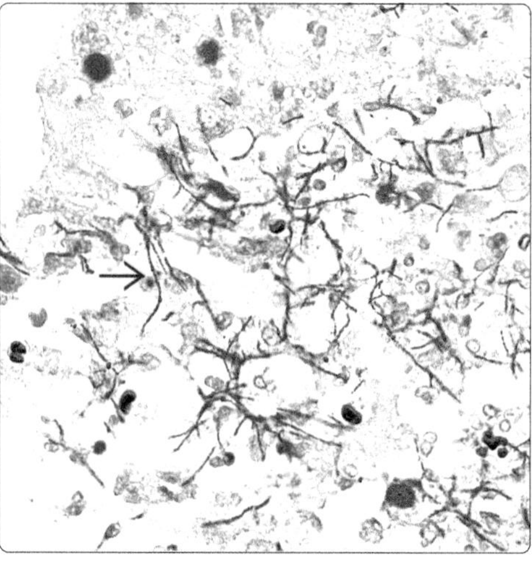

Nocardia **spp. GMS Stain**

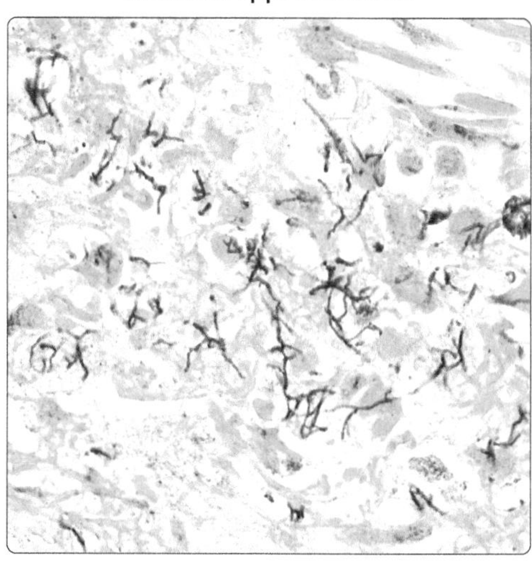

(Left) *Nocardia are weakly positive on modified acid-fast stains in a beaded pattern →. Mycobacteria spp. are also positive on mAFB stains and can be distinguished by shorter length and presence on standard AFB stains.* **(Right)** *Due to similarities in cell wall components, Nocardia filamentous rods are highlighted by this polyclonal antimycobacterial antibody. With tangential sections, Nocardia may appear as shorter rods similar in length to mycobacteria but can be distinguished by more robust staining on Gram/GMS stains.*

Nocardia **spp. mAFB Stain**

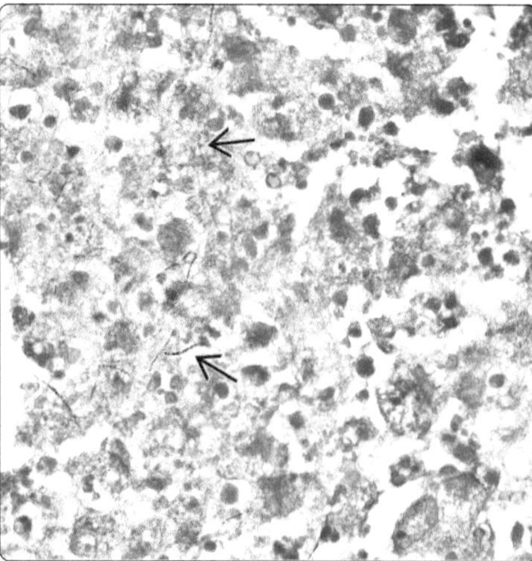

Nocardia **spp. Immunohistochemistry**

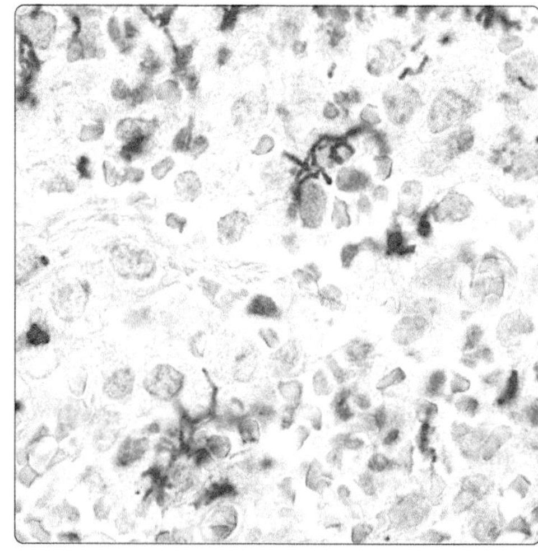

MR: *Nocardia* Brain Abscess

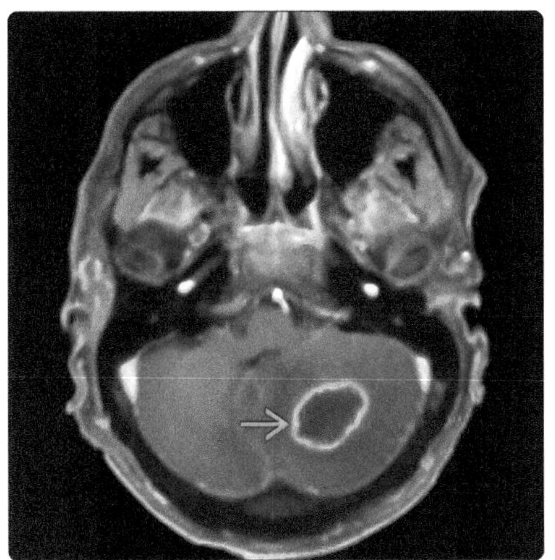

Nocardia Brain Abscess

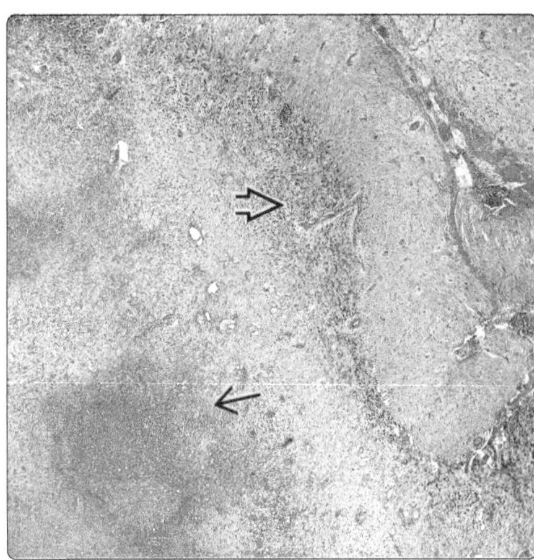

(Left) *Brain MR shows a ring-enhancing lesion ⇨ present in the left cerebellum. Single or multiple lesions in a patient with a lung mass need to be distinguished from metastatic carcinoma.* **(Right)** *Histologic sections of a cerebellar abscess resection show a dense neutrophilic infiltrate in the subcortical white matter ⇨ and a markedly depleted granule cell layer ⇨. Nocardia asteroides was isolated in cultures from concurrently collected brain tissue.*

Nocardia Brain Abscess

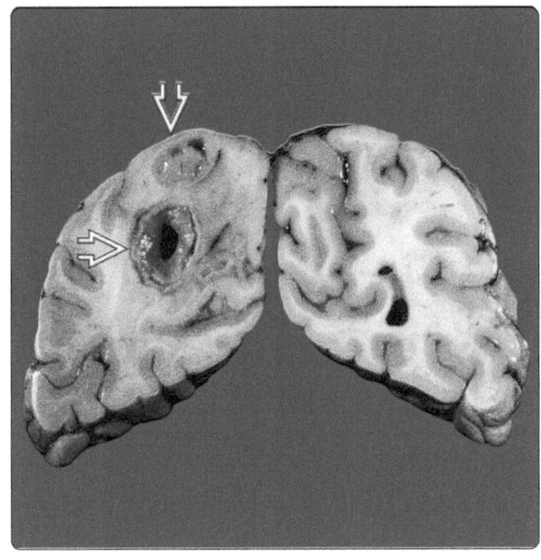

Nocardia Brain Abscess

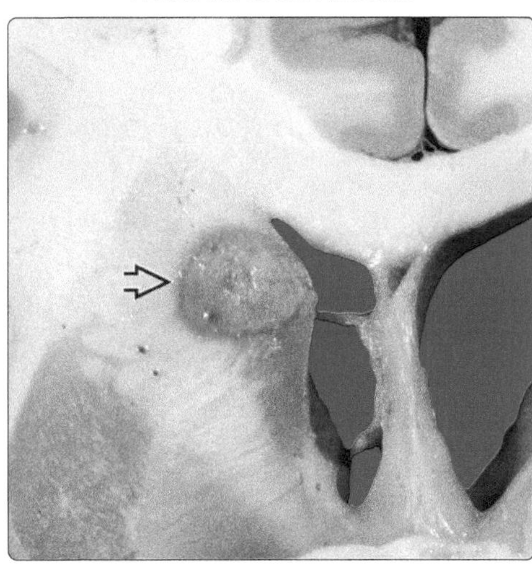

(Left) *A cross section of the brain at autopsy demonstrates multiple large abscesses ⇨, which showed nocardiosis, consistent with disseminated disease.* **(Right)** *A solitary abscess ⇨ in the basal ganglia due to nocardiosis is shown at autopsy on this brain section. The differential diagnosis includes other bacterial abscess, toxoplasmosis, and metastatic cancer.*

Nocardia Meningitis

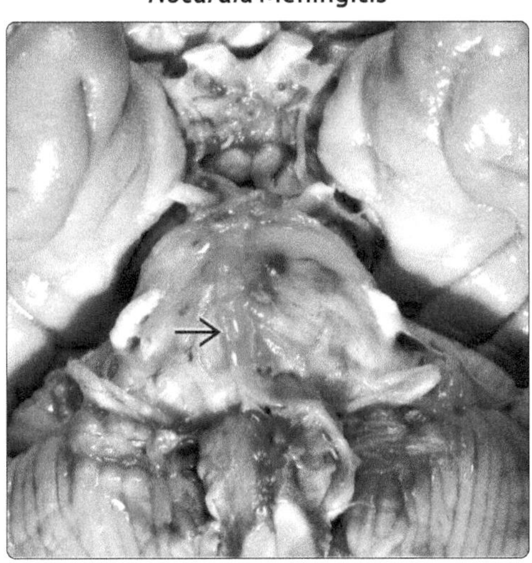

Nocardia Involving Kidney

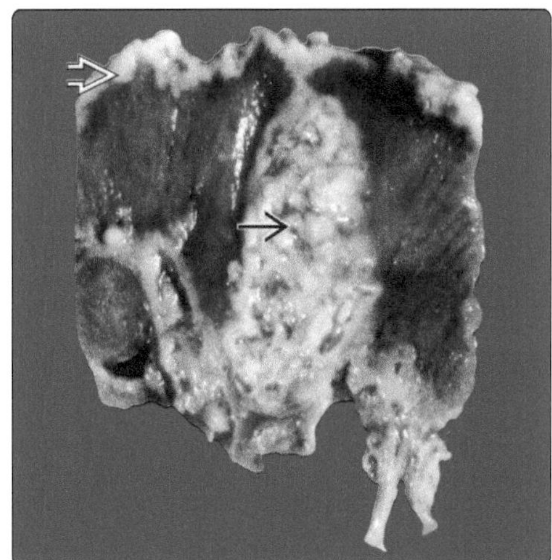

(Left) *Pus ⇨ is found on the base of the brain in a case of CNS nocardiosis. Meningitis is less common than solitary abscess.* **(Right)** *Abscess ⇨ and subcapsular inflammation ⇨ of the kidney are shown in a disseminated case of nocardiosis.*

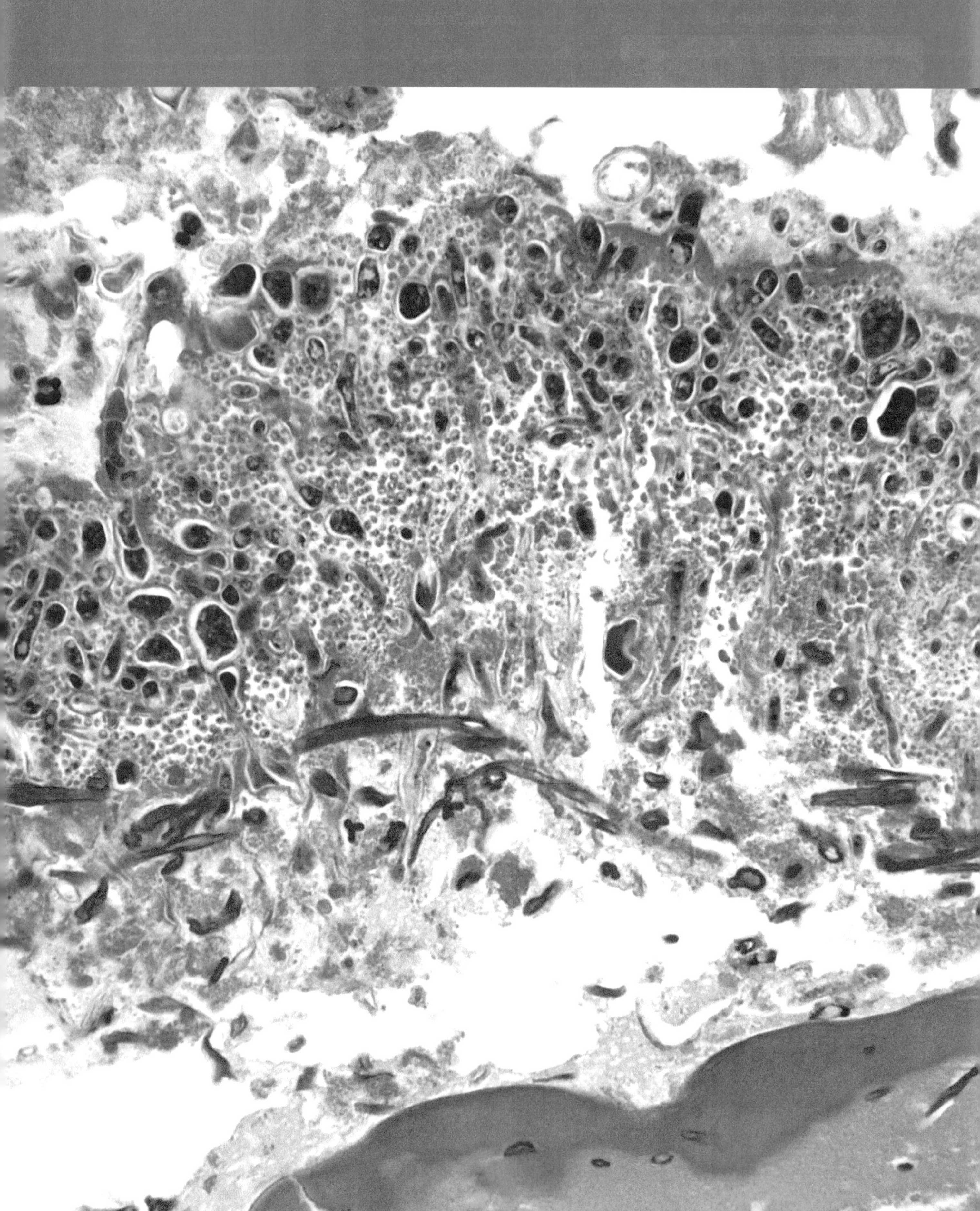

SECTION 5

Fungal Infections

TERMINOLOGY

Definitions

- Fungus: Spore-producing organisms feeding on organic matter, including molds, yeast, mushrooms, and toadstools
- Yeast: Fungus growing as single cells that multiply by budding of daughter yeast cells
  - May form pseudohyphae
- Mold: Fungus growing as multicellular, often branching, hyphae
- Hyphae: Branching filaments of molds, which have morphology and growth patterns useful for diagnosis
  - May be septate or nonseptate
- Conidia: Asexual, nonmotile spores often produced at ends of conidiophores (specialized hyphae, a.k.a. conidiogenous cells)
  - Morphology useful in fungal identification
- Anamorph: Asexual form of fungus
- Teleomorph: Sexual form of fungus
- Holomorph: Fungus with both sexual and asexual forms present

CLINICAL ISSUES

General

- Policies regarding approach to fungal disease should be created (in collaboration with multidisciplinary team) and provided via institutional messaging
- Findings of invasive fungal elements should be considered emergency and reported immediately to care team (i.e., critical value)
  - This should include necrotizing granulomatous inflammation, which may represent fungus, mycobacteria, etc.
- Taxonomy of medically important fungi continues to be updated; clinical microbiology laboratories may choose to report both current and outdated but more recognized names

Immunocompetent Hosts

- Fungal organisms, with few exceptions, do not cause severe or life-threatening infections in humans with competent immune systems

Hyphae in Tissue

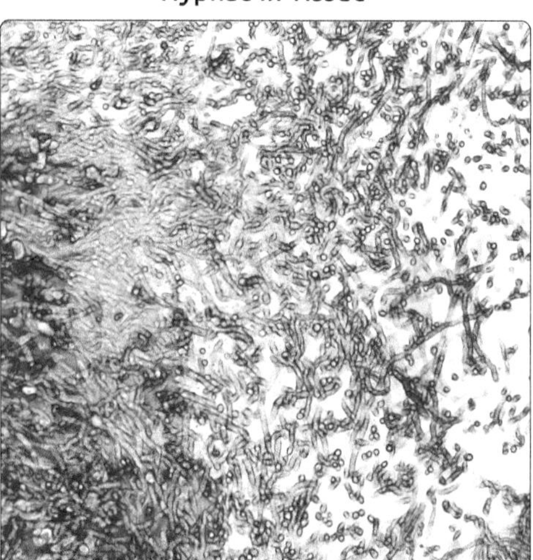

Gram-Positive Yeast

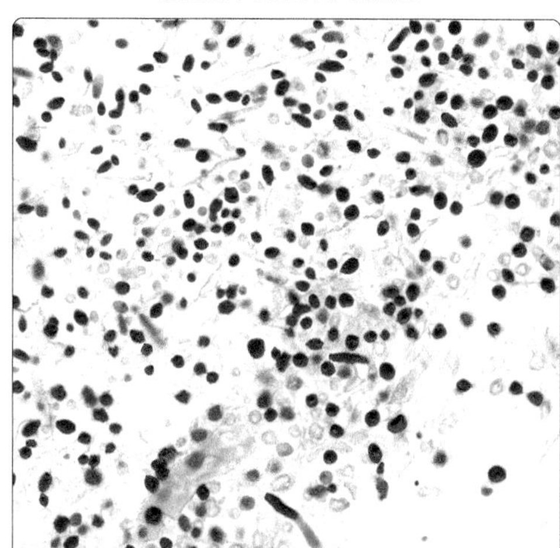

(Left) *Aspergillus species on routine histology is very difficult to distinguish from other hyphae-forming organisms and requires special stains &/or culture for definitive diagnosis. Note the variation in hematoxylin, representing dead-vs.-viable hyphae.* **(Right)** *Gram staining of Candida tropicalis highlights yeast and some filamentous (pseudohyphae) forms, while true hyphae are gram negative.*

PAS With Diastase

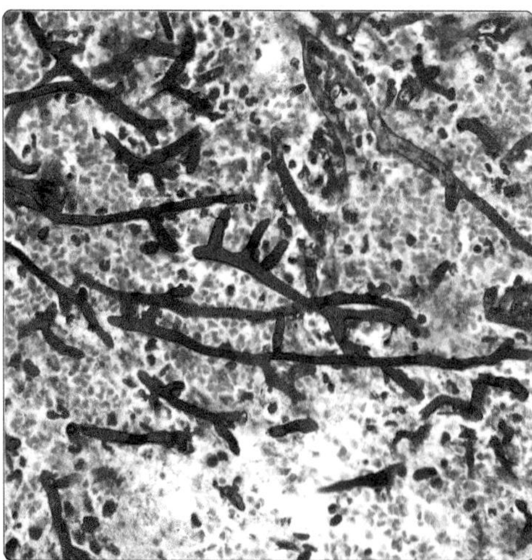

Yeast Morphology: GMS Stain

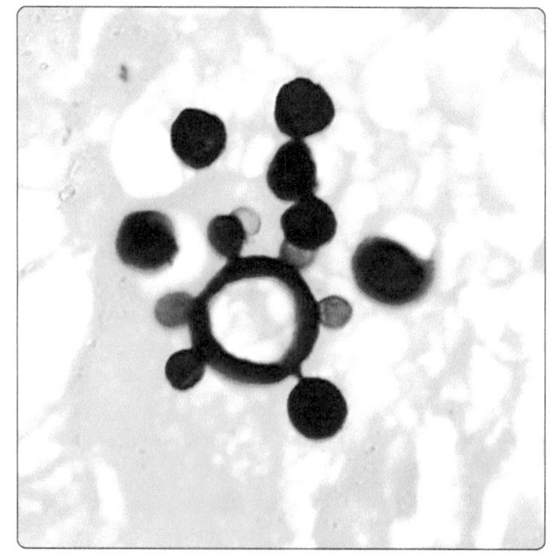

(Left) *PAS-D staining of a pulmonary artery mass highlights broad, pauciseptate hyphae with 90° angle branching, as seen in the Mucorales fungi.* **(Right)** *Grocott methenamine silver staining is frequently used to assess fungal morphology in tissue sections. In a subset of infections, a specific diagnosis can be made without the need for culture or molecular confirmation. In this example, budding yeast forms with a ship's wheel appearance is diagnostic of paracoccidioidomycosis.*

- Common mild fungal infections in immunocompetent hosts: Cutaneous candidiasis, genital yeast infections, thrush, paronychia, onychomycosis, dermatophytosis, dermatophytes (e.g., tinea infections)
- Moderate to severe infections in immunocompetent hosts: Sporotrichosis, mycetoma, chromoblastomycosis, phaeohyphomycosis, coccidioidomycosis, blastomycosis

Immunocompromised Hosts

- Vast majority of significant fungal disease in humans occurs in immunocompromised hosts
- Severe localized infections, as well as small breaks in tissue barriers, can result in dissemination and fungal sepsis
- Mucormycosis, other hyalohyphomycoses, *Cryptococcus* species, *Talaromyces marneffei*, and others are primarily observed in immunocompromised hosts as symptomatic infections
- Depending on severity of immune suppression, **any** fungal species may be able to cause disseminated infection
  - Proper identification of unknown fungus in these hosts may result in rare species without treatment guidelines
  - Length of time required to identify these species may exceed clinical window for treatment
  - Part of institutional policies regarding approach to fungal infections should include empiric antifungal guidance based on patient type and historic data

FUNGAL CLASSES

Yeasts

- By far, most common fungal organisms (*Candida* species) isolated from humans
- Typically grow more rapidly in culture than molds and can grow on many microbiology agarose plates that are for bacteria
- Examples: *Cryptococcus* species, *Candida* species

Molds

- By far most common fungal organisms to which humans are exposed
  - Present in environment, households, food supply, airborne, etc.
  - Inhalation and ingestion are most common exposure mechanisms
  - Disease states can include allergies, chronic pulmonary conditions, mass-forming lesions, invasive disease, and dissemination
- Examples: *Aspergillus* species, *Mucor* species, *Fusarium* species

Thermally Dimorphic Fungi

- Small group of human pathogens that grow as yeast in human tissue at 37 °C or as mold at 25 °C in environment or laboratory
- Commonly cause human skin infections &/or pulmonary lesions with dissemination in immunocompromised hosts
- Typically have endemic or geographically restricted distributions
- Examples: *Coccidioides* species, *Blastomyces* species, *T. marneffei*, *Histoplasma* species, *Paracoccidioides* species

Dematiaceous Fungi

- Naturally pigmented yeasts and molds causing cutaneous and disseminated disease
- Commonly found in environment with history of traumatic penetrations before infection
- Cause disease spectrum depending on mechanism of exposure and immune status (tinea nigra, chromoblastomycosis, phaeohyphomycosis)

PATHOLOGIC PATTERNS

No Tissue Response

- Yeast and molds infecting immunocompromised hosts can invade and spread to tissue with minimal tissue reaction
- Necrosis of tissue secondary to blood vessel compromise &/or infarction may occur
- Special stains to look for fungus in unexplained lesions of immunocompromised are required

Necrosis

- Angioinvasion: Leads to vessel compromise and local destruction of tissue
- Infarction: Upstream vessel occlusion or destruction leads to downstream infarction

Acute Suppurative Inflammation

- Neutrophils are primarily responsive to all fungal elements in immunocompetent hosts
- Can progress to abscesses

Chronic Inflammation

- Mononuclear inflammation
  - Macrophages &/or lymphocytes may join neutrophils after initial response
- Granulomatous inflammation
  - As acute lesions persist, mononuclear inflammation may form granulomata
  - Can present as small disseminated granuloma or large masses (which can form cavities)
- Eosinophilic inflammation
  - Although uncommon, some fungal infections produce eosinophilia (*Coccidioides* species)
  - Fungal elements in tissue can cause Splendore-Hoeppli phenomenon (sporotrichosis, basidiobolomycosis)

Fungus Ball

- Molds and other fungi may colonize preexisting spaces or cavities and form noninvasive fungal masses (lung, nasal passages)
- There is no hyphal growth into tissue (invasion) surrounding cavity
- In immunocompetent hosts with existing fungus ball who become immunosuppressed, invasion and dissemination can occur

DIAGNOSTIC APPROACHES TO FUNGUS

Blood/Body Fluid Examination

- Macrophages containing yeast (*Histoplasma* species) can be seen in blood, body fluids, and bone marrow aspirates
- Cerebrospinal fluid examination for yeast (*Cryptococcus* species) using India ink prep (less sensitive than antigen testing)

- *Candida* species commonly isolated from blood and urine, most often as contaminant
- Positive blood culture bottles for fungus can demonstrate organisms on Gram stain

Cytology and Fine-Needle Aspiration

- Suspected fungal elements (yeast or hyphae) seen on cytology should be confirmed with culture &/or cell block review
- Can be ideal sample to obtain material for culture &/or molecular analysis for large lesions

Tissue Biopsy

- Identification of fungal elements in biopsies or surgical resection specimens should be categorized into saprobic or invasive
  - Correlation with clinical appearance, clinical history, and surgical appearance
  - Contamination of samples prior to processing and cross contamination from other samples should be excluded
  - Depending on body site, fungal forms may be normal flora
- Invasive fungal elements, regardless of inflammatory response, should be communicated as critical value
  - Frozen section and routine H&E may or may not show fungal elements
  - Silver stains (GMS, MSS) are generally better for morphology (exception: So-called zygomycetes, which may not stain well)
  - PAS-D is generally better for epithelial surfaces and for certain species (i.e., zygomycetes)
  - Mucicarmine and Fontana-Masson stains may be positive in *Cryptococcus* species (vs. *Histoplasma* species)
    - Larger yeasts, such as *Blastomyces* and *Coccidioides*, may stain with melanin but are morphologically distinct
- Yeast can be diagnosed with some degree of confidence based on size, budding, and histochemical staining properties
- Morphology of hyphal forms is **never** sufficient to provide diagnosis and should only be used to guide empiric therapy and direct additional testing
  - Immunohistochemistry, in situ hybridization, &/or immunofluorescence, when available, can confirm some species
  - Differential diagnosis for hyphae may represent organisms with completely different treatment and variable outcomes
  - Confirmation with culture, special stains, molecular testing, or mass spectrometry is required

Rapid Diagnostic Tests

- In acute setting, rapid diagnostic tests (RDTs) can be valuable to guide therapy or monitor outcomes of therapy
  - Cryptococcal latex agglutination: Positive in *Cryptococcus* species and trichosporonosis
  - (1,3)-β-D-glucan: Positive in *Aspergillus* species, *Pneumocystis jirovecii*, *Candida* species, and many other fungi (nonspecific)
  - Galactomannan: Positive in *Aspergillus* species and, rarely, in other organisms
    - False-positive may occur in presence of certain β-lactam antibiotics

Culture

- Fungal culture using variety of media has been gold standard for diagnosis
  - Requires media that differentiates fungal forms into morphologically identifiable sexual and asexual forms (evaluated on lactophenol cotton blue-stained slides)
  - Requires variable temperature growth of same fungus to accelerate differentiation
  - May take several days to weeks to get growth sufficient for identification
  - Due to acuity of immunocompromised patients, may not represent most optimal method for diagnosis
  - Rapid assessment using molecular techniques or mass spectroscopy when colony first forms is highly valuable but requires growth

Molecular Diagnostics

- Specific PCR assays (single genus or species detection), inclusion on multitarget syndromic panels, as well as PCR with sequencing, is new gold standard for identification
- Internal transcribed spacer (ITS) and D1/D2 region of 28S rRNA gene are primary targets for broad spectrum fungal sequencing; may require genus-specific targets for speciation
- In primary samples, may be hindered by contaminants (careful interpretation)
- In culture samples, may be challenging for extraction (validated methods required)
- Molecular analysis of tissue after morphologic confirmation of fungal elements is ideal

Mass Spectroscopy

- Highly specific method of identification of fungi using rapid assay based on protein signature
- Typically requires cultured colony (not on primary samples)
- Significantly less time consuming and less reagent cost for detection (high initial capital cost)

SELECTED REFERENCES

1. Borman AM et al: Name changes for fungi of medical importance, 2020 to 2021. J Clin Microbiol. 61(6):e0033022, 2023
2. Hata DJ et al: Candida auris: An emerging yeast pathogen posing distinct challenges for laboratory diagnostics, treatment, and infection prevention. Arch Pathol Lab Med. 144(1):107-14, 2020
3. Lau AF et al: Multicenter study demonstrates standardization requirements for mold identification by MALDI-TOF MS. Front Microbiol. 10:2098, 2019
4. Schwartz IS et al: Emergomyces: the global rise of new dimorphic fungal pathogens. PLoS Pathog. 15(9):e1007977, 2019
5. Arnoni MV et al: Infections caused by Fusarium species in pediatric cancer patients and review of published literature. Mycopathologia. 183(6):941-9, 2018
6. Beardsley J et al: Responding to the emergence of antifungal drug resistance: perspectives from the bench and the bedside. Future Microbiol. 13:1175-91, 2018
7. Wickes BL et al: Molecular diagnostics in medical mycology. Nat Commun. 9(1):5135, 2018
8. Prakash PY et al: Online databases for taxonomy and identification of pathogenic fungi and proposal for a cloud-based dynamic data network platform. J Clin Microbiol. 55(4):1011-24, 2017
9. Douglas AP et al: Emerging infections caused by non-Aspergillus filamentous fungi. Clin Microbiol Infect. 22(8):670-80, 2016
10. Garcia Garcia SC et al: Coccidioidomycosis and the skin: a comprehensive review. An Bras Dermatol. 90(5):610-9, 2015
11. Ritter JM et al: Exserohilum infections associated with contaminated steroid injections: a clinicopathologic review of 40 cases. Am J Pathol. 183(3):881-92, 2013
12. Guarner J et al: Histopathologic diagnosis of fungal infections in the 21st century. Clin Microbiol Rev. 24(2):247-80, 2011

Tissue Stains for Fungal Organisms

Stain	Organisms	Stain Characteristics	Benefits	Pitfalls
H&E	Fungus balls, dead/calcified hyphae, inflammation	Pink and purple with pale pink to purple fungal elements	Evaluation of inflammatory pattern, visualize pigmented fungi	Fungi may be invisible
PAS-D	Most yeasts and molds	Pale pink and pale blue with bright pink fungal elements	High contrast of fungi vs. background for easy screening	Routine PAS may obscure fungi in skin, liver, or other glycogen-rich organs
Silver (GMS, MSS)	Most yeasts and molds	Green background with gray to dark black fungi	Morphology is ideal for identification	Mucormycosis do not stain well on silver
Gram	*Candida* species	Yellow background with dark purple yeast and hyphal forms	Demonstrates bacteria as well	Filamentous bacteria may mimic fungi
Mucicarmine	*Cryptococcus*, *Blastomyces*, *Rhinosporidium* species	Pale yellow background with bright pink fungal elements	Capsule of *Cryptococcus* species, wall of *Blastomyces* species	Capsular (-) *Cryptococcus* species do not stain
Fontana-Masson	*Cryptococcus* species and other fungi with melanized walls	Pale pink background with dark brown to dark black elements	*Histoplasma* (-) vs. *Cryptococcus* (+) species	Some larger fungi also stain with Fontana-Masson
Giemsa	*Histoplasma*, *Penicillium* species	Pink-violet-blue background with dark blue fungal elements	Bone marrow and blood smear visualization	

Classification of Fungi

Ascomycota/Hyphomycetes	Dimorphic Fungi	Dermatophytes	Zygomycota	Yeast and Yeast-Like
Aspergillus species *Bipolaris* species *Chrysosporium* species *Curvularia* species *Exophiala* species *Fonsecaea* species *Fusarium* species *Geotrichum* species *Graphium* species *Madurella* species *Penicillium* species *Scopulariopsis* species *Sporothrix* species *Talaromyces* species > 50 total genera	*Blastomyces dermatitidis* *Coccidioides* species *Histoplasma* species *Paracoccidioides* species *Talaromyces marneffei* *Sporothrix* species *Emergomyces* species	*Epidermophyton* species *Trichophyton* species > 10 total genera	*Basidiobolus* species *Cunninghamella* species *Mucor* species *Rhizomucor* species *Rhizopus* species > 10 total genera	*Candida* species *Cryptococcus* species *Malassezia* species *Pneumocystis jirovecii* *Saccharomyces* species *Torulaspora* species *Trichosporon* species > 25 genera

Aspergillosis

KEY FACTS

ETIOLOGY/PATHOGENESIS

- Infection with *Aspergillus* spp., ubiquitous environment fungi, primarily via inhalation of airborne conidia
- Most common species of clinical significance includes *A. fumigatus*, *A. flavus*, *A. niger*, and *A. terreus*

CLINICAL ISSUES

- Allergic bronchopulmonary aspergillosis (ABPA), chronic pulmonary aspergillosis, invasive (systemic/disseminated) aspergillosis, rhinosinusitis, endocarditis, and central nervous system involvement
- Serum positive for galactomannan and (1,3)-β-D-glucan

MICROSCOPIC

- Regular septate hyaline (nonpigmented) hyphae (3-6 μm in diameter) with dichotomous 45° angle branching; highlighted by GMS and PAS-D stains
- Angioinvasion is commonly present in invasive disease; tends to grow radially from hematogenous lesions in tissue
- Neutrophilic inflammation is often present in invasive disease; lesions may show little inflammatory reaction in neutropenic patients

TOP DIFFERENTIAL DIAGNOSES

- Candidiasis: Gram-positive yeast, pseudohyphae, and occasional hyphae; positive serum (1,3)-β-D-glucan; negative galactomannan
- Mucormycosis: Broad, paucisepate, ribbon-like hyphae; negative serum galactomannan and (1,3)-β-D-glucan
- Hyalohyphomycosis (e.g., fusariosis, scedosporiosis): Hyphae appear similar (lack fruiting bodies); negative serum galactomannan; typically requires culture/PCR to distinguish
- Concurrent infections with other fungi, including *Mucor* spp., *Candida* spp., etc., require molecular/culture, serologic, and histologic correlation

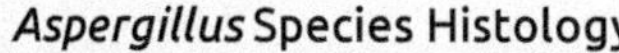
Aspergillus Species Histology

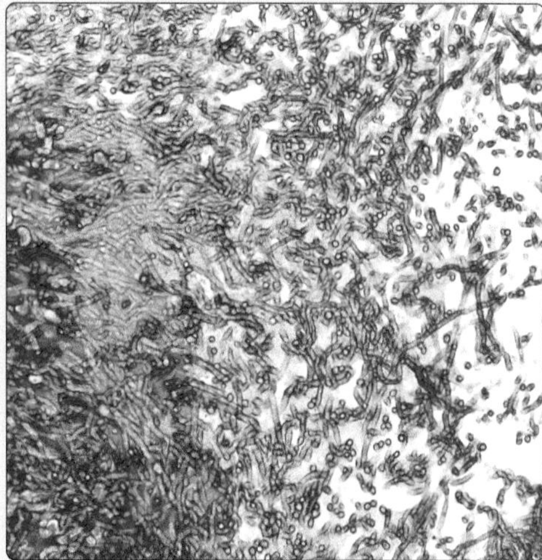

Aspergillus Species GMS Stain

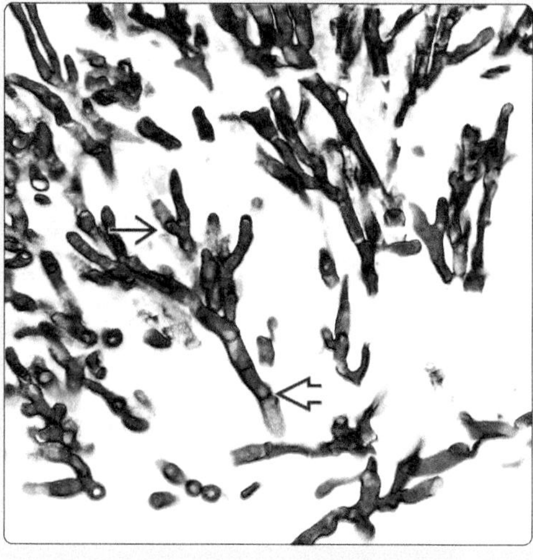

(Left) *Aspergillus spp. on routine histology can be very difficult to distinguish from other hyphae-forming organisms and requires special stains &/or culture for definitive diagnosis. Note the variation in hematoxylin, representing dead vs. viable hyphae.* **(Right)** *High-magnification GMS-stained bronchoalveolar lavage (cell block preparation) shows hyphae with acute-angle branching ➡ and septa ⇨. Other fungi, e.g., agents of hyalohyphomycosis, may be indistinguishable from Aspergillus spp. in this setting.*

Aspergillus Species PAS-D Stain

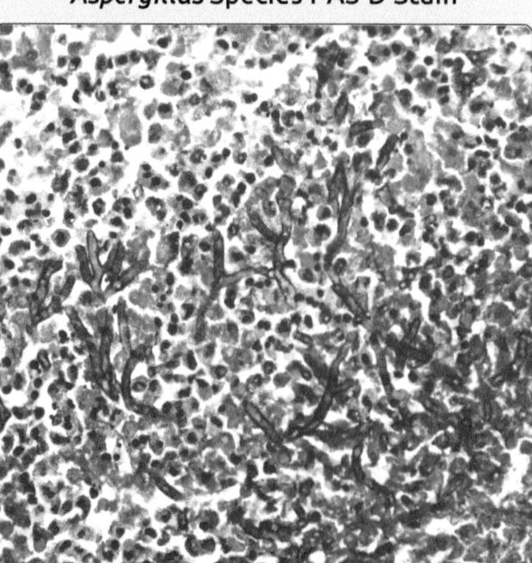

Aspergillus Species Fruiting Body

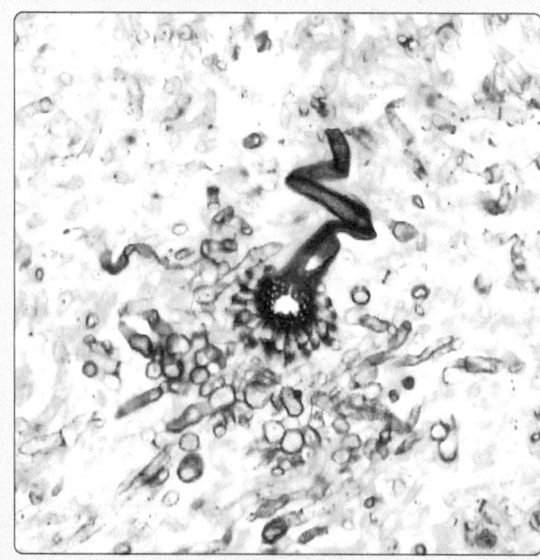

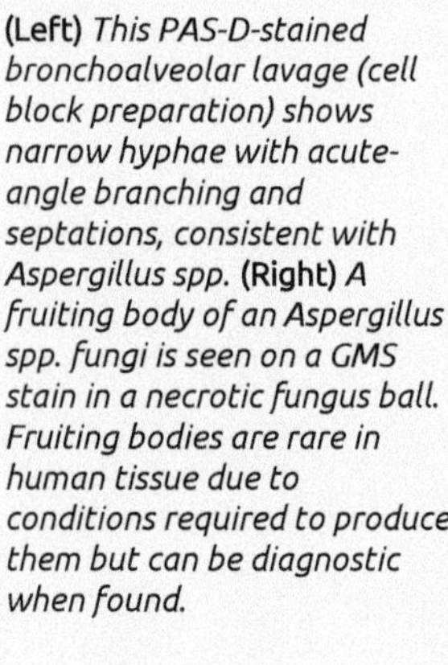

(Left) *This PAS-D-stained bronchoalveolar lavage (cell block preparation) shows narrow hyphae with acute-angle branching and septations, consistent with Aspergillus spp.* **(Right)** *A fruiting body of an Aspergillus spp. fungi is seen on a GMS stain in a necrotic fungus ball. Fruiting bodies are rare in human tissue due to conditions required to produce them but can be diagnostic when found.*

TERMINOLOGY

Definitions

- Latin: From "aspergillum" (liturgical instrument to sprinkle holy water)

ETIOLOGY/PATHOGENESIS

Infectious Agents

- Infection with *Aspergillus* spp., ubiquitous environment fungi, spread primarily via inhalation of airborne conidia with deposition in bronchioles or alveolar spaces
- Member of phylum, Ascomycota
- > 180 known species, ~ 20 of which are known pathogens to humans and other animals
- Most common species of clinical significance: *A. fumigatus* followed by *A. flavus*, *A. niger*, and *A. terreus*

CLINICAL ISSUES

Epidemiology

- Worldwide distribution
- Invasive infection most common in immunocompromised
- Increasing recognition of pulmonary infection in critically ill patients with influenza [influenza-associated pulmonary aspergillosis (IAPA)] and SARS-CoV-2 infection [COVID-19-associated pulmonary aspergillosis (CAPA)]

Presentation

- Pulmonary aspergillosis
  - Allergic bronchopulmonary aspergillosis (ABPA)
    - Hypersensitivity reaction to *Aspergillus* spp., *A. fumigatus* most common
    - Primarily in patients with cystic fibrosis or steroid-dependent asthma
    - Characterized by mucoid impaction of bronchi, eosinophilic pneumonia, and bronchocentric granulomatosis; patients can be asymptomatic in early stage with only infiltrates on chest x-rays
    - Disease is irreversible once patient has reached fibrotic stage
    - *Aspergillus* spp. are cultured from sputum in up to 2/3 of patients with ABPA
  - Tracheobronchitis: Risk factors include solid organ transplant, hematologic malignancies, HIV infection
  - Chronic pulmonary aspergillosis (CPA): Evolves slowly; duration of disease is usually > 3 months; most common sign is hemoptysis, but some patients can be asymptomatic
    - Aspergilloma: Fungus ball with *Aspergillus* hyphae, fibrin, and cellular debris within preexisting pulmonary cavity
    - Chronic cavitary pulmonary aspergillosis: Infection and expansion of ≥ 1 pulmonary cavities over months
    - Chronic fibrosing pulmonary aspergillosis: Disease progression to marked and extensive lung fibrosis
    - Chronic necrotizing pulmonary aspergillosis: Usually associated with immunocompromised states, e.g., diabetes, HIV infection, advanced age, chronic steroid use, malnutrition
- Invasive (systemic/disseminated) aspergillosis
  - Mostly in severely immunocompromised patients (prolonged neutropenia, no remission of underlying hematologic malignancy, use of systemic glucocorticoids)
  - Endophthalmitis may be presenting feature
- Rhinosinusitis: Infection of paranasal sinuses
- Endocarditis: 2nd to *Candida* spp. as most frequent cause of fungal endocarditis
  - Primarily seen in intravenous drug users or in patients with prosthetic heart valves or indwelling central venous catheters
  - Blood cultures are rarely positive
- Cutaneous aspergillosis: Primarily from direct inoculation in setting of trauma, e.g., burn victims
- Gastrointestinal aspergillosis: Relatively rare, but risk factors include neutropenia, glucocorticoid use, and mucosal breakdown
- Central nervous system involvement
  - Occurs in setting of disseminated infection or from local extension from paranasal sinuses
  - Mycotic aneurysms develop in some cases and can rupture, resulting in hemorrhagic cerebrovascular accident, subarachnoid hemorrhage, &/or empyema formation

Laboratory Tests

- PCR: ~ 80% sensitivity/specificity to detect invasive aspergillosis from blood/serum/plasma; consecutive positive results can improve specificity
- PCR with sequencing (ITS region or 28S rRNA gene) from fresh or FFPE tissue may be considered if hyphae detected by histochemistry and cultures are negative
- Skin test: In cases of allergic aspergillosis, positive skin reactivity to *Aspergillus* antigens can be detected
- (1,3)-β-D-glucan: Cell wall component of many fungi; positive in serum in patients with invasive aspergillosis
  - Not specific for aspergillosis; can be detected in patients with other invasive fungal infection (e.g., candidiasis, pneumocystosis)
  - Typically negative in patients with mucormycosis or cryptococcosis
  - False-positive results common in patients receiving IVIg, albumin, or blood products filtered through cellulose filters containing (1,3)-β-D-glucan antigen, hemodialysis with cellulose membranes, or with serosal exposure to gauze packs containing (1,3)-β-D-glucan
  - Serial monitoring not predictive of treatment response
- Galactomannan antigen present on cell walls of *Aspergillus* spp.: Positive in serum in patients with invasive aspergillosis, sometimes prior to presence of clinical symptoms
  - 40-100% sensitive and 56-100% specific; sensitivity of serum detection decreased by concomitant administration of antifungal drugs
  - FDA-approved assays only for serum and broncho-alveolar lavage fluid (BAL); also detectable in other samples (e.g., pleural fluid and CSF)
  - BAL may be positive in colonization; higher optical density cutoffs may be preferred for BAL compared to serum

- Other fungi can produce positive results due to presence of galactomannans or polysaccharides containing galactofuranose residues on their cell walls (e.g., *Penicillium*, *Paecilomyces*, *Alternaria*, and *Histoplasma*)
- False-positive results associated with blood products collected in bags containing galactomannan antigen from single manufacturer (Fresenius Kabi, Germany) and sodium gluconate food additive
- Serial testing may be used to monitor response to therapy
- Serum galactomannan level at time of diagnosis and 1-week galactomannan decay were found to be predictive of all-cause mortality in cases of invasive aspergillosis

- *Aspergillus* antibodies (precipitins)
  - ABPA: Elevated serum IgE and IgG antibodies specific to *Aspergillus* spp. can be detected; total serum IgE is also elevated
  - Chronic pulmonary aspergillosis: Elevated specific IgG detected in most cases and elevated specific IgE detected in ~ 50% of cases; however, standardization of this testing is not well established for this indication
  - No role in diagnosis of invasive aspergillosis
- Lateral flow device (LFD) that detects extracellular antigen secreted by *Aspergillus* spp. using monoclonal JF5 antibody has been approved for use in Europe
- Detection of secondary metabolites in human breath using thermal desorption-gas chromatography/mass spectrometry

Treatment

- Azoles, polyenes, and echinocandins are active against *Aspergillus* spp.
- Initial therapy: Voriconazole (1st line), posaconazole, or isavuconazole; amphotericin B in patients with azole intolerance, or empiric treatment with suspected invasive mucormycosis or aspergillosis prior to definitive diagnosis
- Salvage therapy: Azole plus echinocandin
- Surgical debridement or resection helpful in cases in which drugs cannot be delivered to large symptomatic lesions or when there is imminent threat to vessels
- ABPA: Oral steroids needed for prolonged period of time
- cyp51A mutations conferring pan-azole resistance more common in Europe due to azole use in commercial fungicides; azole resistance is low in USA
- Novel antifungals emerging with in vitro and in vivo activity against *Aspergillus* spp. currently in clinical trials (olorofim, fosmanogepix, ibrexafungerp, etc.), none yet FDA approved for aspergillosis

Prognosis

- Invasive aspergillosis carries poor prognosis (up to 90% in some groups)
- Successful treatment depends on site of lesion and immune status of host

IMAGING

Radiographic Findings

- Invasive lung infection can manifest on CT scan as lung nodule
- Halo sign: Ground-glass opacity surrounding nodule; not specific for aspergillosis and can also be seen with neoplasia and other fungal or bacterial infections (e.g., *Pseudomonas aeruginosa* or mycobacteria)
- Air crescent sign when there is fungal vascular invasion and hemorrhage

MICROBIOLOGY

Culture Isolation and Identification

- Direct examination (e.g., with calcofluor white, lactophenol blue stain) may demonstrate hyaline septate hyphae
- Grows well on standard fungal media; notably inhibited by media containing cycloheximide
  - *A. fumigatus* differentiated from other species by its ability to grow at 45 °C
  - Colony surfaces various shades of green with narrow white border, tan white reverse; color is species dependent
    - *A. fumigatus*: Green
    - *A. flavus*: Yellow-green
    - *A. niger*: Black
- Positive culture from normally sterile site or positive culture in combination with presence of tissue invasion provides good evidence of invasive aspergillosis
- Cultures from BAL fluids may reflect colonization and not actual infection; histopathology is very useful to make distinction
- Commercially available agar to detect azole resistance available

MICROSCOPIC

Histologic Features

- Regular, septate hyphae (3-6 μm in diameter) with acute-angle branching at 45°; vesicles with conidia ("fruiting bodies") can be observed when fungi are in oxygenated areas, such as cavitary lung lesions or paranasal sinuses
- Tend to grow from hematogenous lesions in tissues in radial fashion (especially when infarcted/necrotic)
- Angioinvasion is commonly present, resulting in thrombosis, hemorrhagic lesions, and tissue infarction
- Presence of dark brown or black pigments may be present in infection caused by *A. niger*, which produces pigmented conidiospores; this nonspecific finding can be seen with dematiaceous fungi
- Calcium oxalate crystalloids can be present if primary lesion is longstanding (primarily *A. niger*, also *A. fumigatus*)
- Invasive disease associated with neutrophilic inflammation and necrotic debris; little inflammatory reaction in neutropenic patients; granulomatous response occasionally present
- Allergic or hypersensitivity aspergillosis: Hypersecretion of mucus with neutrophils and eosinophils; Charcot-Leyden crystals sometimes seen
- Aspergilloma (fungal ball): Colonization of preexisting cavity with dense collection of fungi; cavity wall may contain inflammatory granulation tissue, fibrous tissue, granulomas, or eosinophils

ANCILLARY TESTS

Special Stains

- Hyphae highlighted by silver stains Gomori methenamine silver (GMS) stain and periodic acid-Schiff stain with diastase (PAS-D)

Immunohistochemistry and In Situ Hybridization

- *Aspergillus* spp. antibodies are commercially available but not widely used for diagnosis due to cross reactivity within and outside of genus
- Genus- or species-specific RNA/DNA probes may be used to distinguish from other hyaline molds

DIFFERENTIAL DIAGNOSIS

Candidiasis

- Predominantly present as gram-positive yeast forms and pseudohyphae (not present in *Aspergillus* spp.); occasional hyphae
- Hyphae of *Aspergillus* spp. may be mistaken for nonbudding yeast cells when cut transversely
- *Aspergillus* hyphae may show terminal swellings (vesicles), which may be confused with terminal chlamydospores of candida; distinguished by intercalary chlamydospores when present
- Positive for serum (1,3)-β-D-glucan in disseminated disease; negative for galactomannan
- Correlation with culture or PCR is often needed for determination of species

Mucormycosis

- Angioinvasion is commonly present in invasive disease of mucormycosis and aspergillosis
- Mucorales exhibit broad, irregular hyphae with few septations and right-angle branching
- Negative for serum galactomannan and (1,3)-β-D-glucan

Hyalohyphomycosis

- *Fusarium, Scedosporium, Penicillium* spp., and other hyaline septate molds, such as dermatophytes, may present as dichotomous fungi similar to *Aspergillus* spp.
- *Aspergillus* spp. can be distinguished by presence of fruiting heads, but these are usually present only in well-oxygenated lesions or cavities
- Typically requires culture or PCR to identify species

Concurrent Infections With Other Fungi

- Concurrent infection with *Aspergillus* spp., *Candida* spp., or *Mucor* spp. have been reported
- Alternative diagnostic testing of tissues, such as immunohistochemistry, in situ hybridization, or PCR, may be needed for definitive classification

SELECTED REFERENCES

1. Kanaujia R et al: Aspergillosis: an update on clinical spectrum, diagnostic schemes, and management. Curr Fungal Infect Rep. 1-12, 2023
2. Freeman Weiss Z et al: The evolving landscape of fungal diagnostics, current and emerging microbiological approaches. J Fungi (Basel). 7(2), 2021
3. Koehler P et al: Defining and managing COVID-19-associated pulmonary aspergillosis: the 2020 ECMM/ISHAM consensus criteria for research and clinical guidance. Lancet Infect Dis. 21(6):e149-62, 2021
4. Thompson GR 3rd et al: Aspergillus infections. N Engl J Med. 385(16):1496-509, 2021
5. Chen P et al: Uncovering new mutations conferring azole resistance in the Aspergillus fumigatus cyp51A gene. Front Microbiol. 10:3127, 2019
6. Cruciani M et al: Polymerase chain reaction blood tests for the diagnosis of invasive aspergillosis in immunocompromised people. Cochrane Database Syst Rev. 9(9):CD009551, 2019
7. Jenks JD et al: Point-of-care diagnosis of invasive aspergillosis in non-neutropenic patients: Aspergillus galactomannan lateral flow assay versus Aspergillus-specific lateral flow device test in bronchoalveolar lavage. Mycoses. 62(3):230-6, 2019
8. Springer J et al: Identification of Aspergillus and mucorales in formalin-fixed, paraffin-embedded tissue samples: comparison of specific and broad-range fungal qPCR assays. Med Mycol. 57(3):308-13, 2019
9. Chavez JA et al: Practical diagnostic approach to the presence of hyphae in neuropathology specimens with three illustrative cases. Am J Clin Pathol. 149(2):98-104, 2018
10. Ketai L et al: Radiology of chronic cavitary infections. J Thorac Imaging. 33(5):334-43, 2018
11. Suzuki Y et al: Visceral mycoses in autopsied cases in Japan from 1989 to 2013. Med Mycol J. 59(4):E53-62, 2018

***A. fumigatus* Culture Isolate**

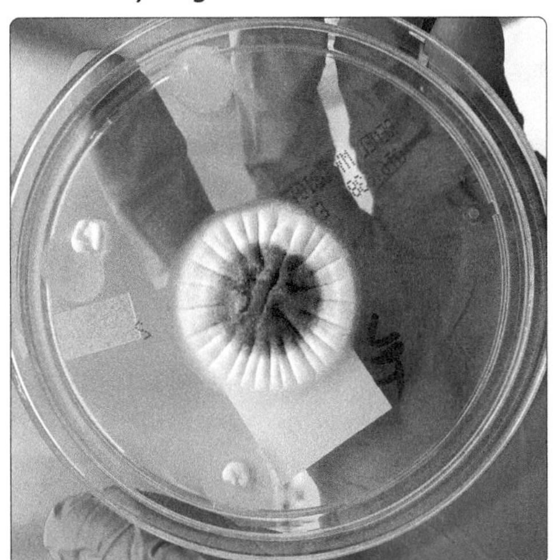

***A. fumigatus* Lactophenol Cotton Blue**

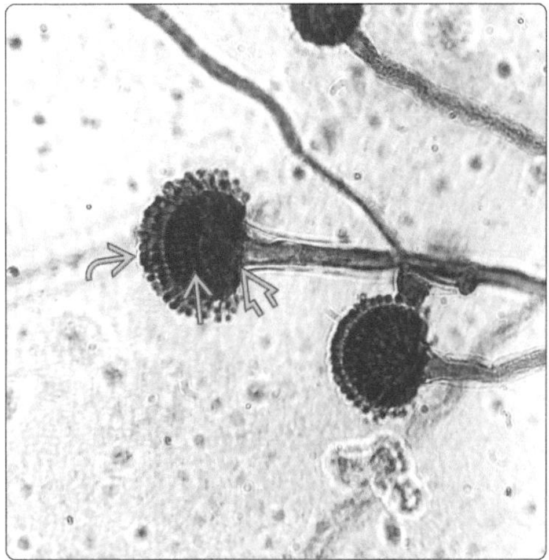

(Left) *Blue-green colonies with a suede-like surface are typically observed on Czapek-Dx agar in cases of Aspergillus fumigatus. (Courtesy J. Crothers, MD.)* **(Right)** *Hyphae with swollen vesicles ➡ give rise to phialides ➡, which produce conidia ➡ in chains. (Courtesy J. Crothers, MD.)*

(Left) *Chest CT of the lungs shows the presence of an irregular nodule surrounded by ground-glass opacity (halo sign) ⇨. Biopsy and ancillary testing confirmed the presence of an aspergilloma.* **(Right)** *Narrow septate hyphae ⇨ with acute-angle branching ⇨ are present in a bronchoalveolar lavage (ThinPrep). Culture confirms the presence of A. fumigatus.*

Chest CT: Aspergilloma

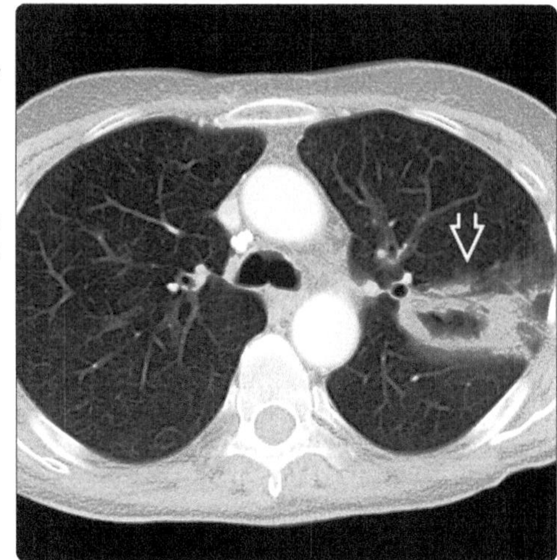

A. fumigatus in Bronchoalveolar Lavage

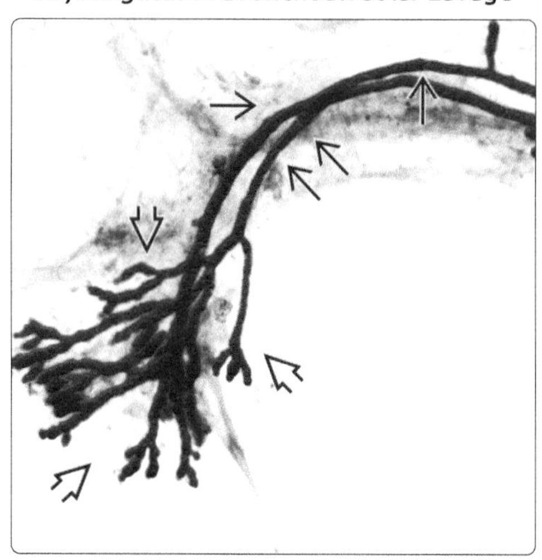

(Left) *A well-defined fungal aggregate is present within the airway, containing narrow, acute-angle branching, septated fungal hyphae morphologically consistent with Aspergillus spp.* **(Right)** *This H&E-stained section from a patient with severe burns shows narrow fungal hyphae with acute angle branching, identified as A. flavus in concurrent cultures.*

Aspergillus Lung Nodule

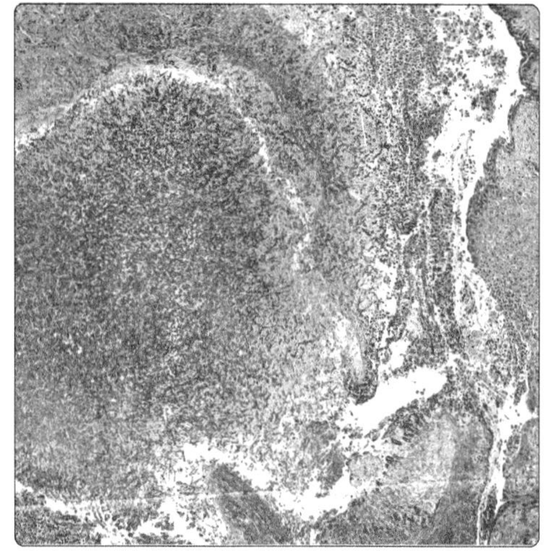

A. flavus

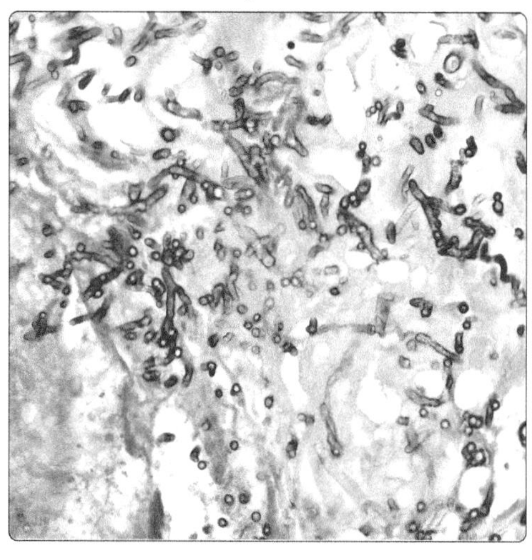

(Left) *This brain MR shows a ring-enhancing mass ⇨, confirmed to be disseminated aspergillosis following surgical biopsy. While fungal abscess can be caused by direct extension from sinuses, the more posterior location in this is consistent with hematogenous spread.* **(Right)** *Numerous narrow hyphae ⇨ are present in this H&E-stained brain section, which may appear yeast-like in cross sections ⇨.*

Aspergillus Brain Abscess

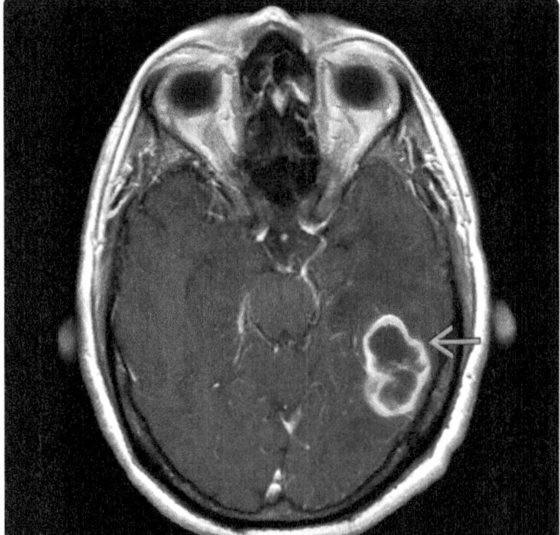

A. fumigatus in Brain

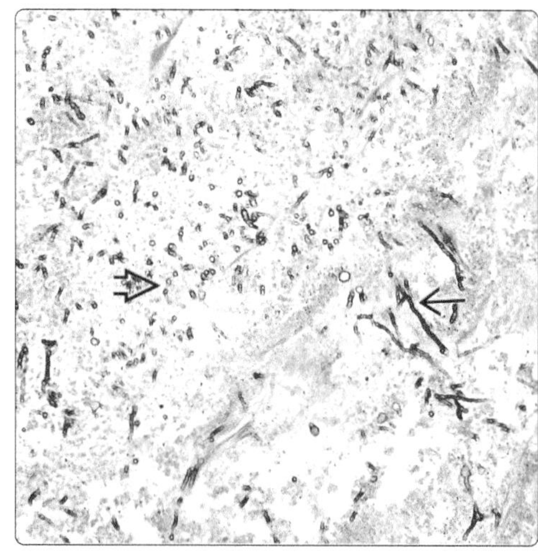

Fungal Sinusitis

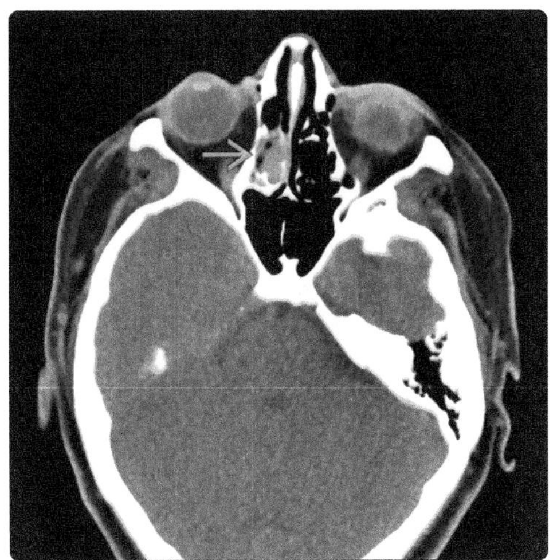

A. niger

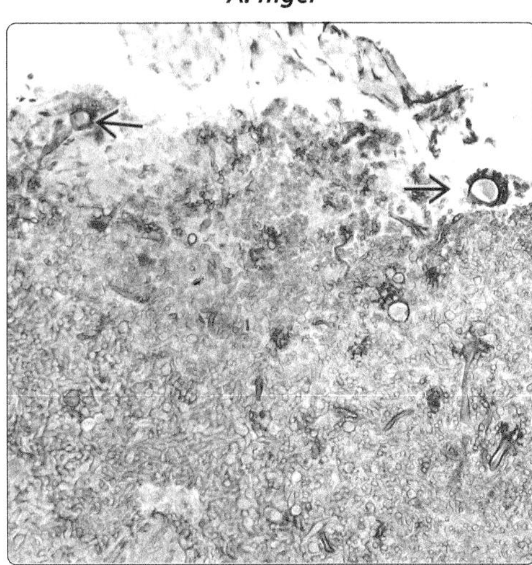

(Left) *On this CT of the face, a soft tissue mass was identified in the sinuses on the right side ➡, identified as fungal sinusitis due to Aspergillus spp.* **(Right)** *This section of sinus contents from a patient with fungal sinusitis shows a dense mass of fungal hyphae with scattered pigmented forms and fruiting bodies ➡, confirmed in culture to be Aspergillus niger. These pigmented hyphae may be confused with dematiaceous fungi if present in a majority of the specimen.*

Calcium Oxalate: *Aspergillus* Species

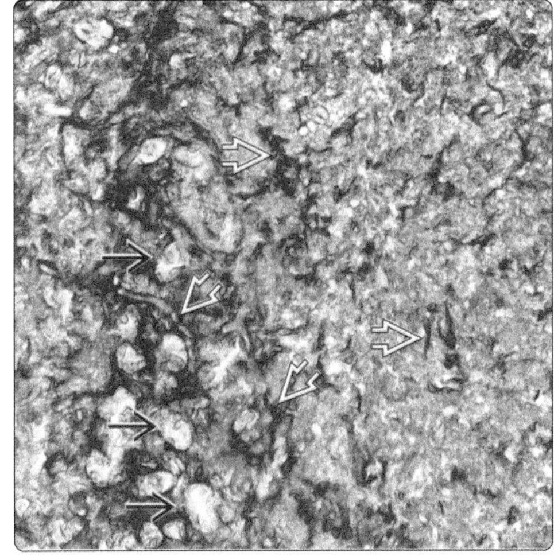

Polarized Calcium Oxalate

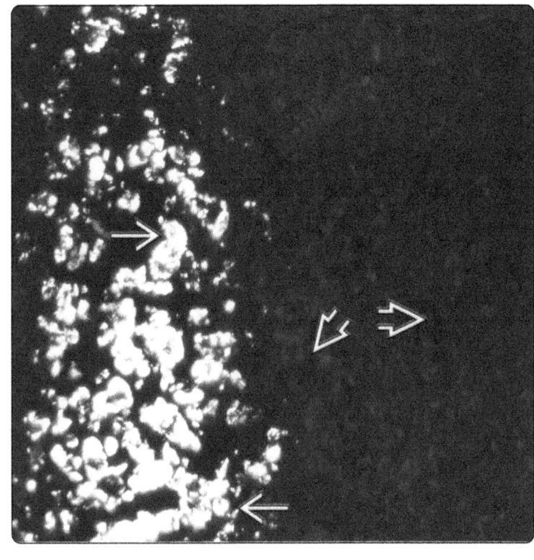

(Left) *Tissue section shows necrosis associated with large hyphal forms ➡ and a collection of calcium oxalate crystals ➡, consistent with Aspergillus spp. (typically A. niger or A. fumigatus).* **(Right)** *Tissue section shows hyphal forms ➡ and collections of Aspergillus-associated calcium oxalate crystals ➡ under polarized light microscopy.*

A. fumigatus

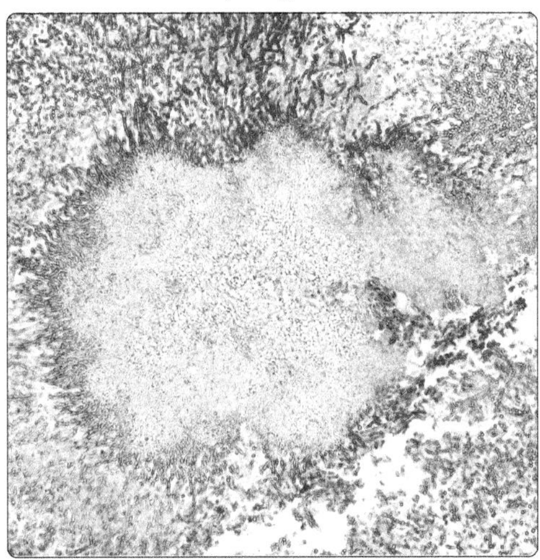

***A. fumigatus*: GMS Stain**

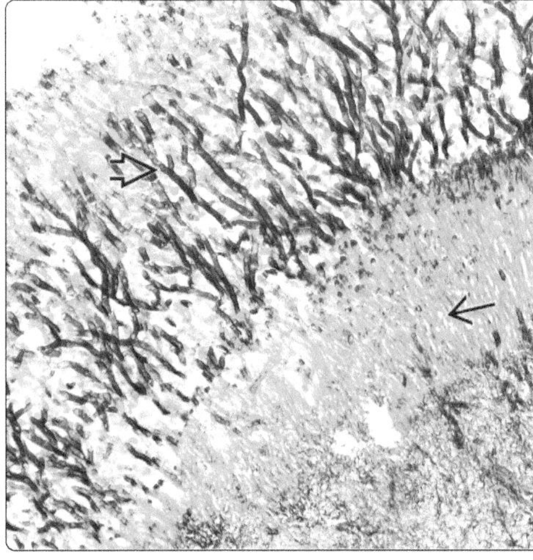

(Left) *This section of tissue from an ear mass shows a dense collection of eosinophilic-appearing fungi surrounded by more basophilic branching forms at the periphery. ITS and 28S rRNA sequencing of the FFPE tissue identified A. fumigatus.* **(Right)** *GMS-stained section of an ear mass shows poor staining in the dense center ➡, and stronger staining at the periphery ➡, allowing for the identification of narrow hyphae with acute angle branching and septations, consistent with Aspergillus spp.*

KEY FACTS

ETIOLOGY/PATHOGENESIS

- Infection with the entomphtoralean fungi *Conidiobolus* spp. and *Basidiobolus* spp., capable of infecting insects and mammalian hosts
- Infections rarely disseminate from initial lesion to other regions of body but rather spread locally

CLINICAL ISSUES

- Conidiobolomycosis: Typically confined to central face (rhinofacial) and presents with nasal discharge, obstruction, and paranasal sinus pain
- Basidiobolomycosis: Presents as subcutaneous, visceral or intestinal mass, mimicking sarcoma or colon cancer; can be large and is typically slowly growing, painless, and firm

MICROBIOLOGY

- *Conidiobolus spp.*: Beige to brown colonies, aerial white hyphae over time; discharged conidia cause plate cloudiness; conidia may have villous projections
- *Basidiobolus spp.*: Gray to beige waxy colonies; discharged club-shaped spores with knob-like tip cover plate; zygospores with beak-like appendage

MICROSCOPIC

- Hyphae are large (8-20 µm wide), irregular, have thin walls, are pauciseptate; highlighted by GMS and PAS-D stains
- Fragments of hyphae are surrounded by granulomatous inflammation, intense eosinophilic inflammation, and Splendore-Hoeppli phenomenon

TOP DIFFERENTIAL DIAGNOSES

- Mucormycosis: Rapidly progressive infection, frequently angioinvasive; irregular, pauciseptate hyphae are similar in appearance but may stain poorly with GMS; confirm with cultures/PCR
- Pythiosis: Rapidly progressive disease with irregular, pauciseptate hyphae with Splendore-Hoeppli phenomenon similar to entomophthoromycosis; confirm with cultures/PCR

(Left) *Centrofacial involvement with swelling and induration of the lower eyelids, bridge of the nose, and upper lips are characteristic of conidiobolomycosis. (Courtesy L. Georg, PhD, CDC/PHIL.)* **(Right)** *Conidiobolus coronatus primary conidia are globose-shaped and have a characteristic basal papilla, corresponding to the residual hyphal segment after conidial ejection. (Courtesy M. Renz, CDC/PHIL.)*

Conidiobolomycosis (Rhinofacial Entomophthoramycosis)

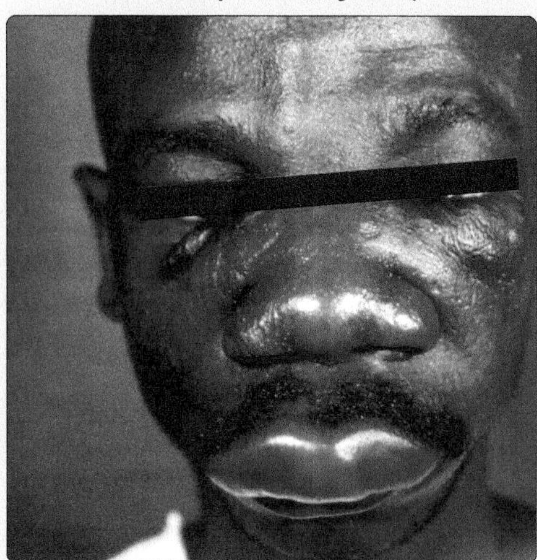

***Conidiobolus coronatus* Primary Conidia**

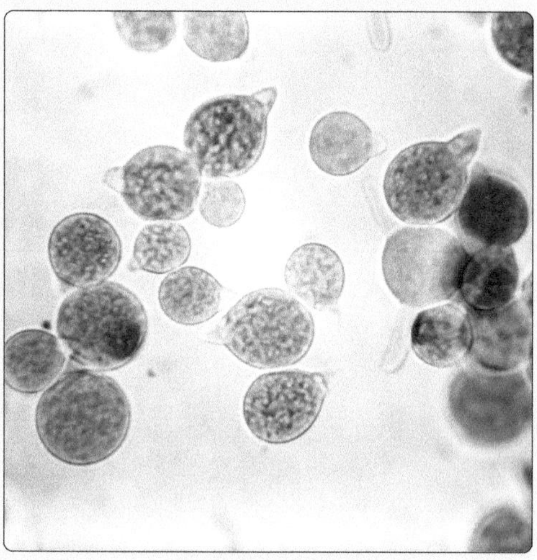

(Left) *A linear tract is highlighted by intense eosinophilic degranulation and proteinaceous material (Splendore-Hoeppli phenomenon) delineating the contours of a large, irregular hypha in a bridge nose mass in a young man believed to be a neoplasm.* **(Right)** *Irregular coenocytic hyphae similar to those seen in mucormycosis are shown in this biopsy from a subcutaneous nasal mass from a young man with conidiobolomycosis.*

Conidiobolomycosis

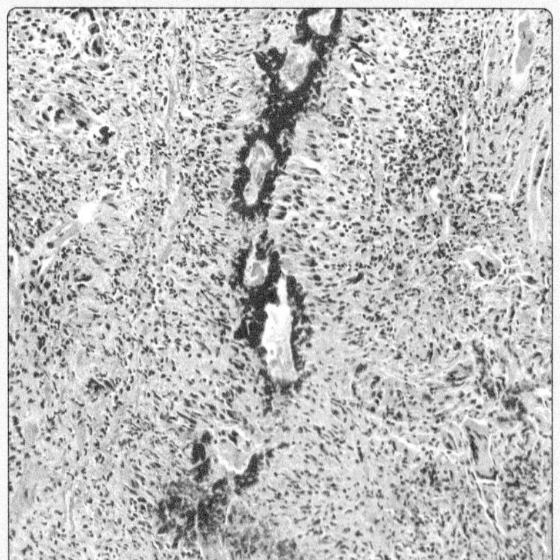

***Conidiobolus* Hyphae**

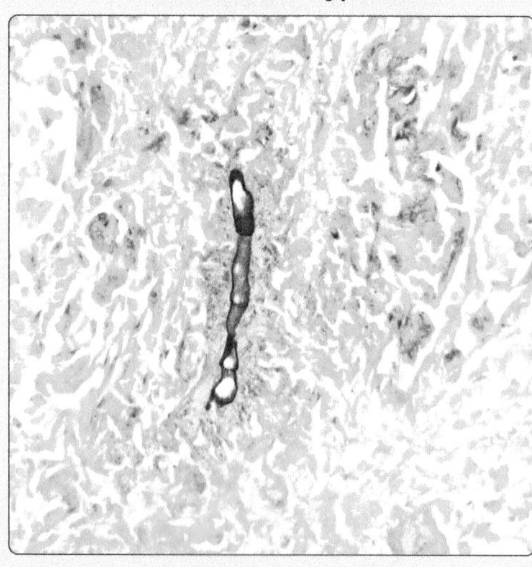

TERMINOLOGY

Synonyms

- Conidiobolomycosis, basidiobolomycosis, rhinofacial entomophthoromycosis, subcutaneous zygomycosis

Definitions

- Greek: Entomo (insect) + phthora (destruction) "insect destroyer"

ETIOLOGY/PATHOGENESIS

Infectious Agents

- Infection with entomophthoralean fungi *Conidiobolus coronatus* (most common species), *C. incongruous*, *C. laprauges*, and *Basidiobolus ranarum*, which are capable of infecting insects and mammalian hosts
- Fungi found in soil and reptile, amphibian, and insect droppings in tropical and subtropical areas
- Mechanism of infection unknown but presumably traumatic inoculation into skin (e.g., insect bite; basidiobolomycosis) or via inhalation of fungal spores (conidiobolomycosis)
- Infections tend to spread locally; rare dissemination from initial lesion to other regions of body; disseminated *C. lamprauges* described in immunocompromised patient

CLINICAL ISSUES

Epidemiology

- Higher prevalence in tropical and subtropical regions
- More common in males than females and in children/young adults
- *Conidiobolus* spp. found in soil and decaying plant matter in high-humidity areas, including beaches of UK., eastern coast of USA, India and Western Africa; disease reported mainly in West Africa
- *B. ranarum* is endemic in India, Pakistan Uganda, Kenya, Ivory Coast, Ghana, Myanmar, and South America; autochthonous cases reported in Arizona

Presentation

- Conidiobolomycosis: Typically confined to central face (rhinofacial) and presents with nasal discharge, obstruction and paranasal sinus pain; advanced stages include involvement of upper lip and eyelids
- Basidiobolomycosis: Presents as subcutaneous, visceral or intestinal mass, mimicking sarcoma or colon cancer; mass may be large and is typically slowly growing, painless and firm

Laboratory Tests

- Peripheral eosinophilia frequently present
- Speciation by PCR/sequencing of ITS, 28S rRNA genes

Treatment

- Prolonged antifungal therapy with triazole and surgical debridement are mainstays of treatment

Prognosis

- Good prognosis with cure after prolonged antifungal therapy and debridement
- Early diagnosis results in better outcome and less sequelae (e.g., scarring, tissue laxitude)

MICROBIOLOGY

Culture and Microbiologic Identification

- *Conidiobolus spp.*: Glabrous, flat, beige to brown colonies that develop aerial white hyphae over time; plate becomes cloudy from conidia discharged from short sporangiospores; conidia may have villous projections
- *Basidiobolus spp.*: Glabrous, gray to beige waxy colonies; plate becomes covered with discharged club-shaped spores with knob-like tip; zygospores (20- to 50-μm diameter) have beak-like appendage

MICROSCOPIC

Histologic Features

- Conidiobolomycosis and basidiobolomycosis histologically indistinguishable; however, distribution of lesions (i.e., rhinofacial for *Conidiobolus* spp. and subcutaneous or gastrointestinal for *B. ranarum*) can help distinguish
- Hyphae are large (8-20 μm wide), irregular, have thin walls, are pauciseptate, and frequently exhibit Mucorales-like wrinkling
- Fragments of hyphae are surrounded by granulomatous inflammation, intense eosinophilic inflammation, and Splendore-Hoeppli phenomenon
- No evidence of angioinvasion, necrosis, or tissue infarction

ANCILLARY TESTS

Special Stains

- Hyphae highlighted by GMS and PAS-D stains

DIFFERENTIAL DIAGNOSIS

Mucormycosis

- May be cutaneous, pulmonary, gastrointestinal, or rhinocerebral; frequently angioinvasive and associated with tissue infarction
- Irregular, pauciseptate hyphae are similar in appearance and may poorly stain with GMS; confirm with cultures/PCR

Pythiosis

- Orbital or vascular occlusive disease but rapidly progressive and not insidious
- Irregular, pauciseptate hyphae with Splendore-Hoeppli phenomenon very similar to entomophthoromycosis

SELECTED REFERENCES

1. Acosta-España JD et al: An old confusion: entomophthoromycosis versus mucormycosis and their main differences. Front Microbiol. 13:1035100, 2022
2. Pezzani MD et al: Gastrointestinal basidiobolomycosis: an emerging mycosis difficult to diagnose but curable. Case report and review of the literature. Travel Med Infect Dis. 31:101378, 2019
3. Vilela R et al: Human pathogenic entomophthorales. Clin Microbiol Rev. 31(4), 2018
4. Shaikh N et al: Entomophthoramycosis: a neglected tropical mycosis. Clin Microbiol Infect. 22(8):688-94, 2016
5. Blumentrath CG et al: Classification of rhinoentomophthoromycosis into atypical, early, intermediate, and late disease: a proposal. PLoS Negl Trop Dis. 9(10):e0003984, 2015
6. Mendoza L et al: Human fungal pathogens of Mucorales and Entomophthorales. Cold Spring Harb Perspect Med. 5(4), 2014
7. Vikram HR et al: Emergence of gastrointestinal basidiobolomycosis in the United States, with a review of worldwide cases. Clin Infect Dis. 54(12):1685-91, 2012

Basidiobolomycosis ("Woody" Cellulitis)

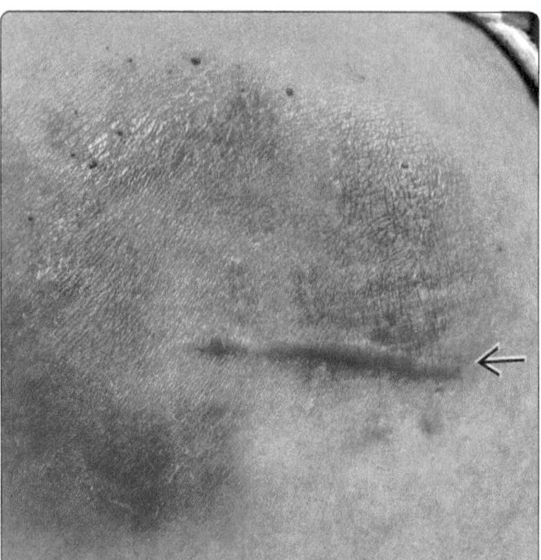

Basidiobolus ranarum Culture Isolate

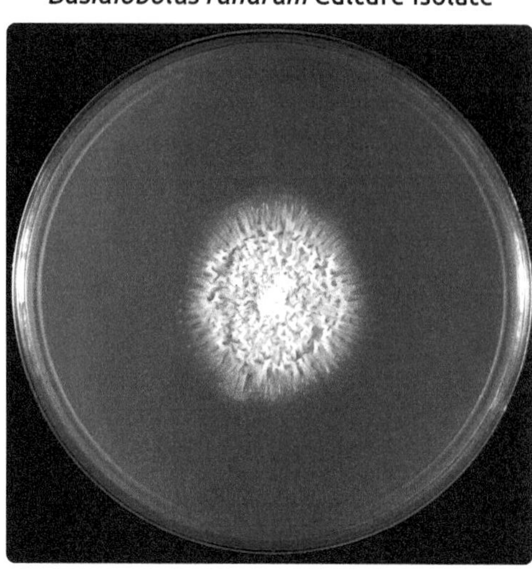

(Left) *Large (10-cm) solitary indurated plaque on the right upper thigh of an otherwise healthy young man is shown. The lesion grew slowly over 2 years and was asymptomatic. Notice the excisional biopsy scar ⊡. (Courtesy P. Pattanaprichakul, MD.)* **(Right)** *Basidiobolus colonies are white and powdery with a roughened appearance and surface mycelium. Notice the folded or ruffled periphery. (Courtesy L. Ajello, PhD, CDC/PHIL.)*

Basidiobolus ranarum Zygospore

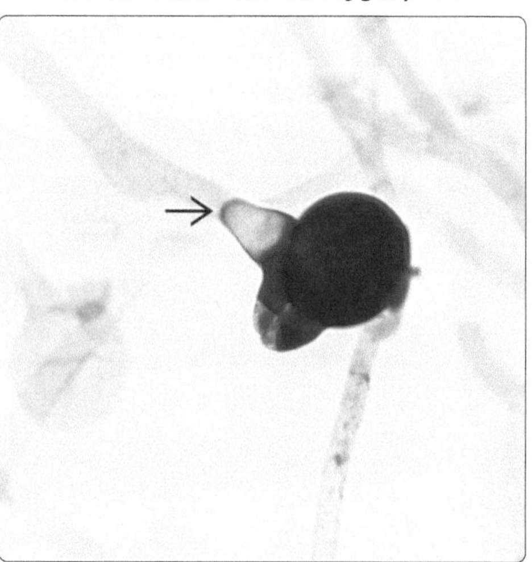

Basidiobolus ranarum Zygospore

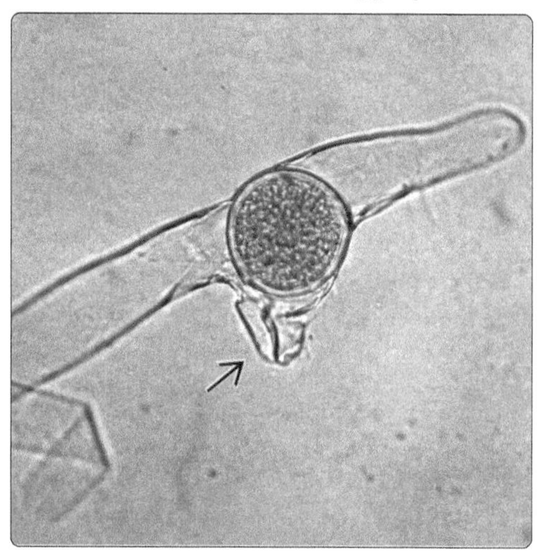

(Left) *A diploid zygospore, formed at the site of fusion between 2 opposite sex hyphal filaments, is noted in this lactophenol cotton blue preparation. After the exchange of genetic material, a characteristic beak is formed ⊡. (Courtesy L. Ajello, PhD, CDC/PHIL.)* **(Right)** *Basidiobolus ranarum (a.k.a. Basidiobolus meristosporus) zygospores are created when 2 haploid hyphae fuse together ⊡. (Courtesy L. Georg, PhD, CDC/PHIL.)*

Eosinophilic Cellulitis in Basidiobolomycosis

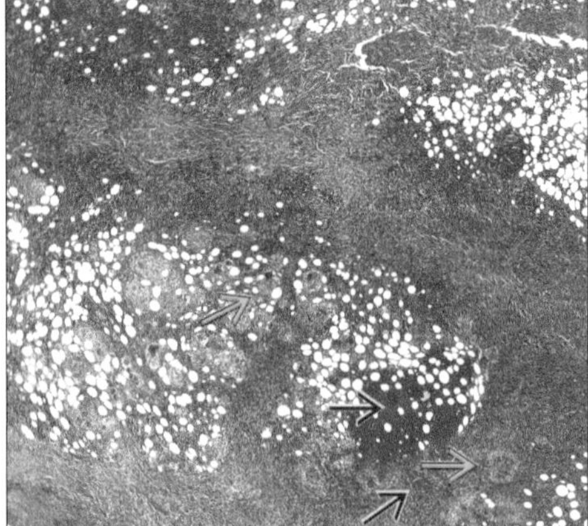

Granulomatous Inflammation in *Basidiobolus* Cellulitis

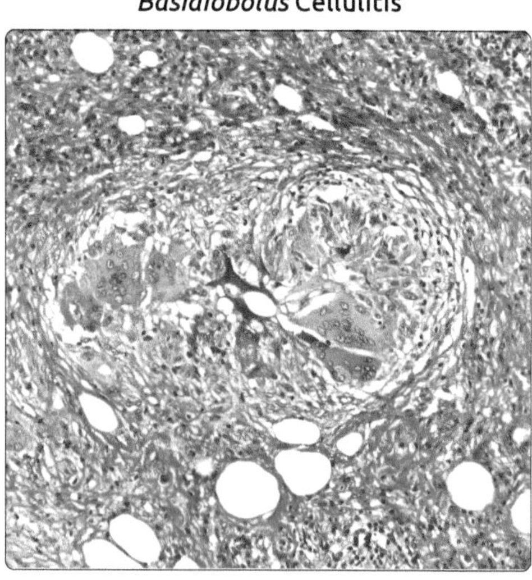

(Left) *Diffuse inflammation of the subcutis with numerous eosinophils ⊡ and granulomas ⊡ should alert histopathologist to the possibility of basidiobolomycosis. (Courtesy P. Pattanaprichakul, MD.)* **(Right)** *Florid granulomas with multinucleate giant cells surrounding irregular, pauciseptate hyphae are shown in a case of "woody" cellulitis due to B. ranarum. (Courtesy P. Pattanaprichakul, MD.)*

Basidiobolomycosis PAS Stain

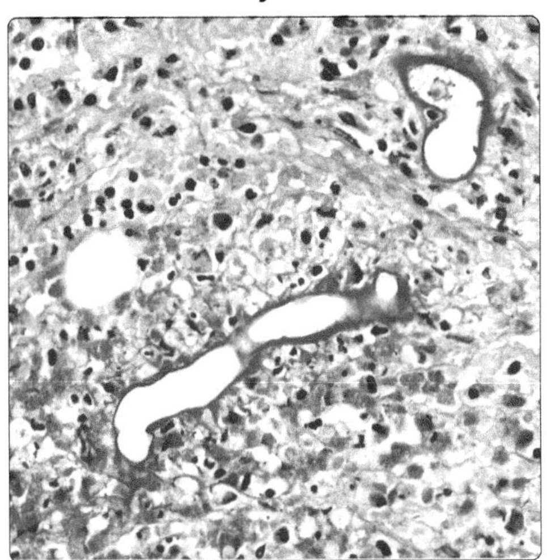

Basidiobolomycosis GMS Stain

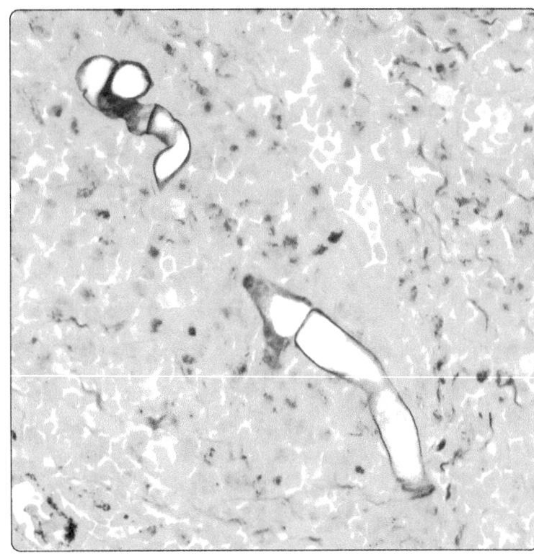

(Left) *Large, irregular hyphae eliciting a prominent eosinophilic response are characteristic of basidiobolomycosis. Interestingly, although identical histologically, Conidiobolus affects the centrofacial region. (Courtesy P. Pattanaprichakul, MD.)* **(Right)** *Fragments of large, irregular hyphae with thin walls are highlighted by the Grocott methenamine silver reaction in this case of "woody" cellulitis due to B. ranarum. (Courtesy P. Pattanaprichakul, MD.)*

Splendore-Hoeppli Phenomenon in Basidiobolomycosis

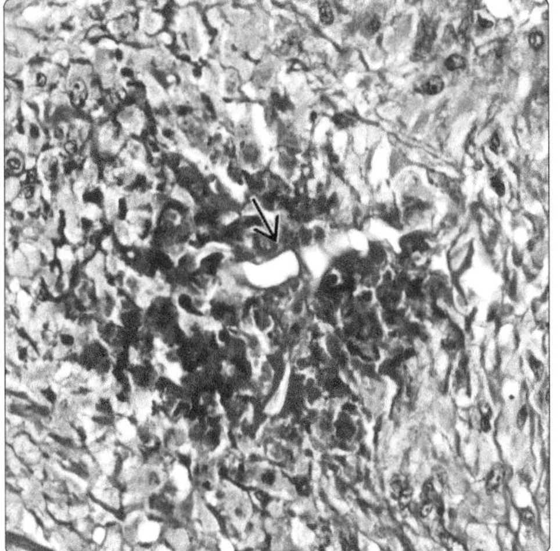

***Basidiobolus* Cecal Mass Mimicking Colon Cancer**

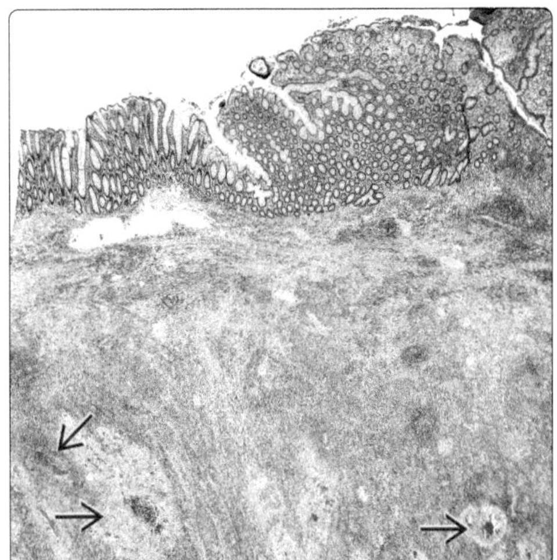

(Left) *The "negative" image of an irregular hypha ⇒ is delineated by the intense eosinophilic granules of the Splendore-Hoeppli reaction in this case of Basidiobolus cellulitis. (Courtesy P. Pattanaprichakul, MD.)* **(Right)** *Dense transmural inflammation with eosinophilic aggregates at the deep aspect of the colonic muscular wall ⇒ are shown in this case of basidiobolomycosis in a patient with acute ileocecal obstruction clinically suspected to have colon cancer.*

Basidiobolomycosis

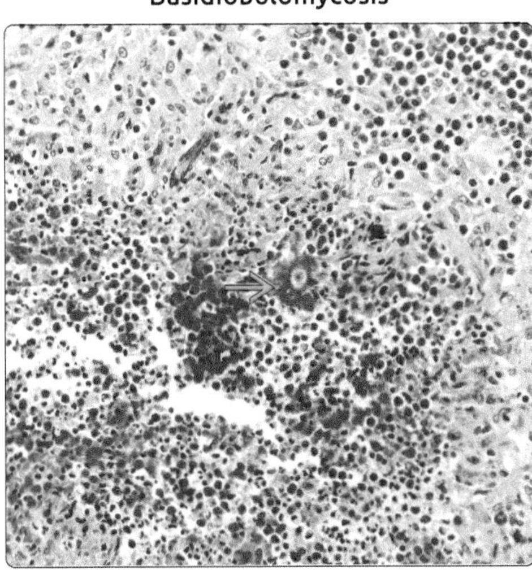

Colonic Basidiobolomycosis PAS-D Stain

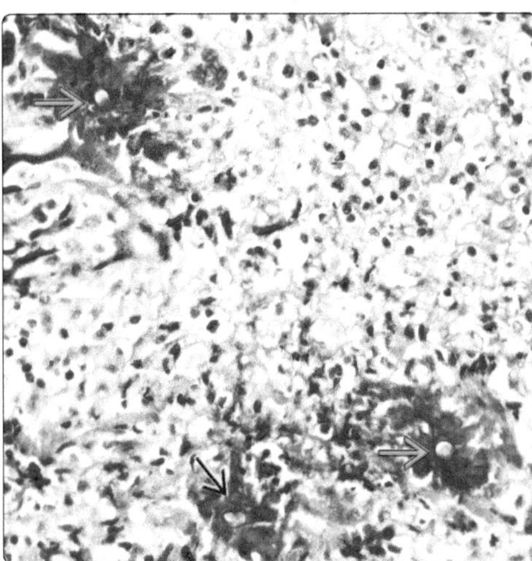

(Left) *Basidiobolomycosis is characterized by necrotizing granulomatous inflammation with multinucleated giant cells, abundant eosinophils, and the Splendore-Hoeppli phenomenon (asteroid body) surrounding a cross section of a hypha ⇒.* **(Right)** *The PAS reaction highlights round cross ⇒ and tangential ⇒ sections of hyphae at the center of asteroid bodies (Splendore-Hoeppli phenomenon) in this case of ileocecal basidiobolomycosis.*

Fusariosis

KEY FACTS

ETIOLOGY/PATHOGENESIS

- Rare infections of humans, hyaline hyphae-forming fungi (nondematiaceous)
- *Fusarium*, *Paecilomyces*, *Acremonium*, and others

CLINICAL ISSUES

- Often limited to keratitis or onychomycosis in immunocompetent patients
- Severe neutropenia with fever on antibiotic therapy
- Can present with cutaneous (papular/nodular lesions), sinus, or pulmonary involvement
- Voriconazole is 1st-line agent (resistant infections reported)
- High mortality, especially with disseminated disease, due to severe host immunosuppression and delays in identification
- ITS or 28S rRNA sequencing can be helpful with cultured or FFPE specimens

MICROBIOLOGY

- Culture is primary tool for definitive identification
- In cases of disseminated fusariosis, peripheral aerobic blood cultures may be positive

MICROSCOPIC

- Variable neutrophilic infiltrates (depending on level of neutropenia) or granulomatous
- Invasive fungal hyphal forms are same size/appearance as *Aspergillus* with vascular invasion; infarction common
- Canoe- or banana-shaped conidia may be present (difficult to detect)
- PAS-D and GMS highlight fungal forms

TOP DIFFERENTIAL DIAGNOSES

- Aspergillosis: Hyphae in tissue are indistinguishable; diagnose with cultures, galactomannan, PCR
- Mucormycosis: Occurs same clinical population but usually more rapid; less inflammatory and have wide, thick, ribbon-like hyphal forms
- Candidiasis: Challenging to distinguish when hyphal forms predominate; yeast forms (when present) are gram positive

Disseminated Hyalohyphomycoses: Skin

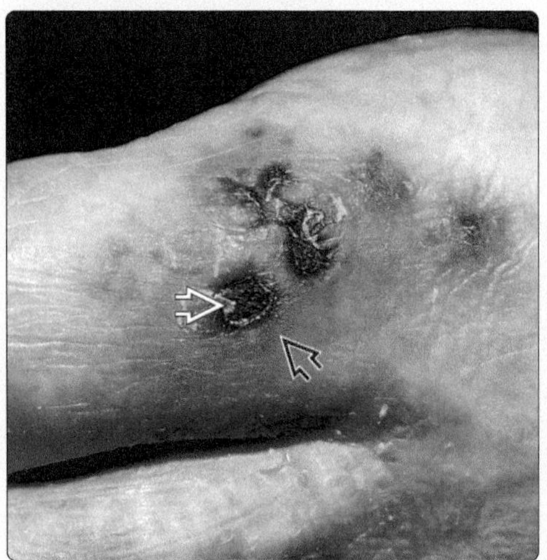

***Fusarium* spp. Hyphae**

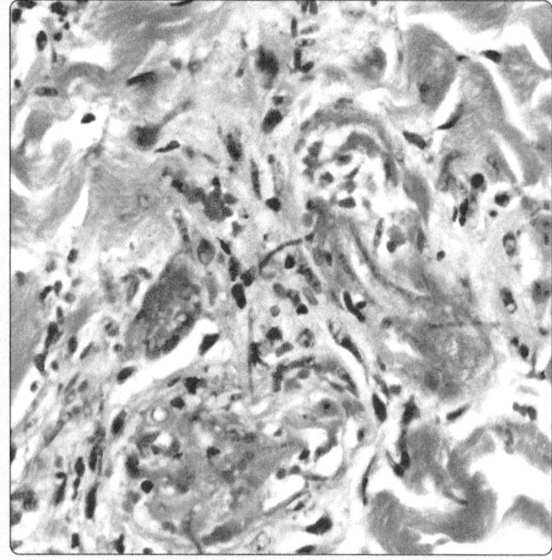

(Left) *Gross photograph shows ecthyma gangrenosum over a toe, which may be seen in disseminated fusariosis. Black gangrenous changes are seen on a red, indurated base. (From DP: Nonneoplastic Derm.)* **(Right)** *Regular hyphae (3-8 μm in width) with readily noted septations and vascular invasion, although nonspecific, are commonly seen in fusariosis.*

***Fusarium* spp. Cytology**

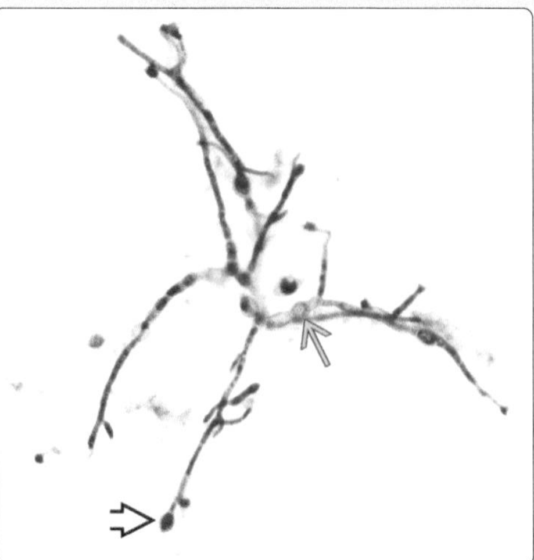

***Fusarium* spp. Conidia: GMS Stain**

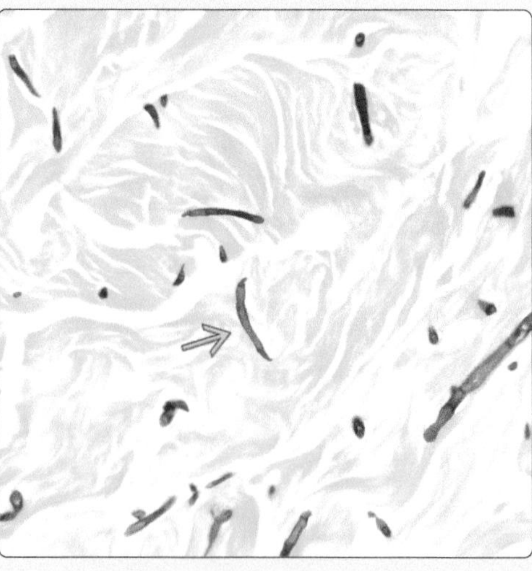

(Left) *Globose swellings in the middle (intercalary) or a the end of hyphae (terminal) representing chlamydospores may be seen in fusariosis but are not specific.* **(Right)** *Sporulation in tissues (adventitious sporulation) is frequent in fusariosis, yielding canoe- or banana-shaped fusiform conidia, which are useful for identification of species when detected.*

TERMINOLOGY

Synonyms

- Derived from Latin "fusus" (spindle)

ETIOLOGY/PATHOGENESIS

Infectious Agents

- Hyalohyphomycosis: Infection of humans caused by any nondematiaceous hyaline fungi where tissue form is mycelial (hyphal) in appearance
- Genera include *Fusarium, Paecilomyces, Purpureocillium, Trichoderma, Chrysosporium, Acremonium*
- Other important genera include *Penicillium, Scopulariopsis,* and *Scedosporium/Lomentospora*
- *Fusarium* species associated with human disease predominantly in *F. solani, F. oxysporum,* and *F. fujikuroi* complexes

CLINICAL ISSUES

Epidemiology

- Fungi are found worldwide

Presentation

- Keratitis with abscess formation after traumatic introduction or cataract surgery
- Onychomycosis of fingernails and toenails
- Invasive disease in immunosuppressed patients (leukemia/lymphoma patients; recipients of bone marrow transplantation, corticosteroids, cytotoxic chemotherapy)
  - Severe neutropenia with fever on antibiotic therapy
  - Skin (erythematous plaque with eschar): Multiple lesions; disseminated disease (60-80% of patients with invasive fusariosis)
  - Localized swelling or pain in face (sinus involvement)
  - Respiratory symptoms: Pneumonia or cavitary mass
  - Neurologic symptoms: Meningoencephalitis or solitary/multiple abscesses
  - Disseminated disease: Sepsis-like syndrome with multiple organs involved

Laboratory Tests

- (1,3)-β-D-glucan: Highly suggestive of invasive fungal disease of any type (except *Mucorales* infection)
- Galactomannan: Highly suggestive of invasive *Aspergillus* infection, though may cross react with *Fusarium* species
- ITS or 28S rRNA for rapid identification to genus and complex; EF-1α, RPB1 &/or RPB2 may be needed to distinguish species
- Sequencing from FFPE tissue has low yield and high rate of false positivity in absence of observable organisms

Treatment

- Voriconazole is 1st-line agent; posaconazole and amphotericin may be used (resistant infections reported)

Prognosis

- High mortality, especially with disseminated disease, due to severe host immunosuppression and delays in identification

MICROBIOLOGY

Culture

- Primary tool for definitive identification
- Routine fungal culture media (Sabouraud dextrose agar): Growth and further differentiation
- Morphologic diagnosis of most species is possible on fungal culture with visualization of macroconidia and other culture-formed structures
- Growing role for matrix-assisted laser desorption/ionization (MALDI) in identification
- Peripheral aerobic blood cultures for fungi occasionally positive in disseminated fusariosis
- May be detected using dedicated fungal blood cultures (e.g., Wampole Isolator tubes)

MICROSCOPIC

Histologic Features

- Inflammation may be variable neutrophilic infiltrates (depending on level of neutropenia) or granulomatous
- Fungal hyphal forms are invasive, smaller size, but similar appearance as *Aspergillus*, and can display vascular destruction with infarction
- Canoe- or banana-shaped conidia may be present but difficult to detect

ANCILLARY TESTS

Special Stains

- PAS and methenamine silver stains highlight fungal hyphae and allow for better morphologic assessment
- Gram stain should be negative in conidia

DIFFERENTIAL DIAGNOSIS

Aspergillosis

- *Aspergillus* hyphae in tissue are morphologically indistinguishable from most species that cause hyalohyphomycoses; culture results, galactomannan, and PCR are primary tools for distinguishing

Mucormycosis

- *Mucorales* infections occur in same clinical population but are usually more rapid; wide, thick, ribbon-like hyphal forms with 90° angle branching; less inflammation

Candidiasis

- Candidal infections with mostly hyphal forms can be challenging to distinguish, but yeast forms (when present) are gram positive

SELECTED REFERENCES

1. Hoenigl M et al: Global guideline for the diagnosis and management of rare mould infections: an initiative of the European Confederation of Medical Mycology in cooperation with the International Society for Human and Animal Mycology and the American Society for Microbiology. Lancet Infect Dis. 21(8):e246-57, 2021
2. Pérez-Nadales E et al: Invasive fusariosis in nonneutropenic patients, Spain, 2000-2015. Emerg Infect Dis. 27(1):26-35, 2021
3. Lockhart SR et al: Emerging and reemerging fungal infections. Semin Diagn Pathol. 36(3):177-81, 2019
4. Moretti ML et al: Airborne transmission of invasive fusariosis in patients with hematologic malignancies. PLoS One. 13(4):e0196426, 2018

Mucormycosis

KEY FACTS

ETIOLOGY/PATHOGENESIS

- Infection with Mucorales, ubiquitous environmental fungi associated with decaying organic matter, via inhalation of spores or though damaged skin

CLINICAL ISSUES

- Most cases have rapid course; disseminated infection carries poor prognosis
- Risk factors include immunosuppression, diabetes mellitus, injection drug use, trauma, burns, malnutrition, iron overload, treatment with deferoxamine
- Most frequent primary clinical manifestations include rhinocerebral, pulmonary, and cutaneous infections
- Serum galactomannan and 1,3-β-D-glucan are typically negative

MICROSCOPIC

- Nonpigmented, wide (5- to 20-μm), thin-walled, ribbon-like hyphae with few septations and right-angle branching; highlighted by GMS and PAS-D stains
- Fragmentation and degeneration of fungal elements can make it hard to assess septation and branching
- Hyphae are angioinvasive, causing tissue necrosis, hemorrhage, and blood vessel thrombosis, particularly in immunocompromised hosts

TOP DIFFERENTIAL DIAGNOSES

- Aspergillosis: Narrow hyphae with septations and acute-angle branching; positive serum galactomannan and 1,3-β-D-glucan
- Candidiasis: Gram-positive yeast, pseudohyphae, and true hyphae; serum 1,3-β-D-glucan positive, galactomannan negative
- Hyalohyphomycosis (e.g., *Fusarium* and *Scedosporium* spp.): narrow hyphae with abundant septations; often positive for 1,3-β-D-glucan, galactomannan negative
- Concurrent infections with other fungi: Confirmation by cultures, molecular testing, IHC/ISH

(Left) *This patient presented with periorbital mucormycosis, which causes damage to the eye and nose through growth and tissue destruction and may result into invasion into brain. (Courtesy L. Ajello, PhD, CDC/PHIL.)* **(Right)** *Numerous broad, irregular, pauciseptate hyphae with wrinkling are present in this section of sinonasal tissue, characteristic of invasive mucormycosis. PCR from FFPE identified Rhizopus oryzae as the causative organism.*

Periorbital Mucormycosis

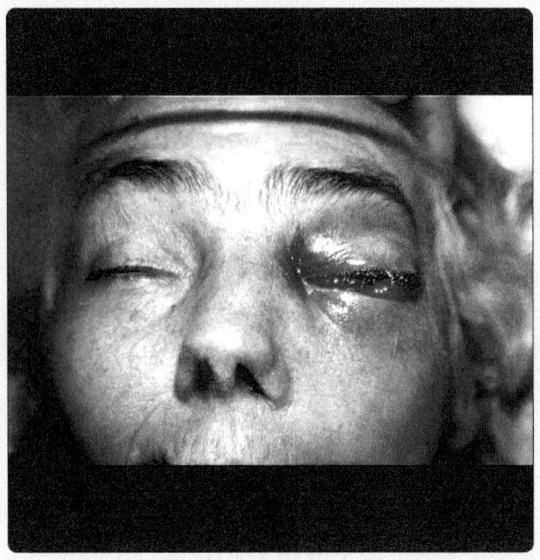

Sinonasal Mucormycosis

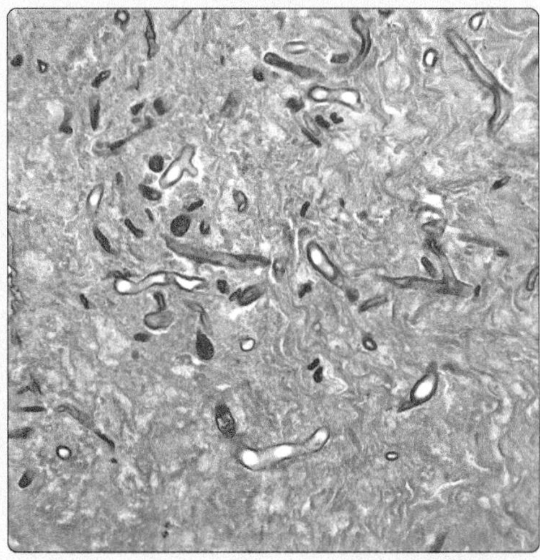

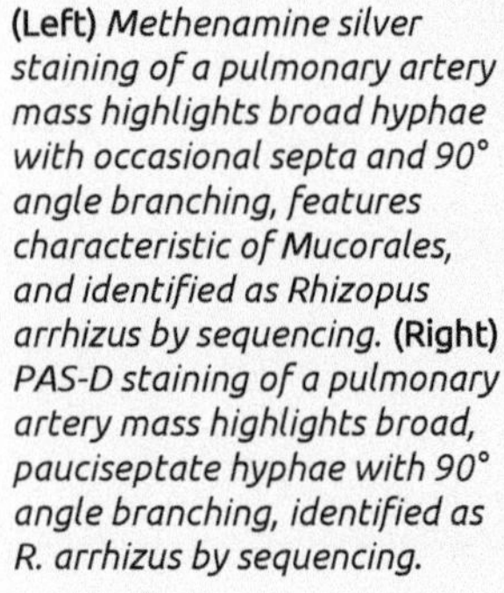

(Left) *Methenamine silver staining of a pulmonary artery mass highlights broad hyphae with occasional septa and 90° angle branching, features characteristic of Mucorales, and identified as Rhizopus arrhizus by sequencing.* **(Right)** *PAS-D staining of a pulmonary artery mass highlights broad, pauciseptate hyphae with 90° angle branching, identified as R. arrhizus by sequencing.*

Methenamine Silver Stain

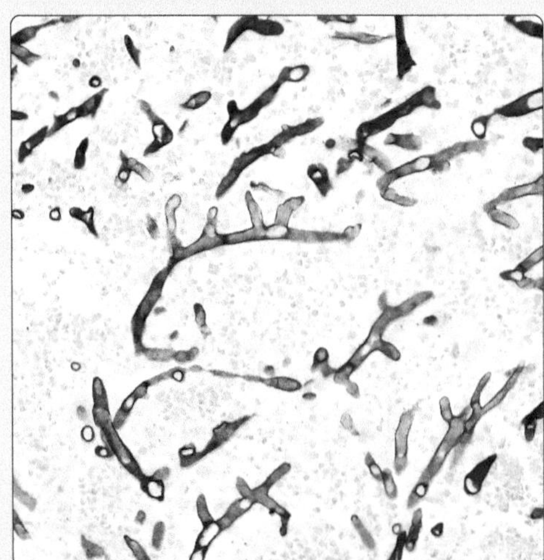

Periodic Acid-Schiff With Diastase Stain

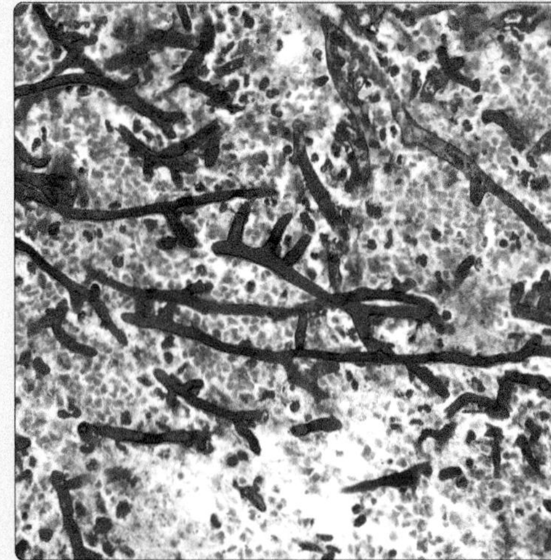

TERMINOLOGY

Definitions

- Latin: "Mucor" (bread mold, wine must)
- Zygomycosis (previous name) from Greek "zygon" (yoke) + "mykes" (mushroom)

ETIOLOGY/PATHOGENESIS

Infectious Agents

- Infection with Mucorales, ubiquitous environmental fungi associated with decaying organic matter, via inhalation of spores or though damaged skin
- Inhaled spores are cleared through GI tract in immunocompetent hosts, while spores persist in immunocompromised individuals, and infection usually begins in nasal sinuses or pulmonary alveoli
- Angioinvasion of fungus results in dissemination, tissue infarction, and necrosis
- *Rhizopus* spp. and *Mucor* spp. most common, followed by *Rhizomucor* spp., *Syncephalastrum* spp., *Cunninghamella bertholletiae*, *Apophysomyces* spp., *Saksenaea* spp., and *Lichtheimia* spp. (formerly *Absidia*)

CLINICAL ISSUES

Epidemiology

- Major risk factors include immunosuppression (e.g., AIDS, hematologic malignancies, solid organ and stem cell transplant recipients, glucocorticoid recipients), and diabetes mellitus with poor glycemic control
- Increased incidence in patients with severe COVID-19 infection, typically with concurrent hyperglycemia
- Iron overload or treatment with deferoxamine; acts as siderophore for *Rhizopus* spp., stimulating fungal growth by increasing iron uptake
- Other risk factors include injection drug use, prematurity, malnutrition, 3rd-degree burns

Presentation

- Most cases have rapid course; rarely indolent
- Rhinocerebral infection is most common clinical presentation, particularly in patients with DKA or neutropenia (most commonly *Rhizopus* spp.); contiguous spread to palate, orbit, and brain, and can progress rapidly
- Rapidly progressive pneumonia with tissue infarction and necrosis, which may ultimately lead to cavitation or hemoptysis; contiguous spread to mediastinum and heart, or hematogenous dissemination
- Cutaneous infection due to inoculation of spores into dermis (e.g., trauma or contaminated wounds) or, rarely, with disseminated disease; deep tissue involvement from cutaneous infection is relatively unusual
- Disseminated infection (from any primary manifestation) usually seen in severely immunocompromised patients, burn patients, premature infants, and transplant recipients; most commonly involving brain
- Gastrointestinal infection is rare, arising from ingestion of fungal organism, and has been described in stomach, colon, and ileum; mostly in transplant recipients and in severely malnourished patients

Laboratory Tests

- Serum galactomannan and 1,3-β-D-glucan are negative
- Mucorales PCR from serum or plasma may detect infection prior to onset of symptoms

Treatment

- Combination of antifungal therapy and surgical debridement of infected tissues
- Predisposing factors should be actively managed, e.g., metabolic acidosis, hyperglycemia, immunosuppressive drugs
- Liposomal amphotericin B is 1st-line therapy
- Intravenous or posaconazole can be used in patients who cannot tolerate or do not respond to amphotericin B
- Combination antifungal therapy (e.g., with echinocandins) may be used in refractory cases, though supportive clinical data is limited
- Voriconazole, fluconazole, and flucytosine are not effective against Mucorales
- Surgical debridement should be made as soon as diagnosis of rhinocerebral or orbital mucormycosis is suspected
- Pulmonary mucormycosis often present with multilobar involvement that precludes surgical resection

Prognosis

- Mortality ~ 50% with sinonasal infections, 75% for pulmonary infections, and > 95% for disseminated mucormycosis
- Early diagnosis and combined surgical and medical therapy are key to improved prognosis

IMAGING

Chest Radiographs or CT Scans

- Focal consolidation, masses, or nodules
- Halo sign: Ground-glass attenuation surrounding nodule, seen with angioinvasive fungi, mycobacteria, or in cases of neoplasia causing tissue infarction or hemorrhage
- Reversed halo sign: Focal area of ground-glass attenuation surrounded by ring of consolidation; mucormycosis most common cause of reversed halo sign in immunocompromised hosts

MICROBIOLOGY

Culture

- Grows on all routine fungal media, inhibited by cycloheximide
- Fast-growing (< 3 days), fluffy colonies rapidly fills agar plate in all directions, called lid lifters
- Yield of culture is low, and grinding tissue specimens can reduce likelihood of recovery
- Airborne spores can cause contamination of laboratory media; hence, positive cultures have to be correlated with clinical and histologic findings
- Tape prep, tease prep, or slide culture and lactophenol blue or calcofluor stains used to visualize microscopically

Microscopic Identification

- Wide hyphae with rare septations, sporangia (large round sac structure), and root-like rhizoids may be present

- Appearance and location of root-like rhizoids used for genus determination: *Mucor* (no rhizoids), *Rhizopus* (nodal rhizoids in line with sporangiophores), *Rhizomucor* (internal rhizoids offset from sporangiophores)

MICROSCOPIC

Histologic Features

- Nonpigmented, wide (5-20 μm in diameter), thin-walled, ribbon-like hyphae with few septations (pauciseptate) and right-angle branching
- Hyphae may vary in width, appear folded, fragmented, crinkled, or degenerated on tissue or cytologic specimens; lack of regular septations makes hyphae fragile and prone to damage during tissue processing
- Fungal elements often seen invading blood vessel wall or within lumen, associated with tissue necrosis, hemorrhage, and blood vessel thrombosis

ANCILLARY TESTS

Special Stains

- Hyphae highlighted by methenamine silver and PAS stains; stains may be faintly positive or negative due to fragmentation and degeneration
- Hyphae highlighted by Papanicolaou and calcofluor white stains on cytologic specimens
- Hyphae are negative with Gram stains

Molecular Diagnostics

- PCR with sequencing targeting ITS and 28S rRNA

Immunohistochemistry/In Situ Hybridization

- Immunohistochemistry not widely used due to antibody cross reactivity and low specificity
- In situ hybridization for specific genera or spp. may be useful for fragmented hyphae that lack classic morphology

DIFFERENTIAL DIAGNOSIS

Aspergillosis

- *Aspergillus* hyphae are narrow with septations and acute-angle branching and strong signal with silver staining
- Serum galactomannan and 1,3-β-D-glucan are typically positive in cases of invasive aspergillosis and negative in cases of invasive mucormycosis

Candidiasis

- *Candida* spp. produce gram-positive yeast forms admixed with pseudohyphae and true hyphae
- Serum 1,3-β-D-glucan positive and galactomannan negative with disseminated candidiasis

Hyalohyphomycosis

- Hyaline molds, such as *Fusarium* and *Scedosporium* spp., generally produce abundant septations and may be positive for 1,3-β-D-glucan in disseminated disease

Concurrent Infections With Other Fungi

- Mix of narrow hyphae with frequent septations adjacent to or intermixed with classic Mucorales morphology often represents infections with additional fungal spp.; less commonly due to antifungal treatment effects
- Confirmation by cultures, molecular testing, IHC/ISH

SELECTED REFERENCES

1. Tahiri G et al: Mucorales and mucormycosis: recent insights and future prospects. J Fungi (Basel). 9(3), 2023
2. Darwish RM et al: Mucormycosis: the hidden and forgotten disease. J Appl Microbiol. 132(6):4042-57, 2022
3. Garre V: Recent Advances and future directions in the understanding of mucormycosis. Front Cell Infect Microbiol. 12:850581, 2022
4. Sharma R et al: Mucormycosis in the COVID-19 environment: a multifaceted complication. Front Cell Infect Microbiol. 12:937481, 2022
5. Steinbrink JM et al: Mucormycosis. Infect Dis Clin North Am. 35(2):435-52, 2021
6. Cornely OA et al: Global guideline for the diagnosis and management of mucormycosis: an initiative of the European Confederation of Medical Mycology in cooperation with the Mycoses Study Group Education and Research Consortium. Lancet Infect Dis. 19(12):e405-21, 2019
7. Jeong W et al: The epidemiology and clinical manifestations of mucormycosis: a systematic review and meta-analysis of case reports. Clin Microbiol Infect. 25(1):26-34, 2019
8. Lecointe K et al: Polysaccharides cell wall architecture of Mucorales. Front Microbiol. 10:469, 2019
9. Guarner J et al: Histopathologic diagnosis of fungal infections in the 21st century. Clin Microbiol Rev. 24(2):247-80, 2011

***Rhizopus oryzae* Culture Isolate**

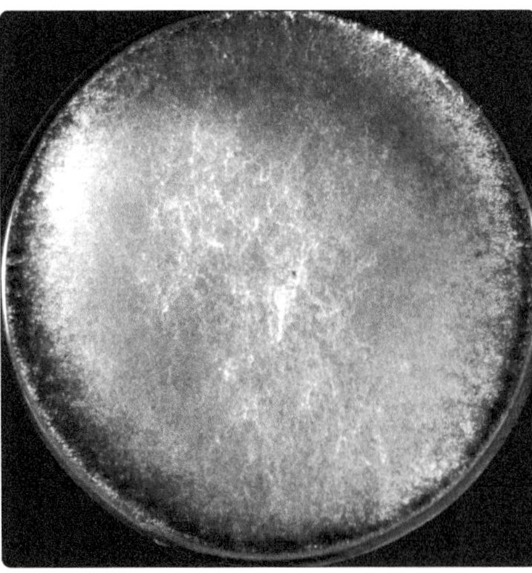

***Rhizopus oryzae* Lactophenol Cotton Blue**

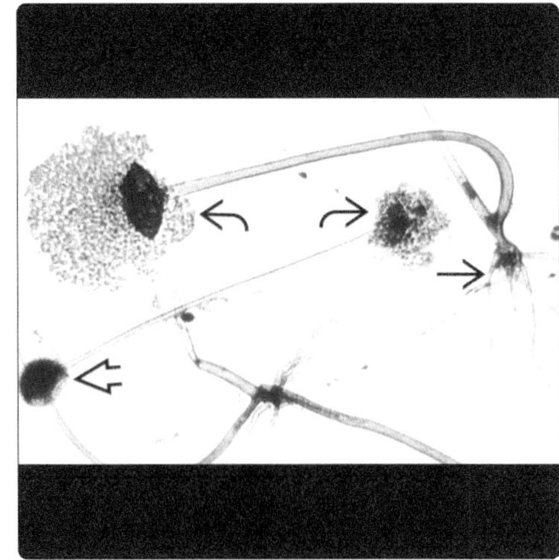

(Left) *This photograph shows a Petri dish filled with rapidly growing grayish yellow fungus with cotton candy-like texture identified as R. oryzae and sometimes referred to as a lid lifter. (Courtesy L. Georg, MD, CDC/PHIL.)* **(Right)** *This slide of an R. oryzae isolate shows characteristic features, including pauciseptate hyphae, root-like rhizoids ➙, developing sporangium ➙, and ruptured mature sporangia releasing their spores ➙. (Courtesy Dr. Hardin, CDC/PHIL.)*

Brain MR: Cerebral Mucormycosis

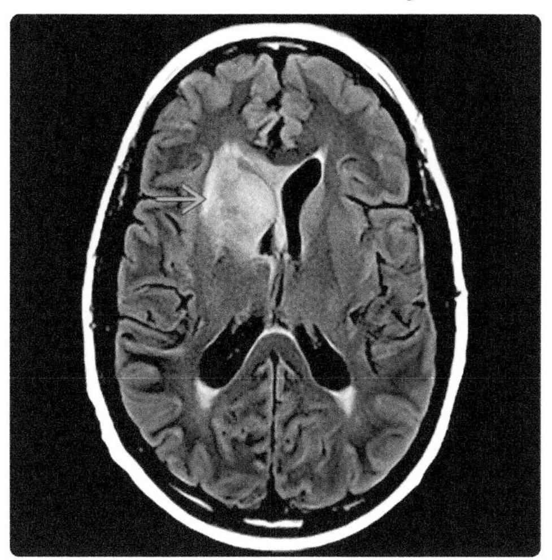

Cerebral Mucormycosis

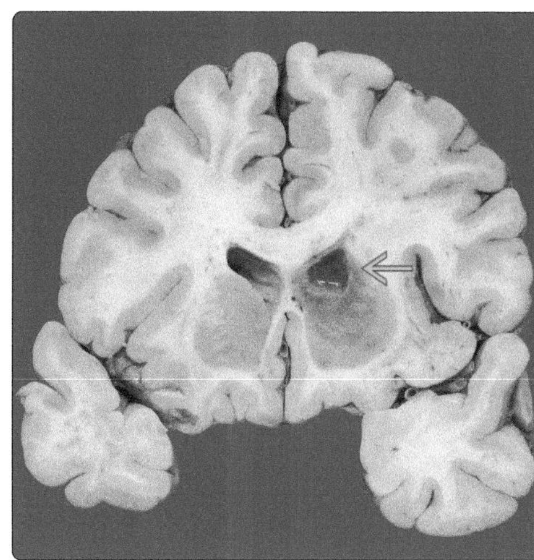

(Left) *This T2 FLAIR MR axial brain image shows a hyperintense mass localized to the right basal ganglia ⊡, subsequently biopsied and found to represent an infection with Rhizomucor spp.* **(Right)** *This autopsy brain slice shows a purulent mass in the right basal ganglia ⊡, corresponding to a fungal abscess caused by disseminated Rhizomucor spp.*

***Mucor* spp.**

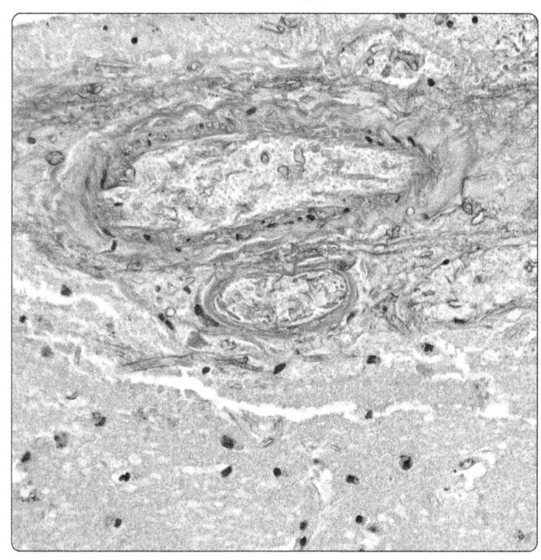

***Rhizomucor* spp.**

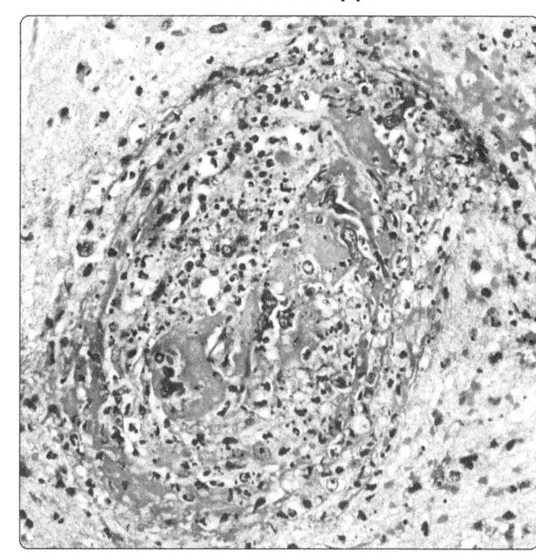

(Left) *Autopsy brain section from a patient status post stem cell transplantation shows broad, ribbon-like hyphae present in the blood vessel lumina and invading the surrounding brain parenchyma, identified as Mucor spp. in culture.* **(Right)** *This section of autopsy brain tissue from a patient status post bone marrow transplantation shows fragments of ribbon-shaped hyphae within this vessel lumen and invading surrounding parenchyma. Concurrent cultures were positive for Rhizomucor spp.*

Lichtheimia corymbifera

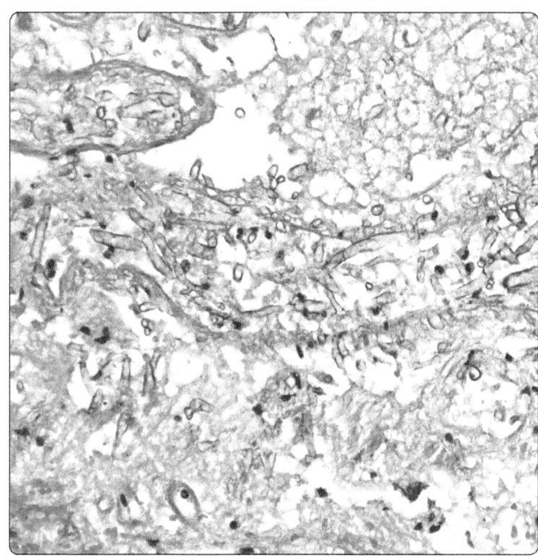

Mixed *Rhizopus* and *Aspergillus*

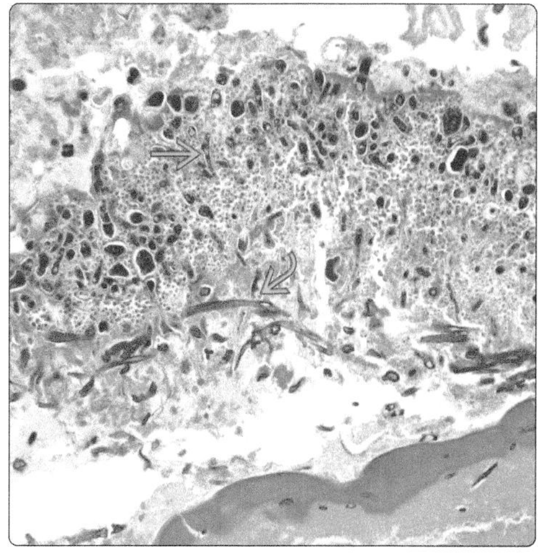

(Left) *Broad, ribbon-like hyphae are present in this occipital lobe mass resection, identified as Lichtheimia corymbifera by ITS sequencing of FFPE tissue.* **(Right)** *Sinonasal resection specimen exhibits abundant organisms, consistent with mucormycosis ⊡; however, broad fungal PCR was positive for Aspergillus section flavi, identified in 1 small focus ⊡ and considered an incidental finding. More focused sequencing identified R. oryzae complex, highlighting the importance of molecular histologic correlation.*

Mycetoma

KEY FACTS

ETIOLOGY/PATHOGENESIS

- Skin and subcutaneous infection (feet > > hands, legs, and knees) occurs via direct inoculation of bacteria (actinomycetoma) or fungi (eumycetoma)

CLINICAL ISSUES

- Worldwide but endemic in tropical and subtropical areas
- Clinical triad: Swollen tissue, draining sinuses, presence of grains from draining discharge

MACROSCOPIC

- Small, subcutaneous skin nodules become flocculent with time; purulence may ooze with grains from skin surface as swellings break open
- Chronic lesions become firmer with fibrosis and sclerosis

MICROSCOPIC

- Actinomycetoma: Colored grains with fine (≤ 1 µm-wide) radially oriented filaments; gram-negative centers with gram-positive fringes
- Eumycetoma: Colored grains with septate hyphae (2-6 µm wide) accompanied by numerous chlamydoconidia and swollen cells; gram negative
- Draining sinus tracts with abscesses containing grains and necrotic debris ± fibrosis (chronic)
- GMS and PAS stains highlight both types of organisms

TOP DIFFERENTIAL DIAGNOSES

- Botryomycosis: Suppurative/granulomatous inflammation; grains of bacterial cocci or nonfilamentous rods
- Dermatophytic pseudomycetoma: Fungal scalp infection with grains but no draining sinuses
- Sporotrichosis: Yeast with mixed suppurative and granulomatous inflammation; no grains
- Chromoblastomycosis: Pigmented sclerotic bodies; no grains
- Phaeohyphomycosis: Pigmented septate hyphae, granulomatous inflammation, suppurative exudate; no grains

Clinical: Mycetoma

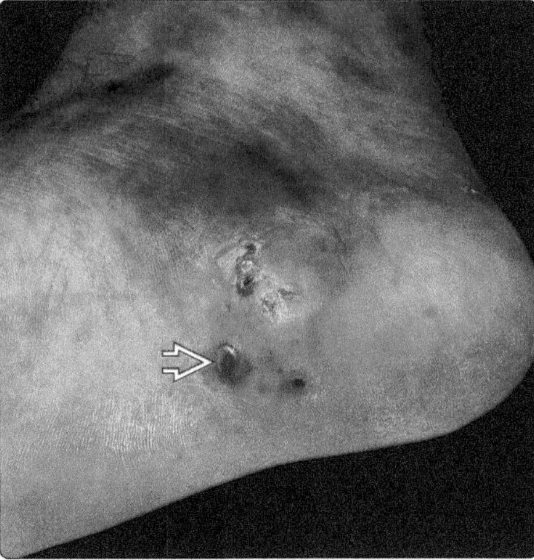

Eumycetoma Granules

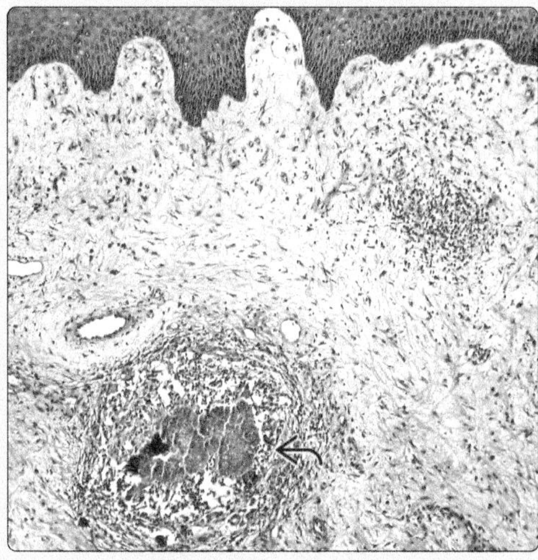

(Left) *Mycetoma of the foot from a patient stationed in Guam demonstrates several draining sinus tracts ➡ (present for months) with tissue swelling and slight hyperpigmentation. (Courtesy J. Steger, MD.)* **(Right)** *Although usually more deep seated, characteristic pale grains of eumycetoma ↗ are seen surrounded by inflammation. (Courtesy S. Florell, MD.)*

Eumycetoma: Pigmented Granules

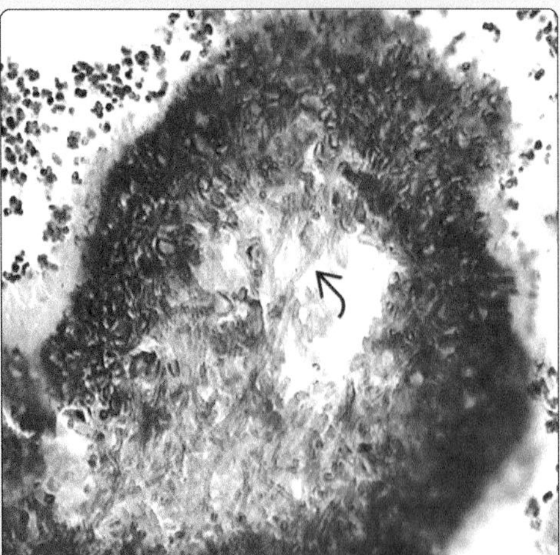

Actinomycetoma

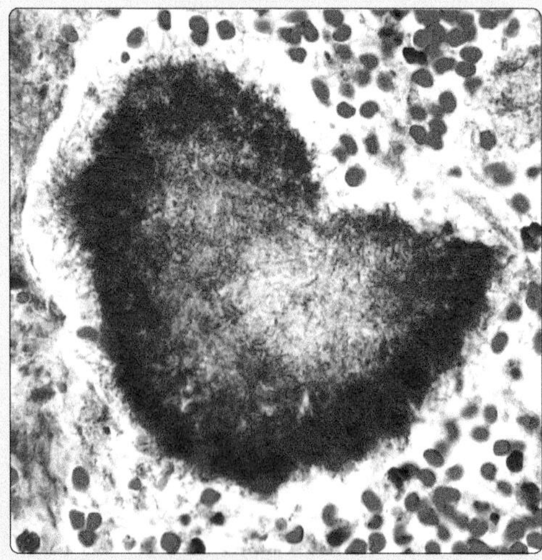

(Left) *This image shows characteristic black grains (brown on H&E) of eumycetoma surrounded by acute inflammation. Note how the filamentous fungi ↗ form a thick mass. (Courtesy C. Rosales, MD.)* **(Right)** *High magnification of a grain shows very fine radiating filaments. Differentials include actinomycosis (acid-fast negative) vs. actinomycotic mycetoma caused by Nocardia spp. (partially acid-fast).*

TERMINOLOGY

Definitions

- Greek: "Mykes" (fungus, mushroom) + "oma" (morbid growth)
- Eumycetoma (fungal origin): Eumycotic mycetoma, mycotic mycetoma, madura foot
- Actinomycetoma (bacterial origin): Actinomycotic mycetoma

ETIOLOGY/PATHOGENESIS

Infectious Agents

- Skin and subcutaneous infection via direct inoculation of organisms through contact with contaminated materials
- Actinomycetoma (grains of various colors but not black) caused by bacteria, including *Nocardia* spp., *Actinomadura* spp., *Streptomyces* spp.
- Eumycetoma: Caused by at least 30 hyaline and pigmented spp. of fungi
  - Black grains/granules caused typically (90%) caused by *Madurella mycetomatis*, *Madurella grisea*, *Leptosphaeria senegalensis*; less common spp. include *Pyrenochaeta romeroi*, *Cladophialophora bantiana*, *Exophiala jeanselmei*
  - White/yellow/green/brown grains/granules most commonly caused by *Scedosporium boydii*; less common spp. include *Acremonium* spp., *Fusarium* spp., *Aspergillus* spp.

CLINICAL ISSUES

Epidemiology

- Worldwide but endemic in tropical and subtropical areas
- Risk factors: Environmental exposure, genetic predisposition to infection, immunosuppression

Presentation

- Feet > > hands, legs, and knees
- Clinical triad: Swollen tissue, draining sinuses, presence of grains from draining discharge
- Secondary bacterial infection and local lymphadenopathy are common

Laboratory Tests

- PCR-based assays can be used for spp. determination

Treatment

- Actinomycetoma: Antibacterials, determined by spp.
- Eumycetoma: Both medical (usually ketoconazole or itraconazole) and surgical interventions

Prognosis

- Actinomycetoma: More rapid clinical progression
- If no treatment is given, severe local tissue destruction involving bone, tendon, and nerve may occur, requiring surgical amputation

MICROBIOLOGY

Culture

- Routine fungal cultures (eumycetoma) and anaerobic and aerobic bacterial cultures (actinomycetoma) for speciation

MACROSCOPIC

Gross Appearance

- Small, subcutaneous skin swellings become flocculent with time; purulence admixed with grains ooze from skin surface as swellings break open
- Chronic lesions firmer with fibrosis and sclerosis

MICROSCOPIC

Histologic Features

- Actinomycetoma: Colored grains composed of fine (≤ 1 μm-wide) radially oriented filaments
- Eumycetoma: Colored grains containing variously shaped septate hyphae (2-6 μm wide) accompanied by numerous chlamydoconidia and swollen fungal cells
- Draining sinus tracts with abscesses containing grains and necrotic debris ± fibrosis (chronic)

Cytologic Features

- Smears of grains may reveal bacteria or fungi

ANCILLARY TESTS

Histochemistry

- Actinomycetoma: Grains have gram-negative centers with gram-positive radiating fringes
- Eumycetoma: Gram negative
- GMS and PAS stains highlight both types of organisms

DIFFERENTIAL DIAGNOSIS

Botryomycosis

- Mixed suppurative and granulomatous inflammation with grains composed of bacterial cocci or nonfilamentous rods

Dermatophytic Pseudomycetoma

- Fungal scalp infection that presents with grains but no draining sinuses

Sporotrichosis

- Round to oval yeast (2-6 μm); mixed suppurative and granulomatous inflammation with lack of grains

Chromoblastomycosis

- Pigmented sclerotic bodies (5-12 μm) with lack of grains

Phaeohyphomycosis

- Pigmented septate hyphae; granulomatous inflammation with suppurative exudate but no grain formation

SELECTED REFERENCES

1. Baby P et al: Madurella mycetoma: a neglected tropical disease. Clin Microbiol Infect. 28(3):375-6, 2022
2. Christodoulou E et al: Mycetoma trichophyton. Pan Afr Med J. 40:121, 2021
3. Oladele RO et al: Mycetoma in West Africa. Trans R Soc Trop Med Hyg. 115(4):328-36, 2021
4. Verma P et al: Mycetoma: reviewing a neglected disease. Clin Exp Dermatol. 44(2):123-9, 2018
5. Arenas R et al: Actinomycetoma: an update on diagnosis and treatment. Cutis. 99(2):E11-5, 2017
6. Fahal AH: Mycetoma: a global medical and socio-economic dilemma. PLoS Negl Trop Dis. 11(4):e0005509, 2017
7. Sampaio FM et al: Review of 21 cases of mycetoma from 1991 to 2014 in Rio de Janeiro, Brazil. PLoS Negl Trop Dis. 11(2):e0005301, 2017
8. Sato T: Practical management of deep cutaneous fungal infections. Med Mycol J. 58(2):E71-7, 2017

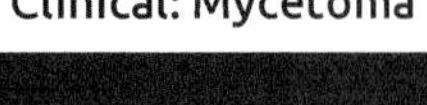

Clinical: Mycetoma

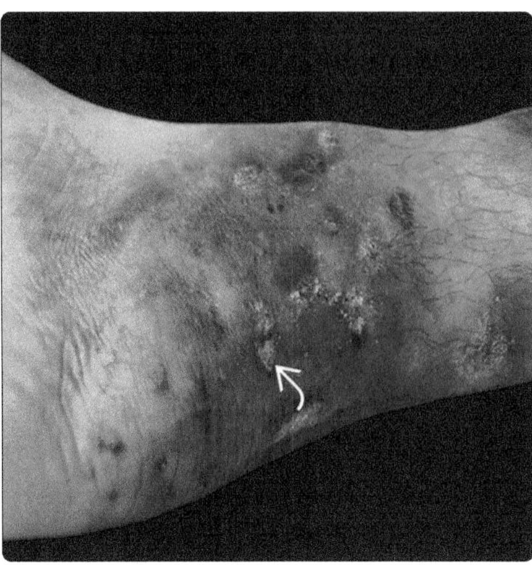

Abscess and Giant Cells

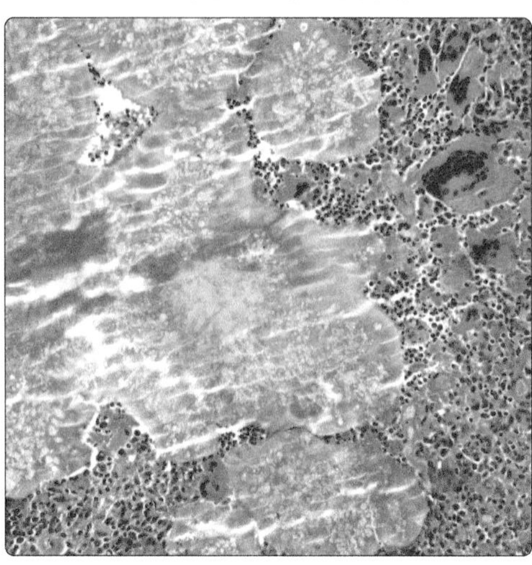

(Left) *This patient with mycetoma presented with a hyperpigmented, edematous, boggy medial ankle with multiple sinus tracts indicative of madura foot. (From DP: Nonneoplastic Derm.)* **(Right)** *Medium magnification of a scalp mass excision shows pale grains associated with abscess formation and giant cell granulomatous inflammation. Irregular hyphal and yeast-like forms are present within the granules. These findings are consistent with eumycetoma.*

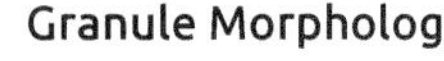

Granule Morphology

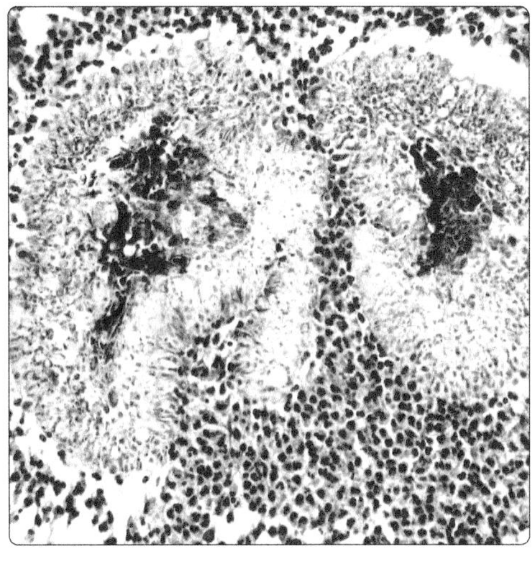

Eumycetoma: Pale Granules

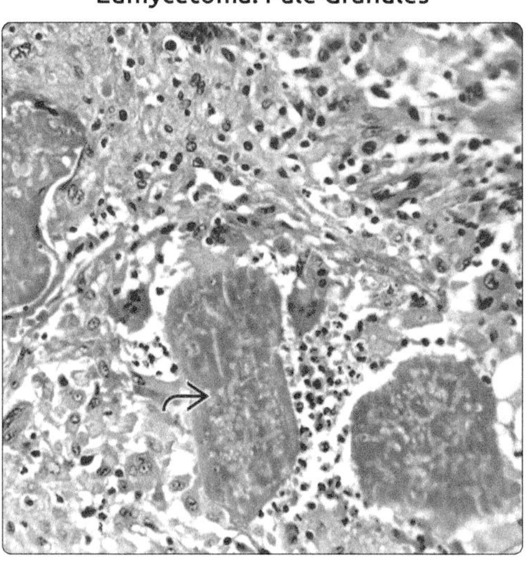

(Left) *Medium magnification of a skin section shows grains composed of thick, short hyphae mixed with numerous swollen cells, consistent with eumycotic mycetoma. Culture is needed for speciation.* **(Right)** *High-power view of a eumycetoma reveals neutrophils and chronic inflammatory cells in association with pale grains, which usually stain light pink or light purple on H&E. (From DP: Nonneoplastic Derm.)*

Eumycetoma: Pale Granules

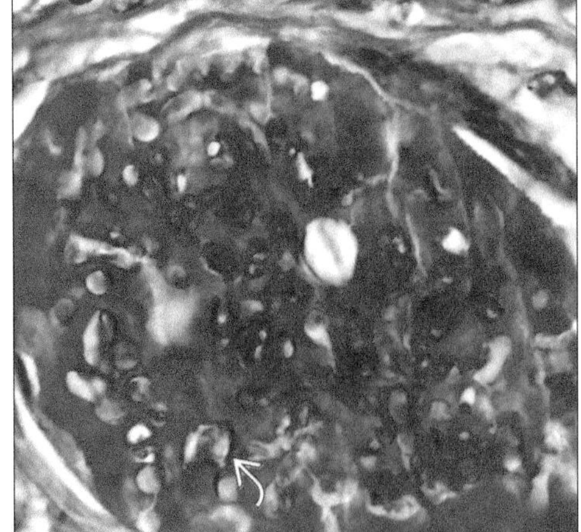

Eumycetoma Granule

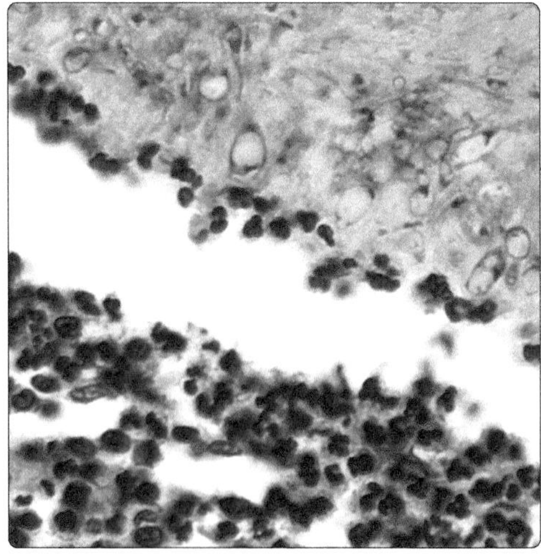

(Left) *High-power view of a pale grain of eumycetoma demonstrates a dense mass of intermeshing hyphae in intercellular cement. (From DP: Nonneoplastic Derm.)* **(Right)** *This image shows the interface between a Scedosporium boydii eumycetoma granule, a dense collection of fungal elements, and surrounding inflammation. (Courtesy Dr. Hardin, CDC/PHIL.)*

Eumycetoma

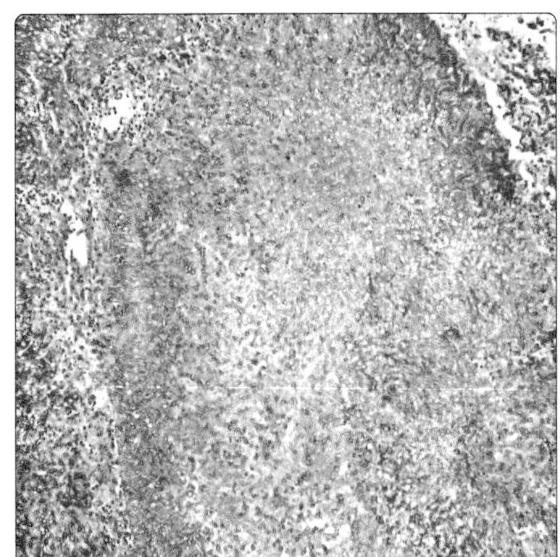

Eumycetoma: PAS Stain

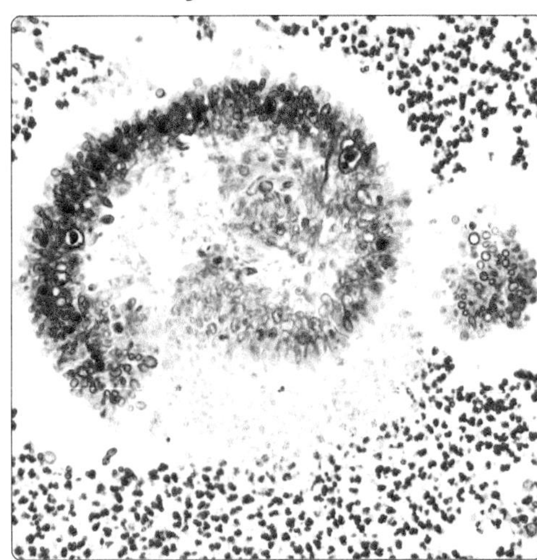

(Left) *Low magnification of a foot mass shows a fungal granule with narrow hyphae and round yeast forms. Culture reveals a mix of Aspergillus spp. and Candida spp.* **(Right)** *PAS stain highlights numerous swollen cells/chlamydoconidia and short hyphae in this fungal grain.*

Eumycetoma: GMS Stain

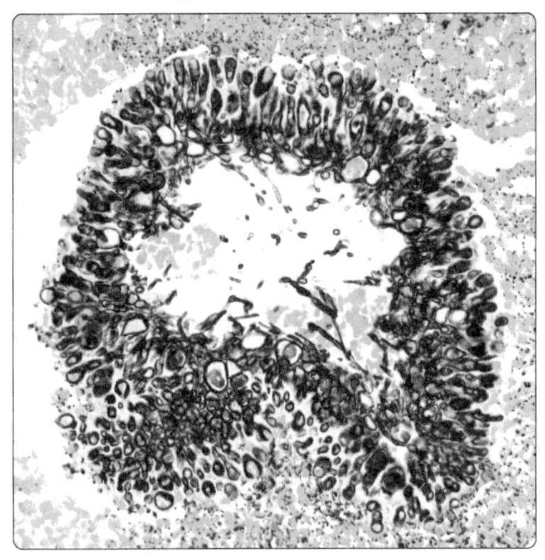

Nocardia Actinomycetoma

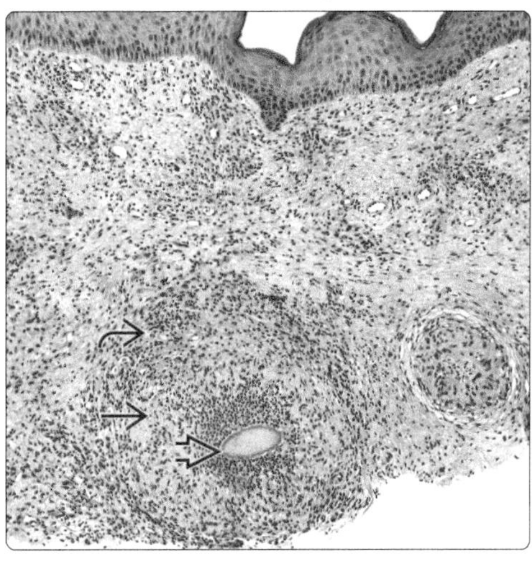

(Left) *Medium magnification of a skin biopsy on GMS stain highlights a grain with numerous swollen cells and hyphae with closely spaced septations. Speciation requires cultures or sequencing.* **(Right)** *Low-power view from a patient with actinomycetoma due to Nocardia spp. shows several nodules in the middermis with layered neutrophilic (suppurative) ⮫ and granulomatous ➔ inflammation surrounding sulfur granules ⇒. (From DP: Nonneoplastic Derm.)*

Actinomycetoma

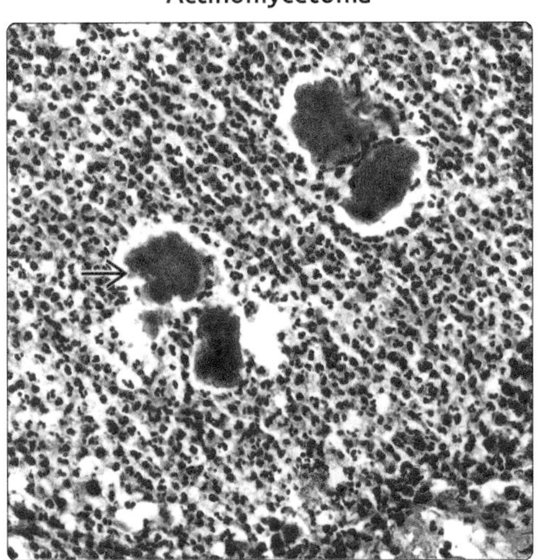

Differential Diagnosis: Dermatophytic Pseudomycetoma

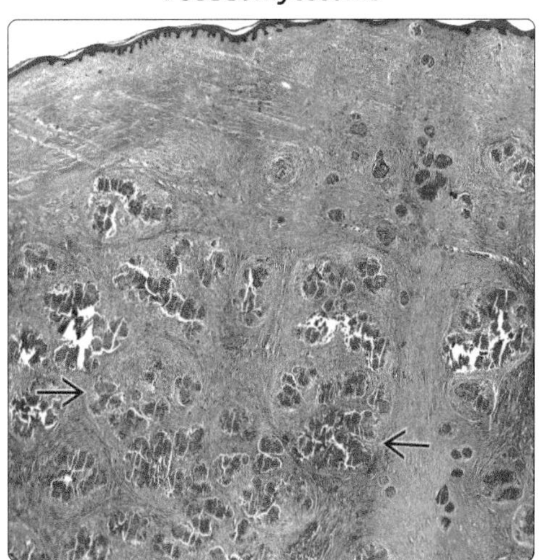

(Left) *Mycetoma can be caused by actinomycetes (actinomycetoma), filamentous bacteria ➔ (usually ≤ 1 μm wide) highlighted by Gram, PAS, and GMS stains. (Courtesy M. Chaffins, MD.)* **(Right)** *This scalp biopsy shows numerous dermatophyte fungal grains present throughout the dermis ➔ and is distinguished from true mycetoma by the lack of draining sinuses.*

KEY FACTS

ETIOLOGY/PATHOGENESIS

- Infection with dematiaceous (melanin-pigmented) fungi via inoculation with splinters or plant fragments or inhalation

CLINICAL ISSUES

- Skin infections: Swelling, induration, or mass with trauma
- Disseminated infections: Neurologic symptoms
- Treated with surgical removal/debridement/drainage and antifungals (itraconazole or amphotericin B)

MICROBIOLOGY

- Due to large number of potential organisms (> 100 spp.), culture or PCR required for speciation
- Colonies exhibit dark coloration due to melanin production
- Molecular identification by 28S rRNA or ITS sequencing

MICROSCOPIC

- Pigmented yeast in chains to hyphal forms; highlighted by GMS and PAS-D but not strictly needed given brown (melanized) color
- Granulomatous inflammation, often cystic, with necropurulent debris
- Brain with reactive gliosis/fibrosis and perivascular arrangement of organisms
- Fragments of foreign material (wood or plant) are often found in primary lesions

TOP DIFFERENTIAL DIAGNOSES

- Chromoblastomycosis: Dematiaceous fungi with "copper pennies" or double septate forms; does not disseminate
- Mycetoma: Dematiaceous fungi with grains/granules
- Aspergillosis: Some pigmented spp. (e.g., *Aspergillus terreus*); positive serum galactomannan in angioinvasive/disseminated disease
- Cryptococcosis: Narrow based-budding yeast with mucicarmine-positive capsule; Fontana-Masson highlights melanin, but yeast lack pigmentation on H&E-stained slides

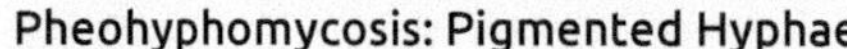

Pheohyphomycosis: Pigmented Hyphae

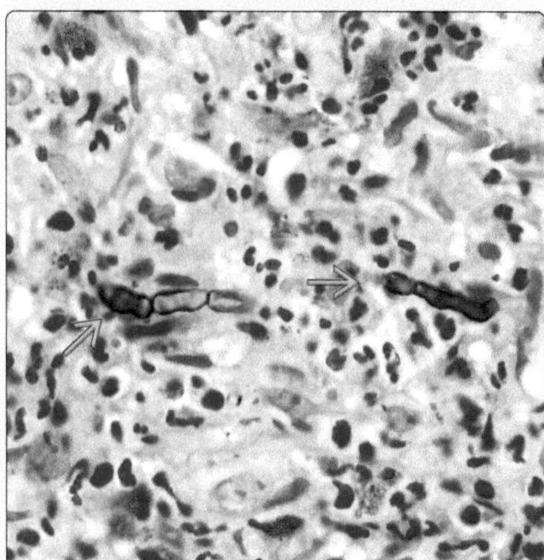

Foreign Material: GMS Stain

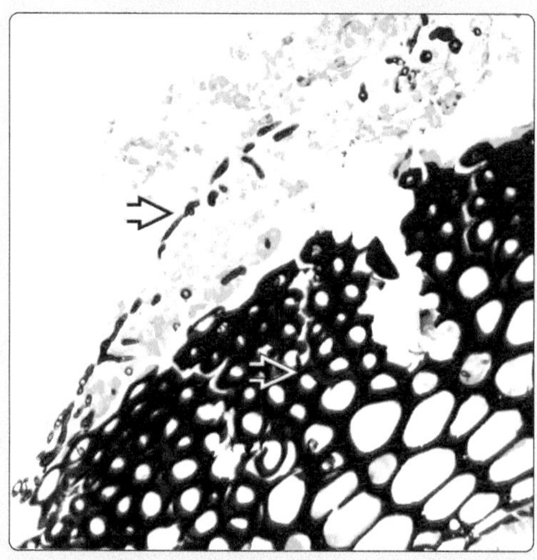

(Left) *Granulomatous inflammation, including suppurative granulomas with eosinophils, is commonly seen in pheohyphomycosis. Note that pigmented (brown) fungal hyphae ⇨ are readily seen on H&E sections.* **(Right)** *Methenamine silver stain from a phaeohyphomycotic cyst demonstrates a large fragment of woody plant matter ➡ with proliferating fungal elements ⇨ adjacent.*

Phaeohyphomycosis: PAS-D Stain

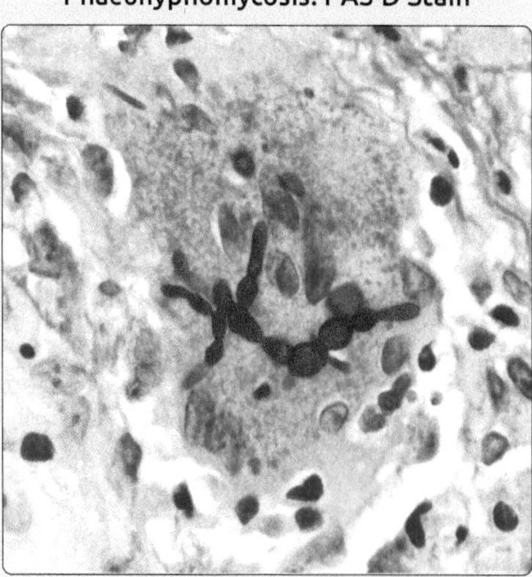

Phaeohyphomycosis: Fontana-Masson Stain

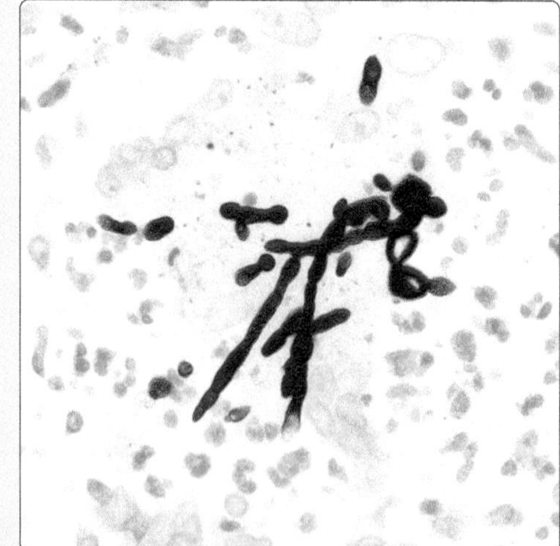

(Left) *PAS stain with diastase highlights chains of yeast inside a multinucleated giant cell in a skin biopsy from a patient with phaeohyphomycosis.* **(Right)** *Fontana-Masson staining highlights fungus-produced melanin pigment characteristic of phaeohyphomycosis-causing organisms. Fungi that are nonpigmented on H&E sections but positive with Fontana-Masson (e.g., Cryptococcus spp. and Coccidioides spp.) should not be interpreted as dematiaceous.*

TERMINOLOGY

Synonyms

- Phaeosporotrichosis, phaeohyphomycotic cyst, cutaneous or subcutaneous pheohyphomycosis

Definitions

- Derived from Greek: "Phaeo" (dusky, dark, twilight) + "hypho" (net) + "mykos" (fungus)

ETIOLOGY/PATHOGENESIS

Infectious Agents

- > 100 spp. of dematiaceous (pigmented, specifically with melanin) fungi can cause phaeohyphomycosis
- Important genera include *Alternaria, Exophiala, Phialophora, Wangiella, Bipolaris, Curvularia, Exserohilum, Lasiodiplodia, Scedosporium/Pseudallescheria, Cladophialophora*, and *Rhinocladiella*
- Ubiquitous organisms associated with soil and wood
- Inoculation can occur with splinters or plant fragments in lesions and typically results in localized disease
- Disseminated disease and cerebral disease associated with inhalation of organisms from environment, ingestion, catheter contamination, or iatrogenic immunosuppression

CLINICAL ISSUES

Presentation

- Localized disease of skin presents with swelling, induration, or mass (history of trauma); resembles epidermoid cyst
- Disseminated disease most commonly presents with neurologic symptoms, but other organs can be involved
- May also present with keratitis, rhinosinusitis, or pneumonia

Laboratory Tests

- Due to large number of potential organisms, culture (or PCR) required for speciation
- Molecular identification by 28S rRNA or internal transcribed spacer (ITS) PCR with sequencing

Treatment

- Surgical removal/debridement/drainage of localized skin disease or brain lesions aids in diagnosis and therapy
- Antifungals (itraconazole &/or amphotericin B)

Prognosis

- Localized disease responds to antifungal therapy &/or surgical intervention
- Disseminated disease may be difficult to treat and fatal

MICROBIOLOGY

Culture

- Routine fungal cultures (Sabouraud dextrose agar, brain-heart infusion agar, corn meal agar, potato dextrose agar) are primary media at multiple temperatures
- Colonies exhibit dark coloration due to melanin production

MICROSCOPIC

Histologic Features

- Granulomatous inflammation, often cystic, with necropurulent debris
- Organisms appear as pigmented yeast in chains to hyphae and present around granulomatous reaction or within multinucleated giant cells
- Brain also exhibits reactive gliosis and fibrosis with fungal hyphae in and around blood vessels
- Fragments of foreign material (wood or plant) are often found in primary lesions
- Disseminated lesions (brain, sites other than skin) will not contain foreign material

ANCILLARY TESTS

Special Stains

- Fungal elements will be positive on standard fungal stains, including methenamine silver and PAS, but brown (melanized) color is best appreciated on H&E
- Melanin in walls of fungi may stain strongly with Fontana-Masson stain, but only fungi that appear brown on H&E should be classified as dematiaceous on tissue sections, since many nondematiaceous fungi will have positive Fontana-Masson reaction

DIFFERENTIAL DIAGNOSIS

Chromoblastomycosis

- Also caused by dematiaceous fungi
- "Copper pennies" or double septate forms; does not disseminate

Mycetoma

- Also can be caused by dematiaceous fungi
- Contain grains or granules

Aspergillosis

- Some spp. of *Aspergillus* are pigmented in tissue (usually *Aspergillus terreus*)
- Positive serum galactomannan in angioinvasive/disseminated infections

Cryptococcosis

- Narrow based-budding yeast with mucicarmine-positive capsule
- Fontana-Masson highlights melanin, but yeast lack pigmentation on H&E-stained slides

SELECTED REFERENCES

1. Bejarano JIC et al: Pediatric phaeohyphomycosis: a 44-year systematic review of reported cases. J Pediatric Infect Dis Soc. 12(1):10-20, 2023
2. Lo Porto D et al: Phaeohyphomycosis in solid organ transplant recipients: a case series and narrative review of the literature. J Fungi (Basel). 9(3), 2023
3. Ferrándiz-Pulido C et al: Cutaneous infections by dematiaceous opportunistic fungi: diagnosis and management in 11 solid organ transplant recipients. Mycoses. 62(2):121-7, 2019
4. Moreno LF et al: Black yeasts in the omics era: achievements and challenges. Med Mycol. 56(suppl_1):32-41, 2018
5. McCarthy MW et al: Molecular diagnosis of invasive mycoses of the central nervous system. Expert Rev Mol Diagn. 17(2):129-39, 2017
6. Revankar SG et al: A mycoses study group international prospective study of phaeohyphomycosis: an analysis of 99 proven/probable cases. Open Forum Infect Dis. 4(4):ofx200, 2017
7. Wong EH et al: Dematiaceous molds. Infect Dis Clin North Am. 30(1):165-78, 2016
8. Revankar SG et al: Primary central nervous system phaeohyphomycosis: a review of 101 cases. Clin Infect Dis. 38(2):206-16, 2004

Scedosporiosis and Lomentosporiosis

KEY FACTS

ETIOLOGY/PATHOGENESIS

- Fungal infections caused by *Scedosporium apiospermum* complex and *Lomentospora prolificans* via direct traumatic skin inoculation or inhalation of airborne conidia
- Ubiquitous saprophytic, filamentous molds found in soil, sewage, compost, and polluted water

CLINICAL ISSUES

- 25% of non-*Aspergillus* transplant-associated mold infections
- Disseminated infection can lead to brain abscess, meningitis, endocarditis, and osteomyelitis
- Marked antifungal resistance (including amphotericin B)
- Mortality 50-100% in immunocompromised
- Elevated serum (1,3)-β-D-glucan; negative galactomannan

MICROSCOPIC

- Hyaline or dematiaceous septated hyphae with acute angle branching (slightly more irregular than *Aspergillus* spp.)
- May display angioinvasion
- *S. apiospermum* conidia (4-12 μm) are unicellular and obovoidal with truncate base
- Teleomorph form (*P. boydii*) has large cleistothecia (50-250 μm) that release ascospores when ruptured
- *L. prolificans* conidia unicellular and obovoidal with truncate base; short flask-shaped conidiogenous cells with annelids
- Background tissue displays neutrophilic and monocytic infiltrates, granulomatous inflammation, or necrosis
- Hyphae and conidia highlighted by PAS-D and GMS stains

TOP DIFFERENTIAL DIAGNOSES

- Other causes of hyalohyphomycosis (e.g., *Aspergillus*, *Fusarium*): Hyphae indistinguishable histologically; serum positive for (1,3)-β-D-glucan (*Aspergillus* is galactomannan positive); identify with culture or sequencing
- Mucormycosis: Broader, thin-walled, ribbon-like hyphae with few septations and right-angle branching; (1,3)-β-D-glucan negative

(Left) *Lactophenol cotton blue stain of a culture isolate shows mature cleistothecium* ⇨ *and ascospores* ➡ *in the sexual teleomorph of Scedosporium (previously known as Pseudallescheria boydii).* **(Right)** *H&E shows numerous thin, nonpigmented hyphae of Scedosporium with septations and acute-angle branching, shared morphologic features with Aspergillus. (Courtesy M. DeSimone, MD, MPH.)*

Sexual Teleomorph of *Scedosporium* spp.

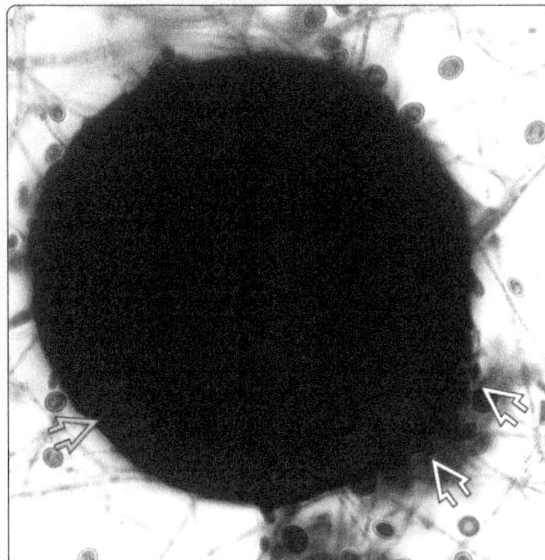

***Scedosporium* spp. Hyphae**

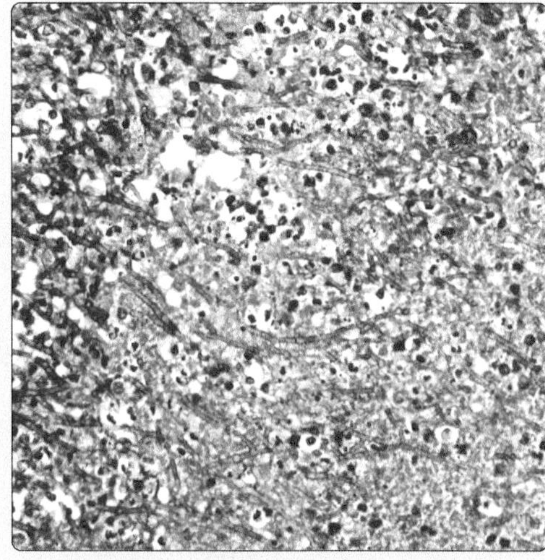

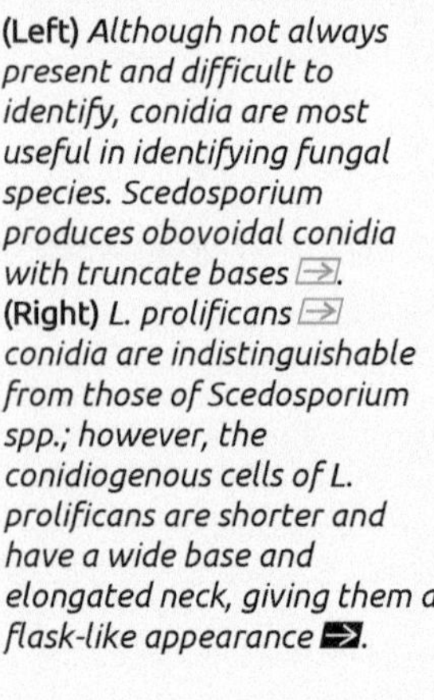

(Left) *Although not always present and difficult to identify, conidia are most useful in identifying fungal species. Scedosporium produces obovoidal conidia with truncate bases* ⇨. **(Right)** *L. prolificans* ⇨ *conidia are indistinguishable from those of Scedosporium spp.; however, the conidiogenous cells of L. prolificans are shorter and have a wide base and elongated neck, giving them a flask-like appearance* ➡.

***Scedosporium* spp. Conidia**

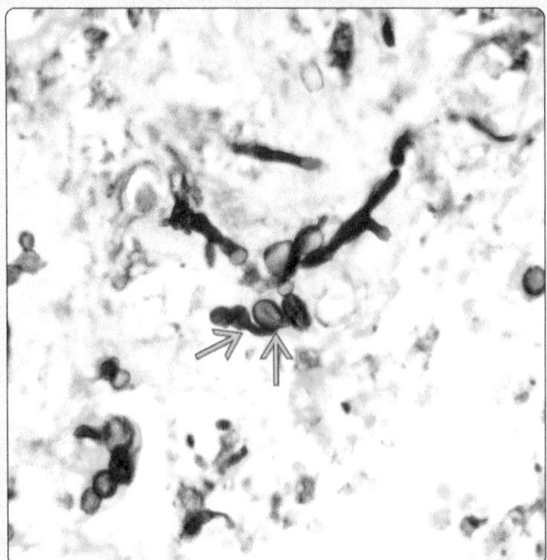

***Lomentospora prolificans* Conidia and Conidiogenous Cells**

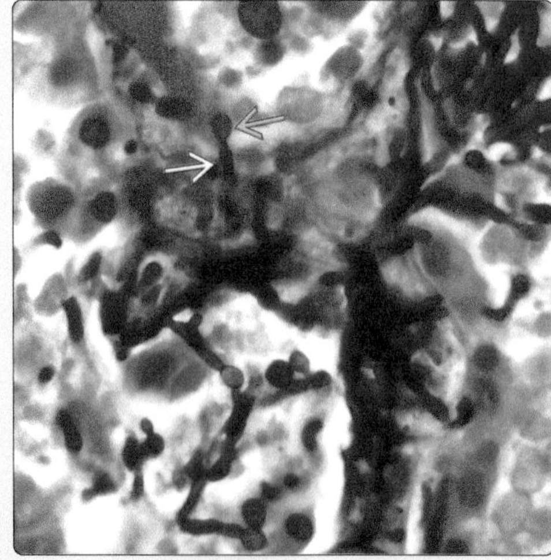

TERMINOLOGY

Definitions

- *Scedosporium* derived from Latin "scedo" (leaf of paper) and Greek "sporium" (seed); a*pio* (Latin: Fasten or join); *prolificans* (Latin: Descendent)

ETIOLOGY/PATHOGENESIS

Infectious Agents

- Fungal infection caused by members of *Scedosporium apiospermum* complex: *S. apiospermum sensus stricto, S. boydii, S. aurantiacum, S. dehoogi, and S. minutispora*
  - Teleomorph state, *Pseudallescheria boydii* (sexual form)
- *Lomentospora prolificans* (previously known as *Scedosporium prolificans*) frequently grouped together due to phenotypic similarities despite being genetically unrelated
- Ubiquitous saprophytic, filamentous molds found in soil, sewage, compost, and polluted water
- Infection can be from direct traumatic inoculation into skin (mycetoma) or through inhalation of airborne conidia

CLINICAL ISSUES

Epidemiology

- Increasingly recognized as cause of infection in solid organ transplant patients (25% of non-*Aspergillus* mold infections)

Presentation

- Patients may be colonized in upper respiratory tract without active infection (confirm histologically)
- Rare cause of skin infection in immunocompetent
- Mycetoma: Most commonly on feet and lower limbs
- In immunocompromised: Pulmonary infection, disseminated infection leading to brain abscess, meningitis, endocarditis, osteomyelitis, and sepsis
- May be 1st presentation of underlying hematopoietic malignancy

Laboratory Tests

- Elevated serum (1,3)-β-D-glucan; negative galactomannan
- Sequencing using conserved fungal primers (28S rRNA)
- β-tubulin sequencing to differentiate species within *S. apiospermum* complex

Treatment

- Extremely resistant to variety of antifungals, including amphotericin B; susceptibility pattern varies with species
- Voriconazole remains 1st-line therapy; combination therapies with terbinafine &/or an echinocandin
- Surgical debridement when possible

Prognosis

- Mortality 50-100% in immunocompromised, worse with disseminated disease and with *L. prolificans* infections

MICROBIOLOGY

Culture Characteristics

- Hyaline or rarely dematiaceous (containing melanin in cell wall), especially in aged cultures
- Septate hyaline hyphae branching at 45° angles
- *S. apiospermum* grows in cornmeal agar or potato dextrose (PDA), reaching maturity in 7 days; spreading white colony, which turns gray-brown with spider web surface
- *L. prolificans* grows on Sabouraud dextrose medium or PDA, reaching maturity in 5 days; cotton-like, light gray becoming gray-black fluffy colony
- Unicellular adventitious forms may be visible in blood cultures, which is not seen in *Aspergillus* infection

MICROSCOPIC

Histologic Features

- Hyaline or dematiaceous septated hyphae with acute angle branching (slightly more irregular than *Aspergillus* spp.); may display angioinvasion
- *S. apiospermum* conidia (4-12 μm) are unicellular and obovoidal with truncate base
- Teleomorph form (*P. boydii*) has large cleistothecia (50-250 μm) that release ascospores when ruptured
- *L. prolificans* conidia are unicellular and obovoidal with truncate base, short flask-shaped (swollen base and elongated neck) conidiogenous cells with annelids (difficult to see on tissue sections); conidia may grow singly or in clusters along hyphae
- Background tissue displays neutrophilic and monocytic infiltrates, granulomatous inflammation, or necrosis

ANCILLARY TESTS

Special Stains

- Hyphae and conidia highlighted by periodic-acid Schiff and methenamine silver stains

DIFFERENTIAL DIAGNOSIS

Other Causes of Hyalohyphomycosis

- e.g., *Aspergillus, Fusarium, Acremonium, Paecilomyces*
- Hyphae are indistinguishable histologically; also positive for serum (1,3)-β-D-glucan; culture or sequencing typically required to make definitive diagnosis
- *Aspergillus* spp.: Rarely exhibits fruiting bodies in tissue sections; serum positive for galactomannan

Mucormycosis

- Nonpigmented, broader, thin-walled, ribbon-like hyphae with few septations and right-angle branching; (1,3)-β-D-glucan negative

SELECTED REFERENCES

1. Jacobs SE et al: Non-Aspergillus hyaline molds: a host-based perspective of emerging pathogenic fungi causing sinopulmonary diseases. J Fungi (Basel). 9(2), 2023
2. Chen SC et al: Scedosporium and Lomentospora infections: contemporary microbiological tools for the diagnosis of invasive disease. J Fungi (Basel). 7(1), 2021
3. DeSimone MS et al: Scedosporium and Lomentospora infections are Infrequent, difficult to diagnose by histology, and highly virulent. Am J Clin Pathol. 156(6):1044-57, 2021
4. Hedayati MT et al: Fungal epidemiology in cystic fibrosis patients with a special focus on Scedosporium species complex. Microb Pathog. 129:168-75, 2019
5. Seidel D et al: Prognostic factors in 264 adults with invasive Scedosporium spp. and Lomentospora prolificans infection reported in the literature and FungiScope®. Crit Rev Microbiol. 1-21, 2019

Scopulariopsis Infections

KEY FACTS

ETIOLOGY/PATHOGENESIS

- Filamentous fungi with intrinsic resistance to antifungal drugs that can be hyaline or dematiaceous
- *Scopulariopsis* spp. associated with human disease include *S. brevicaulis* (most common, hyaline), *S. brumptii* (pigmented), *S. gracilis, Microascus* (*Scopulariopsis*) *cinereus, S. candida* complex, *Microascus* (*Scopulariopsis*) *cirrosus*

CLINICAL ISSUES

- Most common cause of onychomycosis
- Opportunistic infections and invasive disease in immunosuppressed patients involve respiratory tract, sinuses, and endocarditis
- Overall, treatment is poorly effective (relapses and death are common)
- Elevated (1,3)-β-D-glucan
- Real-time PCR targeting β-tubulin gene (TUBB)
- Sequencing of 28S rRNA gene D1/D2 region or EF1-α

MICROBIOLOGY

- Culture: Rapid growth (mature in 5 days); colonies are initially white before becoming tan
- Septate hyphae with short conidiophores; single/groups of annellides; large, round, rough-appearing conidia

MICROSCOPIC

- Granulomatous reactions and necrosis
- Narrow hyphae with acute angle branching; conidia and nonbuddying, yeast-like structures (ascospores)

TOP DIFFERENTIAL DIAGNOSES

- Aspergillosis: Distinctive fruiting bodies rarely present; positive for serum galactomannan
- Scedosporiosis: Conidiogenous cells may be identified; distinguished by culture/molecular testing
- Fusariosis: No pathognomonic morphologic features; distinguished by culture/molecular testing
- Phaeohyphomycosis: Pigmented fungal forms

***Scopulariopsis brevicaulis* Culture Plate**

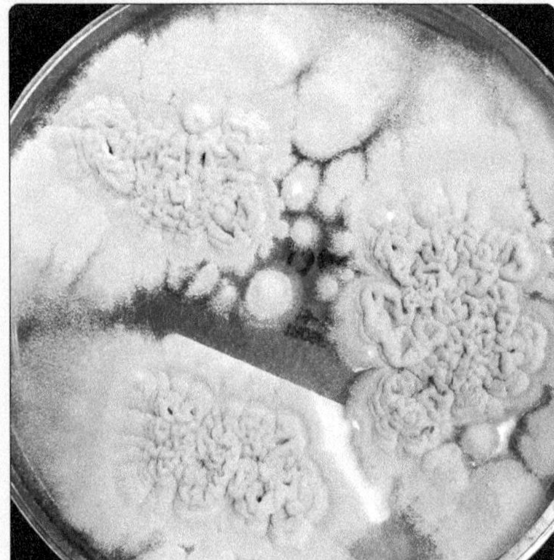

Lactophenol Cotton Blue Preparation

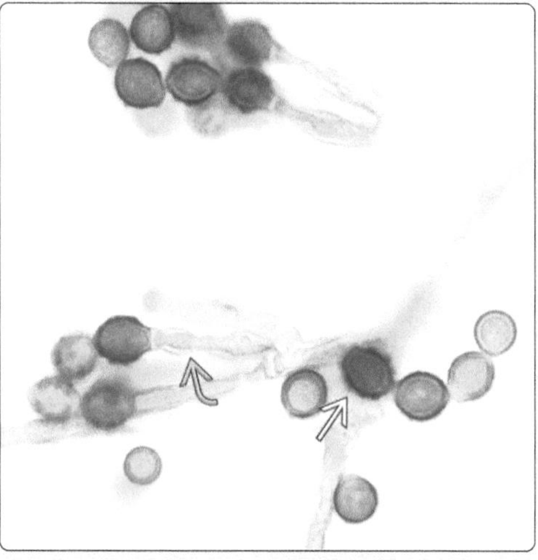

(Left) *The initially white mold of Scopulariopsis brevicaulis becomes powdery and cinnamon colored with age, as shown on this potato dextrose agar plate.* **(Right)** *Scopulariopsis hyphae with conidiogenous cells ⇨ (annellides) bearing conidia are depicted. Conidia ➡ are globose to pyriform, truncate, and spiny (echinulate).*

Skin and Soft Tissue Infection

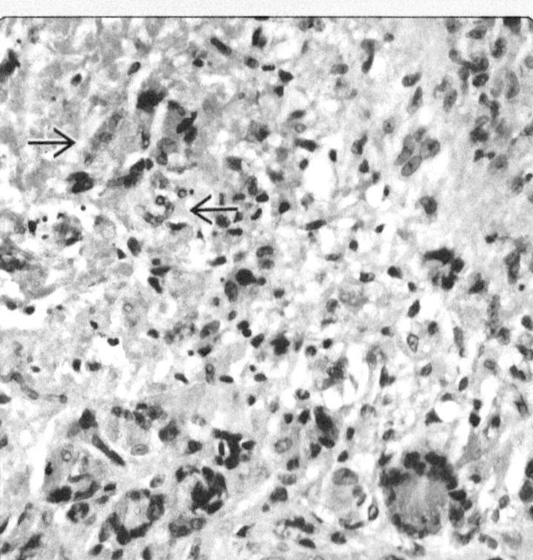

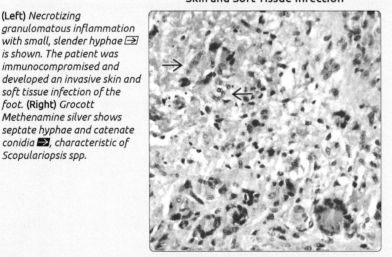

Fungal Morphology in Tissue

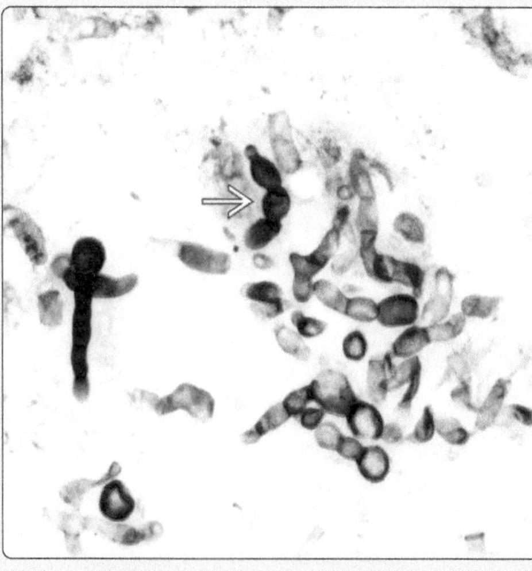

(Left) *Necrotizing granulomatous inflammation with small, slender hyphae ⇨ is shown. The patient was immunocompromised and developed an invasive skin and soft tissue infection of the foot.* **(Right)** *Grocott Methenamine silver shows septate hyphae and catenate conidia ➡, characteristic of Scopulariopsis spp.*

TERMINOLOGY

Definitions

- Latin: "Scopula" (twigs or branches)
- *Scopulariopsis* spp. are anamorphs of *Microascus* spp.

ETIOLOGY/PATHOGENESIS

Infectious Agents

- Infection with *Scopulariopsis* spp., filamentous fungi with intrinsic resistance to antifungal drugs that can be hyaline or dematiaceous depending on spp.
- Frequently regarded as colonizer or laboratory contaminant but increasingly recognized as cause of human disease
- *Scopulariopsis* spp. associated with human disease include *S. brevicaulis* (most common, hyaline), *S. brumptii* (pigmented), *S. gracilis, Microascus* (*Scopulariopsis*) *cinereus, S. candida* complex, *Microascus* (*Scopulariopsis*) *cirrosus*

CLINICAL ISSUES

Epidemiology

- Saprophytes found worldwide in soil (primarily), plant debris, air and moist environments, feathers, and insects

Site

- Nails and skin (immunocompetent), respiratory tract, broadly invasive (immunosuppressed)

Presentation

- Most common cause of nondermatophytic onychomycosis
- Increasingly recognized in opportunistic infections (*S. brevicaulis* most common)
  - Respiratory tract infection (fungal ball and pneumonia); sinusitis
  - Endophthalmitis and brain abscesses
  - Case reports of endocarditis and fatal disseminated infection following bone marrow transplant

Laboratory Tests

- Elevated (1,3)-β-D-glucan

Treatment

- Surgical debridement of infected and necrotic tissue if feasible
- Significant in vitro resistance of nearly all agents; echinocandins show some activity in one study
- Combination antifungal therapies may be used (e.g., amphotericin B and voriconazole)

Prognosis

- Overall, treatment is poorly effective (relapses and death are common)
- Estimated cure rate is ~ 40%
- Mortality depends on site of infection and host immunologic profile

IMAGING

Radiographic Findings

- Brain abscesses: Ring-enhancing lesions on CT
- Pulmonary fungus ball

MICROBIOLOGY

Culture

- Saprophytic mold with rapid growth (mature in 5 days)
- Colonies are initially white and become light brown with tan periphery ("buff colored")
  - Reverse of colonies are tan/brown
  - *S. candida* remains white throughout

Microscopic Features

- Septate hyaline or pigmented hyphae (depending on spp.) with short conidiophores
- Annellides (cells that extrudes conidia) can be single or groups; can be tenpin-shaped
- Conidia are large, round, and may be rough in appearance

MICROSCOPIC

Histologic Features

- Granulomatous reactions and necrosis most common inflammatory patterns
- Fungi typically appear as narrow hyphae with acute angle branching, similar in appearance to other hyaline molds
- Conidia and nonbuddying, yeast-like structures, consistent with ascospores may be present

ANCILLARY TESTS

Histochemistry

- Fungal morphology highlighted by GMS and PAS-D stains

PCR

- Real-time PCR targeting β-tubulin gene (TUBB)
- D1/D2 region of 28S rRNA gene or EF1-α sequencing

DIFFERENTIAL DIAGNOSIS

Aspergillosis

- Distinctive fruiting bodies rarely present; positive for serum galactomannan

Scedosporiosis

- Conidiogenous cells may be identified; distinguished by culture/molecular testing

Fusariosis

- No pathognomonic morphologic features; distinguished by culture/molecular testing

Phaeohyphomycosis

- Pigmented fungal forms

SELECTED REFERENCES

1. Pérez-Cantero A et al: Current knowledge on the etiology and epidemiology of Scopulariopsis infections. Med Mycol. 58(2):145-55, 2020
2. Arroyo MA et al: Closing the brief case: Scopulariopsis endocarditis-a case of mistaken Takayasu's arteritis. J Clin Microbiol. 55(9):2872-3, 2017
3. Kordalewska M et al: Rapid assays for specific detection of fungi of Scopulariopsis and Microascus genera and Scopulariopsis brevicaulis species. Mycopathologia. 181(7-8):465-74, 2016
4. Sattler L et al: Sinusitis caused by Scopulariopsis brevicaulis: case report and review of the literature. Med Mycol Case Rep. 5:24-7, 2014
5. Sandoval-Denis M et al: Scopulariopsis, a poorly known opportunistic fungus: spectrum of species in clinical samples and in vitro responses to antifungal drugs. J Clin Microbiol. 51(12):3937-43, 2013

KEY FACTS

ETIOLOGY/PATHOGENESIS

- Superficial fungal infections of skin and skin appendages acquired by contact
- Most commonly due to 3 genera of dermatophytes: *Trichophyton*, *Microsporum*, and *Epidermophyton*

CLINICAL ISSUES

- Ringworm, tinea corporis, tinea capitis, tinea faciei, tinea barbae, tinea cruris (jock itch), tinea unguium (onychomycosis), tinea gladiatorum, tinea imbricata, tinea manuum, tinea pedis (athlete's foot), tinea incognito
- Affects 20-25% of world population; common in children
- Immunocompromised state increases risk, including dissemination, which may be severe and lead to fatalities

MACROSCOPIC

- Annular plaque with scale at advancing border

MICROSCOPIC

- Fungal hyphae may be difficult to appreciate on H&E (highlighted by PAS-D and GMS)
- Nonspecific changes in skin: Parakeratosis, acanthosis/psoriasiform hyperplasia, inflammation
- Neutrophilic, granulomatous, or necrotizing inflammation with fungal hyphae in disseminated cases

TOP DIFFERENTIAL DIAGNOSES

- Spongiotic/eczematous processes: Similar reactive changes (acanthosis, hyperkeratosis) without fungal forms
- Disseminated fungal infection: Morphologically similar to hyalohyphomycoses and candidiasis; differentiate with cultures/sequencing
- Phaeohyphomycosis: Pigmented fungal forms with granulomatous inflammation

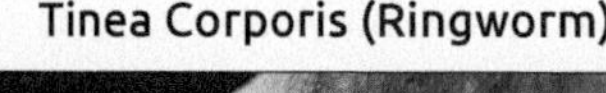

Tinea Corporis (Ringworm)

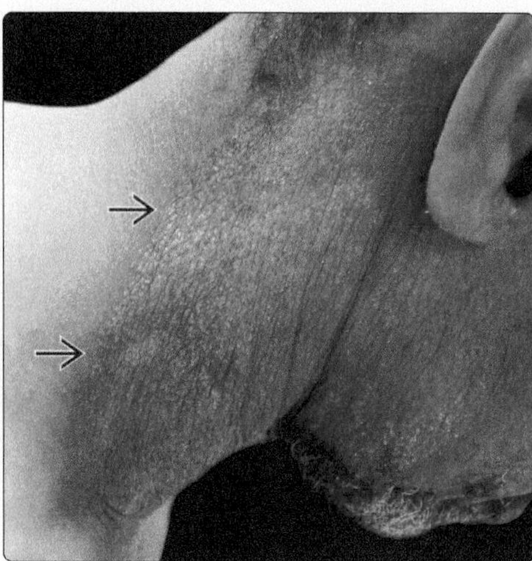

Tinea Corporis: Histology

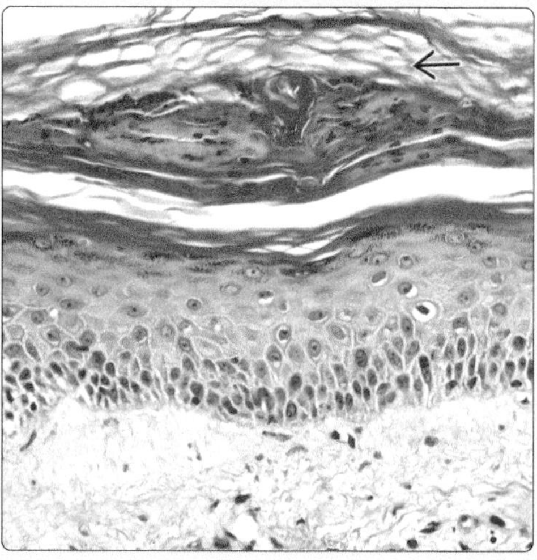

(Left) *There is an erythematous, scaly plaque ⇒ with lichenification on the neck and jawline of this patient. Potassium hydroxide (KOH) examination of the scale showed fungal hyphae. (From DP: Nonneoplastic Derm.)* **(Right)** *This skin biopsy shows perakeratosis, neutrophils, and subtle fungal hyphae oriented horizontally within the stratum corneum ⇒, consistent with the diagnosis of tinea corporis. (Courtesy A. Laga, MD, MMSc.)*

Tinea Corporis: PAS-D

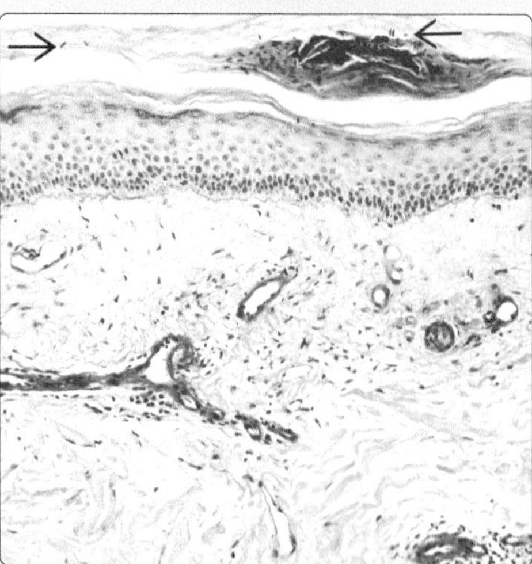

Tinea Corporis: Hair Shaft Involvement

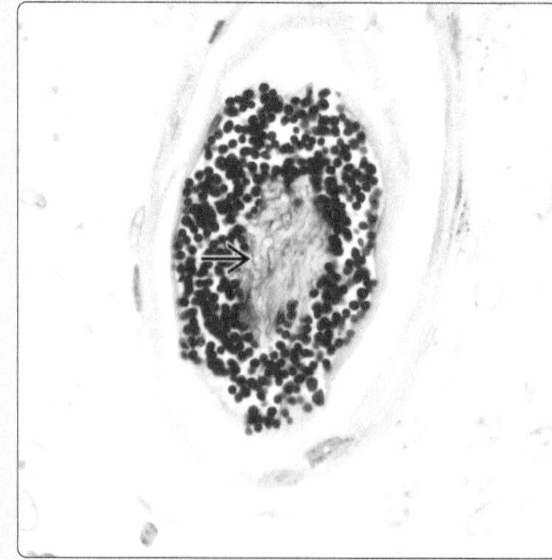

(Left) *Special stains, including Periodic acid-Schiff and Grocott methenamine silver, can be used to highlight fungal forms ⇒, which may be difficult to see on H&E alone. (Courtesy A. Laga, MD, MMSc.)* **(Right)** *This image shows fungal hyphae ⇒ involving a hair follicle from a case of tinea corporis. (Courtesy A. Laga, MD, MMSc.)*

TERMINOLOGY

Definitions

- Latin: "Tinea" (worm)

ETIOLOGY/PATHOGENESIS

Infectious Agents

- Superficial fungal infection of skin and skin appendages acquired by by contact with infected humans (anthropophilic), infected animals (zoophilic), or contaminated soil or fomites (geophilic)
- Most commonly due to 3 genera of dermatophytes: *Trichophyton*, *Microsporum*, and *Epidermophyton*

CLINICAL ISSUES

Epidemiology

- Affects 20-25% of world population

Presentation

- **Tinea corporis (ringworm)** (most commonly due to *Trichophyton* species): Itchy, annular patch or plaque of erythema with scale at advancing edge and central clearing; less commonly, vesicles, bullae, or pustules
- **Tinea pedis (athlete's foot)**: Pruritus, erythema, scale ± vesicles and pustules commonly centered on interdigital clefts; moccasin distribution less common (hyperkeratosis along soles, heels, and sides of feet); risk factors include adolescence, moist skin, maceration
- **Tinea capitis**: Scaly scalp, alopecia, pustules, and "black dots" representing hairs broken at scalp; most common dermatophyte infection in children
    - Endothrix: Invasion of hair shaft by fungi
    - Ectothrix: Coating of hair shaft by fungi
    - Kerion celsi: Superimposed bacterial folliculitis on scalp
- **Tinea unguium (onychomycosis)**: Nail dystrophy; *Candida* and nondermatophytes are other causes; risk factors include Tinea pedis, improperly fitting shoes, diabetes
- **Nodular granulomatous perifolliculitis (Majocchi granuloma)**: Infection of hair follicle (commonly due to *T. rubrum*) affecting legs; erythematous coalescing papules and pustules
- **Tinea incognito**: Subtle features, including poorly defined border, epidermal atrophy, telangiectasia in setting of use of topical immunosuppressants (e.g., corticosteroids)
- **Tinea imbricata** (*T. concentricum*): Multiple concentric annular plaques with thick rims of peripheral scale; Polynesia, Southeast Asia, India, and Central America
- **Tinea gladiatorum**: From skin-to-skin contact in wrestlers (head, neck, and arms); morphology may resemble tinea corporis or numerous erythematous scaling papules and plaques
- **Tinea cruris (jock itch)**: Pruritic, burning red symmetric macules with well-demarcated borders and pustules/vesicles at edge; young men or obese women
- **Disseminated dermatophytosis**: Severely immunosuppressed patients; hematogenous spread may cause signs/symptoms in any organ

Laboratory Tests

- In-office KOH preparation of scrapings is 77% sensitive

Treatment

- Topical or oral antifungals

Prognosis

- Most clinical forms are responsive to therapy
- Tinea unguium/onychomycosis can be difficult to cure; transition from topical to oral therapies requires biopsy/culture confirmation due to hepatotoxicity
- Immunocompromised states (HIV, diabetes, etc.) associated with increased risk, dissemination, and fatal disease

MICROBIOLOGY

Fungal Cultures

- *Trichophyton rubrum*: White colonies with wine-red reverse; pyriform/peg-shaped microconidia along unbranched hyphae (birds on wire); rare macroconidia are thin and cylindrical/clavate with 3-8 septa
- *Microsporum canis*: Whitish colonies with yellow pigment along periphery; septate hyphae; numerous macroconidia are long, spindle-shaped, rough, and thick-walled, usually > 6 cells; rare microconidia
- *Epidermophyton floccosum*: Brownish yellow to olive-gray colonies; abundant macroconidia are clustered, club-shaped, with broadly rounded apex and < 6 cells; hyphae are septate with no microconidia

MICROSCOPIC

Histologic Features

- Skin: Hyperkeratosis, parakeratosis, acanthosis/psoriasiform hyperplasia, neutrophils in stratum corneum, variable dermal mixed inflammatory infiltrate and spongiosis
    - Fungal hyphae in stratum corneum of epidermis, hair shaft, hair follicle, or nail matrix
- Disseminated disease: Neutrophilic, granulomatous, or necrotizing inflammation with fungal hyphae

ANCILLARY TESTS

Histochemistry

- Fungal forms are positive for PAS-D and GMS

DIFFERENTIAL DIAGNOSIS

Spongiotic/Eczematous Processes

- May show similar reactive changes (acanthosis, hyperkeratosis); no fungal organisms present

Disseminated Fungal Infection

- Morphologically similar to hyalohyphomycoses and candidiasis requiring cultures/sequencing to differentiate

Phaeohyphomycosis

- Pigmented fungal forms associated with granulomatous reaction; foreign material at primary site; can disseminate

SELECTED REFERENCES

1. Gold JAW et al: Epidemiology of tinea capitis causative species: an analysis of fungal culture results from a major U.S. national commercial laboratory. J Am Acad Dermatol. 89(2):382-4, 2023
2. Shalin SC et al: PAS and GMS utility in dermatopathology: review of the current medical literature. J Cutan Pathol. 47(11):1096-102, 2020
3. Woo TE et al: Diagnosis and management of cutaneous tinea infections. Adv Skin Wound Care. 32(8):350-7, 2019

Trichosporonosis

KEY FACTS

ETIOLOGY/PATHOGENESIS

- Fungal infection with *Trichosporon* species, yeast that have no teleomorphic (sexual) stage

CLINICAL ISSUES

- White piedra: Asymptomatic soft white nodules at hair base
- Localized cutaneous disease with ulceration and erythema
- Invasive/disseminated trichosporonosis with fever, malaise, skin lesions, hepatosplenomegaly, abdominal pain
  - Hematologic malignancy patients (acute myeloid leukemia) with iron overload
  - Excessive blood transfusions, hemochromatosis, or hemosiderosis with immunosuppression
- Laboratory testing
  - Positive cryptococcal latex agglutination assay (cross reactive)
  - Positive (1-3)-β-D-glucan; negative galactomannan

MICROSCOPIC

- Skin (immunocompromised): Fungal yeast/hyphal elements, lacks inflammation
- Liver/spleen: Large necrotic masses without inflammation, proliferating fungus
- Other organs: Minimal inflammation with proliferating fungal elements and necrosis
- PAS-D and MSS stains highlight hyphal forms
- Arthroconidia may be present in skin and disseminated infections but difficult to reliably identify

TOP DIFFERENTIAL DIAGNOSES

- Aspergillosis: Lacks arthroconidia; positive for galactomannan
- Candidiasis: Pseudohyphae and gram-positive yeast
- Hyalohyphomycosis: Lacks arthroconidia; negative for galactomannan
- Mucormycosis: Thick hyphae, less inflammation, negative for (1,3)-β-D-glucan

White Piedra (Tinea Blanca)

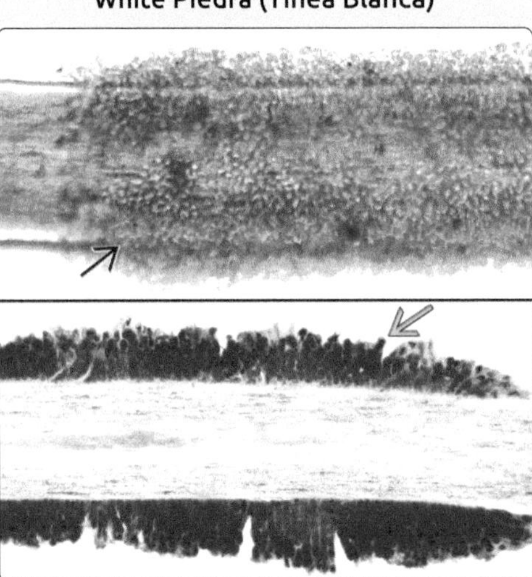

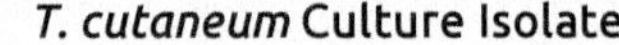

T. cutaneum Culture Isolate

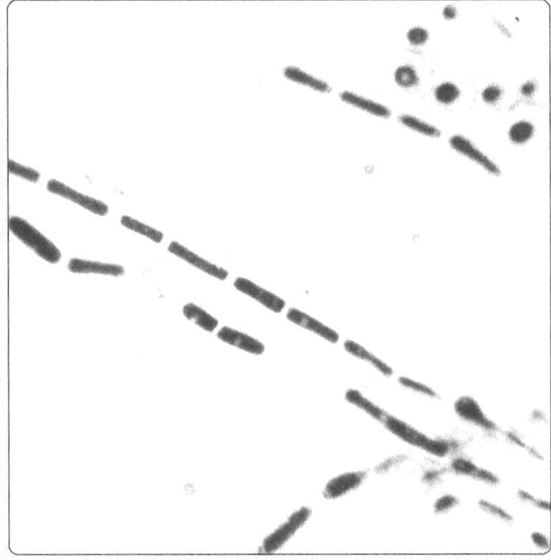

(Left) *This hair shaft exhibits nodular deformation and the presence of numerous Trichosporon beigelii spores* ⇨. *(Courtesy Dr. Hardin.) Periodic acid-Schiff staining of a hair shaft from a different case shows numerous spores coating the surface* ⇨. **(Right)** *Lactophenol cotton blue staining of Trichosporon cutaneum reveals hyphae and cylindrical to ellipsoidal arthroconidia. (Courtesy L. Georg, CDC/PHIL.)*

Disseminated Trichosporonosis

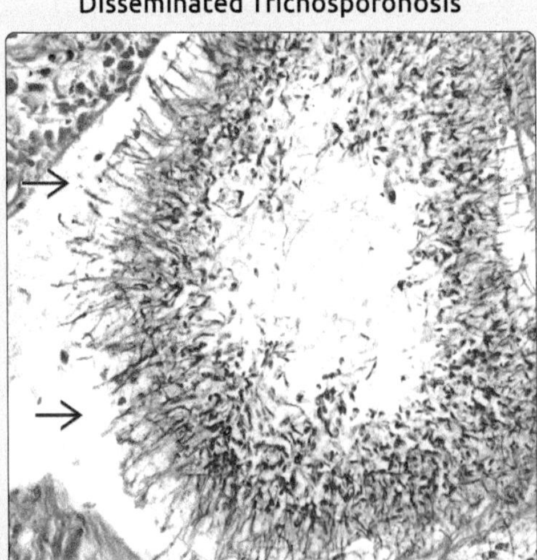

Disseminated Trichosporonosis: GMS Stain

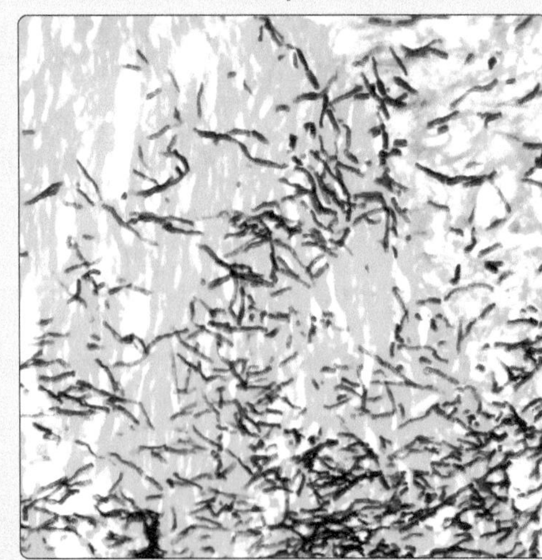

(Left) *A colony of Trichosporon within human tissue in disseminated disease shows hyphal forms* ⇨, *which are morphologically difficult to distinguish from Aspergillus spp. and other hyaline molds. Note the lack of inflammation.* **(Right)** *Medium-power view shows a collection of Trichosporon fungus hyphae highlighted by GMS staining. Correlation with cultures or molecular testing is typically required for definitive diagnosis.*

TERMINOLOGY

Definitions

- Derived from "tricho" (hair) + "spora" (seed)

ETIOLOGY/PATHOGENESIS

Infectious Agents

- Fungal infection with *Trichosporon* species, yeast that have no teleomorphic (sexual) stage, including *T. asahii* (formerly *beigelli*), *T. asteroides*, *T. cutaneum*, *T. dermatis*, *T. dohaense*, *T. inkin*, *T. loubieri*, *T. mucoides*, and *T. ovoides*
- Ubiquitous fungus found on human skin as colonizing organism that has been isolated from soil, cheese, insects, bird feces, and water sources
- Spread by close contact (including sexual transmission), bathing in stagnant waters, long hair, humidity

CLINICAL ISSUES

Presentation

- White piedra: Soft white nodules of fungus at bases of human hair, asymptomatic (any host)
- Summertime hypersensitivity pneumonitis presents as respiratory asthma-like illness associated with sauna usage, particularly in Japan (any host)
- Localized cutaneous trichosporonosis demonstrates localized ulceration with erythema (any host)
- Invasive/disseminated trichosporonosis with fever, malaise, skin lesions, hepatosplenomegaly, abdominal pain
  - Occurs in hematologic malignancy patients (acute myeloid leukemia) with iron overload due to transfusions
  - Any patient with excessive blood transfusions, hemochromatosis, or hemosiderosis with immunosuppression is at risk

Laboratory Tests

- Cryptococcal latex agglutination assay: Positive in trichosporonosis (cross reactive)
- Elevated serum (1,3)-β-D-glucan; Negative galactomannan
- Peripheral blood &/or urine (often 1st) fungal culture usually positive in disseminated disease
- Internal transcribed spacer (ITS) region or D1/D2 28S rRNA sequencing

Treatment

- Voriconazole and posaconazole

Prognosis

- White piedra and localized disease are easily treated with low morbidity and mortality
- Disseminated trichosporonosis, due to host setting, has high fatality rate

MICROBIOLOGY

Culture

- Grows as white, dry to creamy colonies at 25 °C with deep transverse fissures on Sabouraud dextrose agar or malt yeast agar
- Microscopically exhibit hyaline septate hyphae, hyphae breaking up into oval or rectangular arthroconidia 2-4 μm in diameter, and occasional blastoconidia
- Speciate by sequencing or MALDI-TOF MS

MICROSCOPIC

Histologic Features

- Skin
  - Hair shafts: Nodular deformation with numerous *Trichosporon* spp. spores
  - Immunocompetent: Necrotic neutrophilic dermatitis/cellulitis with granulomatous inflammation (later) admixed with fungal elements
  - Immunocompromised: Fungal yeast/hyphal elements often lacking inflammatory component
- Liver/spleen: Large necrotic masses without inflammation, containing proliferating fungus
- Other organs: Minimal inflammation with proliferating fungal elements and necrosis
- Arthroconidia may be present in skin and disseminated infections but difficult to reliably identify

ANCILLARY TESTS

Special Stains

- Periodic acid-Schiff stain (variable depending on viability) and methenamine silver positive in hyphal forms
- Gram stain should be negative

DIFFERENTIAL DIAGNOSIS

Aspergillosis

- Morphologically very similar to trichosporonosis but lacks arthroconidia; positive for (1,3)-β-D-glucan and galactomannan

Candidiasis

- Yeast and pseudohyphae should be present; positive on Gram stain (yeast); positive for (1,3)-β-D-glucan and negative for galactomannan

Hyalohyphomycosis

- Morphologically very similar to trichosporonosis but lacks arthroconidia; positive for (1,3)-β-D-glucan and negative for galactomannan

Mucormycosis

- Thick hyphae with variable branching, less inflammatory reaction; negative for (1,3)-β-D-glucan and galactomannan

SELECTED REFERENCES

1. Nobrega de Almeida J et al: Epidemiology, clinical aspects, outcomes and prognostic factors associated with Trichosporon fungaemia: results of an international multicentre study carried out at 23 medical centres. J Antimicrob Chemother. 76(7):1907-15, 2021
2. Sadamoto S et al: Histopathological study on the prevalence of trichosporonosis in formalin-fixed and paraffin-embedded tissue autopsy sections by in situ hybridization with peptide nucleic acid probe. Med Mycol. 58(4):460-8, 2020
3. de Almeida JN Jr et al: Evaluating and improving Vitek MS for identification of clinically relevant species of Trichosporon and the closely related genera Cutaneotrichosporon and Apiotrichum. J Clin Microbiol. 55(8):2439-44, 2017
4. Duarte-Oliveira C et al: The cell biology of the Trichosporon-host interaction. Front Cell Infect Microbiol. 7:118, 2017
5. Dotis J et al: Non-Aspergillus fungal infections in chronic granulomatous disease. Mycoses. 56(4):449-62, 2013
6. Obana Y et al: Differential diagnosis of trichosporonosis using conventional histopathological stains and electron microscopy. Histopathology. 56(3):372-83, 2010

KEY FACTS

ETIOLOGY/PATHOGENESIS

- Cutaneous fungal infections limited to stratum corneum, hair, and nails, causing minimal inflammation

CLINICAL ISSUES

- Tinea versicolor (*Malassezia* spp.): Hypochromic or hyperchromic macules with irregular borders that coalesce into patches with fine scale
- Tinea nigra (*Hortaea werneckii*): Chronic, hyperpigmented irregular patches
- Black piedra (*Piedraia hortae*): Brown or black, fusiform, hard concretions on hair shafts
- Direct examination with 10-20% potassium hydroxide (KOH) solution and Parker blue ink of skin scrapings or infected hairs

MICROSCOPIC

- Tinea versicolor: Basophilic, round yeast and thin, septate hyphae in stratum corneum with spaghetti and meatballs appearance; typically no inflammation present
- Tinea nigra: Brown pigmented hyphae and blastoconidia in stratum corneum; typically no inflammation present
- Black piedra: Pseudoparenchymatous mass composed of thick-walled septate hyphae, mimicking arthroconidia, oriented perpendicular to long axis of hair shaft
- Fungal elements typically visible on H&E-stained sections (can be highlighted by PAS-D)

TOP DIFFERENTIAL DIAGNOSES

- Dermatophytosis (tinea): In contrast to *Malassezia* spp., dermatophytes appear transparent and are difficult to detect on H&E-stained sections and frequently elicit neutrophilic and eosinophilic inflammation
- Pediculosis capitis: Concretions on hair shaft due to nits and lice; lack fungal elements
- Melanocytic nevus or melanoma: Neoplasm composed of nevomelanocytes; lack pigmented yeast and hyphae in stratum corneum

Tinea Versicolor

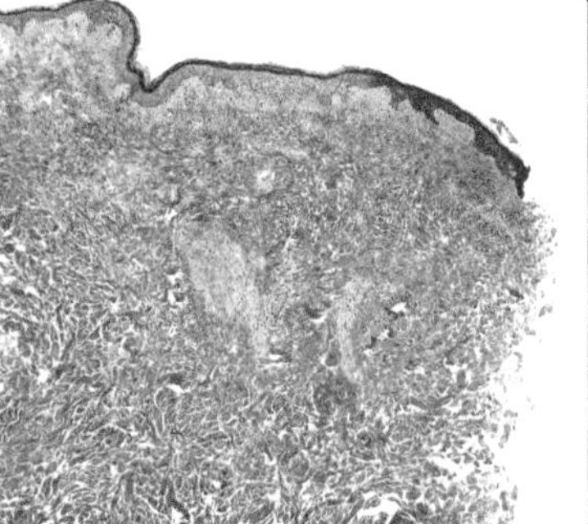

Tinea Versicolor

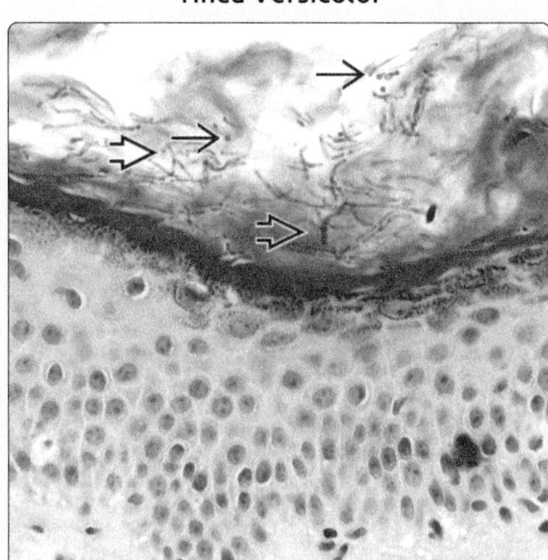

(Left) *Biopsies of tinea versicolor appear essentially "normal" on scanning magnification and require a high index of suspicion &/or careful examination of the stratum corneum to detect fungal elements.* **(Right)** *Numerous, somewhat basophilic, thin septate hyphae ⇨ and blastoconidia → are readily evident in the stratum corneum on routine H&E-stained sections with an appearance that has been likened to spaghetti and meatballs.*

Tinea Nigra

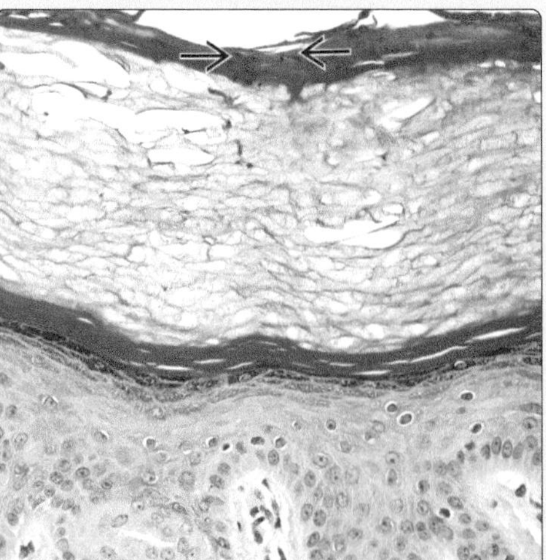

Tinea Nigra

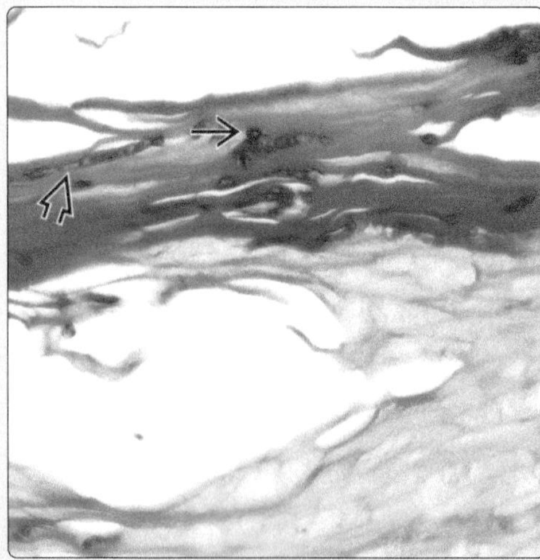

(Left) *Tinea nigra shows noninflamed skin with fungal elements in the stratum corneum →, readily evident on routine H&E-stained sections.* **(Right)** *Tinea nigra, caused by the halophilic fungus Hortaea werneckii, is pigmented and typically shows brown hyphae ⇨ and blastoconidia →.*

ETIOLOGY/PATHOGENESIS

Infectious Agents

- Cutaneous fungal infections limited to stratum corneum, hair, and nails, causing minimal inflammation
- Most frequent are tineas, tinea versicolor, and piedras (white and black)
- Tinea versicolor (pityriasis versicolor) is caused by various lipophilic fungi of genus *Malassezia*: *M. furfur*, *M. globosa*, and *M. sympodialis* are most common
- Tinea nigra is caused by *Hortaea werneckii* (previously *Phaeoannellomyces werneckii*), pigmented, polymorphic, halophilic fungus
- Black piedra is chronic asymptomatic infection of hair shafts of scalp caused by pigmented fungus *Piedraia hortae*

CLINICAL ISSUES

Epidemiology

- Tinea versicolor: Reported worldwide but most commonly in tropical climates
  - Typically in young adults and equally distributed in women and men
  - Heat, humidity, and use of oily tanning lotions, creams, and corticosteroids are predisposing factors
- Tinea nigra: Mostly in tropical regions, particularly in coastal zones
  - Affects young women and men and frequently children
  - Hyperhidrosis of hands and feet is considered essential for disease development
- Black piedra: Most common in tropical climates with high rainfall
  - Affects young women and men and children
  - High humidity and poor personal hygiene are main predisposing factors

Presentation

- Tinea versicolor: Hypochromic or hyperchromic macules with irregular borders that coalesce into patches with fine scale; most patients are otherwise asymptomatic with few complaining of pruritus
- *Malassezia* spp. also implicated in seborrheic dermatitis, folliculitis, and onychomycosis
- Tinea nigra: Chronic, hyperpigmented irregular patches predominantly in hands and, sometimes, feet, arms, legs, neck, and trunk; patches are otherwise asymptomatic, range in color from tan to dark brown or black, and are covered with fine scale
- Black piedra: Brown or black, fusiform, hard concretions on hair shafts of scalp, beard, and, sometimes, axillary and pubic hair; otherwise asymptomatic and similar to white piedra

Laboratory Tests

- Direct examination with 10-20% potassium hydroxide (KOH) solution and Parker blue ink of skin scrapings or infected hairs
- Tinea versicolor: Clusters of small, round blastoconidia or round, budding yeast cells and short, septate, and, occasionally, branching hyphae
- Tinea nigra: Dark septate hyphae with occasional clusters of blastoconidia
- Black piedra: Brown ochre masses of pseudoparenchyma tissue composed of septate, thick-walled hyphae mimicking arthroconidia; asci with 2 or more ascospores sometimes observed

Treatment

- Tinea versicolor: Topical antifungals when limited and systemic antifungals when extensive or recurrent; noncream preparations are preferred and include imidazoles (e.g., miconazole, clotrimazole, ketoconazole)
- Tinea nigra: Control of hyperhidrosis, keratolytics, and topical antifungals (e.g., ketoconazole); oral itraconazole also effective
- Black piedra: Clipping of infected hairs and application of keratolytics and topical antifungals; if disease is disseminated, shaving whole area is recommended

Prognosis

- Excellent; cure after appropriate treatment expected for all 3 conditions
- Recurrences may be observed if predisposing factors are not modified

MICROBIOLOGY

Cultures

- *Malassezia* spp. are fastidious and slow-growing yeasts that need selective culture media to grow
  - On modified Dixon agar, *M. furfur* colonies are cream to yellowish, smooth or lightly wrinkled
  - Clusters of thick-walled, round, budding, yeast-like cells and short hyphal forms are commonly seen
- *H. werneckii* grows on Sabouraud glucose agar in 2 phases
  - Yeast-like phase with slowly growing, shiny, black mucoid colonies and filamentous phase with grayish green hyphae at periphery and olive-colored center due to thin layer of mycelium
  - Brown septate hyphae with lateral annellides and ellipsoidal 2-celled, septate blue and brown annelloconidia are seen in lactophenol cotton blue preparation
- *P. hortae* is slow growing
  - Small, compact, adherent, somewhat raised dark green to black colonies with reddish brown, diffusible pigment
  - Closely septate hyphae with dark, thick walls and many intercalary chlamydoconidia-like cells; ascospores more likely to be seen on direct microscopic examination of specimens than culture

MICROSCOPIC

Histologic Features

- Tinea versicolor
  - Somewhat basophilic, round yeast and thin, septate hyphae in stratum corneum with characteristic spaghetti and meatballs appearance
  - High index of suspicion and careful examination of stratum corneum are needed; no inflammation is typically present
- Tinea nigra
  - Brown pigmented hyphae and blastoconidia in stratum corneum
  - No inflammatory infiltrate present typically

Salient Features of Superficial Mycoses

Superficial Mycosis	Etiology	Distribution	Clinical Features	Treatment
Tinea versicolor	*Malassezia globosa, Malassezia sympodialis, Malassezia furfur*	Face, neck, upper trunk, arms	Hypo- and hyperpigmented macules and patches with fine scale	Topical (imidazoles, terbinafine) and oral antifungals (itraconazole, ketoconazole)
Tinea nigra	*Hortaea werneckii* (previously *Phaeoannellomyces werneckii*)	Palms and soles	Brown to gray, irregular patches	Control of hyperhidrosis
Black piedra	*Piedraia hortae*	Hairs in scalp, beard, axilla, and pubis	Asymptomatic, hard, black fusiform concretions on hair shaft	Hair clipping of affected hairs, topical antifungals, keratolytics
White piedra	*Trichosporon cutaneum, Trichosporon ovoides, Trichosporon inkin, Trichosporon beigelii, Trichosporon asahii*	Hairs in scalp, beard, axilla, and pubis	Asymptomatic, hard, white 1- to 3-mm concretions with well-defined borders; palpable but not visible initially	Hair clipping of affected hairs, topical antifungals, keratolytics
Tinea	*Trichophyton* spp. (primarily *Microsporum* spp., *Epidermophyton* spp., *Nannizzia* spp.)	Skin anywhere in body, including palms, soles, hair, and nails	Annular, erythematous patches and plaques with raised border and scale, onychodystrophy	Topical (butenafine, ciclopirox, tolnaftate) or systemic antifungals (terbinafine, itraconazole, griseofulvin)
Mucocutaneous candidiasis	*Candida albicans, Candida lusitaniae, Candida parapsilosis, Nakaseomyces glabratus* (previously *Candida glabrata*), *Candida kefyr, Candida famata, Candida africana, Candida orthopsilosis*	Oral cavity, genital skin, intertriginous areas	Oral thrush, erythematous itchy papules and plaques with characteristic satellite lesions	Nystatin, clotrimazole, miconazole, amphotericin B

- Black piedra
    - Pseudoparenchymatous mass composed of thick-walled septate hyphae
    - Hyphae are frequently septate mimicking arthroconidia, oriented perpendicular to long axis of hair shaft

ANCILLARY TESTS

Special Stains

- PAS-D highlights *Malassezia* spp. yeast and hyphae (typically not required), *H. werneckii* hyphae and blastoconidia (obscuring brown pigment), and *P. hortae* hyphae

DIFFERENTIAL DIAGNOSIS

Dermatophytosis (Tinea)

- Dermatophytes appear transparent and are difficult to detect on H&E-stained sections, while blastoconidia and hyphae of *Malassezia* spp. usually basophilic and readily evident on H&E
- Dermatophytosis frequently elicit neutrophilic and eosinophilic inflammation, absent in tinea versicolor

Pediculosis Capitis

- Presents with concretions on hair shaft, which upon close/microscopic examination are nits and lice and not fungi

Melanocytic Nevus or Melanoma

- Neoplasm composed of nevomelanocytes in contrast to pigmented yeast and hyphae in stratum corneum

SELECTED REFERENCES

1. Chanyachailert P et al: Cutaneous fungal infections caused by dermatophytes and non-dermatophytes: an updated comprehensive review of epidemiology, clinical presentations, and diagnostic testing. J Fungi (Basel). 9(6), 2023
2. Leung AK et al: Tinea versicolor: an updated review. Drugs Context. 11, 2022
3. Saraswat N et al: Tinea nigra palmaris. JAMA Dermatol. 158(12):1439, 2022
4. Saunte DML et al: Malassezia-associated skin diseases, the use of diagnostics and treatment. Front Cell Infect Microbiol. 10:112, 2020
5. Eksomtramage T et al: Tinea nigra mimicking acral melanocytic nevi. IDCases. 18:e00654, 2019
6. Veasey JV et al: White piedra, black piedra, tinea versicolor, and tinea nigra: contribution to the diagnosis of superficial mycosis. An Bras Dermatol. 92(3):413-6, 2017
7. Harada K et al: Malassezia species and their associated skin diseases. J Dermatol. 42(3):250-7, 2015
8. Hawkins DM et al: Superficial fungal infections in children. Pediatr Clin North Am. 61(2):443-55, 2014
9. Bonifaz A et al: Tinea versicolor, tinea nigra, white piedra, and black piedra. Clin Dermatol. 28(2):140-5, 2010
10. Schwartz RA: Superficial fungal infections. Lancet. 364(9440):1173-82, 2004

Tinea Versicolor

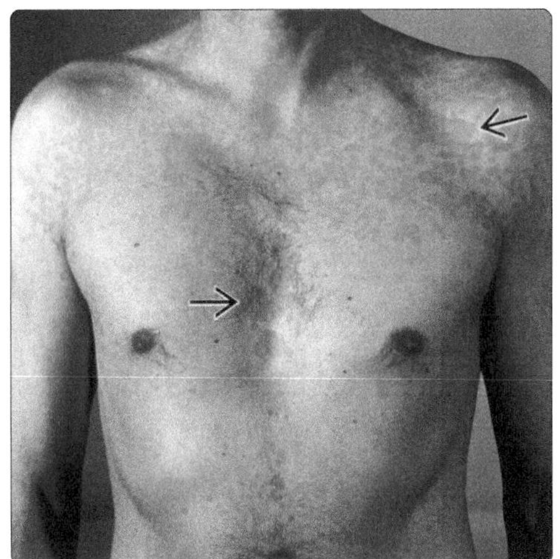

Tinea Versicolor

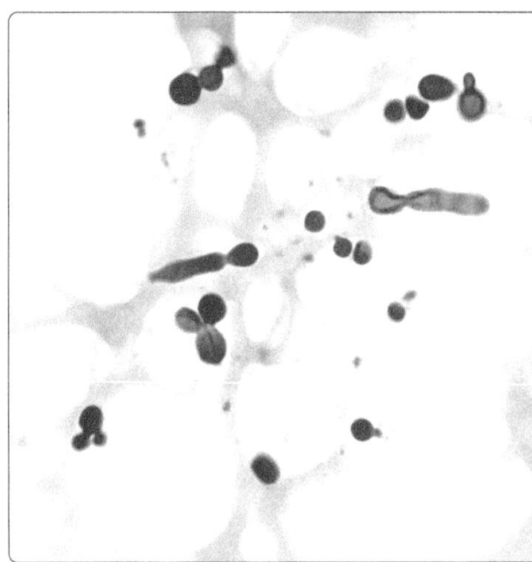

(Left) *In fair-skinned individuals, tinea (pityriasis) versicolor presents with irregular hyperpigmented macules coalescing into patches ⇒, which may have a fine scale.* **(Right)** *Skin scrapings show blastoconidia and small hyphae in this scale from a patient with tinea versicolor due to Malassezia furfur. (Courtesy L. Georg, PhD, CDC/PHIL.)*

Tinea Nigra

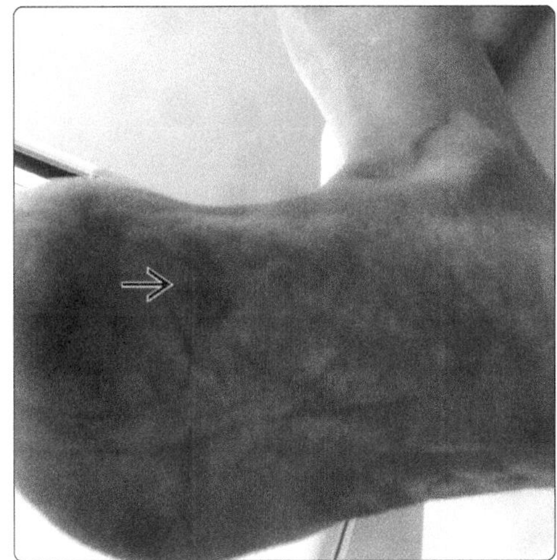

Piedraia hortae

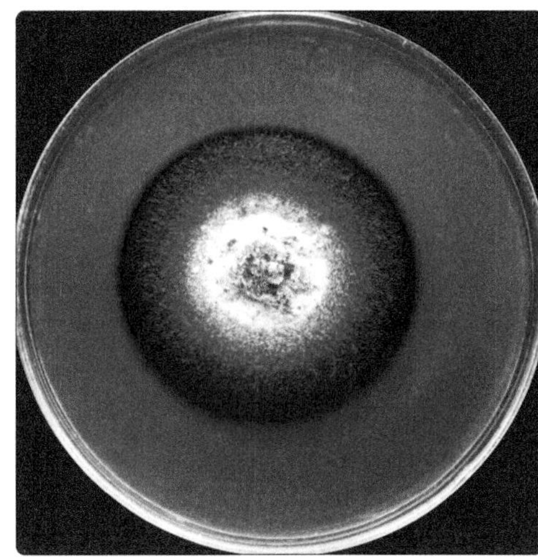

(Left) *Tinea nigra typically affects the palms and soles and presents with irregular, dark brown to gray patches ⇒ simulating an atypical melanocytic neoplasm.* **(Right)** *P. hortae give rise to white, powdery colonies with a dark brown to black outer perimeter. Note the characteristic reddish discoloration of the agar at the colony's perimeter. (Courtesy L. Georg, PhD, CDC/PHIL.)*

Black Piedra

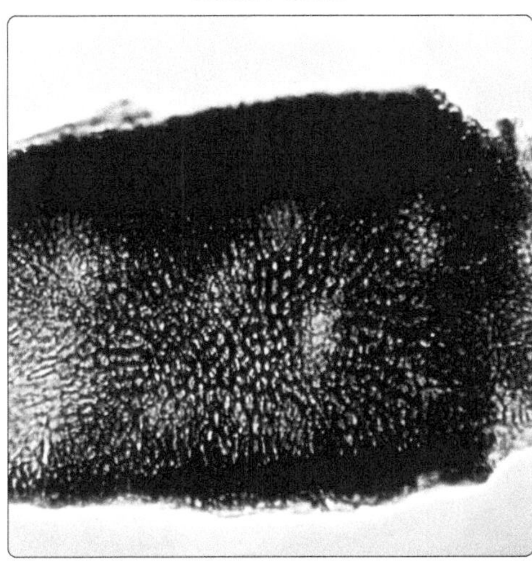

Black Piedra Ascospores

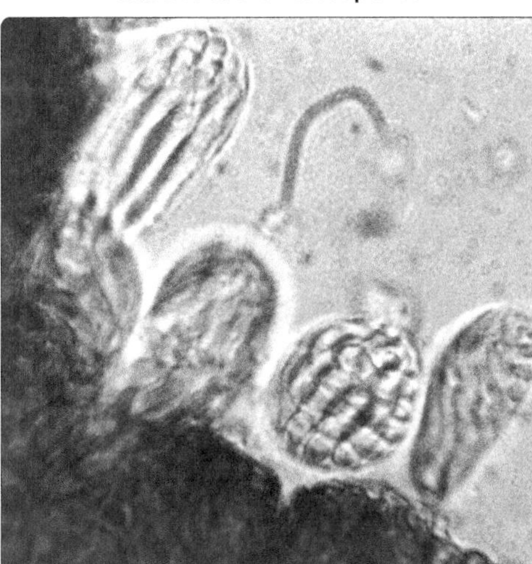

(Left) *Numerous fungal elements coating a hair shaft are shown in this hair from a patient with black piedra. (Courtesy L. Georg, PhD, CDC/PHIL.)* **(Right)** *Sac-like asci with ascospores of P. hortae are noted in this sample of black piedra. (Courtesy L. Georg, PhD, CDC/PHIL.)*

Blastomycosis

KEY FACTS

ETIOLOGY/PATHOGENESIS

- Infection via inhalation of *Blastomyces* spp. fungal conidia
- Predominantly *Blastomyces dermatitidis*; other spp. include *Blastomyces gilchristii, Blastomyces helicus, Blastomyces percursus*, and *Blastomyces emzantsi*
- Endemic areas in North America: Southeastern USA, Mississippi and Ohio River Valleys, USA and Canadian provinces around Great Lakes and St. Lawrence River

CLINICAL ISSUES

- Most common sites: Pulmonary, cutaneous, osseous
- No clinical or radiographic features are specific, and spectrum of disease overlaps with those of other fungal pathogens, mycobacteria, and malignancy
- Immunocompromised patients have more aggressive clinical course
- Visualization of characteristic yeast forms or growth of fungus in culture is necessary for definitive diagnosis

MICROSCOPIC

- Spherical multinucleated yeast cells (8-15 μm) with single broad-based budding, thick refractile wall
- Pyogranulomatous inflammation

ANCILLARY TESTS

- Positive for GMS, PAS-D, Congo red stains
- Variable for Fontana-Masson stain
- Negative for Gram stain

TOP DIFFERENTIAL DIAGNOSES

- Histoplasmosis: Small yeast with narrow-based budding
- Candidiasis: Gram-positive yeast, pseudohyphae, lack of broad-based budding
- Cryptococcosis: Variably sized yeast with narrow-based budding and mucicarmine-positive capsule
- Paracoccidioidosis: Yeast with multiple points of budding
- Coccidioidomycosis: Large spherules with endospores, no budding

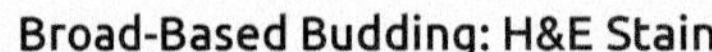

Broad-Based Budding: H&E Stain

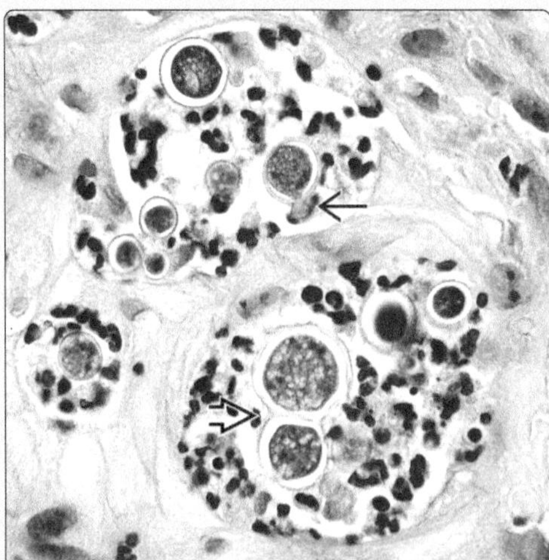

Broad-Based Budding: Silver Stain

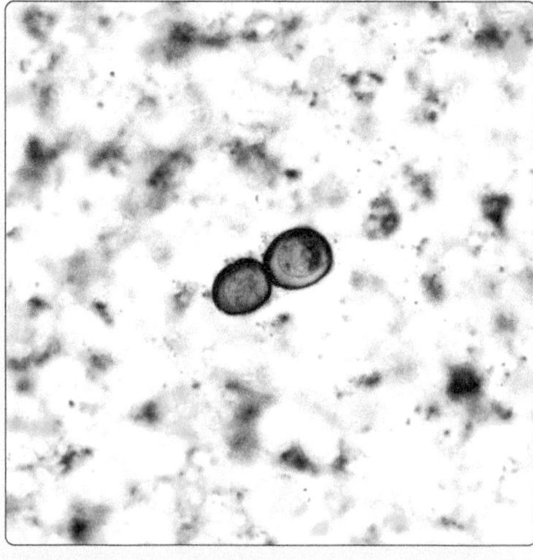

(Left) *High magnification of a skin section on an H&E stain shows multiple multinucleate Blastomyces yeast cells. Thick cell wall as well as broad-based budding at early ⇒ and late ⇒ stages are seen.* **(Right)** *High magnification of this tissue section on GMS stain shows Blastomyces yeast forms with characteristic broad-based budding and a thick cell wall.*

Fine-Needle Aspiration: Papanicolaou Stain

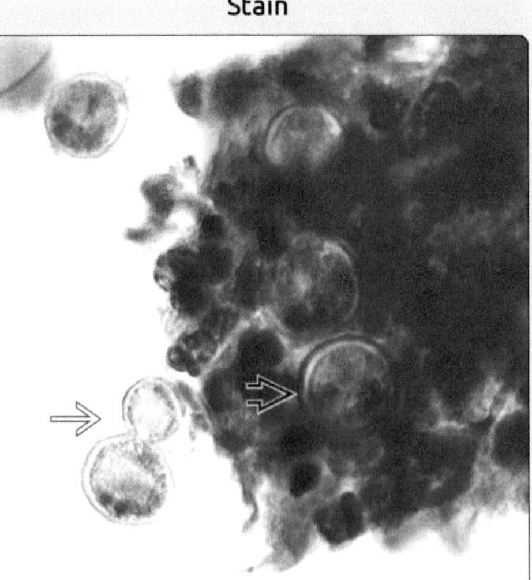

Primary Specimen: Calcofluor White Stain

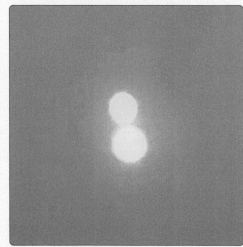

(Left) *Broad-based budding ➡ and double contour cell wall ⇒ observed on Papanicolaou staining of lung cytology specimen are shown.* **(Right)** *Budding yeast identified in direct microscopy of primary clinical specimen is shown. Calcofluor white is a nonspecific fluorochrome that binds cellulose and chitin in the cell walls of fungi.*

TERMINOLOGY

Synonyms

- Gilchrist disease

Definitions

- Greek: "Blasto" (bud, sprout, embryo) + "myces" (fungi)

ETIOLOGY/PATHOGENESIS

Infectious Agent

- Infection most often occurs via inhalation of *Blastomyces* spp. conidia (asexual spores), thermally dimorphic fungus
- Endemic areas in North America predominantly along fresh water drainage basins, including Southeastern, South Central (Mississippi and Ohio River Valleys), Midwestern, New England, and New York state in USA; Canada around Great Lakes and St. Lawrence River Valley
- Majority of cases in USA caused by *Blastomyces dermatitidis* complex composed of *B. dermatitidis* (sexual state formerly known as *Ajellomyces dermatitidis*) and more recently described *Blastomyces gilchristii*
- Additional spp. reported to cause human disease include *Blastomyces helicus* (Western USA, Canada), *Blastomyces percursus* (Africa, Middle East), *and Blastomyces emzantsi* (South Africa)

CLINICAL ISSUES

Presentation

- Range from subclinical infection to fatal disseminated disease
- Disseminated disease occurs in both immunocompromised and immunocompetent hosts
- Pulmonary infection is most common site of involvement
  - Acute pneumonia often indistinguishable from acute bacterial or viral pneumonia; subset of patients have self-limited disease
  - Chronic pneumonia with mass-like infiltrates mimicking pulmonary tuberculosis, malignancy, or other fungal infections, such as histoplasmosis
  - Adult respiratory distress syndrome (ARDS) presents with diffuse bilateral pulmonary infiltrates and is associated with high mortality, particularly in patients requiring mechanical ventilation
- Extrapulmonary infection more common in men
  - Cutaneous infection (2nd most common site of involvement) from direct inoculation or dissemination
    - Typically presents as ulcerative lesions or raised/crusted verrucous lesions with irregular borders, grossly mimicking squamous cell carcinoma, basal cell carcinoma, pyoderma gangrenosum, or giant keratoacanthoma
    - Microabscesses are present
    - Mucosal lesions of nose, mouth, pharynx, or larynx can occur; verrucous lesions can mimic squamous cell carcinoma
    - Can extend to subcutaneous tissues and fistulize to bone or joints
  - Osseous infection (3rd most common site)
    - Can involve any bone; vertebrae, pelvis, and sacrum are most common sites of involvement
    - Extension from osteomyelitis to adjacent joint can cause purulent arthritis
    - Extension into soft tissue can lead to formation of abscesses that track through soft tissues, forming subcutaneous masses at any spinal level and draining through skin, resulting in discharging sinus or ulcer
    - Vertebral osteomyelitis frequently complicated by paravertebral or psoas abscesses
  - Other sites of involvement (any organ can be involved)
    - e.g., genitourinary system: Most common sites of disease are prostate, testicle, and epididymis
    - e.g., CNS: Uncommon in immunocompetent hosts and can present as meningitis, epidural abscess, or intracranial abscesses

Laboratory Tests

- Wet mount preparations
  - Fresh wet preparations of clinical specimens can be examined directly for organisms
  - Calcofluor white fluorochrome staining is useful when organisms are sparse, as it allows yeast cells to fluoresce
  - Potassium hydroxide (KOH) can enhance visibility of yeast organisms by dissolving tissue materials
  - Specimens that can be examined clinically include sputum, bronchoalveolar lavage fluid, pleural fluid, cerebrospinal fluid (CSF), urine, skin scrapings, or purulent material
- Antigen testing: Overall sensitivity 93% and specificity 79%
  - Commercial enzyme immunoassay (EIA) antigen assay is available for testing bronchoalveolar lavage fluid, CSF, serum, urine and can be used to follow response to treatment
    - Cross reactivity reported in patients with histoplasmosis; hence, simultaneous testing for *Histoplasma* spp. should be done
    - Cross reactivity has also been reported in patients with paracoccidioidomycosis and penicilliosis
  - Cross reactivity reported for *Aspergillus* galactomannan serum antigen testing
  - Serum 1,3-Beta-D glucan negative
- Serologic testing generally not used in routine practice
  - Complement fixation and immunodiffusion: Poor sensitivity and specificity
  - Radioimmunodiffusion and EIAs: Better sensitivity (77-83%) and specificity (95%) but are not commercially available
- DNA hybridization
  - To confirm identification from culture-based growth, commercially available chemiluminescent DNA probe (AccuProbe; Gen-Probe, Inc.) that hybridizes to rRNA of *B. dermatitidis* can provide rapid results with good sensitivity (> 87%) and specificity (100%)
  - Can be used to identify organism from both phases of growth regardless of sporulation
  - Cross reacts with *Paracoccidioides brasiliensis* as well as rare human pathogens, *Gymnascella hyalinospora* and *Emmonsia parva*
- Molecular
  - PCR-based assays can be used to confirm isolate identification from culture-based growth

- PCR-based testing of primary clinical specimens, such as bronchial washings, bronchoalveolar fluid, pleural fluid, sputum, blood, in development; utility still needs to be confirmed in large prospective studies

Treatment

- Most patients require therapy, although some immunocompetent patients with acute pulmonary infection spontaneously clear infection and may not need treatment
- Azole (e.g., itraconazole) for mild to moderate pulmonary disease and disseminated disease without CNS involvement
- Amphotericin B (lipid formulation preferred to avoid nephrotoxicity) for moderate to severe pulmonary disease and moderate to severe disseminated disease without CNS involvement
- CNS involvement: Initial therapy with amphotericin B and step-down therapy of voriconazole (good CNS penetration)
- Immunocompromised patients: Amphotericin B followed by itraconazole (if no CNS involvement)
- Supportive therapy may include mechanical ventilation or extracorporeal membrane oxygenation (ECMO)

Prognosis

- Blastomycosis has been reported to have more aggressive course and more likely to relapse in immunocompromised patients
- ARDS caused by pulmonary blastomycosis is associated with high mortality
- Prognosis worsens when infection spreads beyond lungs without treatment
- Bone disease is more likely to relapse than other forms of blastomycosis

IMAGING

Radiographic Findings

- Radiographic features are not specific and can mimic other pathologies, including tuberculosis, histoplasmosis, and coccidioidomycosis
- Lung involvement: Alveolar or mass-like infiltrates are most common findings
  - Reticulonodular and miliary patterns are less common and usually associated with ARDS
  - Cavitation of lung parenchyma can be seen but is rare
- Bone involvement: Can appear as clearly demarcated osteolytic lesion or as diffuse, destructive process with periosteal new bone formation

MICROBIOLOGY

Culture

- White or tan mold grows on sabouraud dextrose agar or brain heart infusion agar
- *B. dermatitidis* typically grows in 5-10 days but can take up to 3 weeks or may not grow at all in culture, depending on clinical specimen
- Sensitivity varies depending on sample and may range from 62-100%

MACROSCOPIC

Lungs

- Single, few, or numerous multifocal lesions ± regions of consolidation
- Lesions variably sized, irregular, and firm
- Dissemination may include draining lymph nodes

Skin

- Isolated lesion or hundreds of lesions may be present
- Central ulceration, abscess formation, &/or violaceous nodules
- Papulopustular lesions often progress to verrucous plaques with heaped margins
- Mucous membranes less commonly affected, although laryngeal, oral, and nasal lesions are reported

MICROSCOPIC

Histologic Features

- Associated with pyogranulomatous reaction
  - Acute infection: Neutrophilic inflammation predominates and yeast organisms easily detected
  - Chronic infection: Granulomata, which are usually noncaseating, may form, and yeast organisms can be difficult to find
- Skin and mucosal specimens associated with microabscess formation and pseudoepitheliomatous hyperplasia
- Spherical yeast cells (8-15 μm in diameter) with thick, double-contoured walls; display single broad-based budding
  - Smaller yeast forms (2-4 μm in diameter) have been reported in cases of blastomycosis
  - Thick refractile wall may give appearance of space between fungal cell contents and surrounding tissue
  - Multiple nuclei of yeast may be seen inside yeast cells
  - Unusual yeast-like cells and hyphal fragments reported in cases of atypical blastomycosis outside USA (e.g., *B. percursus*, *B. emzantsi*)

ANCILLARY TESTS

Histochemistry

- Positive for Grocott methenamine silver (GMS), periodic acid-Schiff (PAS), and Congo red stains
- Variably positive for Fontana-Masson stain (~ 50%)
- Negative for Gram stain
- Negative or weakly positive for mucicarmine, Alcian blue (pH 2.5), and acid-fast stains

PCR

- PCR and broad-range sequencing-based approaches can be used to speciate organism from formalin fixed paraffin-embedded (FFPE) tissue
- Broad-range sequencing assays target combination of internal transcribed spacer 1 and 2 regions (ITS1, ITS2), and conserved nuclear ribosomal RNA (rRNA) genes (D1/D2 28S, 18S)

DIFFERENTIAL DIAGNOSIS

Candidiasis

- Distinguished by presence of gram-positive yeast, pseudohyphae, and lack of broad-based budding

Coccidioidomycosis

- Usually presents as spherules with multiple endospores
- Pairs of endospores may mimic broad-based budding
- Negative for Alcian blue (pH 2.5) and acid-fast stain

Paracoccidioidosis

- Yeast phase distinguished by presence of multiple, narrow-based buds arranged around periphery of mother cell

Cryptococcosis

- Narrow-based budding with mucicarmine-positive capsule
- *Blastomyces* spp. can be positive on Fontana-Masson stain

Histoplasmosis

- Small (2- to 4-μm) yeast forms with narrow-based budding
- Negative for Congo red

SELECTED REFERENCES

1. Smith DJ et al: Surveillance for coccidioidomycosis, histoplasmosis, and blastomycosis - United States, 2019. MMWR Surveill Summ. 71(7):1-14, 2022
2. McBride JA et al: Clinical manifestations and outcomes in immunocompetent and immunocompromised patients with blastomycosis. Clin Infect Dis. 72(9):1594-602, 2021
3. Schwartz IS et al: Blastomycosis in Africa and the Middle East: a comprehensive review of reported cases and reanalysis of historical isolates based on molecular data. Clin Infect Dis. 73(7):e1560-9, 2021
4. Linder KA et al: Current and new perspectives in the diagnosis of blastomycosis and histoplasmosis. J Fungi (Basel). 7(1):12, 2020
5. Scuderi S et al: Heterogeneity of blastomycosis-like pyoderma: a selection of cases from the last 35 years. Australas J Dermatol. 58(2):139-41, 2017
6. He S et al: A systematic review and meta-analysis of diagnostic accuracy of serum 1,3-β-D-glucan for invasive fungal infection: focus on cutoff levels. J Microbiol Immunol Infect. 48(4):351-61, 2015
7. Bishop JA et al: Evaluation of the detection of melanin by the Fontana-Masson silver stain in tissue with a wide range of organisms including Cryptococcus. Hum Pathol. 43(6):898-903, 2012
8. Guarner J et al: Histopathologic diagnosis of fungal infections in the 21st century. Clin Microbiol Rev. 24(2):247-80, 2011
9. Axelson GK et al: Evaluation of the use of Congo red staining in the differential diagnosis of Candida vs. various other yeast-form fungal organisms. J Cutan Pathol. 35(1):27-30, 2008
10. Wages DS et al: Acid-fastness of fungi in blastomycosis and histoplasmosis. Arch Pathol Lab Med. 106(9):440-1, 1982

Pulmonary Blastomycosis: Chest CT

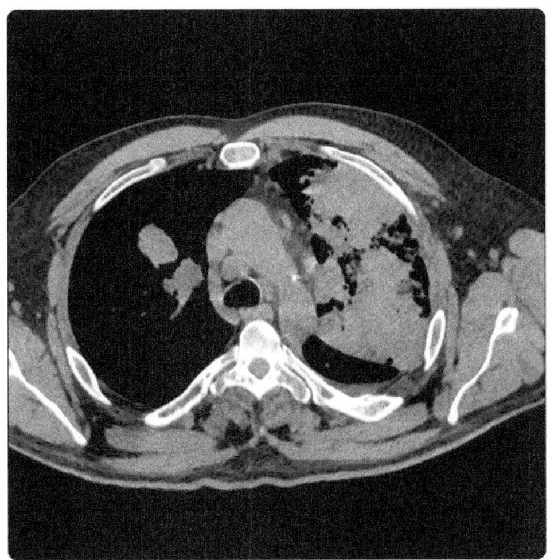

Fine-Needle Aspiration: Rapid Stain

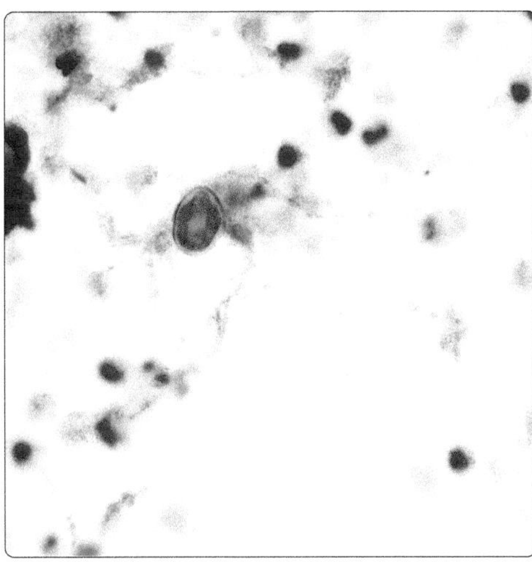

(Left) *CT of pulmonary blastomycosis shows bilateral opacities and an area of large patchy consolidation in the left upper lobe.* **(Right)** *High magnification of a fine-needle aspiration specimen on Diff-Quik stain shows a large yeast form with a thick cell wall. No budding is detected. The findings raise the differential of blastomycosis, which was confirmed on subsequent biopsy and culture.*

Pulmonary Blastomycosis: Fine-Needle Aspiration

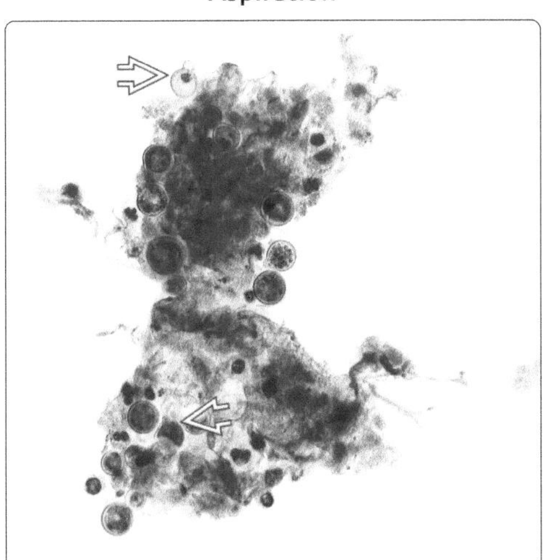

Pulmonary Blastomycosis Tissue Section

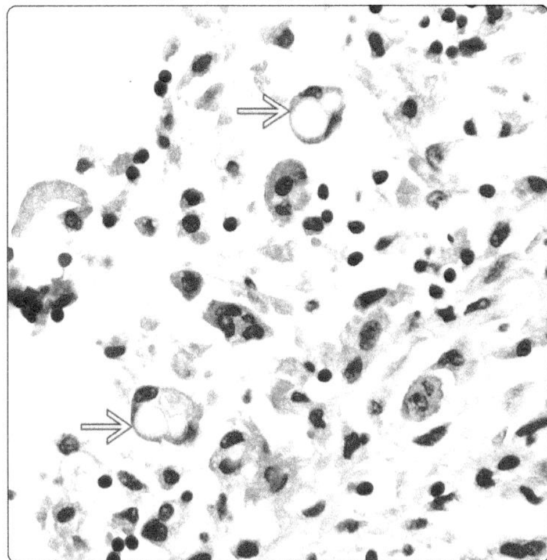

(Left) *This cytology specimen of a left upper lobe mass identified on CT shows necrotic debris and numerous large yeast forms with refractile cell walls and broad-based budding ➡.* **(Right)** *This lung autopsy section shows yeast forms with broad-based budding and clear intracytoplasmic connections ➡.*

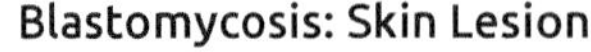

Blastomycosis: Skin Lesion

Blastomycosis: Skin Biopsy

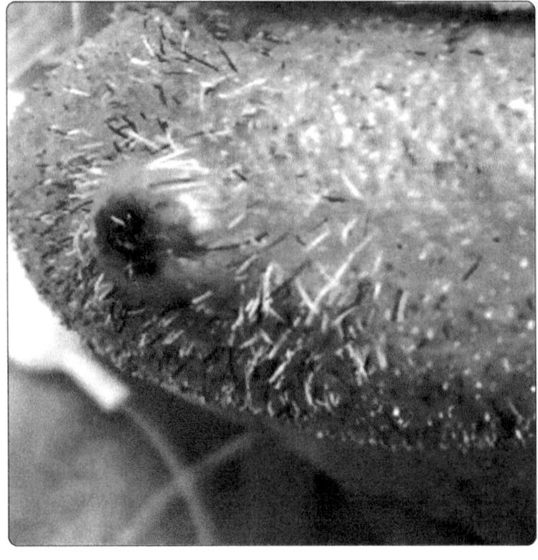

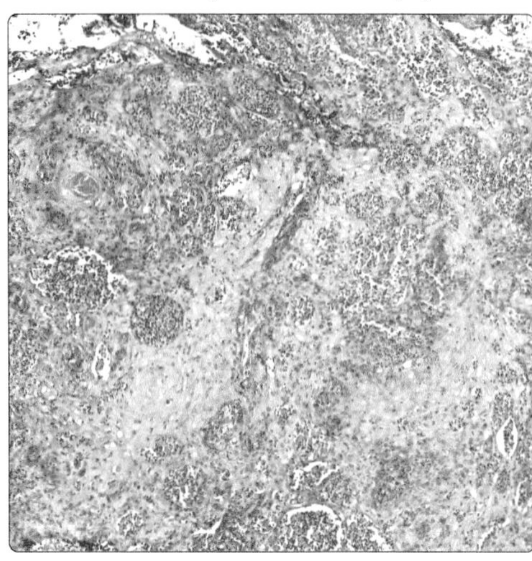

(Left) *Clinical photograph shows a skin infection presenting as a firm, pink nodule with central hemorrhagic crust. Biopsy showed involvement by blastomycosis.* **(Right)** *Biopsy of a skin lesion shows marked acute inflammation and microabscess formation.*

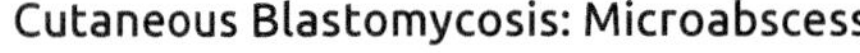

Cutaneous Blastomycosis: Microabscess

Cutaneous Blastomycosis: H&E

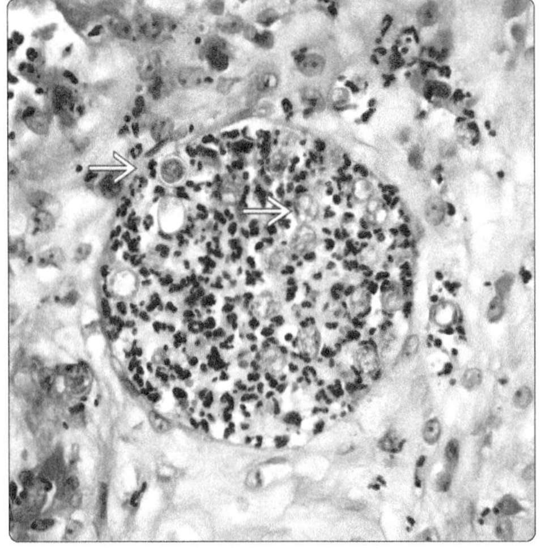

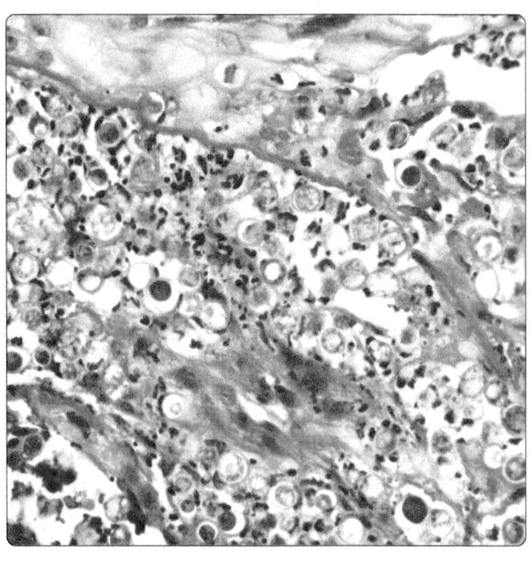

(Left) *Higher magnification (60x) reveals large yeast forms visible by H&E within microabscesses, many with thick, refractile double contour cell walls* →. **(Right)** *Sheets of large yeast forms (8-15 μm) with retractile double contour cell walls are highlighted on this H&E-stained skin biopsy section.*

Cutaneous Blastomycosis: PAS-D

Cutaneous Blastomycosis: GMS

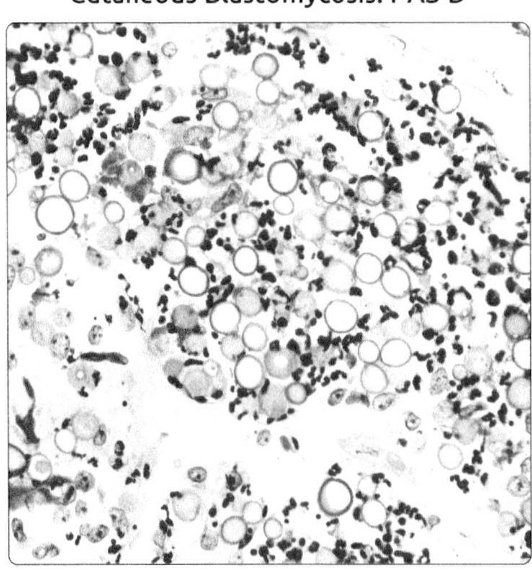

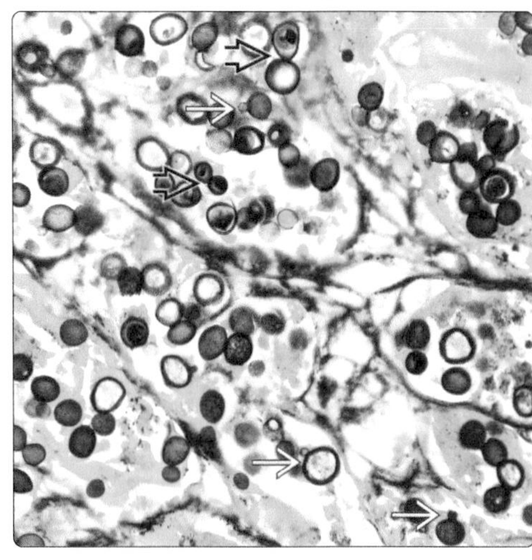

(Left) *Staining of this skin biopsy section with PAS-D highlights numerous yeast forms of Blastomyces dermatitidis.* **(Right)** *Staining of this skin biopsy section with GMS highlights numerous large yeast forms of B. dermatitidis. Multiple examples of early* → *and late* ⇨ *budding are shown.*

Blastomycosis Geographic Distribution

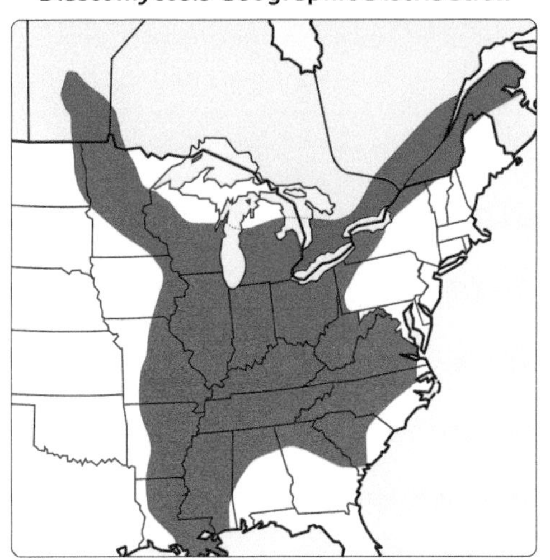

Lactophenol Blue: Hyphae and Conidiophores

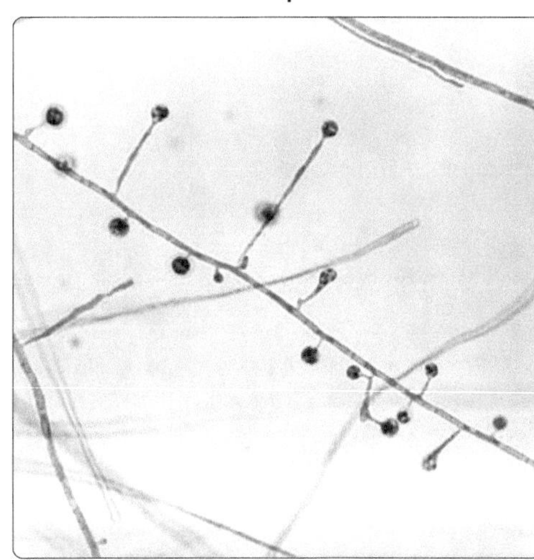

(Left) *The geographic distribution of blastomycosis in the Eastern USA is shown. Blastomycosis, paracoccidioidomycosis, and coccidioidomycosis are New World fungal infections. (Courtesy CDC/PHIL.)* **(Right)** *Lactophenol cotton blue staining of culture isolate shows conidiophores sprouting perpendicularly from the filamentous hyphae, each topped by a spherical-shaped conidium. (Courtesy L. Ajello, PhD, CDC/PHIL.)*

Blastomycosis: Nasal Mass

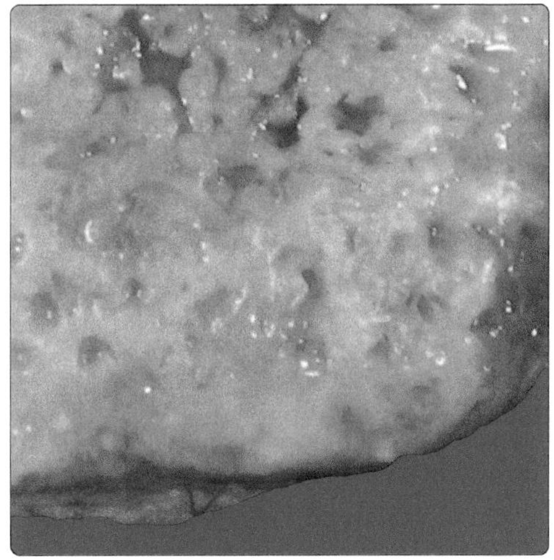

Blastomycosis: Nasal Mass Histology

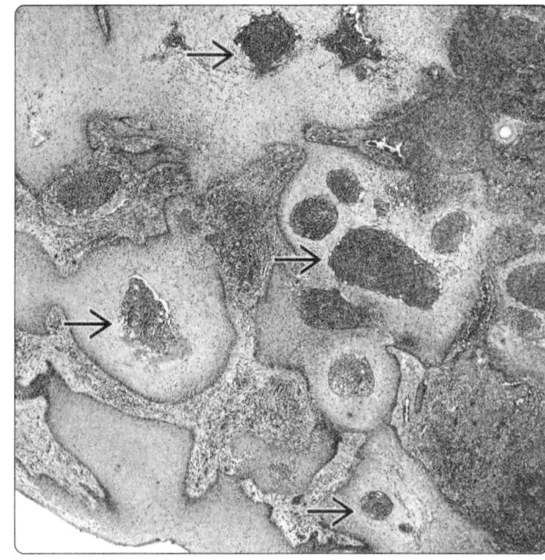

(Left) *Gross photograph shows a cross section of a nasal mass with pseudoepitheliomatous hyperplasia on microscopic examination. Culture confirms presence of blastomycosis.* **(Right)** *Low magnification of a nasal mass on H&E stain shows massive pseudoepitheliomatous hyperplasia mimicking squamous cell carcinoma. Multifocal microabscesses ➔ are noted. The presence of Blastomyces spp. associated with the microabscesses was revealed by higher magnification, follow-up GMS stain, and culture findings.*

Disseminated Blastomycosis: Spleen

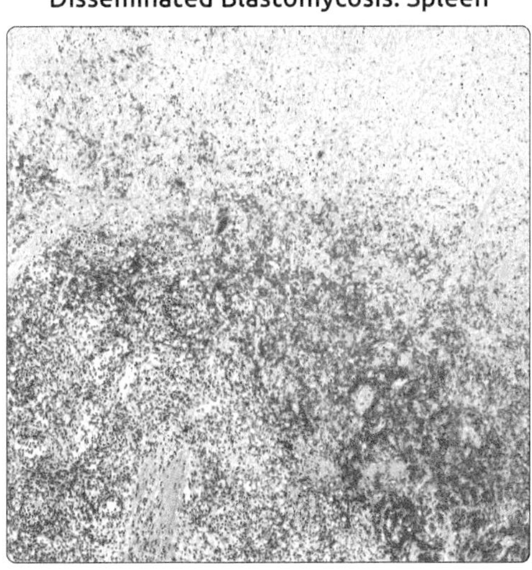

Disseminated Blastomycosis: Brain

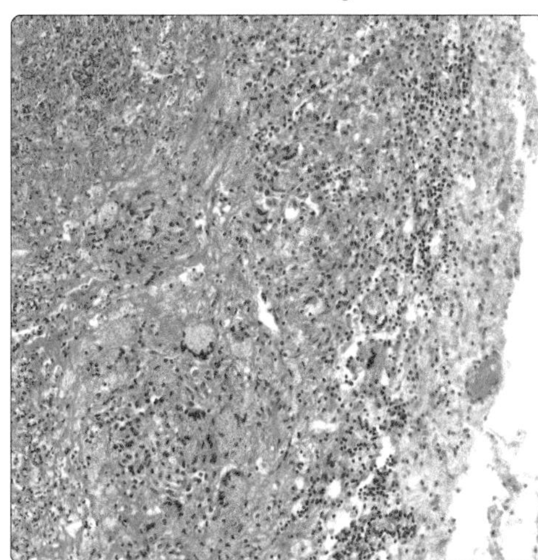

(Left) *Tissue section of autopsy spleen from a patient with disseminated blastomycosis shows destruction of normal parenchymal architecture. Visualization of organisms often requires GMS or PAS-D staining.* **(Right)** *Section of an autopsied brain from a fatal case of disseminated blastomycosis shows diffuse inflammatory infiltrates and necrosis involving brain parenchyma.*

Candidiasis

KEY FACTS

ETIOLOGY/PATHOGENESIS

- Commensal organisms associated with skin and gastrointestinal and genitourinary tracts of humans
- > 20 different species associated with disease, including *Candida albicans*, *Nakaseomyces glabratus* (previously *C. glabrata*), *C. parapsilosis*, *C. tropicalis*, *Pichia kudriavzevii* (previously *C. krusei*), *C. dubliniensis*, and *C. auris*
- Yeast form associated with dissemination; hyphal form associated with adhesion and tissue invasion

CLINICAL ISSUES

- Diseases range from superficial, invasive, to disseminated infections, depending on host immune status
- Treated with amphotericin B, azoles, and echinocandins
- (1,3)-β-D-glucan elevated in candidemia/dissemination
- Most species grow within 3-5 days; MALDI-TOF MS increasingly used for identification

MICROSCOPIC

- Gram-positive yeast (2-6 μm in diameter), pseudohyphae, and septate hyphae highlighted by PAS-D and GMS stains
- Suppurative inflammation and necrosis is often seen, but inflammation can be minimal; giant cells and granulomas are sparse

TOP DIFFERENTIAL DIAGNOSES

- Aspergillosis: Septate hyphae; positive galactomannan
- Trichosporonosis: Yeast-like cells (3-8 μm), pseudohyphae, hyphae with arthroconidia
- Histoplasmosis: Frequently intracellular yeast (2-4 μm), narrow-based budding, granulomatous inflammation
- Cryptococcosis: Yeast (4-10 μm), narrow-based budding, Fontana-Masson and mucicarmine positive
- Sporotrichosis: Yeast (2-6 μm), narrow-based or tube-like budding; Splendore-Hoeppli phenomena common
- *Saccharomyces* spp. infection: Gram-positive budding yeast, short pseudohyphae

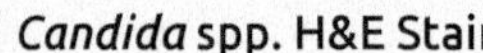

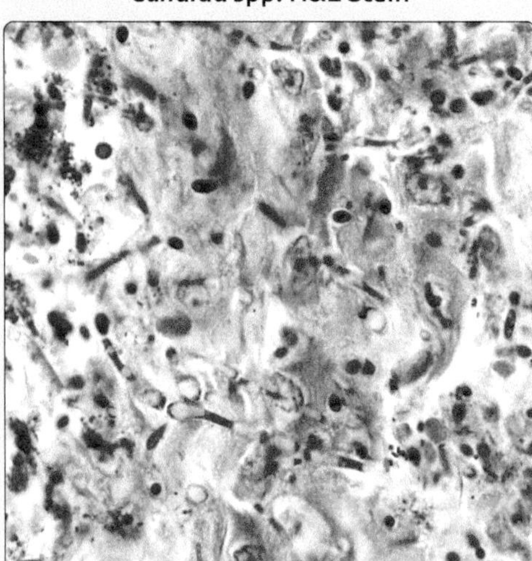

***Candida albicans* Lactophenol Cotton Blue**

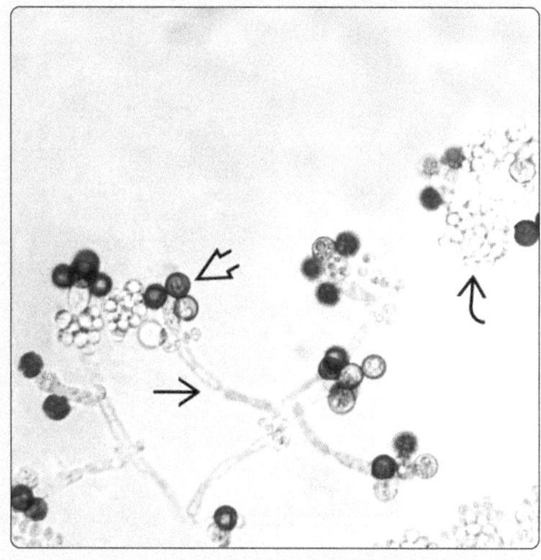

(Left) *H&E section of esophageal mucosa shows abundant Candida yeast forms and hyphal/pseudohyphal forms, diagnostic of Candida esophagitis.* **(Right)** *This lactophenol cotton blue-stained slide from a Candida albicans culture isolate shows pseudohyphae ➡, chlamydospores ➡, and blastospores ➡. (Courtesy G. Roberstad, CDC/PHIL.)*

***Candida* spp. GMS Stain**

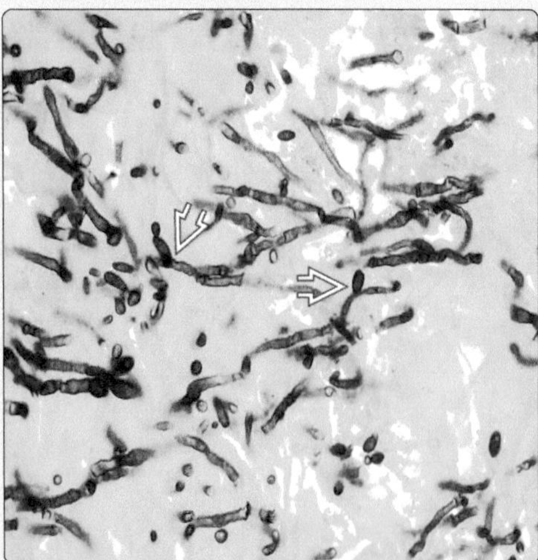

***Candida* spp. Gram Stain**

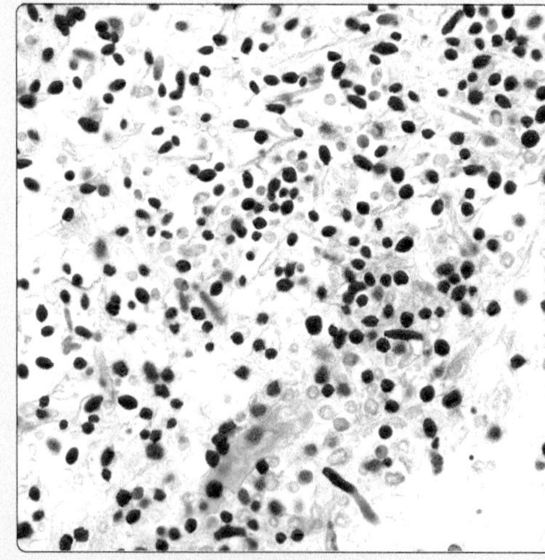

(Left) *GMS stain of esophageal mucosa shows numerous yeast forms, pseudohyphae, and true hyphae with septa, consistent with Candida. Germinating Candida blastospores ➡ can appear to be branching.* **(Right)** *Gram stain of a skin lesion highlights Candida spp. yeast forms and occasional pseudohyphae but is negative in true hyphae.*

TERMINOLOGY

Definitions

- Derived from Latin: "Candidatus" (candidate for public office, who dressed in white)

ETIOLOGY/PATHOGENESIS

Infectious Agents

- Infection with *Candida* spp., normal flora associated with skin and gastrointestinal and genitourinary tracts of humans
- Superficial infections occur when there are microbial imbalances caused by fluctuations in reproductive hormones, antibiotic use, and immunosuppression
- Invasive infections can involve any organ with various inflammatory responses depending on host immune status
- > 20 different species reported as etiologic agents of invasive candidiasis in humans; genus is highly polyphyletic, and several taxonomic rearrangements have recently occurred
- *Candida albicans* is most common (up to 2/3 of invasive cases) followed by *Nakaseomyces glabratus* (previously *C. glabrata*), *C. parapsilosis*, *C. tropicalis*, *Pichia kudriavzevii* (previously *C. krusei*)
- *C. dubliniensis* infection associated with HIV-positive patients
- *C. auris* is emerging multidrug-resistant species associated with outbreaks in healthcare facilities

CLINICAL ISSUES

Epidemiology

- Ubiquitous organisms with global distribution
- Global incidence rate of 2-14 cases per 100,000 persons; most common cause of fungal infection
- Common in ICU, cancer, and transplant populations

Presentation

- Superficial skin infections: Commonly seen in immunosuppressed patients
- Oropharyngeal candidiasis (thrush): White plaques on buccal mucosa; commonly seen in patients with immunodeficiency
- Esophagitis: Most common in HIV-infected patients and patients with hematologic malignancies
- Vulvovaginitis: Most common form of mucosal candidiasis
- Mastitis: Lactating women with injured nipples are at increased risk
- Invasive candidiasis: Often health care associated; risk factors include broad-spectrum antibiotics, immunosuppressants, malignancy, neutropenia, total parenteral nutrition, vascular access devices (biofilm formation)
  - *C. albicans* most common species isolate from blood
  - *C. parapsilosis* associated with hyperalimentation and indwelling devices in neonates
- Urinary tract infections: Often secondary to hematogenous seeding in setting of disseminated candidiasis
  - Candiduria may represent colonization and not infection; microscopic, culture, and clinical correlation needed to determine clinical relevance and need for antifungals
- Osteoarticular infections: Hematogenous seeding in cases of candidemia; inoculation during trauma, intraarticular injection, surgical procedures, or intravenous drug use
- Meningitis: Manifestation of disseminated candidiasis or in premature neonates as complication of contaminated ventricular drainage devices
- Endocarditis: Most common cause of fungal endocarditis; seen in intravenous drug users or patients with prosthetic heart valves, indwelling central venous catheters, or fungemia
- Peritonitis and intraabdominal infections: Often exists in polymicrobial infections that occur following gastrointestinal tract perforation or acute necrotizing pancreatitis
- Pneumonia: Rare
- Empyema: Most common in patients with malignancies
- Pericarditis: Rare; often complication of thoracic surgery, contiguous spread from adjacent focus, or hematogenous spread
- Endophthalmitis: Develops following trauma or eye surgery; hematogenous seeding in cases of candidemia
- Chronic disseminated candidiasis: Persistent microabscesses in liver, spleen, and, occasionally, kidneys; risk factors include acute leukemia, neutropenia, intravascular catheters
- Chronic mucocutaneous candidiasis: Heterogeneous group of syndromes with autoimmune manifestations associated with chronic noninvasive *Candida* infections of skin, nails, and mucous membranes

Laboratory Tests

- KOH preparation on skin scrapings to evaluate for hyphae and pseudohyphae
- (1,3)-β-D-glucan in serum (or CSF)
  - Marker of fungemia or disseminated disease
  - Useful in patients with deep-seated invasive candidiasis for which blood cultures may be insensitive
  - Sensitivity: 57-90%; specificity: 44-92%
- Direct PCR using blood samples has better sensitivity/specificity for invasive candidiasis than culture

Treatment

- Different species have slightly different intrinsic susceptibilities to antifungal agents
- Multidrug-resistance noted in *C. auris*, *N. glabratus*, and *P. kudriavzevii*
- Mucocutaneous infections: Therapy dominated by azoles
- Invasive infections: Amphotericin B-based preparations, azoles, and echinocandin antifungal agents

Prognosis

- Successful treatment depends on site of lesion and immune status of host
- Invasive candidiasis mortality as high as 50%

MICROBIOLOGY

Culture and Speciation

- White to cream-colored smooth, glabrous colonies that mature in 3-5 days
- Species identified according to macroscopic colony morphology on agar and microscopic morphology on specific medium

- Differential chromogenic agars can be used for species-level identification
- Microscopic morphology on cornmeal-Tween 80 agar
  - Distinguishing characteristics include formation of terminal chlamydospores, pseudohyphae, true hyphae, and clusters of round blastoconidia (blastospores)
  - Pseudohyphae formation: *C. albicans, C. dubliniensis, C. parapsilosis, C. tropicalis*
  - No pseudohyphae formation: *C. auris, N. glabratus, C. haemuloni*
  - Germ tube test: Positive in *C. albicans, C. dubliniensis*
- Matrix-assisted laser desorption/ionization time-of-flight (MALDI-TOF) mass spectrometry increasingly incorporated into microbiology laboratory workflow
- Sequencing of D1/D2 region of 28S rRNA and internal transcribed spacer can confirm speciation of unusual isolates
- Peptide nucleic acid fluorescent in situ hybridization can identify most frequent *Candida* spp. directly from positive blood culture bottles without need for subcultures
- *C. auris* may be misidentified using many conventional phenotypic and biochemical methods

MICROSCOPIC

Histologic Features

- Round to oval yeast cells (2-6 μm in diameter) with narrow-based multilateral budding; size varies according to species
- In many species, intermixed with pseudohyphae (filamentous forms) and occasionally true hyphae
- *N. glabratus* only forms small (2-4 μm in diameter) oval yeast cells; no pseudohyphae are formed
- Identification of tissue invasion (versus surface colonization) important
- Neutrophilic inflammation with some lymphocytes and macrophages, fibrin, and coagulative necrosis
- Giant cells and granulomas can be present but are sparse
- Mycotic aneurysms or thrombophlebitis can occur in cases of vascular invasions; necrotizing vasculitis described

Cytologic Features

- Superficial mucosal infections can be associated with enlarged hyperchromatic nuclei with perinuclear halos in gynecologic specimens or Pap smears
- Changes can be confused with low-grade squamous intraepithelial lesions

ANCILLARY TESTS

Histochemistry

- Gram stain: *Candida* spp. yeast stain purple/blue (gram positive)
- Fungal silver stains (methenamine silver stains): Fungal cell wall appears black or dark brown
- PAS: Fungal cell wall appears pink to red-purple

DIFFERENTIAL DIAGNOSIS

Aspergillosis

- Nonpigmented (hyaline), uniform, septate hyphae with dichotomous branching at 45° angles; may appear yeast-like in cross sections
- Confirm by presence of fruiting bodies (rare in tissue sections), culture, PCR, serum galactomannan

Trichosporonosis

- Pleomorphic gram-negative yeast-like cells (3-8 μm in diameter) intermingled with pseudohyphae, septate true hyphae without predominant dichotomous branching
- Distinguished by presence of arthroconidia (formed by fragmentation of true hyphae), which can be sparse or absent on tissue sections

Histoplasmosis

- Small frequently intracellular in macrophages gram-negative yeast forms (2-4 μm in diameter) with narrow-based budding, typically associated with granulomatous inflammation
- Confirm with culture, PCR, antigen testing

Cryptococcosis

- Narrow-based budding pleomorphic gram-negative yeast forms (4-10 μm in diameter) positive with Fontana-Masson stain with mucicarmine positive capsule

Sporotrichosis

- Round, oval, or cigar-shaped gram-negative yeasts (2-6 μm) with narrow-based or tube-like budding; no psuedohyphae, best visualized with PAS-D and GMS stains
- Splendore-Hoeppli phenomena (astroid bodies) common

Saccharomyces spp. Infection

- *Saccharomyces cerevisiae* ("baker's yeast") is typically commensal organism but can cause invasive infections, especially in immunocompromised
- Multilateral budding round to oval gram-positive yeast, short pseudohyphae, and ascospores; confirm by culture or PCR

SELECTED REFERENCES

1. Furuya K et al: A case of bloodstream co-infection of Saccharomyces cerevisiae and Candida glabrata while using micafungin. BMC Infect Dis. 23(1):329, 2023
2. Soriano A et al: Invasive candidiasis: current clinical challenges and unmet needs in adult populations. J Antimicrob Chemother. 78(7):1569-85, 2023
3. Takashima M et al: Taxonomy of pathogenic yeasts Candida, Cryptococcus, Malassezia, and Trichosporon. Med Mycol J. 63(4):119-32, 2022
4. Chavez JA et al: Practical diagnostic approach to the presence of hyphae in neuropathology specimens with three illustrative cases. Am J Clin Pathol. 149(2):98-104, 2018
5. Pappas PG et al: Invasive candidiasis. Nat Rev Dis Primers. 4:18026, 2018
6. Giuliano S et al: Candida endocarditis: systematic literature review from 1997 to 2014 and analysis of 29 cases from the Italian Study of Endocarditis. Expert Rev Anti Infect Ther. 15(9):807-18, 2017
7. Lockhart SR et al: Candida auris for the clinical microbiology laboratory: not your grandfather's Candida species. Clin Microbiol Newsl. 39(13):99-103, 2017
8. Westblade LF et al: Multicenter study evaluating the Vitek MS system for identification of medically important yeasts. J Clin Microbiol. 51(7):2267-72, 2013
9. Guarner J et al: Histopathologic diagnosis of fungal infections in the 21st century. Clin Microbiol Rev. 24(2):247-80, 2011
10. Lyon GM et al: Antifungal susceptibility testing of Candida isolates from the Candida surveillance study. J Clin Microbiol. 48(4):1270-5, 2010

Culture Isolate: *Candida auris*

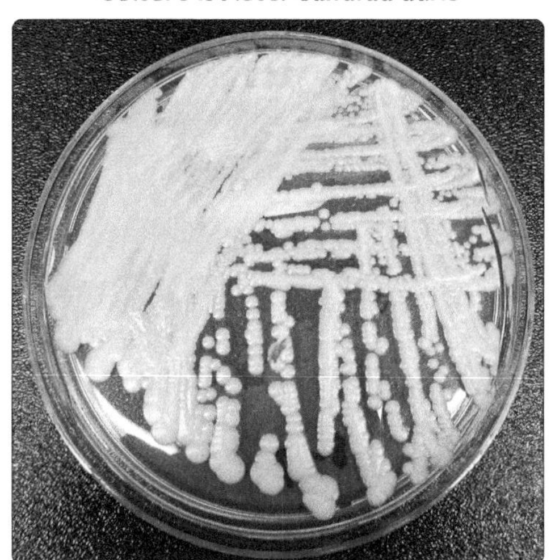

Candida albicans Germ Tubes

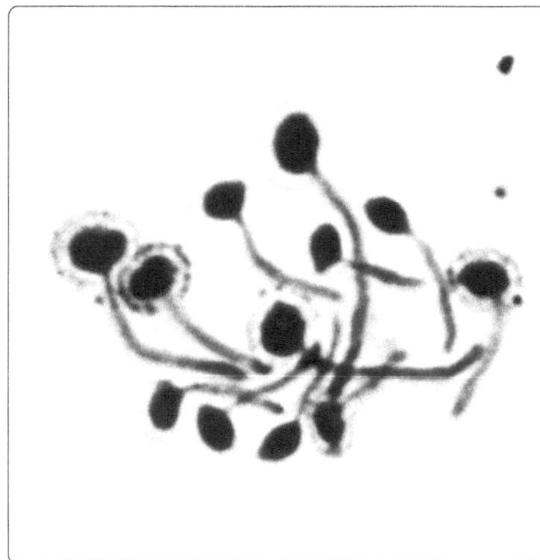

(Left) *Candida spp. typically grow as cream-colored smooth, glabrous colonies, such as this isolate of Candida auris, a multidrug-resistant species that can be difficult to diagnose by standard laboratory methods. (Courtesy S. Lockhart, PhD, CDC/PHIL.)* **(Right)** *Incubation of C. albicans or C. dubliniensis in animal serum results in growth of filamentous germ tubes (highlighted here by Gram stain), used to distinguish from other Candida spp., now largely supplanted by MALDI-TOF MS. (Courtesy Dr. L. Georg, CDC/PHIL.)*

Candida spp. Endocarditis

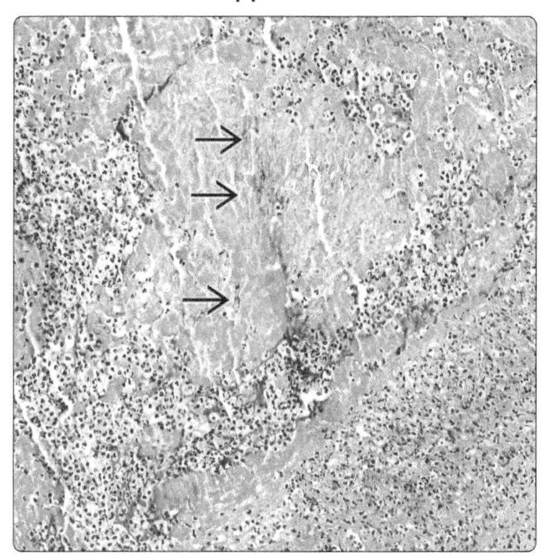

Candida spp. Brain Microabscess

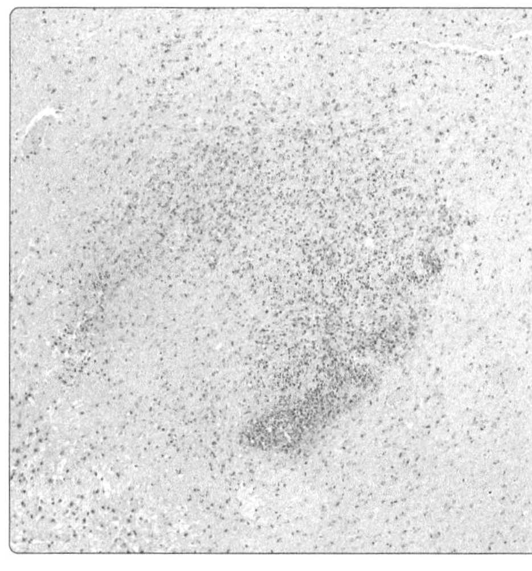

(Left) *This section of a tricuspid valve vegetation shows numerous hyphae/pseudohyphae ➙ in a case of fungal endocarditis.* **(Right)** *This autopsy brain section shows a Nakaseomyces glabratus (formerly Candida glabrata) microabscess resulting from a septic embolus from fungal prosthetic valve endocarditis.*

Candida spp. Deep Skin Infection

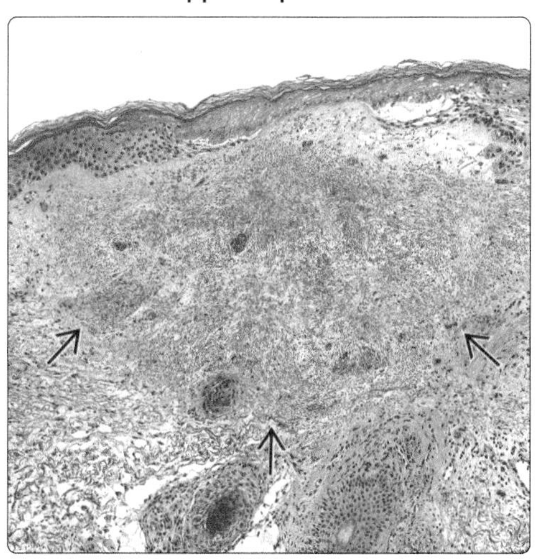

Vulvovaginal Candidiasis

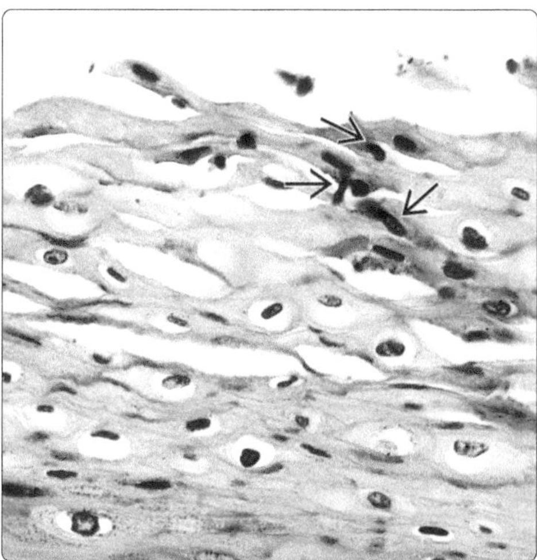

(Left) *This skin biopsy from a neutropenic patient with pink-red tender nodules shows a circumscribed collection ➙ of fugal yeast, hyphae, and pseudohyphae in the dermis, consistent with Candida spp. infection.* **(Right)** *PAS staining highlights occasional pseudohyphal and yeast forms, consistent with Candida spp., in vulvar epithelium ➙. Minimal inflammation is present.*

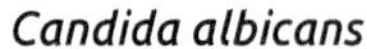

Candida albicans

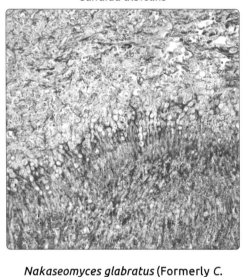

Candida albicans GMS Stain

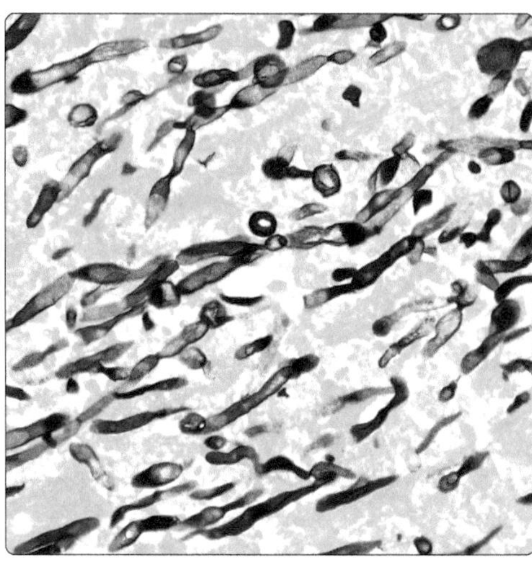

(Left) *This H&E-stained section of a C. albicans-infected valve vegetation shows a dense eosinophilic mass of fungal hyphae, pseudohyphae, and yeast forms that could be overlooked as thrombus.* **(Right)** *GMS staining of C. albicans endocarditis valve vegetation highlights numerous pseudohyphae.*

Nakaseomyces glabratus (Formerly *C. glabrata*)

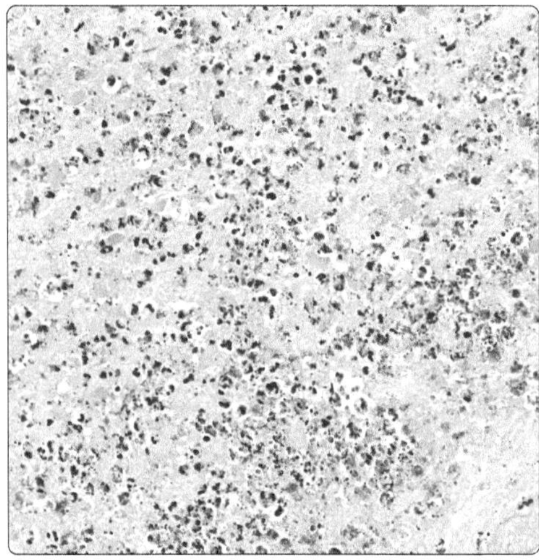

Nakaseomyces glabratus Gram Stain

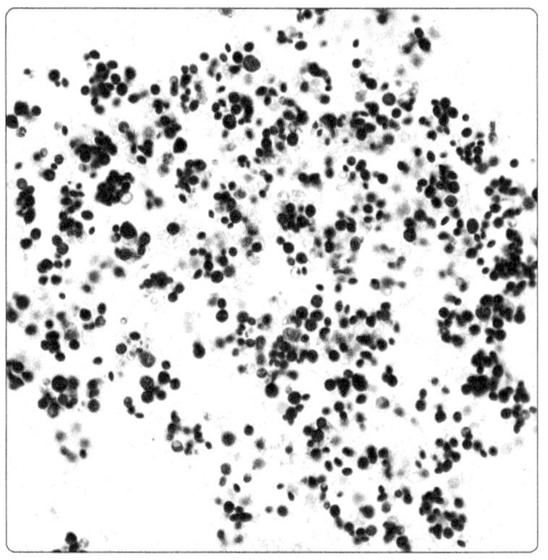

(Left) *This autopsy brain section shows necroinflammatory debris, consistent with a microasbcess secondary to septic embolus from fungal endocarditis due to Nakaseomyces glabratus (formerly Candida glabrata). Palely staining yeast forms may be inconspicuous on H&E sections.* **(Right)** *Gram stain of N. glabratus reveals small positively staining yeast forms without pseudohyphae.*

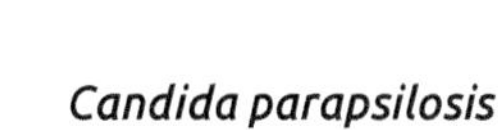

Candida parapsilosis

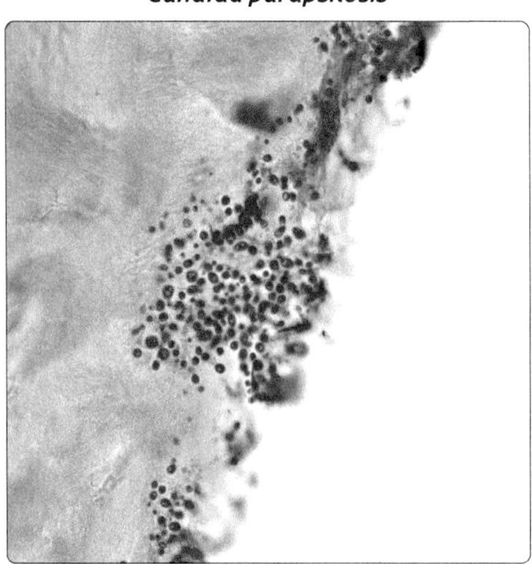

Candida parapsilosis Gram Stain

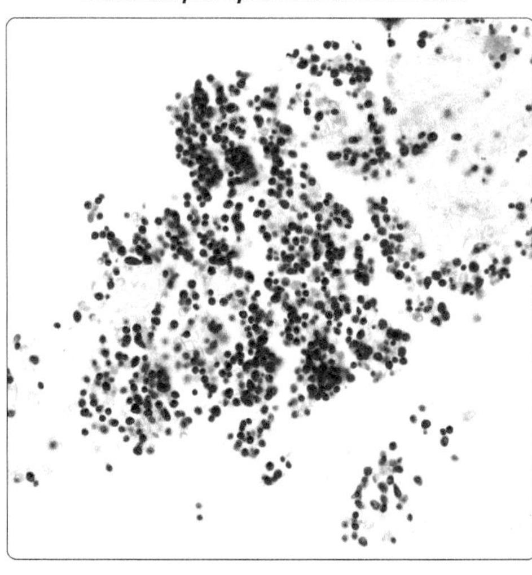

(Left) *H&E-stained section from a Candida parapsilosis wound infection due to foreign object shows a collection of small yeast infiltrating the edge of the tissue.* **(Right)** *Gram staining of C. parapsilosis wound infection shows small gram-positive yeast.*

Candida tropicalis

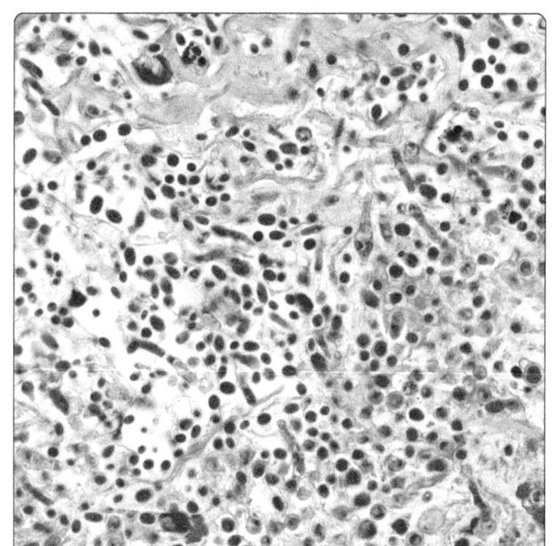

Candida tropicalis PAS-D Stain

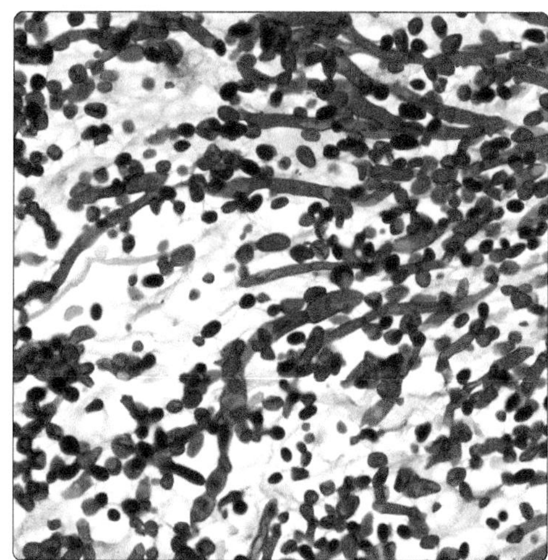

(Left) *This H&E-stained section from a Candida tropicalis skin infection shows a dense collection of hyphae, pseudohyphae, and yeast forms located within the dermis.* **(Right)** *PAS-D staining of C. tropicalis highlights filalmentous (pseudohyphae) and yeast forms.*

Pichia kudriavzevii (Formerly *Candida krusei*)

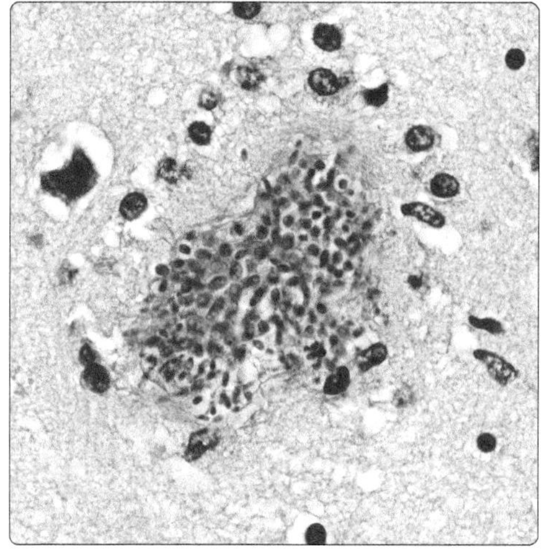

Pichia kudriavzevii Gram Stain

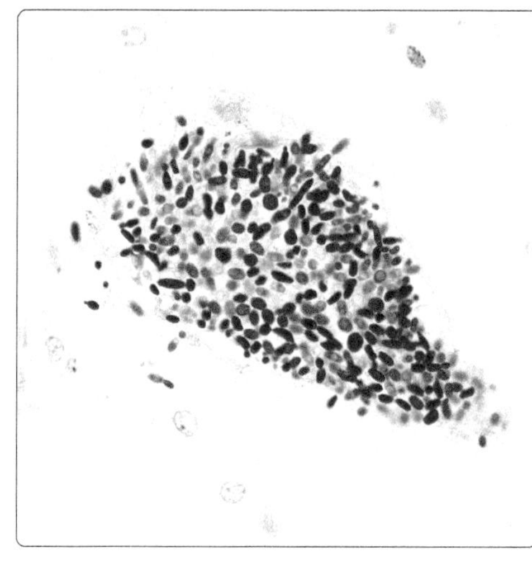

(Left) *Pichia kudriavzevii (formerly Candida krusei) is present intravascularly as yeast and pseudohyphae in the brain of a patient who died of septic shock.* **(Right)** *Gram staining of Pichia kudriavzevii (formerly C. krusei) highlights small yeast and pseudohyphae focally infiltrating outside the blood vessel lumen.*

Candida dubliniensis

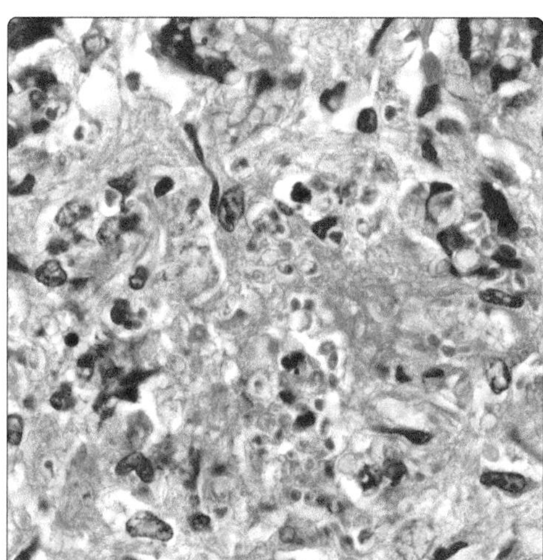

Candida dubliniensis GMS Stain

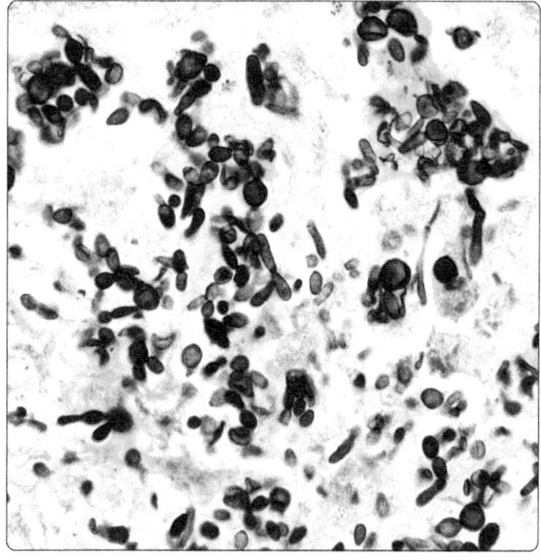

(Left) *This H&E-stained brain section shows pale, eosinophilic-appearing yeast and pseudohyphae of C. dubliniensis in a neutropenic patient.* **(Right)** *GMS staining highlights small to medium-sized yeast and pseudopyphae of C. dubliniensis.*

KEY FACTS

ETIOLOGY/PATHOGENESIS

- Dematiaceous fungi that cause skin and subcutaneous infection via traumatic inoculation
- Common causes include *Fonsecaea pedrosoi*, *Cladophialophora carrionii*, and *Phialophora verrucosa*

CLINICAL ISSUES

- Occurs worldwide, but most cases are reported in tropical and subtropical areas of Americas, Asia, and Africa
- Most common sites are distal limbs; mostly confined to skin and subcutaneous fat and does not invade into underlying muscle or bone

MICROBIOLOGY

- May be grown in standard fungal media (Sabouraud dextrose agar), but histopathology adequate for diagnosis

MACROSCOPIC

- Characteristic "black dots" can form in skin lesion due to migration of fungi to skin surface and keratin scales

MICROSCOPIC

- Brown, thick-walled Medlar bodies (5-12 μm in diameter) with horizontal &/or vertical septations
- Associated with granulomatous inflammation, accompanied by suppurative reaction and pseudoepitheliomatous hyperplasia
- Fungi positive for GMS, PAS, and Fontana-Masson stains

TOP DIFFERENTIAL DIAGNOSES

- Phaeohyphomycosis: Skin/subcutaneous infection with brown-pigmented septate hyphae and large vesicular swellings, sometimes admixed with yeast-like cells
- Blastomycosis: Large nonpigmented yeast forms with broad-based budding
- Coccidioidomycosis: Large nonpigmented spherules with endospores
- Hemosiderosis: Macrophages with round iron collections
- Foreign body: Fragments of wood or plant matter with pigment and morphology reminiscent of yeast

Chromoblastomycosis Skin Lesion

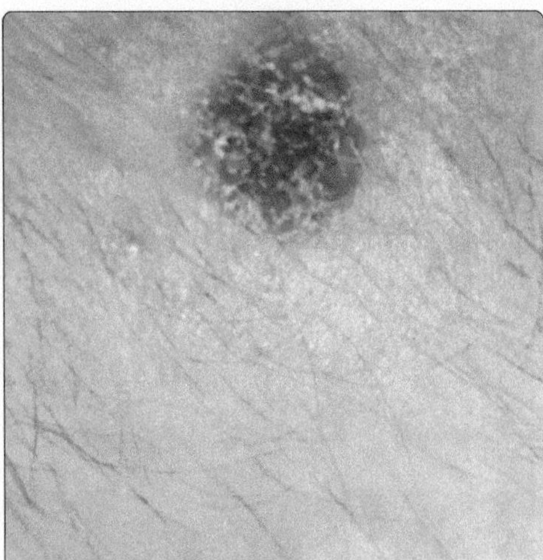

"Copper Pennies"

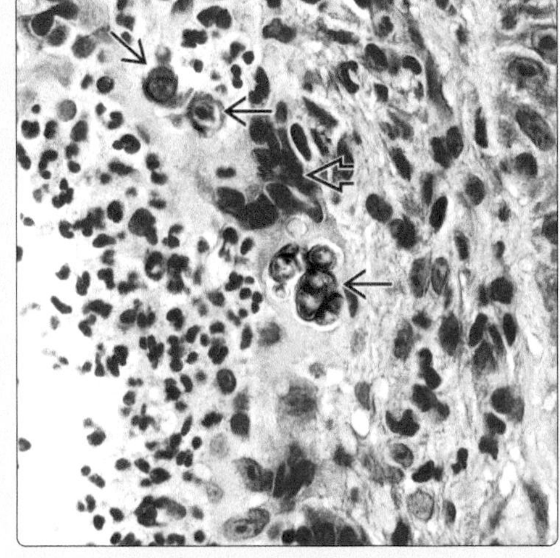

(Left) *This verrucous plaque was determined to be caused by chromoblastomycosis. (Courtesy L. Georg, CDC/PHIL.)* **(Right)** *High-power H&E of skin shows thick-walled, brown sclerotic bodies → in association with microabscess and a multinucleated giant cell ⇒, consistent with chromoblastomycosis.*

Medlar Bodies in Suppurative Granuloma

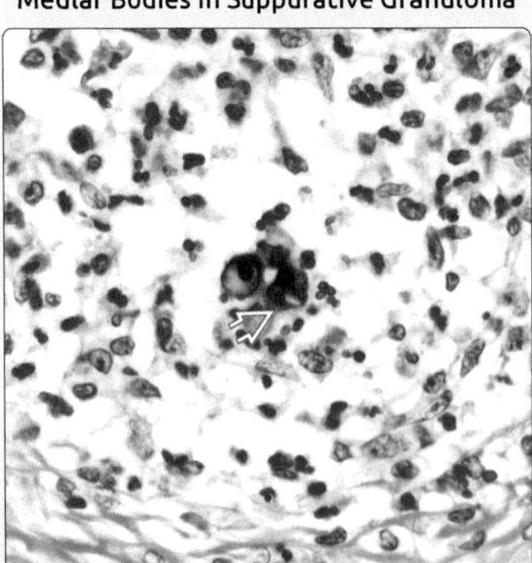

Pigmented Forms

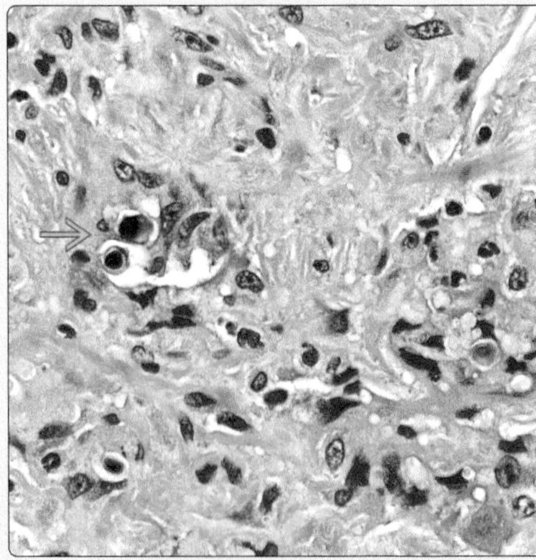

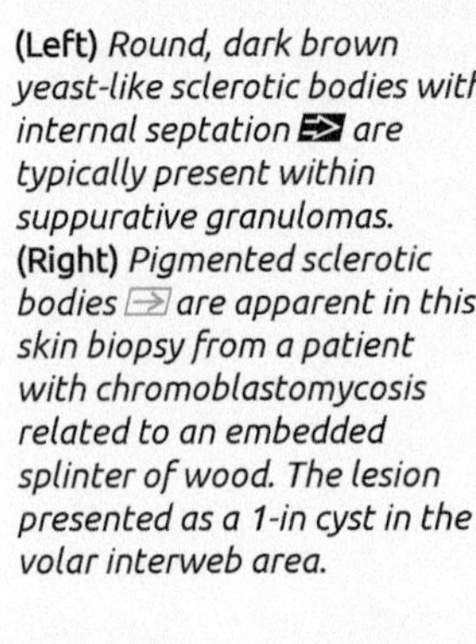

(Left) *Round, dark brown yeast-like sclerotic bodies with internal septation ➡ are typically present within suppurative granulomas.* **(Right)** *Pigmented sclerotic bodies ⇒ are apparent in this skin biopsy from a patient with chromoblastomycosis related to an embedded splinter of wood. The lesion presented as a 1-in cyst in the volar interweb area.*

TERMINOLOGY

Synonyms

- Chromomycosis

Definitions

- Greek: "Khroma" (color) + "blastos" (sprout, germ) + "mykes" (fungus, mushroom)

ETIOLOGY/PATHOGENESIS

Infectious Agents

- Dematiaceous (melanized or brown pigment-producing) fungi that cause skin and subcutaneous infection via traumatic inoculation through contact with wood, soil, plants, or water
- Common causes include *Fonsecaea pedrosoi*, *Cladophialophora carrionii*, and *Phialophora verrucosa*
- Less common agents include *Fonsecaea compacta*, *Rhinocladiella aquaspersa*, *Exophiala dermatitidis*, and *Exophiala jeanselmei* complex

CLINICAL ISSUES

Epidemiology

- Occurs worldwide but most cases are found in tropical and subtropical areas of Americas, Asia, and Africa; species vary by region and climate
    - *F. pedrosoi* is associated with humid areas with tropical and subtropical climate and causes most cases in Brazil, Mexico, northern Madagascar, and Japan
    - *C. carrionii* is associated with semiarid climate and causes most cases in Australia, southern Madagascar, South Africa, and Cuba
- In tropical and subtropical countries, infection more commonly affects male agricultural workers in rural regions, possibly due to increased chance of injury with plant matter

Presentation

- Most common sites of infection are distal limbs, especially feet; other sites have also been reported, including cornea, face, and trunk
- Primary lesion is verrucous papule or nodule, which can grow or proliferate to form verrucous plaques upon coalescence
- Infection mostly confined to skin (including subcutis) and does not invade into underlying muscle or bone
- Dissemination may occur via scratching autoinoculation, resulting in satellite lesions from fungal spread through lymphatic system
- Possible complications (some controversial due to potential misdiagnosis as chromoblastomycosis rather than phaeohyphomycosis): Secondary bacterial infections and ulcerations, lymphedema and elephantiasis, squamous cell carcinoma, dissemination to lung and brain

Laboratory Tests

- Serologic tests have been developed to detect *F. pedrosoi* and *C. carrionii*; sensitivities range from 78-100% and specificities range from 83-99%
- Pan-fungal PCR targeting ITS regions can speciate agents from both fresh and formalin-fixed, paraffin-embedded specimens

Treatment

- Treatment depends on etiologic agent, clinical presentation, and complications
- Common antifungal drugs include itraconazole and terbinafine; emerging use of posaconazole
- *F. pedrosoi* is less sensitive to antifungal therapy than *C. carrionii* or *P. verrucosa*
- Cryosurgery and thermotherapy to eradicate skin lesions
- Combination of laser vaporization and thermotherapy for relapses
- Excisional surgery for small lesions with antifungal therapy

Prognosis

- Morality rare, but low cure rates and high relapse rates, especially in chronic and extensive disease

MICROBIOLOGY

Culture

- Routine fungal cultures (Sabouraud dextrose agar)
- Fungal species are slow growing and require > 2 weeks to mature

MACROSCOPIC

General Features

- Characteristic "black dots" can form in skin lesion due to migration of fungi to skin surface and keratin scales (highest yield for diagnosis)

MICROSCOPIC

Histologic Features

- Characteristic pigmented, round to polyhedral thick-walled sclerotic bodies (5-12 μm in diameter) with horizontal &/or vertical internal septations, known as Medlar bodies, muriform cells, sclerotic bodies, or "copper pennies"
- Pseudoepitheliomatous hyperplasia with granulomatous inflammation and neutrophilic microabscesses are characteristic and frequently observed

ANCILLARY TESTS

Histochemistry

- GMS, PAS, and Fontana-Masson stains highlight fungal forms but are rarely performed due to visualization of intrinsically pigmented fungi
- Determination of pigment should be made on H&E-stained slides, since Fontana-Masson reaction will highlight many nonpigmented fungi

Direct Examination of Clinical Specimens

- Skin scrapings from lesion can be treated with 10% potassium hydroxide for direct microscopy and visualization of brown Medlar bodies

DIFFERENTIAL DIAGNOSIS

Phaeohyphomycosis

- Skin or subcutaneous infection caused by brown-pigmented hyphae with constricted septations and large vesicular swellings, sometimes admixed with yeast-like cells; Medlar bodies are absent

- Encapsulated cystic granulomatous reaction associated with suppurative exudate present in dermis and subcutaneous tissue; epidermis is often spared
- Common genera: *Bipolaris*, *Cladophialophora*, *Coniothyrium*, *Curvularia*, *Exophiala*, *Exserohilum*, *Lasiodiplodia*, *Phialophora*, *Ochroconis*, and *Wangiella*

Blastomycosis

- Large yeast forms with broad-based budding; distinguished by lack of pigmentation in yeast forms, although can be Fontana-Masson positive

Coccidioidomycosis

- Distinguished by lack of pigmentation in yeast forms and may have large spherules with endospores, which can be Fontana-Masson positive

Hemosiderosis

- Excessive iron in macrophages may produce round to oval collections mimicking pigmented yeast

Foreign Body

- Fragments of wood or plant matter may have pigment and morphology suggestive of yeast and produce similar lesions after traumatic introduction

SELECTED REFERENCES

1. Baka JLCES et al: Urban chromoblastomycosis: a diagnosis that should not be neglected. An Bras Dermatol. 98(3):422-5, 2023
2. Gajurel K et al: Medlar bodies of chromoblastomycosis. Transpl Infect Dis. e14047, 2023
3. Seas C et al: Mycetoma, chromoblastomycosis and other deep fungal infections: diagnostic and treatment approach. Curr Opin Infect Dis. 35(5):379-83, 2022
4. Guevara A et al: Chromoblastomycosis in Latin America and the Caribbean: epidemiology over the past 50 years. Med Mycol. 60(1), 2021
5. Passero LFD et al: Reviewing the etiologic agents, microbe-host relationship, immune response, diagnosis, and treatment in chromoblastomycosis. J Immunol Res. 2021:9742832, 2021
6. Santos DWCL et al: The global burden of chromoblastomycosis. PLoS Negl Trop Dis. 15(8):e0009611, 2021
7. da Silva Hellwig AH et al: In vitro susceptibility of chromoblastomycosis agents to antifungal drugs: a systematic review. J Glob Antimicrob Resist. 16:108-14, 2018
8. Queiroz-Telles F et al: Chromoblastomycosis. Clin Microbiol Rev. 30(1):233-76, 2017

Severe Chromoblastomycosis

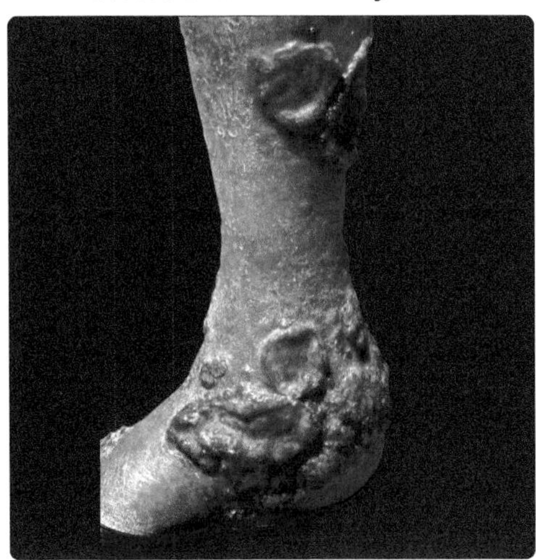

Chromoblastomycosis: GMS Stain

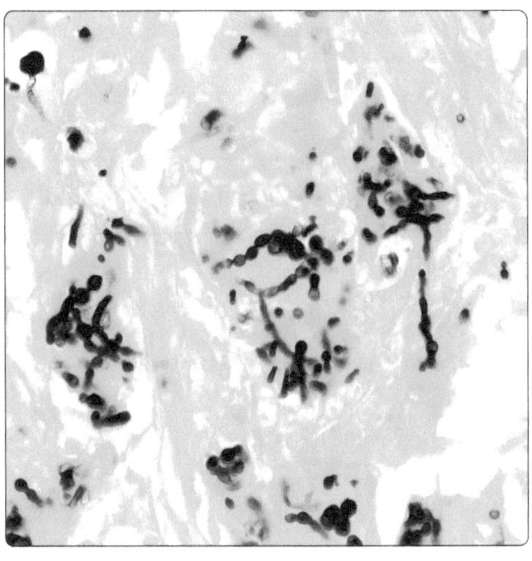

(Left) *This image depicts numerous, rough textured cutaneous nodules, dry, scaly skin, and marked swelling due to chromoblastomycosis of the foot, ankle, and lower right extremity. (Courtesy L. Georg, CDC/PHIL.)* **(Right)** *GMS stain of this specimen from a volar cyst demonstrates multiple chains of conidia. ITS sequencing from FFPE tissue indicated the causative agent to be either Rhinocladiella or Exophiala spp., known agents of chromoblastomycosis.*

F. pedrosoi **Lactophenol Cotton Blue**

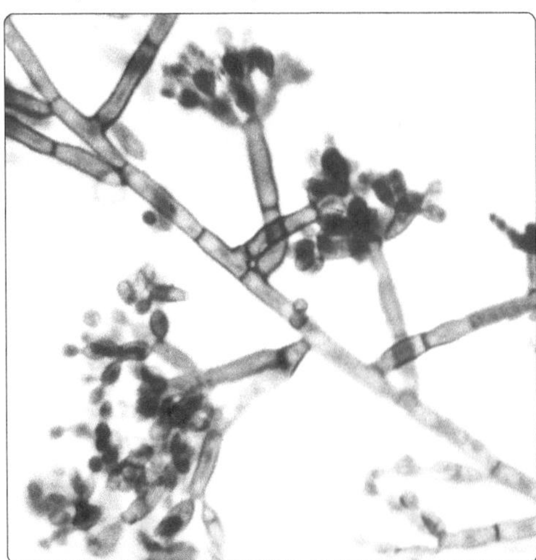

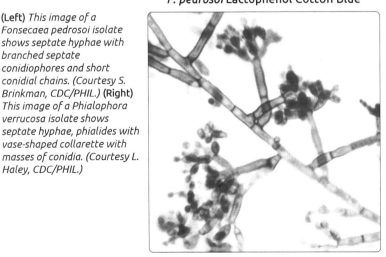

P. verrucosa **Lactophenol Cotton Blue**

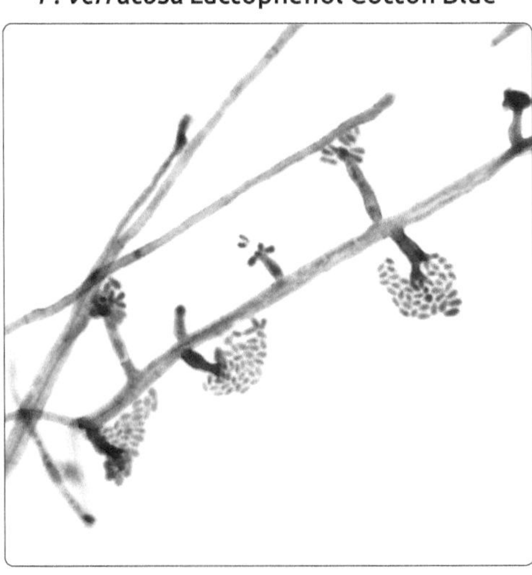

(Left) *This image of a Fonsecaea pedrosoi isolate shows septate hyphae with branched septate conidiophores and short conidial chains. (Courtesy S. Brinkman, CDC/PHIL.)* **(Right)** *This image of a Phialophora verrucosa isolate shows septate hyphae, phialides with vase-shaped collarette with masses of conidia. (Courtesy L. Haley, CDC/PHIL.)*

Pseudoepitheliomatous Hyperplasia

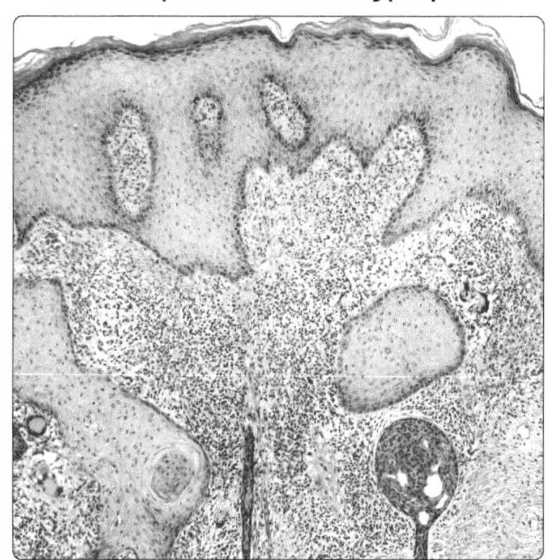

Pigmented Fungus

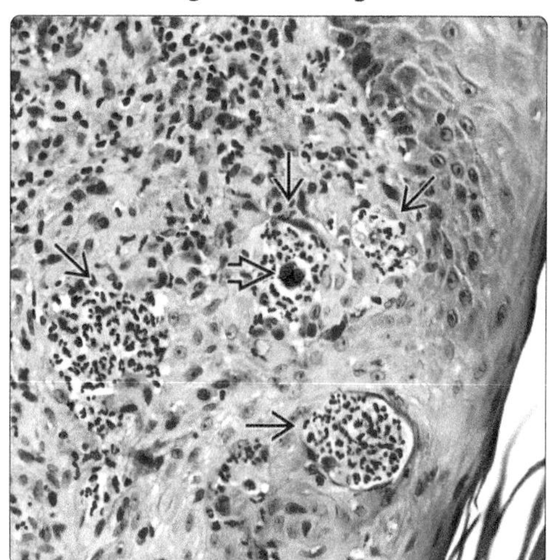

(Left) *Pseudoepitheliomatous hyperplasia and focal granulomatous reaction are characteristic of chromoblastomycosis.* **(Right)** *High-power H&E of the skin shows multifocal microabscesses ⇒ in the epidermis and dermis. Medlar bodies ⇒ are readily identified. These findings are diagnostic of chromoblastomycosis.*

Chromoblastomycosis: PAS Stain

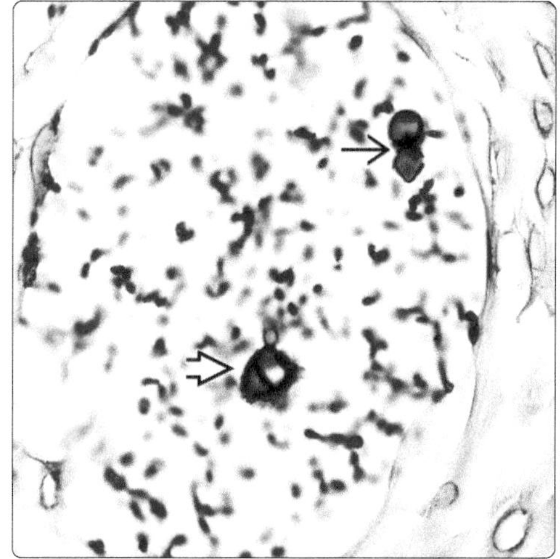

Chromoblastomycosis: GMS Stain

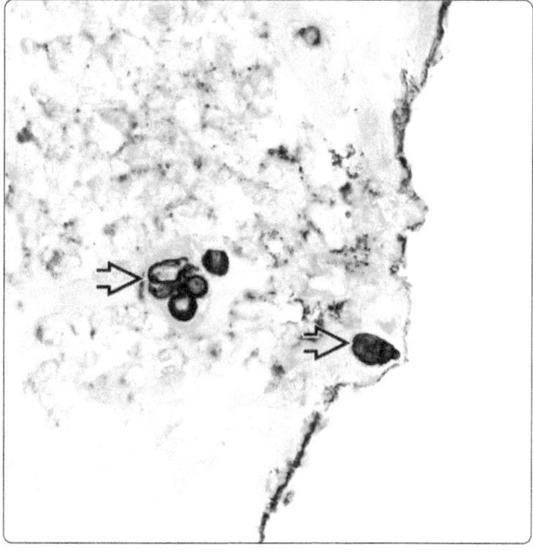

(Left) *High-power PAS of the skin highlights a characteristic thick-walled sclerotic body ⇒ with septation in a patient with chromoblastomycosis. The other fungal form ⇒ may represent a short segment of septate hyphae or daughter cells that are undergoing binary fission.* **(Right)** *High-power GMS of the skin shows thick-walled sclerotic bodies ⇒ with septations, consistent with chromoblastomycosis.*

Differential Diagnosis: Pheohyphomycotic Cyst

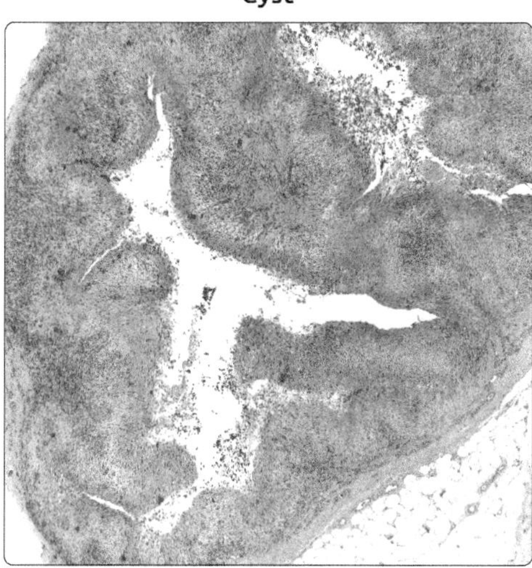

Differential Diagnosis: Pigmented Hyphae of Pheohyphomycosis

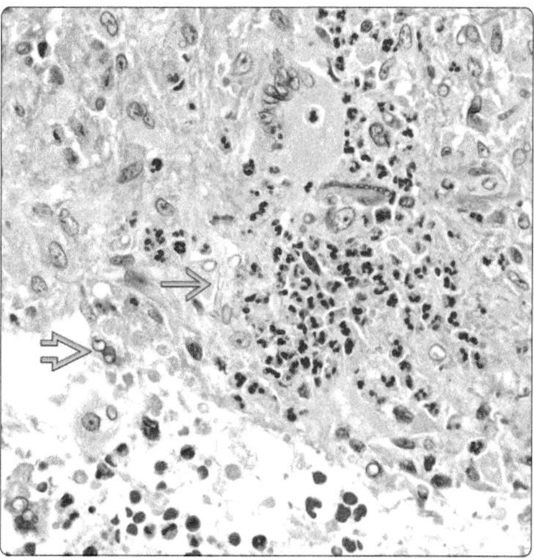

(Left) *This section shows a cavitated subcutaneous cyst typical of pheohyphomycotic cyst.* **(Right)** *Suppurative granulomatous inflammation with pigmented hyphae ⇒ and yeast-like cells ⇒ are readily noted upon closer inspection of a pheohyphomycotic cyst wall. The presence of hyphae defines pheohyphomycosis, which also lacks Medlar bodies of chromoblastomycosis.*

Coccidioidomycosis

KEY FACTS

ETIOLOGY/PATHOGENESIS

- Caused by dimorphic fungi, *Coccidioides immitis* and *Coccidioides posadasii*
- Found in soil in southwestern USA and parts of Mexico and Central and South America
- At body temperature, spores develop into endospore-containing spherules, which enlarge and rupture

CLINICAL ISSUES

- Incidence (USA): 8,232-22,634 reported cases/year
- Primary pulmonary disease is often self-limiting
- Symptomatic persons present after 1-3 weeks with fatigue, cough, dyspnea, headache, night sweats, myalgias, and rash
- Disseminated disease is rare, affecting musculoskeletal, soft tissues, and meninges in immunocompromised
- Treated with oral azoles or amphotericin B

MICROBIOLOGY

- Hyphae are thin and septate with 5- to 8-μm arthroconidia
- High risk for inhalation exposure for laboratory personnel

MICROSCOPIC

- Necrotizing granulomatous inflammation with large, thick-walled spherules (100 μm, containing endospores up to 5 μm)
- Surrounding infiltrate is often rich in chronic inflammatory cells, eosinophils, neutrophils, and giant cell reactions
- Pseudoepitheliomatous hyperplasia and granulomatous dermal inflammation are common in cutaneous disease
- GMS stains highlight spherules, endospores, and hyphae (if present)
- Endospores are PAS positive, but larger/mature spherules are negative

TOP DIFFERENTIAL DIAGNOSES

- Rhinosporidiosis and adiaspiromycosis: Larger spherules
- Histoplasmosis, cryptococcosis, and blastomycosis: Overlap in size with endospores but exhibit budding yeast

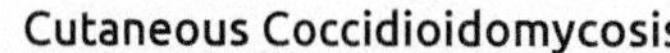

Cutaneous Coccidioidomycosis

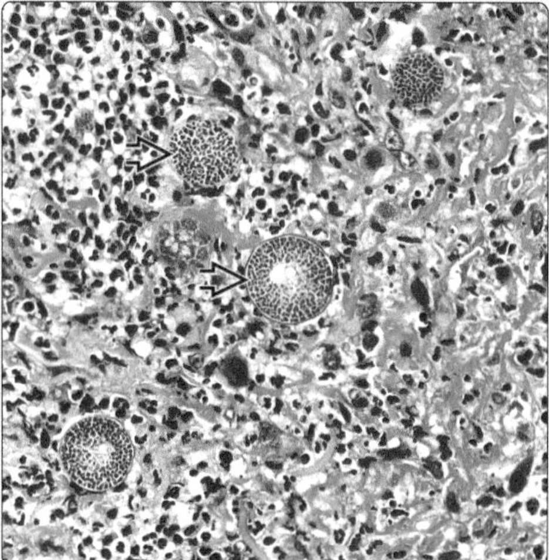

Giant Cell-Engulfed Spherule

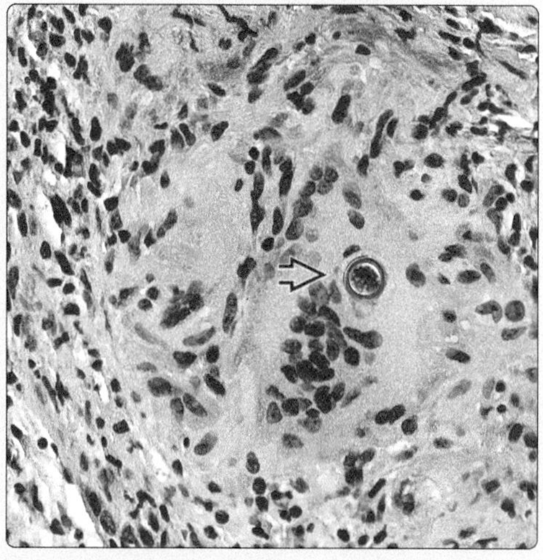

(Left) *Skin biopsy of coccidioidomycosis demonstrates several large spherules ⮊ containing numerous small endospores amidst acute and chronic inflammation. (From DP: Nonneoplastic Derm.)* **(Right)** *High-magnification H&E from a lung biopsy shows a single fungal form with a distinctive refractile, "double-contour" membrane ⮊, consistent with Coccidioides infection.*

Spherules and Endospores: GMS Stain

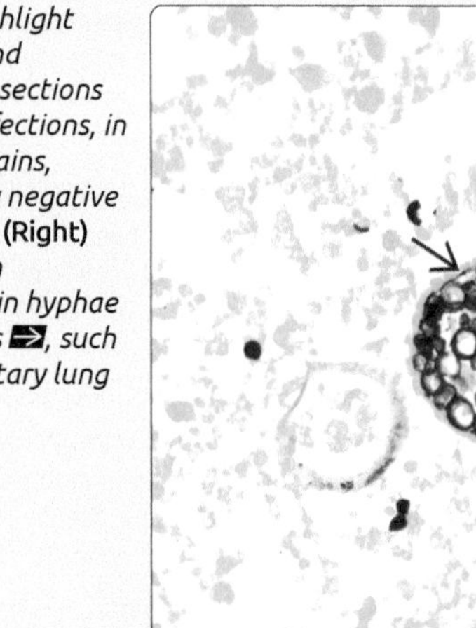

Septate Hyphae: GMS Stain

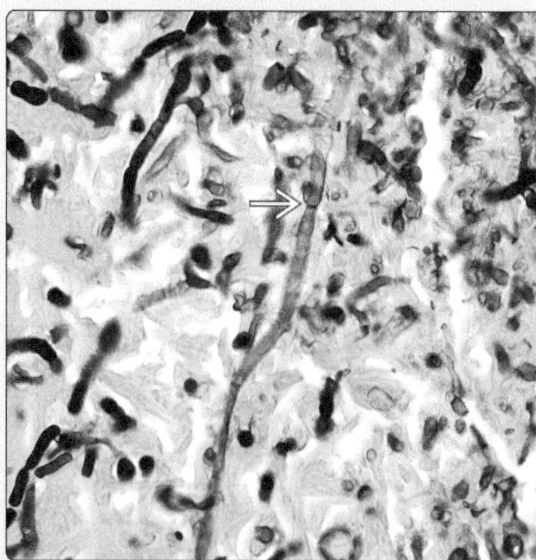

(Left) *GMS stains highlight both spherules ➔ and endospores in tissue sections with Coccidioides infections, in contrast to PAS-D stains, which are frequently negative in mature spherules.* **(Right)** *Coccidioides spp. can occasionally appear in hyphae form with septations ➡, such as this case of a cavitary lung mass.*

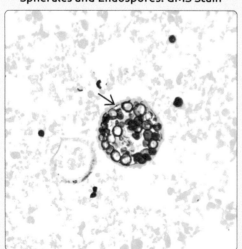

TERMINOLOGY

Synonyms

- Valley fever, San Joaquin Valley fever, desert rheumatism

Definitions

- Derived from Greek "coccidio" (little berry) + "ido" (resemblance); resembles Coccidia (protozoan parasites)

ETIOLOGY/PATHOGENESIS

Infectious Agents

- Caused by dimorphic fungi, *Coccidioides immitis* and *Coccidioides posadasii* (2 species are morphologically identical)
- Found in soil in southwestern USA (and south central Washington), and in parts of Mexico, Central America, and South America
- Inhalation of aerosolized fungal spores (arthroconidia) due to construction, earthquakes, etc. causes disease in minority of exposed individuals
- At body temperature, spores develop into spherules, which enlarge and rupture, releasing endospores, which form new spherules

CLINICAL ISSUES

Epidemiology

- Incidence (USA): 8,232-22,634 reported cases/year (2010-2019)
- Affects all ages; most common in adults ≥ 60 years
- Immunocompromised individuals (i.e., HIV infection, organ transplantation, corticosteroid use, pregnant women, and diabetics) are at higher risk for severe disease
- SARS-CoV-2 infection may cause reactivation of latent coccidioidomycosis
- Risk of dissemination is greater in Filipino and Black populations

Presentation

- Primary pulmonary disease is often self-limiting
- Symptomatic patients (40% of cases) usually present 1-3 weeks after exposure with fatigue, cough, dyspnea, headache, night sweats, myalgias, and rash
- Disseminated disease occurs in estimated 1% of cases and commonly affects musculoskeletal, soft tissues, and meninges in high-risk patients

Laboratory Tests

- Enzyme immunoassay (EIA): Sensitive method for diagnosing coccidioidomycosis (IgM and IgG)
- Immunodiffusion (ID): Detects IgM; positive early in disease
- Complement fixation (CF): Detects IgG; assessment of disease severity
- Urinary antigen detection: Not widely used
- PCR: FDA-approved assays for lower respiratory specimens
- Skin test: Delayed-type hypersensitivity against *C. immitis* spherule-derived antigen

Treatment

- Oral azoles are popular 1st-line therapy
- Amphotericin B: Severe disease
- No vaccine currently available; infection generally causes immunity

MICROBIOLOGY

Culture

- Sabouraud dextrose agar; 2-3 weeks for growth
- At 25-30 °C, colony morphology ranges from moist, glabrous, and grayish to abundant, floccose, and white
- Hyphae are thin and septate with 5- to 8-μm arthroconidia
- Inhalation risk to laboratory personnel is high; therefore, specimens must be handled with extreme caution and inside approved biological safety hood or cabinet

MICROSCOPIC

Histologic Features

- Necrotizing granulomatous inflammation with large, thick-walled spherules (100 μm, containing endospores up to 5 μm)
- Surrounding infiltrate is often rich in chronic inflammatory cells, eosinophils, neutrophils, and giant cell reactions
- Pseudoepitheliomatous hyperplasia and granulomatous dermal inflammation are common in cutaneous disease

ANCILLARY TESTS

Histochemistry

- Methenamine silver stains highlight coccidioidomycosis spherules, endospores, and hyphae (if present)
- Endospores are PAS positive, but larger/mature spherules are negative
- Endospores frequently positive for Fontana-Masson

DIFFERENTIAL DIAGNOSIS

Rhinosporidiosis

- Spherules are much larger (up to 300 μm) with thicker walls

Adiaspiromycosis

- Spherules are much larger (200-400 μm), refractile walls, appear empty

Histoplasmosis

- Yeast forms (2-4 μm) with narrow-based budding; lacks spherules

Cryptococcosis

- Yeast forms (5-10 μm) with narrow-based budding; lacks spherules
- Fontana-Masson and mucicarmine (capsule) positive

Blastomycosis

- Larger organism (12 μm), spherical, double-contoured yeast with broad-based budding; lacks spherules

SELECTED REFERENCES

1. McHardy IH et al: Review of clinical and laboratory diagnostics for coccidioidomycosis. J Clin Microbiol. 61(5):e0158122, 2023
2. Thompson GR et al: Controversies in the management of central nervous system coccidioidomycosis. Clin Infect Dis. 75(4):555-9, 2022
3. Chaturvedi S et al: Real-time PCR assay for detection and differentiation of Coccidioides immitis and Coccidioides posadasii from culture and clinical specimens. PLoS Negl Trop Dis. 15(9):e0009765, 2021
4. Reyna-Rodríguez IL et al: Primary cutaneous coccidioidomycosis: An Update. Am J Clin Dermatol. 21(5):681-96, 2020

(Left) *This patient presented with a 1.2-cm right upper lobe nodule ⮕ of unclear etiology that was biopsied to rule out neoplasia and was determined to be positive for Coccidioides spp.* **(Right)** *Fine-needle aspiration of a pulmonary nodule reveals multiple large spherules containing endospores, diagnostic of pulmonary coccidioidomycosis.*

Pulmonary Coccidioidomycosis

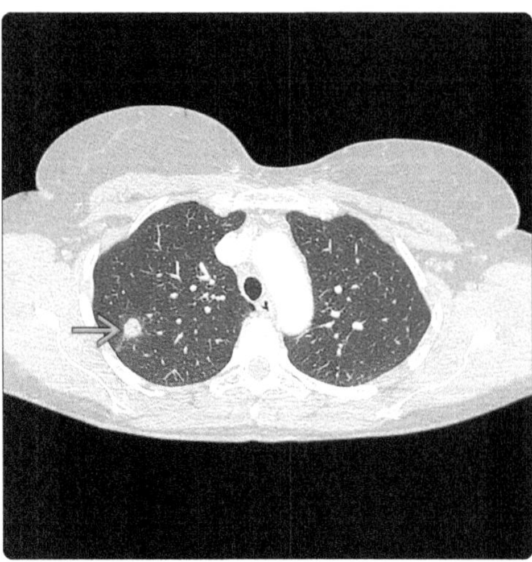

Coccidioides spp. Spherule: FNA

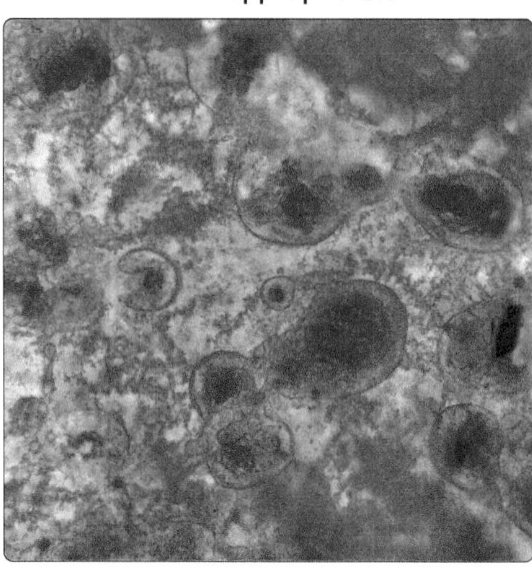

(Left) *This lactophenol cotton blue stain of a Coccidioides immitis spherule (sporangium) shows the distinctive double-contour membrane surrounding developing endospores. (Courtesy L. Georg, PhD, CDC/PHIL.)* **(Right)** *This culture plate contains 2 large grayish-white, downy-textured colonies isolated from soil samples, identified as C. immitis. (Courtesy L. Ajello, PhD, CDC/PHIL.)*

Coccidioides immitis Spherule

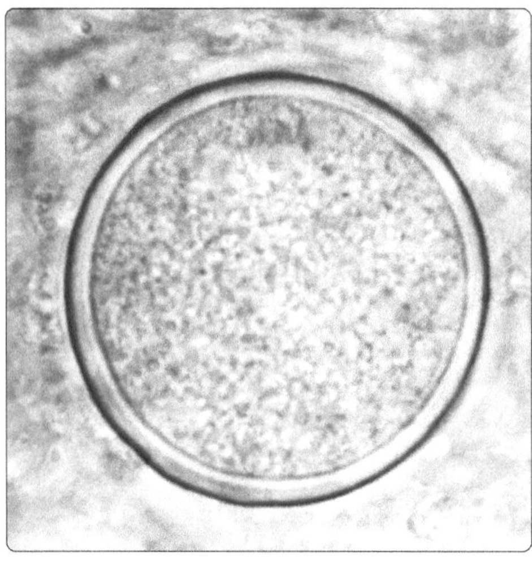

Culture Isolate

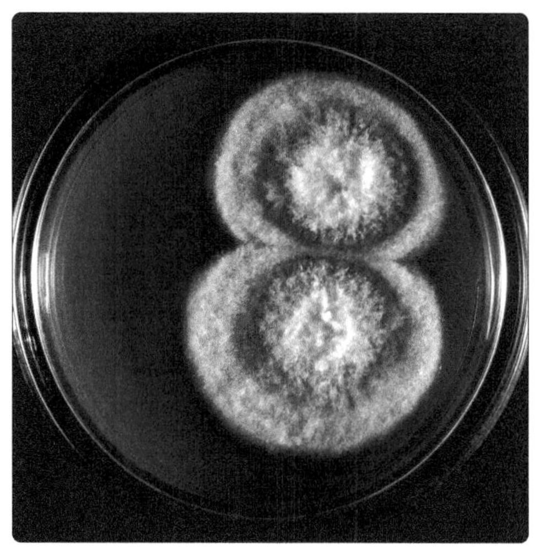

(Left) *This lactophenol cotton blue stain of a C. immitis culture isolate shows barrel-shaped arthroconidia that alternate with empty cells.* **(Right)** *Fluorescent antibody staining of this soil sample reveals the presence of a short chain of C. immitis arthroconidia (arthrospores), which can lead to symptomatic disease when inhaled. (Courtesy Dr. Kaplan, CDC/PHIL.)*

Coccidioides immitis Arthroconidia

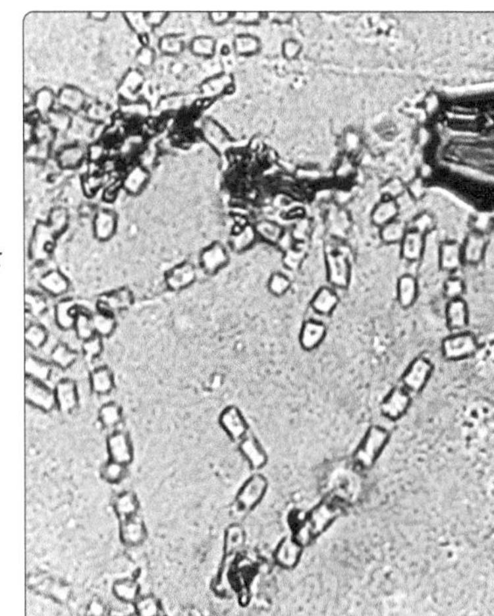

Coccidioides immitis Arthroconidia

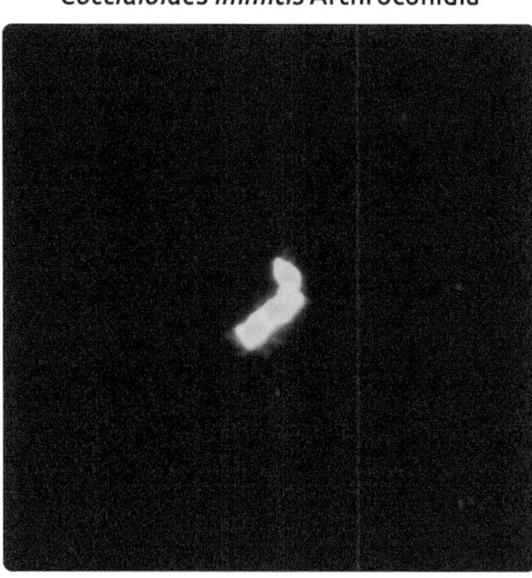

Spherule Within Giant Cell

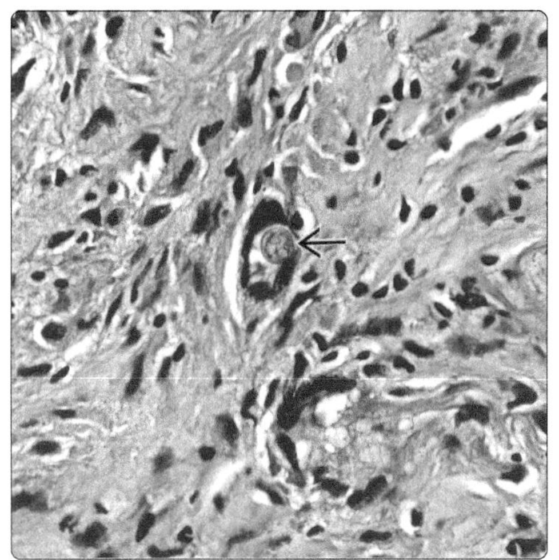

Ruptured Spherule

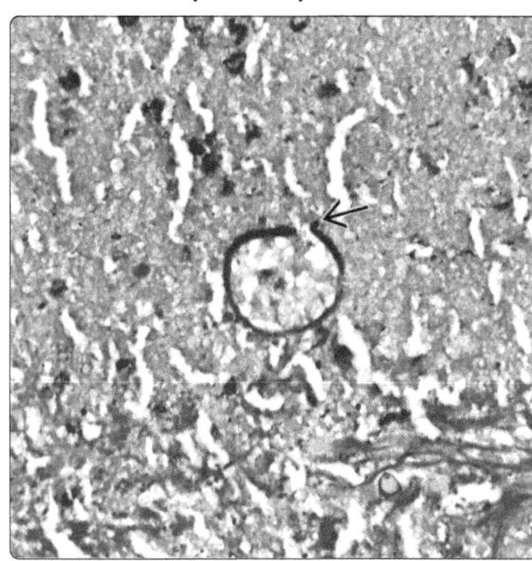

(Left) *Multinucleated giant cells may engulf individual Coccidioides spp. endospores or spherules* ⇨*, as shown in this section of lung from a wedge resection.* **(Right)** *This section of necrotic lung tissue shows a disrupted-appearing spherule* ⇨*, which has released its endospores.*

Ruptured Spherule: GMS Stain

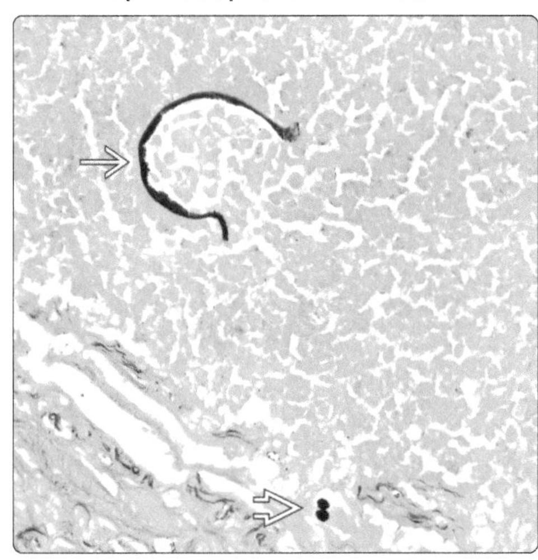

Endospore Within Giant Cell

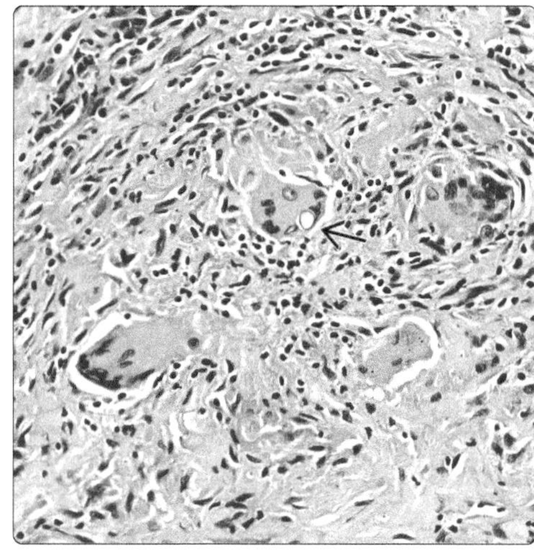

(Left) *GMS stain highlights a pair of adjacent endospores* ➡ *that have an appearance reminiscent of budding. The presence of a ruptured spherule* ➡ *confirms the diagnosis of coccidioidomycosis in this case.* **(Right)** *This section shows several multinucleated giant cells, including one containing a Coccidioides spp. endospore* ⇨*. These features are not unique to coccidioidomycosis, requiring a broader differential diagnosis.*

Endospores: PAS-D Stain

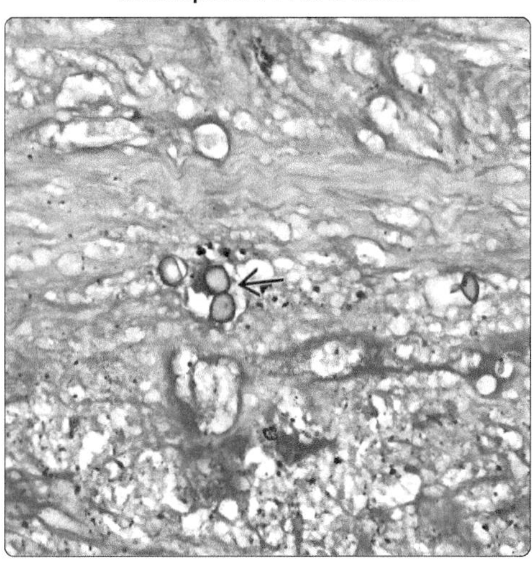

Endospores: GMS Stain

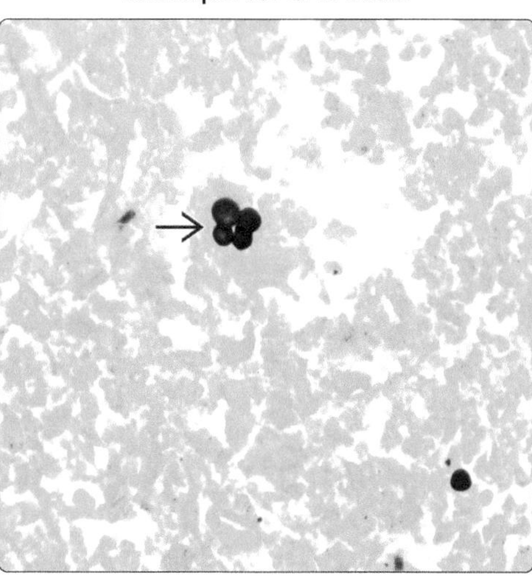

(Left) *PAS-D stain highlights several Coccidioides spp. endospores, including a pair with an appearance reminiscent of budding* ⇨*. In the absence of spherules, these features are not unique to coccidioidomycosis, requiring a broader differential diagnosis.* **(Right)** *GMS stain highlights several Coccidioides spp. endospores, including a cluster with an appearance reminiscent of budding* ⇨*.*

KEY FACTS

ETIOLOGY/PATHOGENESIS

- Infection with *Cryptococcus neoformans* and *Cryptococcus gattii* via inhalation of spores

CLINICAL ISSUES

- Most cases are seen in immunocompromised patients: HIV infection, prolonged use of glucocorticoids or immunosuppressants, history of stem cell and organ transplants, malignancies
- Lung (primary) and central nervous system and skin (secondary) are most common sites of infection
- Untreated disseminated *Cryptococcus* infection has mortality rate of up to 100%
- Cryptococcal antigen (CRAG) testing (CSF, serum) have false-positives due to *Trichosporon* spp.

MICROBIOLOGY

- Culture differentiates between *C. neoformans* and *C. gattii* (usually 3-5 days to grow)

MICROSCOPIC

- Encapsulated, spherical to oval yeast cells (5-10 μm in diameter) with narrow-based budding and polysaccharide capsule
- Yeast cells are positive for GMS, PAS, Fontana-Masson stains
- Mucicarmine and Alcian blue stain polysaccharide capsule
- Granulomatous, mixed suppurative and granulomatous, and minimal/absent inflammatory reactions (immunocompromised) may be observed

TOP DIFFERENTIAL DIAGNOSES

- Candidiasis: Gram positive, Fontana-Masson negative, pseudohyphae common
- Histoplasmosis: Fontana-Masson and mucicarmine negative; more regular in size
- Blastomycosis: Larger in size (8-15 μm in diameter) with broad-based budding; may be Fontana-Masson positive with weak mucicarmine staining

Lung Cryptococcosis

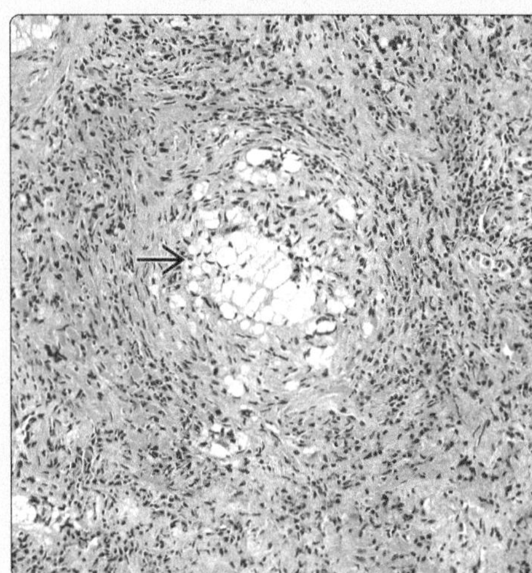

Methenamine Silver Stain

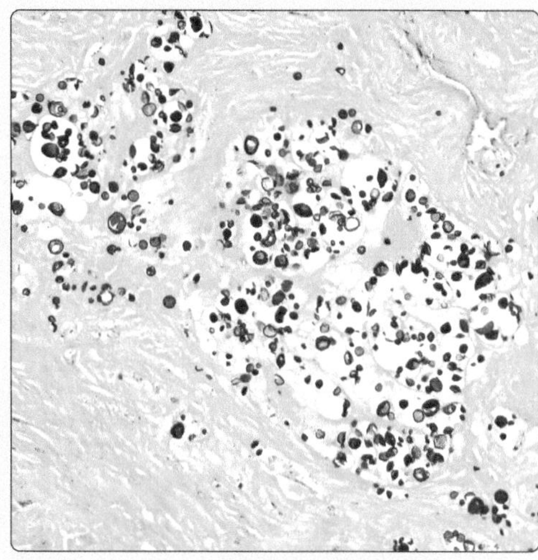

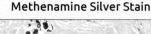

(Left) *This section from a lung wedge resection undertaken to rule out metastatic carcinoma shows granulomatous inflammation and numerous yeast forms* → *identified by a retractile appearance with minimal H&E staining surrounded by an empty halo.* **(Right)** *Methenamine silver staining highlights numerous yeasts of varying sizes, including many with crushed appearances, and occasional narrow-based budding, features typical of Cryptococcus spp.*

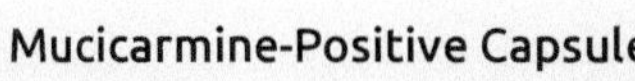

Mucicarmine-Positive Capsule

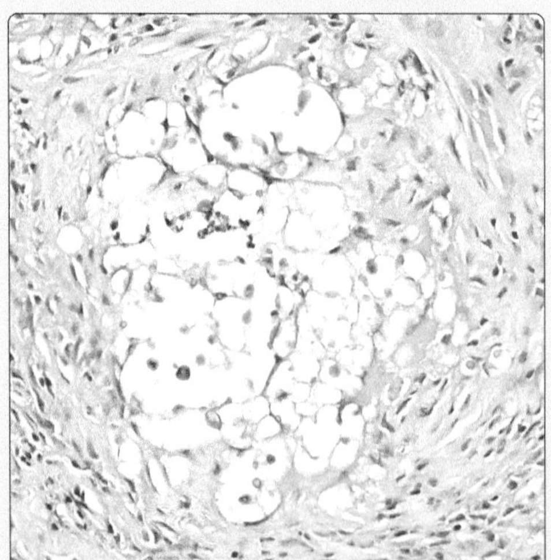

Fontana-Masson

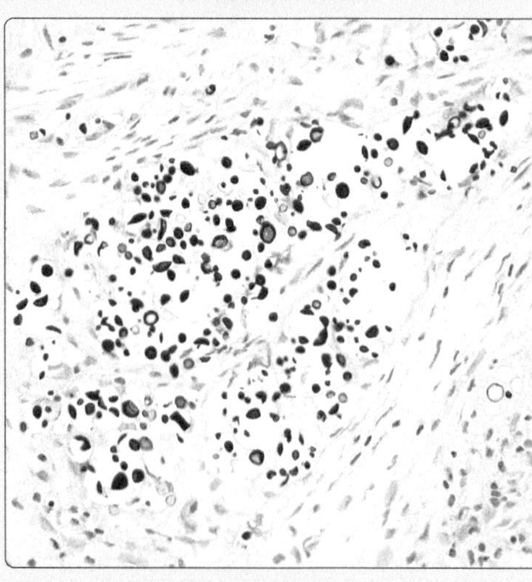

(Left) *The diagnosis of cryptococcosis can typically be confirmed by staining of the yeast polysaccharide capsule with mucicarmine, resulting in a red appearance.* **(Right)** *Fontana-Masson highlights melanin-producing Cryptococcus yeast forms. This property is helpful in identifying capsule-deficient strains but must be used cautiously and in conjunction with other morphologic features.*

TERMINOLOGY

Definitions

- Derived from Greek: "Crypto" (hidden) + "kokkus" (berry, grain)

ETIOLOGY/PATHOGENESIS

Infectious Agents

- Infection with *Cryptococcus neoformans* and *Cryptococcus gattii* (formerly *C. neoformans* var. *gattii*) basidiomycetous encapsulated yeast via inhalation of spores; yeasts may persist within macrophages in lymph nodes and disseminate systemically upon immunosuppression
- *C. neoformans*: Corresponds to serotypes A, D, and AD; found in rotting vegetation and soil samples with excreta of pigeons and chickens
- *C. gattii*: Corresponds to serotypes B and C; associated with several species of eucalyptus trees in tropical and subtropical climates and fir and oak trees in temperate climates

CLINICAL ISSUES

Epidemiology

- Risk factors: HIV (most common), prolonged use of glucocorticoids and other immunosuppressants, underlying lung disease, malignancy, stem cell and solid organ transplantation
- *C. neoformans*: Worldwide distribution; majority of infections (95%) in immunocompromised patients
- *C. gattii*: Present in tropical/subtropical regions, including Australia, Papua New Guinea, parts of Africa, Mexico, and Southern California, British Columbia, and Pacific Northwest of USA; typically in immunocompetent but HIV testing is recommended

Presentation

- Pulmonary involvement: Clinical course determined by host immune status, inoculum size, and innate virulence of organism
  - Pulmonary involvement can be due to primary infection in naïve host, reactivation of latent infection, or reinfection with new strain
  - Immunocompromised patients more likely to have extrapulmonary disease
  - CNS involvement should be ruled out in immunocompromised patients presenting with pulmonary cryptococcosis
- CNS symptoms are nonspecific, and clinical course can vary from indolent, subacute, to acute presentations depending on species causing infection and host immune status
  - Brain parenchyma is often involved in addition to meningeal infection
  - Involvement more commonly seen in immunocompromised patients
  - Lumbar puncture criteria: Neurologic symptoms, high serum cryptococcal antigen (CRAG) titer, and underlying condition that predisposes to CNS dissemination (e.g., immunosuppression)
- Cutaneous involvement
  - Primary infection due to traumatic inoculation is less common than secondary infection
    - Factors suggesting primary infection: Solitary lesion, regional lymph node involvement, lesions on uncovered parts, history of primary inoculation
    - Cases of rarer species, such as *C. laurentii* and *C. albidus*, have been reported
  - Secondary infection due to dissemination
    - Cutaneous signs may be 1st indication of cryptococcosis and precede diagnosis of disseminated disease
    - Factors suggesting secondary infection: Presence of systemic symptoms, multicentric skin lesions, deep dermal or subcutaneous lesions, lesions on covered parts
- Other sites reported include osteomyelitis, hepatitis, pyelonephritis, prostatitis, and peritonitis
- Infection caused by *C. gattii* vs. infection caused by *C. neoformans*
  - Large mass lesions (i.e., cryptococcomas) of lungs &/or brain are more likely to be caused by *C. gattii* than *C. neoformans*
  - Infections due to *C. gattii* are more likely to be associated with neurologic complications

Laboratory Tests

- Direct examination of clinical specimens
  - Encapsulated yeast forms may be visualized in sputum, bronchoalveolar lavage, CSF, or tissue smears
  - Capsule highlighted by India ink in body fluid or tissue smears as halo against black background
- CRAG testing
  - Latex agglutination or enzyme-linked immunosorbent assay (ELISA) to detect cryptococcal polysaccharide antigen
  - CSF: Sensitivity: 93-100%; specificity: 93-98%
  - Serum (immunocompromised patients)
    - Negative serum CRAG result does not exclude diagnosis of cryptococcosis
    - Positive serum CRAG result should prompt investigation for disseminated infection
    - Positive in essentially all patients with HIV infection and pulmonary cryptococcosis and up to 84% of patients with other underlying immunocompromising conditions
  - Antigen titer generally correlates with burden of organisms
  - Limitations
    - False-positive results have been reported with serologic assays in cases of fungal infection due to *Trichosporon asahii* and bacterial infections due to *Stomatococcus* spp. or *Capnocytophaga* spp.
    - False-negative results can occur due to low fungal burden or prozone effect
    - Most serologic tests detect antigens present in capsule; therefore, tests may not be helpful in cases caused by capsule-deficient cryptococcal organisms
    - Assays do not allow distinction of different *Cryptococcus* spp.
    - No role for monitoring serum CRAG titers to determine duration of therapy in either immunosuppressed or immunocompetent hosts
  - CRAG lateral flow immunochromatographic assay
    - Semiquantitative

- Can be used as rapid point-of-care test with CSF, serum, and plasma samples
- Compared with culture: 99.5% sensitivity and 98% specificity
- Molecular testing: RT-PCR, targeted panels, and broad-spectrum (28S rRNA or mNGS) assays available

Treatment

- CNS disease
  - In general: Induction therapy with amphotericin B plus flucytosine followed by consolidation and maintenance therapy with fluconazole
  - Dosages and duration of treatments vary based on patient's immune status and clinical conditions
- Nonmeningeal pulmonary disease
  - Generally treated with fluconazole
  - Severe pulmonary disease presenting with acute respiratory distress syndrome (ARDS) or extrapulmonary manifestations should be treated like CNS disease
  - Patients who have negative cultures and undetectable CRAG titers may not require antifungal therapy
- Nonmeningeal nonpulmonary disease
  - Single site: Generally treated with fluconazole
  - Multiple sites or high serum fungal titer: Treated like CNS disease
- Surgery may be considered for large, accessible lesions with mass effect or for lesions not responding to antifungal therapies

Prognosis

- Untreated disseminated cryptococcal infection has mortality rate of up to 100%
- ARDS is often associated with disseminated infection and high mortality
- High rate of extrapulmonary disease is seen among immunocompromised patients with cryptococcal pneumonia
- Cerebral cryptococcomas are associated with delayed or poor response to therapy and substantial neurologic sequelae

IMAGING

Radiographic Findings

- Chest
  - Most common findings: Solitary or few well-defined nodules; cavitations within nodules/masses are more commonly seen in immunocompromised patients
  - Other findings: Lobar infiltrates, hilar and mediastinal adenopathy, and pleural effusions
- Brain
  - Mass lesions &/or hydrocephalus have been reported but are rare
  - Brain mass lesions seen in HIV or immunocompromised patients should prompt consideration of alternative diagnoses, such as toxoplasmosis, lymphoma, or tuberculosis
- Cryptococcomas may mimic neoplasia or pyogenic abscesses

MICROBIOLOGY

Culture

- Sabouraud dextrose agar, bird seed agar, or canavanine glycine bromothymol blue (CGB) agar (*C. neoformans* appear yellow, and *C. gatti* are blue)
- *C. neoformans* and *C. gattii* usually take 3-5 days to grow in culture
- Cultures are specific, but sensitivity can vary depending on sample and fungal load
- Blood, respiratory samples, CSF, and other body fluids can be collected for cultures
- Species identification can be confirmed by MALDI-TOF MS or molecular testing

MACROSCOPIC

Brain Lesions

- In patients with severe immunosuppression and disseminated disease, classic "soap bubble" lesions with clear gelatinous capsule can be present dissecting through brain tissue without inflammation

MICROSCOPIC

Histologic Features

- Encapsulated, variably sized spherical to oval yeast cells (5-10 μm in diameter) with narrow-based budding and polysaccharide capsule (organisms may be capsule deficient)
- Different *Cryptococcus* spp. cannot be distinguished by histologic features
- Immunocompetent patients
  - Granulomatous or mixed suppurative and granulomatous reaction
  - Granulomas and cryptococcomas can be seen in chronic pulmonary infection; organisms may be found inside macrophages and giant cells
  - Pseudotumoral spindle cell reactions to cryptococcal organisms have been reported in rare cases
- Immunocompromised patients
  - Inflammatory reaction may be minimal or absent
  - Proliferation of organisms forms cyst-like gelatinous lesions packed with cryptococci that appear as soap bubbles (most commonly seen in brain)

ANCILLARY TESTS

Histochemistry

- Yeast cells are positive by methenamine silver and PAS stains and negative by Gram stain
- Fontana-Masson stain highlights melanin contained by yeast cells
- Mucicarmine and Alcian blue stain polysaccharide capsule

Molecular Diagnostics

- Molecular tests, such as DNA hybridization and PCR-based assays, are useful in cases when clinical isolates do not grow in culture or when distinction among *Cryptococcus* spp. is needed

DIFFERENTIAL DIAGNOSIS

Candidiasis

- Yeast forms of *Candida* spp. can be confused with capsule-deficient forms of *Cryptococcus* spp.
- *Candida* spp. are negative on Fontana-Masson stains, positive on Gram stains, and frequently contain pseudohyphae
- *Candida* spp. commonly elicits pyogenic tissue reaction, while *Cryptococcus* spp. generates granulomatous or mixed suppurative granulomatous inflammation

Histoplasmosis

- *Histoplasma* spp. can be mistaken with capsule-deficient forms of *Cryptococcus* spp.
- Yeast cells of *Cryptococcus* spp. show larger variety of sizes and shapes, while *Histoplasma* yeast cells are more uniform in size
- *Histoplasma* spp. are negative on Fontana-Masson and mucicarmine stains

Blastomycosis

- *Blastomyces* spp. are larger in size (8-15 μm in diameter) and usually exhibit broad-based budding, while *Cryptococcus* spp. are generally smaller (5-10 μm in diameter) with narrow-based budding
- *Blastomyces* spp. may exhibit weak cell wall positivity for mucicarmine while strongly positive for capsules of *Cryptococcus* spp.
- Fontana-Masson stain is positive for melanin in *Cryptococcus* spp. and in some cases of *Blastomyces* spp.

Tissue Autolysis

- Autolysis of human cells surrounded by capsule-like vacuolated spaces mimicking *Cryptococcus* spp. in inflammatory infiltrate has been reported in patients with malignancies and immune dysregulations
- Special stains and cultures are needed to rule out fungal infection

SELECTED REFERENCES

1. Misra A et al: The brief case: the cryptic Cryptococcus. J Clin Microbiol. 61(2):e0054822, 2023
2. Zhao Y et al: Cryptococcus neoformans, a global threat to human health. Infect Dis Poverty. 12(1):20, 2023
3. Beardsley J et al: What's new in Cryptococcus gattii: from bench to bedside and beyond. J Fungi (Basel). 9(1), 2022
4. Saidykhan L et al: The Cryptococcus gattii species complex: unique pathogenic yeasts with understudied virulence mechanisms. PLoS Negl Trop Dis. 16(12):e0010916, 2022
5. Marr KA et al: A multicenter, longitudinal cohort study of cryptococcosis in HIV-negative people in the United States. Clin Infect Dis. 70(2):252-61, 2020
6. McHugh KE et al: Sensitivity of cerebrospinal fluid cytology for the diagnosis of cryptococcal infections: a 21-year single-institution retrospective review. Am J Clin Pathol. 151(2):198-204, 2019
7. Setianingrum F et al: Pulmonary cryptococcosis: a review of pathobiology and clinical aspects. Med Mycol. 57(2):133-50, 2019
8. Siqueira LPM et al: Evaluation of Vitek MS for differentiation of Cryptococcus neoformans and Cryptococcus gattii genotypes. J Clin Microbiol. 57(1), 2019
9. Elsegeiny W et al: Immunology of cryptococcal infections: developing a rational approach to patient therapy. Front Immunol. 9:651, 2018
10. Du L et al: Systemic review of published reports on primary cutaneous cryptococcosis in immunocompetent patients. Mycopathologia. 180(1-2):19-25, 2015
11. Hansen J et al: Large-scale evaluation of the immuno-mycologics lateral flow and enzyme-linked immunoassays for detection of cryptococcal antigen in serum and cerebrospinal fluid. Clin Vaccine Immunol. 20(1):52-5, 2013
12. Bishop JA et al: Evaluation of the detection of melanin by the Fontana-Masson silver stain in tissue with a wide range of organisms including Cryptococcus. Hum Pathol. 43(6):898-903, 2012
13. Sing Y et al: Cryptococcal inflammatory pseudotumors. Am J Surg Pathol. 31(10):1521-7, 2007

Cryptococcus **sp. Isolated in Culture**

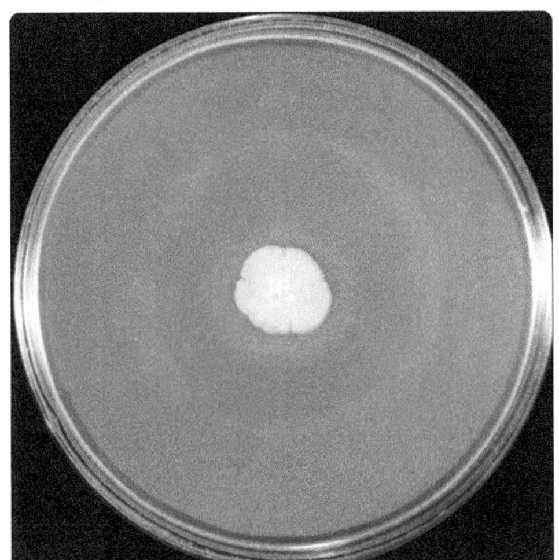

***C. neoforms*: Lactophenol Cotton Blue**

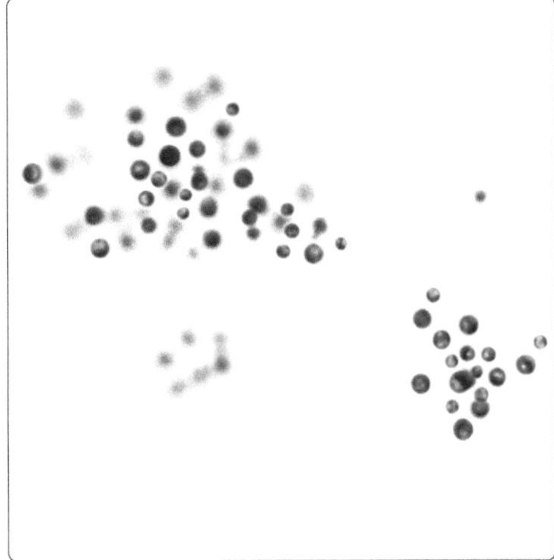

(Left) *This frontal view of a Sabouraud dextrose agar plate shows a single off-white, cottony colony, which was diagnosed as Cryptocccus sp. (Courtesy H. Hardin, CDC/PHIL.)* **(Right)** *This image of a culture isolate stained with lactophenol cotton blue shows small yeast forms with occasional narrow-based budding, consistent with Cryptococcus neoformans. (Courtesy L. Haley, PhD, CDC/PHIL.)*

(Left) *High magnification of this bronchial wash specimen on ThinPrep shows multiple intracellular yeasts, consistent with cryptococci within the cytoplasm of macrophages. The yeasts vary from round* → *to teardrop-shaped* ⇒*. Vague clearing around the yeast cells corresponds to the presence of a capsule.* **(Right)** *High magnification of this bronchial brush specimen on Diff-Quik stain demonstrates numerous round yeast forms* → *in a patient with known pulmonary cryptococcosis.*

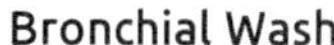

Bronchial Wash

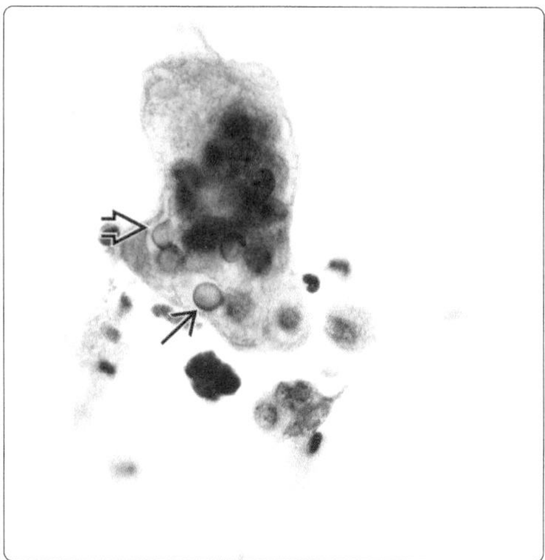

Bronchial Brush

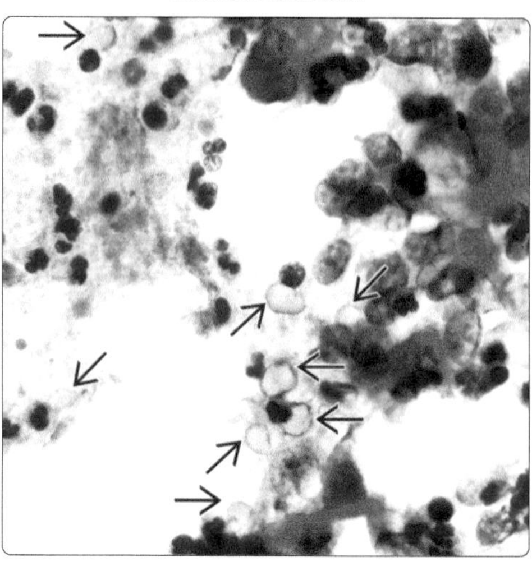

(Left) *India ink staining of CSF demonstrates a halo, or lack of staining, surrounding yeast forms due to the presence of a capsule. (Courtesy L. Haley, PhD, CDC/PHIL.)* **(Right)** *Autopsy brain section from a woman with HIV and CD4 count < 50 cells/μL shows scattered yeast forms within the leptomeninges, which were also positive for mucicarmine, morphologically consistent with Cryptococcus spp.*

Cryptococcal Meningitis: India Ink

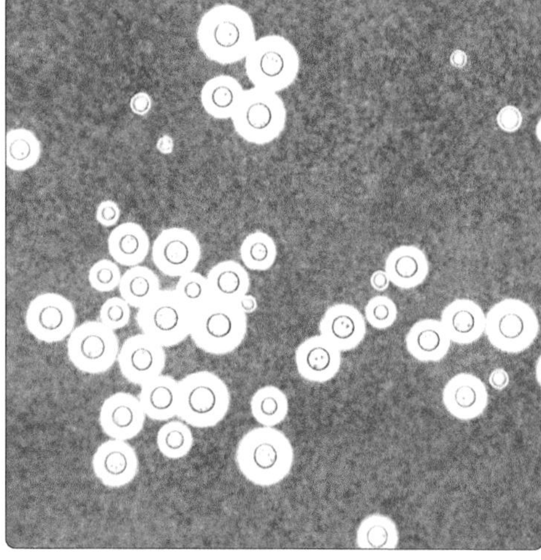

Cryptococcal Meningoencephalitis

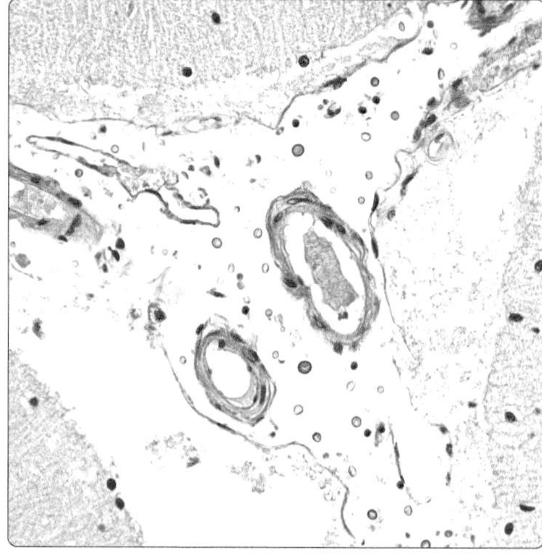

(Left) *A large mount brain section from a patient with disseminated cryptococcosis in the setting of severe immunosuppression shows classic "soap bubble" lesions* ⇒*, which are large colonies of cryptococci with thick mucoid capsules.* **(Right)** *Low magnification of a brain section on H&E stain from a patient with disseminated Cryptococcus infection shows classic "soap bubble" lesions, which are large colonies of encapsulated yeast cells. No inflammation is present.*

Cryptococcal Brain Abscess

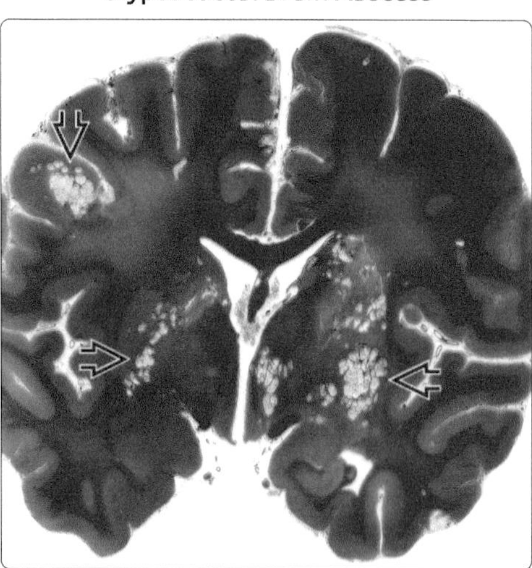

"Soap Bubble" Lesions

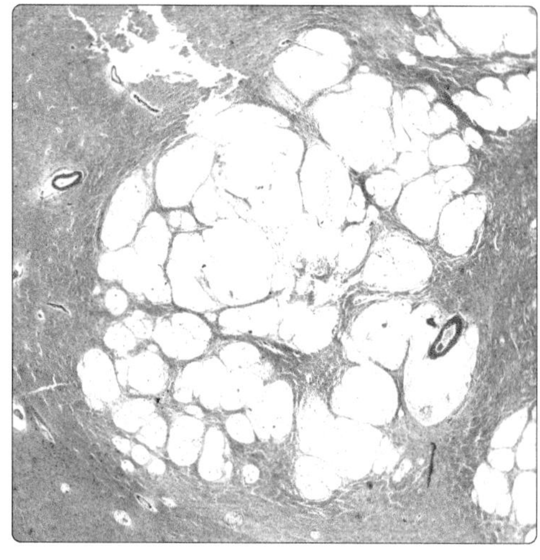

Laryngeal Cryptococcosis

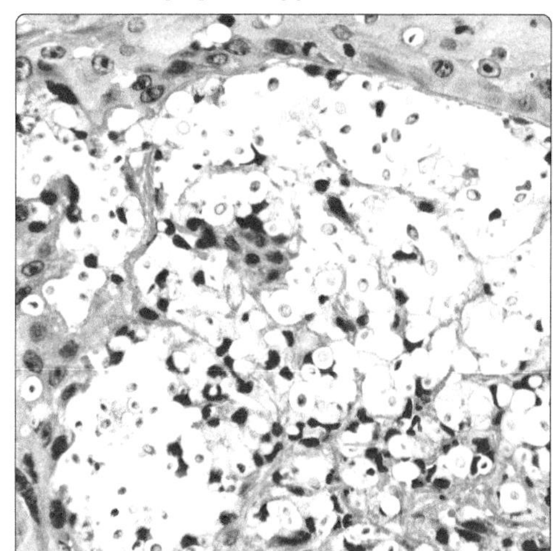

Laryngeal Cryptococcosis: Mucicarmine

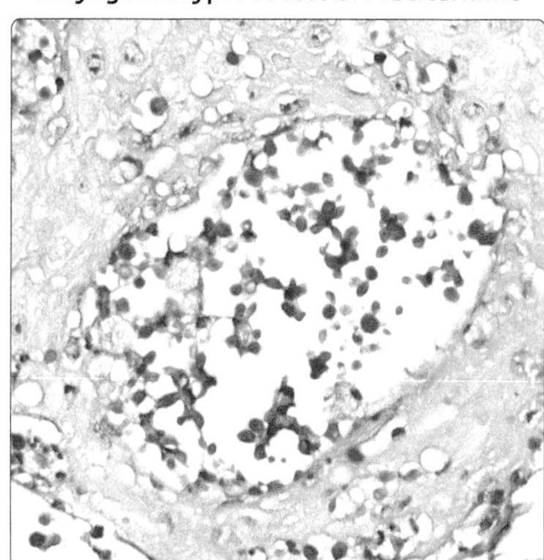

(Left) *Numerous ovoid yeast forms of variable size are readily noted in the submucosa in this H&E-stained laryngeal biopsy. Note the prominent "clearing" around the yeasts, conferring a gelatinous appearance due to the characteristic mucilaginous capsule.* **(Right)** *The yeast capsules are highlighted in red by the mucicarmine stain, characteristic of Cryptococcus spp. Laryngeal cryptococcosis is typically observed in patients with prolonged use of inhalable steroids (e.g., for asthma).*

Cryptococcal Lymphadenitis

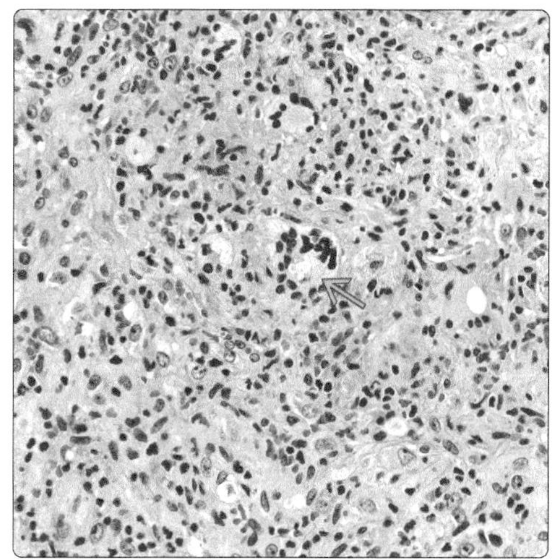

Disseminated Cryptococcosis

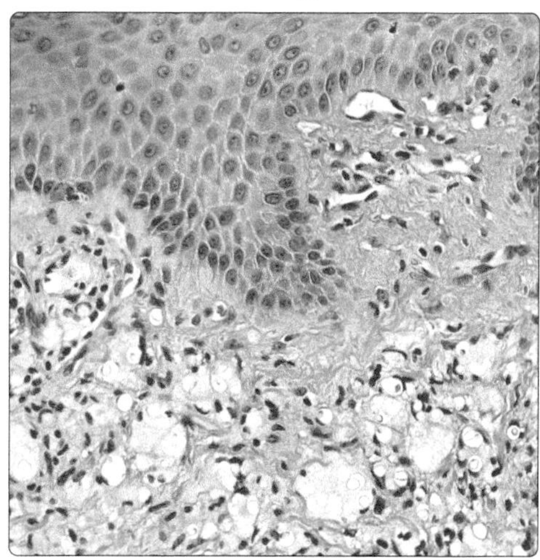

(Left) *This axial lymph node biopsy shows architectural effacement by granulomatous inflammation, including multinucleate giant cells containing yeast forms ⇒, morphologically consistent with Cryptococcus spp.* **(Right)** *This skin biopsy from a lung transplant patient shows a deep fungal infection with intracellular yeast forms, morphologically consistent with Cryptococcus spp.*

Cryptococcal Prostatitis

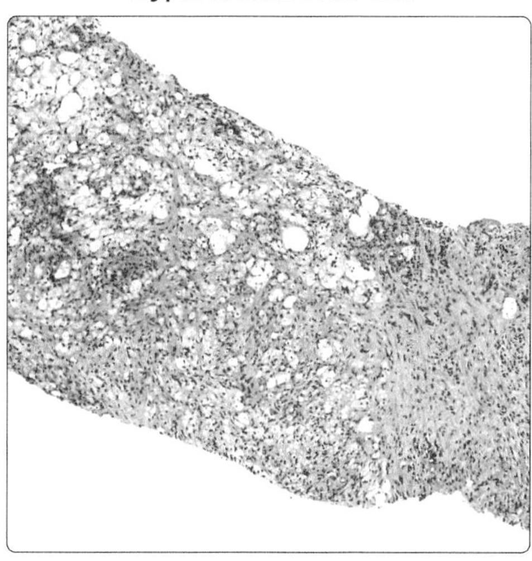

Cryptococcal Prostatitis: PAS-D

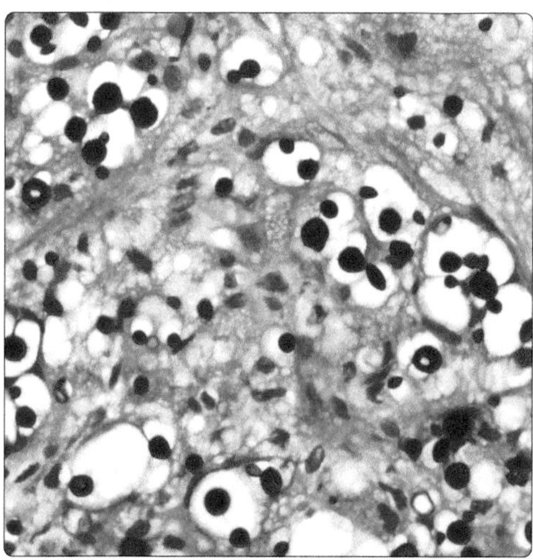

(Left) *This prostate core biopsy taken to evaluate for recurrent prostatic carcinoma shows numerous yeast forms, morphologically consistent with Cryptococcus spp. Fungal prostatitis is rare but can be seen in cases of disseminated cryptococcosis.* **(Right)** *Periodic acid-Schiff with diastase highlights medium to large yeast forms with narrow-based budding in this prostate core biopsy.*

Histoplasmosis

KEY FACTS

ETIOLOGY/PATHOGENESIS

- Infections caused by dimorphic fungi *Histoplasma capsulatum* or *Histoplasma duboisii* via inhalation of microconidia

CLINICAL ISSUES

- Most prevalent endemic mycosis in USA: Mississippi and Ohio River valleys
- Most infections in immunocompetent patients are asymptomatic or self-limited
- Disseminated disease mostly occurs in immunocompromised individuals
- Enzyme immunoassays are available to detect *Histoplasma* antigens in urine or serum

MICROSCOPIC

- Oval small yeast cells (2-4 μm in diameter) with narrow-based budding
- Yeasts tend to cluster within macrophages
- Associated with granulomatous inflammation
- GMS positive; Gram and melanin stains negative

TOP DIFFERENTIAL DIAGNOSES

- Emergomycosis: Similar size with narrow-based budding; distinguish by culture/molecular testing
- Candidiasis: Similar size, gram positive, pseudohyphae
- Cryptococcosis: More size variability; Fontana-Masson and mucicarmine positive
- Coccidioidomycosis (endospores): Similar size, no budding
- Blastomycosis: Large with broad-based budding; distinguish from by *H. duboisii* culture/molecular testing
- Pneumocystosis: Cysts lacks budding, focal thickenings in cyst wall
- Penicilliosis: Yeast-like cells within macrophages, binary fission with central septum
- Leishmaniasis, toxoplasmosis, Chagas disease: No budding, negative GMS/PAS-D

Pulmonary Histoplasmosis: Chest CT

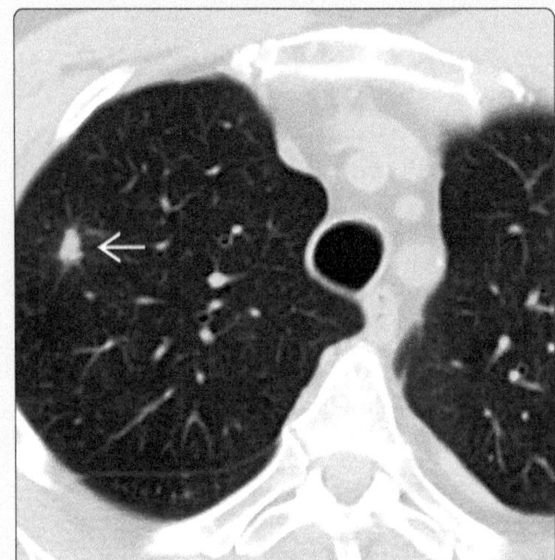

***H. capsulatum*: Lactophenol Cotton Blue**

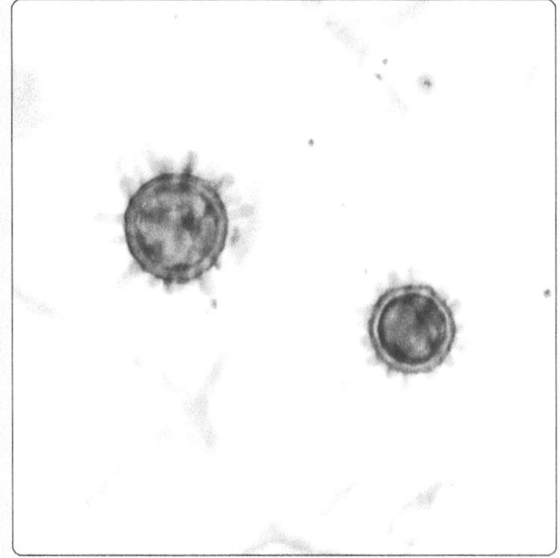

(Left) *Chest CT shows a nodule in the right lung →, raising the concern for neoplastic vs. infectious diseases. Positron emission tomography may be mildly to strongly avid. Wedge resection of the nodule revealed a calcified necrotic mass containing Histoplasma yeast forms.* **(Right)** *This lactophenol cotton blue stain of a culture isolate shows thick-walled, round macroconidia covered with short cylindrical projections, features consistent with H. capsulatum. (Courtesy J. Crothers, MD.)*

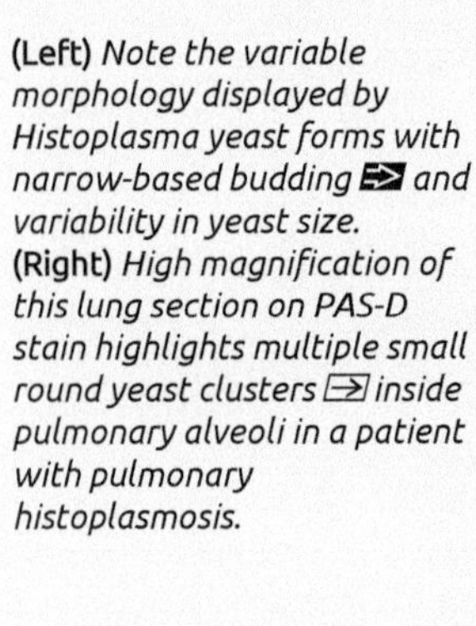

Pulmonary Histoplasmosis: GMS Stain

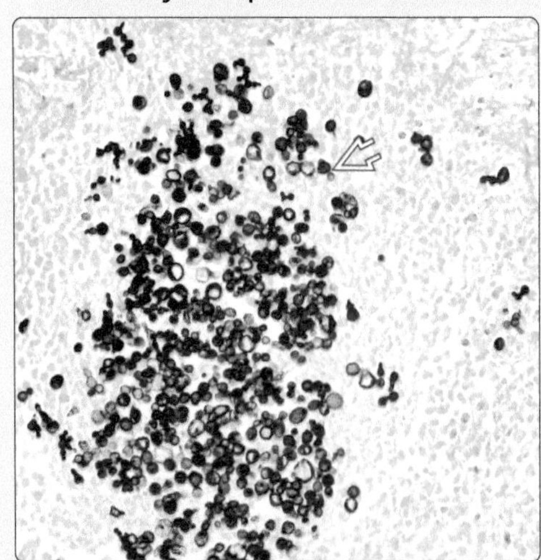

Pulmonary Histoplasmosis: PAS-D Stain

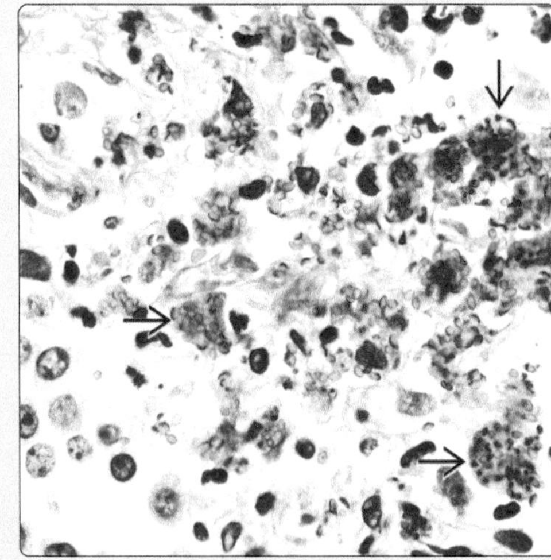

(Left) *Note the variable morphology displayed by Histoplasma yeast forms with narrow-based budding ⇨ and variability in yeast size.* **(Right)** *High magnification of this lung section on PAS-D stain highlights multiple small round yeast clusters → inside pulmonary alveoli in a patient with pulmonary histoplasmosis.*

TERMINOLOGY

Synonyms

- Cave disease, Darling disease, spelunker's disease

Definitions

- Greek: "Histos" (warp, web, from tissue) + "plasma" (something molded or formed)

ETIOLOGY/PATHOGENESIS

Infectious Agents

- Infection with *Histoplasma capsulatum* strains *H. capsulatum* var. *capsulatum* and *H. capsulatum* var. *duboisii* via inhalation of microconidia
- Thermally dimorphic fungus that exists as mold in environment (25 °C) and converts into yeast phase in vitro and in tissues (37 °C)
- Conidia are ingested by lung alveolar macrophages and convert into yeast forms existing as intracellular pathogens until being eliminated by specific cell-mediated immunity
- Phagocytized organisms can disseminate to other body sites, causing disease as macrophages travel in reticulolymphatic system
- Reactivation of latent histoplasmosis has been associated with immunocompromise
- Case reports of transmission through cadaveric kidney transplantation
- Rare transplacental transmission of *H. capsulatum* has been reported

CLINICAL ISSUES

Epidemiology

- Most prevalent endemic mycosis in USA: 22% of population has positive skin test and 50 million individuals infected
- *H. capsulatum* most commonly seen in North America and Central America, but cases have been reported worldwide; organisms mostly found in soil or caves containing bird or bat guano
  - Endemic in Mississippi and Ohio River valleys; also reported in localized foci in Maryland, Pennsylvania, Delaware, West Virginia, Virginia, and North Carolina
- *H. duboisii* (*H. capsulatum* var. *duboisii*) is endemic to Central and West Africa; cases reported elsewhere acquired in Africa
- Risk factors for disseminated infection
  - HIV infection
  - Congenital T-cell immunodeficiencies
  - Hematopoietic stem cell or solid organ transplant recipients on corticosteroids or tumor necrosis factor antagonists
  - Use of other immunosuppressive drugs
  - Hematologic malignancies
  - Infants and older adults

Presentation

- Vast majority of infected persons have either no symptoms or mild self-limited illness; < 5% of individuals who have low-level exposure to *H. capsulatum* develop symptomatic disease
- Pulmonary histoplasmosis
  - Acute disease mostly seen in infants and heavily immunocompromised hosts
    - Hilar and mediastinal lymphadenopathy is common
    - Severe infection occurs in cases with exposure to large fungal inoculum or in immunosuppressed patients
  - Chronic disease seen mostly in patients with underlying lung disease
    - Pleural thickening and apical cavitary lesions are common
    - Clinical and radiographic findings resemble those seen in tuberculosis and sarcoidosis
    - Mycobacterial infection, aspergilloma, blastomycosis, chronic or recurrent bacterial pneumonia may develop in areas of lung damaged by chronic pulmonary histoplasmosis and should be excluded in work-up
  - Extrapulmonary manifestations
    - Granulomatous mediastinitis: Enlarged caseous mediastinal lymph nodes
    - Fibrosing (sclerosing) mediastinitis: Following infection of mediastinal lymph nodes, excessive fibrosis progressively develops and envelops structures of mediastinum
    - Broncholithiasis: Occurs when calcified node erodes into bronchus, causing obstruction, inflammation, and bronchial scarring
- Disseminated histoplasmosis mostly in immunocompromised patients and can involve virtually any organ system
  - Adrenal involvement: Relatively common (up to 80-90% in studies)
    - Patients with adrenal masses, adrenal insufficiency, or electrolyte imbalances should have disseminated histoplasmosis excluded in work-up
  - Gastrointestinal involvement: Relatively common (up to 70% in studies) but rarely produces clinical symptoms
  - Skin involvement: Seen in up to 15% of cases in studies; more common in patients with AIDS
  - Central nervous system (CNS) involvement: Seen in 5-20% of cases; more common in patients with underlying immunosuppression

Laboratory Tests

- Antigen detection
  - Enzyme immunoassays are available to detect *Histoplasma* antigens in urine or serum
  - Sensitivity: 90% in disseminated disease and 75% in acute pulmonary disease
  - False-positive results reported with other endemic mycoses, e.g., blastomycosis, paracoccidioidomycosis, penicilliosis
  - Positive serum antigen assay but negative urine assay are uncommon; false-positive serum assay has been reported in transplant recipients who received rabbit antithymocyte globulin
- Serologic antibody detection
  - Antibodies may take 2-6 weeks to appear in circulation; therefore, serologic assays are less useful for detecting acute infection and in immunosuppressed patients, who mount poor immune response
  - Useful in CSF specimens with negative culture, as presence of antibodies allows one to make diagnosis of *Histoplasma* meningitis in proper clinical context

- Complement fixation test: Cross reactions have been reported in cases caused by *Blastomyces dermatitidis* (up to 40%), *Coccidioides immitis* (up to 16%), and *Aspergillus fumigatus* (up to 2%)
- Immunodiffusion assay: Detects H and M antigens from mycelial and yeast phases; ~ 80% sensitive; more specific than complement fixation assay
- False-positive results for both complement fixation and immunodiffusion have also been reported in cases of tuberculosis

- Molecular testing: RT-PCR and broad-spectrum (ITS, 28S rRNA and mNGS) assays

Treatment

- Most infections in immunocompetent patients are self-limited with no therapy required
- Treatment needed for immunocompromised patients and those who are exposed to large fungal inoculum
- Antifungal regimens vary according to according to clinical presentation
- In general, itraconazole is preferred for mild to moderate histoplasmosis, and amphotericin B is needed in treating disseminated, CNS, or severe infections

Prognosis

- Most infections are asymptomatic and self-limited in immunocompetent individuals
- Immunocompromised patients are more likely to present with disseminated disease; pulmonary disease can progress rapidly to involve multiple lung lobes; patients can develop acute respiratory distress syndrome within days if not treated

IMAGING

Radiographic Findings

- Pulmonary histoplasmosis
  - Most common: Diffuse reticulonodular pulmonary infiltrates
  - Coalescence of nodules can be seen in discrete areas of lung
  - Cavitations are mostly seen in chronic cavitary pulmonary histoplasmosis
  - Mediastinal or hilar lymphadenopathy often present
- Extrapulmonary disease
  - Radiographic findings are highly variable and not specific

MICROBIOLOGY

Culture

- Sabouraud dextrose agar or brain-heart infusion agar
- Organisms grow slowly; 4-6 weeks are needed to determine whether culture is positive or negative
- At 25-30 °C, colonies are white to brown with dense cottony surface; septate hyphae with smooth, pear-shaped microconidia (2-5 μm) present early; thick-walled, round macroconidia (7-15 μm) covered with short cylindrical (tuberculate) projections with older cultures
- At 37 °C, white, moist yeast-like colonies with small, oval budding cells
- Lysis-centrifugation is needed to release organisms from phagocytic cells in clinical samples
- Yield from culture is generally good when respiratory samples are taken from patients who have chronic cavitary pulmonary histoplasmosis, acute pulmonary histoplasmosis, or disseminated infection following exposure to large fungal inoculum
- Cultures are usually negative in respiratory samples taken from cases of mild pulmonary infection, granulomatous mediastinitis, mediastinal fibrosis

MACROSCOPIC

General Features

- Heavy infections may cause marked enlargement of involved organs, e.g., lymph nodes, adrenal glands, liver, spleen

MICROSCOPIC

Histologic Features

- Oval small yeast cells (2-4 μm in diameter) with narrow-based budding
- Not encapsulated; however, it may appear to be surrounded by clear zone/pseudocapsule in tissue
- Yeasts tend to cluster and reproduce within macrophages, monocytes, and occasionally neutrophils
- When yeasts are released from cells into surrounding tissue, such as alveoli in lungs, they often remain in clusters
- Acute histoplasmosis
  - Nodular areas of parenchymal and vascular necrosis associated with lymphohistiocytic vasculitis
  - Scattered small epithelioid and giant cell granulomas with small yeasts in parenchyma can be present
  - Over time, granulomas may turn into fibrocaseous nodules, which can become calcified
- Chronic histoplasmosis
  - Granulomatous inflammation with central necrosis and occasionally calcification
  - Yeasts are usually present in necrotic calcified material, which can be lost during tissue processing
- Disseminated disease: Sheets of macrophages parasitized with yeast cells can be seen
- Organisms may primarily be seen extracellularly, making it more difficult to make diagnosis

ANCILLARY TESTS

Histochemistry

- Yeast cells are positive for Gomori methenamine silver (GMS) and periodic acid-Schiff (PAS) stains (may be weaker); staining is best on extracellular yeast; intracellular yeast may not pick up silver staining to same degree
- Negative for Gram and Fontana-Masson stains

Molecular Diagnostics

- Chemiluminescent DNA probe for *H. capsulatum* (AccuProbe; GenProbe, Inc.)
  - Can be used as confirmatory test for definitive identification in culture
  - Highly sensitive (up to 100%) and specific (up to 100%)
  - False-positive tests have been reported with *Chrysosporium* spp. but are rare
- PCR-based assays

- Commercially available for testing CSF, respiratory, and tissue samples
- Can be detected in formalin-fixed, paraffin-embedded (FFPE) tissue by either universal fungal [internal transcribed spacer (ITS)] assays or specific *Histoplasma* spp. assays

DIFFERENTIAL DIAGNOSIS

Candidiasis

- *Histoplasma* spp. can be confused easily with *Candida* spp., particularly *Nakaseomyces glabratus* (formerly *Candida glabrata*), due to similar size and lack of pseudohyphae
- *Candida* spp. are gram positive, exhibit more size variability, lack pseudocapsule on H&E stain, and predominantly produce neutrophilic inflammation rather than granulomatous reaction seen with histoplasmosis

Cryptococcosis

- Cryptococcal yeast cells are rounder and exhibit more size variation than *Histoplasma* spp.
- Have capsules that are positive for mucicarmine; capsule-deficient cryptococci, however, can be mistaken for *Histoplasma* yeast cells
- Positive for Fontana-Masson, which stains melanin in their cell walls, whereas *Histoplasma* spp. are negative for melanin stains

Coccidioidomycosis

- *Coccidioides* endospores are about same size as *Histoplasma* spp., but they are usually present within intact spherule or associated with ruptured spherule in surrounding tissue
- *Coccidioides* endospores show no budding, while *Histoplasma* spp. exhibit narrow-based budding

Blastomycosis

- *Blastomyces* yeast cells are larger than *Histoplasma capsulatum* and have broad-based rather than narrow-based budding
- *Histoplasma duboisii* yeast forms are similar in size to *Blastomyces spp.* and show broad-based budding, making it great mimic; exposure history and cultures/molecular testing to distinguish

Pneumocystosis

- *Pneumocystis jirovecii* cysts lacks budding and usually have focal thickenings in cyst wall, which stain as dark dots not seen with *Histoplasma* spp.

Talaromycosis (Formerly Penicilliosis)

- *Talaromyces* (formerly *Penicillium*) *marneffei* yeast-like cells within macrophages or monocytes may appear as *Histoplasma* spp., but in contrast to *Histoplasma* spp., *T. marneffei* lacks budding, reproduces by binary fission, and shows prominent central septum
- Extracellular *T. marneffei* cells are larger and may manifest several septa

Protozoan Diseases

- Leishmaniasis, toxoplasmosis, Chagas disease
  - Protozoa are smaller and do not show halo produced by fungal cell wall, as would be seen with *Histoplasma* spp. on H&E stain
  - Protozoa show no budding, and they are negative for GMS or PAS stains
- Paranuclear bar-shaped kinetoplasts should be observed with amastigotes of *Leishmania* spp. and *Trypanosoma cruzi* (under oil immersion) but not with *Histoplasma* spp.

Emergomycosis

- *Emergomyces* is recently described dimorphic fungus with yeast cells of similar size to *Histoplasma* spp. and narrow-based budding, practically undistinguishable on tissue sections from *Histoplasma capsulatum*
- Should be suspected in patients with AIDS and high-burden cutaneous disease

SELECTED REFERENCES

1. Barros N et al: Pulmonary histoplasmosis: a clinical update. J Fungi (Basel). 9(2), 2023
2. Reddy DL et al: Review: emergomycosis. J Mycol Med. 33(1):101313, 2023
3. Valdez AF et al: Pathogenicity & virulence of Histoplasma capsulatum - a multifaceted organism adapted to intracellular environments. Virulence. 13(1):1900-19, 2022
4. Azar MM et al: Current concepts in the epidemiology, diagnosis, and management of histoplasmosis syndromes. Semin Respir Crit Care Med. 41(1):13-30, 2020
5. Mittal J et al: Histoplasma capsulatum: mechanisms for pathogenesis. Curr Top Microbiol Immunol. 422:157-91, 2019
6. Armstrong PA et al: Multistate epidemiology of histoplasmosis, United States, 2011-2014 Emerg Infect Dis. 24(3):425-31, 2018
7. Azar MM et al: Laboratory diagnostics for histoplasmosis. J Clin Microbiol. 55(6):1612-20, 2017
8. Richer SM et al: Improved diagnosis of acute pulmonary histoplasmosis by combining antigen and antibody detection. Clin Infect Dis. 62(7):896-902, 2016
9. Wheat LJ et al: Histoplasmosis. Infect Dis Clin North Am. 30(1):207-27, 2016
10. Couturier MR et al: Urine antigen tests for the diagnosis of respiratory infections: legionellosis, histoplasmosis, pneumococcal pneumonia. Clin Lab Med. 34(2):219-36, 2014
11. Murthy JM et al: Fungal infections of the central nervous system. Handb Clin Neurol. 121:1383-401, 2014
12. Sizemore TC: Rheumatologic manifestations of histoplasmosis: a review. Rheumatol Int. 33(12):2963-5, 2013
13. Gupta AO et al: Immune reconstitution syndrome and fungal infections. Curr Opin Infect Dis. 24(6):527-33, 2011

(Left) *Mean Histoplasma site suitability score by USA ZIP code is shown. Red reflects greater histoplasmosis suitability and green reflects less suitability. Data for geographic regions in west is due to limited surface water data. [Courtesy Maiga AW et al: Emerging Infectious Diseases. 24(10):1835-9, 2018.]* (Right) *This frontal view of a Sabouraud dextrose culture plate shows a large white, smoothly textured colony identified as Histoplasma capsulatum. (Courtesy L. Georg, MD, CDC/PHIL.)*

USA Environmental Sources

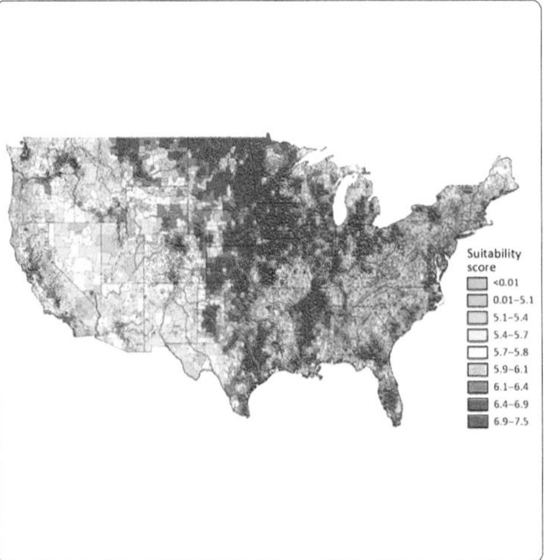

H. capsulatum Isolated in Culture

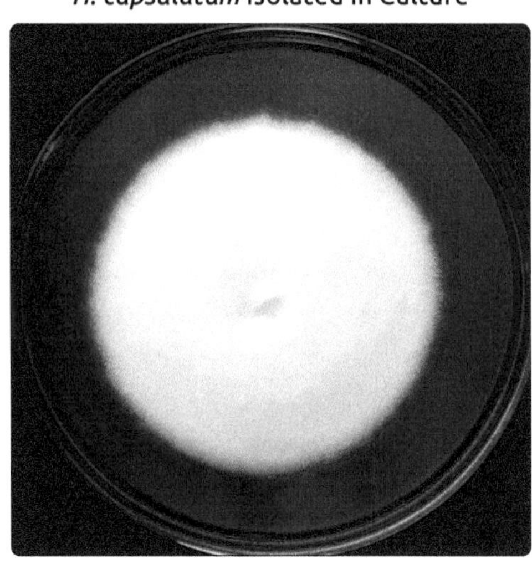

(Left) *High magnification of a lymph node section on H&E stain shows numerous small round to oval yeast forms* → *in clusters. Follow-up Gram stain was negative, consistent with Histoplasma spp.* (Right) *Low magnification of a lung section on H&E stain shows confluent granulomatous inflammation* ⇨ *with necrosis* → *in a patient with acute pulmonary histoplasmosis.*

Histoplasma Lymphadenitis

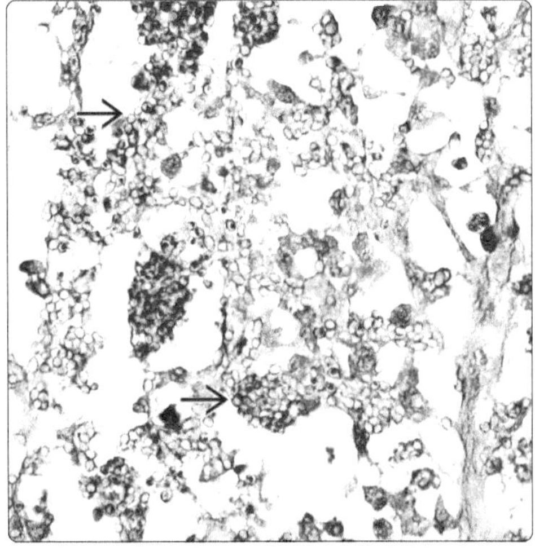

Granulomatous Inflammation

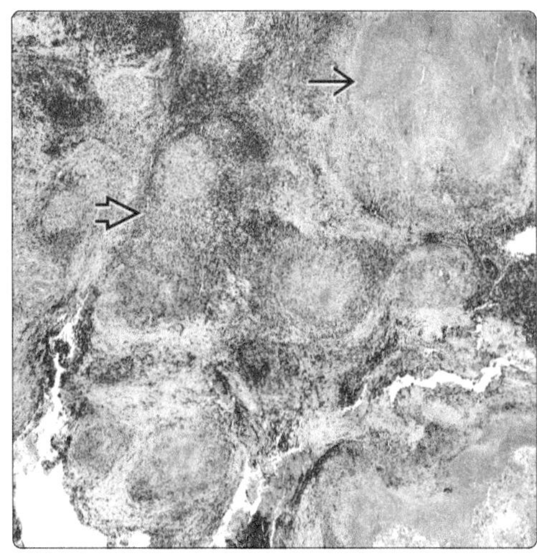

(Left) *High magnification of a lung section on H&E stain shows multiple macrophages and monocytes fully packed with yeast cells* → *in the alveolar spaces in a patient with acute histoplasmosis.* (Right) *High magnification of a lung section on Gram stain shows intracellular* → *and extracellular* ⇨ *round gram-negative yeast cell clusters, consistent with histoplasmosis.*

Alveolar Macrophages

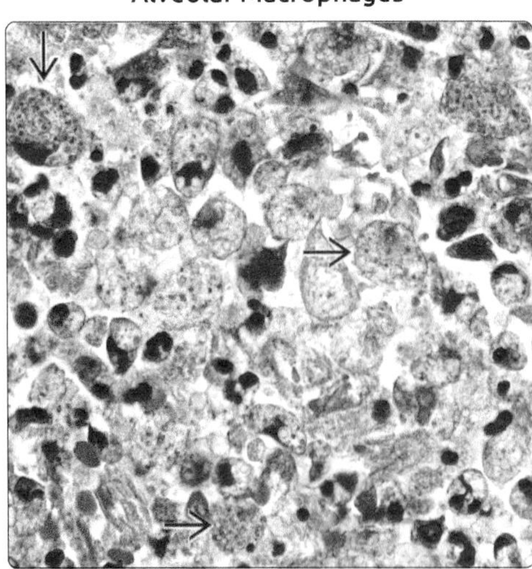

Negative Gram Stain

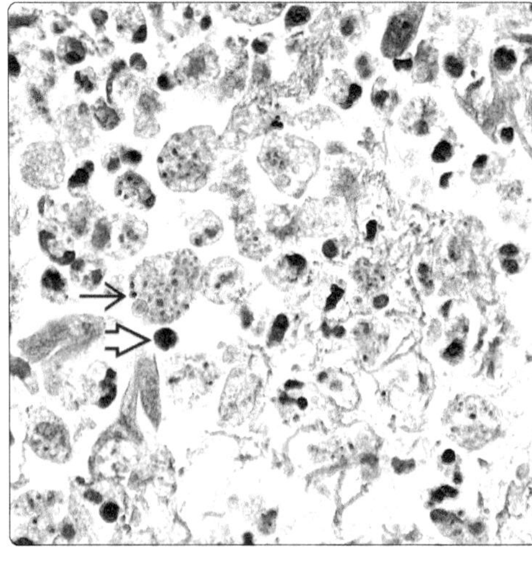

PAS Stain

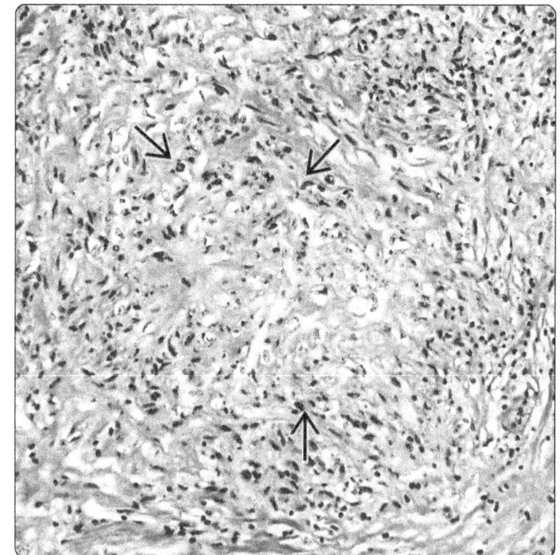

GMS Stain

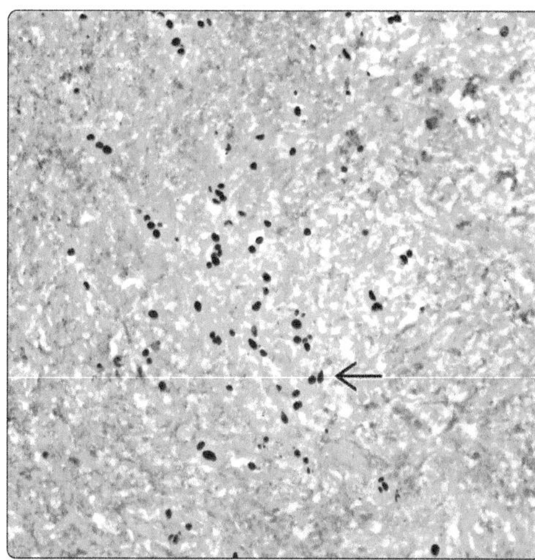

(Left) *This tenosynovial biopsy shows scattered minute clusters of small yeasts* ➡ *on PAS stain, putting histoplasmosis in the differential. The small size of the nonpigmented yeasts makes it challenging to detect on H&E stain.* **(Right)** *GMS stain shows small, variably sized yeast forms with occasional budding* ➡*. A pale halo appears to surround some of the yeast cells, suggesting a pseudocapsule or a capsule, suggesting Cryptococcus spp. A negative Fontana-Masson stain would exclude Cryptococcus spp.*

GMS Stain

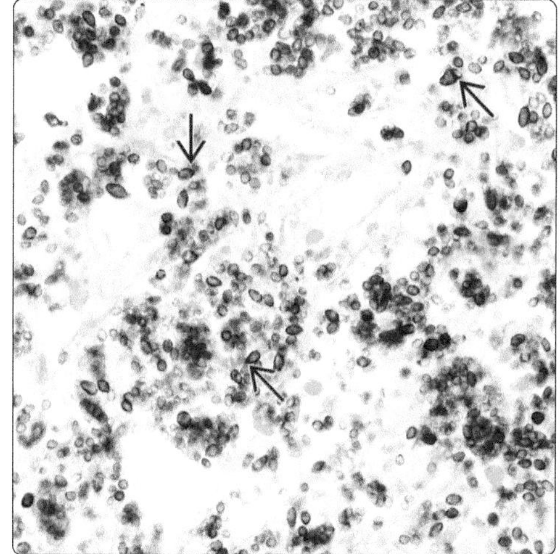

H. duboisii

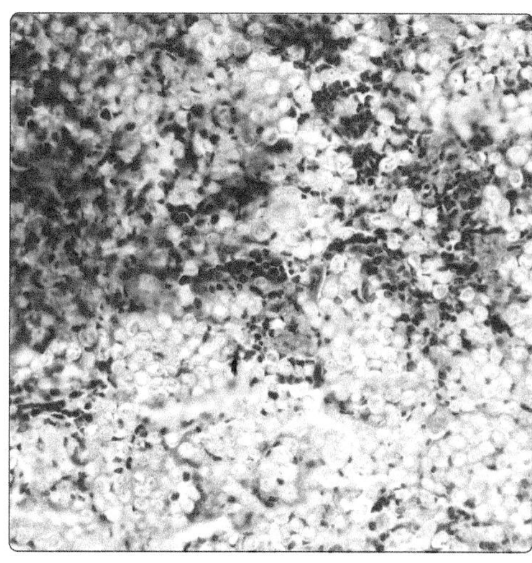

(Left) *High magnification of this tissue section reveals numerous small yeast forms highlighted by GMS stain. A few of the yeast cells appear to exhibit narrow-based budding* ➡*.* **(Right)** *Abundant round yeast forms, larger than those of H. capsulatum, are present and virtually replacing the lymph node parenchyma in a patient with AIDS and African histoplasmosis.*

Cutaneous Histoplasmosis

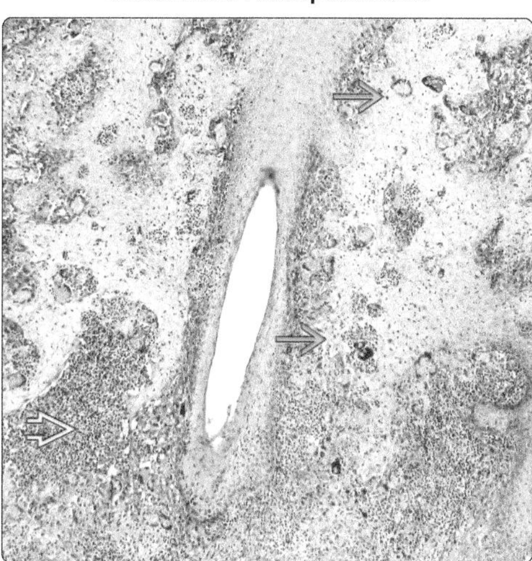

Cutaneous Histoplasmosis

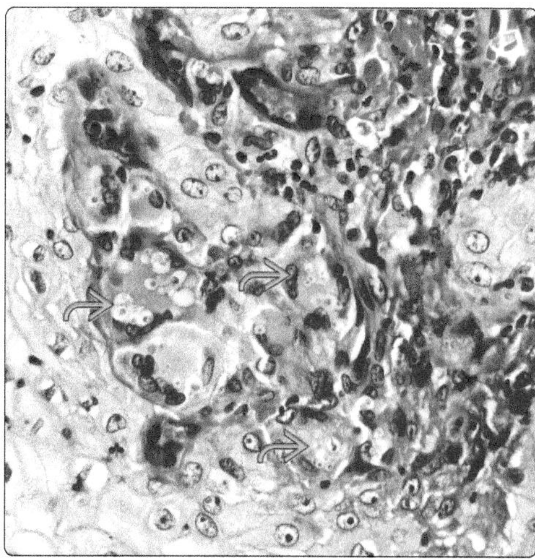

(Left) *Florid pseudocarcinomatous (pseudoepitheliomatous) epidermal hyperplasia is present in cutaneous histoplasmosis. The presence of suppurative inflammation* ➡ *with scattered giant cells* ➡ *should be a clue to fungal infection and not carcinoma.* **(Right)** *Small yeasts with clear halos* ➡ *in the cytoplasm of giant cells are readily seen upon careful examination of H&E-stained sections in cutaneous histoplasmosis.*

Lobomycosis

KEY FACTS

ETIOLOGY/PATHOGENESIS

- Infection with *Paracoccidioides lobogeorgii* (previously *Lacazia loboi*), uncultivable mammalian fungal pathogen, phylogenetically closely related to other, cultivable *Paracoccidioides* species

CLINICAL ISSUES

- Endemic to Central and South America around Amazon basin
- Characteristic cutaneous infections without visceral involvement or systemic dissemination
- Slow-growing, asymptomatic, longstanding verrucous papules and exophytic or subcutaneous nodules resembling keloid scars; ear lobe and extremity involvement is characteristic
- Fungus cannot be cultured in vitro
- Molecular testing with PCR of ITS region or gp43
- Treated with surgical excision and systemic antifungals

MICROSCOPIC

- Diffuse dermal granulomatous inflammation
- Large (15- to 20-μm) spherical, semirefractile yeast forms within sclerotic stroma, readily apparent on H&E, and highlighted by PAS-D and GMS stains

TOP DIFFERENTIAL DIAGNOSES

- Paracoccidioidomycosis: Primarily caused by *Paracoccidioides brasiliensis* and *Paracoccidiodes lutzii*; multiple budding with characteristic captain's wheel appearance, mucosal involvement characteristic
- Blastomycosis: Large yeast forms with characteristic budding with broad neck producing "shoe-print" silhouette
- Histoplasmosis: Small ovoid yeast forms with narrow neck budding within sclerotic mass or necrotizing granulomas

Lobomycosis (*Paracoccidioides lobogeorgii*)

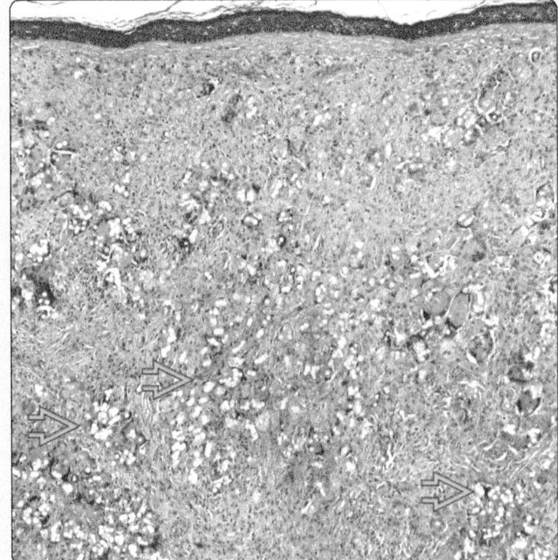

Lobomycosis GMS Stain

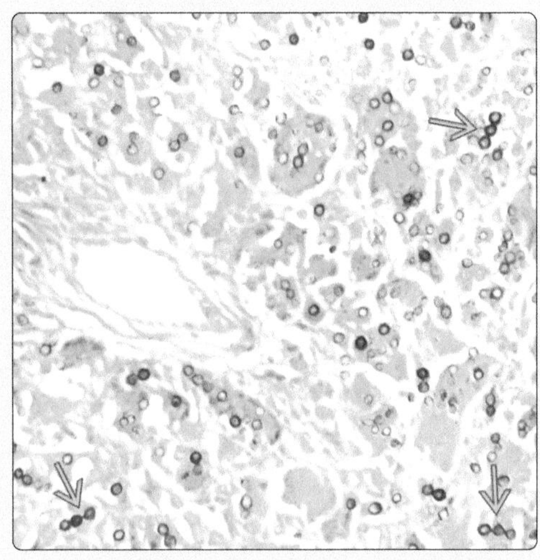

(Left) *Diffuse dermal granulomatous inflammation with evenly dispersed clear ⇨ "vacuoles" is noted on low magnification.* **(Right)** *Several round, argyrophilic yeast forms up to 12 μm in diameter, frequently arranged in short chains ⇨, are shown in this skin biopsy from a patient with lobomycosis. (Courtesy M. Hicklin, CDC/PHIL.)*

Lobomycosis: Chains of Yeast

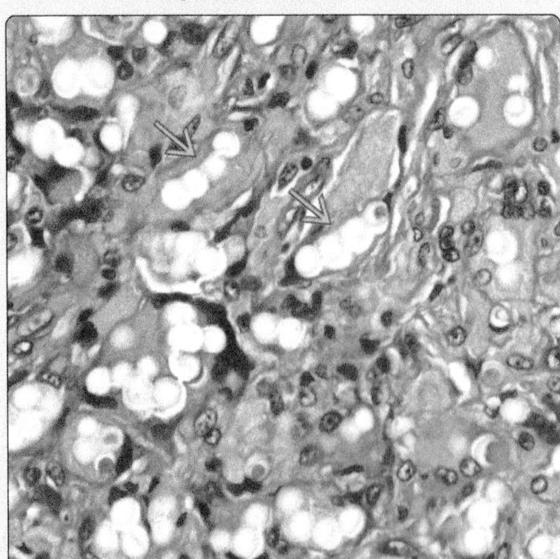

Lobomycosis: Connecting Bridges

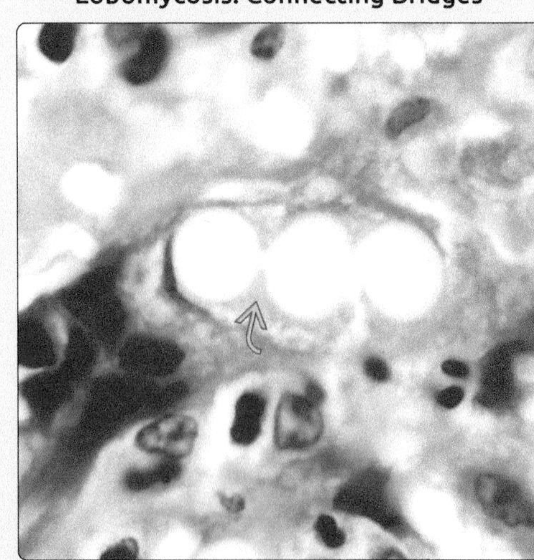

(Left) *Numerous spherical refractile yeast forms are present in this ear biopsy from a patient with lobomycosis. Note the typical catenate beaded distribution ⇨.* **(Right)** *Thin, small bridges ⇨ connecting birefringent yeasts in chains are characteristic.*

TERMINOLOGY

Synonyms

- Keloidal blastomycosis, lacaziosis, (Jorge) Lobo disease, miraip, piraip, Caiabi leprosy, paracoccidioidomycosis lobogeorgii

Definitions

- From para (beside) + *Coccidioides* (another dimorphic fungus) + loboi (Jorge Lobo, who described disease)

ETIOLOGY/PATHOGENESIS

Infectious Agents

- Infection with *Paracoccidioides lobogeorgii* (previously *Lacazia loboi*), uncultivable mammalian fungal pathogen, phylogenetically closely related to other, cultivable *Paracoccidioides* species; presumed implantation mycosis due to traumatic inoculation
- Putative dimorphic fungus with mycelial form in nature switching from hyphae to yeast in mammalian/human hosts
- Previously thought to cause disease in dolphins, but different species causing disease in dolphins now established (*Paracoccidioides cetii*)
- Characteristic cutaneous infections without visceral involvement or systemic dissemination

CLINICAL ISSUES

Epidemiology

- Endemic to Central and South America around Amazon basin (Mexico, Costa Rica, Panama, Brazil, Colombia, Venezuela, Guyana, Ecuador, Peru)
- Unknown natural reservoir and complete life cycle
- Higher prevalence in men, particularly forest rangers, rubber tappers, bushmen, miners, and tropical forest inhabitants

Presentation

- Slow-growing, asymptomatic, longstanding (typically many years) verrucous papules and exophytic or subcutaneous nodules resembling keloid scars
- Incubation period estimated at 3 months to several years; progressive disease over decades is typical
- Involvement of ear lobes and extremities is characteristic (pinna in 38% of cases, upper limbs 28%, and lower limbs 22% according to one study)
- No mucosal involvement or disseminated disease with visceral involvement ever reported

Laboratory Tests

- Fungus cannot be cultured in vitro
- Direct identification on tissue or cytologic preparations based on presence of characteristic spherical, refractile yeast forms forming chains is gold standard
- Molecular testing with PCR of ITS region or gp43

Treatment

- Surgical excision and systemic antifungals (anecdotal improvement with posaconazole or clofazimine and itraconazole for months to years)

Prognosis

- Regional lymph nodes may be affected, but disseminated cutaneous disease is rare, and systemic involvement has not been described
- Protracted course over many years is common with consequent deformities affecting quality of life and decreasing work productivity

MICROSCOPIC

Histologic Features

- Diffuse dermal granulomatous inflammation with multiple round yeast forms readily apparent on H&E
- Large (15- to 20-μm) spherical, semirefractile yeast forms within sclerotic stroma
- Small bridges between yeast forming "pop-bead" linear chains

ANCILLARY TESTS

Special Stains

- Yeast highlighted by PAS and GMS stains

DIFFERENTIAL DIAGNOSIS

Blastomycosis

- Large yeast forms with characteristic budding with broad neck producing "shoe-print" silhouette

Histoplasmosis

- Small ovoid yeast forms with narrow neck budding within sclerotic mass or necrotizing granulomas

Paracoccidioidomycosis

- Primarily caused by *Paracoccidioides brasiliensis* and *Paracoccidioides lutzii*, less commonly by *Paracoccidioides americana*, *Paracoccidioides restrepiensis*, and *Paracoccidioides venezuelensis*
- Multiple budding with characteristic captain's wheel appearance, mucosal involvement characteristic

SELECTED REFERENCES

1. Vilela R et al: A taxonomic review of the genus Paracoccidioides, with focus on the uncultivable species. PLoS Negl Trop Dis. 17(4):e0011220, 2023
2. Vilela R et al: The taxonomy of two uncultivated fungal mammalian pathogens is revealed through phylogeny and population genetic analyses. Sci Rep. 11(1):18119, 2021
3. Pech-Ortiz L et al: Lacaziosis (lobomycosis) from southern Mexico: a case confirmed by molecular biology. Mycopathologia. 185(4):737-9, 2020
4. Arenas CM et al: Lobomycosis in Soldiers, Colombia. Emerg Infect Dis. 25(4):654-60, 2019
5. Beltrame A et al: Case report: molecular confirmation of lobomycosis in an Italian Traveler acquired in the Amazon region of Venezuela. Am J Trop Med Hyg. 97(6):1757-60, 2017
6. Vilela R et al: Cutaneous granulomas in dolphins caused by novel uncultivated Paracoccidioides brasiliensis. Emerg Infect Dis. 22(12):2063-9, 2016
7. Francesconi VA et al: Lobomycosis: epidemiology, clinical presentation, and management options. Ther Clin Risk Manag. 10:851-60, 2014
8. Vilela R et al: Molecular study of archival fungal strains isolated from cases of lacaziosis (Jorge Lobo's disease). Mycoses. 50(6):470-4, 2007
9. Herr RA et al: Phylogenetic analysis of Lacazia loboi places this previously uncharacterized pathogen within the dimorphic Onygenales. J Clin Microbiol. 39(1):309-14, 2001

Paracoccidioidomycosis

KEY FACTS

ETIOLOGY/PATHOGENESIS

- Infection with thermally dimorphic fungi *Paracoccidioides* spp. via inhalation of spores; rarely skin abrasions or trauma

CLINICAL ISSUES

- Present in Central and South America
- More common in men than women
- Juvenile (acute/subacute) form: Skin lesions, lymphadenopathy, hepatosplenomegaly, anemia, eosinophilia
- Chronic form: Lung, mucosal, skin, and CNS involvement; associated with fever, malaise, weight loss, and lymphadenopathy

MICROBIOLOGY

- Yeast at 37 °C: Oval to round yeast with narrow-based, budding conidia
- Mycelial at 22-26 °C: Septate, thin hyphae

MICROSCOPIC

- Large, round yeast cells (20-30 μm) with multiple narrow-based, budding yeasts (ship's wheel appearance)
- Yeast highlighted by GMS and PAS-D stains
- Granulomatous inflammation, multinucleated giant cells, lymphocytes, and few neutrophils
- Fibrosis with chronic infections

TOP DIFFERENTIAL DIAGNOSES

- Blastomycosis: Large yeast with single broad-based budding
- Histoplasmosis: Smaller yeast forms with single narrow-based budding
- Cryptococcosis: Narrow-based budding yeast with mucicarmine-positive capsule
- Tuberculosis: Necrotizing granulomas with acid-fast bacilli
- Sarcoidosis: Noncaseating granulomas with scattered giant cells and asteroid bodies

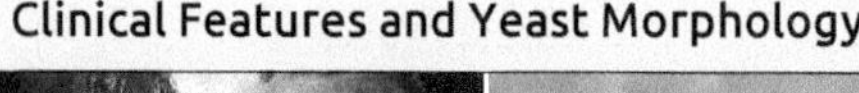

Clinical Features and Yeast Morphology

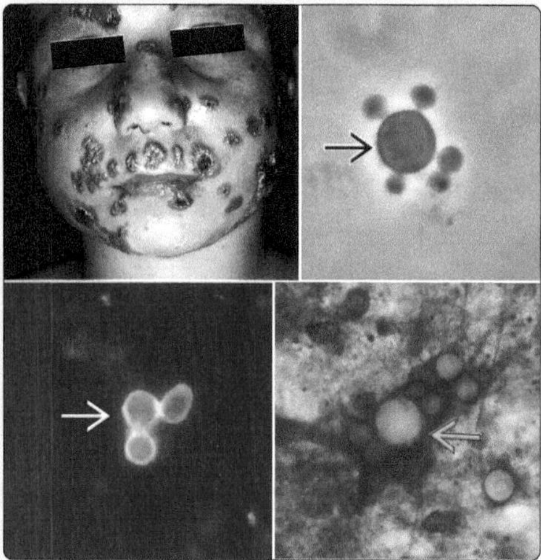

Granulomatous Inflammation

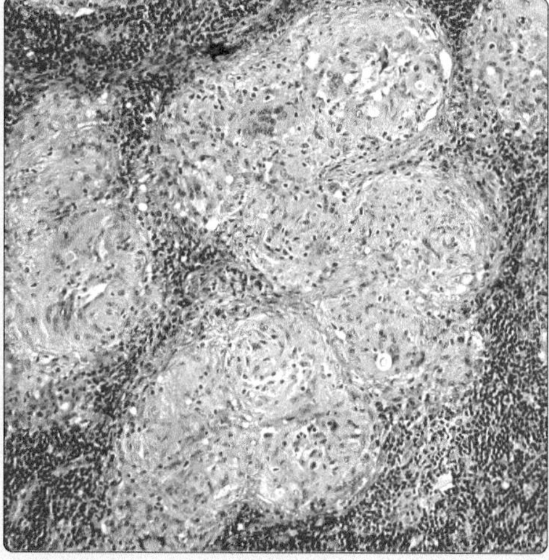

(Left) *Multiple cutaneous lesions are present in this pediatric patient with paracoccidioidomycosis. Characteristic appearance of Paracoccidioides sp. yeast forms are shown by sputum stained with lactophenol cotton blue ➾, pus with fluorescent antibody staining ➡, and brain tissue smear stained with H&E ➾. (Courtesy Dr. Castro, Dr. Harden, and Dr. Georg, CDC/PHIL.)* **(Right)** *Nonnecrotizing granulomatous lymphadenitis is present in a fatal case of paracoccidioidomycosis.*

Multinucleated Giant Cells

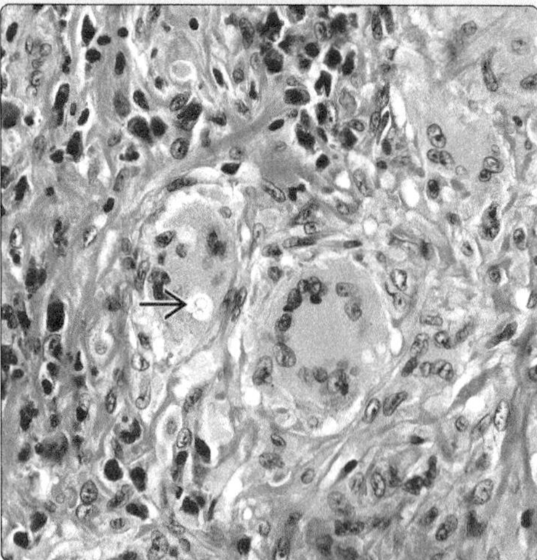

***P. braziliensis*: GMS Stain**

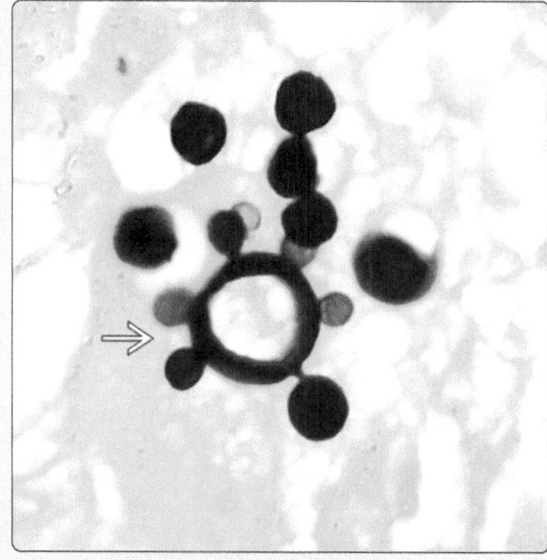

(Left) *Paracoccidioides braziliensis yeast can be seen within multinucleated giant cells and appear white or clear and may show budding ➾.* **(Right)** *Grocott methenamine silver stain of brain tissue shows multiple budding yeast forms of P. braziliensis, including the characteristic ship's wheel appearance ➡.*

TERMINOLOGY

Synonyms

- South American or Brazilian blastomycosis, Lutz-Splendore-de Almeida disease

Definitions

- Derived from "para" (beside) and "coccidioides" (berry)

ETIOLOGY/PATHOGENESIS

Infectious Agents

- Infection with thermally dimorphic fungi in *Paracoccidioides* genus (*P. brasiliensis, P. lutziivia, P. americana, P. restrepiensis, P. venezuelensis*) via inhalation of spores; rarely through skin abrasions or trauma
- Yeasts multiply and spread to mediastinal lymph nodes and become dormant; immunosuppression leads to reactivation with spread via lymphatics and blood to other organs, including adrenal glands, liver, skin, and CNS

CLINICAL ISSUES

Epidemiology

- Present in Central and South America, including Brazil (80% of cases), Columbia, Venezuela, Argentina, and Ecuador
- More common in men possibly due to occupational soil exposure; estradiol may be protective

Presentation

- Typically asymptomatic lung infection following inhalation; positive intradermal paracoccidioidin test
- Juvenile form (acute/subacute): < 10% of all infections, most common < age 30 years; eosinophilia, anemia, skin lesions, lymphadenopathy, hepatosplenomegaly
- Chronic form: Majority have lung involvement; associated with fever, malaise, weight loss, and lymphadenopathy; skin lesions, mucosal involvement, and CNS involvement (typically with HIV coinfection)

Laboratory Tests

- Quantitative immunodiffusion testing and counterimmunoelectrophoresis have high sensitivity and specificity but may be negative for *P. lutziivia*
- Skin scrapings can be examined using KOH preparation

Treatment

- Itraconazole or other azoles (mild to moderate disease)
- Amphotericin B (severe disease, including CNS involvement)
- Terbinafine

Prognosis

- With treatment, vast majority of patients survive
- Sequelae with high morbidity, including pulmonary fibrosis and Addison disease (following adrenal involvement)

IMAGING

CT Findings

- Pulmonary ground-glass opacities (alveolar and interstitial infiltrates), reversed halo sign
- Fibrosis and emphysematous changes may be present in chronic disease

MICROBIOLOGY

Fungal Features

- Yeast form at 37 °C: Oval to round yeast with narrow-based, budding conidia (ship's wheel appearance)
- Mycelial form at 22-26 °C: Septate, thin hyphae (sometimes with conidia)
- White, compact colonies grow on Sabouraud dextrose agar [slow growing (~ 20 days)]

MICROSCOPIC

Histologic Features

- Large, round yeast cells (20-30 μm) with multiple narrow-based, budding yeasts (ship's wheel appearance)
- Granulomatous inflammation with multinucleated giant cells surrounding organisms, lymphocytes, and few neutrophils; fibrosis with chronic infections
- Immunosuppressed may have ill-formed granulomas, foamy histiocytes, and few lymphocytes with greater numbers or organisms
- Skin and oropharyngeal mucosa: Pseudoepitheliomatous hyperplasia, intraepithelial neutrophil microabscesses

ANCILLARY TESTS

Histochemistry

- Methenamine silver stain or PAS-D highlight organisms

DIFFERENTIAL DIAGNOSIS

Blastomycosis

- Large yeast with single broad-based budding

Histoplasmosis

- Smaller yeast forms with single narrow-based budding

Cryptococcosis

- Narrow-based budding yeast with mucicarmine-positive capsule

Tuberculosis

- Necrotizing granulomas with acid-fast bacilli

Noninfectious Causes

- Wegener granulomatosis: Coagulative necrosis with angiitis and palisading histiocytes
- Sarcoidosis: Noncaseating granulomas with scattered giant cells and asteroid bodies
- Lymphoma: Monotonous lymphocytic infiltrate replacing normal lymph node architecture

SELECTED REFERENCES

1. Rodrigues AM et al: Paracoccidioides and paracoccidioidomycosis in the 21st Century. Mycopathologia. 188(1-2):129-33, 2023
2. Vilela R et al: A taxonomic review of the genus Paracoccidioides, with focus on the uncultivable species. PLoS Negl Trop Dis. 17(4):e0011220, 2023
3. Hahn RC et al: Paracoccidioidomycosis: current status and future trends. Clin Microbiol Rev. 35(4):e0023321, 2022
4. de Almeida SM et al: Autopsy and biopsy study of paracoccidioidomycosis and neuroparacoccidioidomycosis with and without HIV co-infection. Mycoses. 61(4):237-44, 2018

Pneumocystosis

KEY FACTS

ETIOLOGY/PATHOGENESIS

- *Pneumocystis jiroveci* is ubiquitous parasitic ascomycetous fungus causing opportunistic disease [i.e., *Pneumocystis* pneumonia (PCP)] associated with HIV infection, immunodeficiencies, and malnourishment
- Asexual trophic (1- to 4-µm) and sexually reproductive cystic (3- to 5-µm) forms

CLINICAL ISSUES

- Presents with dyspnea, dry cough, fever, usually of > 4 weeks duration
- High mortality rate (20-80%) regardless of HIV status
- Immunofluorescence (gold standard), quantitative real-time PCR, serum (1,3)-β-D-glucan
- Cannot be cultured in vitro; serology not useful

IMAGING

- Bat wing appearance on chest x-ray of diffuse bilateral perihilar infiltrates (ground-glass opacities)

MICROSCOPIC

- Intraalveolar eosinophilic foamy proteinaceous material forming alveolar casts, variable interstitial plasma cells, reactive pneumocyte hyperplasia; granulomatous inflammation less common
- GMS stain highlights uniformly sized nonbudding cyst forms (3-5 µm); spherical, boat or crushed ping-pong ball shape with intracystic bodies

TOP DIFFERENTIAL DIAGNOSES

- Noninfectious (e.g., pulmonary edema, alveolar lipoproteinosis): Negative IFA or molecular testing, nonresponsive to antimicrobials, often immunocompetent
- Cryptococcosis: Narrow-based budding yeast forms; Fontana-Masson and mucicarmine (capsule) positive
- Histoplasmosis: Small yeast with narrow based budding, no internal basophilic dots
- Tuberculosis: Necrotizing granulomatous inflammation with positive AFB stain or mycobacterial culture

Pneumocystis jiroveci **Pneumonia**

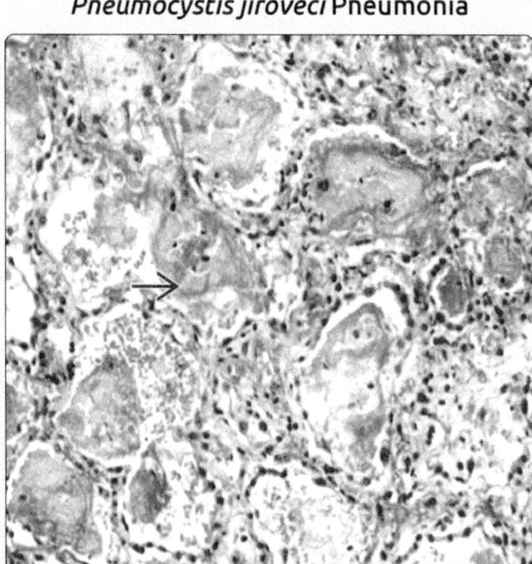

P. jirovecii **Cysts: GMS Stain**

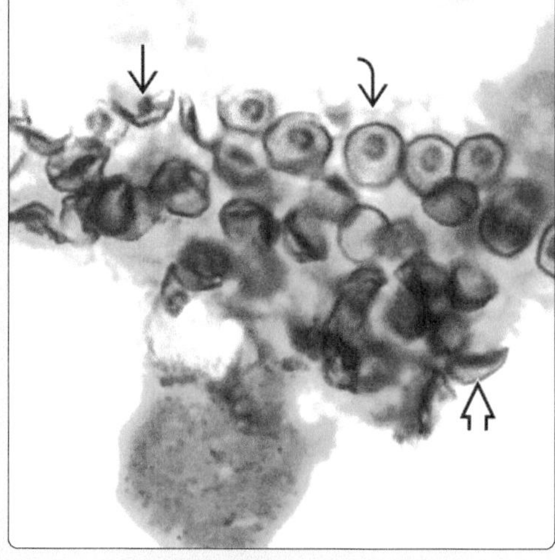

(Left) *The typical appearance of the lung in Pneumocystis jiroveci infection is eosinophilic alveolar foamy plugging → with a limited interstitial inflammatory response. (Courtesy Franz von Lichtenberg Collection of Infectious Disease Pathology, BWH.)* **(Right)** *A bronchial washing with GMS stain demonstrates round ↷ to boat-shaped cysts ⇨ with nuclei adjacent to the cell wall →. (Courtesy R. Brynes, MD, CDC/PHIL.)*

P. jiroveci **Cysts: Immunofluorescence**

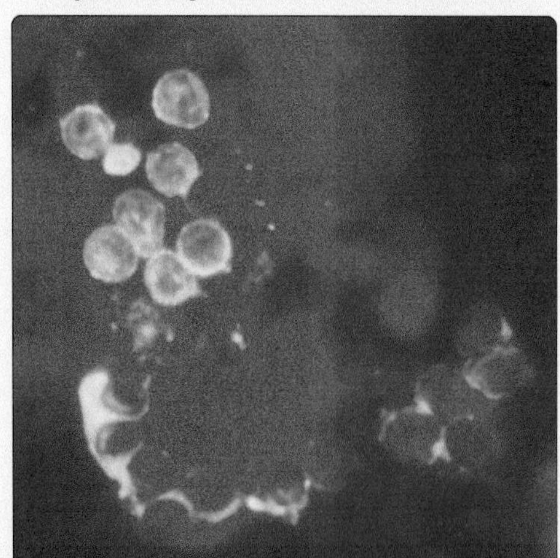

P. jiroveci **Cysts: Toluidine Blue Stain**

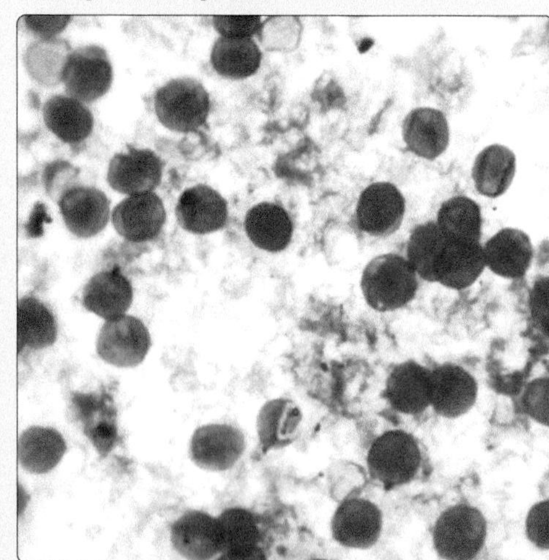

(Left) *P. jiroveci cysts are demonstrated in a bronchoalveolar lavage with immunofluorescence assay. [Courtesy W. Pieciak, Jr., SM (ASCP).]* **(Right)** *Numerous P. jirovecii cysts are highlighted by toluidine blue staining of this lung tissue smear. (Courtesy L. Norman, CDC/PHIL.)*

TERMINOLOGY

Synonyms

- *Pneumocystis* pneumonia (PCP), pneumocystosis, interstitial plasma-cell pneumonia

Definitions

- *Pneumocystis* derived from "pneumo" (breath) and "cystis" (anatomical sac), and *jiroveci* named after Otto Jirovec, who first described PCP in humans in 1952

ETIOLOGY/PATHOGENESIS

Infectious Agents

- Infection with *Pneumocystis jiroveci*, ubiquitous environmental airborne yeast-like parasitic fungus (initially thought to be protozoan)
- Biotrophic parasitic fungi that completes sexual cycle within host; no known nonhuman animal reservoir
- Ascus life-form: Sexually reproductive cystic forms (3-5 μm) (environmental, intraalveolar, transmissible)
- Trophozoite life-form: Asexual troph form (1-4 μm), most abundant form during infection (10:1)

CLINICAL ISSUES

Epidemiology

- Worldwide distribution, most individuals exposed by age 4
- Severe opportunistic disease in immunocompromised patients: HIV infection (CD4 count < 200 cells/mm^3), primary immunodeficiencies, post renal transplant, hematopoietic malignancies, and use of TNF inhibitors, malnourished or premature children

Presentation

- Moderate to severe pulmonary disease in immunocompromised: Dyspnea, dry cough, tachypnea, fever, usually of > 4 weeks duration; low oxygen saturations
- Rare extrapulmonary (lymph nodes, spleen, bone marrow) infection (< 3% of cases), can occur without concomitant pulmonary disease

Laboratory Tests

- Organism cannot be cultured in vitro but may be identified in direct smear of samples sent for fungal culture using calcofluor white (stains cyst wall)
- Direct identification (immunofluorescence) in sputum or bronchoalveolar lavage (rarely on tissue samples) is gold standard for diagnosis; less invasive samples (oral wash, nasopharyngeal aspirate) have reduced sensitivity but high specificity
- In HIV-negative patients or those taking chemoprophylaxis, organism burden may be low, reducing sensitivity of visual detection methods
- Molecular testing with quantitative real-time PCR has increased sensitivity and specificity; enhanced sensitivity results in increased identification of asymptomatic carriage (colonization) with unclear clinical significance
- Serum (1,3)-β-D-glucan can be elevated, found to be 91-95% sensitive and 65-86% specific

Treatment

- Resistant to most antifungals
- 1st-line treatment is trimethoprim-sulfamethoxazole (TMP-SMX); other options include pentamidine, dapsone, atovaquone
- Chemoprophylaxis (with TMP-SMX) recommended for HIV with CD4(+) count < 200, acquired or inherited immunodeficiencies; may develop PCP even while on prophylaxis

Prognosis

- Prognosis directly related to degree of immunosuppression
- Mortality rate can be high (20-80%)

IMAGING

Radiographic Findings

- Bat-wing appearance on chest x-ray of diffuse bilateral perihilar infiltrates (ground-glass opacities)

MICROSCOPIC

Histologic Features

- Intraalveolar eosinophilic foamy proteinaceous material with abundant trophic organisms forming alveolar casts, interstitial plasma cells, and reactive pneumocyte hyperplasia
- Granulomatous response can be present in immune reconstitution syndrome

Cytologic Features

- Alveolar proteinaceous casts appear blue-green, finely granular on Papanicolaou stain
- Both live and dead cyst forms detected in bronchial washings

ANCILLARY TESTS

Special Stains

- Cysts (asci) highlighted by GMS, toluidine blue, and calcofluor white stains
  - Refractile, 3- to 5-μm nonbudding spherical, boat or crushed ping-pong ball shape
  - Intracystic bodies can appear as 2 commas or parentheses or collapsed together as "central dot"
- Troph forms can be detected with Giemsa, Diff-Quik (Romanowsky), Wright-Giemsa, modified Papanicolaou, or Gram-Weigert stains
  - Stippled appearance in casts; less well defined

DIFFERENTIAL DIAGNOSIS

Noninfectious

- PCP eosinophilic exudate resembles pulmonary edema and alveolar lipoproteinosis
- Negative IFA or molecular testing; nonresponsive to antimicrobial therapy; often without coexisting HIV infection or other cause of immunosuppression

Cryptococcosis

- Narrow-based budding pleomorphic yeast forms (4-10 μm in diameter); Fontana-Masson positive with mucicarmine-positive capsule; confirm with cultures, PCR, antigen testing

Histoplasmosis

- Uniformly small yeasts (2-4 μm) with narrow-based budding lacking internal basophilic dots, typically associated with granulomatous inflammation; Confirm with culture, PCR, antigen testing

Tuberculosis

- Necrotizing granulomatous inflammation with positive AFB stain or mycobacterial culture
- Often demonstrates apical cavitary lesion radiologically

SELECTED REFERENCES

1. Szydłowicz M et al: Pneumocystis jirovecii colonization in preterm newborns with respiratory distress syndrome. J Infect Dis. 225(10):1807-10, 2022
2. Le Gal S et al: The shift from pulmonary colonization to Pneumocystis pneumonia. Med Mycol. 59(5):510-3, 2021
3. Tan SJ et al: Quantitative Pneumocystis jirovecii real-time PCR to differentiate disease from colonisation. Pathology. 53(7):896-901, 2021
4. Bateman M et al: Diagnosing Pneumocystis jirovecii pneumonia: a review of current methods and novel approaches. Med Mycol. 58(8):1015-28, 2020
5. Cissé OH et al: Humans are selectively exposed to Pneumocystis jirovecii. mBio. 11(2), 2020
6. Del Corpo O et al: Diagnostic accuracy of serum (1-3)-β-D-glucan for Pneumocystis jirovecii pneumonia: a systematic review and meta-analysis. Clin Microbiol Infect. 26(9):1137-43, 2020
7. Guegan H et al: Molecular diagnosis of Pneumocystis pneumonia in immunocompromised patients. Curr Opin Infect Dis. 32(4):314-21, 2019
8. Hauser PM et al: Is sex necessary for the proliferation and transmission of Pneumocystis? PLoS Pathog. 14(12):e1007409, 2018
9. Ma L et al: A molecular window into the biology and epidemiology of pneumocystis spp. Clin Microbiol Rev. 31(3), 2018
10. White PL et al: Therapy and management of pneumocystis jirovecii infection. J Fungi (Basel). 4(4), 2018
11. Rabodonirina M et al: Molecular evidence of interhuman transmission of Pneumocystis pneumonia among renal transplant recipients hospitalized with HIV-infected patients. Emerg Infect Dis. 10(10):1766-73, 2004
12. Powers CN: Diagnosis of infectious diseases: a cytopathologist's perspective. Clin Microbiol Rev. 11(2):341-65, 1998

Ultrastructural Features

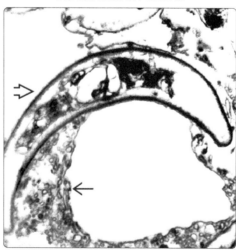

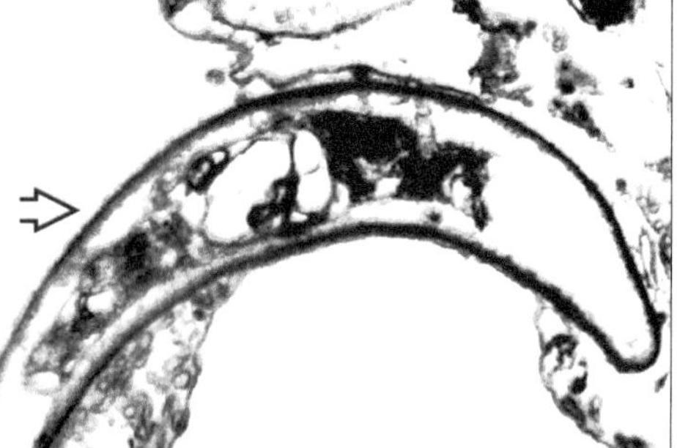

P. jirovecii Cysts and Trophozoites

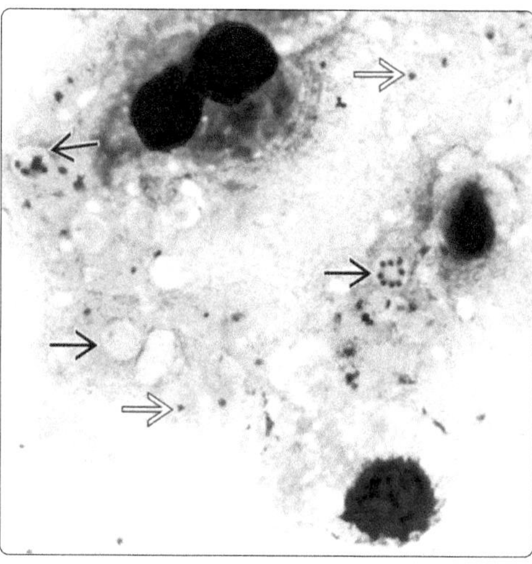

(Left) *Electron microscopy demonstrates a boat-shaped P. jiroveci cell ⇨. The membranotubular extensions ⇨ contribute to the alveolar infiltrate. (Courtesy Franz von Lichtenberg Collection of Infectious Disease Pathology, BWH.)* **(Right)** *This Giemsa-stained lung smear shows scattered P. jirovecii cysts ⇨ and numerous trophozoites ➡. (Courtesy M. Melvin, PhD, CDC/PHIL.)*

Intraalveolar *P. jiroveci* Organisms

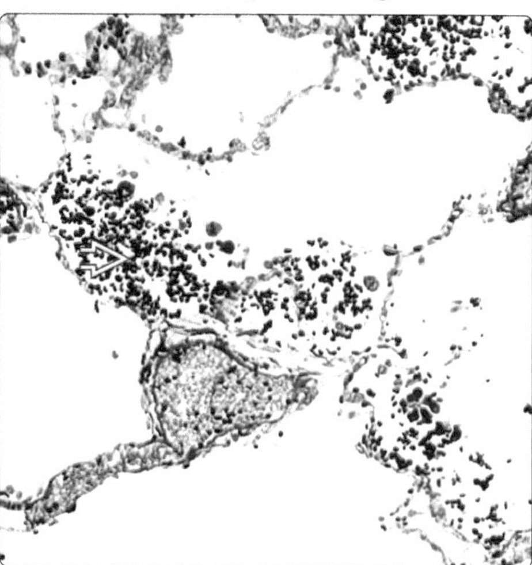

Variable Appearances of *P. jiroveci*

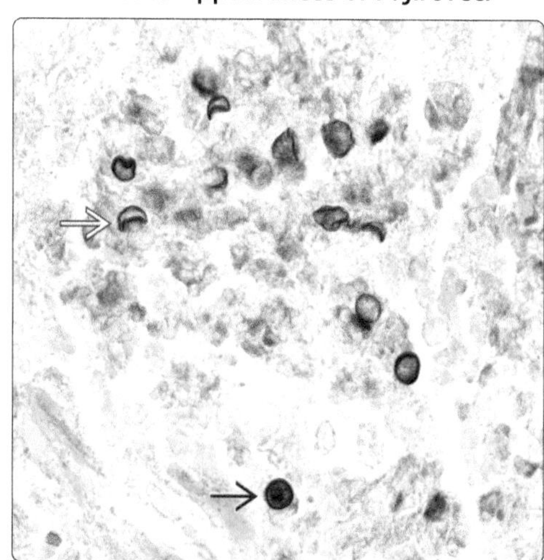

(Left) *A lung section from a case of disseminated P. jiroveci infection is shown. The alveolar spaces are empty except for the presence of P. jiroveci organisms ➡, as seen on this GMS stain. (Courtesy Franz von Lichtenberg Collection of Infectious Disease Pathology, BWH.)* **(Right)** *GMS stain of a lung section highlights variable appearances of P. jiroveci, including spheres with prominent dots ⇨ and crushed helmet or ping-pong ball forms ➡.*

Pneumocystis Pneumonia: Chest CT

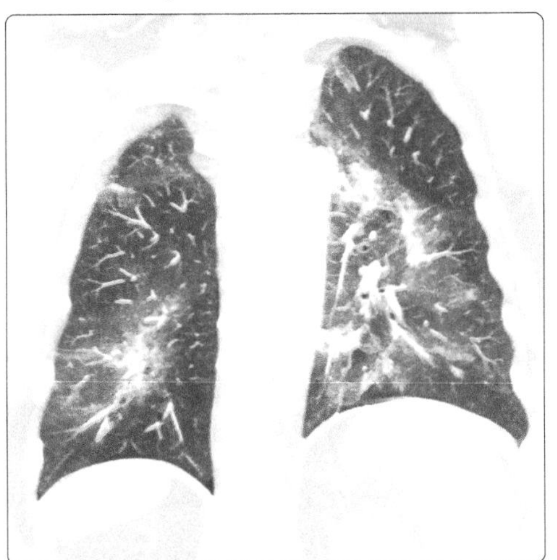

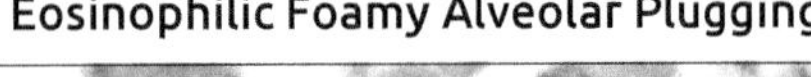

Eosinophilic Foamy Alveolar Plugging

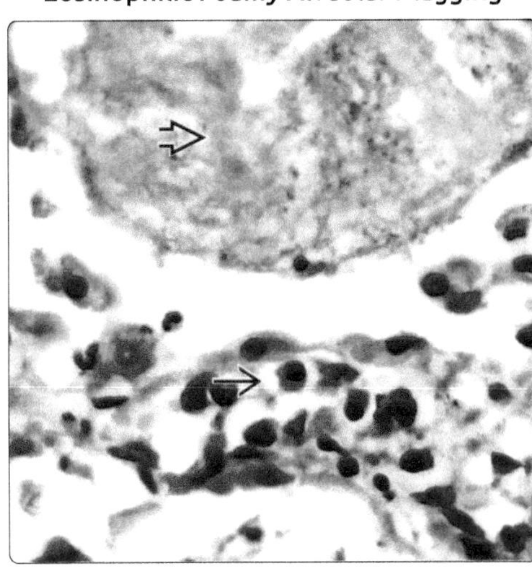

(Left) *Ground-glass opacities are considered a principal finding in Pneumocystis pneumonia, which predominantly involves the perihilar or mid zones.* **(Right)** *Eosinophilic foamy alveolar plugging ⇨ is shown with a plasma cell inflammatory infiltrate →. (Courtesy Franz von Lichtenberg Collection of Infectious Disease Pathology, BWH.)*

Alveolar Plugging With Eosinophilic Exudate

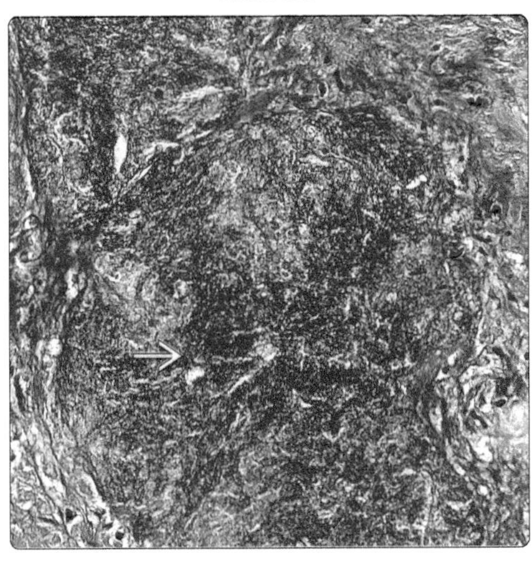

Interstitial Inflammatory Infiltrates

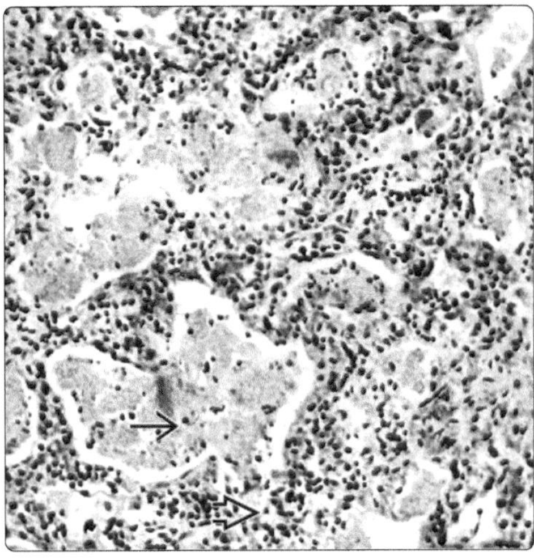

(Left) *Extensive alveolar plugging with eosinophilic exudate ➡ is demonstrated in the lung of an infected patient. (Courtesy Franz von Lichtenberg Collection of Infectious Disease Pathology, BWH.)* **(Right)** *Eosinophilic foamy alveolar plugging → and interstitial infiltrates ⇨ are shown in the lung of an infected patient. Note the prominent interstitial inflammatory response, which is atypical. (Courtesy Franz von Lichtenberg Collection of Infectious Disease Pathology, BWH.)*

Granulomatous Inflammation

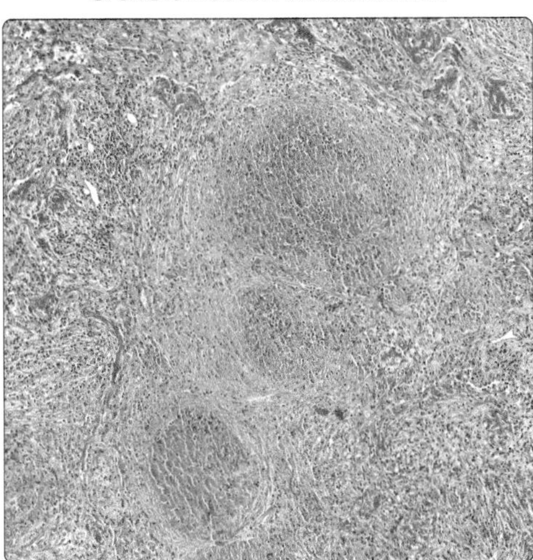

Kidney Involvement

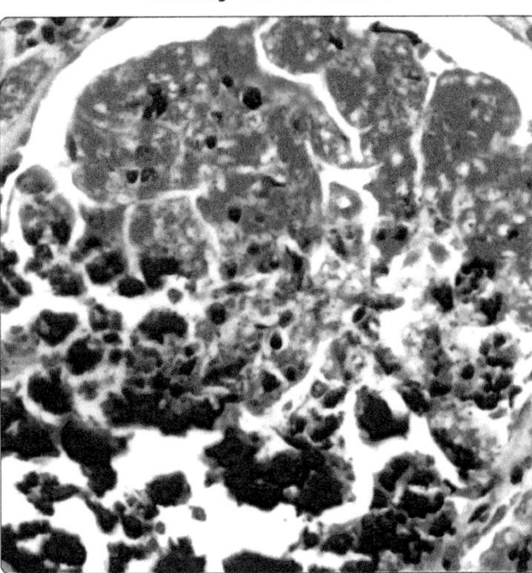

(Left) *Necrotizing granulomatous inflammation is occasionally present in patients with P. pneumonia.* **(Right)** *Disseminated pneumocystosis is demonstrated involving the kidney glomerulus. (Courtesy Franz von Lichtenberg Collection of Infectious Disease Pathology, BWH.)*

Sporotrichosis

KEY FACTS

ETIOLOGY/PATHOGENESIS

- Infection with thermally dimorphic fungi in *Sporothrix schenckii* complex via direct inoculation into skin or inhalation
- Plants (roses); mosses, hay, and oil (farmers); animals (veterinary risk)

CLINICAL ISSUES

- Skin: Begin as small, inoculation site lesions that enlarge in size, become discolored (dark red to purple) with crusting, "boils"
- Sporotrichoid pattern of nodules on extremity is nonspecific but should elicit thorough work-up for organisms
- Lungs: Inhalational exposure with cough and lesions on chest x-ray; chronic disease with fibrosis, large nodules ± cavitation, and hilar adenopathy

MICROSCOPIC

- Mixed neutrophilic and granulomatous lesions with round to oval yeast, narrow-based budding, teardrop configuration (highlighted by GMS and PAS-D)
- Splendore-Hoeppli phenomenon useful but not always present
- 28S rRNA for genus and calmodulin gene for species

TOP DIFFERENTIAL DIAGNOSES

- Histoplasmosis: Small yeast with narrow-based budding; confirm by serology, antigen testing, culture, PCR
- Mycobacterial infections: Acid-fast bacilli; speciated by culture, molecular testing
- Cat-scratch disease: Gram-negative bacilli; confirm with serologic testing, PCR
- Syphilis: Dense plasma cell infiltrates with spirochetes on silver stain or IHC
- Sarcoidosis: Nonnecrotizing granulomas; may have asteroid bodies but lack yeast forms

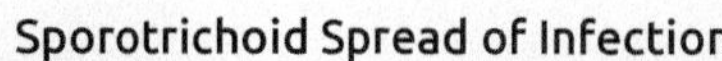

Sporotrichoid Spread of Infection

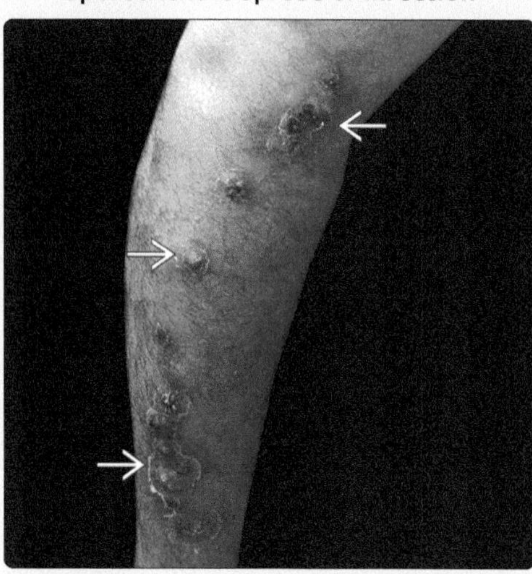

Sporotrichosis With Splendore-Hoeppli Phenomenon

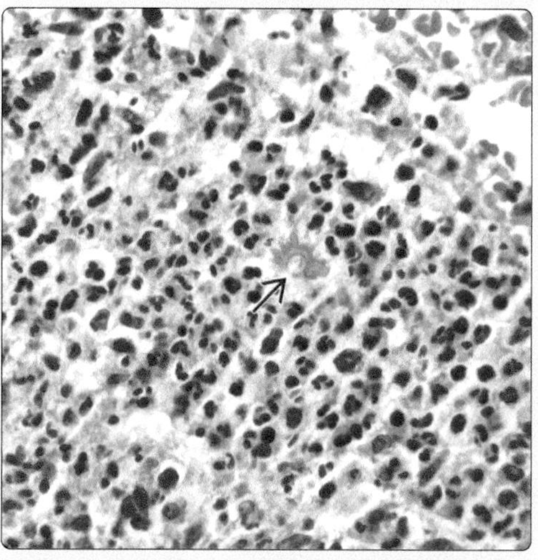

(Left) *Sporotrichosis (forearm) shows ulcerative spread up lymphatic channels ➡. The pattern, called sporotrichoid, can be seen in other diseases (e.g., leishmaniasis, mycobacteria).* **(Right)** *This skin biopsy shows suppurative granulomatous inflammation and a Sporothrix spp. yeast form surrounded by eosinophilic material ➡, characteristic of Splendore-Hoeppli phenomenon.*

Giant Cells in Sporotrichosis

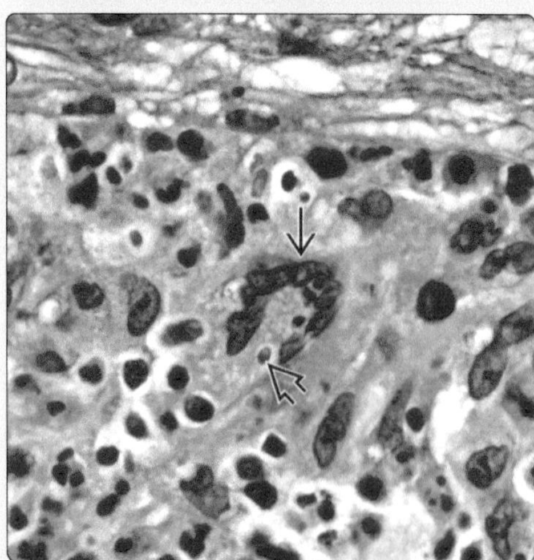

PAS Stain for Sporotrichosis

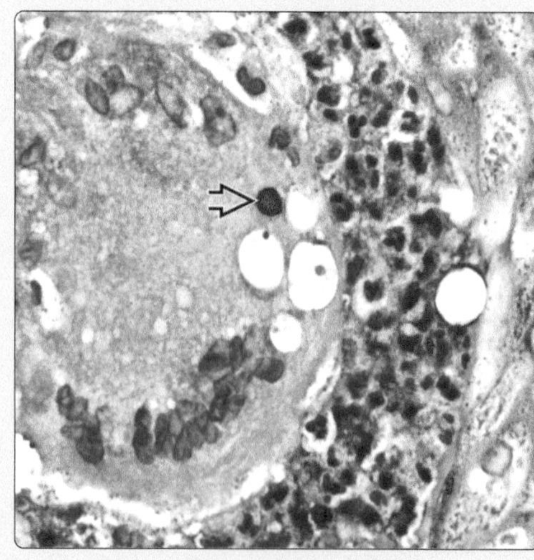

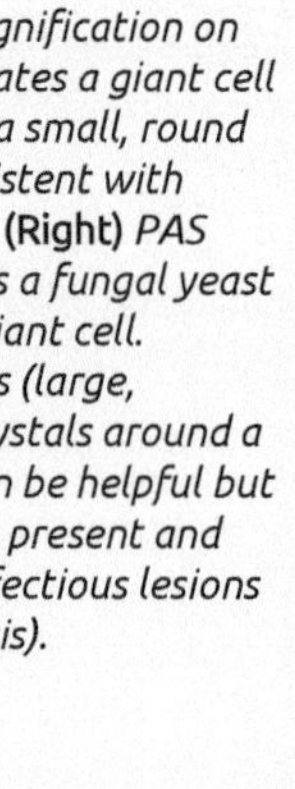

(Left) *High magnification on H&E demonstrates a giant cell ➡ containing a small, round yeast ➡, consistent with sporotrichosis.* **(Right)** *PAS stain highlights a fungal yeast ➡ in a large giant cell. Asteroid bodies (large, eosinophilic crystals around a yeast form) can be helpful but are not always present and occur in noninfectious lesions (e.g., sarcoidosis).*

TERMINOLOGY

Synonyms

- Rose thorn or rose gardener's disease

Definitions

- Greek: "Spora" (seed) + "thrix" (hair)
- "*schenckii*" from Benjamin Schenck, who first isolated fungus from patient

ETIOLOGY/PATHOGENESIS

Infectious Agents

- Infection with thermally dimorphic fungi in *Sporothrix schenckii* complex via direct inoculation into skin or inhalation
  - From plants (roses): *S. schenckii, S. globosa*
  - Mosses, hay, and oil (farmers): Inhalational
  - In cats (veterinary/owner risk): *S. brasiliensis*
- Clinical clade
  - *S. brasiliensis*: Severe clinical disease
  - *S. schenckii*: Benign subcutaneous mycosis
  - *S. globosa*: Similar to *S. schenckii*
  - *S. pallida* (formerly *S. albicans*)
  - *S. mexicana*
  - *S. luriei* and *S. chilensis* rare human infections
- > 37 nonclinically important species
  - e.g., *S. inflata, S. sternoceras, S. gossypina, S. candida*

CLINICAL ISSUES

Epidemiology

- Worldwide distribution of fungus
  - *S. schenckii*: Western South America, Central and North America, Australia, and South Africa
  - *S. brasiliensis*: Southeastern South America
  - *S. globosa*: Asia
- No racial or sex predilections

Presentation

- Cutaneous sporotrichosis
  - Initial inoculation (distal extremities) with small entry site lesions (1 week to several months) that enlarge in size; discolored (dark red to purple) with crusting, "boils"
  - New nodule(s) proximal to initial lesion spread along lymphatics beginning 2 weeks after initial lesion
  - Ulceration of any lesion can occur with risk of secondary bacterial infection
- Pulmonary sporotrichosis
  - Inhalational exposure with cough and lesions on chest x-ray
  - Chronic disease with fibrosis, large nodules ± cavitation, and hilar adenopathy
  - Secondary infections, including bacterial pneumonia, atypical mycobacterial infections, and tuberculosis
- Disseminated sporotrichosis
  - Spread to other organs (especially bone &/or brain) occurs with anorexia
  - More common in immunosuppressed patients

Laboratory Tests

- ELISA and immunoblotting (blood, synovial fluid, CSF)
- Culture of lesions (skin), sputum (pulmonary), cerebrospinal fluid (disseminated), or joint/bone aspirates (disseminated)
- Intradermal test (sporotrichin): Primarily for epidemiologic studies
- 28S rRNA PCR (ITS) and sequencing can distinguish *Sporothrix* from other fungi
- Sequencing β-tubulin, calmodulin, elongation factor 1-α may also be used to distinguish between species

Treatment

- Skin lesions treated with topical antifungals (potassium iodide)
- Pulmonary and disseminated infections treated with itraconazole, posaconazole, &/or amphotericin B
- Deep mycoses, including lung nodules and bone involvement, may require surgical removal

Prognosis

- Most patients recover with antifungal treatment
- Immunosuppressed patients with disseminated disease have worse prognosis

MICROBIOLOGY

Culture

- Rapidly maturing colonies produced within 5 days (varies with species)
- Malt extract agar or potato dextrose agar yield smooth/wrinkled colonies that go from white to black
  - Growth at 25 °C yields mycelium, including dark-cell-walled conidia, which distinguish *Sporothrix* from other species
- Brain-heart infusion agar for transition from mold to yeast, Sabouraud dextrose agar to maintain yeast
  - Growth at 37 °C yields yeast forms that are similar in appearance to tissue forms
- Assimilation of sucrose, raffinose, and ribitol can assist with speciation
- MALDI-TOF MS has similar reliability and accuracy to currently used molecular methods

MACROSCOPIC

Skin Lesions

- Nodules are large, indurated, crusting, ulcerated, and appear in linear fashion on extremity (sporotrichoid growth pattern)
- "Sporotrichoid" is often used by dermatologists but may refer to several diseases (i.e., not specific for sporotrichosis)

MICROSCOPIC

Histologic Features

- Mixed neutrophilic and granulomatous inflammation (all sites), frequently with lymphocytes and plasma cells
- Yeast forms are round to oval (2-6 μm) with narrow budding or show teardrop configuration; occasionally club-shaped "cigar bodies" (4-10 μm in length); hyphae rarely present
- Splendore-Hoeppli phenomenon with asteroid bodies: Crystalline host proteins surrounding yeast (nonspecific)
- Cutaneous lesions associated with hyperkeratosis, parakeratosis, and pseudoepitheliomatous hyperplasia

Sugar Assimilation and Colony Size

Species (Cl)	Sucrose/Raffinose/Ribitol (%)	At 20°, 30°, 35°, and 37° C (mm ± SD)
Sporothrix brasiliensis (I)	0/0/19	25 ± 6, 25 ± 6, 17 ± 7, 8 ± 2
Sporothrix schenckii (IIa)	100/100/100	29 ± 5, 36 ± 6, 21 ± 7, 6 ± 3
S. schenckii (IIb)	100/100/33	30 ± 3, 34 ± 3, 21 ± 4, 6 ± 2
Sporothrix globosa (III)	100/0/91	29 ± 7, 31 ± 5, 12 ± 5, < 1
Sporothrix mexicana (IV)	100/100/100	54 ± 1, 68 ± 2, 11 ± 1, 2 ± 1
Sporothrix albicans (V)	100/0/50	51 ± 3, 67 ± 4, 28 ± 1, 4 ± 1

The pattern of sugar assimilation by fungus in culture as well as the relative sizes of the colonies at various temperatures is shown for the species, representing the 6 clades of Sporothrix. The clades (Cl) are based on molecular analysis of the calmodulin gene. (Adapted from Marimon R et al, 2007.)

ANCILLARY TESTS

Histochemistry

- GMS and PAS-D stains highlight yeast forms

DIFFERENTIAL DIAGNOSIS

Histoplasmosis

- Pulmonary and disseminated forms
- Small yeast with narrow-based budding associated with granulomatous inflammation
- Confirm by serology, antigen, culture, PCR

Nocardiosis

- Cutaneous, pulmonary, and disseminated forms
- Gram-positive, weakly acid-fast bacilli identified histologically; speciated by culture, molecular testing

Mycobacterial Infections

- e.g., *Mycobacterium marinum* infection and leprosy (skin), tuberculosis (skin, lung, disseminated)
- Granulomatous lesions with necrosis lacking neutrophils or plasma cells
- Acid-fast bacilli identified histologically; speciated by culture, molecular testing

Syphilis

- Dense plasma cell infiltrates without granulomas
- *Treponema pallidum* spirochetes on silver stain or immunohistochemistry

Leishmaniasis

- Macrophages filled with organisms showing dot-dash (nucleus-kinetoplast) appearance
- Giemsa stains highlight organisms

Tularemia

- Francisella tularensis (gram-negative bacilli)
- History of exposure; confirm with serologic testing, PCR

Melioidosis

- *Burkholderia pseudomallei* (gram-negative bacilli)
- History of exposure; confirm with serologic testing, PCR, or culture

Cat-Scratch Disease

- *Bartonella henselae* (gram-negative bacilli); identify with Warthin-Starry stain and confirm with serologic testing, PCR
- Involves lymph nodes (uncommon in sporotrichosis)

Sarcoidosis

- May have asteroid bodies but lack yeast forms
- More granulomatous (without necrosis) and less suppurative

Malignancy

- Ulceration may disrupt upper layers of tumor
- Malignant cells with mitoses, pleomorphism, and invasion

SELECTED REFERENCES

1. Izoton CFG et al: Sporotrichosis in the nasal mucosa: a single-center retrospective study of 37 cases from 1998 to 2020. PLoS Negl Trop Dis. 17(3):e0011212, 2023
2. Orofino-Costa R et al: Human sporotrichosis: recommendations from the Brazilian Society of Dermatology for the clinical, diagnostic and therapeutic management. An Bras Dermatol. 97(6):757-77, 2022
3. Rabello VBS et al: The historical burden of sporotrichosis in Brazil: a systematic review of cases reported from 1907 to 2020. Braz J Microbiol. 53(1):231-44, 2022
4. Ramos V et al: Bone sporotrichosis: 41 cases from a reference hospital in Rio de Janeiro, Brazil. PLoS Negl Trop Dis. 15(3):e0009250, 2021
5. Hayashi S et al: Diagnostic value of a nested polymerase chain reaction for diagnosing cutaneous sporotrichosis from paraffin-embedded skin tissue. Mycoses. 62(12):1148-53, 2019
6. Lopes-Bezerra LM et al: Sporotrichosis between 1898 and 2017: the evolution of knowledge on a changeable disease and on emerging etiological agents. Med Mycol. 56(suppl_1):126-43, 2018
7. Espinel-Ingroff A et al: Multicenter, international study of MIC/MEC distributions for definition of epidemiological cutoff values for sporothrix species identified by molecular methods. Antimicrob Agents Chemother. 61(10), 2017
8. He Y et al: Disseminated cutaneous sporotrichosis presenting as a necrotic facial mass: case and review. Dermatol Online J. 23(7), 2017
9. Shimizu T et al: Sporotrichal tenosynovitis diagnosed helpfully by musculoskeletal ultrasonography. Intern Med. 56(10):1243-6, 2017
10. Fischman Gompertz O et al: Atypical clinical presentation of sporotrichosis caused by Sporothrix globosa resistant to itraconazole. Am J Trop Med Hyg. 94(6):1218-22, 2016
11. McGuinness SL et al: Epidemiological investigation of an outbreak of cutaneous sporotrichosis, Northern Territory, Australia. BMC Infect Dis. 16:16, 2016
12. Freitas DF et al: Sporotrichosis in the central nervous system caused by Sporothrix brasiliensis. Clin Infect Dis. 61(4):663-4, 2015

Gross Lesion: Skin

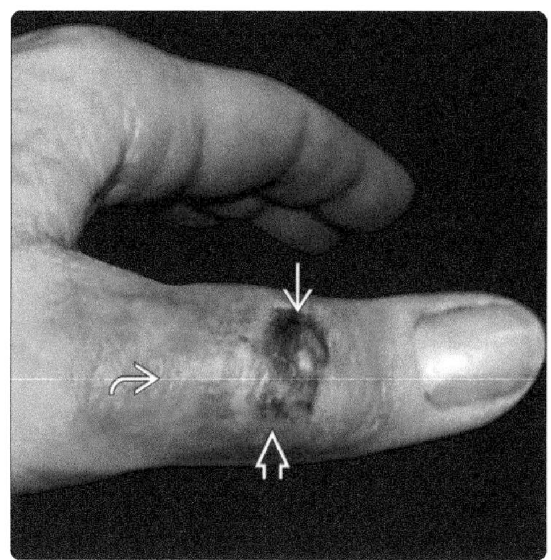

Culture Isolate

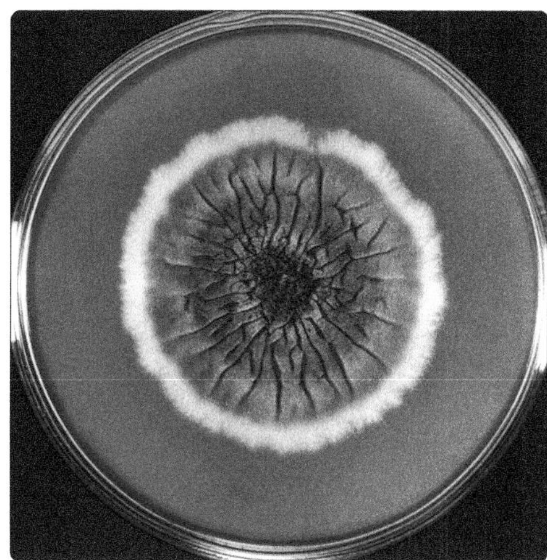

(Left) *An isolated lesion of sporotrichosis on the left thumb demonstrates ulceration ➡, induration ➡, and adjacent inflammation ➡. (Courtesy K. Gardiner.)* **(Right)** *This Sabouraud dextrose agar culture plate shows a wrinkled colony with a leathery, moist appearance, ranging from beige-yellow at its periphery to a darker, brownish-purple in its more central, older areas, characteristic of Sporothrix schenckii. (Courtesy Dr. L. Georg, CDC/PHIL.)*

Sporothrix schenckii Culture Isolate

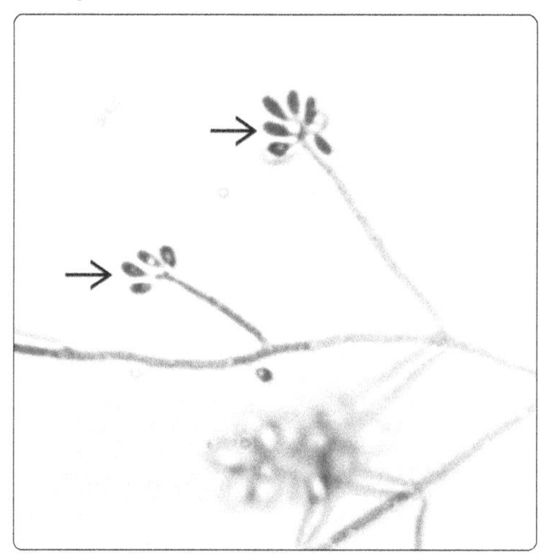

Sporotrichosis in Skin

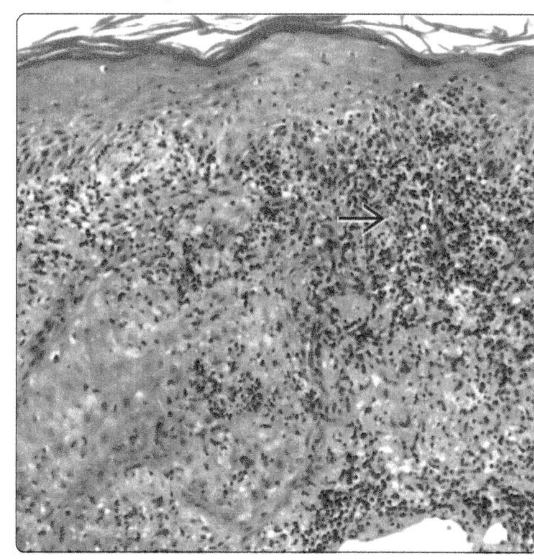

(Left) *This lactophenol cotton blue stain of a S. schenckii isolate shows narrow fungal hyphae and clusters of oval-shaped conidia ➡. (Courtesy Dr. Kaplan, CDC/PHIL.)* **(Right)** *H&E shows low magnification of the skin in sporotrichosis with prominent inflammation ➡.*

Inflammation in Sporotrichosis

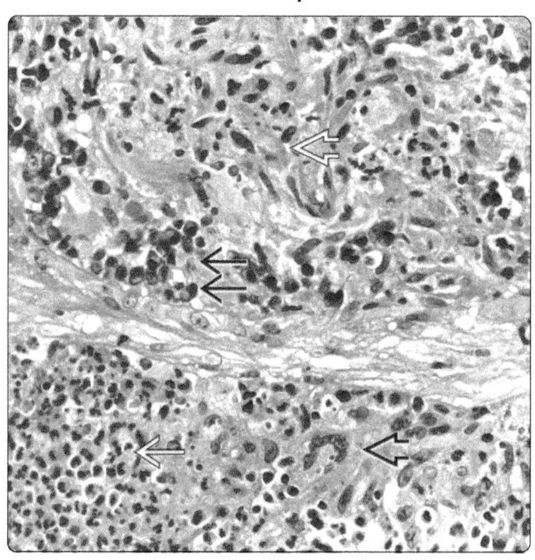

Silver Stain for Sporotrichosis

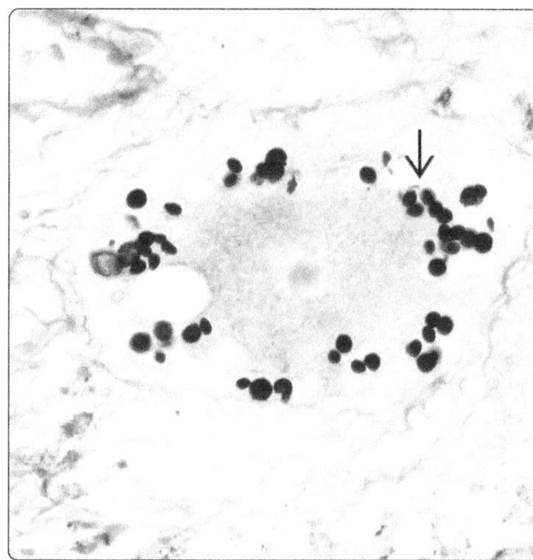

(Left) *H&E shows sporotrichosis in the skin with neutrophils and eosinophils ➡, epithelioid histiocytes ➡, giant cells ➡, and plasma cells ➡. The chronicity of the lesion, spread via lymphatics, and acute response lead to a mixed inflammatory pattern.* **(Right)** *High magnification of sporotrichosis shows yeast forms ➡ within a large, multinucleated giant cell. (Courtesy L. Thompson, MD.)*

Talaromycosis

KEY FACTS

ETIOLOGY/PATHOGENESIS

- Infection with *Talaromyces* (formerly *Penicillium*) *marneffei*, thermally dimorphic saprophytic fungus endemic to tropical and subtropical Asia

CLINICAL ISSUES

- HIV patients commonly present with fever, weight loss, weakness, anemia, and umbilicated skin papules; commonly misdiagnosed as tuberculosis
- Disseminated disease involves skin, joints, and bone

MICROBIOLOGY

- At 25-30 °C, on Sabouraud dextrose agar, produces flat, powdery to velvety colonies within 3 days
- Produces red pigment, which diffuses into agar and stains colony within 1 week
- Microscopically composed of conidiophores with several metulae that end in multiple phialides

MICROSCOPIC

- ~ 5-µm, capsular-shaped, yeast-like arthroconidia that divide by binary fission with prominent central septa, highlighted by GMS and PAS-D stains
- Macrophage (early), acute inflammation/necrosis/abscess, chronic granulomatous inflammation

TOP DIFFERENTIAL DIAGNOSES

- Histoplasmosis: Small round yeast forms with narrow-based budding, distinct halo in macrophages, and produces calcifications in chronic lesions
- Leishmaniasis: Kinetoplastid parasites found within macrophages and have distinctive dot-dash (nucleus-kinetoplast) morphology
- Leprosy: Foamy macrophages with abundant acid-fast bacilli (globi)

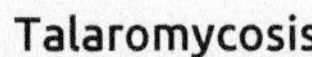

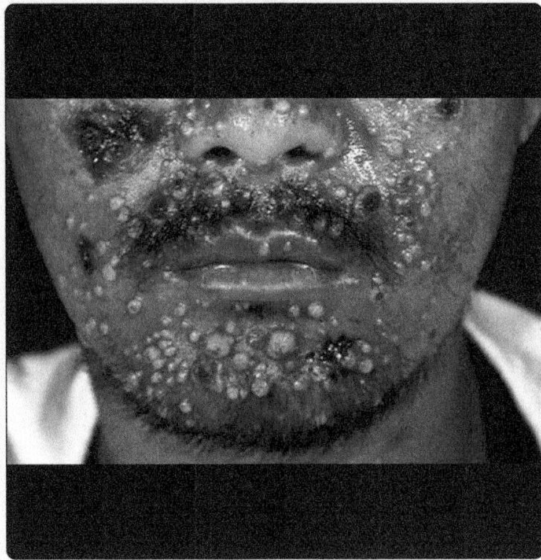

Talaromycosis Histology

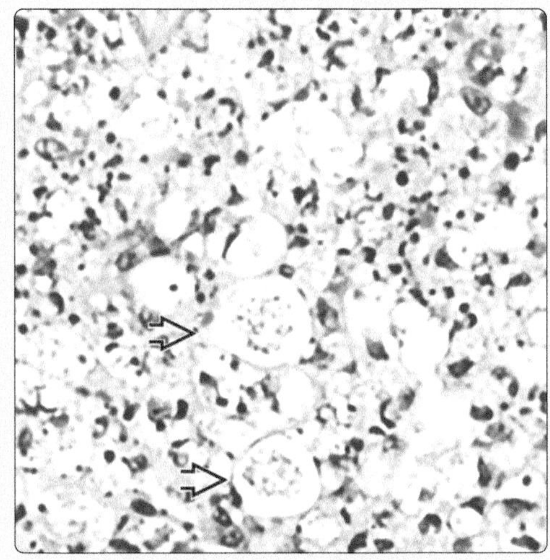

(Left) *Multiple umbilicated (molluscoid) papules are commonly seen in patients with cutaneous involvement in disseminated talaromycosis. (Courtesy P. Pattanprichakul, MD.)* **(Right)** *Multiple histiocytes with abundant intracellular fungal spores* ⇨ *imparting a characteristic parasitized appearance is typical of talaromycosis. (Courtesy P. Pattanprichakul, MD.)*

Yeast Within Multinucleated Giant Cell

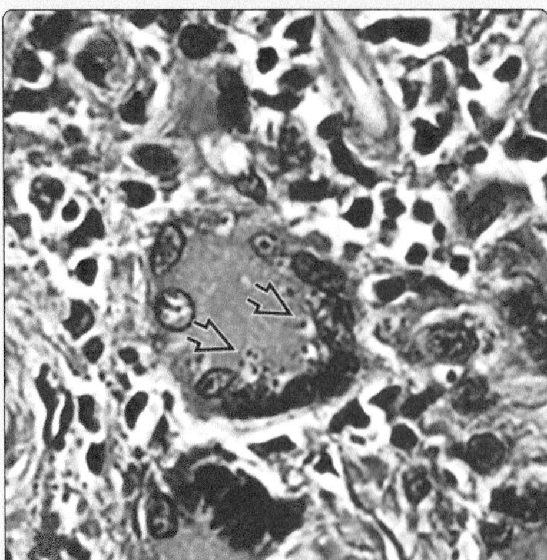

Septate Yeast Forms: GMS Stain

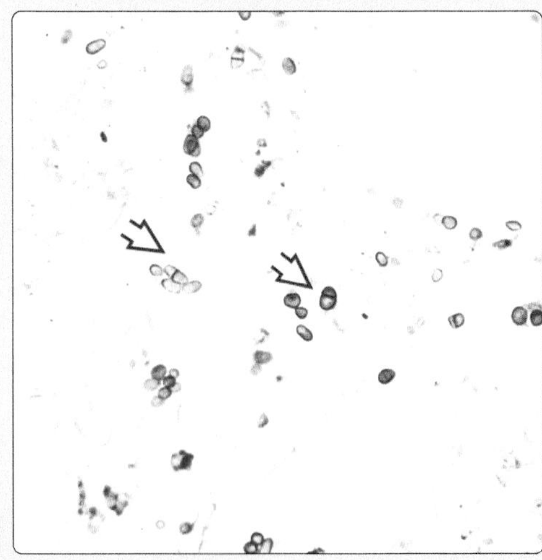

(Left) *A multinucleate giant cell with multiple small, round Talaromyces marneffei yeast forms* ⇨*, some with a clear halo, are shown in talaromycosis. This finding raises a differential diagnosis with histoplasmosis. (Courtesy P. Pattanprichakul, MD.)* **(Right)** *GMS staining reveals characteristic yeast forms of T. marneffei showing central septation* ⇨*, making them resemble a capsule. (Courtesy P. Pattanprichakul, MD.)*

TERMINOLOGY

Definitions

- *Talaromyces marneffei* derived from Greek "tálaros" (basket) and "múkēs" (mushroom) + Marneffe (from Hubert Marneffe, director of Pasteur Institute)

ETIOLOGY/PATHOGENESIS

Infectious Agents

- Infection with *T.* (formerly *Penicillium*) *marneffei,* thermally dimorphic saprophytic fungus
- Environmental source is soil and bamboo rats

CLINICAL ISSUES

Epidemiology

- Estimated > 17,000 cases per year (~ 4,900 deaths)
- Systemic disease almost exclusively in immunosuppressed patients; limited local disease in immunocompetent
- Endemic to tropical and subtropical Asia, including Indonesia, China, Vietnam, and Thailand; possibly also in Cambodia, Laos, Myanmar, and Malaysia
- Early indicator disease of HIV/AIDS infection in endemic regions (CD4 < 100)
- Cases in Europe and USA are typically in immunosuppressed patients with travel to endemic areas
- Other *Talaromyces* spp. have produced < 30 total cases of infection in literature

Presentation

- HIV patients commonly present with fever, weight loss, weakness, anemia, and umbilicated skin papules
  - Dyspnea, cough, fever, generalized lymphadenopathy, hepatosplenomegaly, diarrhea may also be seen
  - Commonly misdiagnosed as tuberculosis
- Disseminated disease: Skin, joints, and bone infected
  - Papules on face, chest, arms, and legs may occur in ~ 70% of patients with disseminated disease
  - HIV-negative patients develop arthritis and bone lesions

Laboratory Tests

- Molecular identification: Internal transcribed spacer (ITS) sequencing, metagenomic next-generation sequencing (mNGS)

Treatment

- Initially amphotericin B followed by long-term itraconazole

Prognosis

- 60-80% response to treatment; ~ 33% mortality

MICROBIOLOGY

Culture

- At 25-30 °C, on Sabouraud dextrose agar, produces flat, powdery to velvety colonies within 3 days
  - Produces red pigment, which diffuses into agar and stains colony within 1 week
  - Microscopically composed of conidiophores with several metulae that end in multiple phialides
  - Growth is inhibited by cycloheximide
- At 35-37 °C, inhibitory mould agar or brain heart infusion agar produces soft, dry, yeast-like colonies
  - Hyphal elements with fragmenting ends that produce arthroconidia (yeast-like capsules)
  - Blood cultures with disseminated disease may only show hyphal elements
  - Arthroconidia (3-5 μm) are present in human tissue infections and divide by binary fission (no budding) but may elongate to 9 μm before separating
  - Conversion from mold to yeast-like colony within 2 weeks
  - *T. marneffei* is only dimorphic species in genus

MICROSCOPIC

Histologic Features

- Organisms are ~ 5-μm, capsular-shaped, yeast-like arthroconidia that divide by binary fission with prominent central septa; routine H&E stain may produce halo (mimicking *Histoplasma*)
- Affected tissue may have variable inflammatory reaction, depending on immunosuppressed state
- Affected organs include skin, bone marrow, lung, gastrointestinal tract, lymph nodes, and most other organs
- Macrophages are usually present in early lesions
- Acute inflammation with necrosis may develop with frank abscesses
- Chronic inflammation produces granulomatous lesions with scarring/fibrosis without calcification

ANCILLARY TESTS

Special Stains

- GMS and PAS-D stains highlight arthroconidia

DIFFERENTIAL DIAGNOSIS

Histoplasmosis

- *Histoplasma capsulatum* produces small round yeast forms with narrow-based budding, distinct halo in macrophages, and produces calcifications in chronic lesions

Leishmaniasis

- *Leishmania* species are kinetoplastid parasites found within macrophages and have distinctive dot-dash (nucleus-kinetoplast) morphology

Leprosy

- Foamy macrophages with abundant *Mycobacterium leprae* bacilli (globi), best visualized in acid-fast, alcohol-resistant stains (e.g., Fite-Faraco)

SELECTED REFERENCES

1. Wang F et al: An overlooked and underrated endemic mycosis-talaromycosis and the pathogenic fungus Talaromyces marneffei. Clin Microbiol Rev. 36(1):e0005122, 2023
2. Narayanasamy S et al: A global call for talaromycosis to be recognised as a neglected tropical disease. Lancet Glob Health. 9(11):e1618-22, 2021
3. Borman AM et al: Rapid and robust identification of clinical isolates of Talaromyces marneffei based on MALDI-TOF mass spectrometry or dimorphism in Galleria mellonella. Med Mycol. 57(8):969-75, 2019
4. Cao C et al: Talaromycosis (penicilliosis) due to Talaromyces (Penicillium) marneffei: insights into the clinical trends of a major fungal disease 60 years after the discovery of the pathogen. Mycopathologia. 184(6):709-20, 2019
5. Limper AH et al: Fungal infections in HIV/AIDS. Lancet Infect Dis. 17(11):e334-43, 2017
6. Nor NM et al: Skin and subcutaneous infections in south-east Asia. Curr Opin Infect Dis. 28(2):133-8, 2015

KEY FACTS

ETIOLOGY/PATHOGENESIS

- Infection with *Rhinosporidium seeberi* (class Mesomycetozoea) via direct contact with infected, stagnant water

CLINICAL ISSUES

- More prevalent in India, Sri Lanka, and Southeast Asia
- Nasal cavity and conjunctiva are most infected sites
- Often presents as red/pink sessile or pedunculated polyps
- Generally benign clinical course; it may recur
- Surgical excision is mainstay of treatment; no effective antibiotic therapy

MICROSCOPIC

- Round, thick-walled, mature sporangia (100-450 μm in diameter) containing lobulated sporangiospores (1-10 μm)
- Young spores form crescent-like mass at one pole of sporangium, at periphery along inner wall; larger mature spores are centrally located
- Mixed chronic inflammatory tissue response with granulation tissue formation
- GMS and PAS highlight walls of sporangiospores and mature sporangia
- Mucicarmine stains walls of spores and inner surface of sporangial wall

TOP DIFFERENTIAL DIAGNOSES

- Coccidioidomycosis: Smaller spherules (100 μm) that contain uniform endospores (5 μm in diameter); GMS highlights endospores but not spherule wall
- Adiaspiromycosis: *Emmonsia crescens* infection with similarly sized spherules (200-400 μm in diameter) that usually appear empty
- Myospherulosis: Iatrogenic, benign, tumor-like mass or cyst composed of spherules of damaged erythrocytes and lipogranulomatous reaction

Rhinosporidiosis in Oral Cavity

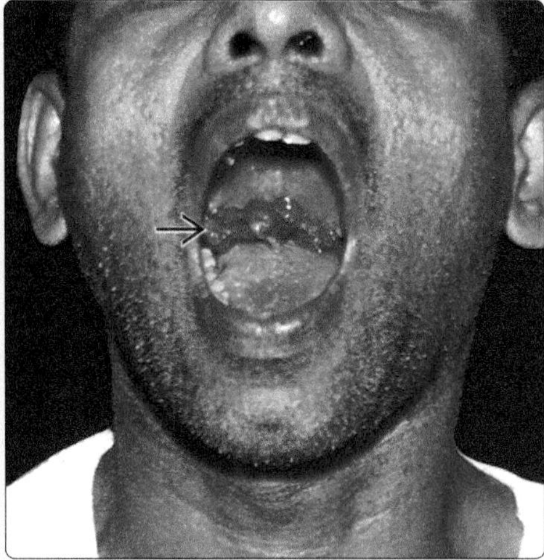

***Rhinosporidium* Juvenile Sporangia**

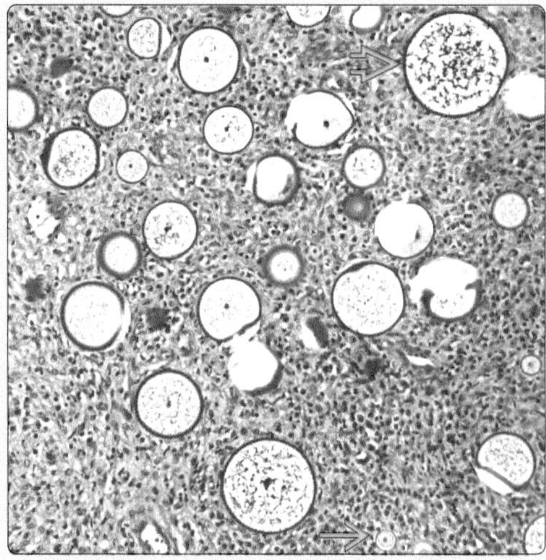

(Left) *Rhinosporidiosis appears as red/pink, sessile, mobile, pedunculated polypoid friable mucocutaneous lesions ➜, most frequently involving tissue in nasopharynx, conjunctiva, or oral cavity, as in this case. (Courtesy C. Satyanarayana, L. Georg, CDC/PHIL.)* **(Right)** *Rhinosporidium juvenile sporangia (a.k.a. trophic cysts or trophocytes) have a central nucleus and are initially very small ➜. Upon maturation, immature endospores ➜ appear.*

***Rhinosporidium seeberi* Mature Sporangium**

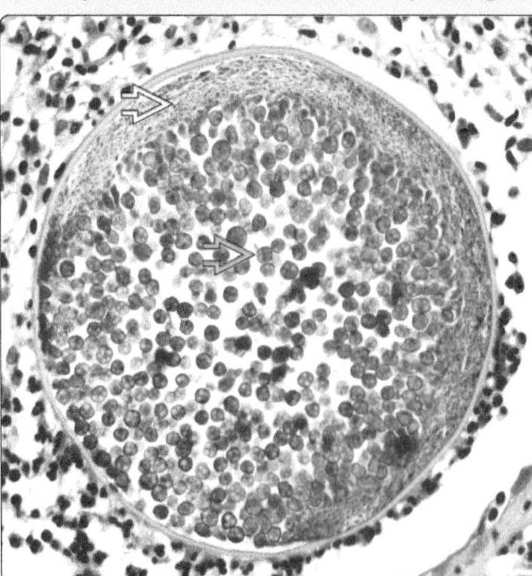

***Rhinosporidium* Mature Sporangium: GMS**

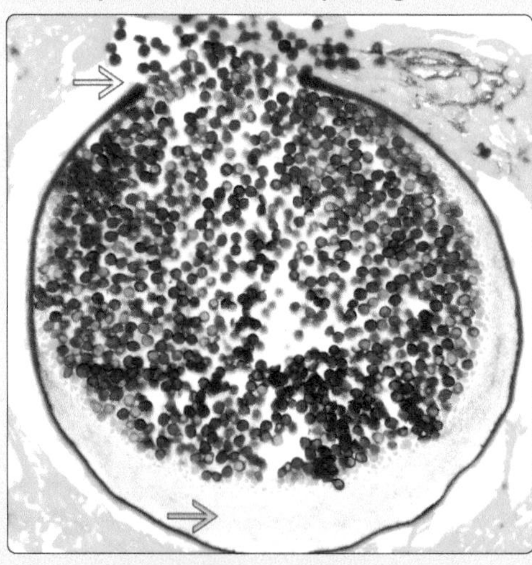

(Left) *Mature sporangia are up to 500 μm in diameter and contain multiple sporangiospores (endospores). Note the endospores mature from the periphery ➜ toward one end. Eosinophilic globular bodies are noted in mature endospores ➜.* **(Right)** *The Grocott methenamine silver reaction highlights the wall and mature endospores of mature sporangia but not the immature sporangiospores ➜. Mature endospores are released through a pore created by focal thinning of the wall ➜.*

TERMINOLOGY

Definitions

- Greek: "Rhino" (of nose) + "sporidiosis" (spore forming)

ETIOLOGY/PATHOGENESIS

Infectious Agents

- Infection with *Rhinosporidium seeberi*, previously thought to be fungus or parasite, now classified in its own taxon: Mesomycetozoea
- Believed to be acquired by exposure to contaminated water: Bathing in ponds, rivers, or lakes contaminated with *Rhinosporidium*
- Transmission is through direct contact with infected water, although dust is thought to harbor organism in arid areas
- There is no human-to-human transmission

CLINICAL ISSUES

Epidemiology

- Associated with warm tropical environments
- More prevalent in India, Sri Lanka, and Southeast Asia
- Occasional cases reported in Africa, South America, Europe, USA (Texas and southwest)
- More common in young males

Site

- Mucocutaneous tissue in nasopharynx (most common), conjunctiva, oral cavity
- Other sites are rare but can include upper airways, salivary glands, urethra, genitals, rectum, ears, skin
- Disseminated disease is rare but has been reported, especially in immunocompromised individuals

Presentation

- Red/pink, sessile, mobile, or pedunculated polypoid friable lesions with easy bleeding upon touch
- Nasal blockage, rhinorrhea, epistaxis, conjunctival or urethral mass sensation
- Clinical course is usually benign

Treatment

- No effective antibiotic therapy
- Surgical excision is mainstay of treatment

Prognosis

- Excellent with surgical excision
- Recurrence not uncommon

MICROSCOPIC

Histologic Features

- Mature sporangia consist of large, round, thick-walled cysts (100-500 μm in diameter) containing sporangiospores (endospores; 1-10 μm in diameter)
- Mature sporangiospores are lobulated due to eosinophilic globular inclusions [electro-dense bodies (EDBs) on electron microscopy]
- Characteristic zonal pattern of sporangiospore development in sporangia with young spores forming crescent-like mass at one pole of sporangium, at periphery along inner wall; larger mature spores are centrally located
- Tissue reaction consists of mixed chronic inflammatory response with granulation tissue formation
- Granulomas can form when sporangia rupture and release sporangiospores

Cytologic Features

- Immature sporangia and endospores may be identified in fine-needle-aspirated material

ANCILLARY TESTS

Special Stains

- GMS and PAS highlight walls of sporangiospores and mature sporangia
- Mucicarmine stains walls of spores and inner surface of sporangial wall

DIFFERENTIAL DIAGNOSIS

Coccidioidomycosis

- Spherules of *Coccidioides* spp. are generally smaller (100 μm in diameter) containing smaller, uniform endospores (5 μm in diameter)
- Grocott methenamine silver stain highlights endospores but not spherule wall

Adiaspiromycosis

- Rare human infection caused by soil fungi *Emmonsia crescens*
- Mostly affects rodents and small mammals; seen as respiratory disease involving lungs
- Spherules have refractile walls, are of similar size (200-400 μm in diameter), and usually appear empty but may contain small globules
- On H&E, thick walls of adiaspores show narrow, eosinophilic outer layer and thicker inner hyaline layer

Myospherulosis

- Iatrogenic, benign, tumor-like mass or cyst composed of spherules mimicking endosporulating fungal infection
- Can occur in any part of body but most frequent sites are paranasal sinus and subcutaneous tissue
- Cysts composed of spherules of damaged erythrocytes and fibrous cystic cavities accompanied by lipogranulomatous reaction to extravasated erythrocytes and lipids

SELECTED REFERENCES

1. Izimukwiye AI et al: Cluster of nasal rhinosporidiosis, eastern province, Rwanda. Emerg Infect Dis. 25(9):1727-9, 2019
2. Vélez A et al: Rhinosporidiosis in Colombia: case series and literature review. Trop Doct. 49475518787123, 2018
3. Thompson LD: Rhinosporidiosis. Ear Nose Throat J. 95(3):101, 2016
4. Prakash M et al: Rhinosporidiosis and the pond. J Pharm Bioallied Sci. 7(Suppl 1):S59-62, 2015
5. Anstead GM et al: Adiaspiromycosis causing respiratory failure and a review of human infections due to Emmonsia and Chrysosporium spp. J Clin Microbiol. 50(4):1346-54, 2012
6. Das S et al: Nasal rhinosporidiosis in humans: new interpretations and a review of the literature of this enigmatic disease. Med Mycol. 49(3):311-5, 2011
7. Madana J et al: Rhinosporidiosis of the upper airways and trachea. J Laryngol Otol. 124(10):1139-41, 2010
8. Fredricks DN et al: Rhinosporidium seeberi: a human pathogen from a novel group of aquatic protistan parasites. Emerg Infect Dis. 6(3):273-82, 2000
9. Herr RA et al: Phylogenetic analysis of Rhinosporidium seeberi's 18S small-subunit ribosomal DNA groups this pathogen among members of the protoctistan Mesomycetozoa clade. J Clin Microbiol. 37(9):2750-4, 1999

Protothecosis

KEY FACTS

ETIOLOGY/PATHOGENESIS

- Infection caused by saprophytic, achlorophyllic microalgae *Prototheca wickerhamii* and *Prototheca zopfii* via exposure to contaminated water or soil

CLINICAL ISSUES

- Global distribution: Southeastern USA and Japan most common
- Cutaneous infection via traumatic inoculation and olecranon bursitis most common presentations
- Rare dissemination in immunocompromised hosts
- Treatment options include surgical excision, topical, and systemic antifungals
- PCR or sequencing-based approaches for speciation

MICROBIOLOGY

- Grows aerobically on standard bacterial and fungal medias
- Gram stain of colonies reveal morula-like structures with internal septations

MICROSCOPIC

- Morula-like sporangia (3-30 μm) with internal septations (soccer ball) that lack budding; highlighted by PAS and GMS stains
- Variable inflammatory background

TOP DIFFERENTIAL DIAGNOSES

- Coccidioidomycosis: Larger sporangia (> 50 μm) with numerous small endospores (2-5 μm); pulmonary involvement common
- Blastomycosis: Uniformly sized (8- to 15-μm) broad-based budding yeast (without internal septations)
- Cryptococcosis: Variably sized (5- to 15-μm) narrow-based budding yeast (without internal septations)
- Chlorellosis: Chlorophyll-containing green algae (8-30 μm) with PAS-positive cytoplasmic granules

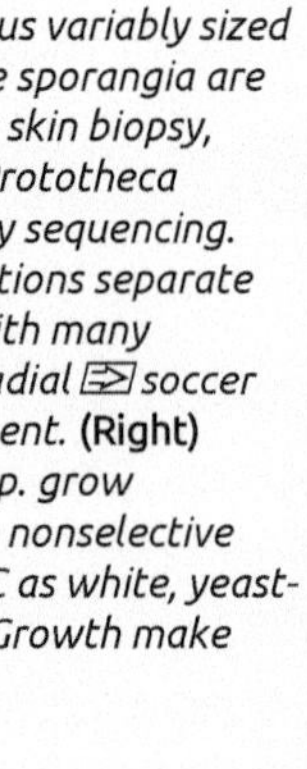

(Left) *Numerous variably sized ➔ morula-like sporangia are present in this skin biopsy, identified as Prototheca wickerhamii by sequencing. Internal septations separate endospores with many displaying a radial ➔ soccer ball arrangement.* **(Right)** *Prototheca spp. grow aerobically on nonselective media at 37 °C as white, yeast-like colonies. Growth make take 3-5 days.*

Cutaneous Protothecosis

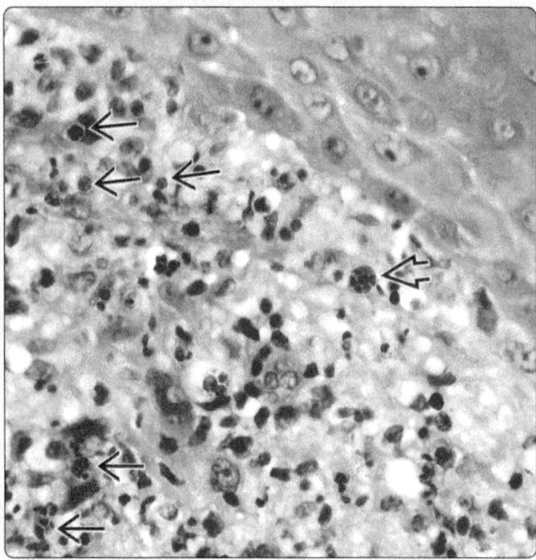

***Prototheca* Colonies: Blood Agar**

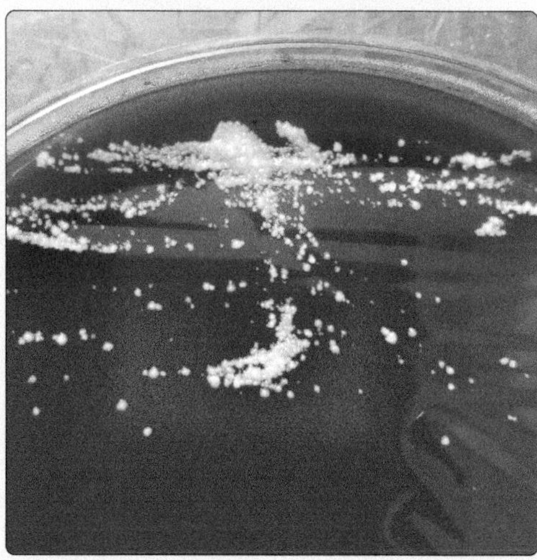

(Left) *Human protothecosis is rare but can be readily identified histologically by the presence of a classic soccer ball or cartwheel arrangement of P. wickerhamii endospores.* **(Right)** *Numerous morula-like sporangia are highlighted by methenamine silver staining. Note variable size and number of internal endospore formation.*

***Prototheca wickerhamii* Endospores**

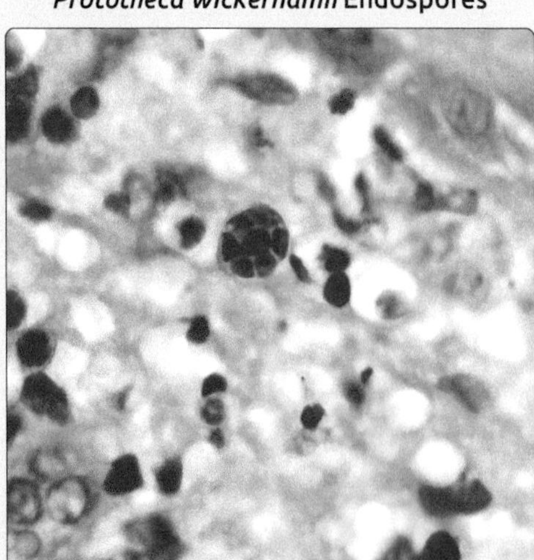

Protothecosis: GMS Stain

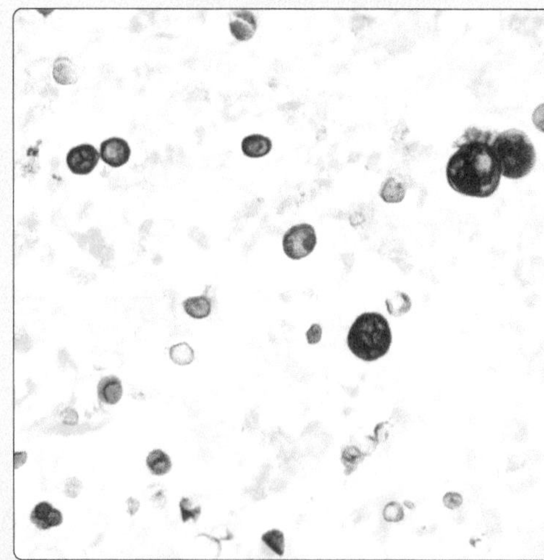

TERMINOLOGY

Definitions

- Greek: "Proto" (1st) + theke (sheath)

ETIOLOGY/PATHOGENESIS

Infectious Agents

- Infection caused by saprophytic microalgae in genus *Prototheca*, family *Chorellaceae* (*P. wickerhamii*, *P. zopfii*)
- Achlorophyllic (unable to photosynthesize); genus is heterotrophic (require external carbon sources)
- Veterinary pathogen (bovine mastitis)
- Unicellular organism reproduces asexually in process of internal cellular division, resulting in formation of classic morula-like sporangia
- Incubation period not well documented (weeks to months)

CLINICAL ISSUES

Epidemiology

- Global distribution, reported in tropical and subtropical regions; Southeastern USA and Japan most common
- Increasing prevalence may be related to increasing rates of immunosuppression and changes in climate

Presentation

- Infection occurs in both immunocompetent and immunocompromised (dissemination more common)
- Major risk factors: Systemic immunosuppression and corticosteroid use
- Cutaneous lesions and olecranon bursitis common
- Cutaneous infection often via traumatic inoculation with contaminated water (not uniformly killed by chlorination); at-risk populations include farmers, fishermen, wastewater workers, pool workers, and aquarium staff
- Rare case reports of meningitis, vaginitis, endocarditis, colitis, pulmonary, and urinary tract infections

Laboratory Tests

- PCR or sequencing-based approaches for speciation

Treatment

- Lack of standardized treatment protocols; in vitro antimicrobial susceptibility testing does not correlate with response
- Combination of systemic azoles, IV amphotericin B, topical agents, &/or surgical excision

Prognosis

- Superficial nail infections have best prognosis (100% treatment success rate), while disseminated infections have worst (33% treatment success rate)
- Attributable mortality rate of 2.2% suggested

MICROBIOLOGY

Culture

- Dull white yeast-like colonies grow aerobically between 3-5 days; optimal growth at 30 °C, will grow at 37 °C
- Overgrowth of bacteria on nonselective medias (blood and chocolate agars) can make identification challenging
- Selective medias may enhance recovery; however, cycloheximide may inhibit growth
- Gram stain: Morula-like structures with internal septations
- Genus-level identification possible using commercially available automated biochemical platforms (e.g., Vitek)

MACROSCOPIC

General Features

- Cutaneous protothecosis: Most commonly erythematous plaques that can be vesicular bullous or ulcerative with crusting and purulent discharge
- Other presentations include: Pustules, papules, nodules, verrucous lesions, pyodermia and herpetiform lesions, vesicles, and hypopigmented or atrophic lesions

MICROSCOPIC

Histologic Features

- Morula-like sporangia appear as yeast-like spherical structures (3-30 μm) with thick double-layer walls
  - *P. wickerhamii*: Symmetric, radially arranged endospores in daisy, cartwheel, or soccer ball configuration
  - *P. zopfii*: Randomly arranged endospores
- Unicellular, reproduces through internal septation followed by release of endospores (lacks budding)
- Variable inflammatory background

ANCILLARY TESTS

Histochemistry

- Highlighted by PAS and GMS stains

DIFFERENTIAL DIAGNOSIS

Coccidioidomycosis

- Larger sporangia (> 50 μm) with numerous small endospores (2-5 μm); pulmonary involvement common

Blastomycosis

- Uniformly sized (8- to 15-μm) broad-based budding yeast (without internal septations)

Cryptococcosis

- Variably sized (5- to 15-μm) narrow-based budding yeast (without internal septations)
- Fontana-Masson and mucicarmine (capsule) positive

Chlorellosis (*Chlorella* spp.)

- Chlorophyll-containing algae (8-30 μm) infection of sheep and, rarely, humans; lesions grossly green (lost during processing); chloroplasts and starch bodies appear as PAS-positive cytoplasmic granules

SELECTED REFERENCES

1. Guo J et al: Genome sequences of two strains of Prototheca wickerhamii provide insight into the protothecosis evolution. Front Cell Infect Microbiol. 12:797017, 2022
2. Riet-Correa F et al: Protothecosis and chlorellosis in sheep and goats: a review. J Vet Diagn Invest. 33(2):283-7, 2021
3. Inoue M et al: Case report of cutaneous protothecosis caused by Prototheca wickerhamii designated as genotype 2 and current status of human protothecosis in Japan. J Dermatol. 45(1):67-71, 2018
4. Todd JR et al: Protothecosis: report of a case with 20-year follow-up, and review of previously published cases. Med Mycol. 50(7):673-89, 2012

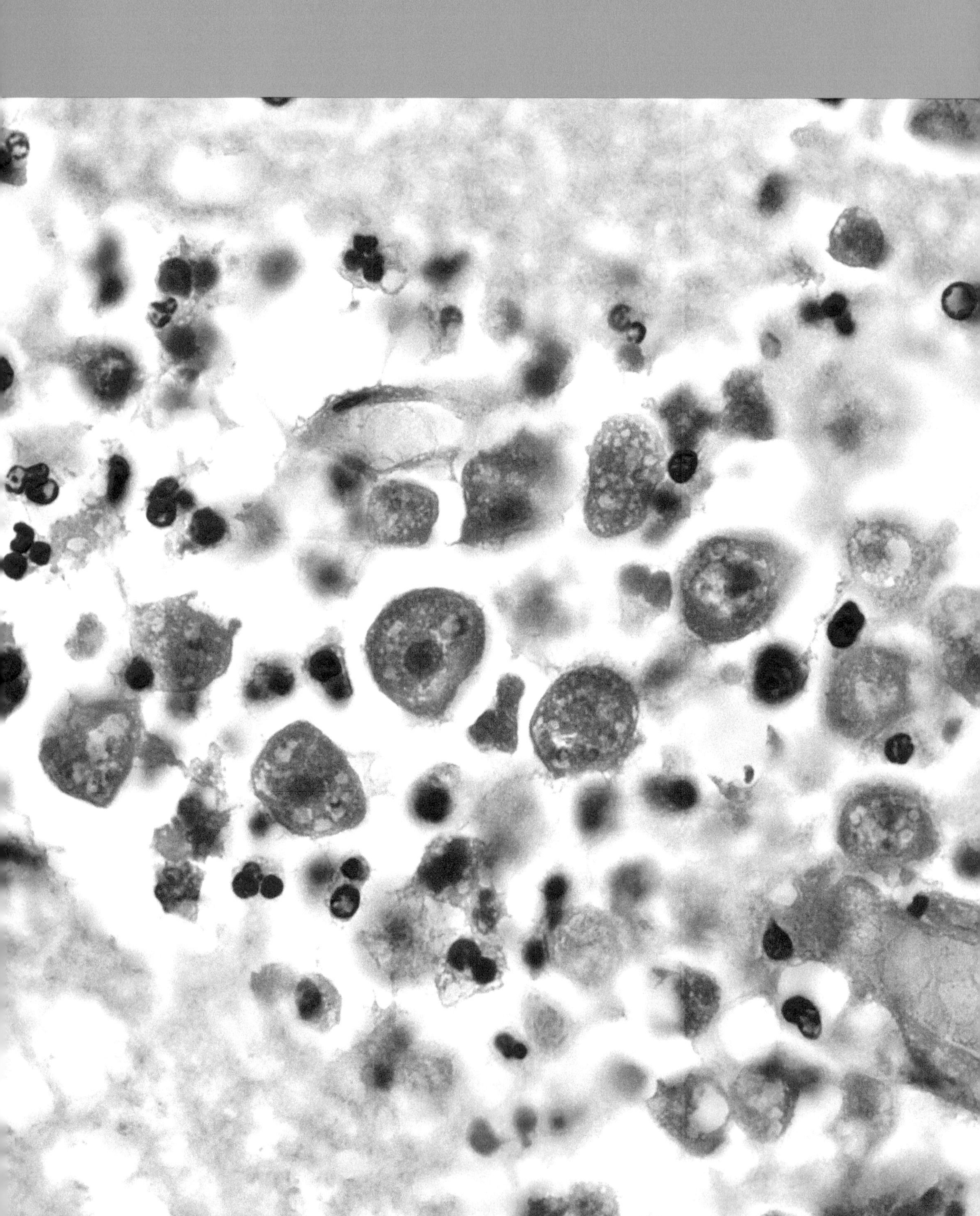

SECTION 6

Protozoan Parasitic Infections

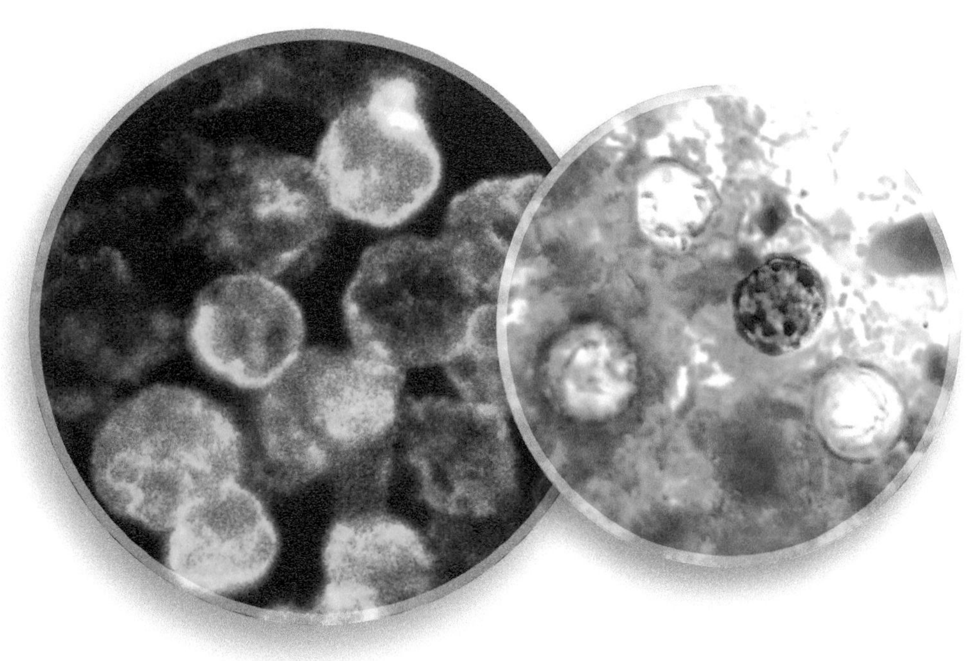

TERMINOLOGY

Definitions

- Protozoan: Single-celled eukaryotic organisms
- Helminth: Worm-like parasite
- Pathogen: Causes human symptomatic disease
- Parasite: Completes part of life cycle within host
- Definitive: Reproduces sexually inside host (also referred to as "final" or "primary")
- Intermediate: Changes stage but reproduces only asexually or not at all inside host
- Direct: Infects single species without intermediate host
- Indirect: Infects several species ± intermediate host
- Obligate: Must pass through specific host
- Facultative: May pass through host
- Accidental: Cannot complete life cycle in host
- Paratenic: Passes through host without reproducing or changing stage
- Free living: Completes life cycle without host

CLINICAL IMPLICATIONS

Parasite &/or Pathogen

- Parasitic infection results in detriment to infected host
    - Direct competition for nutrition (e.g., hypoglycemia): *Plasmodium* spp.
    - Chronic nutritional challenges (e.g., anemia, malnutrition, growth restriction): *Giardia* spp., hookworm
    - Disturbances of immune system (e.g., macrophage dysfunction): *Leishmania* spp.
- Pathogenic infections result in symptomatic disease
    - Direct tissue damage (e.g., liver necrosis, microhemorrhages): *Entamoeba histolytica*, *Toxoplasma* spp., *Toxocara* spp.
    - Space-occupying effects (e.g., hepatosplenomegaly): *Leishmania* spp., *Echinococcus* spp.
    - Failure of immune system (e.g., as opportunistic infection): *Entamoeba* spp., *Balantidium* spp.
- Human host can determine behavior as parasite or pathogen
    - *Toxoplasma* spp.: Asymptomatic disease in normal hosts or mild acute lymphadenopathy; severe necrotizing disease in newborns and immunosuppressed patients
    - *Cryptosporidium* spp.: Asymptomatic in normal host at low concentration; watery diarrhea in normal host at high concentration; severe diarrhea in immunocompromised host
- Pathogens affect host regardless of immune status
    - *Naegleria fowleri*: Free-living ameba incidentally enters human; nearly 100% fatal; limited treatment options
    - *Trypanosoma brucei rhodesiense*: Zoonosis; 100% fatal without treatment

CLINICALLY RELEVANT ORGANISMS

Ciliates

- Protozoa covered with hundreds of cilia
- *Balantidium coli*: Gastrointestinal tract pathogen (only known human ciliate pathogen)
- Many nonpathogen species are ubiquitous in water sources and may be found in human samples

Flagellates

- Protozoan having ≥ 1 flagella
- *Giardia lamblia*: Gastrointestinal tract pathogen
- *Trichomonas tenax*: Oral commensal flagellate

Amebae

- Protozoa without definitive shape, which moves through pseudopodia; cyst and trophozoites
- *E. histolytica*: Gastrointestinal tract pathogen; may invade mucosa and disseminate to liver, brain
- *Entamoeba coli*: Gastrointestinal tract parasites (nonpathogen), one of many nonpathogenic amebae; may indicate exposure to unclean water supply
- Free-living ameba: *N. fowleri*, *Balamuthia mandrillaris*, *Acanthamoeba* spp.: Usually fatal encephalitis

Apicomplexa

- Coccidia: Protozoa that are obligate intracellular parasites, often of gastrointestinal tract

Thin Blood Smear: *Trypanosoma brucei*

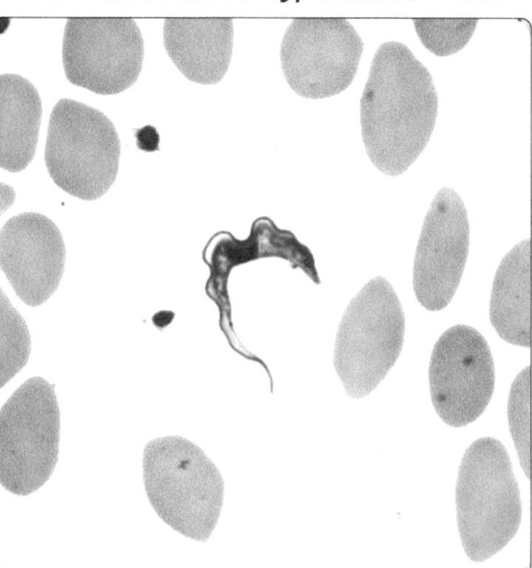

Thick Blood Smear: *Mansonella perstans*

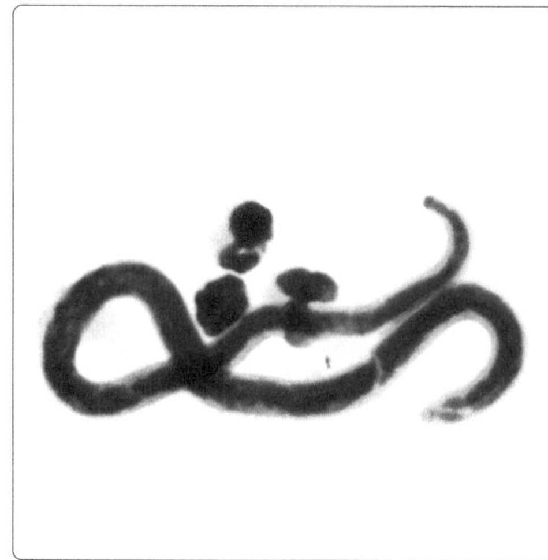

(Left) *Giemsa-stained thin blood smears are useful for quantification and speciation of Plasmodium spp., Babesia spp., Trypanosoma spp., and microfilariae. (Courtesy B. Mathison, BS, M(ASCP), CDC/PHIL.)* **(Right)** *Thick blood smears are useful for rapid screening for organisms. Microfilaria can be morphologically identified by shape, presence or absence of sheath, and arrangement of nuclei. (Courtesy M. Melvin, PhD, CDC/PHIL.)*

- Opportunistic coccidia pathogens: *Cryptosporidium* spp., *Cystoisospora* spp., *Cyclospora* spp.
- Blood-borne protozoans: Obligate intracellular parasites found in peripheral blood
- *Plasmodium* spp.: Cause human malaria
  - *Plasmodium falciparum*: Severe human disease with mortality
  - *Plasmodium vivax*, *Plasmodium ovale*: Recurrent human malaria (liver hypnozoite stage)
- *Babesia* spp.: Cause human babesiosis
  - Increase pathology in splenectomized patients
  - Share *Ixodes* spp. vector with *Borrelia* spp. and *Anaplasma* spp.
- Zoonotic protozoans: Obligate intracellular parasites of other definitive hosts and accidentally found in humans (cannot transmit/complete life cycle)
- *Toxoplasma gondii*: Deep tissue, opportunistic pathogen commonly from feline sources
- *Sarcocystis* spp.: Humans are dead-end host; often incidental finding

Kinetoplastids

- Protozoa having 1 flagellum and kinetoplast organelle causing systemic disease
- Amastigote, promastigote, epimastigote, and trypomastigote stages
- *Trypanosoma* spp.: African sleeping sickness, Chagas disease
- *Leishmania* spp.: Cutaneous, mucocutaneous, and visceral leishmaniasis

Nematodes (Roundworms)

- Adult and larval roundworms are cylindrical and may live in intestinal or extraintestinal sites; eggs may be identified in tissue and feces or microfilariae in blood
- Cuticle, hypodermis (with conspicuous lateral cords), and musculature surrounding pseudocoelom bathing digestive tract and reproductive organs (separate sexes)
- Rhabditiform larvae, filariform larvae, and microfilariae found in humans
- Gastrointestinal: *Ascaris lumbricoides* (largest affecting humans), *Enterobius vermicularis* (pinworm), *Trichuris trichiura* (whipworm), *Necator americanus* and *Ancylostoma duodenale* (hookworm)
- *Trichinella* spp.: Encysted larvae reside in muscle
- *Strongyloides stercoralis*: Predominantly gastrointestinal but can disseminate with autoinfection
- Zoonotic: *Toxocara* spp., *Baylisascaris procyonis*, *Pseudoterranova* spp., *Anisakis* spp., *Angiostrongylus* spp., *Gnathostoma* spp.
- Filarial nematodes: *Wuchereria bancrofti*, *Brugia* spp., *Loa loa*, *Mansonella* spp., *Onchocerca volvulus*, *Dirofilaria* spp., *Dracunculus* spp.

Cestodes (Tapeworms)

- Adults are elongated, flat, segmented, hermaphroditical worms that live in intestinal lumen; eggs/proglottids identified in feces
- Scolex, proglottids (contain male and female reproductive organs and lack digestive tract), parenchymal calcareous corpuscles
- Larvae are cystic or solid and inhabit extraintestinal tissues
- Larval forms found in humans: Cysticercus (*Taenia solium*), coenurus (*Taenia multiceps*), sparganum (*Spirometra* spp.), hydatid (*Echinococcus* spp.)
- *Diphyllobothrium latum* (fish tapeworm), *Hymenolepis nana* (dwarf tapeworm), *Hymenolepis diminuta* (rat tapeworm), *Dipylidium caninum* (dog tapeworm)

Trematodes (Flukes)

- Adults are leaf-shaped, hermaphroditical (except for blood flukes, which have separate sexes) flatworms with prominent ventral suckers
- Tegument, muscle, parenchymal cells, alimentary tract with no anus, reproductive organs (both in same worm)
- Eggs typically identified in feces but may be deposited in unusual locations and cause pathology
- *Schistosoma* spp. (mesenteric blood vessels; blood flukes) affect gastrointestinal and urinary tract and are important cause of cirrhosis
- *Paragonimus* spp. (lung flukes): Pulmonary and extrapulmonary manifestations
- Intestinal flukes: *Fasciolopsis buski*, *Echinostoma* spp., *Heterophyes heterophyes*
- Liver flukes: *Clonorchis sinensis*, *Opisthorchis* spp., *Fasciola* spp.

DIAGNOSTIC APPROACHES

Stool Examination

- Fresh examination (within 1 hour of collection) for trophozoites, cysts, eggs, larvae
- Formalin fixation (no time limitation) for cysts, coccidia, eggs, larvae
- Polyvinyl alcohol (PVA) fixation (no time limitation) for trophozoites, cysts
- Size range of intestinal protozoa is 4 μm (*Cryptosporidium* spp.) to 200 μm (*Balantidium* spp.)
- Iodine stain: Fresh or formalin-fixed stool; rapid for visualization in wet mounts
- Modified acid-fast stain: Fresh or formalin-fixed stool; intestinal coccidia species
- Trichrome stain: Fresh, PVA, or Schaudinn fixative; intestinal protozoa, yeast
- Iron hematoxylin stain: Fresh, sodium acetate-acetic acid formalin (SAF), or PVA; permanent stain for intestinal protozoa
- Modified iron hematoxylin stain: SAF fixative; adds acid-fast detection for coccidia
- Variety of other staining techniques are available for both classes and specific parasites

Peripheral Blood Smear

- Thin smear (20 μL of blood on clean glass slide): Quantification and speciation of *Plasmodium* spp., *Babesia* spp., *Trypanosoma* spp., microfilariae
- Thick smear (20-40 μL of blood on clean glass slide): Rapid screening for parasites
- Wright-Giemsa stain: Standard blood film stain highlights all protozoa; does not optimally highlight Schüffner dots (*Plasmodium* spp.)
- Giemsa stain: Standard stain for blood-stage protozoa; accentuates Schüffner dots for malaria speciation

Parasitic Protozoa and Their Diseases

Phylum	Representative Genera	Human Diseases
Euglenozoa	*Leishmania*	Cutaneous, mucocutaneous, and visceral leishmaniasis
	Trypanosoma	Chagas disease, sleeping sickness
Metamonada	*Giardia*	Diarrhea
	Trichomonas	Vaginitis
	Dientamoeba	Colitis
Amoebozoa	*Entamoeba*	Dysentery, liver abscess
	Acanthamoeba	Meningoencephalitis, keratitis, skin and soft tissue infection
Apicomplexa	*Babesia*	Babesiosis
	Plasmodium	Malaria
	Cystoisospora, Cryptosporidium	Diarrhea
	Sarcocystis	Diarrhea
	Toxoplasma	Toxoplasmosis
Microspora	*Enterocytozoon*	Diarrhea
Ciliophora	*Balantidium*	Dysentery

Cytology and Fine-Needle Aspiration

- Cerebrospinal fluid: Free-living ameba
- Liver mass, brain mass, large abscess: *Entamoeba* spp.
- Bone marrow: *Leishmania* spp.
- Cervical Pap smear: *Trichomonas* spp.
- Skin nodules: *Leishmania* spp. (or touch preps of fresh biopsy)
- Lymph nodes: *Trypanosoma* spp.
- Hepatosplenomegaly: *Leishmania* spp.

Tissue Biopsy

- Gastrointestinal tract (invasive or adherent organisms): *Giardia* spp., *Entamoeba* spp., *Balantidium* spp., *S. stercoralis*
- Skin, liver, spleen: Cutaneous or visceral leishmaniasis
- Lymph node: *Toxoplasma* spp.
- Bladder: *Schistosoma haematobium*
- Brain: *Toxoplasma* spp., cysticercosis
- Heart: *Trypanosoma cruzi*
- Lungs: *Toxoplasma* spp., *Paragonimus spp.*, *Dirofilaria immitis*

Serology

- Presence of antibodies to given pathogen in patient's blood
- Useful for patients without chronic exposure history: Travelers, military personnel
- Not useful for patients with chronic exposure history: Immigrants from endemic areas or history of prior infection
- Invasive infections may produce positive serology

Rapid Diagnostic Tests

- Parasite antigen-based detection for rapid diagnosis
- Lateral flow assays most common; as sensitive or more sensitive than microscopy
- *Plasmodium* spp., *Giardia* spp., *Cryptosporidium* spp., *Entamoeba* spp., *Wuchereia* spp.

Molecular Diagnostics

- Detection of parasite RNA/DNA; targeted, incorporated into multiplex panels, and unbiased metagenomic sequencing assays
- Helpful in difficult differential diagnoses: *Plasmodium* spp. vs. *Babesia* spp.
- Speciation within genus: *Leishmania donovani* vs. *Leishmania mexicana*

SELECTED REFERENCES

1. Centers for Disease Control and Prevention: Diagnostic procedures. DPDx: laboratory identification of parasitic diseases of public health concern. Updated June 16, 2023. Reviewed August 30, 2023. Accessed August 30, 2023. http://www.cdc.gov/dpdx/diagnosticProcedures/index.html
2. Mathison BA et al: The landscape of parasitic infections in the United States. Mod Pathol. 36(8):100217, 2023
3. Al-Tawfiq JA et al: Parasitic lung diseases. Eur Respir Rev. 31(166), 2022
4. Lynn MK et al: Soil-transmitted helminths in the USA: a review of five common parasites and future directions for avenues of enhanced epidemiologic inquiry. Curr Trop Med Rep. 8(1):32-42, 2021
5. Garcia HH et al: Parasitic infections of the nervous system. Semin Neurol. 39(3):358-68, 2019
6. Freire ML et al: Evaluation of a new brand of immunochromatographic test for visceral leishmaniasis in Brazil made available from 2018. Rev Inst Med Trop Sao Paulo. 60:e49, 2018
7. Garcia LS et al: Practical guidance for clinical microbiology laboratories: laboratory diagnosis of parasites from the gastrointestinal tract. Clin Microbiol Rev. 31(1), 2018
8. Norgan AP et al: Parasitic infections of the skin and subcutaneous tissues. Adv Anat Pathol. 25(2):106-23, 2018
9. Sánchez C et al: Molecular detection and genotyping of pathogenic protozoan parasites in raw and treated water samples from southwest Colombia. Parasit Vectors. 11(1):563, 2018
10. Pallen MJ: Diagnostic metagenomics: potential applications to bacterial, viral and parasitic infections. Parasitology. 141(14):1856-62, 2014

Stool Exam: *Entamoeba histolytica* Cyst

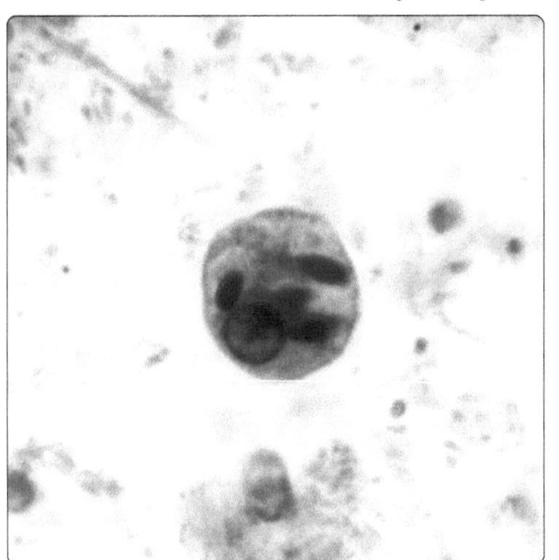

Stool Exam: *Trichuris trichiura* Egg

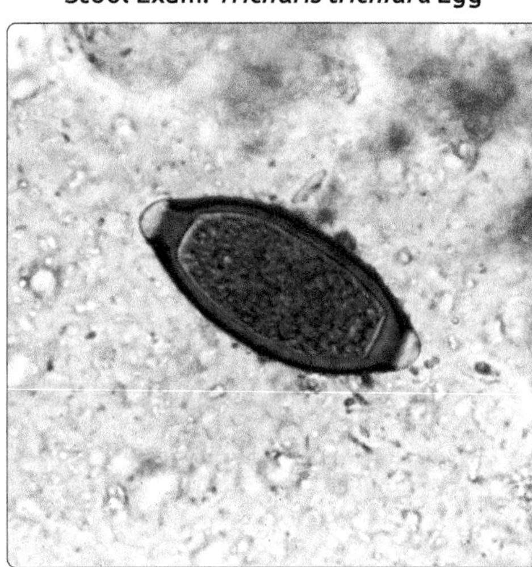

(Left) *Examination of stool specimens with various fixatives and stains can help identify trophozoites, cysts, coccidia, eggs, and larvae. Trichrome staining highlights an Entamoeba histolytica cyst with 4 chromatid bodies and a single nucleus with karyosome. (Courtesy Dr. Green, CDC/PHIL.)* **(Right)** *Stool examination highlights an egg from the parasitic nematode, Trichuris trichiura. (Courtesy M. Melvin, PhD, CDC/PHIL.)*

Skin Biopsy: Leishmaniasis

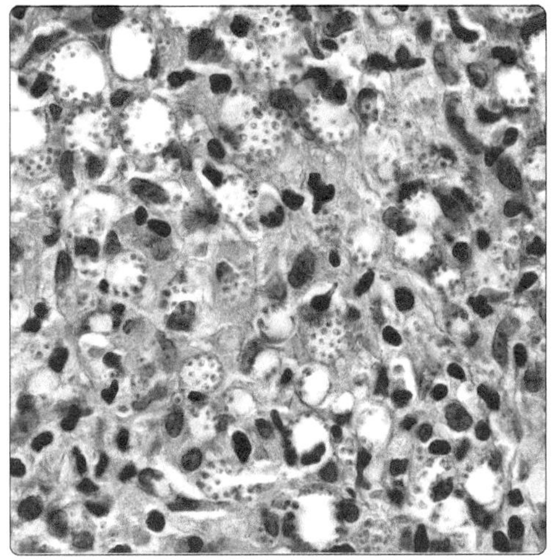

Tissue Nematode: *Trichuris trichiura*

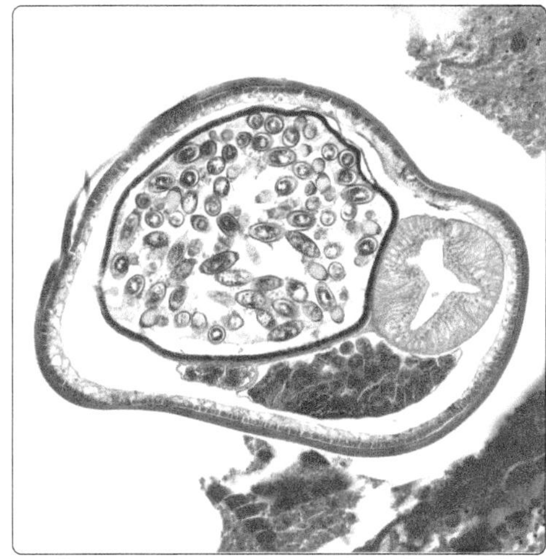

(Left) *Leishmaniasis diagnosis, like many protozoan infections, can be made by morphologic features, in the context of clinical symptoms and travel/exposure history. Identification of specific species typically requires molecular or other ancillary testing.* **(Right)** *Adult (and larvae) nematodes can be identified in tissue sections by empty-appearing body cavity containing gastrointestinal tract and male or female reproductive organs. Presence of eggs and morphology of lateral cords facilitates further classification.*

Tissue Cestode: *Taenia multiceps*

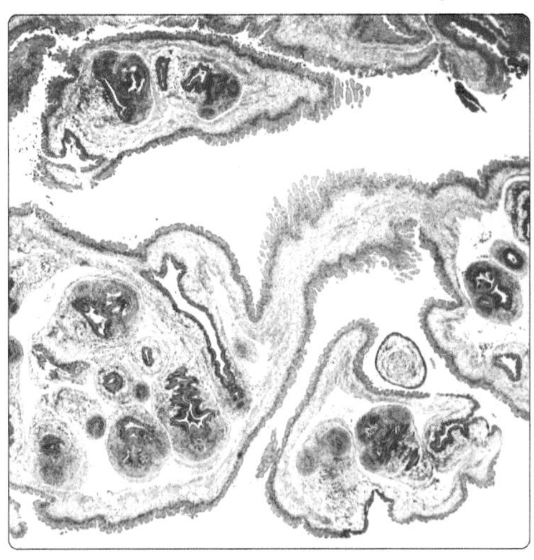

Tissue Trematode: *Clonorchis sinensis*

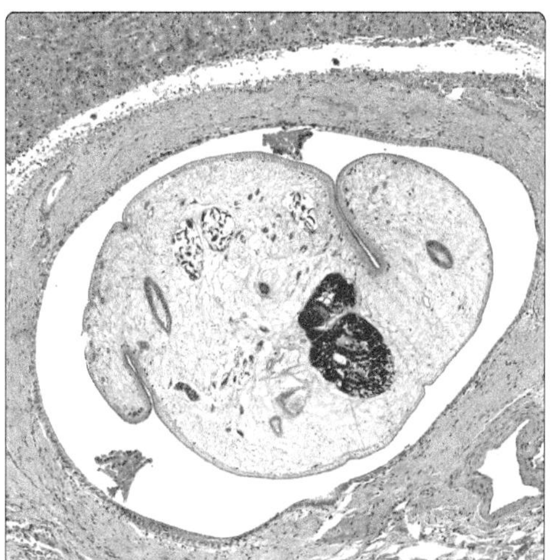

(Left) *Cestode larvae can be identified in tissue sections by thick tegument with underlying muscle and stroma containing calcareous corpuscles. Presence and number of protoscolices and size of hooklets assist in speciation.* **(Right)** *Adult trematodes can be identified in tissue sections by thick tegument, male and female reproductive organs (with eggs), alimentary tract, and a body filled with connective parenchymal cells. Genus and species classification may be difficult without gross examination of intact worm.*

KEY FACTS

ETIOLOGY/PATHOGENESIS

- Infection with *Balantidium coli*, large ciliated protozoan parasite spread via fecal-oral exposure

CLINICAL ISSUES

- Found worldwide (endemic in Philippines)
- Frequent, "explosive," bloody, mucus-containing diarrhea; risk of perforation
- Stool examination for parasites will reveal large, ciliated protozoa as trophozoites or smaller cysts
- Organisms may rarely cause infection in other sites (osteomyelitis, lung, eye, bladder) due to migratory nature

MICROSCOPIC

- Trophozoites (40-200 μm) contain cilia on cell surface, cytostome (mouth/gullet), and bean-shaped macronucleus and smaller micronucleus (often hidden)
- Cysts (50-70 μm) are spherical or ovoid
- Ulcerative colitis with loss of mucosa, severe acute inflammatory infiltrates, edema, and penetration of bowel wall (perforation)
- Appendicitis with neutrophilic infiltrates and neutrophilic peritonitis with organisms in ascitic fluid can occur

TOP DIFFERENTIAL DIAGNOSES

- Entamebiasis: Similar presentation, stool examination with smaller trophozoites/cysts; distinctive flask-shaped lesions histologically with trophozoites showing ingested red blood cells
- Bacillary dysentery: Positive stool cultures, lack of trophozoites in tissue, milder inflammatory reaction
- Ulcerative colitis &/or Crohn disease: Lack of organisms, uniformity of inflammation (± granulomas)

Balantidium Life Cycle

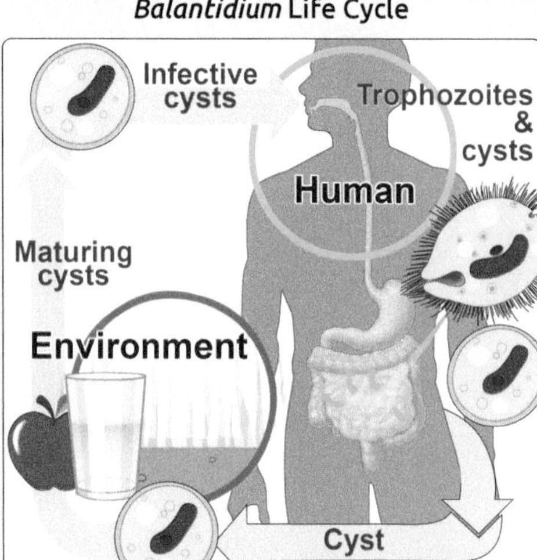

Colonic Appearance

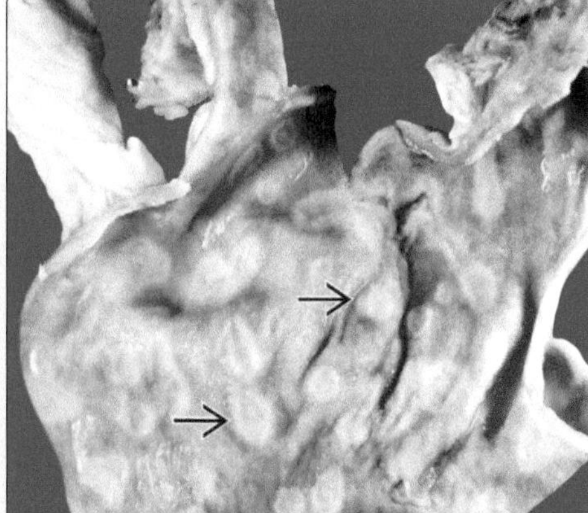

(Left) *Infective cysts are ingested from contaminated food or water (typically with pig exposure) and excyst in the intestine. Typically, infections are asymptomatic. The trophozoites can invade mucosa and cause tissue damage and severe colitis. Immature cyst forms are excreted with feces in the environment.* **(Right)** *The colon of a patient with balantidiasis demonstrates multiple ulcers ➡ in the mucosa. Ulcerations of this size and number are responsible for bloody stool. (Courtesy R. Neafie, MD.)*

B. coli Trophozoite in Stool

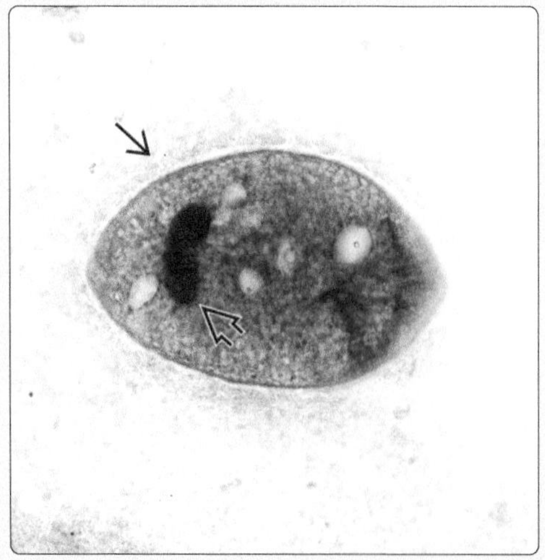

B. coli Trophozoites in Tissue Sections

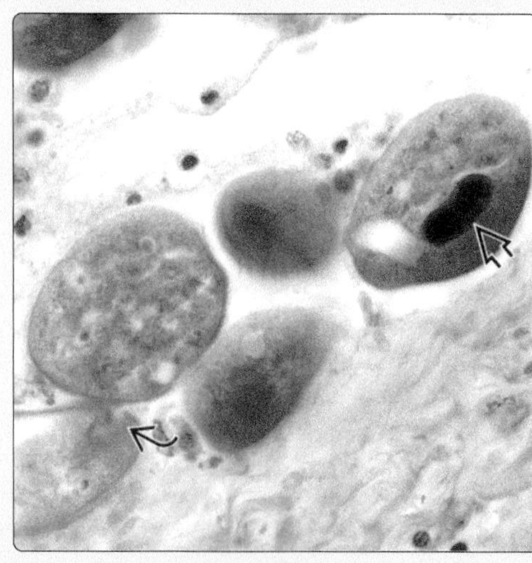

(Left) *Iron-hematoxylin stain of feces shows a trophozoite with a circumferential layer of cilia ➡ and prominent bean-shaped macronucleus ➡.* **(Right)** *This section of human intestine shows several large trophozoites relative to the adjacent inflammatory cells; bean-shaped macronuclei ➡ and cytosomes ➡ can be seen depending on plane of section.*

TERMINOLOGY

Definitions

- Greek: "Balantidion" (little bag) + "kolon" (colon)

ETIOLOGY/PATHOGENESIS

Infectious Agents

- Infection with *Balantidium coli*, large ciliated protozoan parasite spread via fecal-oral exposure; only ciliate that infects humans/causes gastrointestinal disease
- Normal host of parasite is pigs; humans are incidental/accidental hosts; also found in rats and other mammals, which may be source in immunosuppressed
- Natural disasters may lead to increased use of contaminated water and outbreaks in normal hosts
- Cysts pass into environment from feces of infected mammals/humans (triggered by dehydration) and are ingested by next host through contaminated food/water
- Cysts pass through susceptible stomach (usually destroyed by low pH) into small bowel, where they excyst and mature to trophozoites, which infect large intestine, feed on bacteria, and occasionally burrow into intestinal wall
- Organisms predominantly multiply by asexual reproduction (binary fission), but sexual reproduction occurs through conjugation

CLINICAL ISSUES

Epidemiology

- Prevalence of 0.02-1% in human population
- Found worldwide, but endemic focus present in Philippines
- Immunocompromised and patients with malnutrition or other gastrointestinal imbalances at highest risk

Presentation

- Asymptomatic carriage occurs
- Active, acute disease with frequent, "explosive," bloody, mucus-containing diarrhea (2-3x per hour); severe abdominal pain &/or sepsis may indicate bowel perforation
- Chronic disease with nonbloody diarrhea, cramping, halitosis, and abdominal pain

Laboratory Tests

- Stool examination for parasites will reveal large, ciliated protozoa as trophozoites or smaller cysts; yield enhanced by sedimentation or flotation techniques
- Bronchoalveolar lavage can reveal trophozoites, distinguished from ciliated respiratory epithelial cells
- Trophozoites have been isolated from urine in patients with genitourinary involvement (direct spread from colon)

Treatment

- Tetracycline for gastrointestinal diarrheal disease
- Surgical resection may be required for perforation

Prognosis

- Uncomplicated disease is easily treated with medication
- Severe abdominal disease with perforation may be life threatening (30% mortality)

MICROBIOLOGY

Parasite Characteristics

- Trophozoites (40-200 μm) contain cilia on cell surface, cytostome (mouth/gullet), and bean-shaped macronucleus and smaller micronucleus (often hidden); reside in intestines; shed in diarrheal stool and may be visible by naked eye in glass of clean water
- Cysts (50-70 μm) are spherical or ovoid; shed in diarrheal and formed stool

Culture

- No role in diagnosis of balantidiasis

MACROSCOPIC

Gastrointestinal Tract

- Ulcerative colitis, gangrenous appendix, frank perforation with fibrinous peritonitis

MICROSCOPIC

Histologic Features

- Organisms appear as large, round to oval bodies covered in fine cilia layer (similar appearance to brush border of intestine) with large, dark blue to black macronucleus
- Ulcerative colitis with loss of mucosa, severe acute inflammatory infiltrates, edema, and penetration of bowel wall (perforation)
- Appendicitis with neutrophilic infiltrates and neutrophilic peritonitis with organisms in ascitic fluid can occur
- Lung (rare): Hematogenous spread from colon associated with discrete lesions of frank neutrophilic pneumonia with necrosis containing organisms
- Osteomyelitis (extremely rare): Purulent abscess of spine containing *B. coli* trophozoites has occurred

DIFFERENTIAL DIAGNOSIS

Entamebiasis

- Similar presentation with stool examination revealing smaller *Entamoeba histolytica* trophozoites/cysts
- Similar histologically, but with distinctive flask-shaped lesions and trophozoites showing ingested red blood cells

Bacillary Dysentery

- Positive stool cultures, lack of trophozoites in tissue, milder inflammatory reaction

Ulcerative Colitis &/or Crohn Disease

- Lack of organisms, uniformity of inflammation (± granulomas), and clinical history

SELECTED REFERENCES

1. Aninagyei E et al: Prevalence and risk factors of human Balantidium coli infection and its association with haematological and biochemical parameters in Ga West Municipality, Ghana. BMC Infect Dis. 21(1):1047, 2021
2. Byun JW et al: Identification of zoonotic Balantioides coli in pigs by polymerase chain reaction-restriction fragment length polymorphism (PCR-RFLP) and its distribution in Korea. Animals (Basel). 11(9), 2021
3. da Silva RKM et al: Balantidiasis in humans: a systematic review and meta-analysis. Acta Trop. 223:106069, 2021
4. Pinilla JC et al: Comparison between five coprological methods for the diagnosis of Balantidium coli cysts in fecal samples from pigs. Vet World. 14(4):873-7, 2021

KEY FACTS

ETIOLOGY/PATHOGENESIS

- Infections with coccidian intestinal parasites (*Cryptosporidium* spp., *Cyclospora cayetanensis,* and *Cystoisospora belli)* via ingestion of food or water contaminated with oocysts

CLINICAL ISSUES

- Profuse, watery diarrhea
- Stool examination
  - *Cryptosporidium* spp. (4-6 μm) and *Cyclospora* spp. (8-10 μm) have round oocysts
  - *Cystoisospora* spp. (30 x 20 μm) have ellipsoidal-shaped oocysts containing sporoblasts, sporocysts, or sporozoites
  - Modified acid-fast stain (stool) positive for all 3 coccidia (*Cyclospora* variably positive)
- Rapid antigen testing for *Cryptosporidium* spp.
- Immunocompromised have recovery with risk of recurrence

MICROSCOPIC

- Mild villous blunting, surface epithelial cell disarray with apoptosis, and mildly increased surface intraepithelial lymphocytes
- *Cryptosporidium* spp.: Small, round, bluish-purple bodies within cytoplasm present at luminal tips and surfaces of villi
- *Cyclospora* and *Cystoisospora* spp.: Round to oval large inclusions within epithelial cells toward apical surface

TOP DIFFERENTIAL DIAGNOSES

- Microsporidiosis (often small bowel): Intracytoplasmic bodies in epithelial surface; microsporidia cysts in stool; EM on tissue
- Giardiasis (small bowel): Purple, triangular, flagellated bodies on or near epithelial surface; trophozoites or cysts in stool
- Entamebiasis (colon): Trophozoites invasive into lamina propria and submucosa, and with ingested RBCs in stool

Life Cycle of Coccidia

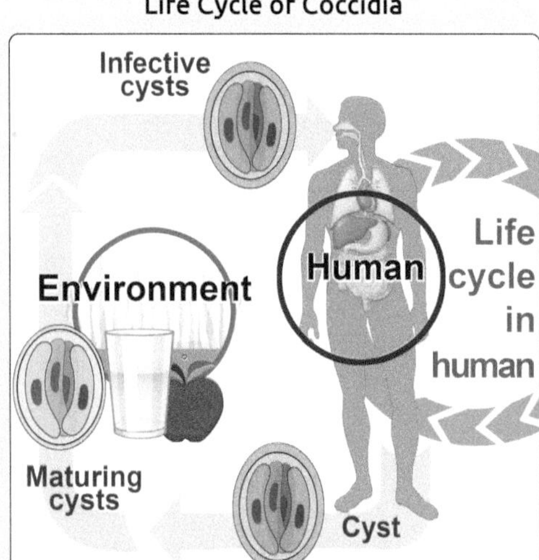

Cryptosporidiosis

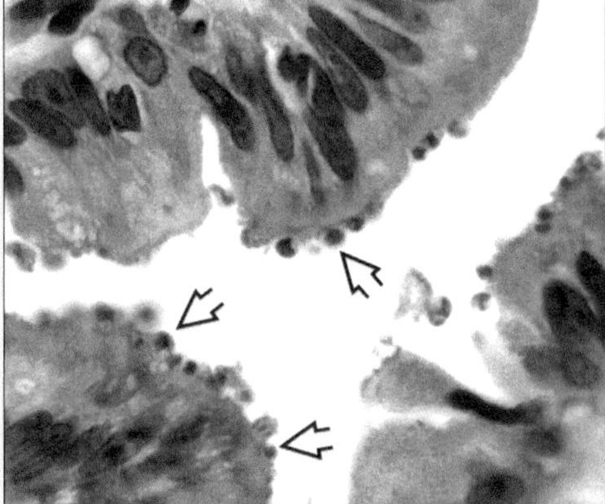

(Left) *Coccidia are ingested from contaminated environmental sources (food and water) and excyst in the human GI tract to invade epithelium. Recurrent cycles of reinvasion of the epithelium (due to immunosuppression or infective load) leads to secretory diarrhea. Immature cysts exit in the stool to the environment.* **(Right)** *Cryptosporidium organisms are basophilic, spherical structures ⊡ (2-5 μm) present intracytoplasmically within the apical brush border of the intestinal epithelial cells.*

Cyclosporiasis

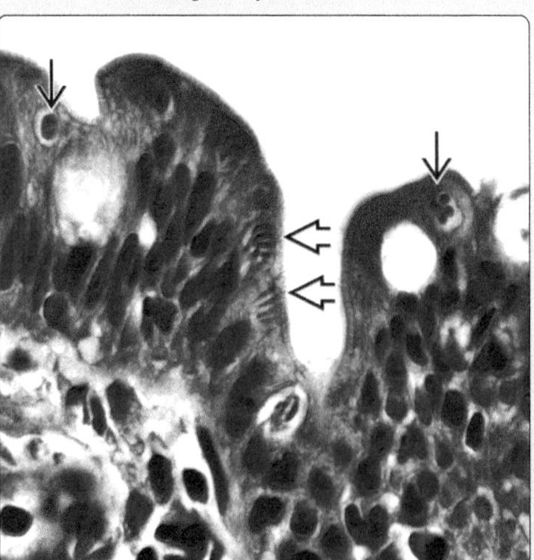

Cystoisosporiasis

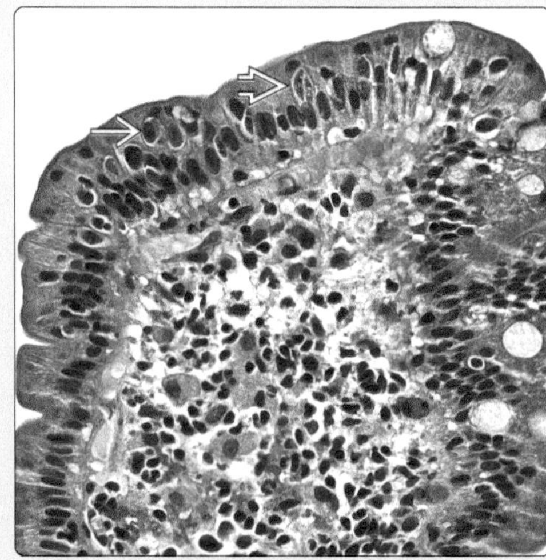

(Left) *Cyclospora (round forms ⊡ and crescent-shaped forms ⊡) in parasitophorous vacuoles are most often present in the surface epithelium in the upper 1/3 of epithelial cells. (From DP: Endoscopic.)* **(Right)** *Tissue section shows crescent-shaped Cystoisospora asexual forms ⊡ and ovoid sexual forms ⊡ within parasitophorous vacuoles. (From DP: GI.)*

TERMINOLOGY

Definitions

- *Cryptosporidium* spp. derived from Greek "crypto" (hidden) + "sporos" (seed)
- *Cyclospora cayetanensis* derived from Greek "cyclo" (round) + "sporos" (seed) and Cayetano Heredia University (Lima, Peru) for Dr. Ortega
- *Cystoisospora belli* derived from Greek "kustis" (cyst) + "isos" (equal) + "sporos" (seed) +"belli" (beautiful)

ETIOLOGY/PATHOGENESIS

Infectious Agents

- Cryptosporidiosis is most common human coccidian intestinal parasite infection via ingestion of water contaminated with *Cryptosporidium* spp. sporulated oocysts
  - Water treatment requires prohibitive levels of chlorine for inactivation; may be inactivated by UV light; primarily removed from drinking water through flocculation
  - *C. parvum* and *C. hominis* leading causes of infection; *C. canis, C. cuniculus, C. felis, C. meleagridis, C. muris, C. ubiquitum*, and *C. viatorum* can also infect humans
- Cyclosporiasis infection from ingestion of food and drink (water, vegetables, fruits) contaminated with *Cyclospora cayetanensis* sporulated oocysts
  - Most cases occur during spring and summer months; 1/3 of cases in USA are acquired from Latin America and Caribbean
- Cystoisosporiasis is least common of 3 human coccidian intestinal parasite infections from water contaminated with *Cystoisospora belli* (formerly *Isospora belli*) mature oocysts with sporozoites

CLINICAL ISSUES

Presentation

- Cryptosporidiosis, cyclosporiasis, cystoisosporiasis: Profuse, watery diarrhea
- Contaminated water during water system failures leads to epidemic outbreaks of cryptosporidiosis due to massive ingestion
- *Cystoisospora* spp. causes eosinophilia
- Individual patient's failing immune system leads to amplified infection
- Coinfection with *Cyclospora, Cryptosporidium*, and other parasites has been described for immunocompetent and immunocompromised individuals

Laboratory Tests

- PCR/molecular testing
  - 18S rRNA targets can detect both human and bovine spp. specifically for *Cryptosporidium* spp.
  - 18S rRNA targets specific for *Cyclospora* spp. (cross reacts with *Eimeria* spp.)
- Rapid antigen testing
  - *Cryptosporidium* spp.: Highly sensitive and specific
  - Not available for other coccidia

Treatment

- *Cryptosporidium* spp.: Usually self-limited, support with fluids, nitazoxanide
- *Cyclospora* and *Cystoisospora* spp.: Trimethoprim-sulfamethoxazole (TS), pyrimethamine (if TS-allergic), ciprofloxacin (less effective)
- Reverse immunosuppression in immunosuppressed hosts
- Uncontrolled HIV leads to chronic diarrhea, corrects with increased antiretrovirals; prevented with prophylaxis (when no antiviral therapy available)

Prognosis

- Immunocompetent have full recovery with no recurrence
- Immunocompromised have recovery with risk of recurrence

MICROBIOLOGY

Stool Examination

- Conventional wet mount
  - *Cryptosporidium* spp. (4-6 μm) and *Cyclospora* spp. (8-10 μm) have round oocysts that may have visible sporozoites
  - *Cystoisospora* spp. (30 x 20 μm) have ellipsoidal-shaped oocyst containing sporoblasts, sporocysts, or sporozoites
- Modified acid-fast stain: All 3 coccidia are acid-fast; *Cyclospora* spp. is variably acid-fast, and organisms in same field may be negative
- Safranin stain: All 3 coccidia are orange to red, although more variable than acid-fast
- Trichrome stain: Highly variable and should not be used for confirmatory diagnosis
- Autofluorescence: *Cyclospora* and *Cystoisospora* spp.

Culture

- No role in diagnosis of coccidian parasites

Sporulation Assay

- For distinguishing *Cyclospora* from other stool organism, assayed over 3 weeks to monitor for evidence of sporulation
- Potassium dichromate (2.5%) reduces bacterial growth

MICROSCOPIC

Histologic Features

- Coccidian infections of small intestine have mild villous blunting, surface epithelial cell disarray with apoptosis, and mildly increased surface intraepithelial lymphocytes
- *Cryptosporidium* spp.
  - Small, round, bluish-purple bodies present at luminal tips and surfaces of villi of small bowel
  - Minimal to mild chronic inflammation may be present in lamina propria
  - Severely immunosuppressed hosts may show multiple infections
- *Cyclospora* spp.
  - Located toward luminal surface of small bowel epithelium but within cytoplasm
  - Round forms (2-3 μm) with parasitophorous vacuole ("halo")
  - Crescentic merozoites (5-6 μm) with parasitophorous vacuole
- *Cystoisospora* spp.
  - Located toward luminal surfaces of epithelial cells but within cytoplasm

- Schizonts and merozoites with crescentic or banana-shaped forms

ANCILLARY TESTS

Electron Microscopy

- In highly suspect cases, tissue submitted for EM can show diagnostic forms of organisms as well as assist with differential diagnosis (primarily excluding microsporidiosis)

DIFFERENTIAL DIAGNOSIS

Microsporidiosis

- Identification of microsporidia cysts in stool in infected patient via stool O&P exam or by EM on biopsy
- On biopsy, microsporidia are small collections of intracytoplasmic bodies in epithelial surface of colon or small intestine with villous blunting

Giardiasis

- Identification of *Giardia intestinalis* trophozoites or cysts in stool of infected patients via stool O&P
- On biopsy, *Giardia* organisms are purple, triangular, flagellated bodies adherent to or floating near epithelial surface of small intestine

Entamebiasis

- Microscopic examination of fresh stool smears for *Entamoeba histolytica* trophozoites that contain ingested RBCs
- On biopsy, *E. histolytica* may be invasive into lamina propria and submucosa with edema and inflammation in colon

SELECTED REFERENCES

1. Love MS et al: Emerging treatment options for cryptosporidiosis. Curr Opin Infect Dis. 34(5):455-62, 2021
2. Mathison BA et al: Cyclosporiasis-updates on clinical presentation, pathology, clinical diagnosis, and treatment. Microorganisms. 9(9), 2021
3. Khurana S et al: Laboratory diagnosis of cryptosporidiosis. Trop Parasitol. 8(1):2-7, 2018
4. Swanson EA et al: Epithelial inclusions in gallbladder specimens mimic parasite infection: histologic and molecular examination of reported Cystoisospora belli infection in gallbladders of immunocompetent patients. Am J Surg Pathol. 42(10):1346-52, 2018
5. Cama VA et al: Infections by intestinal Coccidia and Giardia duodenalis. Clin Lab Med. 35(2):423-44, 2015

(Left) *A wet mount of stool from a patient with cryptosporidiosis shows the very small, round oocysts ⇒ (4-6 μm), which may be difficult to diagnose without modified acid-fast staining. (Courtesy P. Drotman, MD, CDC/PHIL.)* **(Right)** *A small intestine biopsy shows numerous Cryptosporidium organisms ⇒ disrupting the epithelial brush border that are negative for acid-fast staining (in contrast to positive mAFB staining in stool).*

***Cryptosporidium* spp. Stool Preparation**

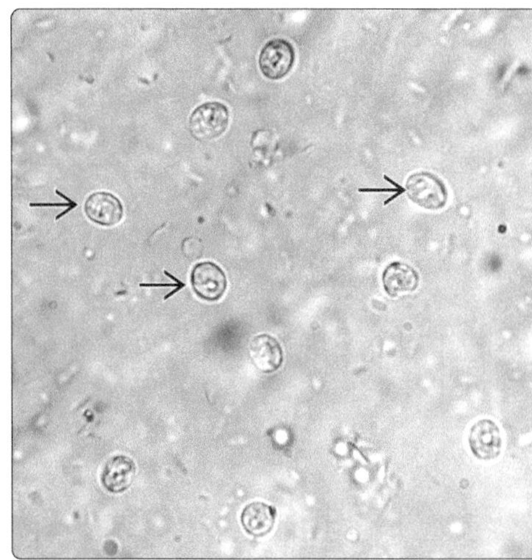

***Cryptosporidium* spp. mAFB Stain in Tissue**

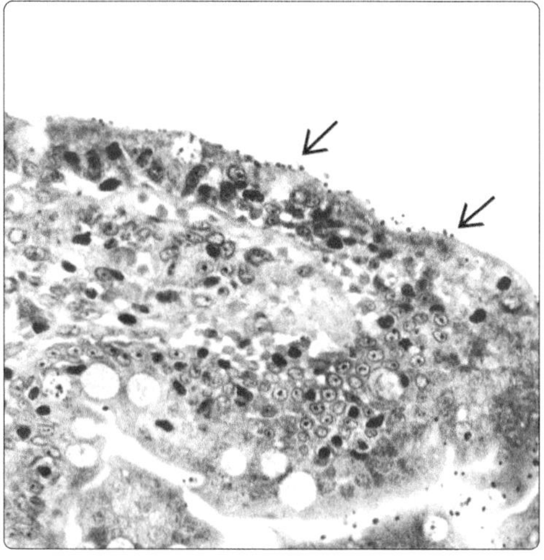

(Left) *A case of cryptosporidiosis in the small intestine stained with PAS shows a uniform, pink brush border interrupted by occasional parasites ⇒ appearing as blue to purple dots.* **(Right)** *Giemsa staining of small intestine tissue shows numerous spherical Cryptosporidium organisms ⇒ within the epithelial brush border.*

***Cryptosporidium* spp. PAS Stain in Tissue**

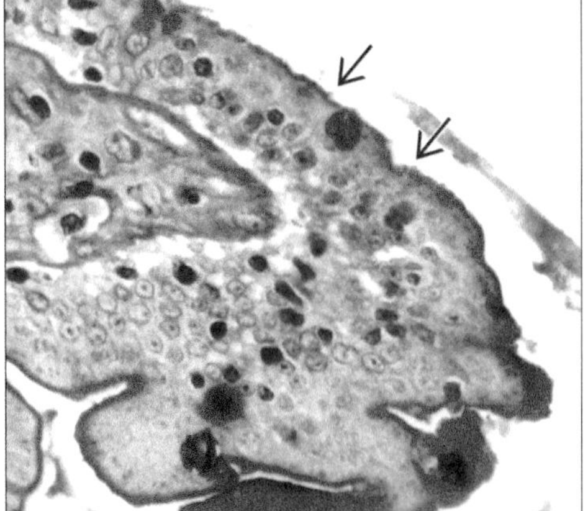

***Cryptosporidium* spp. Giemsa Stain in Tissue**

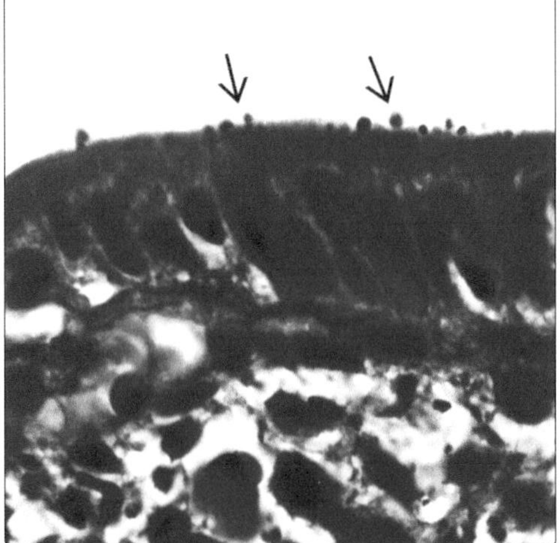

Cryptosporidium parvum: AFB in Stool

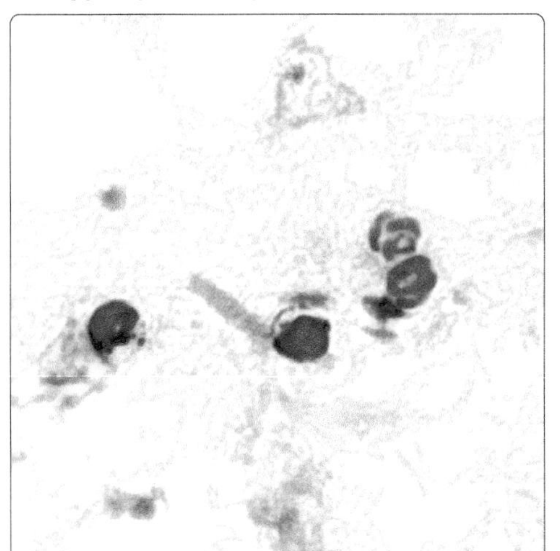

Cryptosporidium spp. in Tissue Sections

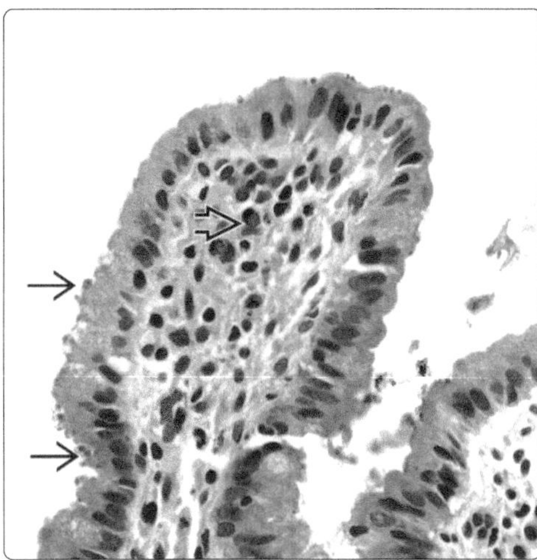

(Left) *Modified acid-fast staining highlights Cryptosporidium parvum oocysts in red (4-6 µm), which contain visible sporozoites. (Courtesy CDC/DPDx.)* **(Right)** *Histologic section of small intestine shows mixed inflammation with prominent eosinophils ➡ and basophilic, spherical forms of a Cryptosporidium spp. infection ➡.*

Cyclospora spp.: AFB in Stool

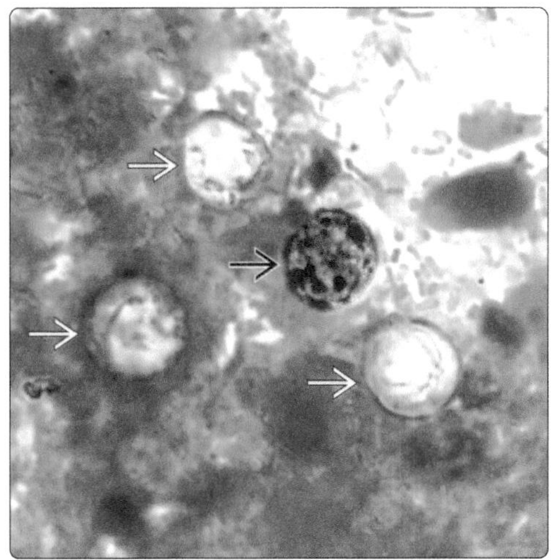

Cyclospora spp. in Tissue Sections

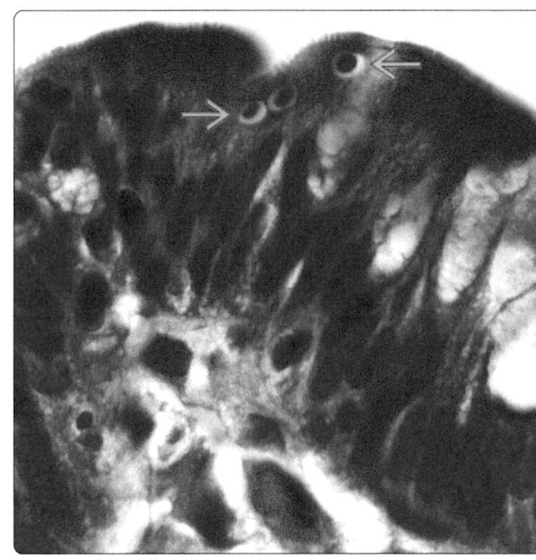

(Left) *Cyclospora spp. on stool smear after AFB staining shows almost perfectly round, variably positive cysts (8-10 µm), some staining red ➡ and others nonstaining ➡. (Courtesy M. Moser, CDC/PHIL.)* **(Right)** *This biopsy shows 3 Cyclospora organisms ➡ present within parasitophorous vacuoles located in the apical cytoplasm of enterocytes beneath the brush border. (From DP: GI.)*

Cystoisospora belli: AFB in Stool

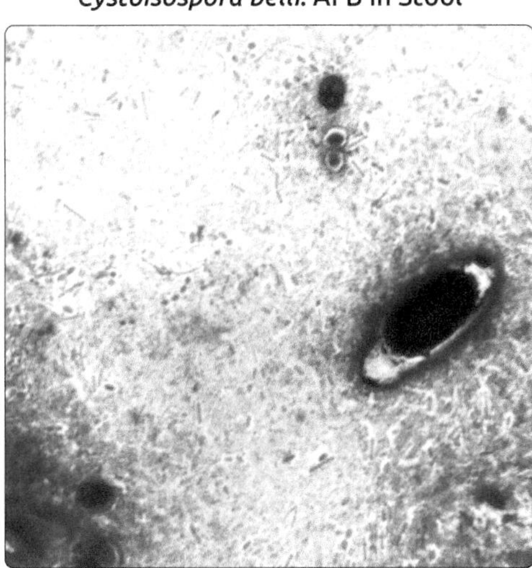

Cystoisospora belli in Tissue Sections

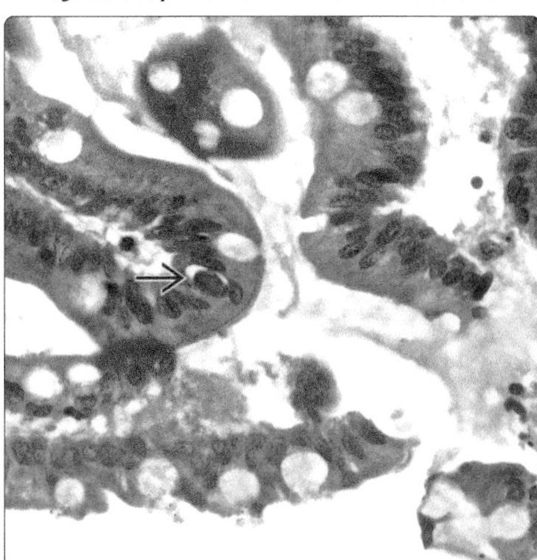

(Left) *Modified acid-fast stain shows positive Cystoisospora belli oocysts (30 x 20 µm) in a stool specimen. (From CP: Medical Microbiology.)* **(Right)** *The asexual and sexual stages of the Cystoisospora spp. ➡ in the epithelium may stain the same as, or slightly paler than, the human epithelial cell nuclei adjacent, which makes distinguishing them very challenging.*

Entamebiasis

KEY FACTS

ETIOLOGY/PATHOGENESIS

- Infection with *Entamoeba histolytica* ("lyser of tissue") via ingestion of cysts through fecal-oral transmission

CLINICAL ISSUES

- Dysentery (bloody diarrhea), fulminant colitis, ameboma, and extraintestinal disease (e.g., liver abscess)
- ~ 50 million cases and ~ 100,000 deaths/year worldwide
- Antigen testing, serology, PCR, and stool examination

MICROBIOLOGY

- Mature cysts (12-15 μm) have 4 nuclei with central karyosomes and uniformly distributed peripheral chromatin
- Trophozoites (usually 15-20 μm) have single nucleus with central karyosome, uniformly distributed peripheral chromatin, and cytoplasm with granular appearance

MICROSCOPIC

- Multiple discrete flask-shaped ulcers separated by regions of normal-appearing colonic mucosa
- Diffusely inflamed and edematous mucosa, necrosis, or wall perforation
- Trophozoites at ulcer base contain single nucleus with karyosome, foamy cytoplasm, and ingested RBCs
- Disseminated disease with acellular abscess containing necrotic debris, trophozoites, and variable rim
- Thick, yellow-brown liver abscess aspirate ("anchovy paste")

TOP DIFFERENTIAL DIAGNOSES

- Enteroinvasive or enterohemorrhagic *Escherichia coli* infections: Absence of parasites; positive stool cultures
- *Shigella* spp. infections: Fecal leukocytes, fresh blood in stool
- *Campylobacter* spp. infections: Positive Gram stain of stool samples for characteristic curved rod organisms; ELISA or PCR are specific for detecting *Campylobacter jejuni*
- Pyogenic hepatic abscesses: Most commonly isolated organisms include *E. coli*, *Bacteroides* spp., and *Streptococcus* spp.; cryptogenic (no identified cause) in 1/2 of cases

Life Cycle of *Entamoeba*

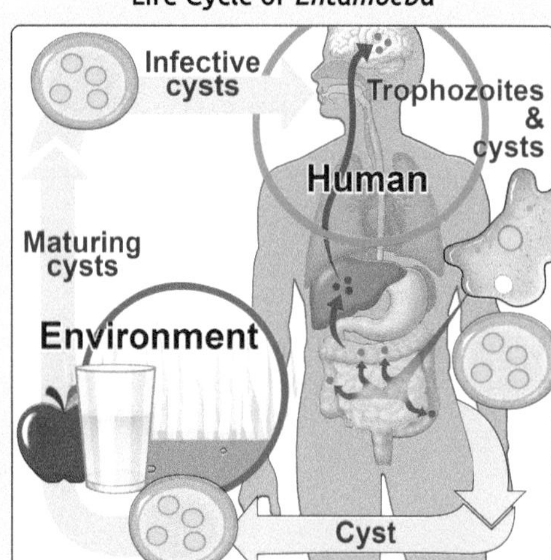

Amebic Colitis

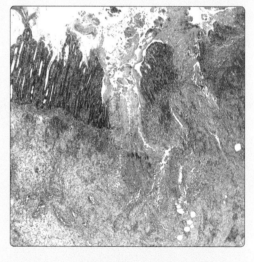

(Left) *Entamoeba histolytica and other ameba share a life cycle of ingested, infective cysts, which excyst in the intestine. For most organisms, trophozoites thrive in the intestine, eventually produce immature cysts, and pass them into stool. E. histolytica, however, can damage tissue, penetrate the wall of the GI tract, and disseminate to liver, lung, brain, etc.* **(Right)** *Multiple discrete flask-shaped ulcers are present in amebic colitis, which are separated by normal-appearing colonic mucosa.*

Entamoeba histolytica Trophozoites

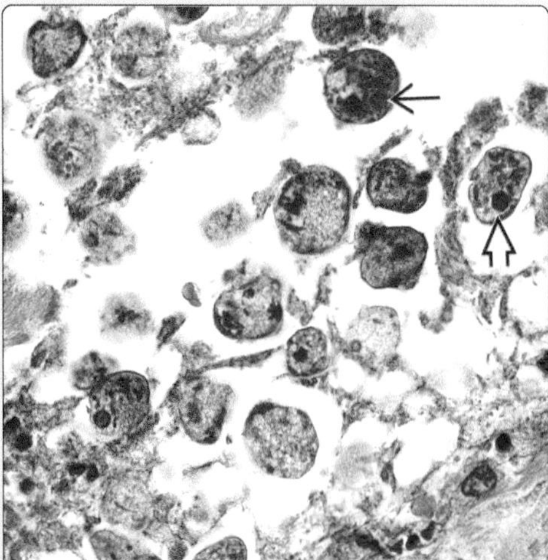

Entamoeba histolytica Trophozoites: Trichome Stain

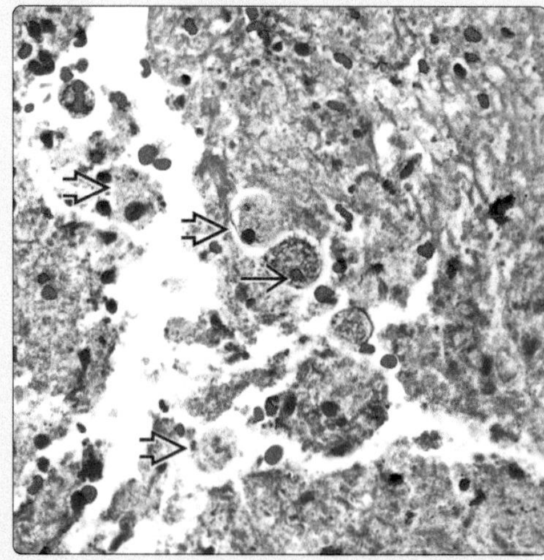

(Left) *In tissue sections, E. histolytica trophozoites (up to 60 μm) appear round, contain a nucleus with central karyosome ⇒, have foamy cytoplasm, and may exhibit ingested RBCs ⇒.* **(Right)** *Trichrome staining of colon with invasive E. histolytica demonstrates numerous trophozoites ⇒, some of which contain ingested RBCs ⇒.*

TERMINOLOGY

Synonyms

- Amebic dysentery, amebiasis

Definitions

- *Entamoeba* derived from Latin "ent" (intestine, internal) + Greek "amoiba" (change, alteration)
- *histolytica* derived from Latin "histo" (tissue) + "lytica" (lyses) named for parasite's ability to destroy host tissues

ETIOLOGY/PATHOGENESIS

Infectious Agents

- Infection with *Entamoeba histolytica,* anaerobic, eukaryotic, parasitic protozoan via ingestion of cysts through fecal-oral transmission
- Infection also occurs through sexual transmission; men who have sex with men (MSM) have higher incidence than general population
- Excystation occurs in terminal ileum or colon, resulting in trophozoites, which can remain luminal, invade intestinal mucosa, or invade blood vessels to reach liver, brain, and lungs
- Mechanism of human cell killing has been unclear but may be through ingestion of distinct pieces of living cells, resulting in intracellular calcium elevation and eventual cell death
- Trophozoites multiply by binary fission and produce cysts; both trophozoites and cysts passed in feces with cysts surviving in environment for days to weeks
- Additional nonpathogenic spp. that can colonize humans, including *E. dispar, E. moshkovskii, E. polecki, E. coli, E. hartmanni, Endolimax nana, Dientamoeba fragilis,* and *Iodamoeba buetschlii*

CLINICAL ISSUES

Epidemiology

- ~ 50 million cases of invasive disease, and ~ 100,000 deaths occur each year worldwide
- Prevalence of amebiasis in USA is ~ 4%
- Commonly affects people in tropical areas with poor sanitary conditions with exposure to water contaminated with human feces
- Humans are only known reservoir for *E. histolytica*

Presentation

- Dysentery (bloody diarrhea)
- Fulminant colitis
- Toxic megacolon
- Ameboma (amebic colonic pseudotumor formation)
- Invasive extraintestinal disease includes liver abscess, pleuropulmonary disease, pericarditis, brain abscess, peritonitis, and GU disease

Laboratory Tests

- Antigen testing
  - Commercially available assays with good sensitivity and specificity; may be able to distinguish between *E. histolytica* and *E. dispar*
  - May require fresh tissue
- Serology: Greatest use for liver and disseminated disease
  - Highly sensitive and specific but may be negative in first 7-10 days
  - Less useful in endemic areas where large percentage of population has positive antibodies
  - Enzyme immunoassays (EIAs) have ~ 95% sensitivity for extraintestinal disease, ~ 70% for intestinal infection, and ~ 10% for asymptomatic infection
- Molecular testing (performed on stool or tissue samples)
  - Single and multiplexed PCR-based assays targeting different genes, including 18S rRNA
  - High sensitivity and specificity but takes longer and can be more costly than antigen testing

Treatment

- Asymptomatic amebiasis: Iodoquinol, paromomycin, or diloxanide furoate
- Amebic colitis: Nitroimidazole derivative, paromomycin
- Amebic liver abscess: Drainage or metronidazole
- Flavonoids represent very promising and innocuous strategy that should be considered for use against *E. histolytica* in era of microbial drug resistance
- There is no effective vaccine; therefore, prevention focuses on sanitation and access to clean water

Prognosis

- Mortality is related to extent of dissemination and lack of treatment
- Toxic megacolon can present with bacteria sepsis with high mortality

IMAGING

Ultrasonographic Findings

- Evaluate amebic liver abscess, which is solitary homogeneous, hypoechoic, round lesion

MICROBIOLOGY

Parasite Features

- Mature cysts (12-15 μm) have 4 nuclei with centrally located karyosomes and fine, uniformly distributed peripheral chromatin
- Trophozoites (usually 15-20 μm; more elongated in diarrheal stool) have single nucleus with centrally placed karyosome, uniformly distributed peripheral chromatin, and cytoplasm with granular or ground-glass appearance

Stool Exam

- Microscopic examination of fresh stool smears for trophozoites that contain ingested RBCs
- Erythrophagocytosis is classically associated with *E. histolytica* but may rarely occur with *E. dispar,* considered diagnostic for *E. histolytica* infection in patients with dysentery
- 3 stool samples over no more than 10 days can improve detection rate to 85-95%
- Motility of *E. histolytica* in fresh preparations usually occurs in linear (not random) fashion with clear hyaline ectoplasm flowing to form blunt-ended pseudopodia, which guide endoplasm that contains nucleus

- If fresh stool specimen cannot be examined immediately, it should be preserved with fixative, such as polyvinyl alcohol, or kept cool (4 °C); motility can cease, and trophozoites can lyse within 20-30 minutes

Culture

- Complex system not used for routine diagnosis with success rate of 50-70%

MICROSCOPIC

Histologic Features

- GI disease
  - Mucosal thickening, multiple discrete ulcers separated by regions of normal-appearing colonic mucosa
  - Diffuse inflammation and edematous mucosa, necrosis, or wall perforation
  - Flask-shaped ulcer of amebic colitis
  - Trophozoites (10-60 μm) appear round with central karyosome-containing nucleus, foamy cytoplasm, and ingested RBCs
  - Trophozoites are present in ulcer base, at adjacent mucosal surface, and, less commonly, in bowel wall and blood vessels
- Disseminated disease
  - Acellular abscess containing necrotic debris, trophozoites, and variable rim
  - Minimal inflammation may be present due to direct cell lysis by parasite

Cytologic Features

- Liver abscess aspirate is usually thick, yellow-brown liquid classically referred to as anchovy paste
- Amebas may be rarely seen, and no inflammatory cells are present in aspirate

ANCILLARY TESTS

Histochemistry

- Masson trichrome highlights trophozoites in red
- PAS stains intracytoplasmic glycogen and complex carbohydrates in trophozoites

Immunohistochemistry

- CD68 generally negative but may show weak staining due to ingested contents
- Anti-*E. histolytica* IHC is available but not widely utilized

DIFFERENTIAL DIAGNOSIS

Enteroinvasive or Enterohemorrhagic *Escherichia coli* Infections

- Absence of parasites; positive stool cultures
- Negative ELISA and PCR for *E. histolytica*

Shigella spp. Infections

- Fecal leukocytes, which are absent or rare in *E. histolytica*
- Fresh blood in stool

Pyogenic Hepatic Abscesses

- Microorganisms most commonly isolated from blood and abscess cultures include *E. coli*, *Bacteroides* spp., *Streptococcus* spp., and others
- Can be cryptogenic in 1/2 of cases (no cause)

Campylobacter spp. Infections

- Positive Gram stain of stool samples for characteristic curved rod organisms
- ELISA or PCR are specific for detecting *Campylobacter jejuni*

SELECTED REFERENCES

1. Guzmán-Arocho YD et al: Multi-institutional 10-year retrospective review of amoeba diagnosed on cytologic evaluation of anal pap tests: what is the significance? J Am Soc Cytopathol. 12(3):197-205, 2023
2. Müller A et al: Colitis caused by Entamoeba histolytica identified by real-time-PCR and fluorescence in situ hybridization from formalin-fixed, paraffin-embedded tissue. Eur J Microbiol Immunol (Bp). 12(3):84-91, 2022
3. König C et al: Taxon-specific proteins of the pathogenic Entamoeba Species E. histolytica and E. nuttalli. Front Cell Infect Microbiol. 11:641472, 2021
4. Ali IKM et al: A real-time PCR Assay for simultaneous detection and differentiation of four common Entamoeba species that infect humans. J Clin Microbiol. 59(1), 2020
5. Saidin S et al: Update on laboratory diagnosis of amoebiasis. Eur J Clin Microbiol Infect Dis. 38(1):15-38, 2019
6. Shirley DT et al: A review of the global burden, new diagnostics, and current therapeutics for amebiasis. Open Forum Infect Dis. 5(7):ofy161, 2018
7. Ralston KS et al: Trogocytosis by Entamoeba histolytica contributes to cell killing and tissue invasion. Nature. 508(7497):526-30, 2014

CT of Amebic Abscess

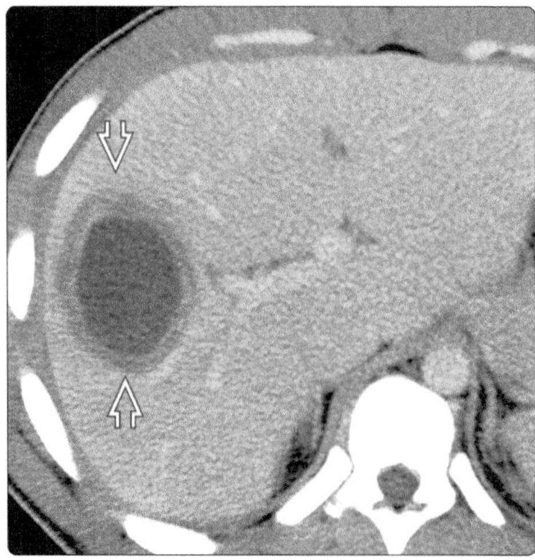

Amebic Liver Abscess

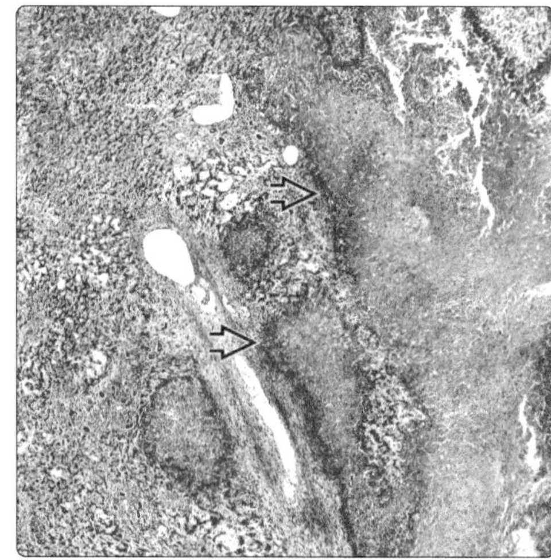

(Left) *Axial CT of the liver shows an amebic abscess with a surrounding rim ⇨. This cavity was filled with thick, tenacious necrotic debris (often compared to anchovy paste). (From DP: Hepatobiliary and Pancreas.)* **(Right)** *A large liver abscess ⇨ from a patient with disseminated E. histolytica shows large areas of necrosis with little inflammatory reaction due to lysis by the protozoa.*

Trophozoite Pseudopodia

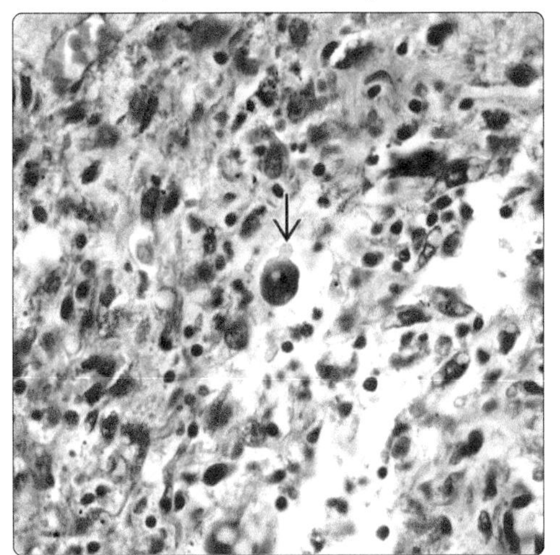

Stool Smear of *Entamoeba histolytica*

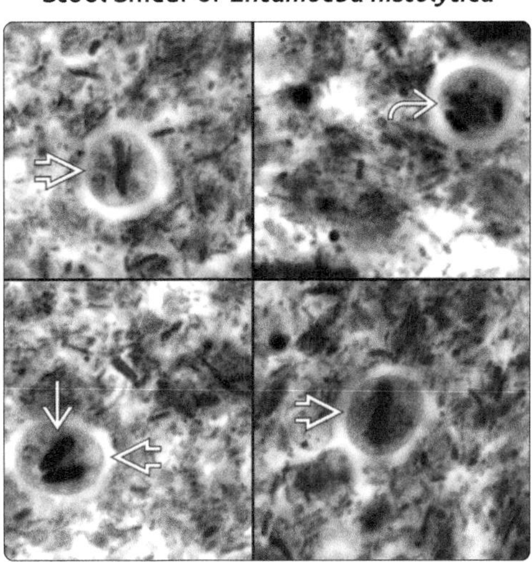

(Left) *An E. histolytica trophozoite is seen at high power within the edema of the colon in an invasive case of infection. The presence of a pseudopodia ➡ on the ameba aids in distinguishing it from inflammatory cells.* **(Right)** *Iron-hematoxylin permanent stool mount from a patient with E. histolytica shows cysts ➡ with chromatid bodies ➡ and trophozoites ➡ with digested RBCs.*

Entamoeba histolytica Trophozoites

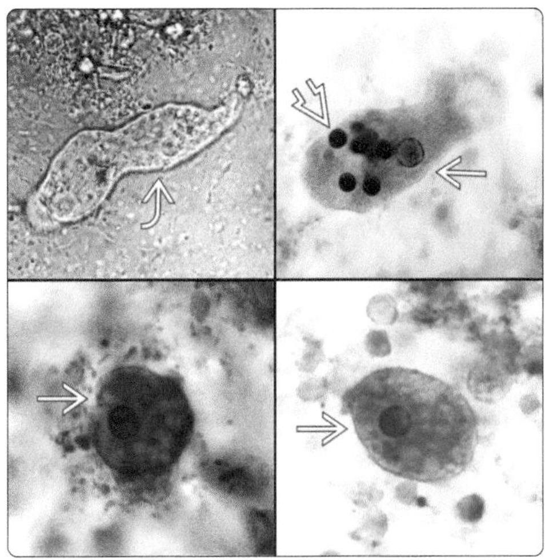

Entamoeba histolytica Cysts

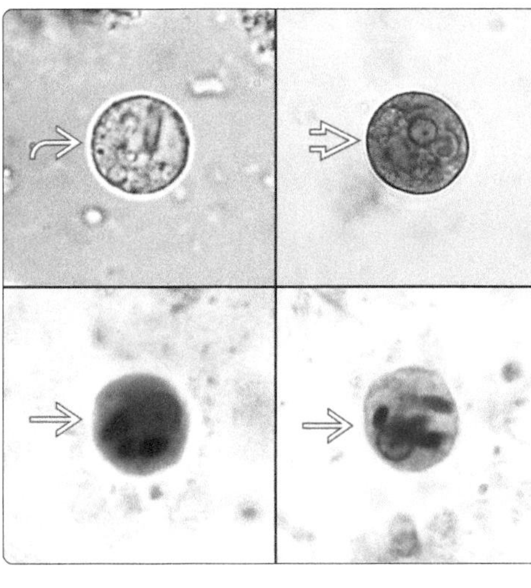

(Left) *Unstained wet mount ➡ and trichrome-stained ➡ E. histolytica trophozoites exhibit single nuclei with centrally placed karyosome (and may exhibit ingested RBCs ➡). (Courtesy Dr. Melvin, Dr. Green, Dr. Healy, and M. Moser, MPH, CDC/PHIL.)* **(Right)** *Unstained ➡, iodine-stained ➡, and trichrome-stained ➡ E. histolytica cysts contain blunt-tipped chromatoid bodies. Mature cysts contain 4 nuclei with central karyosomes. (Courtesy Dr. Melvin, Dr. Moore, Jr., and Dr. Green, CDC/PHIL.)*

Intestinal (Nonpathogenic) Amebae

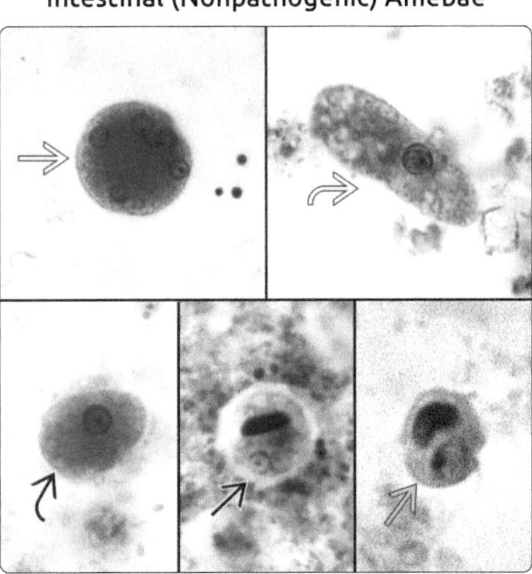

Intestinal (Nonpathogenic) Amebae

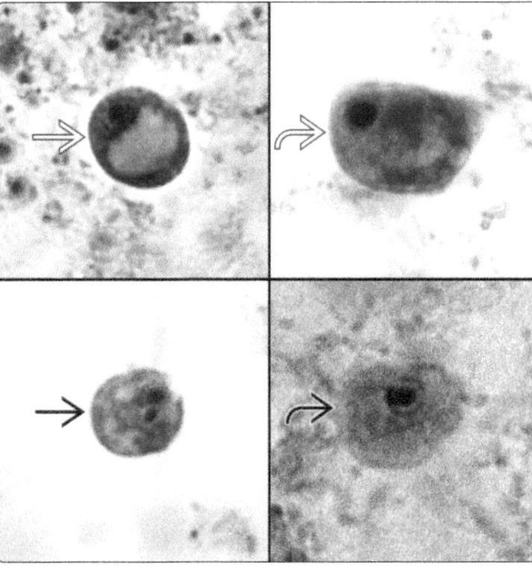

(Left) *Nonpathogenic Entamoeba spp. can colonize the human GI tract and be identified in stool samples, including Entamoeba coli cysts ➡ and trophozoites ➡, E. hartmanni trophozoites ➡ and cysts ➡, and E. polecki cysts ➡. (Courtesy Dr. Melvin, Dr. Healy, and R. K. Carver, CDC/PHIL.)* **(Right)** *Other nonpathogenic amebae identified in stool samples include Iodamoeba buetschlii cysts ➡ and trophozoites ➡ and Endolimax nana cysts ➡ and trophozoites ➡. (Courtesy Dr. Melvin, CDC/PHIL.)*

KEY FACTS

ETIOLOGY/PATHOGENESIS

- Transmission by ingestion of *Giardia lamblia* cysts, which can occur from contaminated food and water
- Infected patients can shed 1-10 billion cysts daily in their feces, which can continue for several months

CLINICAL ISSUES

- Most common intestinal parasitic disease in USA; > 20,000 cases/per year
- Acute infection presents as diarrhea with steatorrhea, flatulence, abdominal pain, nausea, and vomiting
- Chronic infection can lead to chronic steatorrhea and malabsorption with significant weight loss
- Antigen testing by ELISA or immunochromatographic assays; PCR testing
- Treatment with metronidazole; full recovery in vast majority of cases

MICROSCOPIC

- Trophozoites are purple to pink bodies with tapered end; attach to duodenal and jejunal mucosal surface but do not invade
- Cysts visible on fresh iodine-stained wet mounts or trichrome-stained smears

TOP DIFFERENTIAL DIAGNOSES

- Amebiasis: Round cysts (12-15 μm), prominent chromatoid bodies, nuclei with centrally located karyosomes
- Balantidiasis: Trophozoites (40-200 μm) with ciliated surface and bean-shaped macronucleus
- Cryptosporidiosis: Round oocysts (4.2-5.4 μm) in epithelial cell parasitophorous vacuoles
- Strongyloidiasis: Intraepithelial eggs, larvae, and adults (not visible endoscopically)
- Celiac disease: Severe villous atrophy, hyperplastic crypts, lymphocytic infiltrate, and plasma cells in lamina propria; no organisms present

Life Cycle of *Giardia*

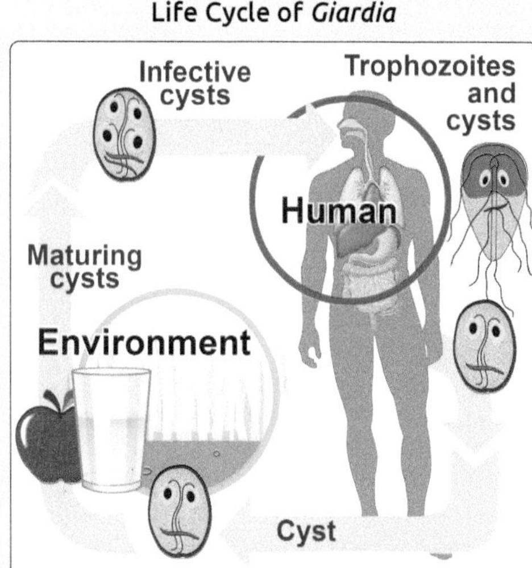

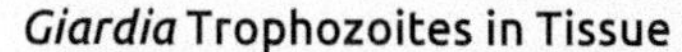
***Giardia* Trophozoites in Tissue**

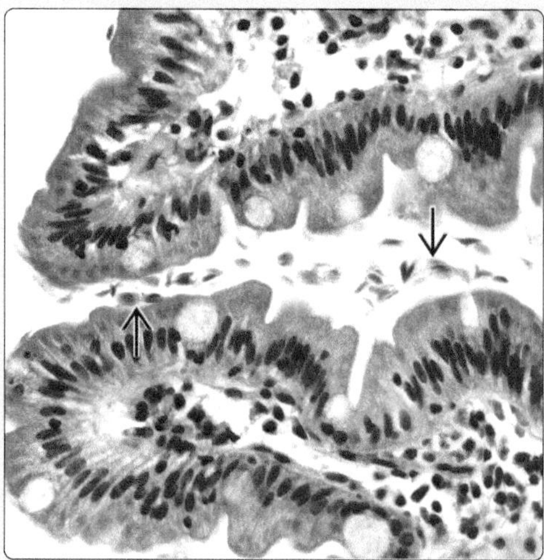

(Left) *Infective cysts are ingested through contaminated water, which then excyst in the intestinal tract and infect the small bowel. Eventually, organisms encyst and are passed into the stool as immature cysts, contaminating water sources. After maturation, the cysts can infect the next host.* **(Right)** *Small bowel biopsy from a young patient with diarrhea demonstrates large numbers of Giardia trophozoites ⇨ around and adherent to the mucosa.*

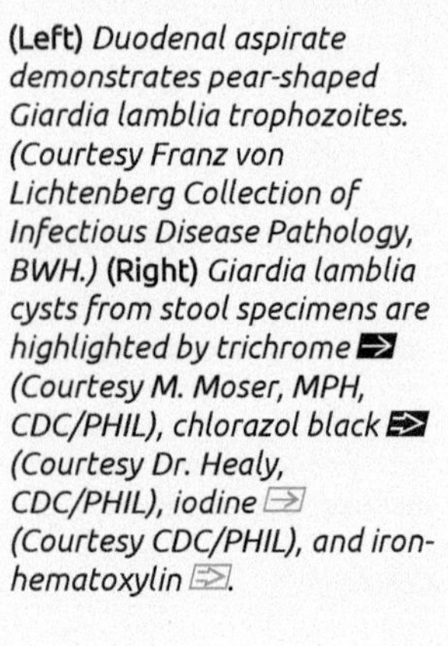

(Left) *Duodenal aspirate demonstrates pear-shaped Giardia lamblia trophozoites. (Courtesy Franz von Lichtenberg Collection of Infectious Disease Pathology, BWH.)* **(Right)** *Giardia lamblia cysts from stool specimens are highlighted by trichrome ➡ (Courtesy M. Moser, MPH, CDC/PHIL), chlorazol black ➡ (Courtesy Dr. Healy, CDC/PHIL), iodine ⇨ (Courtesy CDC/PHIL), and iron-hematoxylin ⇨.*

***Giardia lamblia* Trophozoites on Aspirate**

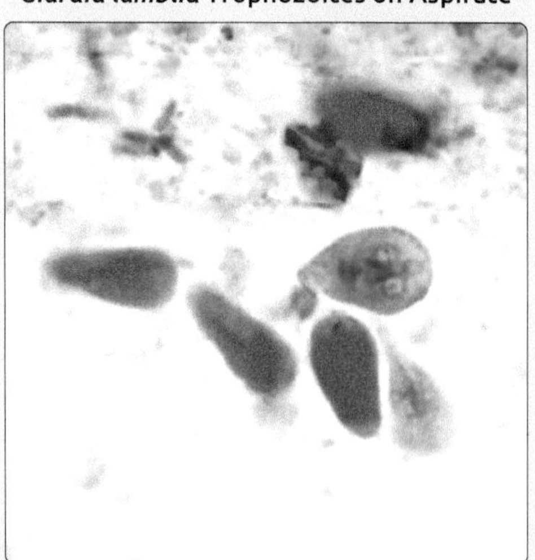

***Giardia lamblia* Cysts**

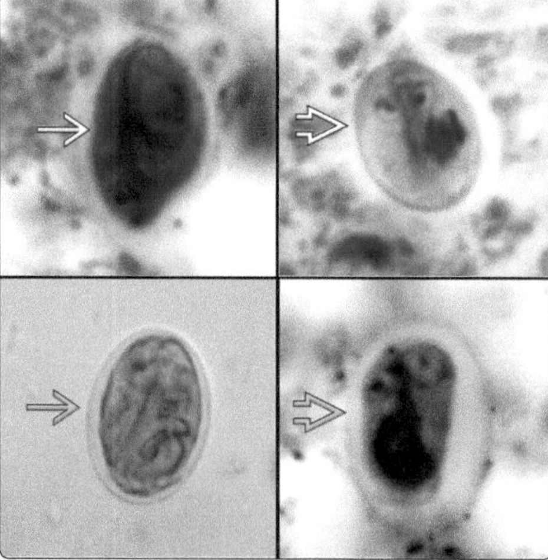

TERMINOLOGY

Synonyms

- Beaver fever

Definitions

- *Giardia lamblia* named after French biologist, Alfred M. Giard, and Czech physician, Vilém Lambl

ETIOLOGY/PATHOGENESIS

Infectious Agents

- Infection with *G. lamblia* cysts by fecal-oral transmission, via ingestion of contaminated food or water (1- to 3-week incubation period)
- Following ingestion, trophozoites excyst in small intestine and attach to mucosal surface via ventral sucking disc but do not invade; diarrhea results from combination of malabsorption and hypersecretion
- Trophozoites multiply by longitudinal binary fission, reencyst in large intestine, and are shed as cysts, resulting in low ratio of trophozoites to cysts in feces
- Infected patients can shed 1-10 billion infectious cysts daily, which can survive in environment for prolonged periods of time; as few as 10 cysts are sufficient to cause infection
- Subdivided into 8 genetic assemblages (A-H); some strains may infect both humans and animals, and human disease mostly caused by A and B groups

CLINICAL ISSUES

Epidemiology

- Risk factors include travel to high-prevalence areas, child care settings, drinking fresh river or lake water
- 1/3 of those in developing countries have been infected
- Affects 2% of adults and 6-8% of children in developed countries
- Most common intestinal parasitic disease in USA: 20,000 cases reported per year (likely much higher)

Presentation

- Many infections asymptomatic, but organisms can still be shed
- Acute infection presents as diarrhea with steatorrhea, flatulence, abdominal pain, nausea, vomiting lasting up to 4 weeks
- Chronic infection can lead to chronic steatorrhea and malabsorption with significant weight loss

Laboratory Tests

- Enzyme-linked immunosorbent assay for antigen detection
- Immunochromatographic assay for antigen detection (rapid test)
- Nucleic acid-based approaches for detection of viable oocysts and cysts of *Cryptosporidium* and *Giardia*

Treatment

- Metronidazole
- Supportive treatment to maintain hydration

Prognosis

- Full recovery in vast majority of cases
- Poorer outcomes associated with severe infection in infants or immunocompromised patients

MICROBIOLOGY

Parasite Features

- Cysts are oval (11-14 μm), contain 4 nuclei, 4 axonemes, and 4 median bodies
- Trophozoites are pear-shaped (10-20 μm), contain 2 nuclei, sucking disc, 4 pairs of flagella, 2 axonemes, and 2 median bodies

Stool Examination

- Light microscopic exam: Cysts &/or trophozoites visible on wet mounts with differential interference contrast (DIC) or iodine staining as well as trichrome-stained smears
- Direct fluorescent antibody (DFA) testing for *Cryptosporidium* and *Giardia*

MICROSCOPIC

Histologic Features

- Biopsies are commonly done in cases of diarrhea to rule out other possible causes of symptoms
- Organisms are seen on surface of mucosa as purple to pink bodies with tapered end
- Changes in mucosa range from subtle to severe (depending on chronicity); rare villous atrophy, increased crypt depth with shortening of microvilli

DIFFERENTIAL DIAGNOSIS

Amebiasis

- *Entamoeba histolytica* cysts (12-15 μm) are round with prominent chromatoid bodies and nuclei containing centrally located karyosomes; trophozoites (15-20 μm) are elongated with granular cytoplasm

Balantidiasis

- *Balantidium coli* trophozoites (40-200 μm) have ciliated surface and contain bean-shaped macronucleus; cysts (50-70 μm) are less frequent

Cryptosporidiosis

- *Cryptosporidium* spp. oocysts (4.2-5.4 μm) are rounded and become embedded in parasitophorous vacuoles within epithelial cells

Strongyloidiasis

- *Strongyloides stercoralis* eggs, larvae, and adults are not visible endoscopically, but are seen in intestinal biopsies

Celiac Disease

- Severe villous atrophy, hyperplastic crypts, lymphocytic infiltrate, and plasma cells in lamina propria; no organisms present

SELECTED REFERENCES

1. Adam RD: Giardia duodenalis: biology and pathogenesis. Clin Microbiol Rev. 34(4):e0002419, 2021
2. Conners EE et al: Giardiasis outbreaks - United States, 2012-2017. MMWR Morb Mortal Wkly Rep. 70(9):304-7, 2021
3. Jothikumar N et al: Detection and identification of Giardia species using real-time PCR and sequencing. J Microbiol Methods. 189:106279, 2021
4. Adeyemo FE et al: Methods for the detection of Cryptosporidium and Giardia: from microscopy to nucleic acid based tools in clinical and environmental regimes. Acta Trop. 184:15-28, 2018

Microsporidiosis

KEY FACTS

ETIOLOGY/PATHOGENESIS

- Infection via ingestion or inhalation of microsporidia resistant spores, obligate intracellular pathogens (currently classified as fungi)

CLINICAL ISSUES

- Opportunistic disease that affects immunocompromised patients (e.g., AIDS and transplant patients)
- GI microsporidiosis: Chronic diarrhea, abdominal pain, nausea, vomiting, and weight loss
- Extraintestinal: Ocular, musculoskeletal, CNS, and skin
- Albendazole; topical fumagillin for keratoconjunctivitis
- Organisms (ovoid, refractile spores 0.7-4 μm) identified in stool and other tissues by modified trichrome, rapid Gram chromotrope, and fluorochrome stains

MICROSCOPIC

- Mild to severe villous blunting with mild lymphoplasmacytic infiltrate
- Organisms (2- to 3-μm spores and larger plasmodia) identified as clusters within supranuclear cytoplasm of epithelial cells
- Organisms poorly staining on H&E but may be birefringent or polarize and highlighted by Gram, Warthin-Starry, Giemsa, and modified trichrome stains
- Electron microscopy or PCR required for speciation

TOP DIFFERENTIAL DIAGNOSES

- Cryptosporidiosis: Larger oocysts (2-5 μm) present at surface of small intestine villi
- Cyclosporiasis: Larger round (2- to 3-μm) and crescentic (5- to 6-μm) forms in cytoplasm parasitophorous vacuoles
- Cystoisosporiasis: Schizonts and merozoites with crescentic or banana-shaped forms (25-30 μm) located in cytoplasm
- Cytomegalovirus infection: Enlarged cells with nuclear and cytoplasmic inclusions; confirm with IHC, PCR, or serology
- Giardiasis: Trophozoites (leaf-shaped with 2 nuclei and 4 pairs of flagella) in small intestine lumen

(Left) *High-power electron micrograph shows the pathognomonic polar tube coils, a unique structure of microsporidia spores. Here, 5 coils are present, typical of Encephalitozoon intestinalis. (From DP: Kidney.)* **(Right)** *Specimen consisting of a plastic-embedded thick section shows spores as well as plasmodial forms of microsporidia. (From DP: GI.)*

Microsporidiosis: Ultrastructural Features

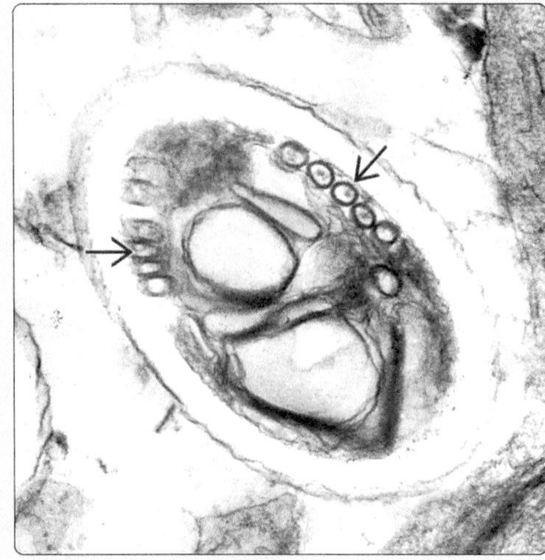

Microsporidiosis in Intestinal Wall

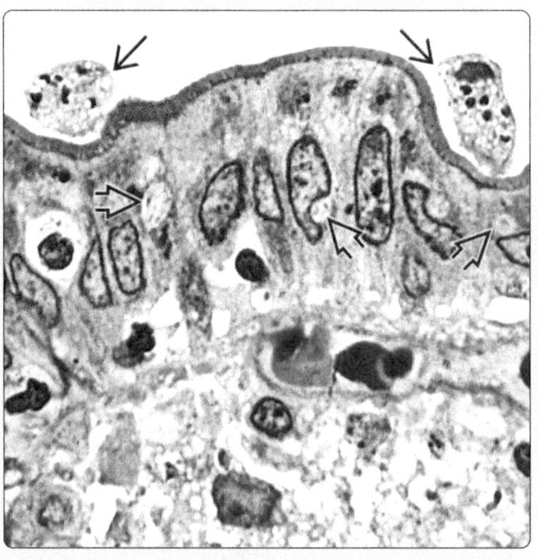

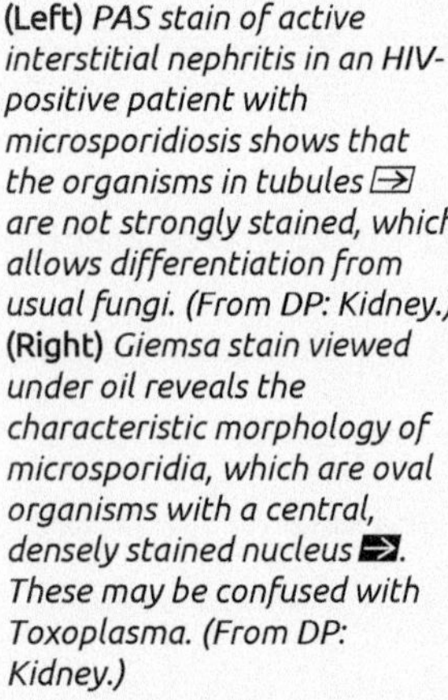

(Left) *PAS stain of active interstitial nephritis in an HIV-positive patient with microsporidiosis shows that the organisms in tubules are not strongly stained, which allows differentiation from usual fungi. (From DP: Kidney.)* **(Right)** *Giemsa stain viewed under oil reveals the characteristic morphology of microsporidia, which are oval organisms with a central, densely stained nucleus. These may be confused with Toxoplasma. (From DP: Kidney.)*

Kidney Tubules With Microsporidiosis

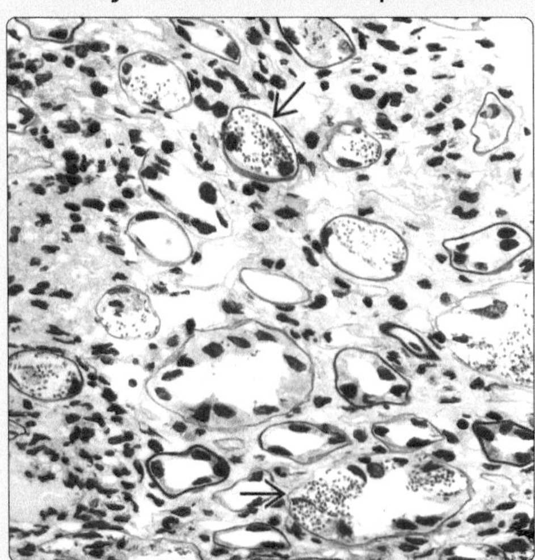

Microsporidiosis: Giemsa Stain

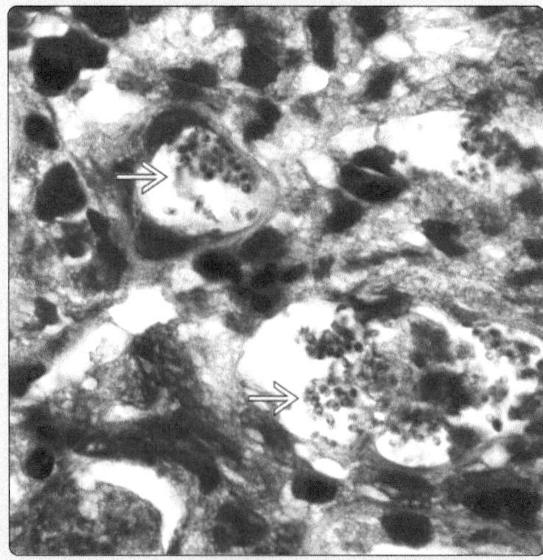

TERMINOLOGY

Definitions

- Greek: "Mikros" (small) + "sporos" (seed)

ETIOLOGY/PATHOGENESIS

Infectious Agents

- Infection with microsporidia, ubiquitous obligate intracellular pathogens via ingestion or inhalation of resistant spores
- Spores extrude polar tubule to infect host cell; sporoplasm then undergoes extensive multiplication by merogony and maturation by sporogony until host cell cytoplasm is filled; cell membrane disruption releases spores shed in feces
- Microsporidia are classified in fungi kingdom (previously thought to be protozoa); they lack mitochondria and flagella, instead possessing mitosomes
- 1,500 species identified; human pathogens include *Anncaliia* (formerly *Brachiola*) *algerae, A. connori, A. vesicularum, Encephalitozoon cuniculi, E. hellem, E. intestinalis, Enterocytozoon bieneusi, Microsporidium ceylonensis, M. africanum, Nosema ocularum, Pleistophora* spp., *Trachipleistophora hominis, T. anthropophthera, Vittaforma corneae*, and *Tubulinosema acridophagus*

CLINICAL ISSUES

Epidemiology

- Opportunistic disease that affects immunocompromised patients (e.g., AIDS and transplant patients); generally occurs when CD4(+) T-cell counts fall below 150 in HIV patients
- Cases have been reported in immunocompetent individuals

Presentation

- GI microsporidiosis: Chronic diarrhea, abdominal pain, nausea, vomiting, and weight loss
- Ocular microsporidiosis: Blurred vision, foreign body sensation, pain, redness, and tearing
- Disseminated microsporidiosis: Musculoskeletal (myalgia, weakness), CNS (headache, seizure), dermatologic (nodular lesions)
- Early diagnosis is essential for preventing significantly associated morbidity and mortality of extraintestinal microsporidiosis

Treatment

- Albendazole
- Topical fumagillin for keratoconjunctivitis
- Thalidomide (unresponsive chronic diarrhea)

MICROBIOLOGY

Stool Examination

- Fecal WBCs are usually absent
- Modified trichrome stain shows ovoid, refractile spores (0.7-4 μm in diameter) with bright red wall
- Rapid Gram chromotrope shows spores that stain dark violet with enhanced equatorial stripe
- Fluorochrome stains can be used in stool as well as urine, mucus, and tissue sections

MICROSCOPIC

Histologic Features

- Mild to severe villous blunting with mild lymphoplasmacytic infiltrate
- Organisms (2- to 3-μm spores and larger plasmodia) identified as clusters within supranuclear cytoplasm of epithelial cells
- Organisms are poorly staining on H&E but may be birefringent or polarize

ANCILLARY TESTS

Histochemistry

- Gram, Warthin-Starry, Giemsa, and modified trichrome stains highlight organisms

PCR

- Species and genus targeted assays available; greater sensitivity and specificity than histology and stool examination

Electron Microscopy

- Can confirm diagnosis and distinguish between organisms

DIFFERENTIAL DIAGNOSIS

Cryptosporidiosis

- Small, round, bluish-purple bodies (2-5 μm) present at luminal tips and surfaces of villi of small intestine

Cyclosporiasis

- Round forms (2-3 μm) and crescentic merozoites (5-6 μm) located toward luminal surface of small bowel epithelium within parasitophorous vacuole ("halo") in cytoplasm

Cystoisosporiasis

- Schizonts and merozoites with crescentic or banana-shaped forms (25-30 μm) located toward luminal surfaces of epithelial cells but within cytoplasm

Cytomegalovirus Infection

- Intracellular inclusions surrounded by clear halo in tissue biopsy; positive IHC, PCR, or antibody tests

Giardiasis

- Stool examination for trophozoites (leaf-shaped with 2 nuclei and 4 pairs of flagella) or cysts (smooth walled and oval with curved median bodies, axonemes, and nuclei)
- Stool antigen ELISA when 3 O&P tests are negative

SELECTED REFERENCES

1. Han B et al: Microsporidiosis in humans. Clin Microbiol Rev. 34(4):e0001020, 2021
2. Matoba A et al: Microsporidial stromal keratitis: epidemiological features, slit-lamp biomicroscopic characteristics, and therapy. Cornea. 40(12):1532-40, 2021
3. Nadelman DA et al: Cutaneous microsporidiosis in an immunosuppressed patient. J Cutan Pathol. 47(7):659-63, 2020
4. Heyworth MF: Molecular diagnosis of human microsporidian infections. Trans R Soc Trop Med Hyg. 111(9):382-3, 2017
5. Field AS et al: Intestinal microsporidiosis. Clin Lab Med. 35(2):445-59, 2015
6. Hocevar SN et al: Microsporidiosis acquired through solid organ transplantation: a public health investigation. Ann Intern Med. 160(4):213-20, 2014
7. Ramanan P et al: Extraintestinal microsporidiosis. J Clin Microbiol. 52(11):3839-44, 2014

Trichomoniasis

KEY FACTS

ETIOLOGY/PATHOGENESIS

- Infection with *Trichomonas* spp. (typically *T. vaginalis*) flagellated protozoans via sexual contact or during birth

CLINICAL ISSUES

- Most common nonviral sexually transmitted disease worldwide; more prevalent in women than in men
- Risk factors include unprotected sexual intercourse, new or multiple sex partners, concurrent or history of other STIs
- Women present with vaginitis with mucosal erythema and greenish yellow, frothy, malodorous discharge; colpitis macularis (strawberry cervix) in ~ 2% of infections
- Men are symptomatic in < 25% of cases: Urethritis with dysuria and urethral discharge
- Commercial immunoassays and PCR-based assays have better sensitivities than culture or wet mount methods
- Treated with metronidazole or other nitroimidazoles; sex partners treated concurrently

MICROSCOPIC

- Oval, round, pear-shaped, or kite-shaped protozoa (length: 10 µm; width: 7 µm) with eosinophilic cytoplasmic granules and vesicular nuclei
- Associated with acute and chronic inflammatory reaction as well as epithelial reactive changes
- On wet mount, motile flagellated trichomonads with jerky and spinning motion are present

TOP DIFFERENTIAL DIAGNOSES

- Sexually transmitted bacterial infections (e.g., *N. gonorrhoeae, C. trachomatis, M. genitalium*): Confirm by special stains, IHC/ISH, culture, molecular testing, antigen testing
- Noninfectious artifacts (e.g., cell fragments with moving cilia, cytoplasmic debris, bare epithelial nuclei): Lack definitive elliptical nucleus or eosinophilic granules
- Giardiasis: Flagellated, pear-shaped binucleate trophozoites in small intestine biopsies (rarely, anal Pap tests)

Trichomonas vaginalis **Wet Mount**

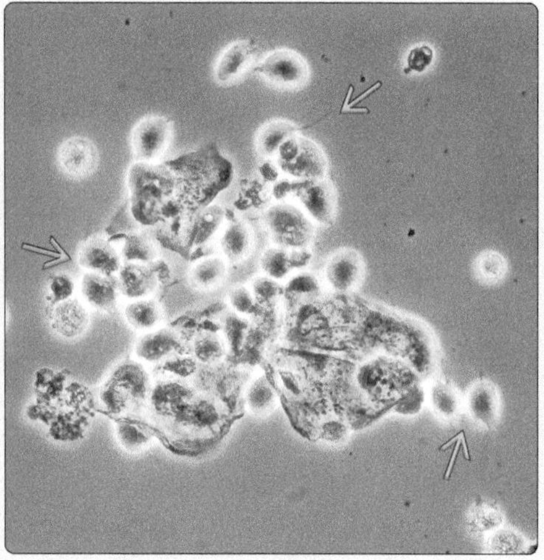

Trichomonas **Cervicitis**

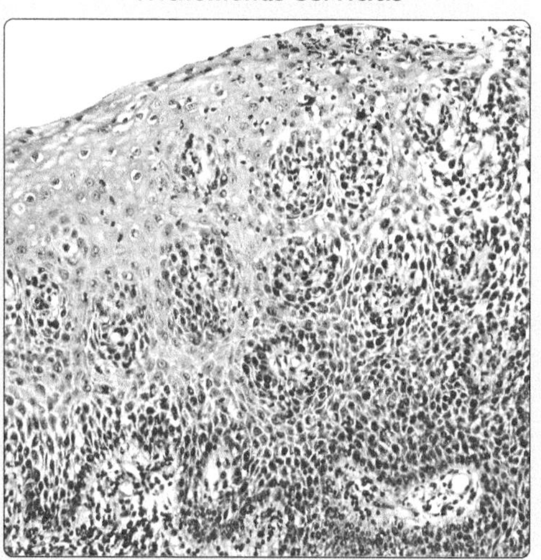

(Left) *Wet-mounted vaginal discharge reveals multiple flagellated trichomonads* →. *(Courtesy J. Miller, CDC/PHIL.)* **(Right)** *Cervical biopsy on H&E stain shows diffuse and florid acute and chronic inflammation associated with reactive epithelial changes. Trichomonad morphology is generally not well preserved in histological section. In this case, concurrent Pap test revealed trichomoniasis.*

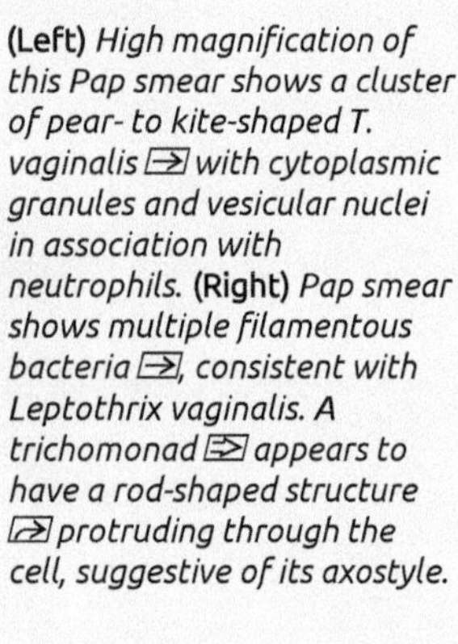

(Left) *High magnification of this Pap smear shows a cluster of pear- to kite-shaped T. vaginalis* → *with cytoplasmic granules and vesicular nuclei in association with neutrophils.* **(Right)** *Pap smear shows multiple filamentous bacteria* →*, consistent with Leptothrix vaginalis. A trichomonad* ⇒ *appears to have a rod-shaped structure* ↗ *protruding through the cell, suggestive of its axostyle.*

Trichomonas vaginalis **With Neutrophils**

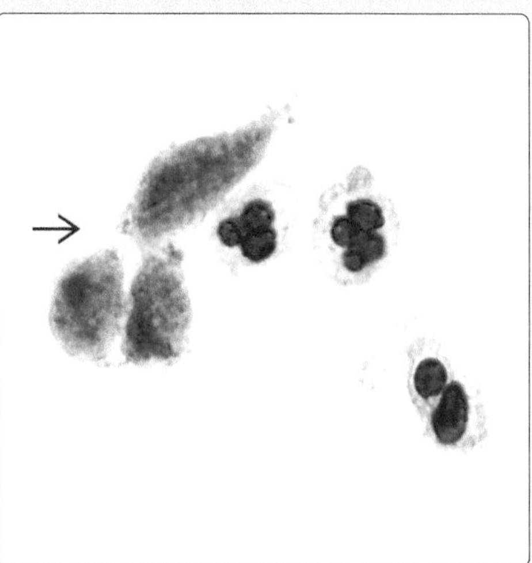

Leptothrix **and** ***Trichomonas***

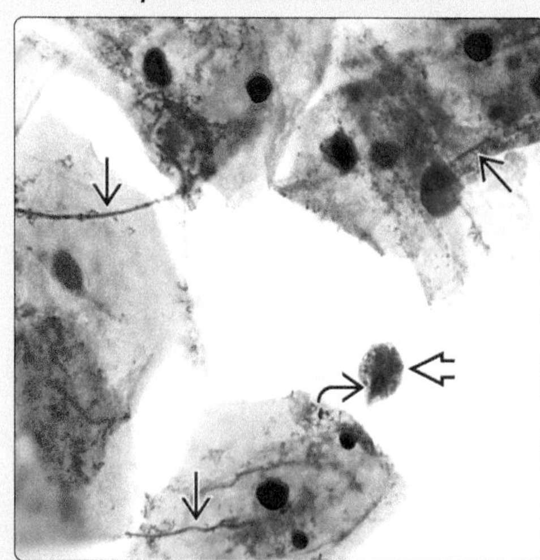

TERMINOLOGY

Definitions

- Greek: "Trikhos" (hair) + "monas" (unit)

ETIOLOGY/PATHOGENESIS

Infectious Agents

- Infection with *Trichomonas* spp. (predominantly *T. vaginalis*) flagellated protozoans via sexual contact or during birth
- Epithelial cells destroyed by direct cell contact and release of cytotoxic substances; flagella internalized and switched to ameboid conformation while adhered to host cells
- *T. tenax* considered oropharyngeal commensal; rare reports of respiratory infection resulting in empyema
- *T. hominis* isolated from human intestinal tract; considered nonpathogenic but may be associated with diarrhea
- *T. foetus* mostly isolated from animals but human peritonitis has been reported

CLINICAL ISSUES

Epidemiology

- Most common nonviral sexually transmitted disease worldwide; estimated > 150 million new infections/year
- More prevalent in women than in men
- Risk factors include unprotected sexual intercourse, new or multiple sex partners, concurrent or history of other sexually transmitted infections

Presentation

- Women are symptomatic in ~ 50% of cases: Vaginitis with mucosal erythema and greenish yellow, frothy, malodorous discharge; colpitis macularis (strawberry cervix) in ~ 2% of infections
- Men are symptomatic in < 25% of cases: Urethritis with dysuria and urethral discharge

Laboratory Tests

- Antigen test: Commercial immunoassays using vaginal swab specimens have good sensitivity (> 80%) and specificity (> 95%)
- Molecular diagnostics: Commercial PCR-based assays have better sensitivities than culture or wet mount methods

Treatment

- Metronidazole or other nitroimidazoles, such as tinidazole
- Sex partners should be treated concurrently

Prognosis

- Women: Untreated infections may progress to urethritis or cystitis and are associated with pelvic inflammatory disease, infertility, increased risk of cervical cancer, and susceptibility to HIV infection
- Men: Untreated infections associated with prostatitis, epididymitis, infertility, and increased risk of prostate cancer

MICROBIOLOGY

Parasite Features

- Trophozoites exhibit 4 anterior flagella, single 5th posterior flagellum, and axostyle (bundle of microtubules) that passes through cell and protrudes from posterior end
- No cyst form identified

Culture

- Culture on traditional Diamond broth medium or its variants generally takes 2-7 days to obtain result
- InPouch culture system combining culture and microscopy is commercially available with high sensitivity (> 80%)

Microscopic Examination of Wet Mount

- Motile flagellated trichomonads with jerky and spinning motion; sensitivity varies depending on inoculum size

MICROSCOPIC

Histologic Features

- Associated with acute and chronic inflammatory reaction as well as epithelial reactive changes
- Protozoa tend to lose morphologic characteristics during fixation and staining

Cytologic Features

- Oval, round, pear-shaped, or kite-shaped protozoa (average length: 10 μm; width: 7 μm)
- Eosinophilic cytoplasmic granules and vesicular nuclei are present
- Adjacent squamous cells may show reactive changes, including hyperchromatic nuclei and small perinuclear halos that mimic LSIL or ASCUS

DIFFERENTIAL DIAGNOSIS

Sexually Transmitted Bacterial Infections

- e.g., *Neisseria gonorrhoeae*, *Chlamydia trachomatis*, *Mycoplasma genitalium*
- Overlap in clinical symptoms and inflammatory infiltrate; confirm by special stains, IHC/ISH, culture, molecular testing, antigen testing

Noninfectious Artifacts

- e.g., cell fragments (including moving cilia in wet mounts), cytoplasmic debris, bare epithelial nuclei
- Lack definitive elliptical nucleus or eosinophilic granules

Giardiasis

- Flagellated, pear-shaped binucleate trophozoites of *Giardia duodenalis* found in small intestine biopsies and occasionally on anal Pap tests

SELECTED REFERENCES

1. Van Gerwen OT et al: Trichomoniasis. Infect Dis Clin North Am. 37(2):245-65, 2023
2. Benchimol M et al: Unusual cell structures and organelles in Giardia intestinalis and Trichomonas vaginalis are potential drug targets. Microorganisms. 10(11), 2022
3. Bisson C et al: Assessment of the role of Trichomonas tenax in the etiopathogenesis of human periodontitis: a systematic review. PLoS One. 14(12):e0226266, 2019
4. Graves KJ et al: Trichomonas vaginalis virus among women with trichomoniasis and associations with demographics, clinical outcomes, and metronidazole resistance. Clin Infect Dis. 69(12):2170-6, 2019
5. Patel EU et al: Prevalence and correlates of Trichomonas vaginalis infection among men and women in the United States. Clin Infect Dis. 67(2):211-7, 2018

KEY FACTS

TERMINOLOGY

- African sleeping sickness; human African trypanosomiasis (HAT)

ETIOLOGY/PATHOGENESIS

- Protozoan infection transmitted by *Glossina* spp. (tsetse flies)
- East African trypanosomiasis due to *Trypanosoma brucei rhodesiense* has rapid progression over weeks
- West African trypanosomiasis due to *Trypanosoma brucei gambiense* has chronic progression over months (98%)

CLINICAL ISSUES

- 1st stage: Hemolymphatic; severe lymphadenopathy and bite site chancre (early)
- 2nd stage: Neurologic phase; symptomatic invasion of CNS; without treatment, disease is 100% fatal; coma → multiorgan failure → death
- Card agglutination test for trypanosomiasis (CATT)
- CSF examination; WBC count correlates with prognosis, dictates treatment

MICROSCOPIC

- Blood smear: Large, extracellular trypomastigotes, flagellum with dark body at base (kinetoplastid)
- Neuropathology: Meningoencephalitis, lymphoplasmacytic inflammation with Mott cells
- Lymph node fine-needle aspiration: Trypomastigote forms admixed with reactive lymphoid cells

TOP DIFFERENTIAL DIAGNOSES

- Cerebral malaria: More rapid onset and clinical course; "ring" hemorrhages confined to white matter with parasite sequestration in vessels
- Arsenic toxicity: Clinical overlap (melarsoprol is arsenic based); demyelination and neuron apoptosis, limited inflammation; lack of plasma cells

Life Cycle of African Trypanosomiasis

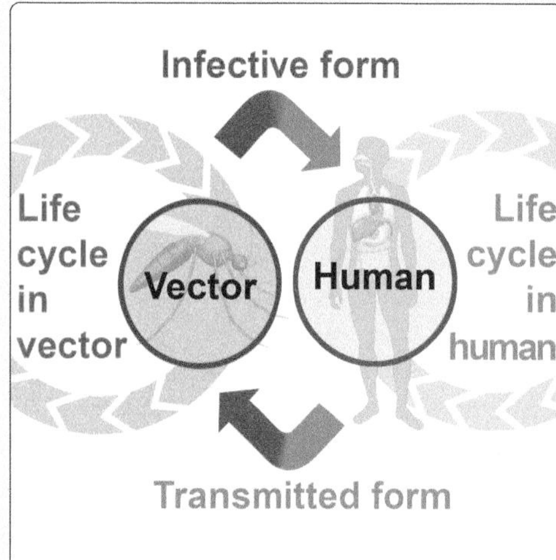

Glossina **(Tsetse) Flies**

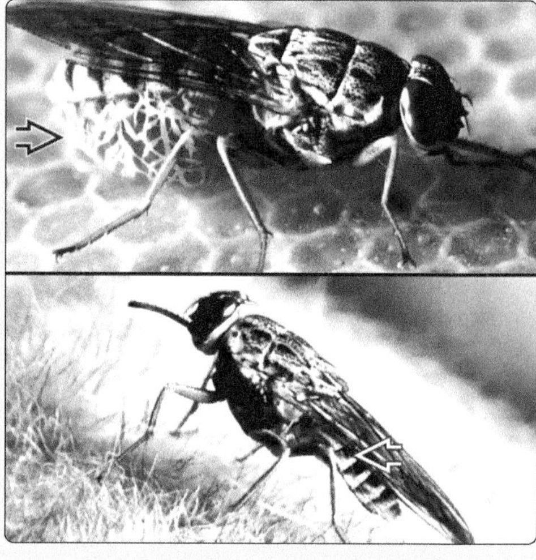

(Left) *Humans become infected with T. brucei when bitten by infected tsetse flies. Although similar vectors, the geographic distribution and the subspecies leads to rapid vs. slow clinical progression. Infected cattle (East African, T. brucei rhodesiense) or infected humans (West African, T. brucei gambiense) serve as the disease reservoir.* **(Right)** *The tsetse fly (engorged ⇨ and not ➡) transmits T. brucei through a painful bite on exposed skin, resulting in a large chancre. Infected flies bite more frequently. (Courtesy WHO.)*

Trypanosoma brucei**: Thin Blood Smear**

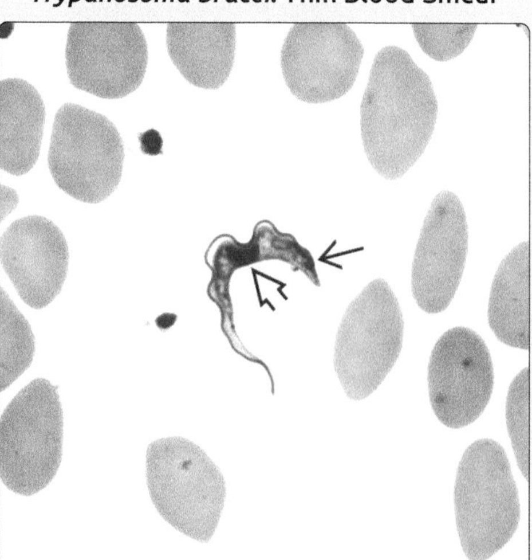

Trypanosoma brucei**: Thick Blood Smear**

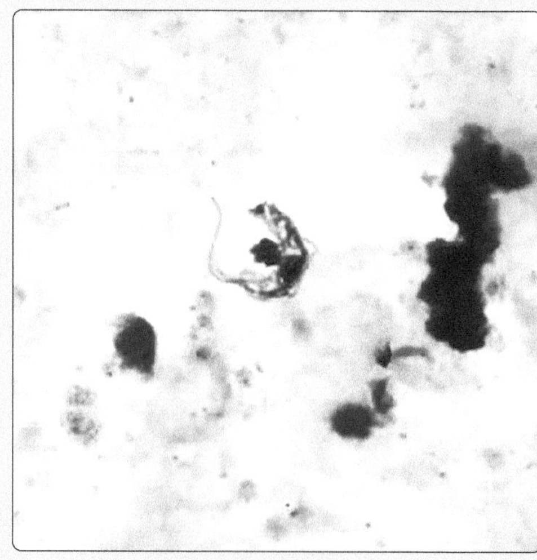

(Left) *Giemsa-stained blood sample reveals the presence of a T. brucei parasite with a prominent central nucleus ⇨, a dark-staining kinetoplast at the base of the flagellum →, and an undulating membrane. (Courtesy B. Mathison, CDC/PHIL.)* **(Right)** *T. brucei is present in a thick blood smear, which increases diagnostic yield compared to thin blood smears. (Courtesy CDC/DPDX.)*

TERMINOLOGY

Definitions

- African sleeping sickness; human African trypanosomiasis (HAT); from Greek "trypano" (borer) and "soma" (body) due to corkscrew-like motion

ETIOLOGY/PATHOGENESIS

Infectious Agents

- Protozoan infection with *Trypanosoma brucei* transmitted by *Glossina* spp. (tsetse flies); rare vertical transmission
- East Africa: *Trypanosoma brucei rhodesiense* is zoonotic transmission; primary reservoir is wild animals; primary vector *Glossina morsitans* transmits rarely to humans; rapid (weeks) progression to death without treatment
- West Africa: *Trypanosoma brucei gambiense* (98%) reservoirs are humans (primary) and animals; primary vector *Glossina palpalis* transmit human to humans; chronic (years) progression to death without treatment
- Trypomastigotes present in various body sites, including bloodstream, lymph nodes, adipose tissue, and CNS

CLINICAL ISSUES

Epidemiology

- 98 cases of East African trypanosomiasis reported to WHO in 2020, 91% in Malawi; also reported in Uganda, Tanzania, and Zambia
- 565 cases of West African trypanosomiasis reported to WHO in 2020, 70% in Democratic Republic of Congo; also reported in Equatorial Guinea, Uganda, Gabon, Congo, South Sudan, Chad, Cameroon, Angola, Guinea, and Central African Republic

Presentation

- 1st hemolymphatic stage: Headache, fever, arthralgias, pruritus, severe lymphadenopathy, bite site chancre; ongoing invasion of deep body tissues
- 2nd neurologic stage: Symptomatic invasion of CNS; psychiatric manifestations, including circadian cycle disturbances, irritability, aggression, bizarre behavior, "demonic possession," "witchcraft"; physical manifestations, including paralysis or hemiparalysis, malaise, weakness, physical apathy, tremors, movement disorders; coma → multiorgan failure → death

Laboratory Tests

- Card agglutination test for trypanosomiasis (CATT)
  - *T. b. gambiense* at-risk population screened for chronic disease
  - *T. b.rhodesiense* test symptomatic patients with acute disease
- CSF: Organisms may be seen; WBC count correlates with prognosis and guides treatment

Treatment

- *T. b. gambiense*: Pentamidine (1st stage), eflornithine ± nifurtimox (2nd stage), fexinidazole (1st/2nd stage)
- *T. b. rhodesiense*: Suramin (1st stage), melarsoprol (2nd stage)
- Melarsoprol carries 5% risk of mortality from treatment due to posttreatment reactive encephalopathy (PTRE)
- Targeted tsetse fly removal for prevention

Prognosis

- Early treatment reduces mortality; without treatment, disease is 100% fatal; damage to CNS is irreversible

IMAGING

MR Findings

- Focal, patchy white matter and gray matter changes

MICROBIOLOGY

Life Cycle

- Within *Glossina* fly, ingested bloodstream trypomastigotes transform into procyclic trypomastigotes, which mature to epimastigotes, then leave fly midgut and enter salivary glands, transform into metacyclic trypomastigote stage, and are injected with next blood meal
- Within human bloodstream, metacyclic trypomastigotes transform back to bloodstream trypomastigotes, which multiply by binary fission, and invade various body spaces, including blood, lymph and lymph nodes, and CSF

MACROSCOPIC

General Features

- Brain: Hemorrhagic leukoencephalopathy
- Lymph nodes: Diffuse reactive lymphadenopathy

MICROSCOPIC

Histologic Features

- Brain: Leptomeningeal, parenchymal, and perivascular lymphoplasmacytic inflammation (with Mott cells), and blood vessel/parenchymal necrosis with fibrin deposition

Cytologic Features

- Peripheral blood smear: Large, extracellular trypomastigotes (14-33 µm long) containing flagellum with dark body at base (kinetoplastid), central nucleus, and undulating membrane along flagellum
- Lymph node FNA: Trypomastigote forms admixed with reactive lymphoid cells

DIFFERENTIAL DIAGNOSIS

Cerebral Malaria

- Significant epidemiologic overlap; more rapid onset and clinical course; "ring" hemorrhages confined to white matter with parasite sequestration in vessels

Arsenic Toxicity

- Clinical overlap in presentation (melarsoprol is arsenic based); demyelination and neuron apoptosis, limited inflammation; lack of plasma cells

SELECTED REFERENCES

1. Pays E et al: The pathogenesis of African trypanosomiasis. Annu Rev Pathol. 18:19-45, 2023
2. Gaillot K et al: Vertical transmission of human African trypanosomiasis: clinical evolution and brain MRI of a mother and her son. PLoS Negl Trop Dis. 11(7):e0005642, 2017
3. Chimelli L et al: Trypanosomiasis. Brain Pathol. 7(1):599-611, 1997

KEY FACTS

ETIOLOGY/PATHOGENESIS

- Infection with apicomplexan protozoa of genus *Babesia*, predominantly though tick bites, as well as blood-transfusions, and transplacental transmission

CLINICAL ISSUES

- *Babesia microti* is endemic in northeastern and upper midwestern USA
- *Babesia divergens*-like strains WA-1 and MO-1 are documented in Washington, California, and Missouri
- Symptoms include fatigue, malaise, weakness, fever, chills, sweats, hemoglobinuria, jaundice, arthralgia
- Coinfections with *Borrelia burgdorferi* and *Anaplasma phagocytophilum* should be evaluated in endemic areas, as all are transmitted by *Ixodes* species
- Babesiosis can be severe, life-threatening disease, particularly in asplenic patients, immunocompromised individuals, and older patients
- 18s rRNA PCR is more sensitive than blood smear
- Serologic testing and xenodiagnosis

MICROSCOPIC

- Diagnosis primarily made by blood smear showing parasites with distinguishing features, including "Maltese cross" (occasional merozoites arranged in tetrads) &/or intraerythrocytic ring forms
- *Babesia* may be mistaken for malarial parasites, such as ring forms of *Plasmodium falciparum* (clinical history is key)

TOP DIFFERENTIAL DIAGNOSES

- Malaria: Parasites may be very difficult to distinguish; *Babesia* lacks hemozoin, is dyssynchronous, shows tetrads, and has extraerythrocytic forms
- Trypanosomiasis: Trypomastigotes have terminal/subterminal kinetoplast, central nucleus, undulating membrane, and flagellum (12-33 μm in length)
- Leishmaniasis: Amastigotes reside in macrophages and are spherical to ovoid (1-5 μm long) with large nucleus, prominent kinetoplast, and short axoneme

Life Cycle of *Babesia*

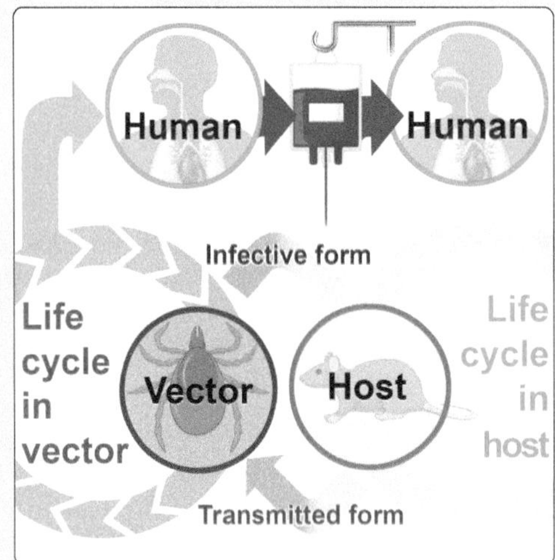

Ixodes scapularis

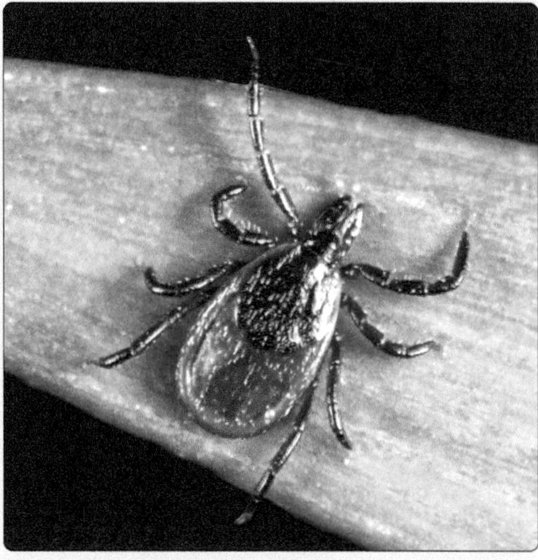

(Left) *Babesia is a zoonotic apicomplexan parasite that cycles between ticks and rodents. Babesia infects human red blood cells and lyses them with maturation. Patients with disruptions of spleen function (trauma, surgery, etc.) are at risk for more severe infection.* **(Right)** *Ixodes scapularis (black-legged tick, deer tick) transmits Babesia spp. as well as Powassan virus, Borrelia burgdorferi, and Anaplasma phagocytophilum. (Courtesy M. Levin, PhD.)*

"Ring" Trophozoites

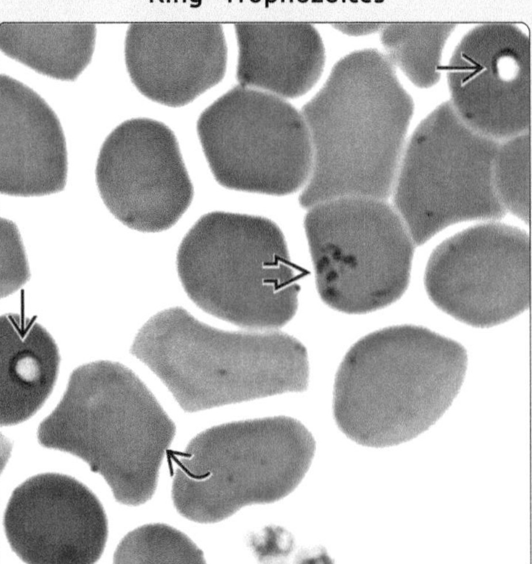

Diagnostic Tetrad Forms

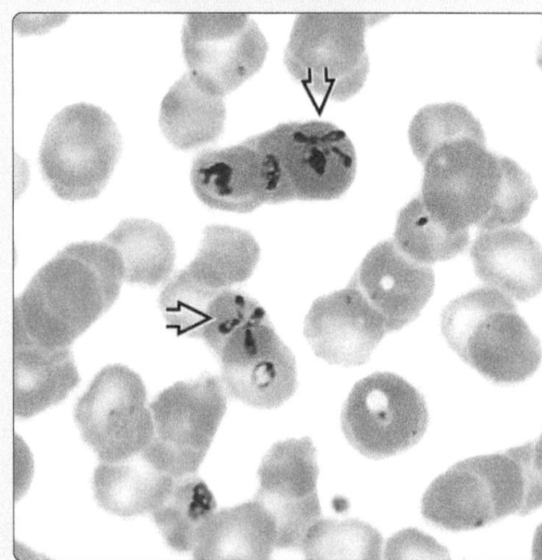

(Left) *Peripheral blood smear with babesiosis demonstrates 4 pear-shaped merozoites ⇨ (small tetrad form) as well as "2 ring" stage trophozoites ➡ within red blood cells. A reticulocyte ↷ is also seen. Without the tetrad or extraerythrocytic forms, confusion with malaria species may occur.* **(Right)** *Babesia parasites in a peripheral blood smear demonstrate the classic tetrad ⇨ appearance of this organism, which is diagnostic. (Courtesy CDC.)*

TERMINOLOGY

Definitions

- *Babesia* (Latin) from Victor Babeș (Romanian bacteriologist, 1854-1926)

ETIOLOGY/PATHOGENESIS

Infectious Agents

- Infection with apicomplexan protozoa of genus *Babesia*, predominantly though tick bites
- *Babesia microti* and *B. microti*-like
  - Primary vector for transmission is deer tick *Ixodes scapularis*
  - Mice exposure is also risk factor
- *Babesia duncani* and *B. duncani*-like
  - Unclear vector
  - Canine exposure is risk factor
- *Babesia divergens* and *B. divergens*-like (WA-1 and MO-1 strains in Washington, California, and Missouri)
  - Primary vector for transmission is cattle tick *Ixodes ricinus*
- *Babesia bovis*
  - Primary vectors for transmission are cattle ticks *Rhipicephalus microplus* and *R. annulatus*
- *Babesia venatorum*
  - Primary vector for transmission is cattle tick *I. ricinus*
- One of most common transfusion-associated infections due to asymptomatic cases
- Cases have been reportedly associated with transplacental transmission

CLINICAL ISSUES

Epidemiology

- Incidence
  - True incidence remains to be determined
  - 2,418 cases were reported in 25 states in 2019 (increasing, majority in northeastern USA)
- Geographical distribution
  - *B. microti* is endemic in northeastern and upper midwestern USA
  - *B. duncani* is found mainly in western USA
  - *B. divergens* is found in Europe
  - *B. venatorum* is found in Europe
  - *B. divergens*-like strains WA-1 and MO-1 are documented in Washington, California, and Missouri
  - *B. bovis* is found in Europe, Australia, African, Central and South America, and Asia
  - > 100 species of *Babesia* worldwide
- Seasonality
  - Transmission mainly from May to September

Presentation

- Symptoms range from mild to severe and usually develop 1-6 weeks post tick bite
  - Fatigue, malaise, weakness, fever, chills, sweats, hemoglobinuria, and jaundice arthralgia
- Parasitemia may be present with lack of symptoms
- Signs include hemolytic anemia, hepatosplenomegaly
- Complications include acute respiratory distress syndrome, disseminated intravascular coagulation, congestive heart failure, renal failure, liver failure, splenic infarcts or rupture
- Complications are associated with severe anemia (hemoglobin < 10 g/dL) and high parasitemia (> 10%)
- Risk factors for severe illness include age > 50 years, asplenic state, and coinfection with HIV or other immunosuppressive conditions
- Coinfections with *Borrelia burgdorferi* and *Anaplasma phagocytophilum* should be evaluated in endemic areas, as all are transmitted by *Ixodes* species
- Presentations of *B. divergens* and *B. duncani* are usually more fulminant than *B. microti*

Laboratory Tests

- Low hematocrit, elevated LDH, low hemoglobin, elevated total bilirubin, low haptoglobin, reticulocytosis, thrombocytopenia, transaminitis
- Parasitemia ranges from 1-20% in patients with functional spleens
  - Mild disease is associated with parasitemia of 4-5%
- PCR: 18s rRNA PCR is more sensitive than blood smear
- Serologic testing
  - Indirect immunofluorescent antibody testing available for asymptomatic individuals
  - Onset of symptoms usually precedes positive serology by 1 week
  - Positive serology can persist for years after infection, though usually returns to < 1:64 within 6-12 months
  - Titers poorly correlated with symptoms
  - Serologies are of little value in patients treated with rituximab where B cells are depleted
  - *B. microti* serologies will not detect WA-1 or MO-1 strains, *B. duncani*, *B. divergens*, or *B. venatorum*
- Xenodiagnosis
  - Antibody analysis of hamsters and gerbils intraperitoneally inoculated with patient blood may be considered for diagnosis of *B. microti* and *B. divergens*, respectively

Treatment

- Adjuvant therapy
  - Red cell exchange transfusion should be considered for patients with parasitemia > 10% at risk for pulmonary, renal, or hepatic complications with goal of 90% reduction in parasitemia
- Drugs
  - Treatment indicated in symptomatic patients with positive smear or PCR and asymptomatic patients with positive smear or PCR > 3 months
  - For *B. microti*, standard therapy is 7- to 10-day regimen of atovaquone plus azithromycin or clindamycin plus quinine
    - 2nd course of treatment (duration > 6 weeks, including 2 weeks after parasites no longer detectable on smear) indicated if symptoms persist > 3 months and *Babesia* DNA or parasites detected by PCR or smear
  - For *B. divergens*, standard therapy is clindamycin and quinine with exchange transfusion, as course is more frequently fulminant

Prognosis

- Estimated death rate is low; < 2% of hospitalized patients

MICROBIOLOGY

Parasite Features

- Pear-shaped (a.k.a. piroplasms) apicomplexan parasites that invade and subsequently lyse red blood cells
- Traditionally classified into 4 clades based on morphology and life cycle characteristics
  - Clade 1: Contains *B. microti* that cause human babesiosis mainly responsible for disease in northeastern and upper midwestern USA and Japan
    - Small trophozoites (1-3 μm) and forms up to 4 merozoites arranged in tetrad, a.k.a. "Maltese cross"
  - Clade 2: Contains *B. duncani* and related organisms mainly responsible for disease in western USA
    - Small trophozoites (1-3 μm) and forms up to 4 merozoites arranged in tetrad, a.k.a. "Maltese cross"
  - Clade 3: Contains *B. divergens*, related organisms, and *B. venatorum* responsible for disease in Europe and USA
    - With exception of *B. divergens*, which appears more similar to organisms in clades 1 and 2 with smaller trophozoites and tetrad of merozoites, clade 3 generally contains larger trophozoites (3-5 μm) and forms 2 merozoites only
  - Clade 4: Contains *Babesia* species that rarely infect humans
    - Larger trophozoites (3-5 μm) and forms 2 merozoites only

Life Cycle

- Tick feeding introducing sporozoites into vertebrate host
- Sporozoites invade host red blood cells and differentiate into trophozoites, which asexually reproduce to produce 2-4 merozoites that egress while lysing red blood cells and invade other red blood cells
- Infected red blood cells are ingested by tick
- Pregametocytes mature into gametocytes and then fuse to form zygotes, which translocate across tick gut and become ookinetes
- Ookinetes enter tick hemolymph and migrate to salivary acini where they hypertrophy into sporoblasts
- Sporoblasts bud into thousands of sporozoites (sporogony) when nymph-stage ticks attach to vertebrate mammals

MACROSCOPIC

Spleen

- Rare complications include splenomegaly, splenic infarct, and splenic rupture

MICROSCOPIC

Histologic Features

- Diagnosis primarily made by blood smear showing parasites with distinguishing features, including "Maltese cross" (occasional merozoites arranged in tetrads) &/or intraerythrocytic ring forms
- Ring forms may be mistaken for *P. falciparum* trophozoites with distinguishing features of *Babesia* to include absence of hemozoin in ring forms and absence of schizonts and gametocytes, occasional exoerythrocytic parasites
- Blood smear may reveal hemolysis

ANCILLARY TESTS

Immunohistochemistry

- Anti-*Babesia* antibodies available at some reference laboratories

DIFFERENTIAL DIAGNOSIS

Malaria (*Plasmodium* Species)

- Peripheral blood smear parasites may be very difficult to distinguish and may require PCR for definitive diagnosis
- *Babesia* lacks hemozoin, is dyssynchronous, shows tetrads, and has extraerythrocytic forms

Trypanosomiasis

- Trypomastigotes in peripheral blood smear with terminal/subterminal kinetoplast, central nucleus, undulating membrane, and flagellum (12-33 μm in length)
- Dividing forms are seen in African trypanosomes but not in American trypanosomes

Leishmaniasis

- Amastigotes reside in macrophages and are spherical to ovoid (1-5 μm long x 1-2 μm wide) with large nucleus, prominent kinetoplast, and short axoneme

Lyme &/or Anaplasmosis

- Because of cotransmission in *Ixodes* vector, these infections should be evaluated when *Babesia* is seen on peripheral smear or suspected due to tick exposure history

SELECTED REFERENCES

1. Swanson M et al: Trends in reported babesiosis cases - United States, 2011-2019. MMWR Morb Mortal Wkly Rep. 72(11):273-7, 2023
2. Waked R et al: Human babesiosis. Infect Dis Clin North Am. 36(3):655-70, 2022
3. Hildebrandt A et al: Human babesiosis in Europe. Pathogens. 10(9), 2021
4. Stanley J et al: Detection of Babesia RNA and DNA in whole blood samples from US blood donations. Transfusion. 61(10):2969-80, 2021
5. Dumic I et al: Splenic complications of Babesia microti infection in humans: a systematic review. Can J Infect Dis Med Microbiol. 2020:6934149, 2020
6. Sanchez E et al: Diagnosis, treatment, and prevention of Lyme disease, human granulocytic anaplasmosis, and babesiosis: a review. JAMA. 315(16):1767-77, 2016
7. Yager PH et al: Case records of the Massachusetts General Hospital. Case 6-2014. A 35-day-old boy with fever, vomiting, mottled skin, and severe anemia. N Engl J Med. 370(8):753-62, 2014
8. Froberg MK et al: Case report: spontaneous splenic rupture during acute parasitemia of Babesia microti. Ann Clin Lab Sci. 38(4):390-2, 2008
9. Krause PJ et al: Persistent and relapsing babesiosis in immunocompromised patients. Clin Infect Dis. 46(3):370-6, 2008
10. Dobroszycki J et al: A cluster of transfusion-associated babesiosis cases traced to a single asymptomatic donor. JAMA. 281(10):927-30, 1999
11. Fitzpatrick JE et al: Human case of piroplasmosis (babesiosis). Nature. 217(5131):861-2, 1968

Trophozoites

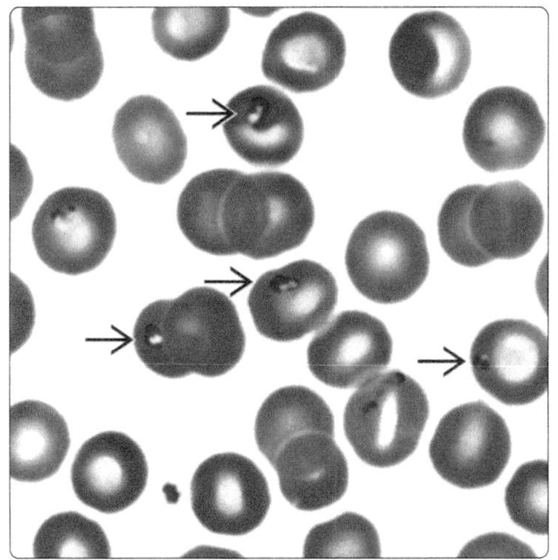

Tiny Ring Trophozoites

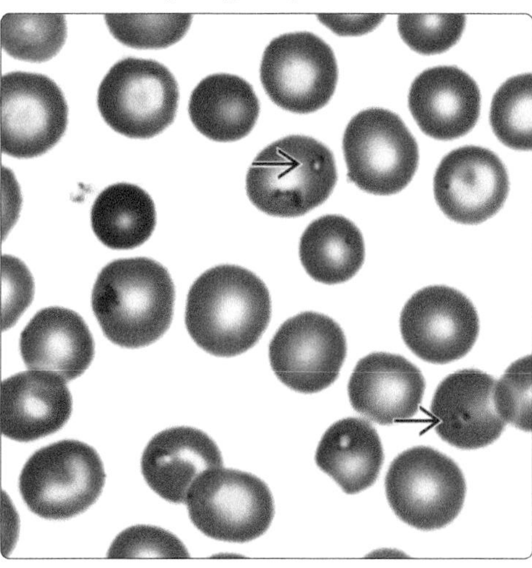

(Left) *Numerous trophozoite forms in various stages of babesiosis are shown. Note the very tiny forms →, which are much smaller than malaria species.* **(Right)** *Very tiny ring forms → are shown, which are much smaller than most malaria species.*

Extraerythrocytic Forms

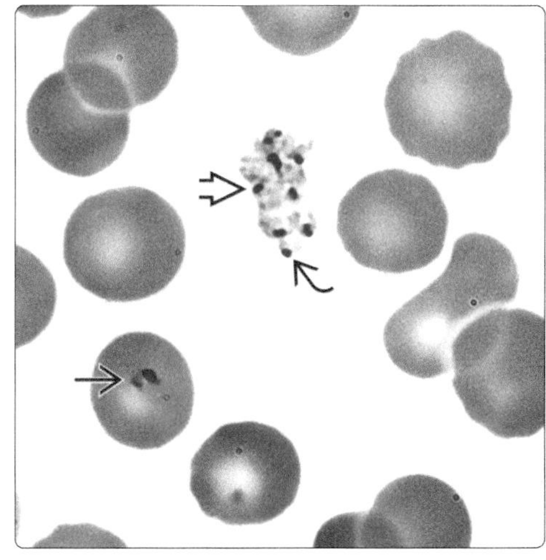

Platelets vs. Trophozoites

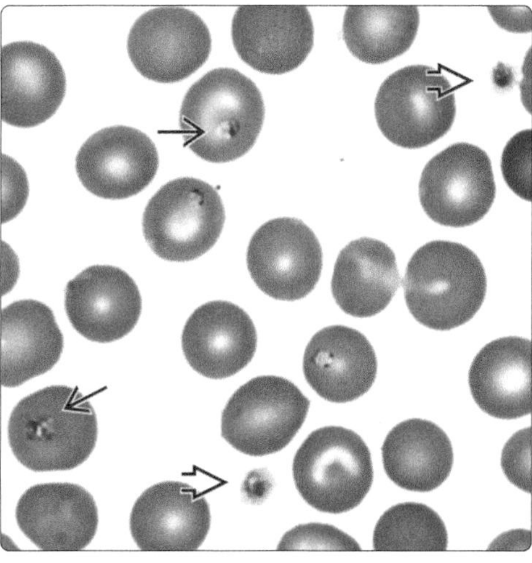

(Left) *Peripheral blood smear demonstrates a nondescript intracellular form → and a clump of extracellular forms ⇨, which are indicative of Babesia infection. Confusion with clumped platelets can be avoided by looking for the distinct, dark nuclei ↶. (Courtesy CDC.)* **(Right)** *Extracellular forms of Babesia are very similar to intracellular forms → but can rarely be confused with platelets. In this example, the platelets ⇨ have larger, less dense granular centers with feathery cytoplasm, which is not a feature of Babesia.*

Challenging Forms

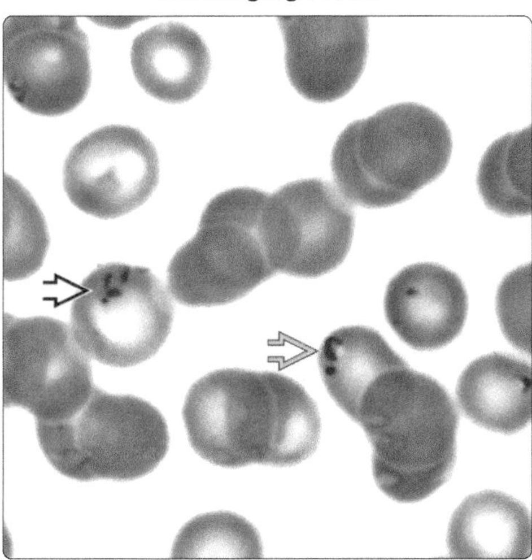

Splenic Rupture

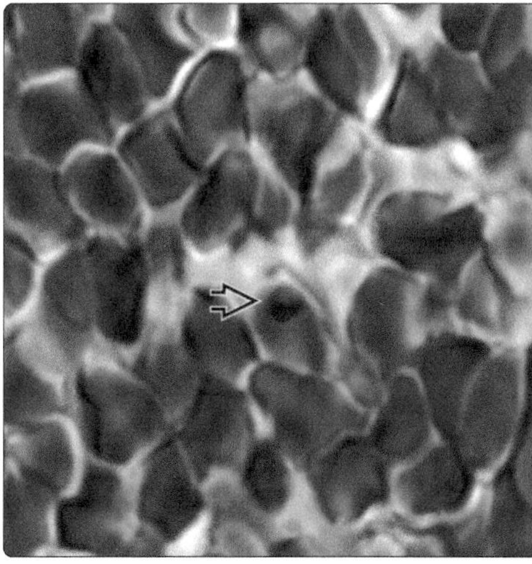

(Left) *Babesia may be challenging on peripheral blood smears when the tetrad is fragmenting ⇨ or if the ring forms are very tiny ⇨. Examining an entire smear and making additional smears when the differential includes malaria or platelet morphology is interfering is recommended.* **(Right)** *Spleen from a patient who presented with spontaneous rupture demonstrates a Babesia parasite within a red blood cell ⇨. A week after the splenectomy, the patient presented with clinical severe babesiosis.*

KEY FACTS

ETIOLOGY/PATHOGENESIS

- Malaria endemicity is closely tied to temperature, rainfall, and mosquito populations
- Organisms are present in peripheral blood (all species) and sequestered in deep endothelial beds (*Plasmodium falciparum*)

CLINICAL ISSUES

- Cerebral malaria (*P. falciparum*): Comatose, peripheral parasitemia, low platelets, high lactate, hypoglycemia
- Placental malaria (*P. falciparum*): Site of sequestration for *P. falciparum* parasites expressing specific type of "knob" protein

MICROSCOPIC

- Brain
  - Sequestration of parasites is present in small vessels from trophozoite to schizont stage
  - > 20% of vessels parasitized = cerebral malaria
  - Ring hemorrhages are associated with current or previous sequestration in cerebral malaria
- Placenta: Parasites of various stages adherent to and within maternal blood space, pigment-laden macrophages, leukocyte infiltration
- Malaria pigment polarizes and does not stain with iron stains (unlike hemosiderin)

TOP DIFFERENTIAL DIAGNOSES

- Babesiosis: Lacks hemozoin, is dyssynchronous, shows tetrads, and has extraerythrocytic forms; may require confirmation by PCR
- Severe hypoglycemia of newborn: Petechial white matter hemorrhages; no exposure history, or parasites/pigment
- Fat embolism after traumatic bone fracture: Petechial white matter hemorrhages associated with lipid; no exposure history or parasites/pigment
- Chronic intervillositis (placental): Idiopathic/autoimmune disease with no parasites

(Left) *Humans are infected when bitten by mosquitos carrying Plasmodium parasites. After a liver stage, asexual parasites circulate and cause disease. Sexual parasites are ingested by mosquitos, go through several stages, and migrate to salivary glands to infect the next human host.* **(Right)** *A female Anopheles gambiae mosquito obtains a blood meal through insertion of its needle-like labrum into the skin of its human host. The labrum and enlarged abdomen are red due to the blood meal contents. (Courtesy J. Gathany CDC/PHIL.)*

Life Cycle of Malaria

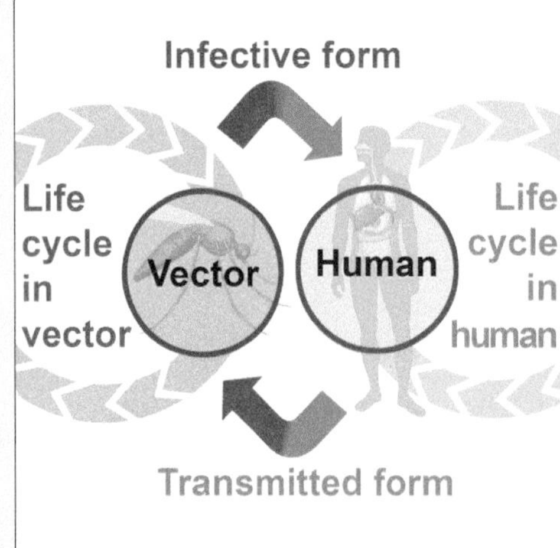

Anopheles gambiae Mosquito

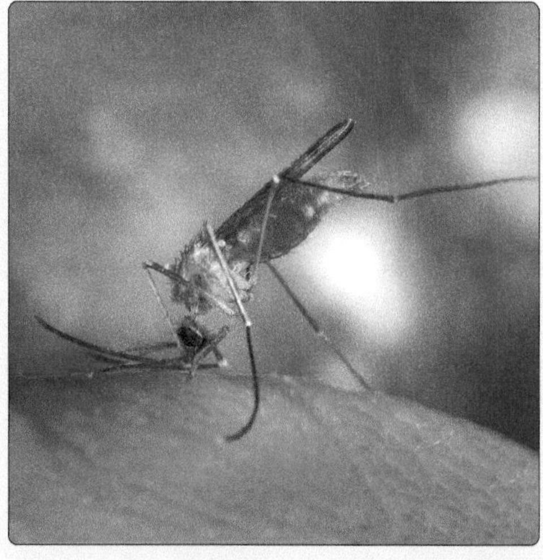

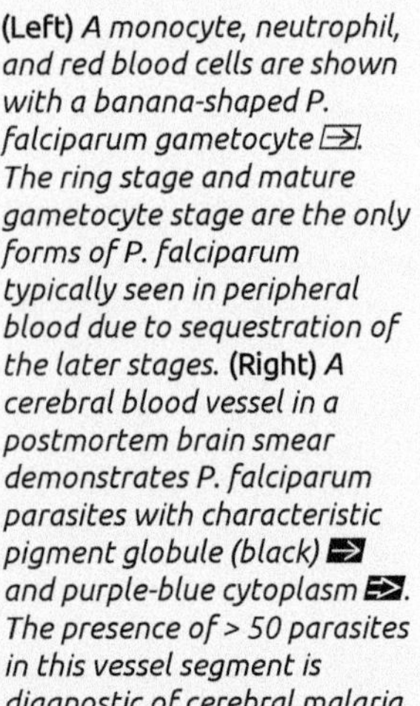

(Left) *A monocyte, neutrophil, and red blood cells are shown with a banana-shaped P. falciparum gametocyte ➩. The ring stage and mature gametocyte stage are the only forms of P. falciparum typically seen in peripheral blood due to sequestration of the later stages.* **(Right)** *A cerebral blood vessel in a postmortem brain smear demonstrates P. falciparum parasites with characteristic pigment globule (black) ➡ and purple-blue cytoplasm ➡. The presence of > 50 parasites in this vessel segment is diagnostic of cerebral malaria.*

Plasmodium falciparum Gametocyte

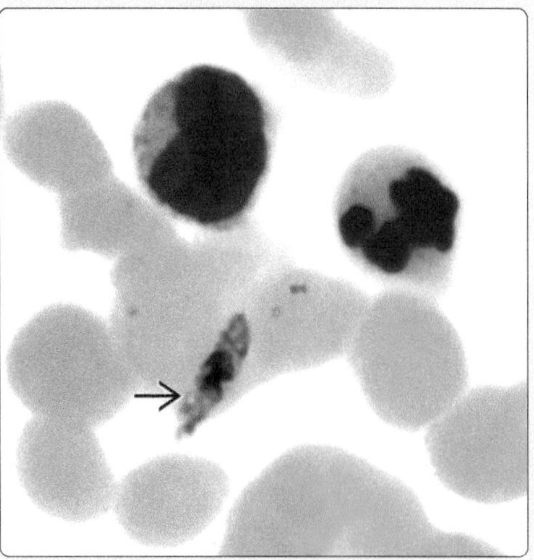

Brain Smear With Sequestered Parasites

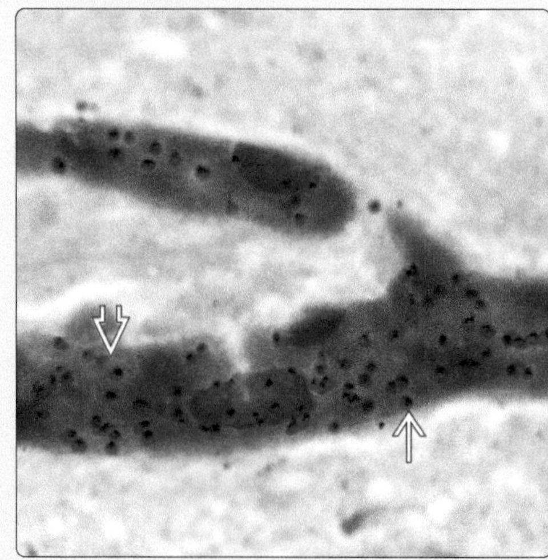

TERMINOLOGY

Synonyms

- Miasma (ancient Greek), Febris tertiana or Febris quartana (Latin), Marsh fever, Tertian ague (Middle French)

Definitions

- Malaria from Italian "mal" (bad) + "aria" (air) due to association with swamps and disease
- *Plasmodium* from Latin "plasma" (mold, formation) from morphologic forms of mass of nuclei (schizont)
- *falciparum* from Latin "falx/flac" (sickle) + "parus" (bearing) from sickle-shaped form of gametocytes
- *vivax* from Latin "vivace" (brisk, lively, long-lived) from its periodic recurrence due to liver reemergence
- *ovale* from Latin "ovalis" (egg-shaped) from oval to egg-shaped deformation of red blood cells during infection
- *knowlesi*, *curtisi*, and *wallikeri* named for from Robert Knowles, Christopher Curtis, and David Walliker

ETIOLOGY/PATHOGENESIS

Infectious Agents

- Infection with single-cell apicomplexan *Plasmodium* species transmitted via mosquito vector
- 6 main species: *P. falciparum*, *P. ovale curtisi*, and *P. ovale wallikeri*, *P. malaria*, *P. vivax*, and *P. knowlesi*
- Organisms present in peripheral blood (all species) and sequestered in deep endothelial beds (*P. falciparum*)
- *P. falciparum* and *P. malariae* cycle through liver once, whereas *P. ovale* and *P. vivax* remain in liver as hypnozoites

CLINICAL ISSUES

Epidemiology

- *P. falciparum* most common in Africa; also present in subtropical areas of Central and South America and Southeast Asia
- *P. vivax* most common outside of Africa, including Central and South America, India, and Southeast Asia; recent resurgence in East Africa
- *P. ovale* found primarily in sub-Saharan Africa (similar distribution to *P. vivax*)
- *P. malariae* found in subtropical areas of Central and South America, Africa, and Southeast Asia
- *P. knowlesi* found in Southeast Asia in areas inhabited by long-tailed macaques
- Travelers not on prophylaxis traveling to regions with malaria and exposed to mosquitos are at risk for mild to severe disease
- In highly endemic regions, children bear bulk of disease and mortality, while adults achieve nonsterile immunity; all ages at risk during epidemics in low-endemicity regions

Presentation

- Asymptomatic infection: Screened individuals from endemic areas may have circulating parasites with no clinical symptoms
- Symptomatic infection: Fever and malaise, abdominal pain, vomiting, diarrhea, headache, somnolence, loss of consciousness, coma
- Severe malaria anemia (*P. falciparum*): Very young children in endemic regions; hemoglobin < 5 g/dL, hematocrit < 15%
- Acidosis (*P. falciparum*): Children in endemic regions; high respiratory rate with respiratory acidosis, high lactate
- Cerebral malaria (*P. falciparum*): Young children in endemic regions, all ages in low-endemicity regions; coma, peripheral parasitemia, low platelets, high lactate, hypoglycemia
- Retinal examination by ophthalmoscopy will reveal malaria-specific retinal changes, including hemorrhages, vessel whitening, and peripheral whitening
- Placental malaria (*P. falciparum*): Primigravid women are more at risk in endemic areas; placental sequestration due to specific type of *P. falciparum* "knob" protein
- *P. vivax* severe infection: Infants to early 20s, respiratory failure
- *P. knowlesi* severe infection: Respiratory symptoms, renal failure, and thrombocytopenia without coagulopathy

Laboratory Tests

- CBC: Thrombocytopenia (*P. falciparum*, *P. knowlesi*)
- Rapid diagnostic tests ("dipsticks"): Lateral flow assay for antigen detection
  - Primarily available for *P. falciparum* and *P. vivax* (usually captures *P. ovale*, *P. malariae*, and *P. knowlesi* nonspecifically)
- Peripheral blood PCR: Single/multispecies primer sets; may remain positive for weeks after successful treatment of disease

Treatment

- *P. falciparum*: 2-drug combination therapy with artemisinin agent (IV artesunate for severe disease)
  - Sulfadoxine/pyrimethamine intermittent preventive therapy (IPT) during pregnancy
- *P. vivax*, *P. ovale* = chloroquine with primaquine (liver stages)
- *P. malariae* = chloroquine
- *P. knowlesi* = chloroquine with primaquine
- Fluid rehydration, respiratory support, dialysis, blood transfusion, red blood cell exchange, and other intensive care measures may be required in severe disease

Prognosis

- Overall mortality from malaria infection is < 1%
- Cerebral malaria is 15-20%, regardless of treatment/intervention

MICROBIOLOGY

Life Cycle

- Sexual cycle (10-18 days): Mosquito ingests male and female gametocytes during human blood meal; micro- and macrogametocytes form ookinete in midgut; ookinete migrates to midgut wall and forms oocysts; infective sporozoites develop in oocysts, which migrate to salivary glands then enter human skin with mosquito saliva
- Asexual cycle (in humans): Sporozoites infect liver hepatocytes and transform into thousands of merozoites within liver schizont (5-16 days); schizont rupture releases merozoites into circulation, which invade red blood cells, which mature, and rupture every 24-72 hours releasing 16-24 merozoites that reinvade red blood cells

Culture

- Primarily for research purposes

Peripheral Blood Smear Examination

- Primary diagnostic tool with quantification and speciation of blood-stage parasites based on morphology; decreasing parasitemia is best estimate of response to therapy
- *P. falciparum* = ring-stage parasites in small infected cells and banana-shaped gametocytes
- *P. vivax* = Schüffner dots, ameboid forms, large infected cells
- *P. ovale* = Schüffner dots, oval, large infected cells with fimbria, "comet" form
- *P. malariae* = small infected cells, "band" forms, "daisy" forms
- *P. knowlesi* = very similar to (often confused with) *P. malariae* (PCR required for definitive diagnosis)

MACROSCOPIC

Gross Features

- Pediatric cerebral malaria: Swollen and congested brain ± purple/gray discoloration (due to malaria pigment) ± petechial hemorrhages in white matter
- Adult cerebral malaria: Congested brain ± purple/gray discoloration ± petechial hemorrhages in white matter; no swelling/edema
- Liver: Dark purple to black discoloration
- Spleen: Enlarged, often massive spleen with dark purple to black discoloration; splenic rupture (more common in travelers)
- Multiorgan failure associated with heavy, infiltrated lungs, boggy, swollen kidneys, and scattered tissue hemorrhages

MICROSCOPIC

Histologic Features

- **Brain**: Sequestration of parasites in small vessels, ring hemorrhages associated with current or previous sequestration, and Dürck granuloma in healing stage
- **Lung**: Substantial amounts of parasite hemozoin pigment within macrophages with limited sequestered parasite biomass
- **Liver**: Macrophages with parasite hemozoin pigment found throughout parenchyma (active infection) or concentrated in portal triads (prior infection)
- **Spleen**: Primary site of parasite clearance with massive loads of hemozoin pigment; red pulp is greatly expanded with macrophages &/or parasites in development; white pulp is normal or may be very prominent/reactive
- **Bone marrow**: Increased numbers of gametocytes in development are found in marrow parenchyma (developmental niche)
- **Heart, kidney, gastrointestinal tract, and other organs**: Sequestration of parasites is present in small vessels from trophozoite to schizont stage
- **Placenta:** Parasites of various stages adherent to and within maternal blood space, pigment-laden macrophages, leukocyte infiltration; fibrin-entrapped collections of malaria pigment (prior infection)
- Malaria pigment polarizes and does not stain with iron stains (unlike hemosiderin)

ANCILLARY TESTS

Immunohistochemistry

- Antibodies to *Plasmodium* lactate dehydrogenase (pLDH) will stain all parasite forms (species specific)

PCR

- Tissue-based PCR to determine genotypes may be helpful in epidemic outbreaks for determining origin in fatal cases

DIFFERENTIAL DIAGNOSIS

Severe Hypoglycemia of Newborn

- Produces petechial hemorrhages in white matter of brain but without exposure history and no parasites/pigment in tissue sections

Fat Embolism After Traumatic Bone Fracture

- Produces petechial hemorrhages in white matter of brain associated with lipid in sections but without exposure history and no parasites/pigment in tissue sections

Babesiosis

- *Babesia* lacks hemozoin, is dyssynchronous, shows tetrads, and has extraerythrocytic forms; may require confirmation by PCR

Chronic Intervillositis (Placental)

- Idiopathic/autoimmune disease with no parasites

SELECTED REFERENCES

1. Daily JP et al: Diagnosis, treatment, and prevention of malaria in the US: a review. JAMA. 328(5):460-71, 2022
2. Duffy PE: Current approaches to malaria vaccines. Curr Opin Microbiol. 70:102227, 2022
3. Joste V et al: Distinction of Plasmodium ovale wallikeri and Plasmodium ovale curtisi using quantitative polymerase chain reaction with high resolution melting revelation. Sci Rep. 8(1):300, 2018
4. Ourives SS et al: Analysis of the lymphocyte cell population during malaria caused by Plasmodium vivax and its correlation with parasitaemia and thrombocytopaenia. Malar J. 17(1):303, 2018
5. Poostchi M et al: Image analysis and machine learning for detecting malaria. Transl Res. 194:36-55, 2018
6. De Niz M et al: Progress in imaging methods: insights gained into Plasmodium biology. Nat Rev Microbiol. 15(1):37-54, 2017
7. Tubman VN et al: Turf wars: exploring splenomegaly in sickle cell disease in malaria-endemic regions. Br J Haematol. 177(6):938-46, 2017
8. Kasetsirikul S et al: The development of malaria diagnostic techniques: a review of the approaches with focus on dielectrophoretic and magnetophoretic methods. Malar J. 15(1):358, 2016
9. Barrera V et al: Severity of retinopathy parallels the degree of parasite sequestration in the eyes and brains of Malawian children with fatal cerebral malaria. J Infect Dis. 211(12):1977-86, 2015
10. Joice R et al: Plasmodium falciparum transmission stages accumulate in the human bone marrow. Sci Transl Med. 6(244):244re5, 2014
11. Milner DA Jr et al: The systemic pathology of cerebral malaria in African children. Front Cell Infect Microbiol. 4:104, 2014
12. Milner DA Jr et al: A histological method for quantifying Plasmodium falciparum in the brain in fatal paediatric cerebral malaria. Malar J. 12:191, 2013
13. Mayor A et al: Placental infection with Plasmodium vivax: a histopathological and molecular study. J Infect Dis. 206(12):1904-10, 2012
14. Daneshvar C et al: Clinical and laboratory features of human Plasmodium knowlesi infection. Clin Infect Dis. 49(6):852-60, 2009
15. Pongponratn E et al: An ultrastructural study of the brain in fatal Plasmodium falciparum malaria. Am J Trop Med Hyg. 69(4):345-59, 2003

Plasmodium vivax in Peripheral Blood

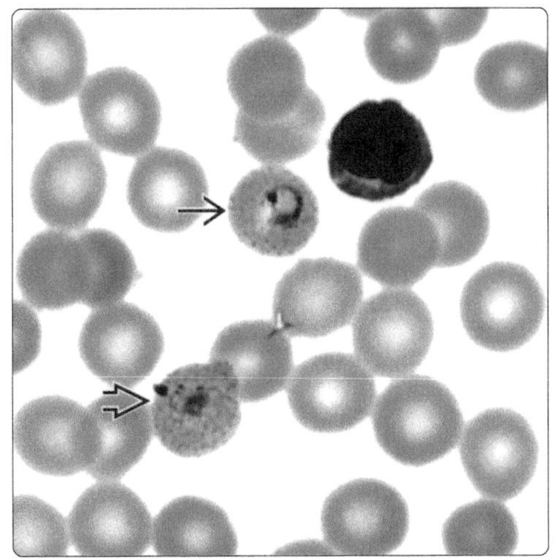

Plasmodium vivax in Peripheral Blood

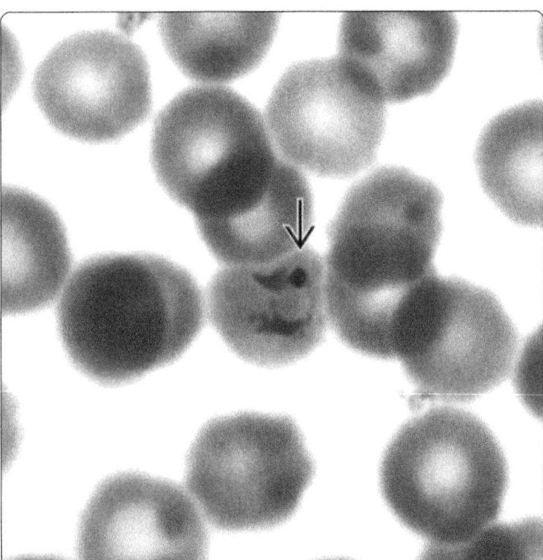

(Left) *A ring stage ➡ and ameboid trophozoite stage ⇨ of Plasmodium vivax are shown with the characteristic Schüffner dots on the red cell. Note that the infected cells are larger than the uninfected cells, as they are reticulocytes (younger). A lymphoid cell is present.* **(Right)** *The ameboid forms ➡ of P. vivax are distinct from the other malaria species' more round trophozoite forms. In this thicker part of the smear, morphology is more difficult to read.*

Plasmodium ovale in Peripheral Blood

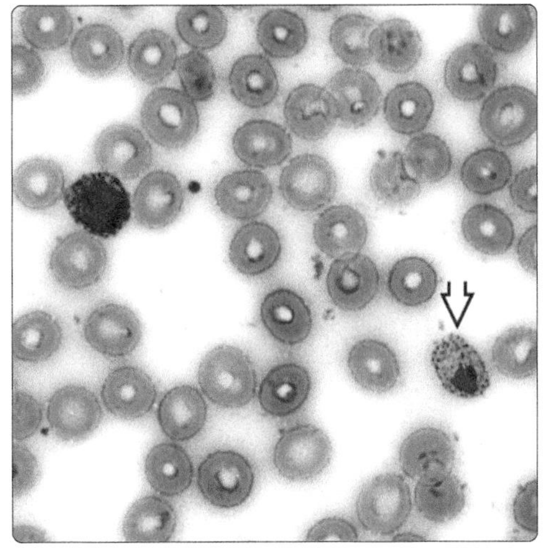

Plasmodium malariae in Peripheral Blood

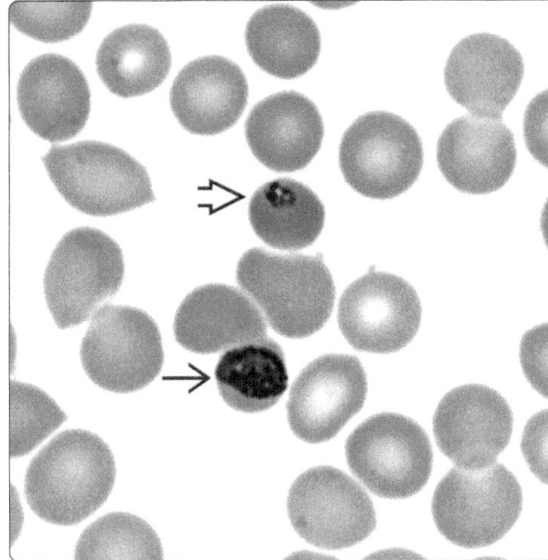

(Left) *Plasmodium ovale typically infects younger cells (reticulocytes) so that the cell appears larger than the uninfected cells around it. Note the oval shape of the infected cell and the Schüffner dots ⇨ on the surface. A gametocyte is also present.* **(Right)** *Plasmodium malariae infection can demonstrate a "band" form ➡ in peripheral blood as well as schizonts with a central golden pigment ("daisy" forms). An early-trophozoite-stage parasite ⇨ is also seen.*

Plasmodium knowlesi in Peripheral Blood

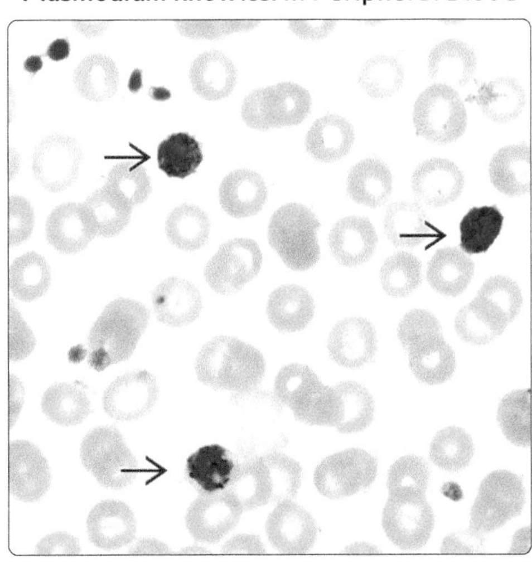

Liver With Malaria Pigment

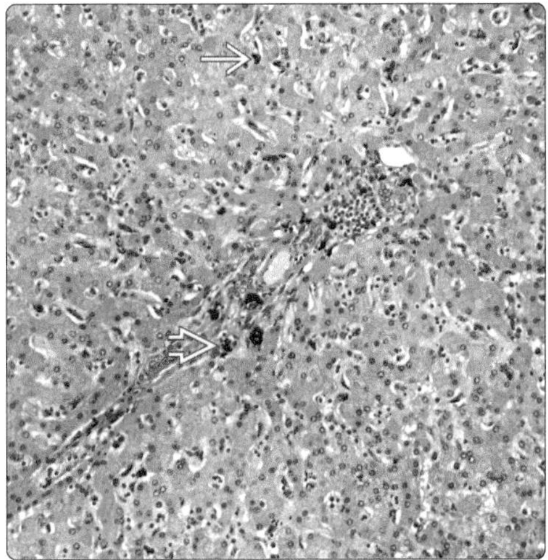

(Left) *P. knowlesi gametocytes ➡ are typically spherical, fill the host RBC, and contain blue cytoplasm, an eccentric red nucleus, and scattered coarse black pigment in cytoplasm. (Courtesy M. Peterson, MD, PhD and M. Galinski, PhD.)* **(Right)** *A section of liver from a patient with multiple episodes of malaria infection shows scattered pigment in macrophages ➡ (recent infection) as well as concentrations of pigment in the portal triad ➡ (remote infection).*

(Left) *A child with retinopathy-positive cerebral malaria is shown on midsagittal T1 FLAIR (TR2100, TE 26) with diffuse brain swelling and effacement of the prepontine cistern. (Courtesy T. E. Taylor, DO.)* (Right) *Cerebral gray-white junction is shown in a patient who died of cerebral malaria with classic petechial hemorrhages → limited to the white matter.*

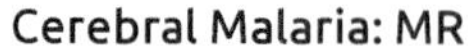

Cerebral Malaria: MR

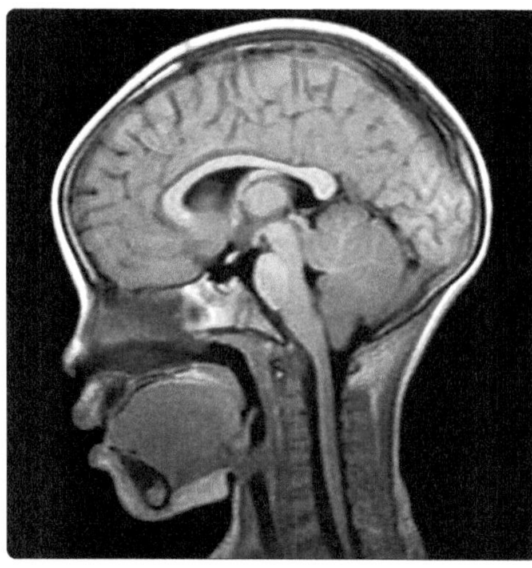

Cerebral Malaria: Gross

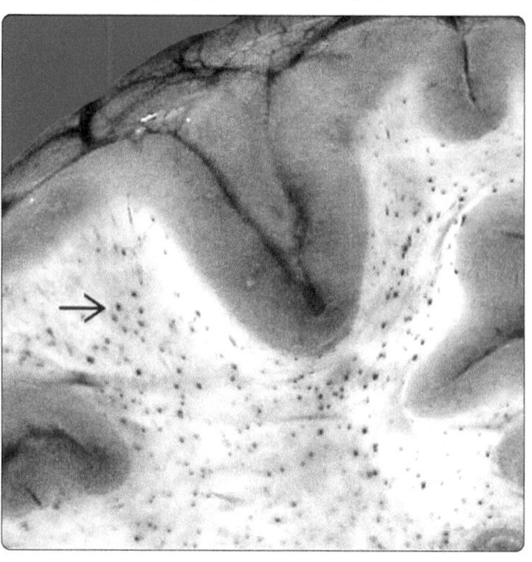

(Left) *Ring hemorrhages ↩ in various stages of evolution are shown in the white matter ⇨ of the cerebrum of a patient who died of cerebral malaria. Note lack of hemorrhages in the gray matter →.* (Right) *Two ring hemorrhages are shown in cerebral malaria, the larger demonstrating a fibrin thrombus →. Coagulation activation occurs in malaria, and local effects through EPCR binding are implicated.*

Cerebral Malaria: Ring Hemorrhages

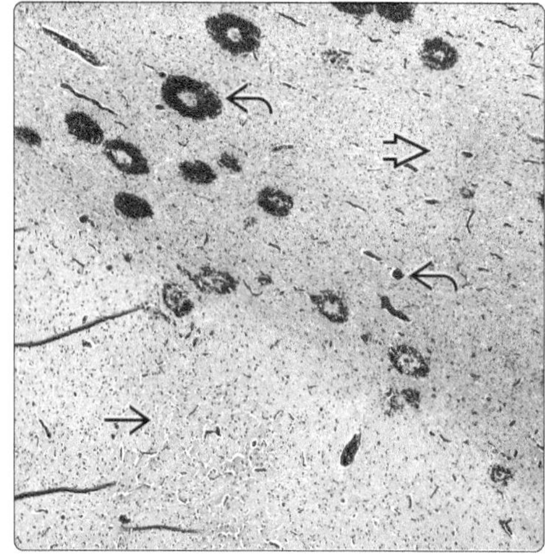

Ring Hemorrhage

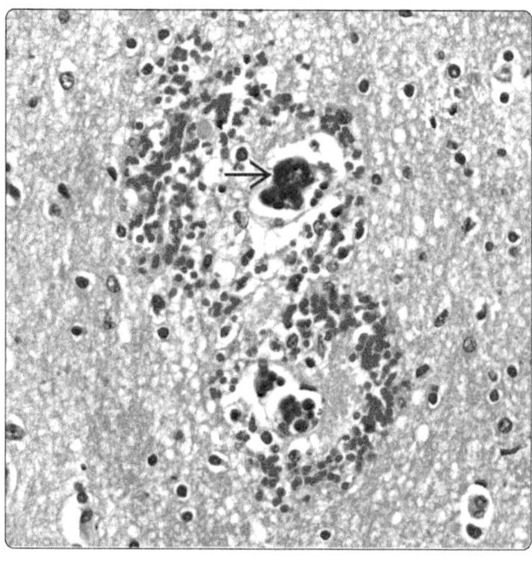

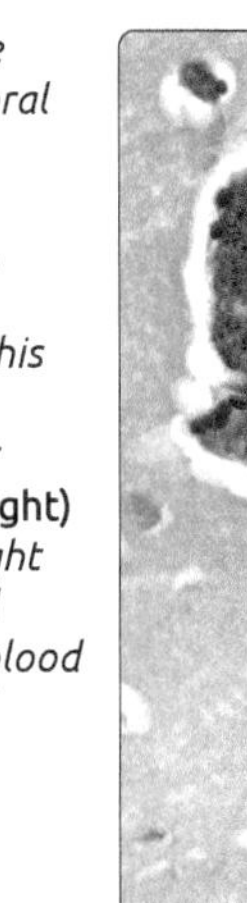

(Left) *A large vessel of the brain from a case of cerebral malaria demonstrates innumerable sequestered parasites → in the lumen. Although difficult to appreciate, all vessels in this section are packed with parasites, evident by their visibility at low power.* (Right) *Polarized light will highlight the hemozoin pigment → within each infected red blood cell, which is a product of hemoglobin digestion.*

Cerebral Vessel Sequestration

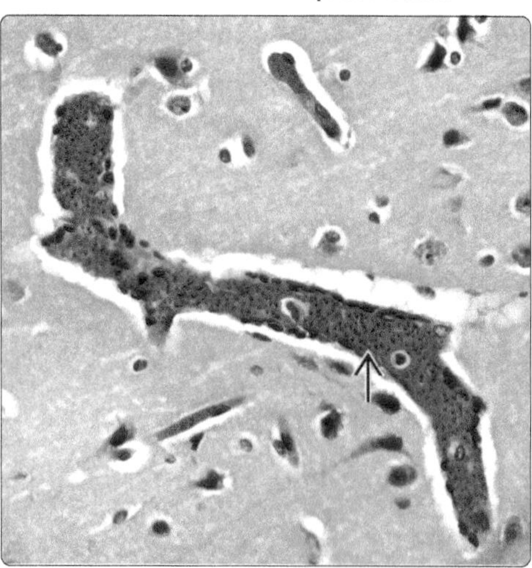

Cerebral Vessel Sequestration: Polarized

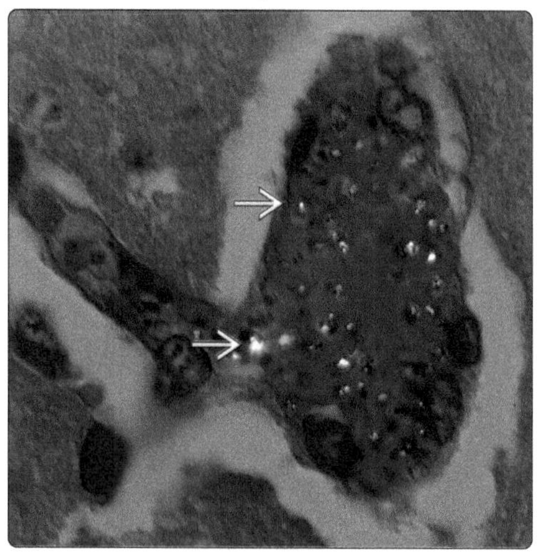

Retinal Hemorrhage in Malaria

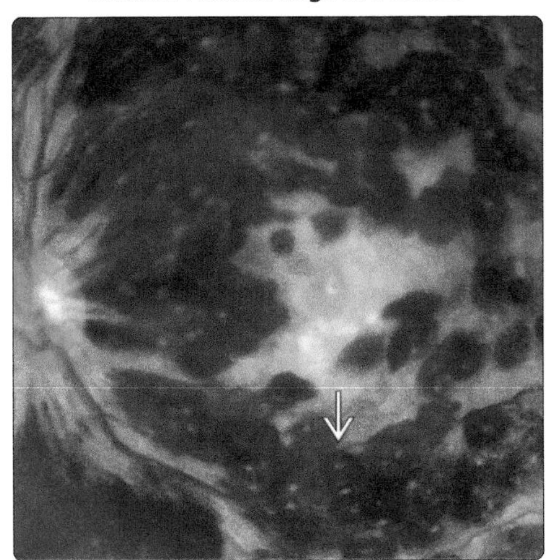

Retinal Histology in Malaria

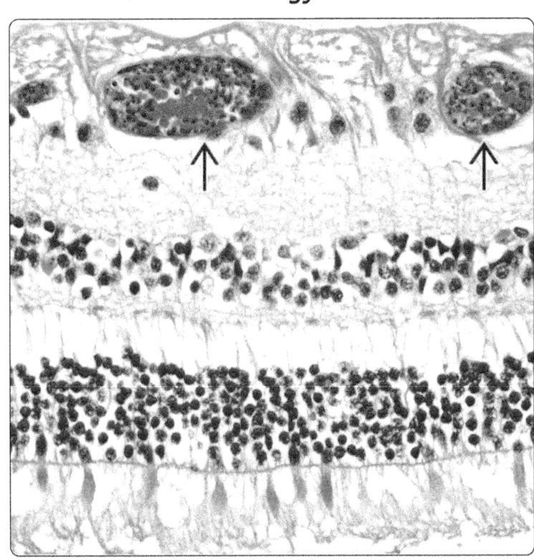

(Left) *Retina in cerebral malaria demonstrates innumerable white, centered hemorrhages ➡ in the retinal vessels that mirror the ring hemorrhages in the brain. (Courtesy I. MacCormick, MD.)* **(Right)** *The retina of a child who died from cerebral malaria demonstrates sequestration ⇨ in the retinal vessels of late-stage parasites, which parallels sequestration in the brain. This sequestration produces changes visible in the retina during life. (Courtesy V. White, MD.)*

Cardiac Sequestration

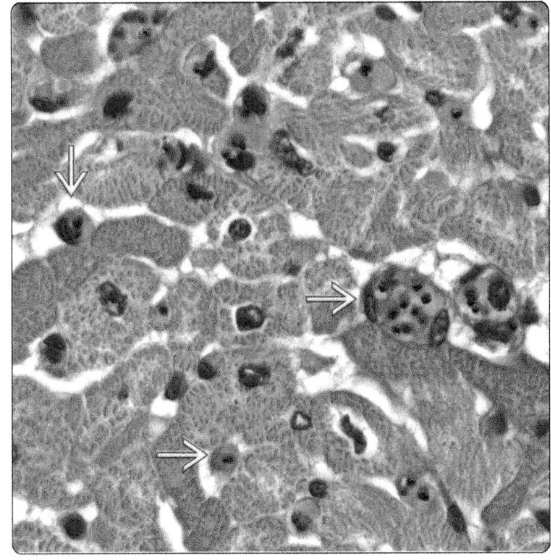

Spleen: Parasite Burden

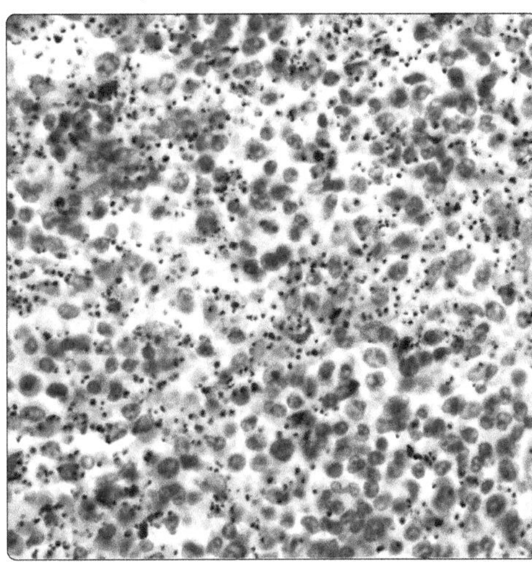

(Left) *Cardiac vessels show sequestered parasites ➡ in a cerebral malaria patient. Although rare events have been reported in experimental malaria infections, no tissue damage is seen in pediatric malaria.* **(Right)** *A section of spleen on CD8 immunohistochemistry from a patient with malaria demonstrates enormous quantities of pigment representing parasites, free pigment, and macrophages. The spleen is the primary parasite clearance site by phagocytosis and digestion.*

Small Bowel Sequestration

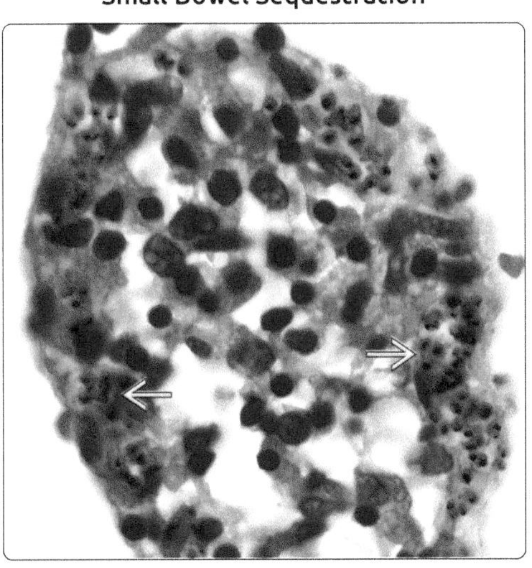

Placental Malaria Sequestration

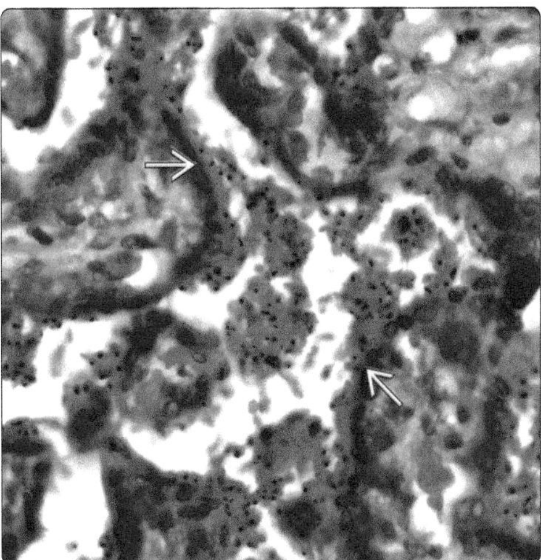

(Left) *Small bowel with denuded epithelium (postmortem artifact) demonstrates dense sequestration ➡ in the capillary that runs along the base of the mucosal surface. The GI tract is a large site for vascular parasite sequestration.* **(Right)** *Dense sequestration of parasitized red blood cells line the villous surface ➡ in this active placental malaria infection. Intermittent preventative therapy during pregnancy works at the population level to prevent placental malaria.*

Free-Living Amebiasis

KEY FACTS

ETIOLOGY/PATHOGENESIS

- *Acanthamoeba*, *Balamuthia*, and *Naegleria* species present worldwide in water and soil, enter body through scrapes or inhalation, and reach brain by hematogenous spread or direct invasion into cribriform plate

CLINICAL ISSUES

- Primary amebic encephalitis (PAM; *Naegleria fowleri*) and granulomatous amebic encephalitis (GAE; *Acanthamoeba* spp. and *Balamuthia mandrillaris*)
- Keratitis, disseminated amebiasis, and skin lesions (± concurrent neurologic involvement)
- Very few patients survive PAM or GAE (> 95% mortality)
- MR: Single or multifocal space-occupying brain masses, ring-enhancing lesions, hydrocephalus, &/or edema

MICROBIOLOGY

- *Acanthamoeba* spp. and *N. fowleri* grow on agarose plates with bacterial lawns, while *B. mandrillaris* requires mammalian cell cultures or inoculation in mice

MICROSCOPIC

- Trophozoites (10-45 µm): Large nuclei with karyosomes; difficult to distinguish between species morphologically; easily overlooked or mistaken for histiocytes
- Cysts (15-20 µm): Walls with 2 (*Acanthamoeba*) or 3 layers (*Balamuthia*; requires EM); no *N. fowleri* cysts in tissue
- GAE: Subacute to chronic meningitis, encephalitis with vasculitis and thrombosed vessels, giant cells, cysts, and trophozoites
- PAM: Trophozoites, mononuclear cells, and neutrophils
- Keratitis: Minimal stromal inflammation, cysts > trophozoites

TOP DIFFERENTIAL DIAGNOSES

- Encephalitis/meningoencephalitis: Bacterial, fungal, viral, and other parasitic infections confirmed by morphology, isolation in culture, or molecular testing
- Other causes of skin lesions: Panniculitis, necrotizing skin and soft tissue infections

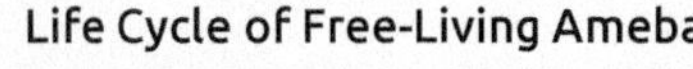

Life Cycle of Free-Living Ameba

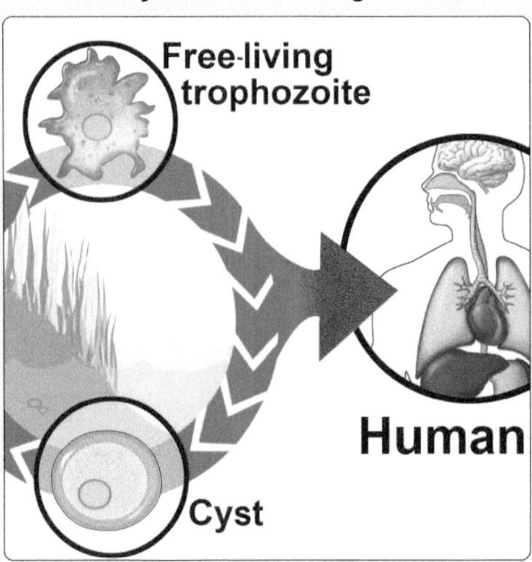

***Acanthamoeba* spp. in Brain**

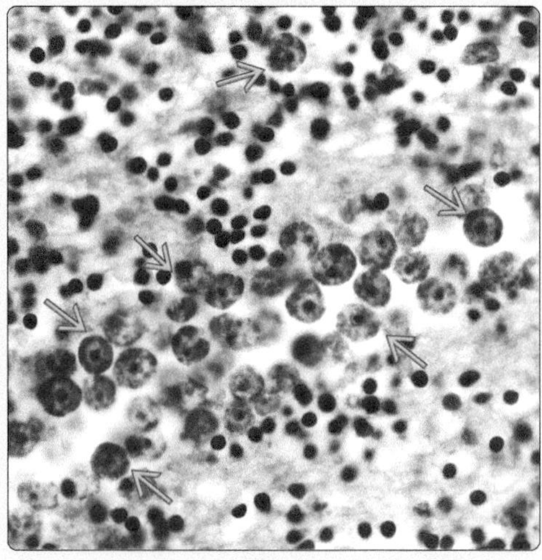

(Left) *Free-living ameba species thrive in warm, wet environments and do not require a human host for completion of their life cycle. Humans become directly infected by pathogenic species or have disseminated disease in the setting of immunosuppression.* **(Right)** *Numerous amebic trophozoites ⇒ with distinctive karyosomes are present in the cerebellum of this case of granulomatous amebic encephalitis (GAE).*

***Balamuthia mandrillaris* in Brain**

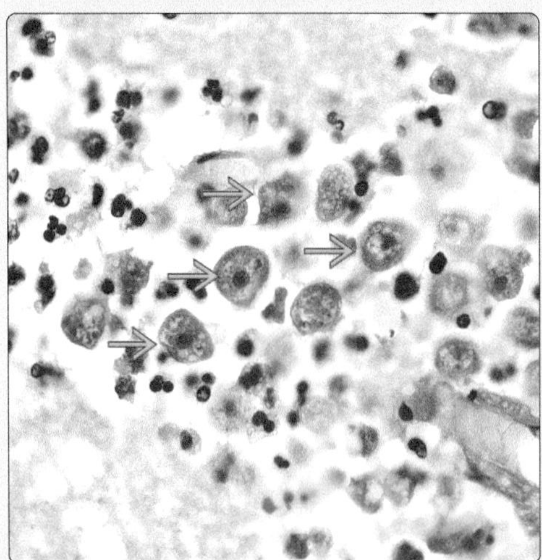

***Naegleria fowleri* in Brain**

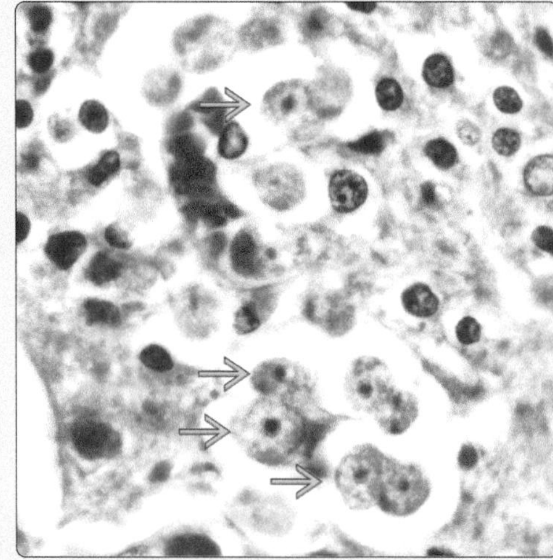

(Left) *Numerous amebic trophozoites ⇒ with distinctive karyosomes are present in the brain of this case of GAE.* **(Right)** *Numerous amebic trophozoites ⇒ are present in the cerebellum in this case of primary amebic meningoencephalitis.*

TERMINOLOGY

Synonyms

- Brain-eating ameba, free-living ameba, amphizoic ameba

Definitions

- *Balamuthia* from Balamuth, parasitologist, + *mandrillaris* from mandrill (baboon, from which it was isolated)
- *Naegleria* from Nägler, Austrian bacteriologist, + *fowleri* from Fowler, who 1st described (with Carter)
- *Acanthamoeba* from Greek: "Akantha" (thorn) + "amoibe" (change)
- *Sappinia pedata* from Mr. Sappin-Trouffy, mycologist at Paris Academy of Sciences, where it was discovered
- *Vermamoeba vermiformis*, formerly *Harmanella vermiformis*, described by Hartmann

ETIOLOGY/PATHOGENESIS

Infectious Agents

- *Acanthamoeba* spp. are ubiquitous organisms found in water sources as well as soil; may enter body via inhaled dust or cutaneous lacerations and disseminate; also associated with contact lens use (does not disseminate)
  - > 20 species of *Acanthamoeba* exist with 11 causing human disease: *A. astronyxis, A. byersi, A. castellanii, A. culbertsoni, A. hatchetti, A. keratitis, A. lugdunensis, A. palestinensis, A. polyphaga, A. quina, A. rhysodes*
  - Cyst form in tissue is resistant to immune clearance and may lead to recurrence of infection
- *B. mandrillaris* may enter body via inhaled dust or cutaneous lacerations; rare reports of transmission through organ donation; incubation time unknown (weeks to months to develop 1st symptoms)
  - Few trophozoites and thus difficult to identify in immunocompetent patients; may also affect immunocompromised patients
- *N. fowleri* is found in warm fresh water sources as well as soil; exposure via nasal passages from water allows direct entry of ameba into cribriform plate (incubation time: 1-12 days); unclear risk from organ donation
  - May be reservoir of *Legionella pneumophila* and other bacteria
- *S. pedata* is found in soil contaminated with bovid and cervid feces
- *V. vermiformis* is ubiquitous in tap water and has been documented in hospital networks
  - Considered important endocytobiont for *L. pneumophila, Bacillus anthracis*, and *Pseudomona aeruginosa*, among others

CLINICAL ISSUES

Epidemiology

- *Acanthamoeba* spp.: 1-33 keratitis cases per million contact lens wearers per year; 173 nonkeratitis infections reported in USA from 1956-2020
- *B. mandrillaris*: > 200 cases of granulomatous amebic encephalitis (GAE) reported since 1993; many in Hispanic Americans for unclear reasons
- *N. fowleri*: 157 cases reported in USA from 1962-2022
- *S. pedata*: 1 known case of amebic encephalitis in previously healthy man
- *V. vermiformis*: Associated with amebic keratitis

Site

- Eye, skin, sinuses, lungs, CNS

Presentation

- GAE (*Acanthamoeba, Balamuthia*, and *Sappinia* spp.) and primary amebic encephalitis (PAM; *N. fowleri*)
  - Headache, fever, fatigue, nausea, and vomiting, followed by neck stiffness and pain, photophobia, then movement and speech disturbances, unilateral paralysis, behavioral changes, seizures, and coma
- Disseminated infection (*Acanthamoeba* or *Balamuthia* spp.) can involve skin, sinuses, lungs, and other organs via hematogenous spread, predominantly in immunocompromised patients
  - Deep skin lesions form erythematous hard nodules (± neurologic involvement)
- Keratitis (*Acanthamoeba* spp., *V. vermiformis*) associated with contact use in healthy individuals: Redness, irritation, and cloudiness of cornea with possible ulceration and blindness

Laboratory Tests

- CSF: Predominantly lymphocytic pleocytosis, normal or low glucose, elevated protein
- Actively moving *N. fowleri* trophozoites (~ 1 μm/s) may be observed in wet mount of CSF sediment
- Indirect immunofluorescence (IIF) staining for antigens
- Indirect immunofluorescence assay (IFA) for antibodies; not used as routine diagnostic test
- RT-PCR (CSF, tissue): Single or multitargeted assays

Treatment

- Early diagnosis treated with miltefosine with hypothermia for *Acanthamoeba* and *Balamuthia* spp.
- Combinations of antibiotics and antiparasitics have been tried but with rare survival (9 cases in USA from 1974-2016)
- No effective treatment for *N. fowleri*

Prognosis

- Very few patients survive PAM or GAE (> 95% mortality)
- Risk of permanent visual impairment or blindness with delayed keratitis treatment

IMAGING

MR Findings

- Single or multifocal space-occupying brain masses, ring-enhancing lesions, hydrocephalus, &/or edema

CT Findings

- Brain edema with diffuse enhancement of meninges

MICROBIOLOGY

Culture

- *Acanthamoeba* spp. and *N. fowleri*: Growth on agarose plates containing bacterial lawns
- *B. mandrillaris*: Growth on mammalian cell cultures (e.g., monkey kidney, human lung fibroblasts) or in mice after intranasal or intraperitoneal inoculation

MACROSCOPIC

Granulomatous Amebic Encephalitis

- Diffuse meningitis with cerebral edema
- Focal softening, hemorrhage, or frank necrosis may be present

Primary Amebic Encephalitis

- Cerebral edema; uncal or cerebellar herniation may be present
- Meninges may appear cloudy and purulent

Skin Lesions

- May appear as reddish nodules, skin ulcers, or abscesses

MICROSCOPIC

Histologic Features

- GAE (*Acanthamoeba* spp. and *B. mandrillaris*)
  - Subacute to chronic meningitis, encephalitis with vasculitis and thrombosed vessels, and giant cells (in immunocompetent hosts) with cysts or trophozoites
  - *Acanthamoeba* spp. cysts are 10-25 µm in diameter, contain 1 nucleus with large karyosome, and 2-layered wall; trophozoites are 15-45 µm, contain large nucleus with large, centrally located karyosome without peripheral chromatin, and multiple acanthopodia
  - *B. mandrillaris* cysts cannot be distinguished from *Acanthamoeba* spp. by light microscopy; trophozoites are also similar, 15-60 µm, have long pseudopodia, with rare binucleate forms; multiple nucleoli may be present
- PAM (*N. fowleri*)
  - Affected areas include olfactory bulbs (site of entry), small to midsize artery perivascular spaces, and frontal and temporal gray matter, which may show mixture of trophozoites, mononuclear cells, and neutrophils
  - *N. fowleri* trophozoites measure 10-35 µm and contain granular cytoplasm with many vacuoles and single large nucleus with large dense karyosome; flagellated form may be found in CSF; cysts are not formed in human tissues
- Skin lesions (*Acanthamoeba* spp. and *B. mandrillaris*)
  - Granulomatous inflammation with infiltrating giant cells, lymphocytes, plasma cells, and eosinophils; trophozoites may be present around blood vessels or within necrotic tissue with limited inflammation
- Keratitis (*Acanthamoeba* spp.)
  - Minimal stromal keratitis with cysts more commonly seen than trophozoites; stromal necrosis may be seen in advanced lesions

ANCILLARY TESTS

Histochemistry

- Trichome stain highlights nucleus in red (vs. dark brown to black of human cells)
- Methenamine silver stain highlights ruffled membrane and internal structure of cysts in black
- Periodic acid-Schiff highlights ruffled membrane and internal structure of cysts in purple

Immunohistochemistry

- Antibodies targeting specific species may be available at reference laboratories
- Amebas resemble histiocytes but are CD68 negative

PCR

- RT-PCR can be used on formalin-fixed, paraffin-embedded tissue

Electron Microscopy

- 3rd cyst wall layer (mesocyst) of *B. mandrillaris* is only visible via EM

DIFFERENTIAL DIAGNOSIS

Other Causes of Encephalitis/Meningoencephalitis

- *Acanthamoeba*, *Balamuthia*, and *Naegleria* species may appear very similar to each other on tissue biopsies and require culture, immunofluorescence, or molecular testing to distinguish
- *Entamoeba histolytica*, when disseminated from bowel, may appear very similar to free-living ameba but forms large, solitary abscesses rather than diffuse processes
- Bacterial, fungal, viral, and other parasitic infections can be confirmed morphologically, by isolation in culture, or by molecular testing

Other Causes of Skin Lesions

- Panniculitis, necrotizing skin and soft tissue infections
- Bacteria, mycobacteria, or fungal organisms identified by histochemical stains, isolation in culture, or molecular testing

SELECTED REFERENCES

1. Haston JC et al: The epidemiology and clinical features of non-keratitis Acanthamoeba infections in the United States, 1956-2020. Open Forum Infect Dis. 10(1):ofac682, 2023
2. McLean AC et al: Sinonasal amoebiasis: an unexpected cause of sinonasal necroinflammatory disease. Am J Surg Pathol. 47(1):102-10, 2023
3. Spottiswoode N et al: Successful treatment of Balamuthia mandrillaris granulomatous amebic encephalitis with nitroxoline. Emerg Infect Dis. 29(1):197-201, 2023
4. Alvarez P et al: Cutaneous balamuthiasis: a clinicopathological study. JAAD Int. 6:51-8, 2022
5. Kofman A et al: Free living amoebic infections: review. J Clin Microbiol. 60(1):e0022821, 2022
6. Norgan AP et al: Detection of Naegleria fowleri, Acanthamoeba spp, and Balamuthia mandrillaris in formalin-fixed, paraffin-embedded tissues by real-time multiplex polymerase chain reaction. Am J Clin Pathol. 152(6):799-807, 2019
7. Shehab KW et al: Balamuthia mandrillaris granulomatous amebic encephalitis with renal dissemination in a previously healthy child: case report and review of the pediatric literature. J Pediatric Infect Dis Soc. 7(3):e163-8, 2018
8. Brondfield MN et al: Disseminated Acanthamoeba infection in a heart transplant recipient treated successfully with a miltefosine-containing regimen: case report and review of the literature. Transpl Infect Dis. 19(2), 2017
9. Neelam S et al: Pathobiology and immunobiology of Acanthamoeba keratitis: insights from animal models. Yale J Biol Med. 90(2):261-8, 2017
10. LaFleur M et al: Balamuthia mandrillaris meningoencephalitis associated with solid organ transplantation--review of cases. J Radiol Case Rep. 7(9):9-18, 2013
11. Cetin N et al: Naegleria fowleri meningoencephalitis. Blood. 119(16):3658, 2012
12. Guarner J et al: Histopathologic spectrum and immunohistochemical diagnosis of amebic meningoencephalitis. Mod Pathol. 20(12):1230-7, 2007

Acanthamoeba Cyst in Culture

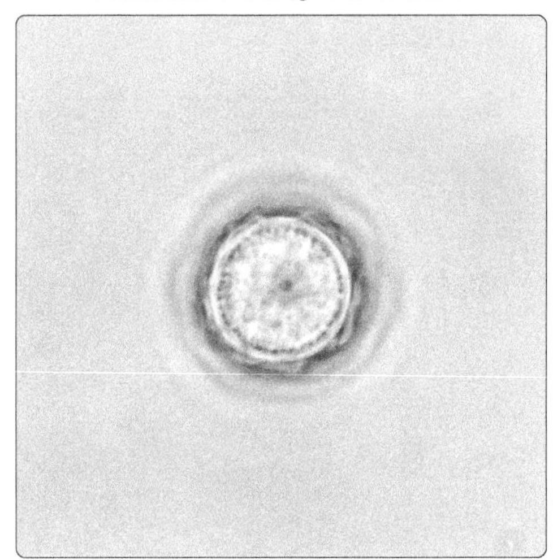

Acanthamoeba Cyst: Electron Microscopy

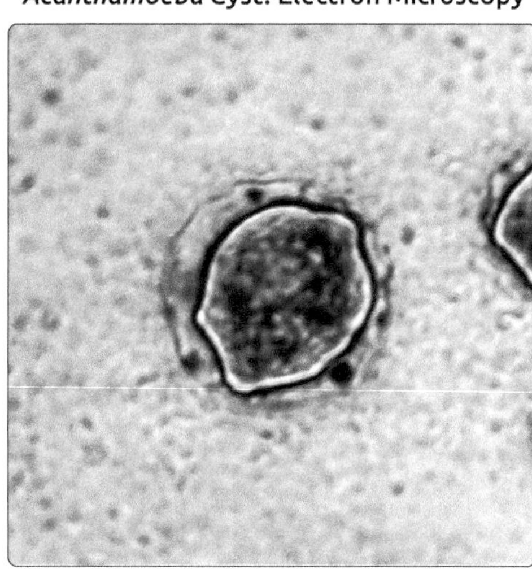

(Left) *Acanthamoeba spp. cysts are 10-25 μm in diameter, contain a single nucleus, large karyosome, and a 2-layered wall consisting of a wrinkled fibrous outer wall (exocyst) and an inner wall (endocyst) that may be hexagonal, spherical, star-shaped, or polygonal. (Courtesy G. Healy, PhD, CDC/PHIL.)* **(Right)** *As shown by electron microscopy, Acanthamoeba spp. cysts contain 2-layered walls, which help to distinguish from the 3-layered walls of B. mandrillaris. (Courtesy J. Hierholzer, MD, CDC/PHIL).*

Acanthamoeba Cyst in Tissue Section

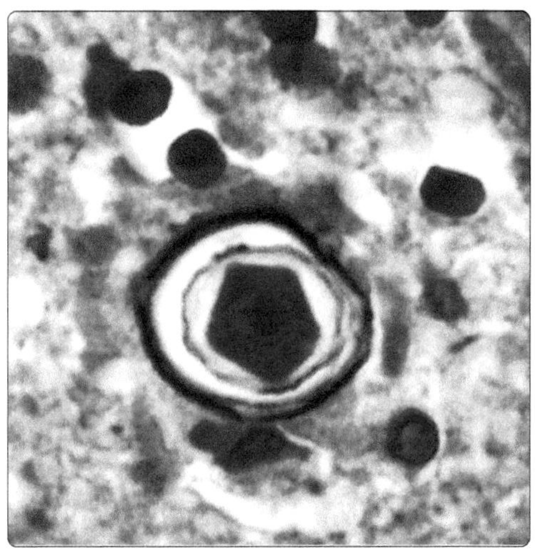

Acanthamoeba Cyst: GMS Stain

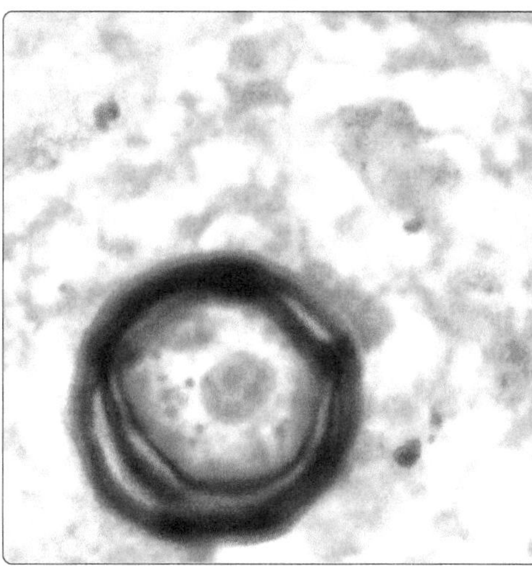

(Left) *Shrinkage artifact produces the artifactual pentagonal shape in an encysted Acanthamoeba. (Courtesy A. Yachnis, MD.)* **(Right)** *GMS highlights cyst walls of Acanthamoeba spp. Cysts are often found in chronic GAE due to Acanthamoeba, occasionally in chronic examples due to B. mandrillaris, but not in primary amebic meningoencephalitis due to N. fowleri. (Courtesy A. Yachnis, MD.)*

Acanthamoeba Trophozoite: Cytology

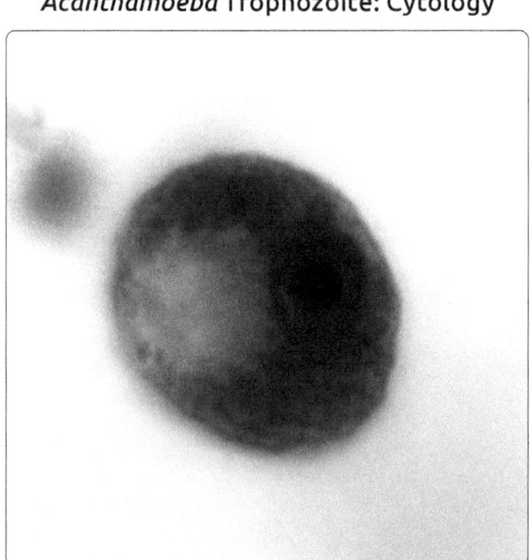

Acanthamoeba Trophozoite: Histology

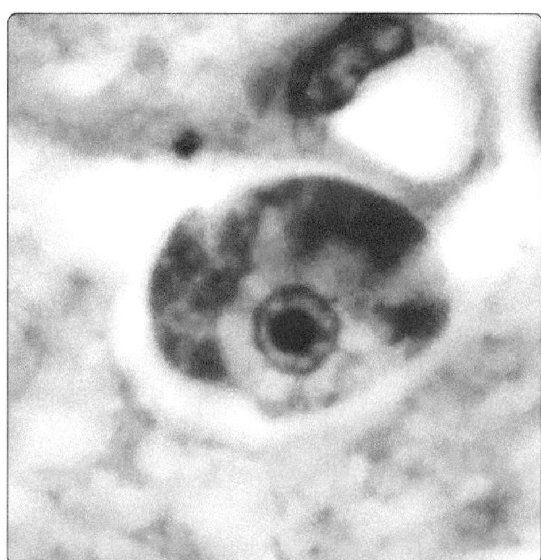

(Left) *High magnification of an Acanthamoeba trophozoite on a Pap stain from a brain FNA shows the heterogeneous cell body and large karyosome. The ruffled membrane cannot be seen.* **(Right)** *Acanthamoeba spp. trophozoites are pleomorphic, 15-45 μm, and contain a large nucleus with a large, centrally located karyosome but no peripheral chromatin, features than can help distinguish from histiocytes in tissue sections.*

(Left) *Numerous cysts and trophozoites are present in necrotic dermal tissue in a biopsy from an immunocompromised patient. Note the lack of inflammation.* (Right) *This section of sinonasal mucosa from a patient with chronic lymphocytic leukemia (CLL) shows necrotic tissue with scattered cysts of Acanthamoeba. The simultaneous presence of skin lesions is consistent with widely disseminated acanthamoebiasis.*

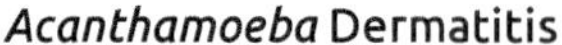

Acanthamoeba Dermatitis

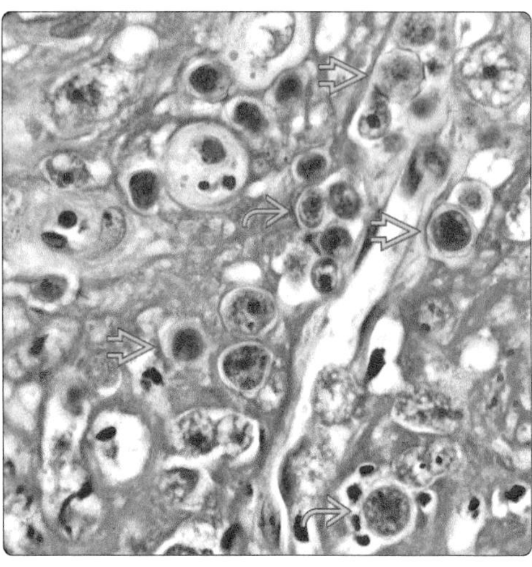

Acanthamoeba Rhinosinusitis

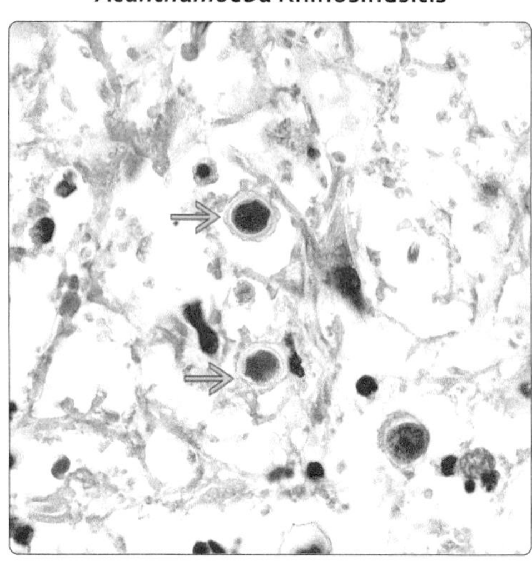

(Left) *Clinical photograph shows an eye with a corneal infiltrate in a ring shape, typical of Acanthamoeba keratitis. Notice the hyperemic conjunctiva. (From DP: Cytopathology.)* (Right) *Contact lens wearers may develop keratitis due to infection by Acanthamoeba spp. Scattered organisms can be see on H&E sections and are also readily highlighted by GMS and PAS-D stains.*

Acanthamoeba Keratitis

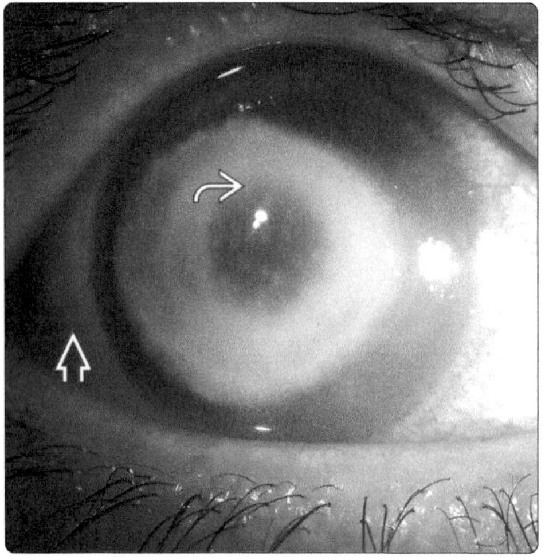

Acanthamoeba Keratitis

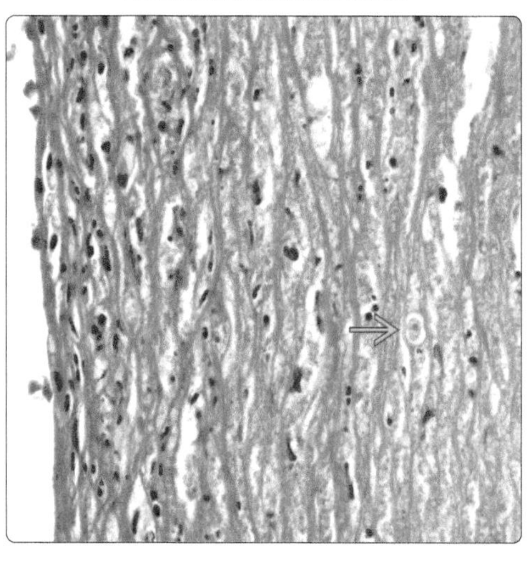

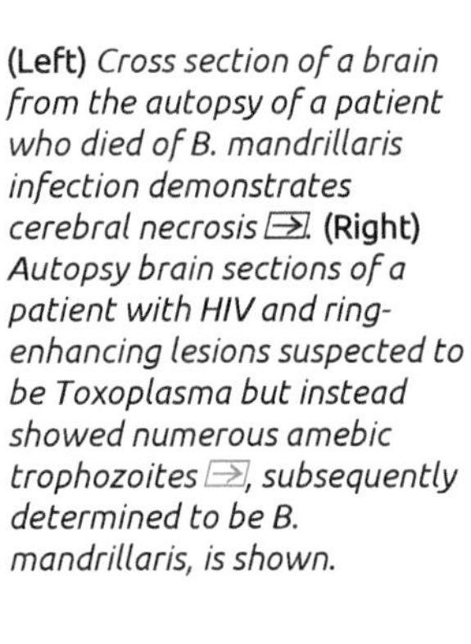

(Left) *Cross section of a brain from the autopsy of a patient who died of B. mandrillaris infection demonstrates cerebral necrosis.* (Right) *Autopsy brain sections of a patient with HIV and ring-enhancing lesions suspected to be Toxoplasma but instead showed numerous amebic trophozoites, subsequently determined to be B. mandrillaris, is shown.*

Balamuthia mandrillaris Brain Abscesses

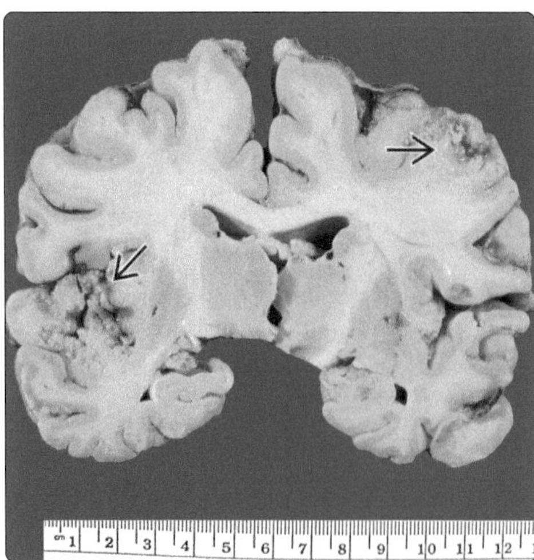

Balamuthia mandrillaris Granulomatous Amebic Encephalitis

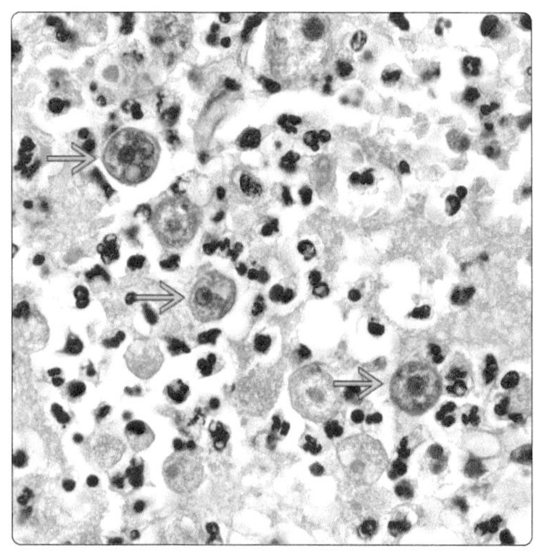

Balamuthia mandrillaris Lung Abscesses

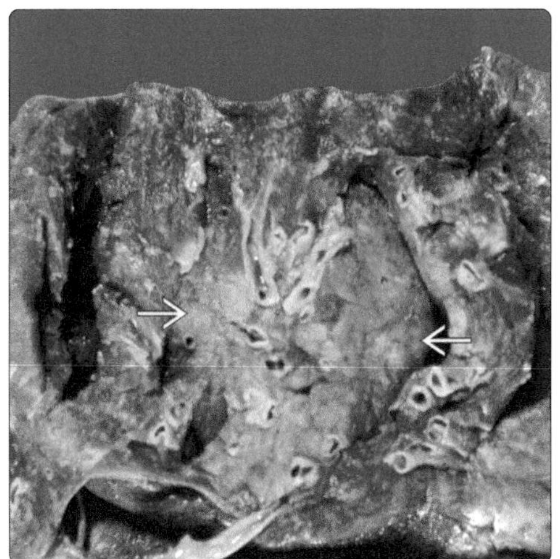

Balamuthia mandrillaris Pneumonitis

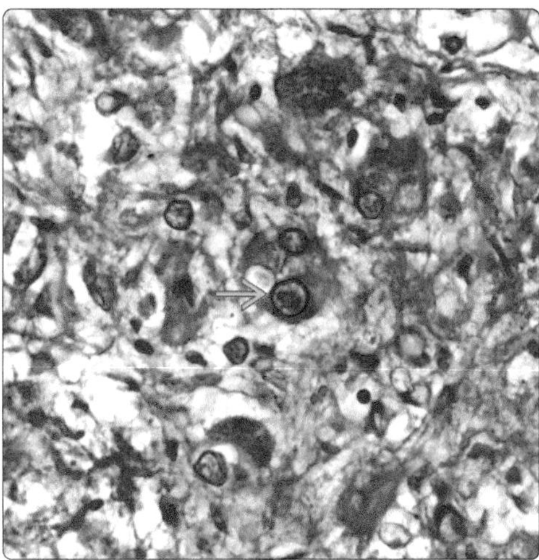

(Left) *Lung tissue from an autopsy of a patient who died of Balamuthia infection demonstrates infiltrates ➔ in the parenchyma, which are mostly trophozoites, necrosis, and limited inflammation.* **(Right)** *High-magnification PAS stain of lung tissue from a disseminated Balamuthia case demonstrates the purple rim of ruffled membrane ➔ surrounding the nucleus of a trophozoite.*

Balamuthia mandrillaris Dermatitis

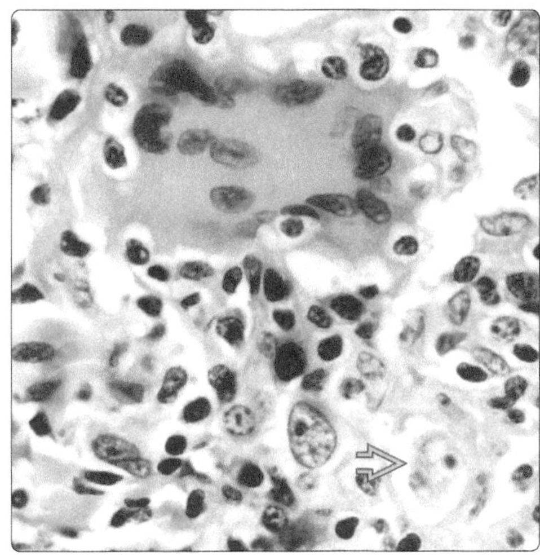

Naegleria fowleri: Direct Fluorescent Antibody

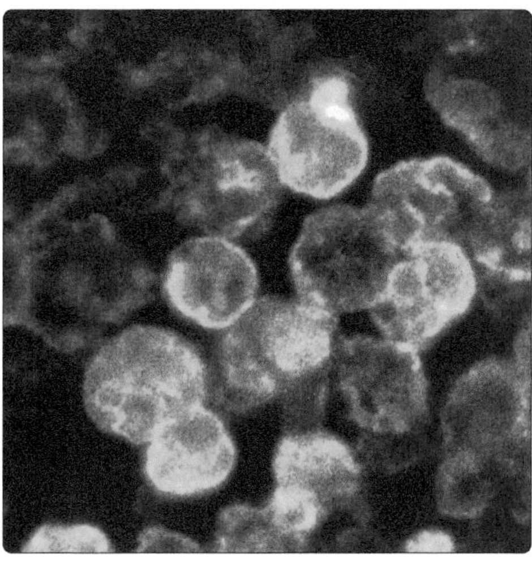

(Left) *A single trophozoite ➔ is noted in this biopsy from a patient with cutaneous balamuthiasis. Trophozoites are scarce and difficult to identify in cutaneous balamuthiasis in immunocompetent patients.* **(Right)** *This image shows direct fluorescent antibody (DFA) staining of amebic meningoencephalitis due to N. fowleri. (Courtesy G. Visvesvara, PhD, CDC/PHIL.)*

Naegleria Species: Cytology

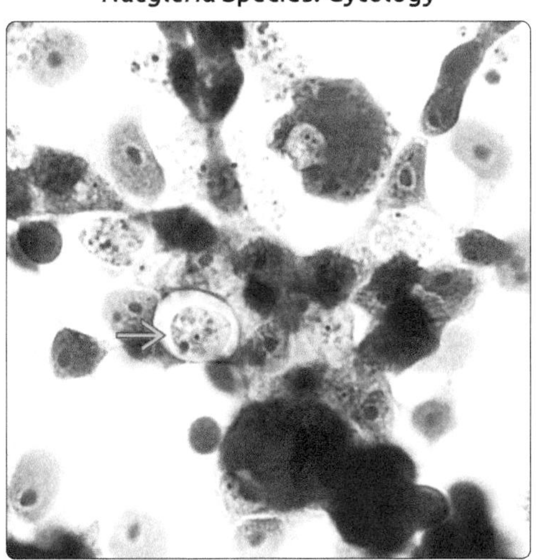

Naegleria fowleri Primary Amebic Meningoencephalitis

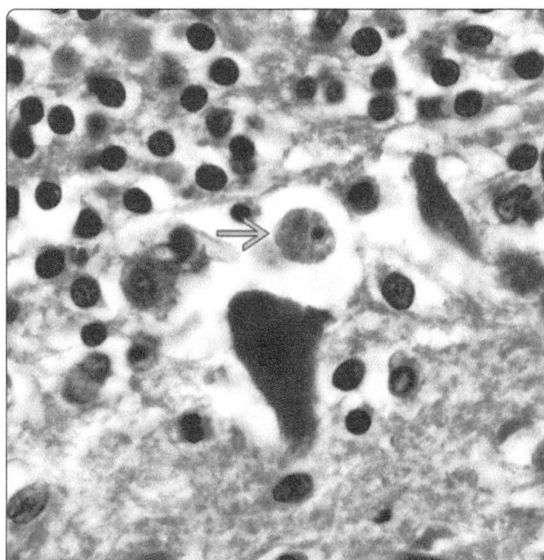

(Left) *Trichrome stain reveals Naegleria trophozoites ➔ in a human brain tissue specimen in this case of primary amebic meningoencephalitis. (Courtesy G. Healy, PHIL.)* **(Right)** *This section of autopsy cerebellum from a patient with primary amebic meningoencephalitis shows occasional N. fowleri trophozoites ➔ in the granule cell and Purkinje cell layers.*

American Trypanosomiasis

KEY FACTS

ETIOLOGY/PATHOGENESIS

- Infection with *Trypanosoma cruzi*, protozoan transmitted by triatomine bug (reduviid bugs) vector

CLINICAL ISSUES

- Acute phase: Nonspecific symptoms, such as malaise and fever; Romaña sign, chagoma
- Chronic phase: Cardiomegaly with ventricular aneurysms, megaesophagus, megacolon
- RT-PCR for acute infection, congenital disease
- Serology for chronic disease, indeterminate phase
- Benznidazole or nifurtimox for acute infection

MICROBIOLOGY

- Trypomastigote (12-30 μm): Large terminal/subterminal kinetoplast, centrally located nucleus, undulating membrane, and flagellum; present in blood, CSF
- Amastigote: Exhibit dot-dash pattern of nucleus and kinetoplast; cytoplasm of infected cells

MACROSCOPIC

- Dilated cardiomyopathy, megaesophagus, megacolon

MICROSCOPIC

- Acute phase: Diffuse parasitemia in tissues and blood, brisk periparasitic inflammatory reaction, myocarditis with necrosis, edema, and vascular dilation, and inflammation and parasitemia in smooth muscle of gastrointestinal tract
- Chronic phase: Mild chronic myocarditis, necrosis, edema

TOP DIFFERENTIAL DIAGNOSES

- Leishmaniasis: Amastigotes are morphologically indistinguishable from *T. cruzi*; confirm with isoenzyme analysis, ITS rRNA PCR
- Toxoplasma: Bradyzoites in brain and cardiac and skeletal muscle; confirm with serology, PCR, IHC
- Sarcocystosis: Bradyzoites in cardiac and skeletal muscle; confirm by stool exam, PCR

(Left) *Trypomastigotes enter host through wound or intact mucosal membranes. Inside the host, they circulate in blood and differentiate into intracellular amastigotes in various tissues. Feeding reduviid bugs ingest the trypomastigotes from blood.* **(Right)** *Periorbital swelling (Romaña sign) → occurs when parasite enters conjunctiva. Triatoma infestans ("kissing bug") transmits Trypanosoma cruzi trypomastigotes through feces after blood meal, which can be seen in Giemsa-stained blood smears →. (Courtesy M. Melvin, CDC/PHIL.)*

Trypanosoma cruzi **Life Cycle**

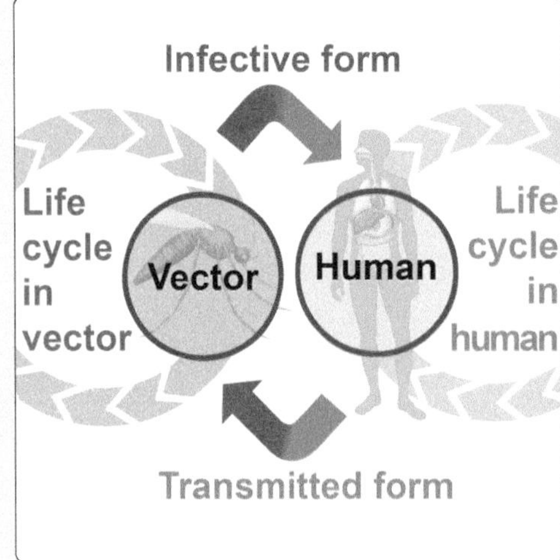

Romaña Sign, Kissing Bug, and Blood Smear Trypomastigote

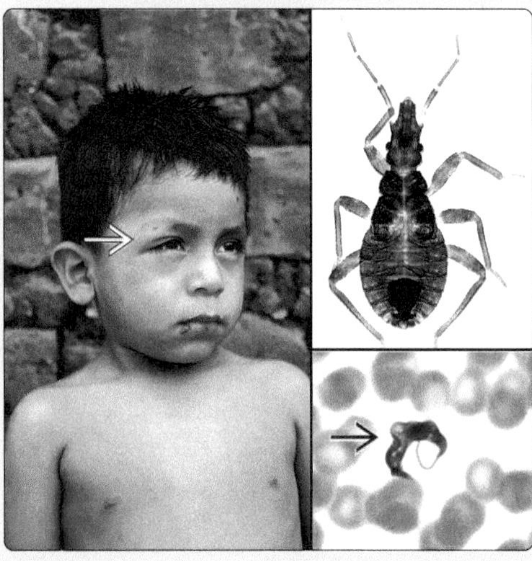

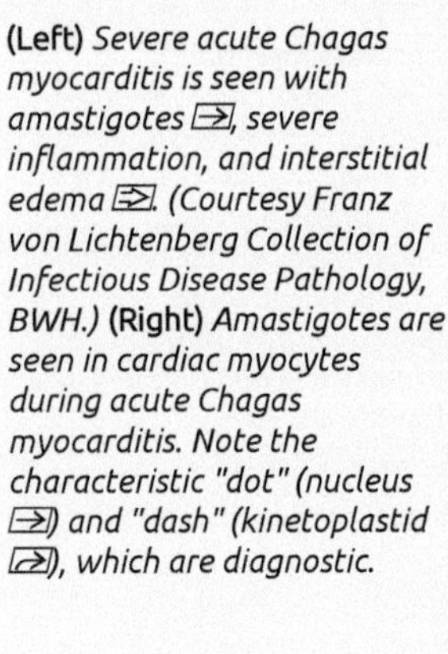

(Left) *Severe acute Chagas myocarditis is seen with amastigotes →, severe inflammation, and interstitial edema →. (Courtesy Franz von Lichtenberg Collection of Infectious Disease Pathology, BWH.)* **(Right)** *Amastigotes are seen in cardiac myocytes during acute Chagas myocarditis. Note the characteristic "dot" (nucleus →) and "dash" (kinetoplastid →), which are diagnostic.*

Chagas Muscle Infiltrates

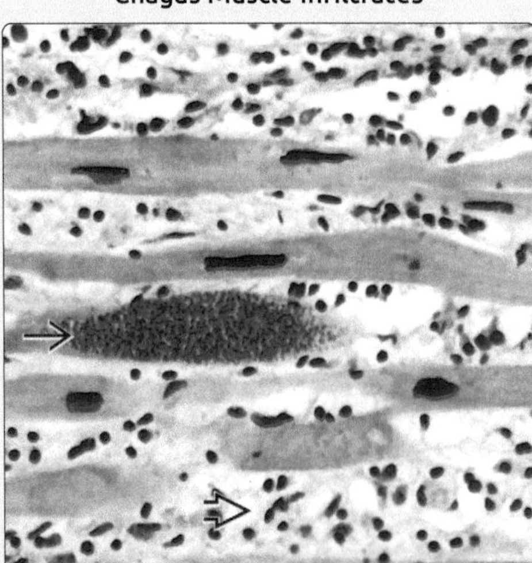

Dot-Dash Pattern: Kinetoplastids

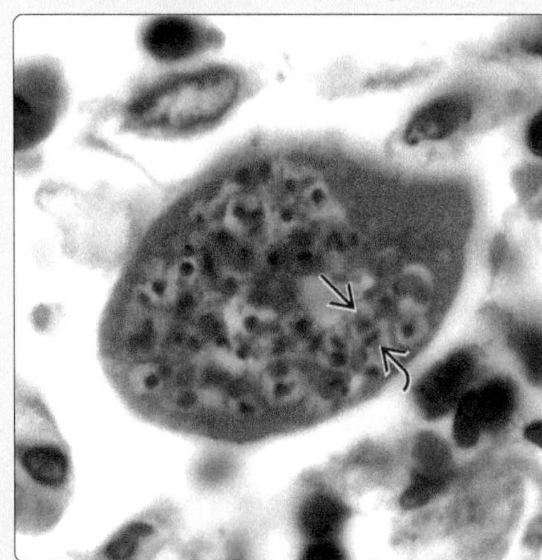

TERMINOLOGY

Definitions

- Chagas disease named after Brazilian physician Carlos Chagas (1909)
- *Trypanosoma cruzi* from Greek "trypano" (borer) + "soma" (body) and Brazilian physician Oswaldo Cruz

ETIOLOGY/PATHOGENESIS

Infectious Agents

- Infection with *T. cruzi*, flagellate protozoa in Kinetoplastida class via triatomine bug (reduviid bugs; "kissing" bug) vector
- Triatomine bugs live in cracks and holes in cement housing, animal kennels, chicken coops, and other areas; rural areas of southern USA, Central America, and South America
- Trypomastigotes enter host through wound or mucosal surface and become amastigotes in infected tissues
- Vector takes up circulating trypomastigotes, which become epimastigotes in midgut, then trypomastigotes in hind gut released in feces near site of bite wound
- Cases are also reported from contaminated food and water, blood transfusions, organ transplants, and vertical transmission from mother to child

CLINICAL ISSUES

Epidemiology

- Estimated 300,000 infected in USA
- Endemic in South America; 8 million infected

Presentation

- Acute phase lasts 8-12 weeks and includes nonspecific symptoms, such as malaise and fever; rarely acute myocarditis, pericardial effusion, or meningoencephalitis
- Chagoma: Swelling at site of inoculation
- Romaña sign: Parasite enters conjunctiva, causing periorbital swelling
- Chronic phase: Cardiomegaly with ventricular aneurysms, megaesophagus, megacolon; any smooth muscle structure may be affected
- Indeterminate phase: Serologic testing is positive without apparent clinical disease; 20-30% will progress to overt clinical disease over years

Laboratory Tests

- RT-PCR (blood, heart tissue, CSF) for acute infection, congenital disease, and laboratory exposures
- Serology for chronic disease, indeterminate phase

Treatment

- Antiprotozoal (benznidazole or nifurtimox) for acute infection
- Treatment is recommended for those < 18 years of age with indeterminate-phase infection
- Symptomatic treatment for symptoms of chronic disease; antiprotozoals do not affect disease outcome at this stage

Prognosis

- 20-30% with chronic infection will develop end-stage cardiac or other parasite-related disease

IMAGING

Radiographic Findings

- Nonspecific radiographic findings include cardiomegaly, megaesophagus on barium swallow, and megacolon on barium enema

MICROBIOLOGY

Parasite Features

- Trypomastigote (12-30 µm): Large terminal/subterminal kinetoplast, centrally located nucleus, undulating membrane, and flagellum; present in blood, CSF
- Amastigote: Exhibits dot-dash pattern of nucleus and kinetoplast; cytoplasm of infected cells
- Epimastigote: Not seen in humans but present in midgut of infected triatomines

Culture

- Although parasites can be cultured in artificial media, it is not necessary for diagnosis and treatment

MACROSCOPIC

Megaorgan Appearance

- Dilated cardiomyopathy with ventricular apical aneurysm is most common cardiac lesion
- Megaesophagus, megacolon, megaureter

MICROSCOPIC

Histologic Features

- Acute phase: Diffuse parasitemia throughout tissues (amastigotes) and in blood (trypomastigotes) with brisk periparasitic inflammatory reaction
    - Myocarditis with necrosis, edema, and vascular dilation
    - Inflammation and parasitemia in smooth muscle and Auerbach plexus of gastrointestinal tract
- Chronic phase: Parasites rarely found; mild chronic myocarditis, necrosis, edema, fibrosis
- Immunosuppression: CNS chagoma (reactivation) may occur; necrosis with numerous amastigotes

DIFFERENTIAL DIAGNOSIS

Leishmaniasis

- *Leishmania* spp. amastigotes are morphologically indistinguishable from *T. cruzi*; confirm with isoenzyme analysis, ITS rRNA PCR

Toxoplasma

- *Toxoplasma gondii* cysts with bradyzoites in brain and cardiac and skeletal muscle; confirm with serology, PCR, IHC

Sarcocystosis

- *Sarcocystis* spp. form sarcocysts with numerous bradyzoites in cardiac and skeletal muscle; confirm by stool exam, PCR

SELECTED REFERENCES

1. Hochberg NS et al: Chagas disease. Ann Intern Med. 176(2):ITC17-32, 2023
2. Forsyth CJ et al: Recommendations for screening and diagnosis of Chagas disease in the United States. J Infect Dis. 225(9):1601-10, 2022

Leishmaniasis

KEY FACTS

ETIOLOGY/PATHOGENESIS

- Vector-borne infection with *Leishmania* and *Endotrypanum* spp. spread by phlebotomine sand flies

CLINICAL ISSUES

- Presentation depends on species, host immune status, and geographic location
- Cutaneous leishmaniasis most common
- Visceral leishmaniasis affects spleen, liver, and bone marrow and can be life threatening
- PCR for speciation and guidance of treatment
- Serology for visceral disease
- Treatment may include miltefosine, amphotericin B

MICROSCOPIC

- Amastigotes are round to oval-shaped (2-4 μm), present within macrophages, demonstrate dot-dash pattern (nucleus-kinetoplast)
- Cutaneous: Ulcerated epidermis with hyperkeratosis, acanthosis, or atrophy; lymphoplasmacytic infiltrate, parasitized macrophages ± eosinophils
- Mucocutaneous: Marked ulceration, pseudoepitheliomatous hyperplasia, suppurative granulomata, and amastigotes
- Visceral: Macrophages, epithelioid cells, lymphoplasmacytic infiltrate, and amastigotes

TOP DIFFERENTIAL DIAGNOSES

- Chagas disease: *Trypanosoma cruzi* amastigotes are indistinguishable; confirm by serology, PCR, or detection of trypomastigotes in blood smear
- Histoplasmosis: Similar size to leishmania but GMS positive with narrow-based budding and periorganism halo
- Rhinoscleroma: *Klebsiella rhinoscleromatis*, rod-shaped gram-negative bacillus within vacuolated macrophages (Mikulicz cells)

Life Cycle of Leishmaniasis

Infective form
Life cycle in vector
Vector
Human
Life cycle in human
Transmitted form

Ulcer of Cutaneous Leishmaniasis

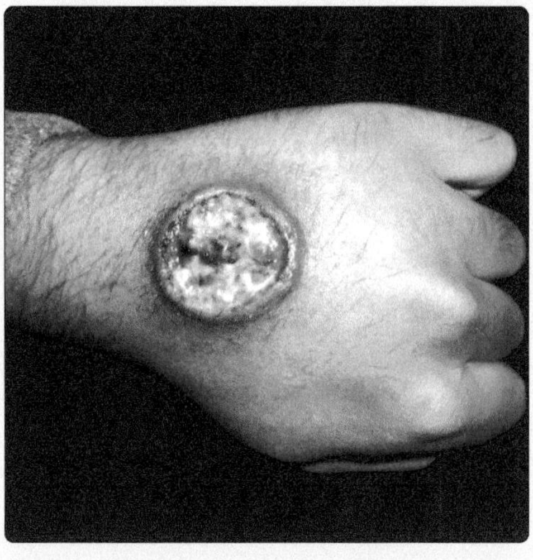

(Left) *Humans are infected by bites of sand flies, which inject organisms into the skin. Macrophages serve as the reservoir for replication and movement to other parts of the body (especially in visceral form). Sand fly bites pick up organisms and continue the life cycle.* **(Right)** *Cutaneous leishmaniasis manifests as a typical, round to oval, painless ulcer with a well-delineated, elevated border on an exposed area of skin. This patient spent 3 months in Peru and did not recall a bite. (Courtesy T. Sofarelli, PA-C.)*

Cutaneous Leishmaniasis

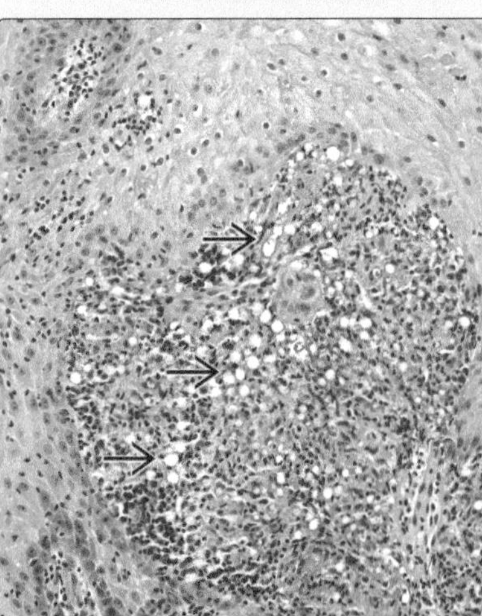

***Leishmania* Amastigotes**

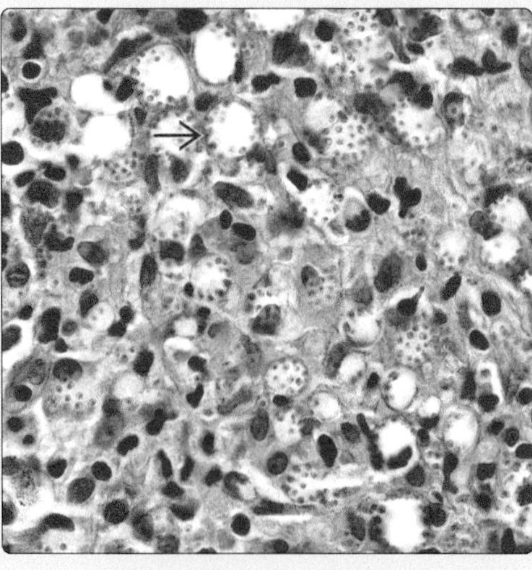

(Left) *Features of cutaneous leishmaniasis include ulcerated epidermis (not pictured) with hyperkeratosis, acanthosis, exuberant inflammatory infiltrate, and parasitized macrophages that may appear empty at low power ⇒.* **(Right)** *Amastigotes (2-4 μm) are round to oval-shaped within macrophages and demonstrate a dot-dash pattern representing the nucleus and kinetoplast. Amastigotes located at periphery of macrophages ⇒ are referred to as the marquee sign.*

TERMINOLOGY

Synonyms

- Cutaneous leishmaniasis: Oriental sore, uta, chiclero ulcer, tropical sore, Bagdad boil, Bauer ulcer, Aleppo button, Delhi boil
- Mucocutaneous leishmaniasis: Forest yaws, espundia, pian bois, American leishmaniasis
- Visceral leishmaniasis: Kala-azar, black fever, dumdum fever

Definitions

- *Leishmania* named for William Leishman (1865-1926)
- *L. donovani* named for Charles Donovan (1863-1951); Leishman-Donovan bodies (protozoa seen in tissue)

ETIOLOGY/PATHOGENESIS

Infectious Agents

- Vector-borne infection with *Leishmania* and *Endotrypanum* spp., obligate intracellular protozoa, via sand flies (*Lutzomyia* and *Phlebotomus*)
- Flagellate phase (promastigote) within vector and retracted flagellum (amastigote) in infected human tissue
- Parasites deactivate phagocytic host cells by inducing specific mammalian phosphatases that are capable of impeding signaling
- Infection in human is caused by > 20 species
  - *Endotrypanum* genus: *E. colombiensis* and *E. equatoriensis*
  - Subgenus *Leishmania*: *L.* (*L*) *aethiopica*, *L.* (*L*) *amazonensis*, *L.* (*L*) *donovani*, *L.* (*L*) *infantum*, *L.* (*L*) *major*, *L.* (*L*) *mexicana*, *L.* (*L*) *tropica*, *L.* (*L*) *venezuelensis*, *L.* (*L*) *waltoni*
  - Subgenus *Mundinia*: *L.* (*M*) *martiniquensis*, *L.* (*M*) *orientalis*
  - Subgenus *Sauroleishmania*: *L.* (*S*) *tarentolae*
  - Subgenus *Viannia*: *L.* (*V*) *braziliensis*, *L.* (*V*) *guyanensis*, *L.* (*V*) *lainsoni*, *L.* (*V*) *lindbergi*, *L.* (*V*) *naiffi*, *L.* (*V*) *panamensis*, *L.* (*V*) *peruvinana*, *L.* (*V*) *shawi*
  - Cutaneous leishmaniasis caused by all species
  - Mucocutaneous leishmaniasis caused by *L.* (*L*) *amazonensis*, *L.* (*V*) *braziliensis*, *L.* (*V*) *guyanensis*, *L.* (*V*) *panamensis*, *L.* (*V*) *peruvinana*
  - Visceral leishmaniasis caused by *L.* (*L*) *donovani*, *L.* (*L*) *infantum*

CLINICAL ISSUES

Epidemiology

- Classified as neglected tropical disease (NTD, WHO)
- 12 million infected worldwide; ~ 1 million new cases and 20,000-40,000 deaths per year
- Occurs more commonly in rural than urban areas; climate and other environmental changes have potential to expand geographic range of sand fly vectors
- Cutaneous leishmaniasis occurs in Afghanistan, Algeria, Brazil, Colombia, Islamic Republic of Iran, Pakistan, Peru, Saudi Arabia, and Syrian Arab Republic
- 90% of mucocutaneous leishmaniasis occurs in Plurinational State of Bolivia, Brazil, and Peru
- 90% of visceral leishmaniasis occurs in 6 countries: Bangladesh, Brazil, Ethiopia, India, South Sudan, and Sudan
- Rare cases reported in southern Texas

Presentation

- Cutaneous leishmaniasis: Skin lesions, which may change in shape and size, and progress up lymphatic tracts (sporotrichoid pattern)
- Mucocutaneous leishmaniasis: Less common form with mucosal manifestations (possibly due to host genetic factors)
- Visceral leishmaniasis: Enlargement of spleen, liver, and bone marrow; fever, weight loss, pancytopenia, hypergammaglobulinemia; onset can be insidious or sudden

Laboratory Tests

- PCR (rRNA ITS2 gene or kinetoplast DNA): Important for exact speciation and guidance of treatment
- Direct agglutination tests (DATs), enzyme immunoassay (EIA), and immunochromatographic test with rK39 antigen have good sensitivity and specificity for visceral disease
- Leishmanin skin test (LST, Montenegro test) detects latent disease: Measures reaction 48-72 hours after intradermal injection of antigen

Treatment

- Treatment decisions should be individualized with expert consultation
- Oral miltefosine FDA approved for treatment of cutaneous, mucosal, and visceral leishmaniasis caused by *L. donovani* in adolescents and adults who are not pregnant or breastfeeding
- Molecular mechanisms known to contribute to resistance to antimonials, amphotericin B, and miltefosine

Prognosis

- Depends on species, host immune status, *Leishmania* forms, and geographic location
- Outcomes of cutaneous and mucocutaneous leishmaniasis much better than visceral (which is often fatal)

MICROBIOLOGY

Parasite Features

- Amastigotes are spherical to ovoid (1-5 μm x 1-2 μm) with large nucleus, prominent kinetoplast, and short axoneme (rarely visible by light microscopy); reside in host macrophages
- Promastigotes are elongate and slender (10-12 μm) with large central nucleus, anterior kinetoplast, and anterior-arising flagellum; present in midgut of sand flies but not in human hosts

Culture

- Required for drug screening, animal inoculation (xenodiagnosis, rarely used)
- Schneider insect, M199, or Grace medium (monophasic)
- Novy-MacNeal-Nicolle or Tobie medium (diphasic)
- Specialized reference labs may provide media to patient site for direct inoculation and complete testing in reference laboratory
- Isoenzyme analysis or PCR for speciation of culture isolates

MACROSCOPIC

General Features

- Cutaneous leishmaniasis: Usually presents as papules, nodules, flat plaques, and wart-like lesion; unusual presentations include paronychial, chancriform, annular, zosteriform, erysipeloid forms, and palmoplantar form

MICROSCOPIC

Histologic Features

- Cutaneous leishmaniasis has acute, chronic, recidivous, and disseminated forms
  - Acute form: Ulcerated epidermis with hyperkeratosis, acanthosis, or atrophy
    - Exuberant infiltrate of lymphocytes, plasma cells, parasitized macrophages ± eosinophils
    - Amastigotes are round to oval-shaped (2-4 μm), present within macrophages, demonstrate dot-dash pattern (nucleus-kinetoplast, best seen with oil immersion); peripheral location within macrophages referred to as marquee sign
  - Chronic form: Few organisms; tuberculoid granulomata ± necrosis
  - Recidivous: Similar to lupus vulgaris
  - Disseminated: Mainly in immunocompromised patients with many parasitized cells
- Mucocutaneous leishmaniasis: Marked ulceration with pseudoepitheliomatous hyperplasia, suppurative granulomata, and amastigotes
- Visceral leishmaniasis: "Post-kala-azar" lesions consist of macrophages, epithelioid cells, and lymphoplasmacytic infiltrate; amastigotes in spleen or liver biopsy/aspirate

ANCILLARY TESTS

Cytology

- Giemsa-stained direct smear can be helpful in identifying free amastigotes

Immunohistochemistry

- G2D10 antibody is more sensitive than H&E

DIFFERENTIAL DIAGNOSIS

Chagas Disease

- *Trypanosoma cruzi* amastigotes are indistinguishable; confirm by serology, PCR, or detection of trypomastigotes in blood smear

Histoplasmosis

- Similar size to leishmania but GMS positive with narrow-based budding and periorganism halo

Rhinoscleroma

- *Klebsiella rhinoscleromatis*, which is rod-shaped bacillus and not oval like *Leishmania*
- Mikulicz cells are vacuolated macrophages often with bacteria inside

Malakoplakia

- Aggregates of histiocytes containing small, round to oval, targetoid structures (Michaelis-Gutmann bodies)

Malignant Neoplasms

- Primary skin lesions or metastases
- Lymphoma (e.g., angiocentric NK-/T-cell lymphoma)
- Lethal midline granuloma
- Negative for classic histologic features and organisms

Ulcers

- Traumatic ulcers, stasis ulcers

SELECTED REFERENCES

1. Mathison BA et al: Review of the clinical presentation, pathology, diagnosis, and treatment of leishmaniasis. Lab Med. 54(4):363-71, 2023
2. Carstens-Kass J et al: A review of the leishmanin skin test: a neglected test for a neglected disease. PLoS Negl Trop Dis. 15(7):e0009531, 2021
3. Cardozo RS et al: Cutaneous leishmaniasis: a pathological study of 360 cases with special emphasis on the contribution of immunohistochemistry and polymerase chain reaction to diagnosis. J Cutan Pathol. 47(11):1018-25, 2020
4. Soulat D et al: Function of macrophage and parasite phosphatases in leishmaniasis. Front Immunol. 8:1838, 2017
5. Aronson N et al: Diagnosis and treatment of leishmaniasis: clinical practice guidelines by the Infectious Diseases Society of America (IDSA) and the American Society of Tropical Medicine and Hygiene (ASTMH). Clin Infect Dis. 63(12):e202-64, 2016

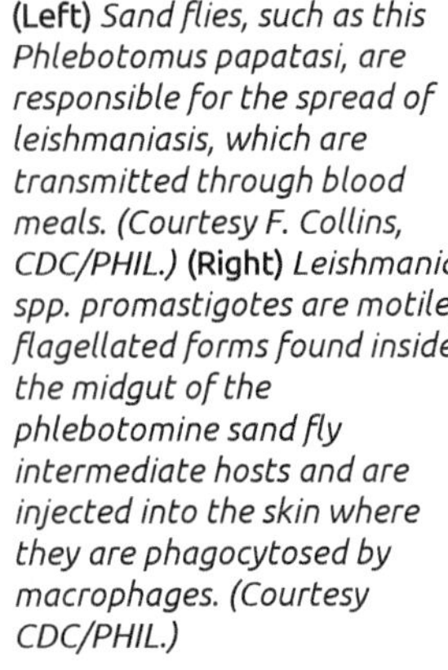

(Left) *Sand flies, such as this Phlebotomus papatasi, are responsible for the spread of leishmaniasis, which are transmitted through blood meals. (Courtesy F. Collins, CDC/PHIL.)* **(Right)** *Leishmania spp. promastigotes are motile, flagellated forms found inside the midgut of the phlebotomine sand fly intermediate hosts and are injected into the skin where they are phagocytosed by macrophages. (Courtesy CDC/PHIL.)*

Phlebotomus papatasi **(Sand Fly)**

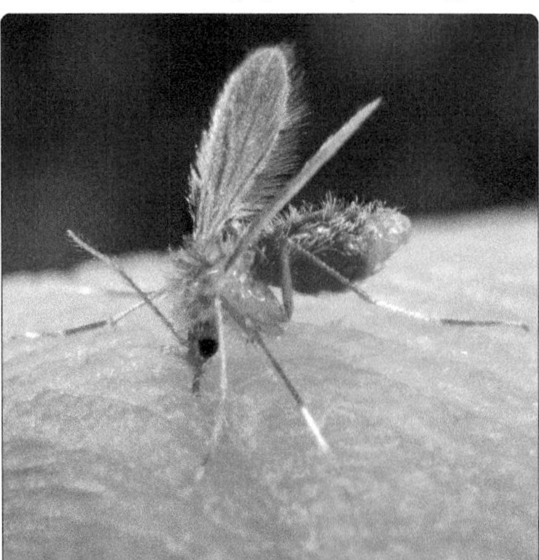

Leishmania **Promastigotes**

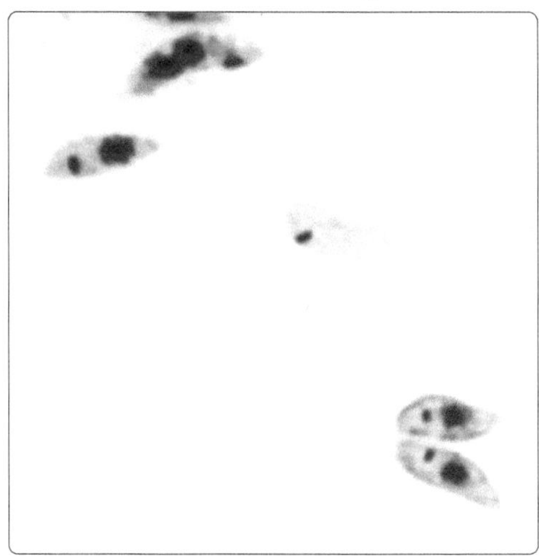

Leishmania Ultrastructural Features

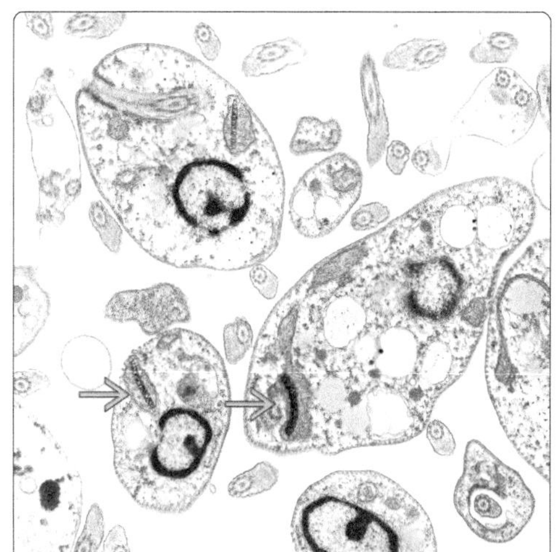

Leishmania Bone Marrow Smear

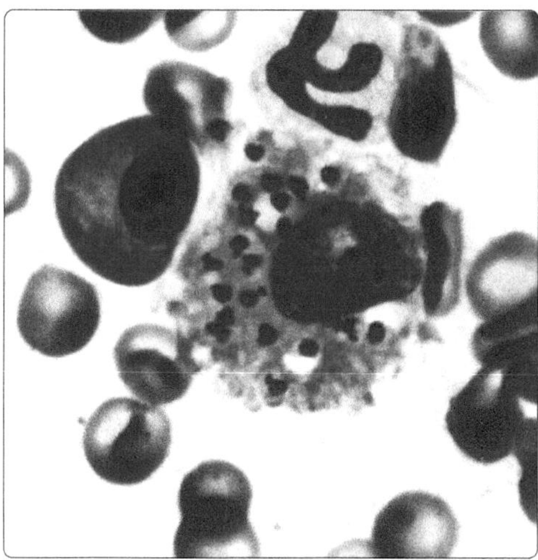

(Left) *This electron micrograph of Leishmania major amastigotes shows dense kinetoplasts ➡ in the cytoplasm. (Courtesy C. Goldsmith, L. Flannery, CDC/PHIL.)* **(Right)** *This Giemsa-stained bone marrow smear shows numerous Leishmania donovani amastigotes contained within a bone marrow histiocyte. (Courtesy Dr. Chandler, CDC/PHIL.)*

Cutaneous Leishmaniasis: Giemsa Stain

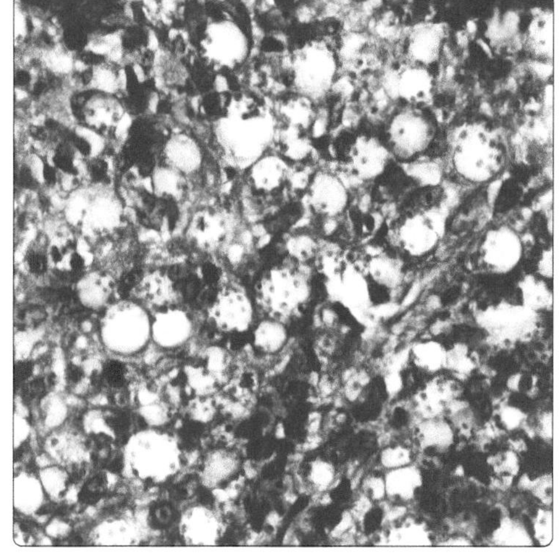

Mucocutaneous Leishmaniasis

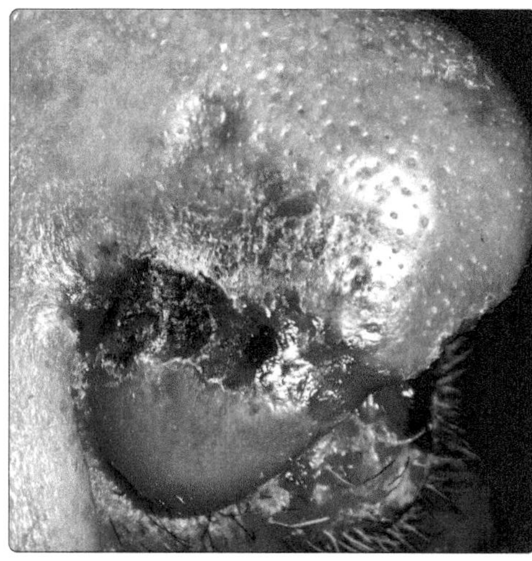

(Left) *Giemsa staining of skin tissue shows numerous parasitized macrophages containing Leishmania spp. amastigotes.* **(Right)** *This photograph shows mucocutaneous leishmaniasis, which is notorious for producing destructive lesions. (From DP: Nonneoplastic Derm.)*

Visceral Leishmaniasis: Liver

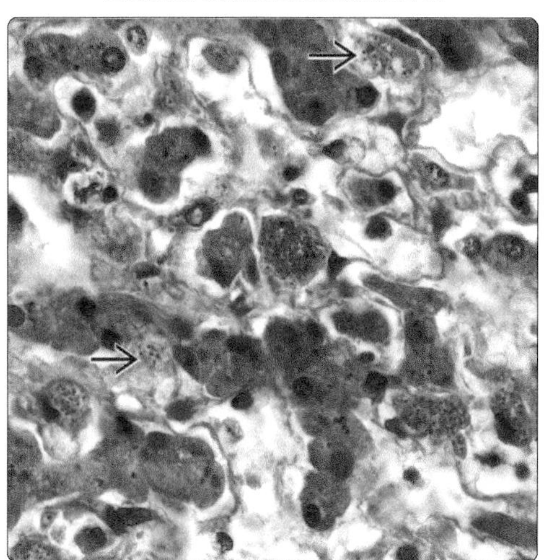

Visceral Leishmaniasis: Spleen

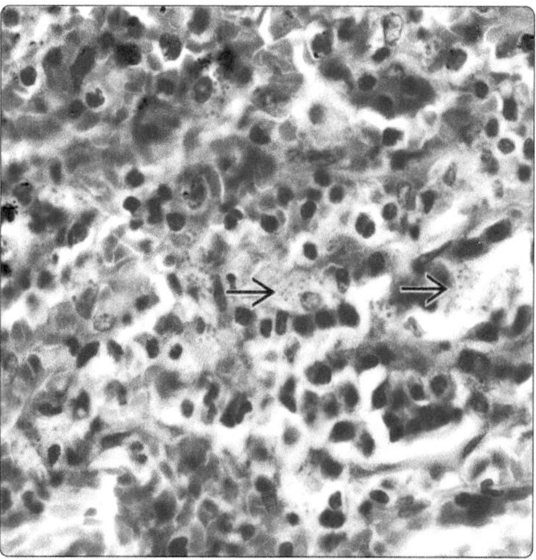

(Left) *Hepatomegaly is frequently seen with visceral leishmaniasis with marked Kupffer cell hyperplasia, parasitized by numerous amastigotes ➡.* **(Right)** *Visceral leishmaniasis is frequently associated with splenomegaly with prominent red pulp expansion. Numerous amastigotes are present within macrophages ➡.*

KEY FACTS

ETIOLOGY/PATHOGENESIS

- Infection caused by obligate intracellular parasite, *Toxoplasma gondii* via eating meat with tissue cysts, water contaminated with oocysts, or transplacentally

CLINICAL ISSUES

- Age-adjusted seroprevalence rate in USA is 11%
- Severe disease with reactivation/dissemination in immunocompromised (e.g., HIV positive)
- IgM and IgG for acute and past exposure
- PCR can be performed on variety of specimen types

MICROSCOPIC

- Tachyzoites (4-8 µm x 2-3 µm): Tapered anterior end, blunt posterior end, large nucleus
- Bradyzoite cysts (5-50 µm): Spherical (brain), elongated (muscle)
- *T. gondii* IHC highlights both bradyzoites and tachyzoites
- Lymphadenitis: Florid follicular hyperplasia, monocytoid B cells, phagocytosing macrophages
- CNS abscess: Coagulative necrosis, bradyzoites at periphery, free tachyzoites, fibrinoid necrosis, variable inflammation
- Diffuse encephalitic: Cortical microglial nodules in absence of necrosis, multifocal bradyzoites and tachyzoites
- Bradyzoites and tachyzoites also identified in skin, heart, lungs, liver, gastrointestinal tract, kidneys, and placenta

TOP DIFFERENTIAL DIAGNOSES

- Chagas Disease: *Trypanosoma cruzi* amastigotes with kinetoplasts; confirm by IHC, serology, PCR, trypomastigotes in blood smear
- Leishmaniasis: Amastigotes with kinetoplasts; confirm with isoenzyme analysis, ITS rRNA PCR
- Sarcocystosis: *Sarcocysts* with numerous bradyzoites in cardiac and skeletal muscle; confirm by stool exam, PCR

***Toxoplasma gondii* Life Cycle**

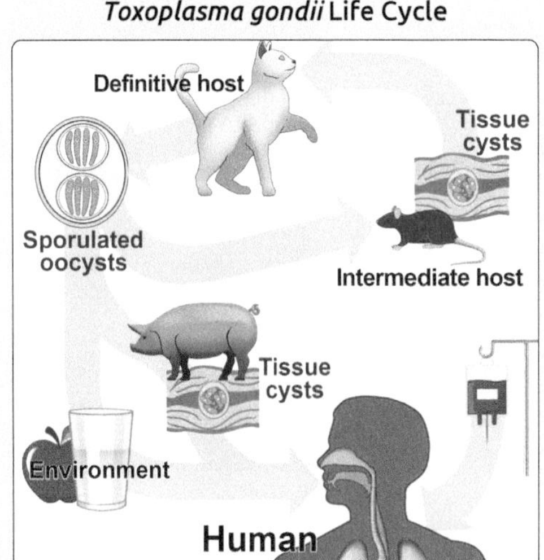

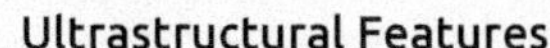
Ultrastructural Features

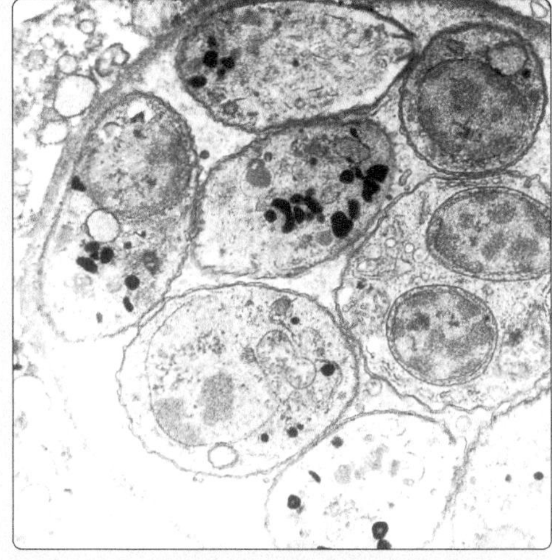

(Left) *Humans infected by eating undercooked meat of animals harboring tissue cysts (intermediate hosts), consuming food/water contaminated with cat feces (sporulated oocysts), blood transfusion, organ transplantation, or transplacentally from mother to fetus.* **(Right)** *This transmission electron micrograph shows multiple developing Toxoplasma gondii bradyzoites within a larger tissue cyst. (Courtesy CDC/PHIL.)*

***T. gondii* Bradyzoites**

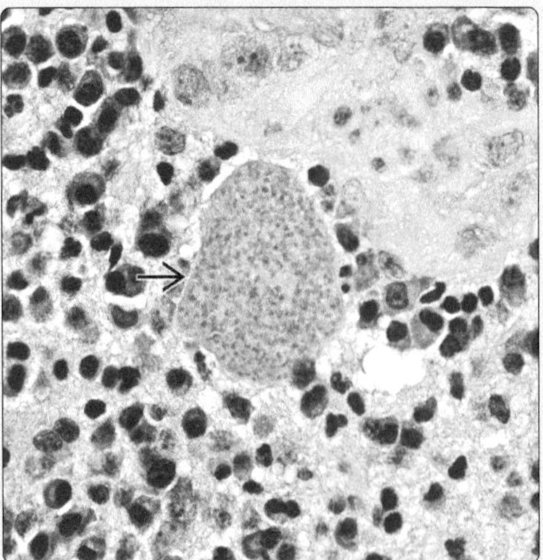

***T. gondii* Tachyzoites**

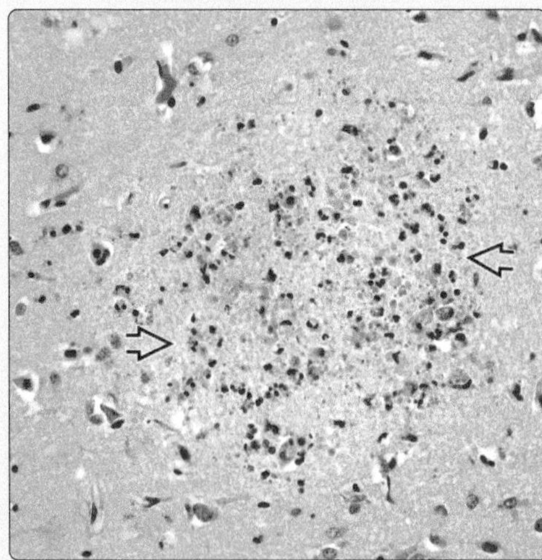

(Left) *This brain biopsy shows a large tissue cyst ➡ containing numerous Toxoplasma gondii bradyzoites, surrounded by lymphoplasmahistiocytic inflammation.* **(Right)** *A less common manifestation of CNS toxoplasmosis is the diffuse encephalitic form, which contains scattered tachyzoites ➡ and microglia in the absence of larger necrotic abscesses.*

TERMINOLOGY

Synonyms

- Piringer-Kuchinka lymphadenitis

Definitions

- Greek: "Toxon" (bow-shaped) + "plasma" (shape or form)

ETIOLOGY/PATHOGENESIS

Infectious Agents

- Infection with *Toxoplasma gondii*, obligate intracellular parasite in phylum Apicomplexa
- Definitive hosts (cats) infected after consuming intermediate hosts harboring tissue cysts, and shed oocysts in feces for 1-3 weeks
- Intermediate hosts (birds, rodents) infected by ingesting oocysts, which transform into tachyzoites, then migrate to neural and muscle tissue and develop into tissue cyst bradyzoites
- Humans infected by eating undercooked meat of animals harboring tissue cysts, consuming food/water contaminated with cat feces, blood transfusion, organ transplantation, or transplacentally from mother to fetus

CLINICAL ISSUES

Epidemiology

- Up to 60% seroprevalence in some populations; highest in hot, humid climates and lower altitudes that allow longer oocyst survival
- Estimated age-adjusted seroprevalence rate in USA is 11%
- Risk of congenital toxoplasmosis infection is lowest in 1st trimester of pregnancy and highest in 3rd trimester, while severity of infection is highest in 1st trimester

Presentation

- Congenital toxoplasmosis characterized by ocular lesions (most common), cerebral calcification, and hydrocephalus; visualization of placenta cysts/pseudocysts in severe cases
- *Toxoplasma* lymphadenitis in immunocompetent adults is usually self-limited; presents as cervical unilateral or bilateral lymphadenopathy
- Cerebral toxoplasmosis in immunocompromised presents as encephalitis and abscess [usually in HIV(+) patients]
- HIV infection has very high burden of *T. gondii* infection, especially in sub-Saharan Africa; highlighting importance of routine surveillance
- Immunodeficient patients are at risk for more severe manifestations and multisystem disease

Laboratory Tests

- Serology: IgM and IgG are diagnostic of acute exposure and past exposure; important screening tool for women prior to pregnancy/childbirth
- PCR of *T. gondii* B1 gene can be performed on brain tissue, CSF, vitreous and aqueous fluid, BAL, urine, amniotic fluid, and peripheral blood

Treatment

- Pyrimethamine and either sulfadiazine or clindamycin are usually used in symptomatic patients
- Treatment of infection in fetus and infants has been demonstrated to significantly improve clinical outcome
- Prevention by cooking food, avoiding untreated drinking water and unpasteurized milk; immunocompromised or pregnant should not change or handle cat litter boxes

Prognosis

- Immunocompetent: Self-limited
- Immunosuppressed: Severe manifestations can result in prolonged neurologic deficits and death
- Congenital: Severe manifestations lead to neurologic deficits, visual problems, and death

IMAGING

Radiographic Findings

- Brain MR: Multiple ring-enhancing lesions
- Fetal ultrasound: Hydrocephalus, intracranial calcifications

MICROBIOLOGY

Parasite Features

- Infective mature oocysts (10-12 µm in diameter) contain 2 sporocysts; present in environment
- Tachyzoites (4-8 µm x 2-3 µm) have tapered anterior end, blunt posterior end, and large nucleus; found in various sites throughout host body
- Bradyzoite cysts (5-50 µm in diameter) are spherical in brain and more elongated in cardiac and skeletal muscles; less commonly present in other sites

MACROSCOPIC

General Features

- Brain: Acute necrotizing, organizing, chronic abscesses

MICROSCOPIC

Histologic Features

- Lymphadenitis: Well-preserved nodal architecture with florid follicular hyperplasia, prominent parasinusoidal and parafollicular monocytoid B cells, clustered macrophages engulfing debris; cysts are rarely identified (~ 1% of cases)
- CNS abscess: Coagulative necrosis, bradyzoites at periphery, free tachyzoites, fibrinoid vascular necrosis, and often minimal inflammation; organizes over time
- Diffuse encephalitic form contains cortical microglial nodules in absence of necrosis with multifocal bradyzoites and tachyzoites
- Lungs: Interstitial or necrotizing pneumonitis with rare organisms
- Liver: Diffuse hepatitis with infiltration of portal tracts and sinusoids by mononuclear cells with focal abscess; bradyzoites in histocytes and granulomata
- Bradyzoites and tachyzoites also identified in heart, skin, gastrointestinal tract, kidneys, and placenta

Cytologic Features

- Pap stain may demonstrate organism on FNA &/or epithelioid microgranulomas
- Reactive lymphoid hyperplasia and tachyzoites

ANCILLARY TESTS

Immunohistochemistry

- Anti-*T. gondii* ab highlights bradyzoites and tachyzoites

- Monocytoid B cells of reactive lymph node are CD20(+), CD5(-), CD23(-), BCL2(-), BCL5(-), and CD10(-)

Electron Microscopy

- Paired organelles, dense bodies, conoid nuclei at rounded posterior end, double-layered pellicles

DIFFERENTIAL DIAGNOSIS

Chagas Disease

- *Trypanosoma cruzi* amastigotes with kinetoplasts; confirm by IHC, serology, PCR, trypomastigotes in blood smear

Leishmaniasis

- *Leishmania* spp. amastigotes with kinetoplasts; confirm with isoenzyme analysis, ITS rRNA PCR

Sarcocystosis

- *Sarcocystis* spp. form sarcocysts with numerous bradyzoites in cardiac and skeletal muscle; confirm by stool exam, PCR

CNS Lymphoma in HIV

- EBV associated; single solidly enhancing lesion on MR

Cat-Scratch Disease

- *Bartonella henselae* infection; history of cat scratch/bite, regional adenopathy; stellate granulomata with central necrosis; confirm with IHC, serology, culture, PCR

Tuberculosis

- Larger epithelioid histiocyte clusters, presence of multinucleated giant cells, and caseation; confirm by AFB stains, IHC, culture, PCR

SELECTED REFERENCES

1. Cova MM et al: How Apicomplexa parasites secrete and build their invasion machinery. Annu Rev Microbiol. 76:619-40, 2022
2. Matta SK et al: Toxoplasma gondii infection and its implications within the central nervous system. Nat Rev Microbiol. 19(7):467-80, 2021
3. Zhou Z et al: Toxoplasmosis and the heart. Curr Probl Cardiol. 46(3):100741, 2021
4. Robert-Gangneux F et al: Toxoplasmosis in transplant recipients, Europe, 2010-2014. Emerg Infect Dis. 24(8):1497-504, 2018
5. Wang ZD et al: Prevalence and burden of Toxoplasma gondii infection in HIV-infected people: a systematic review and meta-analysis. Lancet HIV. 4(4):e177-88, 2017
6. Paquet C et al: Toxoplasmosis in pregnancy: prevention, screening, and treatment. J Obstet Gynaecol Can. 35(1):78-9, 2013

Brain MR

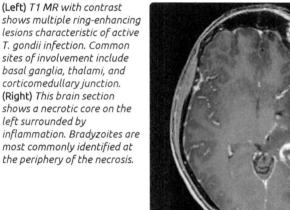

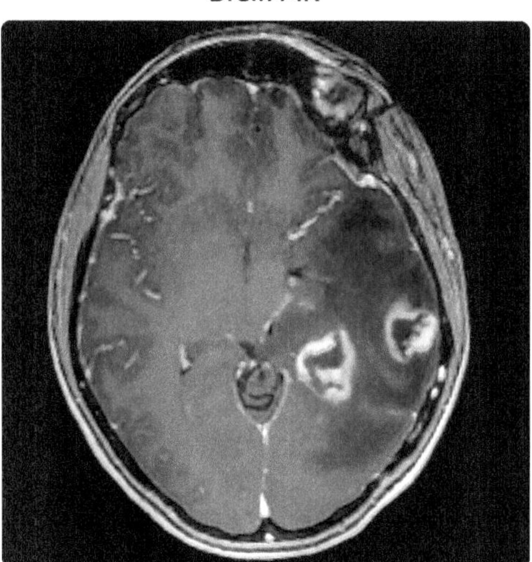

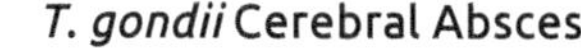

***T. gondii* Cerebral Abscess**

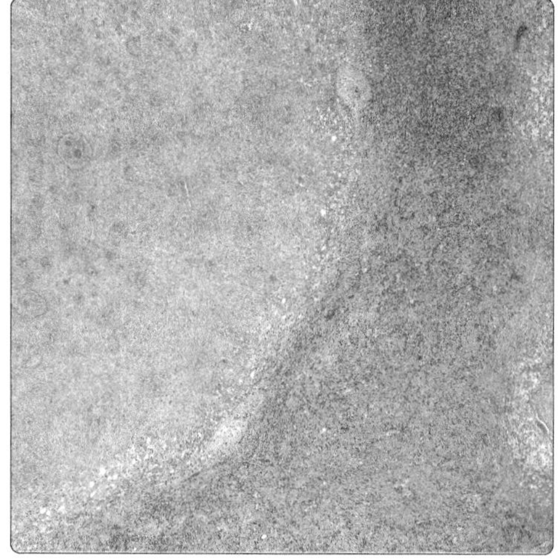

(Left) *T1 MR with contrast shows multiple ring-enhancing lesions characteristic of active T. gondii infection. Common sites of involvement include basal ganglia, thalami, and corticomedullary junction.* **(Right)** *This brain section shows a necrotic core on the left surrounded by inflammation. Bradyzoites are most commonly identified at the periphery of the necrosis.*

***Toxoplasma* Infection in Brain**

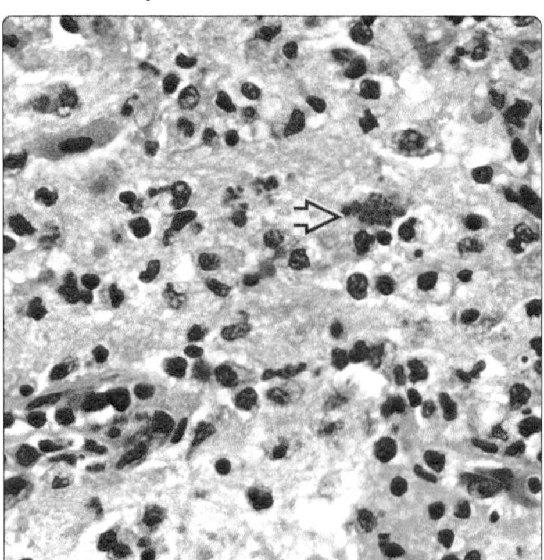

***T. gondii* IHC**

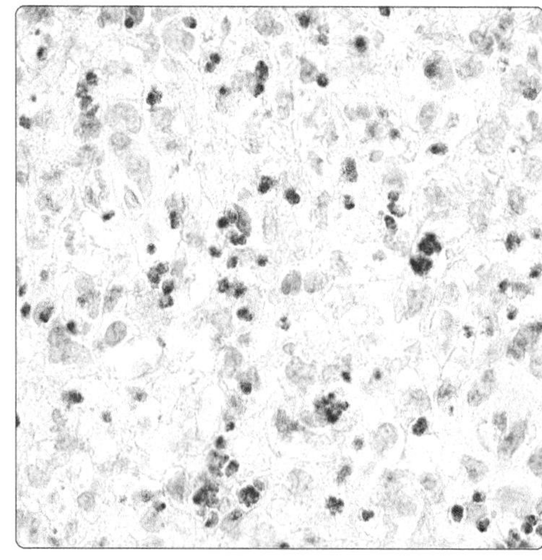

(Left) *H&E section of Toxoplasma encephalitis in an AIDS patient shows a necrotic brain lesion and only a few Toxoplasma cysts ⇒.* **(Right)** *T. gondii IHC highlights organisms in a brain biopsy of an immunocompromised patient. Inflammation can range from frank necrosis to minimal reaction.*

T. gondii Tachyzoites

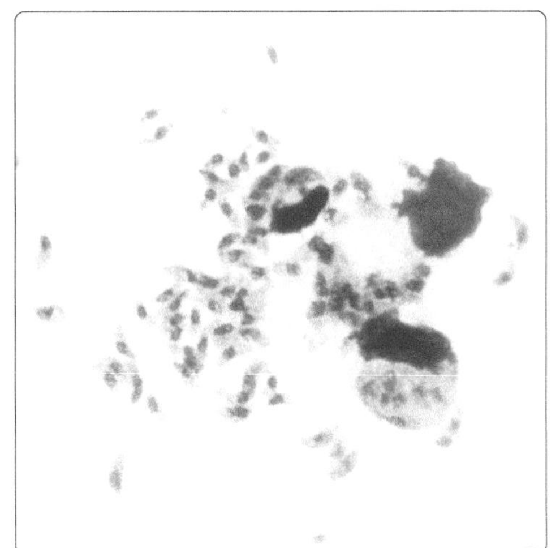

Toxoplasma Lymphadenitis

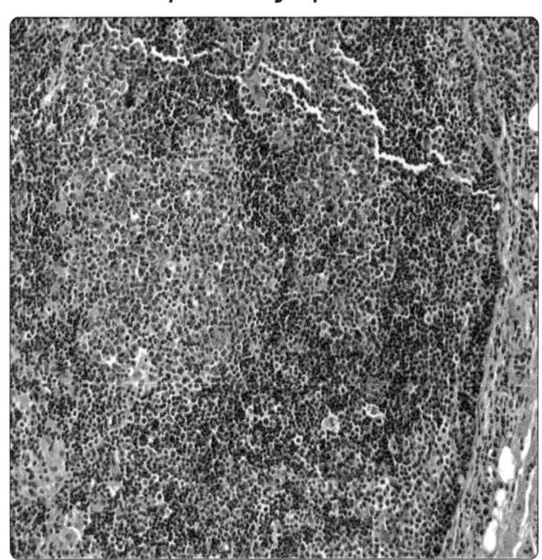

(Left) *This smear of murine ascitic fluid contains numerous crescent-shaped T. gondii tachyzoites. (Courtesy CDC/PHIL.)* **(Right)** *Low-power view of a toxoplasmosis lymphadenitis case shows a reactive follicle with a cluster of epithelioid histocytes within and outside the follicle center. Scattered throughout the lymph node will be macrophages with a moth-eaten appearance and evident phagocytosis of debris. Cysts are occasionally found with careful sectioning but are not required for diagnosis.*

Toxoplasma Lymphadenitis

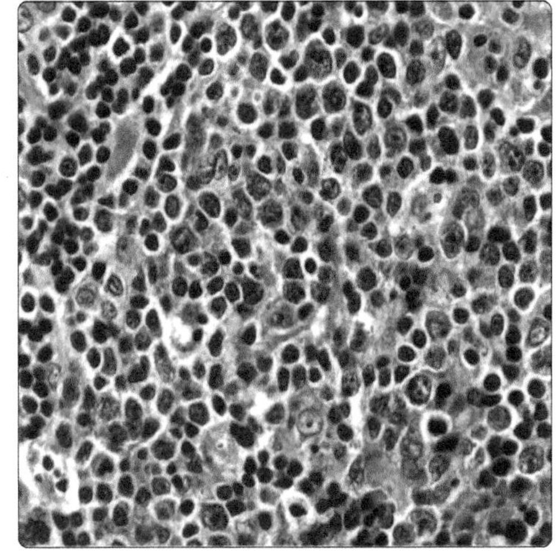

Disseminated Toxoplasmosis in Lungs

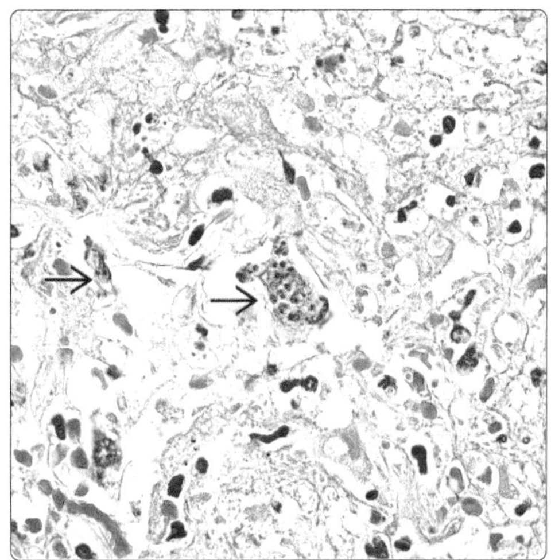

(Left) *High-power view of a toxoplasmosis lymphadenitis case shows the "monocytoid" cells that are actually B cells.* **(Right)** *This lung autopsy section shows occasional clusters of Toxoplasma cysts/pseudocysts ⇒, which can be confirmed with IHC.*

T. gondii Bradyzoites in Heart

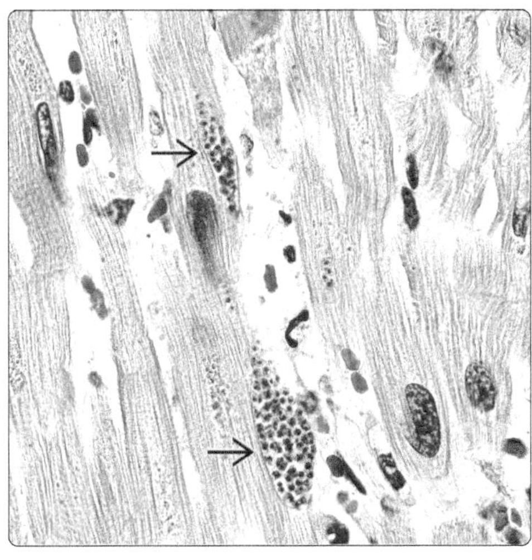

Differential Diagnosis: Sarcocystosis

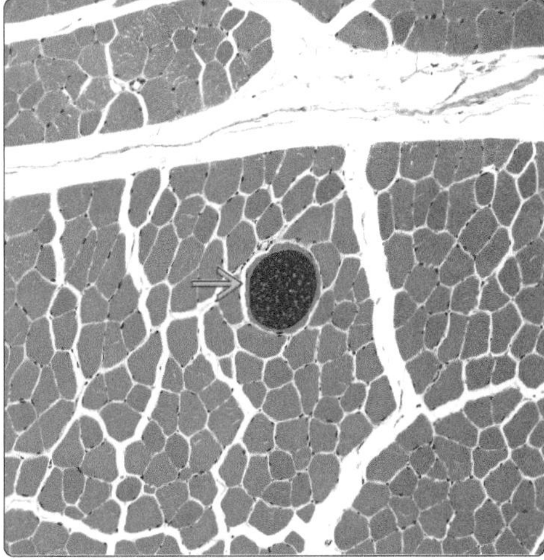

(Left) *Compared to the round cysts seen in brain, T. gondii cysts in cardiac and skeletal muscle tend to be more elongated ⇒. Trypanosoma cruzi amastigotes may appear similar but can be distinguished by presence of kinetoplasts or by organism-specific IHC.* **(Right)** *This skeletal muscle section from a reindeer shows incidental Sarcocystis sarcocysts ⇒, which contain bradyzoites similar in appearance to T. gondii but can be distinguished by IHC. (Courtesy H. Fenton, DVM.)*

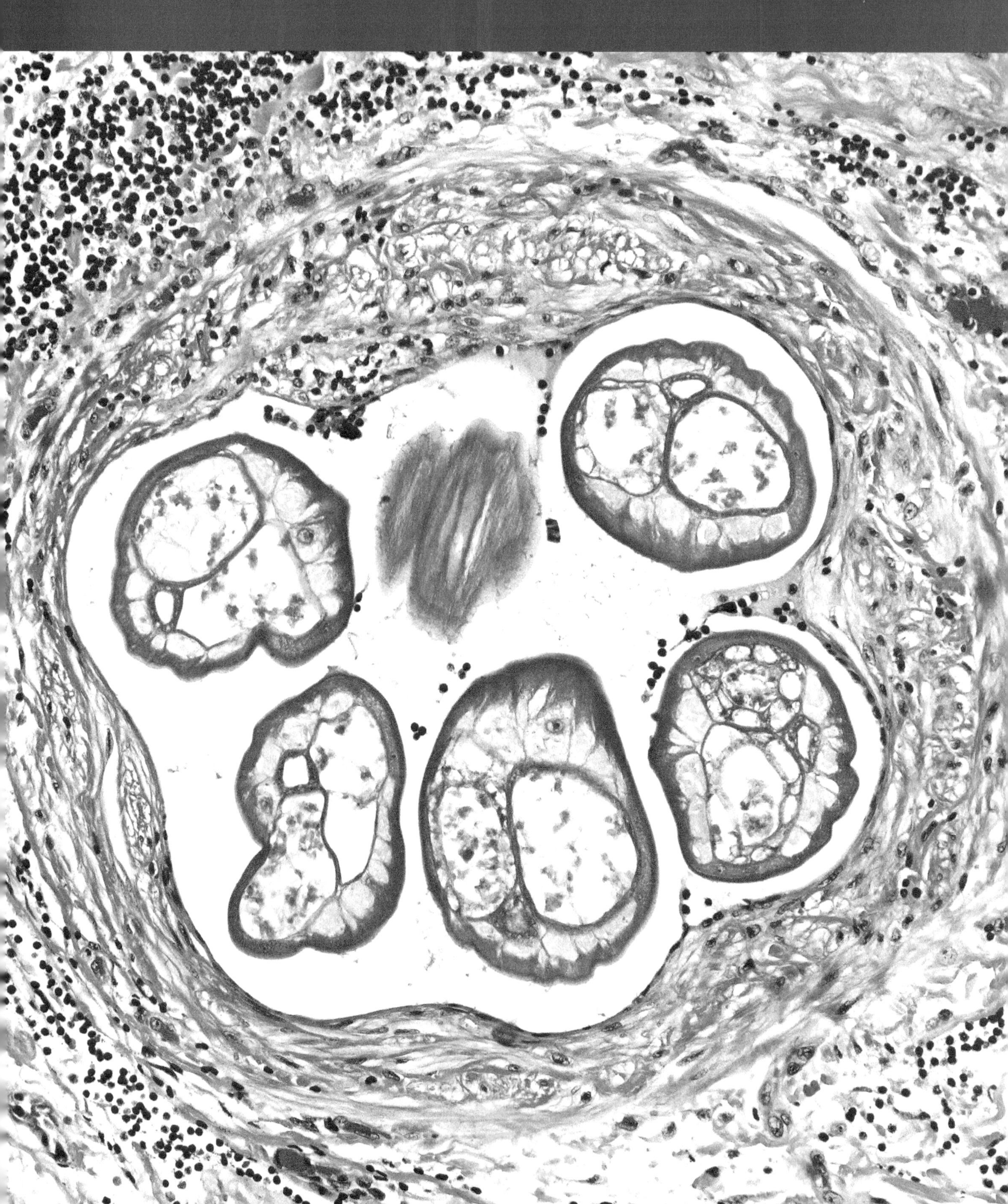

SECTION 7

Helminthic Parasitic Infections

Nematodes

Trematodes

Cestodes

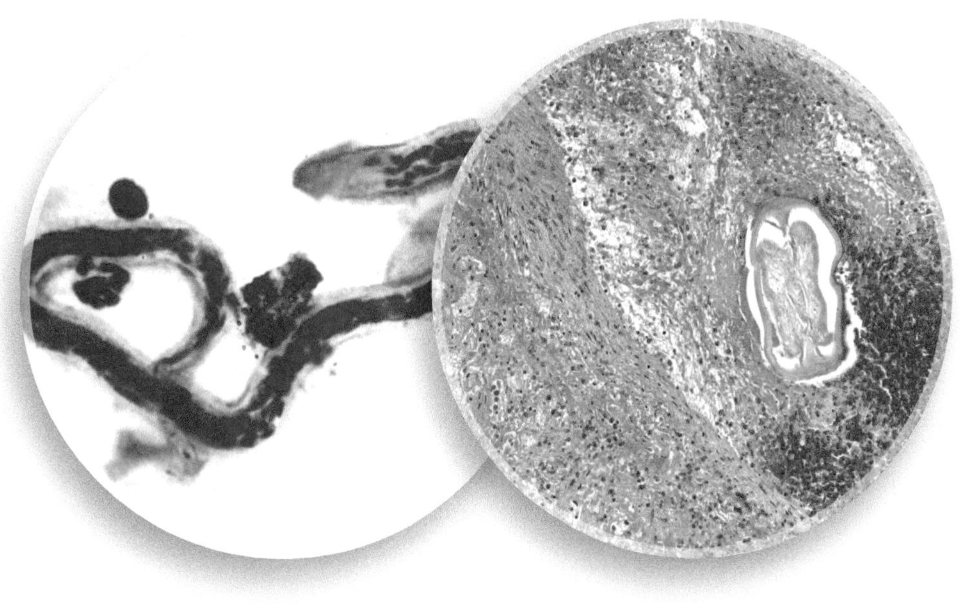

KEY FACTS

ETIOLOGY/PATHOGENESIS

- Infection with filariform larvae of *Necator americanus* (New World hookworm) or *Ancylostoma* spp. (Old World hookworm) via direct penetration of skin

CLINICAL ISSUES

- Worldwide distribution; associated with poor sanitation, bare feet, and poverty
- Loeffler syndrome: Cough, eosinophils in sputum
- Acute infection: Abdominal pain, melena, blood per rectum
- Chronic infection: Anemia, growth stunting, and mental milestone delay
- Albendazole or mebendazole; iron supplements

MACROSCOPIC

- Worms are large, easily visualized, attached to mucosa and do not penetrate wall of small bowel

MICROSCOPIC

- Adult worms in small bowel resections: Damaged mucosa in mouthparts, RBCs in body
- Sections show thick cuticle, thin hypodermis, few muscle cells, lateral cords, esophagus with triradiate lumen, and intestine with microvillus border
- Inflammatory response is variable (limited to diffuse)
- Larvae in skin contain conspicuous double alae

TOP DIFFERENTIAL DIAGNOSES

- Loeffler syndrome also caused by *Ascaris lumbricoides* and *Strongyloides stercoralis*; migrating larvae may not be seen
- Trichuriasis: Long, thin head burrowed into intestinal mucosa, larger posterior in lumen; eggs in epithelium/stool
- Strongyloidiasis: Small adult worms burrowed between intestinal epithelial cells; larvae have short buccal canal and prominent genital primordium; hookworm adults and rhabditiform larvae do not leave gastrointestinal tract

(Left) *Hookworm filariform larvae directly penetrate skin, migrate through the bloodstream to the lungs, are swallowed, and then reside as mature adults in the small intestine. Eggs mature into rhabditiform larvae in the stool, then into infective forms in the environment.* **(Right)** *Duodenum from a patient with hookworm demonstrates the small, 5-mm worms ➡ adherent to the mucosa with minimal changes. These were found on resection for other reasons. (Courtesy R. Cooke, MD.)*

Life Cycle of Hookworms

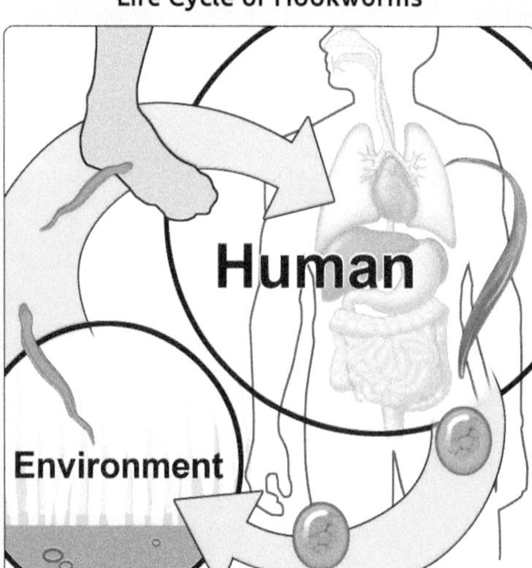

Worms on Mucosal Surface

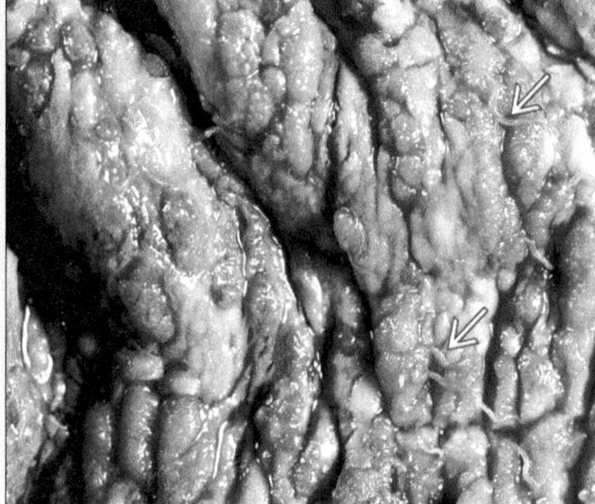

(Left) *This duodenal section shows an adult worm ⇨, which was clamped to the mucosa for feeding, and inflamed, blunted villi ⇨.* *(Courtesy R. Cooke, MD.)* **(Right)** *Hookworm eggs (60 x 40 µm) contain a thin shell ⇨ and are indistinguishable between species. Filariform larva are distinguished from Strongyloides by presence of long buccal canal ⇨. The presence of sharp cutting teeth ➡ helps to distinguish adult Ancylostoma from Nector, which contains cutting plates ⇨. (Courtesy Dr. Melvin, Dr. Moore, CDC/PHIL.)*

Worm in Small Bowel Resection

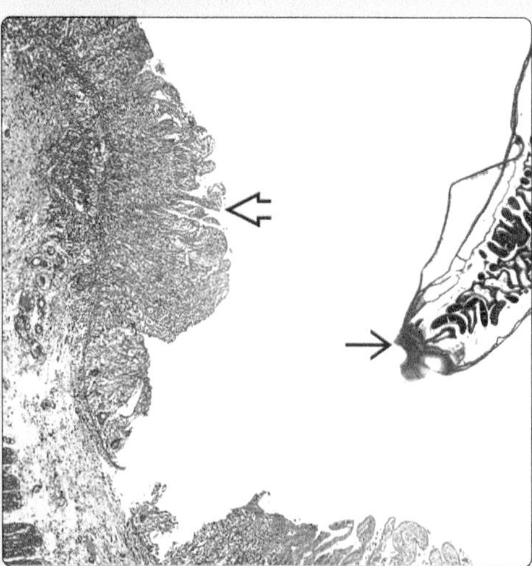

Hookworm Eggs, Larva, and Adults

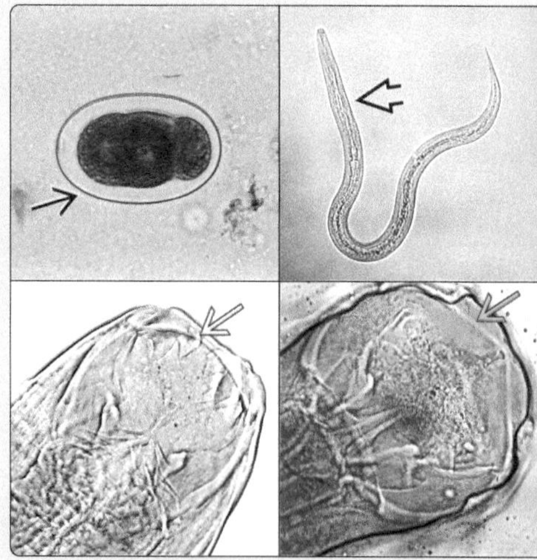

TERMINOLOGY

Synonyms

- Hookworm disease, miner's anemia, tunnel disease, brickmaker's anemia, Egyptian chlorosis

Definitions

- Greek: "Ankylos" (crooked) + "stoma" (mouth)
- Latin: "Necator" (to kill) + "americanus" (American origin)

ETIOLOGY/PATHOGENESIS

Infectious Agents

- Infection with soil-transmitted hookworm filariform larvae via direct skin penetration
- *Necator americanus* (New World hookworm): Live 5 years and produce ~ 10,000 eggs/day
- *Ancylostoma* spp. (Old World hookworm): Live 1 year and produce ~ 30,000 eggs/day
    - *A. duodenale* and *A. ceylanicum* (human hookworm infections), *A. braziliense* (cutaneous larva migrans), *A. caninum*, *A. pluridentatum*, and *A. tubaeforme*
- Unembryonated eggs pass into soil from infected human feces; embryonate, hatch into rhabditiform larvae, molt into juvenile larvae, then infectious filariform larvae
- Filariform larvae pass into human skin directly, migrate to and mature in lungs, are coughed up and swallowed; adult worms clamp onto small bowel mucosa and feed on human blood

CLINICAL ISSUES

Epidemiology

- Worldwide distribution (estimated 700 million infected)
- Associated with poor sanitation, bare feet, and poverty

Presentation

- Mostly asymptomatic
- Primary infection: Penetration of skin by larvae; "ground itch" (more common in zoonotic hookworm acquisition)
- Loeffler syndrome (larvae pass through lungs): Cough, eosinophils in sputum
- Acute infection: Abdominal pain, melena, blood per rectum
- Chronic infection: Anemia (loss 0.2 mL of blood/worm/day), growth stunting, milestone delay

Laboratory Tests

- Stool examination: Eggs and rhabditiform larvae
- Anemia on CBC; eosinophilia uncommon

Treatment

- Albendazole or mebendazole; iron supplements
- Large effort to develop vaccine is underway due to lack of efficacy of mass drug treatment in hookworm disease

Prognosis

- Mortality is extremely rare and most patients recover fully with proper treatment
- Reinfection will occur without exposure prevention
- Chronic disease complications (such as stunted growth) may not revert with treatment

MICROBIOLOGY

Parasite Features

- *Necator americanus*: Adult males 5-9 mm, females 9-11 mm; buccal capsule containing cutting plates
- *Ancylostoma* spp.: Adult males 8-11 mm, females 10-13 mm; buccal capsule containing 2 pairs of teeth
- Eggs: ~ 60 x 40 μm, thin-shelled, colorless (species not distinguishable)
- Rhabditoid larvae: 250-300 μm, long buccal canal, small genital primordium
- Filariform larvae: 500-700 μm, pointed tail, 1:4 ratio of esophagus to intestine; sheath striations more conspicuous in *Necator* than *Ancylostoma*

MACROSCOPIC

Endoscopy/Small Bowel Gross Examination

- Worms are large, easily visualized, attached to mucosa and do not penetrate wall of small bowel

MICROSCOPIC

Histologic Features

- Biopsy is rarely performed
- Larvae in skin contain conspicuous double alae
- Small bowel resections may contain adult worms with damaged mucosa in mouthparts and RBCs in body of worm
- Sections show thick cuticle, thin hypodermis, few muscle cells, lateral cords, esophagus with triradiate lumen, and intestine with microvillus border
- Inflammatory response is variable (limited to diffuse)

DIFFERENTIAL DIAGNOSIS

Helminth Infections of Lung

- Loeffler syndrome (eosinophilic pneumonitis) due to *Ascaris lumbricoides*, hookworm, or *Strongyloides stercoralis*; migrating larvae may not be seen
- Disseminated strongyloidiasis: Hookworm adults and rhabditiform larvae do not leave gastrointestinal tract

Helminth Infections of Small Intestine

- Trichuriasis (or whipworm): Long, thin head burrowed into intestinal mucosa, larger posterior structure in lumen; eggs entrapped in epithelium or stool
- Strongyloidiasis: Small adult worms and larvae (not grossly visible) burrowed between intestinal epithelial cells/into lamina propria with eosinophils; larvae have short buccal canal and prominent genital primordium

SELECTED REFERENCES

1. Quintana TA et al: Genetic characterization of the zoonotic parasite Ancylostoma caninum in the central and eastern United States. J Helminthol. 97:e37, 2023
2. Wong MTJ et al: Soil-transmitted helminthic vaccines: where are we now? Acta Trop. 239:106796, 2023
3. Clements ACA et al: Global distribution of human hookworm species and differences in their morbidity effects: a systematic review. Lancet Microbe. 3(1):e72-9, 2022
4. Loukas A et al: Hookworm infection. Nat Rev Dis Primers. 2:16088, 2016
5. Feldmeier H et al: Mini review: hookworm-related cutaneous larva migrans. Eur J Clin Microbiol Infect Dis. 31(6):915-8, 2012

Angiostrongyliasis

KEY FACTS

ETIOLOGY/PATHOGENESIS

- Parasitic infection caused by *Angiostrongylus* spp. from eating raw or undercooked snails or slugs or raw produce

CLINICAL ISSUES

- *Angiostrongylus cantonensis*: Eosinophilic meningitis, ocular disease
- *Angiostrongylus costaricensis*: Eosinophilic gastroenteritis; masses
- CSF: Eosinophilia (> 10% eosinophils), elevated protein, low/normal glucose; larvae rarely identified

MACROSCOPIC

- Basal/cerebellar meningeal opacification, focal hemorrhage
- Focal brain hemorrhage/necrosis from worm tracks

MICROSCOPIC

- *A. cantonensis*: Living or dead worms in meninges, blood vessels, or perivascular spaces
- *A. costaricensis*: Immature adults, L1 larvae, and thin-shelled eggs in wall of intestine/appendix
- Immature adult worms: Thin cuticle with fine transverse striations, polymyarian and coelomyarian musculature, intestines with few multinucleated cells, prominent dome-shaped lateral chords
- Minimal inflammatory reaction to living worms
- Eosinophils, granulomatous inflammation, giant cells engulfing degenerating worms, Splendore-Hoeppli reaction

TOP DIFFERENTIAL DIAGNOSES

- Gnathostomiasis: Shorter L3 larvae covered in spines
- Strongyloidiasis: Larvae are larger and contain double lateral alae, no granulomatous reaction or thin-shelled eggs
- Other causes of CSF eosinophilia: Other parasitic infections, Hodgkin disease, lymphocytic choriomeningitis virus, fungal infections, bacterial infections, foreign bodies, and allergic reactions

(Left) *A definitive host (rat) produces eggs that mature into larvae. These are consumed by intermediate hosts (slugs/snails) and mature into L3 larvae. Humans become infected when they eat intermediate hosts (raw or undercooked) with adults residing in brain or intestines.* **(Right)** *Cross section of an immature adult female Angiostrongylus cantonensis shows somewhat compressed dome-shaped lateral cords ⇒, paired reproductive tubules ↷, and central GI tract ⇒.*

***Angiostrongylus* spp. Life Cycle**

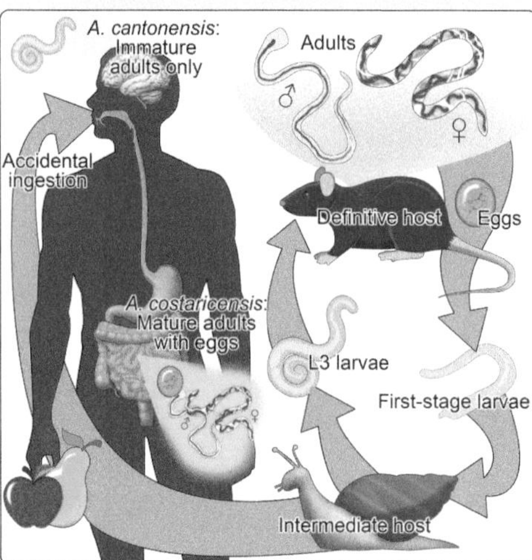

***Angiostrongylus cantonensis* in Meninges**

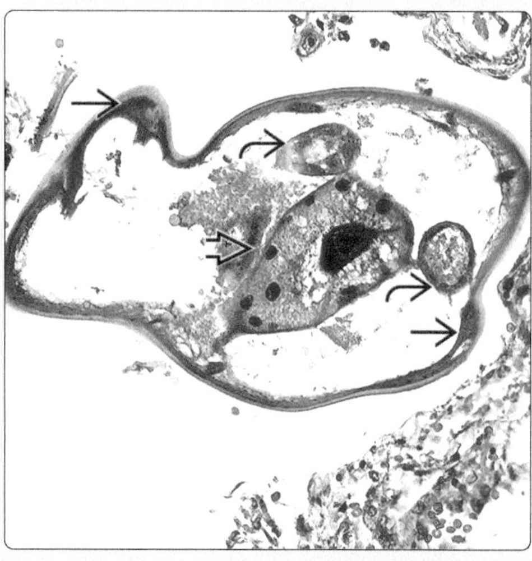

(Left) *Cross section of an immature adult female A. cantonensis shows paired reproductive tubules → and GI tract ↷. Dome-shaped lateral cords are not well visualized in this section.* **(Right)** *Multinucleated giant cells → engulf a degenerating A. cantonensis ⇒ worm, which cannot be reliably identified morphologically in this image.*

Cross Section of Immature Adult Female

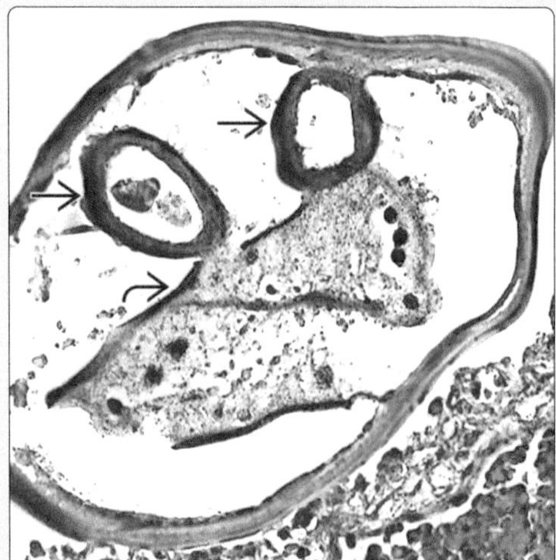

Inflammatory Reaction in Meninges

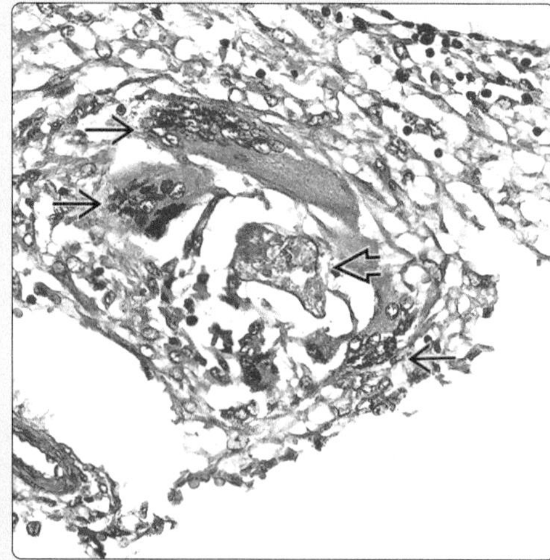

TERMINOLOGY

Synonyms

- Rat lungworm; *Parastrongylus*

Definitions

- Greek: "Angio" (vessel) + "strongylus" (round)

ETIOLOGY/PATHOGENESIS

Infectious Agents

- Parasitic infection caused by *Angiostrongylus* spp. from eating raw or undercooked snails or slugs or raw produce
- Incubation period: 12-28 days
- Eggs excreted by host (rats) into environment, where they are ingested by gastropod (snails, slugs) intermediate host, hatch, molt twice, and are ingested by definitive host
- 3rd-stage larvae migrate to brain or lymphatic vessels of abdominal cavity, develop into young adults, and return to venous system/pulmonary arteries or mesenteric arteries and become sexually mature
- *Angiostrongylus cantonensis*: In aberrant human host, ingested larvae migrate to brain, eyes, or lungs but do not reach reproductive maturity
- *Angiostrongylus costaricensis*: Larvae migrate to intestinal walls and can mature to produce eggs/larvae

CLINICAL ISSUES

Epidemiology

- *A. cantonensis*: Southeast Asia, Pacific Islands
  - Also reported in Africa, Caribbean, Australia, Hawaii, and southern USA
- *A. costaricensis*: Latin America, Caribbean

Presentation

- *A. cantonensis*: Eosinophilic meningitis, ocular disease
- *A. costaricensis*: Eosinophilic gastroenteritis; masses

Laboratory Tests

- CSF: Eosinophilia (> 10% eosinophils), elevated protein, low/normal glucose
- Larvae rarely identified in CSF or brain tissue sections
- RT-PCR (CSF)
- Serologic tests not commercially available
- No role for culture or stool examination in diagnosis

Treatment

- Unclear benefit of anthelminthics
- Corticosteroids to limit inflammatory reaction
- CSF removal in patients with elevated intracranial pressure

Prognosis

- Majority of cases asymptomatic or resolve completely with treatment
- Rare severe cases can result in death without treatment

MICROBIOLOGY

Parasite Features

- Immature adults seen in human tissue are 11-12 mm long with dome-like lateral chords
- Females: Barber pole-like appearance of body due to spiral appearance of paired reproductive tubules twisting around intestines
- Males: Transparent cuticle with 1-mm spicules, well-developed bursa

MACROSCOPIC

General Features

- Basal/cerebellar meningeal opacification, focal hemorrhage
- Focal brain hemorrhage/necrosis from worm tracks

MICROSCOPIC

Histologic Features

- *A. cantonensis:* Living or dead worms in meninges, blood vessels, or perivascular spaces
  - Eye: Larvae in anterior chamber and vitreous, subretinal space, which can lead to retinal detachment
- *A. costaricensis*: Immature adults, L1 larvae, and thin-shelled, unembryonated eggs in wall of intestine/appendix
- Minimal inflammatory reaction to living worms
- Eosinophils, granulomatous inflammation, giant cells engulfing degenerating worms, Splendore-Hoeppli reaction
- Immature adult worms: Thin cuticle with fine transverse striations, polymyarian and coelomyarian musculature, intestines with few multinucleated cells, prominent dome-shaped lateral chords

DIFFERENTIAL DIAGNOSIS

Gnathostomiasis

- Presents with transverse or ascending myelitis
- Shorter L3 larvae covered in spines

Strongyloidiasis

- Larvae are larger and contain double lateral alae
- Lack granulomatous reaction or thin-shelled eggs

Other Causes of Cerebrospinal Fluid Eosinophilia

- Other parasitic infections, Hodgkin disease, lymphocytic choriomeningitis virus, fungal infections, bacterial infections, foreign bodies, and allergic reactions

SELECTED REFERENCES

1. Carvalho MSN et al: Epidemiological, clinical and laboratory aspects of Angiostrongylus cantonensis infection: an integrative review. Braz J Biol. 82:e262109, 2022
2. Morgan ER et al: Angiostrongylosis in animals and humans in Europe. Pathogens. 10(10), 2021
3. Rojas A et al: Abdominal angiostrongyliasis in the Americas: fifty years since the discovery of a new metastrongylid species, Angiostrongylus costaricensis. Parasit Vectors. 14(1):374, 2021
4. Sears WJ et al: AcanR3990 qPCR: a novel, highly sensitive, bioinformatically-informed assay to detect Angiostrongylus cantonensis infections. Clin Infect Dis. 73(7):e1594-600, 2021
5. Feng L et al: The metagenomic next-generation sequencing in diagnosing central nervous system angiostrongyliasis: a case report. BMC Infect Dis. 20(1):691, 2020
6. Sinawat S et al: Ocular angiostrongyliasis in Thailand: a retrospective analysis over two decades. Clin Ophthalmol. 13:1027-31, 2019

Ascariasis

KEY FACTS

ETIOLOGY/PATHOGENESIS

- Infection with *Ascaris lumbricoides*, largest nematode (roundworm) infecting humans via ingestion of embryonated eggs

CLINICAL ISSUES

- Worldwide distribution and more common in areas of poverty with increased soil exposure
- Mostly asymptomatic; can cause malnutrition and stunted growth, Loeffler syndrome, intestinal obstruction with bowel infarction, and liver abscess

MACROSCOPIC

- Adult worms (males 15-30 cm, females 20-35 cm) in lumen of small bowel; seen on colonoscopy or passed in stool

MICROSCOPIC

- Adult worms: Thick acellular cuticle, thin hypodermis, tall polymyarian muscle cells, and pair of lateral cords; coiled ovary and gravid uterus (females)
- Fertilized eggs are rounded (45-75 μm in length) with thick shell and external mammillated layer (may be decorticated)
- Unfertilized eggs are elongated (90 μm) have thinner shell and variable outer layer
- Lung: Eosinophils ± larval forms
- Gastrointestinal tract: Normal or ischemic with necrosis
- Liver: Adult worms and eggs, neutrophilic abscesses, eosinophils, and giant cells

TOP DIFFERENTIAL DIAGNOSES

- Trematode infection of liver: Limited inflammation; size and shape of eggs with opercula for speciation
- Echinococcosis of liver: Contain multiple protoscolices with birefringent hooklets
- Loeffler syndrome: Also caused by *Strongyloides* spp., hookworm; other sources of pulmonary eosinophilia lack larvae/adult worms

Life Cycle of *Ascaris* Species

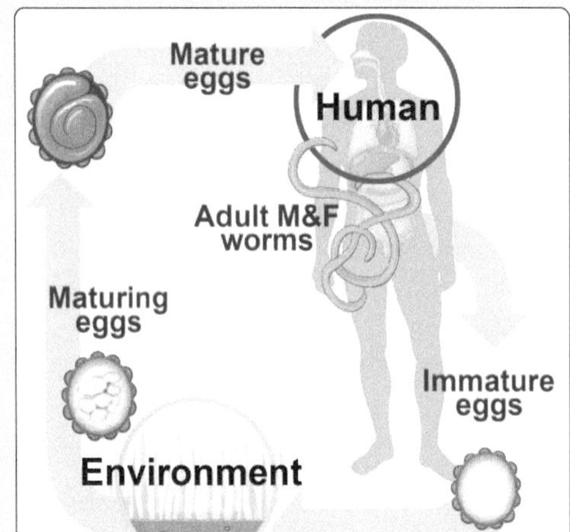

Mass of *Ascaris* Worms

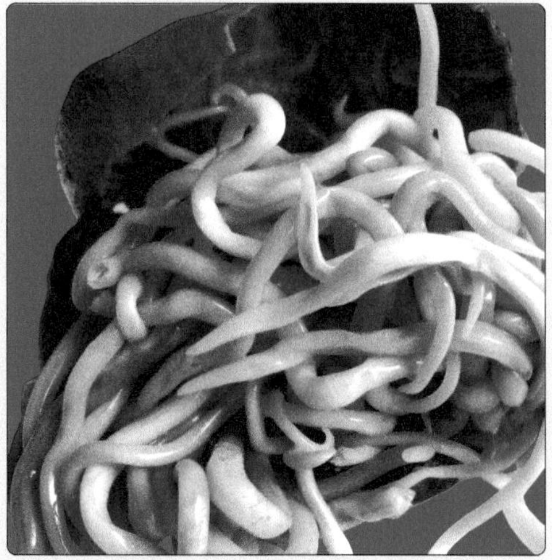

(Left) *Ascaris eggs are ingested from soil exposure and mature into male and female adult worms in the intestinal tract. Female worms lay large numbers of eggs per day, which pass into the stool. These eggs mature in the environment over weeks and become infective.* **(Right)** *A large mass of Ascaris worms removed at surgery demonstrates knotting and compression, consistent with obstruction.*

***Ascaris* Eggs in Stool**

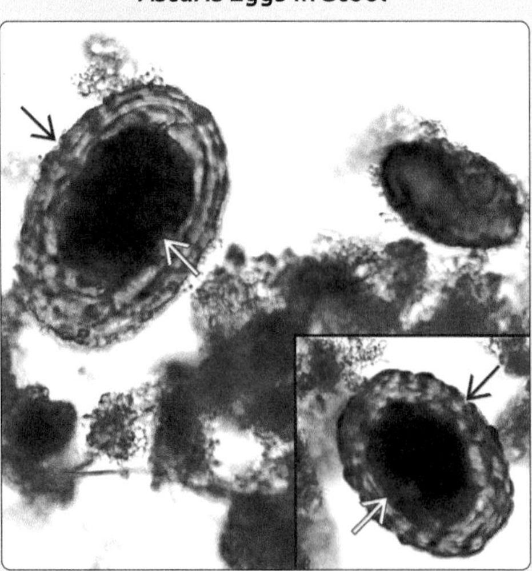

***Ascaris* Eggs in Tissue Section**

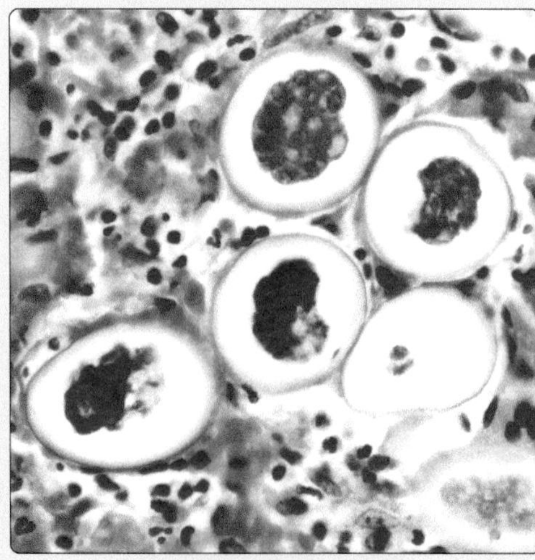

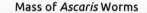

(Left) *Stool examination with iodine demonstrates the rough surface ⇨ and dark center ➡ of the large Ascaris lumbricoides eggs. The fertilized egg is protected by its thick mammillated, albuminous outer coat.* **(Right)** *Ascaris eggs in tissue sections often appear ovoid, depending on the plane of section, and contain a dark center. Mixed inflammation, including neutrophils, eosinophils, and giant cells, may be present.*

TERMINOLOGY

Definitions

- Greek: "Askaris" (intestinal worm)
- Latin: "Lumbricus" (earthworm)

ETIOLOGY/PATHOGENESIS

Infectious Agents

- Infection with *Ascaris lumbricoides* (soil-transmitted helminth), largest nematode (roundworm) infecting humans
- Unembryonated eggs pass out of stool into environment, mature into embryonated eggs in soil, and are ingested by next host
- Larvae hatch in intestinal tract, migrate through tissues/bloodstream to lungs where they mature into adults and are coughed up and swallowed
- Adult worms reside in small bowel, copulate, and release eggs
- Worms secrete molecules to protect against immune clearance, including *Ascaris* carboxypeptidase inhibitor (ACI)
- Links to asthma and allergy through IL13 and STAT6
- *Ascaris* derived from pigs is referred to as *A. suum,* but there is lack of consensus as separate species

CLINICAL ISSUES

Epidemiology

- Estimated 800 million to 1.2 billion people infected
- Worldwide distribution and more common in areas of poverty with increased soil exposure

Presentation

- Vast majority of infections are asymptomatic
- Chronic infection can lead to malnutrition and stunted growth
- Loeffler syndrome: Pulmonary alveolar space eosinophilia in response to larval passage
- Large burden: Abdominal pain, swollen abdomen, intestinal obstruction, bowel infarction, and nausea/vomiting
- Adult worms pass through ampulla of Vater, become trapped in liver, causing right upper quadrant pain, transaminitis, cholestasis, and abscess formation

Laboratory Tests

- Stool exam for ova and parasites is almost always positive if gravid female worms are in patient due to large burden of eggs per day produced (200,000 per female)
  - Presence of only male worms will not produce positive stool exams
  - Presence of only female worms will produce unfertilized eggs at lower numbers than gravid females

Treatment

- Gastrointestinal obstruction/infarction may require surgical decompression/resection
- Liver abscess may require surgical drainage
- Albendazole or mebendazole for intestinal infection

Prognosis

- Most patients return to normal health after treatment
- Obstruction may lead to infarction, sepsis, and death without treatment
- Liver masses may progress to frank hepatitis or lead to scarring

MICROBIOLOGY

Parasite Features

- Adult female worms are 20-35 cm with straight tails, and adult males are 15-30 cm with curved tails; both have 3 "lips" at anterior end of body without teeth/hooklets; inhabit lumen of small intestine, and can migrate elsewhere
- Unfertilized eggs: Elongated (up to 90 μm in length), thinner shell, and variable mammillated layer; mass of retractile granules
- Fertilized eggs: Rounded (45-75 μm in length), thick shell with external mammillated layer; decorticated eggs are fertilized eggs with absent outer layer
- 2nd-stage larvae: 300 μm in length, prominent single lateral alae, intestine with lumen and 3 cells, small excretory columns
- 3rd-stage larvae: 1.6 mm in length, larger excretory columns, prominent alae, and patent gut lined with microvilli

Culture

- No role for culture in diagnosis

MACROSCOPIC

Colonoscopy

- *Ascaris* worms are very large and easily identified on visual inspection of colon

Stool

- These large worms may be passed in stool with high burden, after treatment, or spontaneously, and patients may attest to presence of "common earthworms"

Sputum or Expectorated

- Through lung passage stage, worms may mature into adults and expire in respiratory system to be coughed up whole or in fragments

MICROSCOPIC

Histologic Features

- Adult worm sections contain thick acellular outer cuticle, thin hypodermis, tall polymyarian muscle cells, and pair of prominent lateral cords; short muscular esophagus, simple intestinal tube with columnar cells; paired coiled genital tubes/uteri with developing eggs (in females)
- Eggs (± external mammillated layer) seen in tissue sections with abundant mixed inflammation, including neutrophilic abscesses, eosinophils, and giant cells
- Lung: Eosinophils in alveolar spaces or in interstitium ± larval forms
- Gastrointestinal tract: Resected tissue may appear normal (mechanical obstruction) or ischemic with necrosis
- Liver: Cross sections of adult worms and eggs admixed with inflammation

DIFFERENTIAL DIAGNOSIS

Trematode Infection of Liver

- e.g., *Clonorchis*, *Opisthorchis*, *Fasciola*, and (rarely) *Fasciolopsis*
- Limited inflammation (natural habitat); size and shape of eggs with opercula aid in speciation

Echinococcosis of Liver

- Larval stage of *Echinococcus* spp. cestodes; cystic (*E. granulosus*) and alveolar (*E. multilocularis*) forms
- Contain multiple protoscolices with birefringent hooklets

Loeffler Syndrome

- Also caused by *Strongyloides* spp., hookworm
- Other sources of pulmonary eosinophilia occur

SELECTED REFERENCES

1. Aiadsakun P et al: Comparison of the complete filtration method using an automated feces analyzer with three manual methods for stool examinations. J Microbiol Methods. 192:106394, 2022
2. Gobert GN et al: Clinical helminth infections alter host gut and saliva microbiota. PLoS Negl Trop Dis. 16(6):e0010491, 2022
3. Jõgi NO et al: Ascaris exposure and its association with lung function, asthma, and DNA methylation in Northern Europe. J Allergy Clin Immunol. 149(6):1960-9, 2022
4. Demeke G et al: Effects of intestinal parasite infection on hematological profiles of pregnant women attending antenatal care at Debre Markos Referral Hospital, Northwest Ethiopia: -nstitution based prospective cohort study. PLoS One. 16(5):e0250990, 2021
5. Qazi F et al: Real-time detection and identification of nematode eggs genus and species through optical imaging. Sci Rep. 10(1):7219, 2020
6. Wang J et al: Ascaris. Curr Biol. 30(10):R423-5, 2020
7. Ayana M et al: Comparison of four DNA extraction and three preservation protocols for the molecular detection and quantification of soil-transmitted helminths in stool. PLoS Negl Trop Dis. 13(10):e0007778, 2019
8. Elhadidy T et al: Ascaris lumbricoides through pleural biopsy needle. A rare case of intrapleural ascariasis. Arch Bronconeumol. 53(3):171-2, 2017
9. Silber SA et al: Efficacy and safety of a single-dose mebendazole 500 mg chewable, rapidly-disintegrating tablet for ascaris lumbricoides and trichuris trichiura infection treatment in pediatric patients: a double-blind, randomized, placebo-controlled, phase 3 study. Am J Trop Med Hyg. 97(6):1851-6, 2017
10. Khuroo MS et al: Hepatobiliary and pancreatic ascariasis. World J Gastroenterol. 22(33):7507-17, 2016

A. lumbricoides Unfertilized Egg

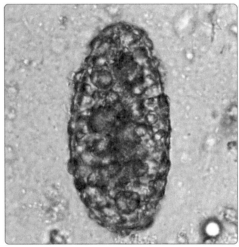

A. lumbricoides Fertilized Egg

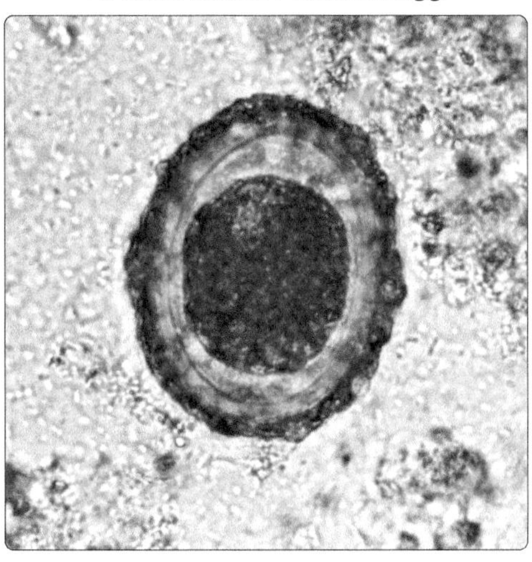

(Left) *Unfertilized Ascaris eggs are elongated (up to 90 µm in length) with thin shells and prominent mammillations. (Courtesy Dr. Moore, B. Partin, CDC/PHIL.)* **(Right)** *Fertilized Ascaris eggs are are round (45-75 µm in length) and have a thick shell with an external mammillated layer that is often stained brown by bile. (Courtesy Dr. Moore, B. Partin, CDC/PHIL.)*

A. lumbricoides Decorticated Egg

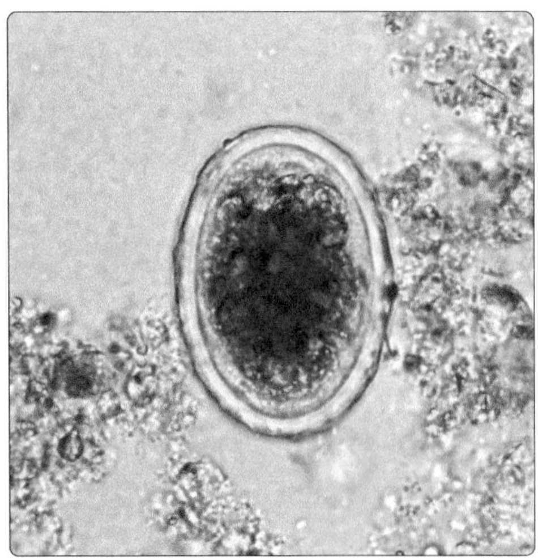

A. lumbricoides Egg With Embryo

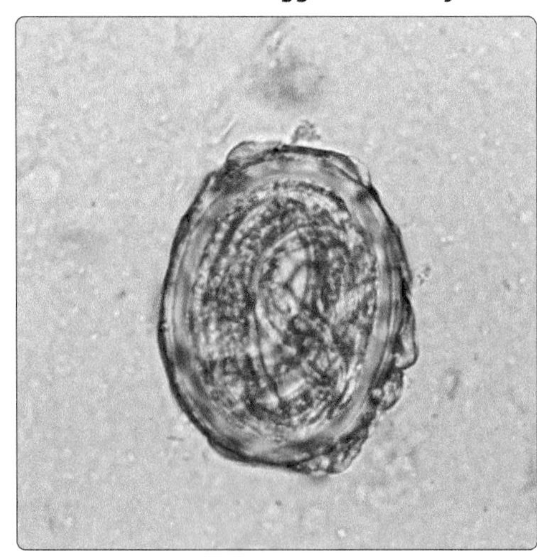

(Left) *Fertilized Ascaris eggs may lose their outer mammillated layer and are referred to as decorticated eggs. (Courtesy B. Partin, CDC/PHIL.)* **(Right)** *Following fertilization, Ascaris embryos develop and will eventually leave the egg as larvae. (Courtesy B. Partin, CDC/PHIL.)*

Anterior End of *Ascaris* Worm

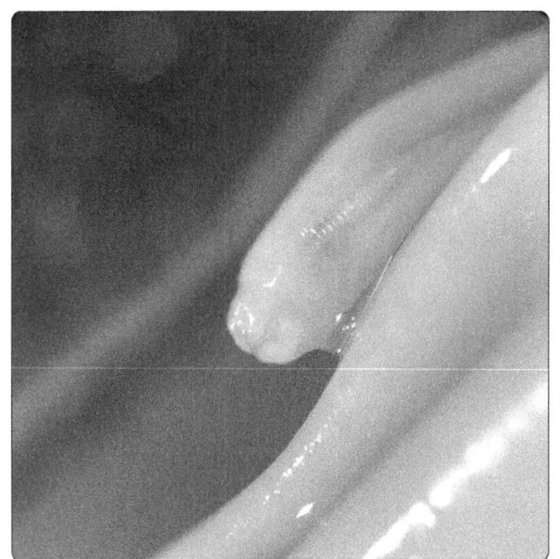

Ascaris Worms in Necrotic Mass

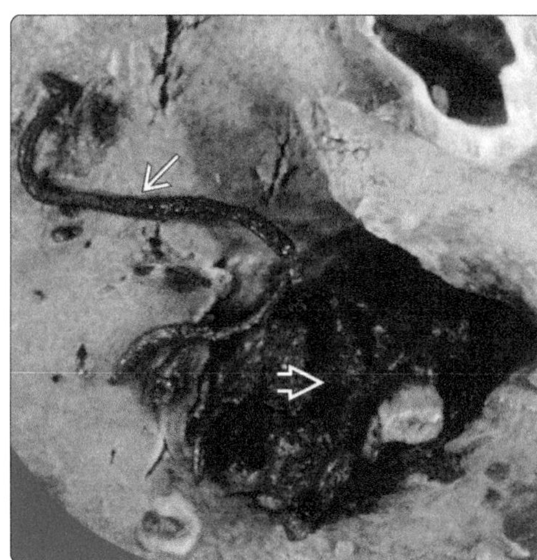

(Left) *This close-up image of the anterior end of an adult Ascaris lumbricoides worm shows 3 "lips," which are seen both in male and female worms. (Courtesy J. Crothers, MD.)* **(Right)** *A liver with a large necrotic mass ➡ demonstrates dead adult Ascaris worms ➡ within the lesions. (Courtesy A. Velez Hoyos, MD.)*

Ascaris Adult in Cross Section

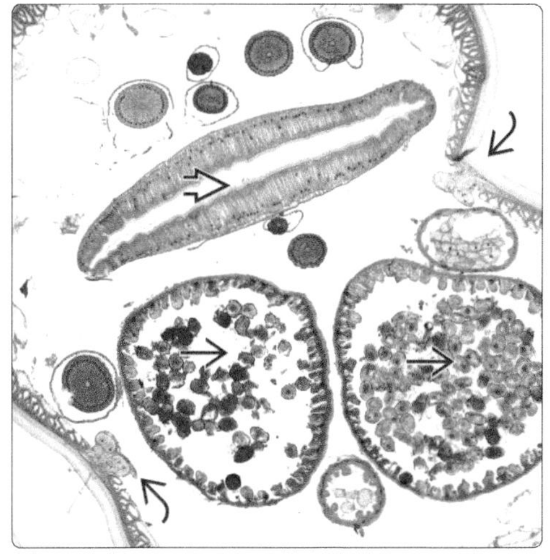

Ascaris Worm in Liver

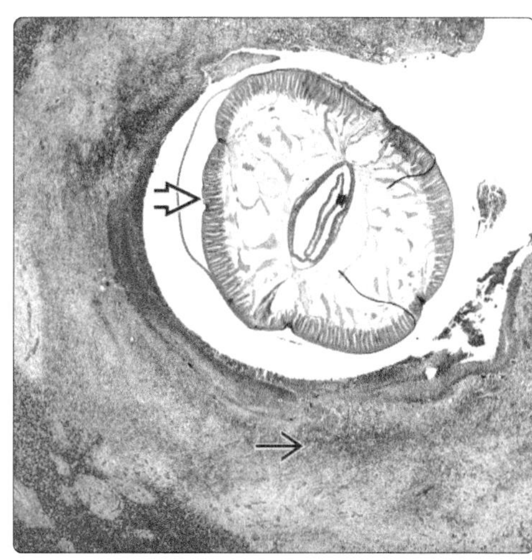

(Left) *A cross section of a gravid female Ascaris worm shows the gastrointestinal tract ➡, the uterus containing eggs ➡, and lateral longitudinal cords ➡.* **(Right)** *A section of liver from a large liver mass demonstrates a cross section of an Ascaris worm ➡ with surrounding dense inflammation ➡. Eggs may be seen in the liver parenchyma.*

Ascaris Worm in Liver

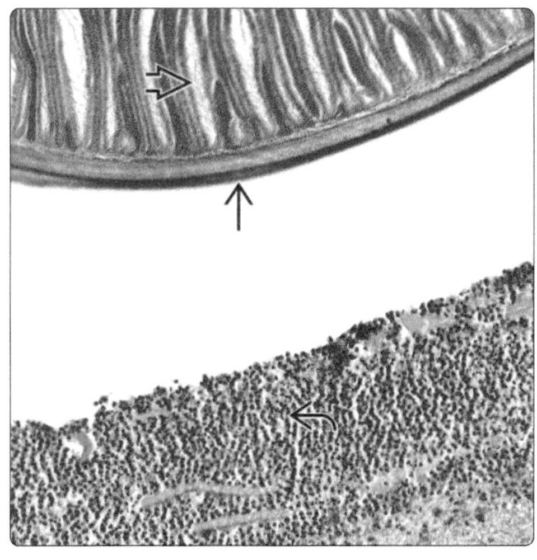

Ascaris Eggs in Tissue Section

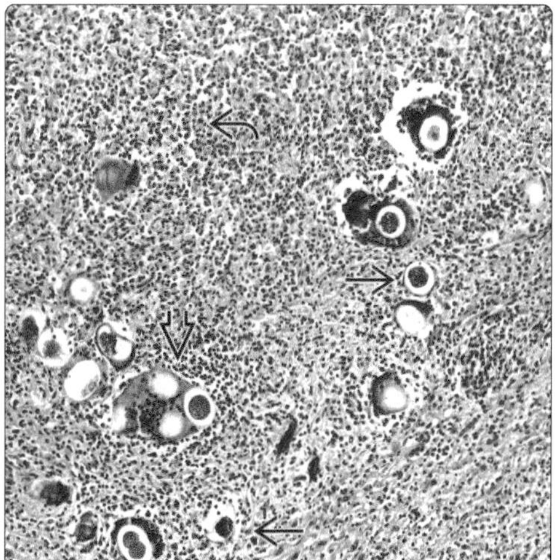

(Left) *High magnification of the interface of an Ascaris worm with the inflamed liver tissue demonstrates the tall polymyarian muscle layer ➡, thin acellular cuticle ➡, and sheet of neutrophils ➡.* **(Right)** *Numerous Ascaris eggs ➡ are seen in this section of liver tissue within sheets of inflammatory cells ➡, which includes giant cell-containing eggs ➡.*

KEY FACTS

ETIOLOGY/PATHOGENESIS

- Extremely common human parasite; prevalence of 20-70%
- Transmission via anus-to-mouth transfer by contaminated hands, directly or indirectly via contaminated surfaces; self-infection and person-to-person transmission may occur
- Gravid female worms migrate from colon to perianal area to deposit eggs; extraintestinal disease mostly due to ectopic migration

CLINICAL ISSUES

- Often asymptomatic
- Perianal pruritus and secondary excoriations, sometimes complicated by bacterial superinfection
- Generally intestinal parasite, but notable disease caused by infections of female genital tract

MICROSCOPIC

- Intraluminal adult worms with minimal inflammation; rare mucosal invasion
- Sections of adult worm contain thin cuticle, platymyarian muscle cells, and prominent lateral cords; esophagus, intestine, ovaries and gravid uterus with eggs (females), or reproductive tubules with spermatozoa (males)
- Eggs (50-60 μm) are ovoid with have refractile double-contour shells, flattened on one side; may be deposited in tissues with granulomas and eosinophils

TOP DIFFERENTIAL DIAGNOSES

- Strongyloidiasis: Not observed endoscopically; embedded within epithelium with marked inflammation; rhabditiform larvae shed in stool
- Ancylostomiasis/necatoriasis: Adult worms (5-13 mm) attached to small intestine; thin-shelled eggs (60-75 μm)
- Trichuriasis: Adult worms (30-50 mm) with thin anterior segment embedded into mucosa; barrel-shaped eggs (50 μm) with pair of polar "plugs" at each end
- Ascariasis: Large intraluminal adults worms (15-35 cm); ovoid eggs (50-70 μm) with prominent mammillations

***Enterobius vermicularis*: Life Cycle**

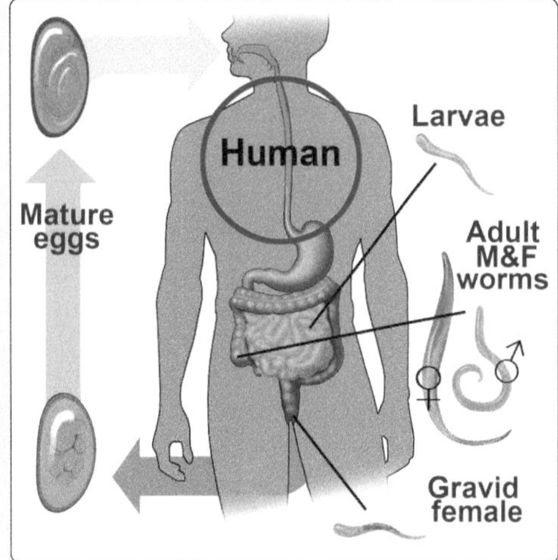

***Enterobius vermicularis* (Pinworm) in Appendix**

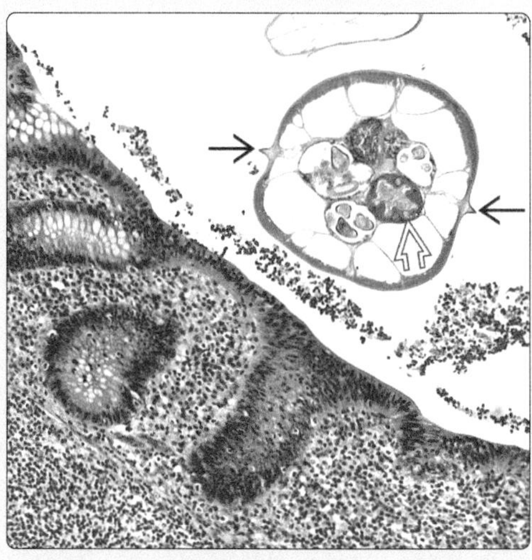

(Left) *Following ingestion of infective eggs, larvae hatch in the small intestine, and adults worms establish themselves in the colon. Gravid females migrate nocturnally outside the anus and deposits eggs on perianal folds. Eggs become infective in 4-6 hours. Newly hatched larvae can migrate back into the rectum (retroinfection).* **(Right)** *Cross section of intraluminal Enterobius vermicularis with prominent lateral alae ⇨ and intestinal tract ➡ stained with H&E is shown.*

***Enterobius vermicularis* Egg in Wet Mount**

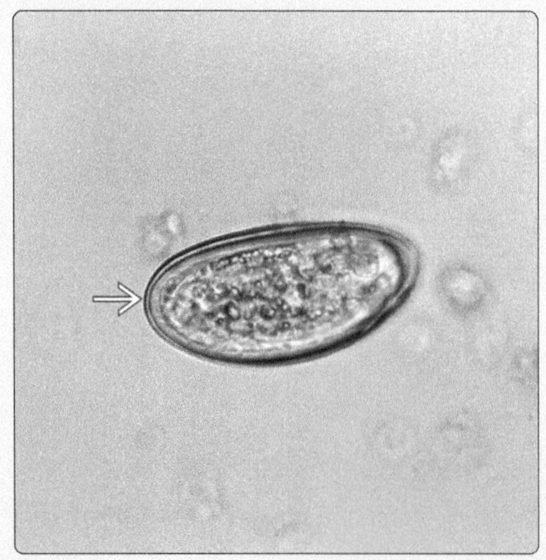

***Enterobius vermicularis* Eggs in Tissue Section**

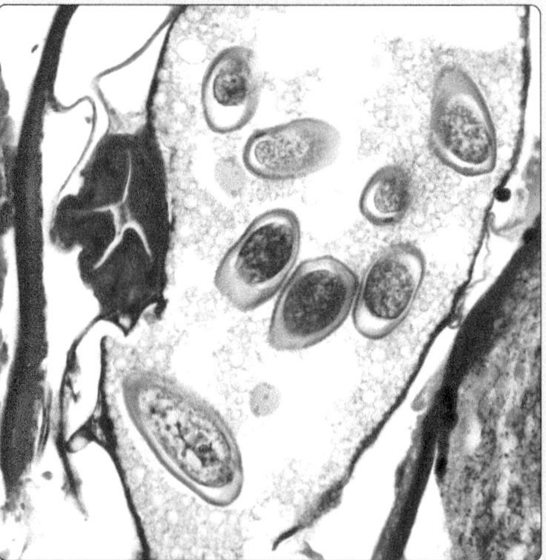

(Left) *Egg of E. vermicularis (50-60 μm in length) in a wet mount shows characteristic flattening on one side and a retractile double-contour shell ➡. (Courtesy of B. Partin, Dr. Moore, CDC/PHIL.)* **(Right)** *Multiple E. vermicularis eggs with a characteristic flattened side are present in the uterus of this gravid female in tissue sections.*

TERMINOLOGY

Synonyms

- Pinworm, oxyuriasis, seatworm, and threadworm

Definitions

- Greek words "enteron" (guts, bowels) and "bíos" (mode of life); "vermiculus" (little worm)

ETIOLOGY/PATHOGENESIS

Infectious Agents

- Infection with oxyurid nematode *Enterobius vermicularis* (*Oxyuris vermicularis*), either through self-inoculation of eggs transferred by fingers from perianal area to mouth or exposure to eggs in environment; airborne transmission of aerosolized eggs can occur
- Larvae hatch from ingested eggs in small intestine, and then adult worms reside in colon; gravid adult females deposit eggs on perianal folds at night while host is asleep, which can be transferred to hands, bedding, and clothing
- Humans are considered only host for *E. vermicularis*
- Rat pinworm (*Syphacia obvelata*) very rarely reported to infect humans

CLINICAL ISSUES

Epidemiology

- Global distribution; estimated incidence > 1 billion worldwide
- More common in temperate climates
- Infections occurring most frequently in school or preschool children and in crowded conditions
- Estimated prevalence ~ 20-70%; infection associated with nail biting (onychophagia/perionychophagia), unsupervised body hygiene, and poor compliance with basic hand hygiene

Presentation

- Frequently asymptomatic
- Most typical symptom is nocturnal perianal pruritus, which may lead to excoriations and bacterial superinfection
- Severe complications include bowel obstruction, perforation, bacterial peritonitis
- Gynecologic disease (vulvovaginitis) likely due to ectopic migration of gravid female worms; severe complications associated with ascending infections (pelvic or peritoneal granulomas, salpingitis, infertility)
- Other extraintestinal sites of disease rare (e.g., urinary tract, ocular, biliary/hepatic)
- Symptomatic infection associated with mental disturbances or nervous disorders
- Symptoms can mimic appendicitis (anorexia, irritability, and abdominal pain)

Laboratory Tests

- Cellulose/scotch tape test for perianal eggs
- Stool examination not recommended due to sparse presence of eggs
- Serologic tests are not available

Treatment

- Mebendazole, pyrantel embonate, and pyrvinium embonate
- For recurrent infections, prolonged treatment (up to 16 weeks with "pulse scheme") recommended
- Treatment of all persons living in patient's household, including sexual partners, recommended to prevent recurrent infection

Prognosis

- Majority of cases successfully resolved following treatment
- Rare case of severe disease due to ectopic infections

MICROBIOLOGY

Parasite Features

- Adult worms are white-tan; females (8-13 mm x 0.3-0.5 mm) have long pointed tail, while adult males are smaller (2-5 mm x 0.1-0.2 mm) and have blunt posterior end with single spicule
  - Identification of adult worms in perianal area via anorectal or vaginal examinations is diagnostic
- Ova (50-60 μm x 20-30 μm) are transparent, elongate to oval, and planoconvex (slightly flattened on one side) with bilayered refractile shell
  - Diagnosis often made by applying cellulose tape to perianal skin of suspected patient followed by microscopic examination (best if performed in morning prior to washing)
  - Eggs also found in stool, urine, vaginal, or cervicovaginal Papanicolaou smear samples
  - Contain coarsely granular embryos or curved larvae in different states of expulsion

MACROSCOPIC

General Features

- Adults worms (size of staple) can be observed during colonoscopy and by direct examination of perianal area

MICROSCOPIC

Histologic Features

- Infection usually localized in large bowel and cecum or appendix; intraluminal adult worms with little to no associated inflammation; rarely mucosal invasion
- Sections of worm exhibit thin cuticle that thickens after death, platymyarian muscle cells, and thin hypodermis and prominent lateral cords; internal structures include esophagus, intestine, ovaries and gravid uterus with eggs (females), or reproductive tubules with spermatozoa (males)
- Extraparasitic eggs may be deposited in tissues with associated granulomas and eosinophils; eggs have retractile double-contour shells and may be embryonated or with partially expelled embryo

Cytologic Features

- Identification of eggs, embryos, and larvae in background of acute inflammatory cells in cervical Papanicolaou test
- May be due to true vaginal infection or contamination of sample with eggs from perineum

DIFFERENTIAL DIAGNOSIS

Strongyloidiasis

- Small nematode not observed endoscopically, embedded within epithelium with marked transmural eosinophilic and neutrophilic infiltrate; rhabditiform larvae (180-380 μm long) shed in stool

Ancylostomiasis/Necatoriasis

- Adult worms (5-13 mm long) attach to small intestine
- Eggs (60-75 μm x 35-40 μm) are thin shelled and colorless

Trichuriasis

- Adult worms (30-50 mm long) with thin anterior segment embedded into mucosa of cecum and ascending colon
- Eggs (50 x 20 μm) are barrel-shaped, thick shelled, and possess pair of polar "plugs" at each end

Ascariasis

- Large adult worms reside in small intestine and are easily identified grossly due to large size (15-35 cm long)
- Eggs (50-70 μm) are ovoid with prominent mammillations

SELECTED REFERENCES

1. Haghshenas M et al: Detection of Enterobius vermicularis in archived formalin-fixed paraffin-embedded (FFPE) appendectomy blocks: It's potential to compare genetic variations based on mitochondrial DNA (cox1) gene. PLoS One. 18(2):e0281622, 2023
2. De Kostha YBNS et al: Characterization of antigens of Enterobius vermicularis (pinworm) eggs. Sci Rep. 12(1):14414, 2022
3. Mendos A et al: Intramural ova of Enterobius vermicularis in the appendix-an egg-topic location! Int J Surg Pathol. 30(2):214-6, 2022
4. Ummarino A et al: A PCR-based method for the diagnosis of Enterobius vermicularis in stool samples, specifically designed for clinical application. Front Microbiol. 13:1028988, 2022
5. Tsai CY et al: Vaginal Enterobius vermicularis diagnosed on liquid-based cytology during Papanicolaou test cervical cancer screening: a report of two cases and a review of the literature. Diagn Cytopathol. 46(2):179-86, 2018
6. Babady NE et al: Enterobius vermicularis in a 14-year-old girl's eye. J Clin Microbiol. 49(12):4369-70, 2011
7. Lamps LW: Infectious causes of appendicitis. Infect Dis Clin North Am. 24(4):995-1018, ix-x, 2010
8. Wu ML et al: Enterobius vermicularis. Arch Pathol Lab Med. 124(4):647-8, 2000
9. Mayers CP et al: Manifestations of pinworms. Can Med Assoc J. 103(5):489-93, 1970

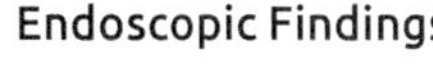

Endoscopic Findings

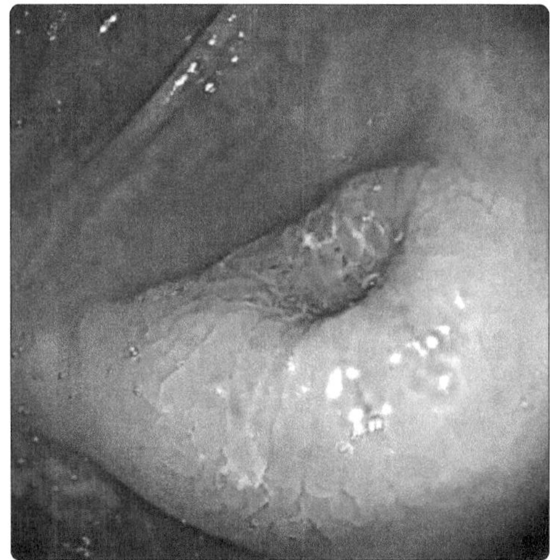

Female and Male Adult Worms

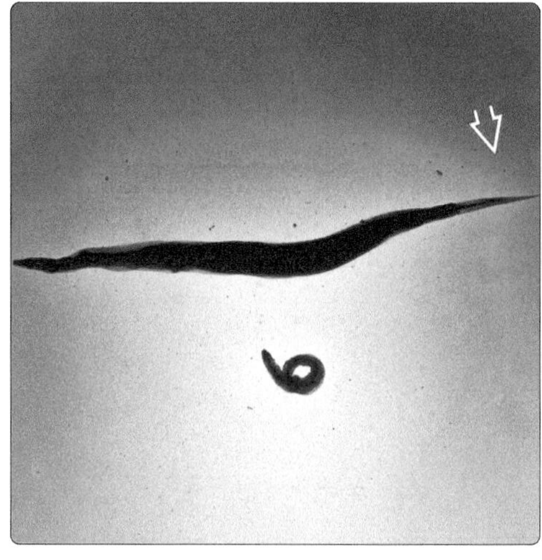

(Left) *Thread-like E. vermicularis adult worms visible at appendiceal opening (yellow arrows) are seen during surveillance colonoscopy.* **(Right)** *This thick-mount section illustrates the marked size difference between adult female worms (8-13 mm long) with a long pointed tail* ➡ *and adult male worms (2-5 mm long) with a blunt posterior end.*

Eggs on Cellulose Tape Test

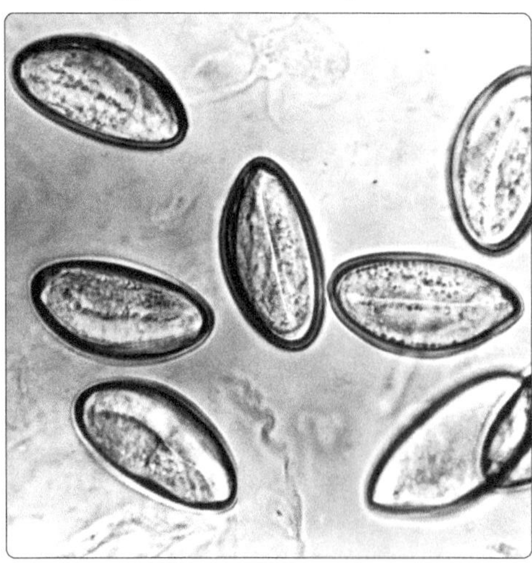

Eggs in Tissue Sections

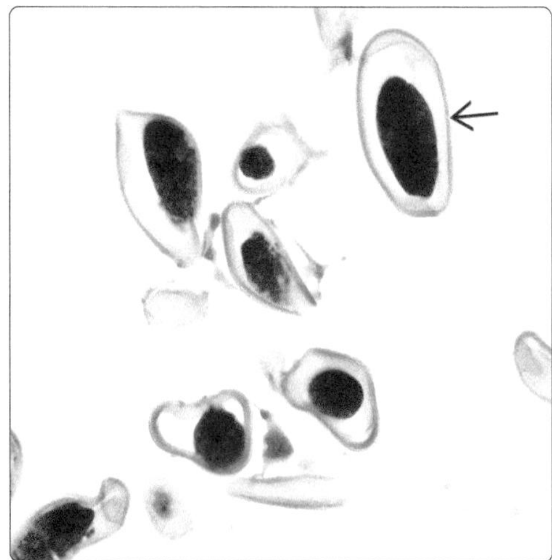

(Left) *This image demonstrates E. vermicularis eggs collected from the perianal folds via application of cellulose tape, which should be performed 1st thing in the morning. (Courtesy CDC/PHIL.)* **(Right)** *E. vermicularis eggs in tissue sections are 50-60 μm in length with a characteristic flattening on one side* → *but can appear irregularly shaped due to orientation and plane of section.*

Adult Female *Enterobius vermicularis*

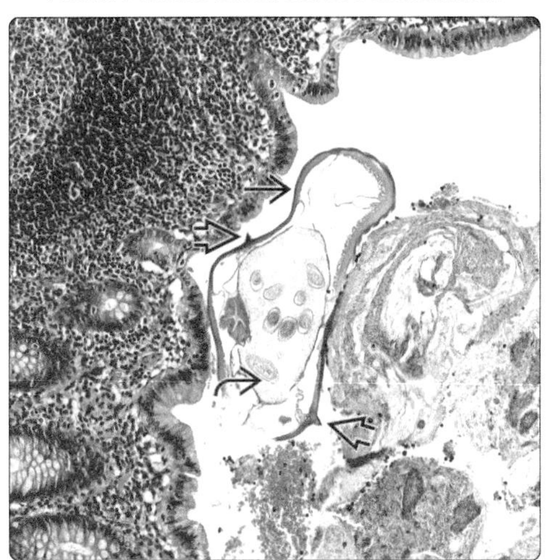

Enterobius vermicularis Lateral Alae

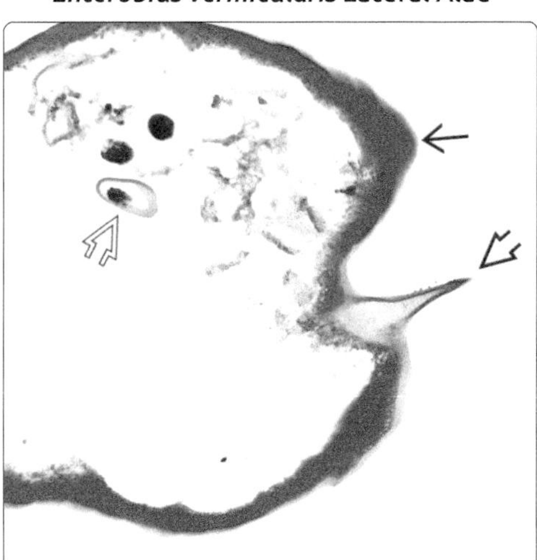

(Left) *This section shows an adult female worm in the lumen of the appendix. The worm contains a thin cuticle* →*, prominent lateral alae* →*, and uterus with multiple characteristic eggs* →*.* **(Right)** *This cross section of degenerating E. vermicularis shows a thickened cuticle* →*. Diagnostic features include a prominent lateral ala* → *and a characteristic planoconvex egg* →.

Enterobius vermicularis Adult Worm

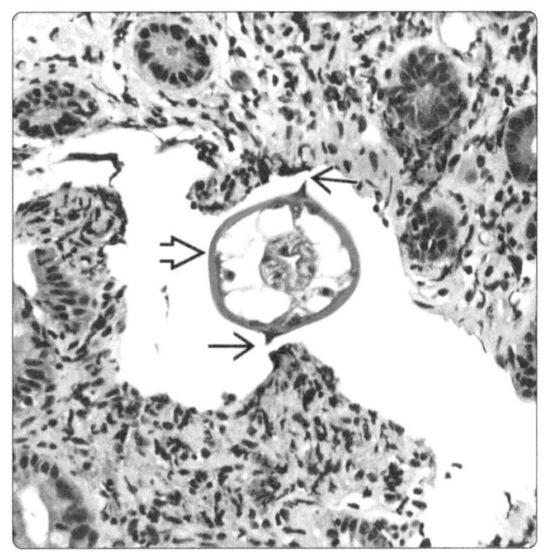

Multiple Sections of Adult *Enterobius vermicularis*

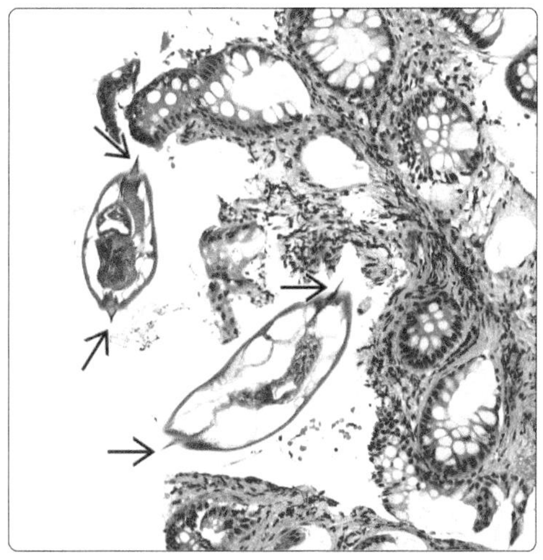

(Left) *This anterior cross section of intraluminal E. vermicularis shows a thin cuticle* → *with underlying platymyarian muscle cells, centrally located esophagus, and prominent lateral alae* →*.* **(Right)** *Multiple E. vermicularis cross sections, identified by prominent lateral alae* →*, may be from a single worm leaving the plane of section or from multiple adjacent worms. The size is most suggestive of adult male worm.*

Tangential Sections of *Enterobius vermicularis*

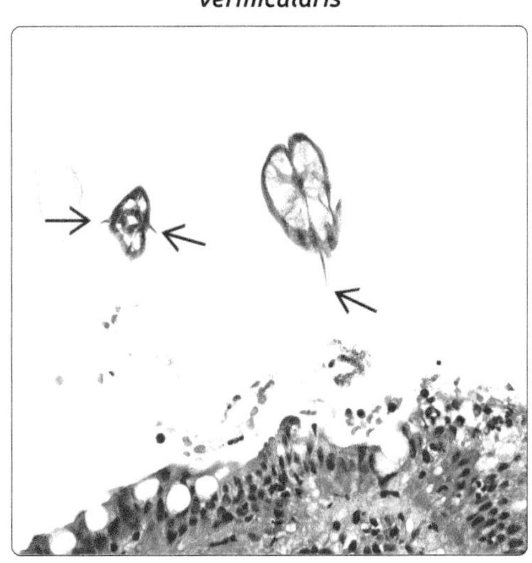

Anterior Cross Section of *Enterobius vermicularis*

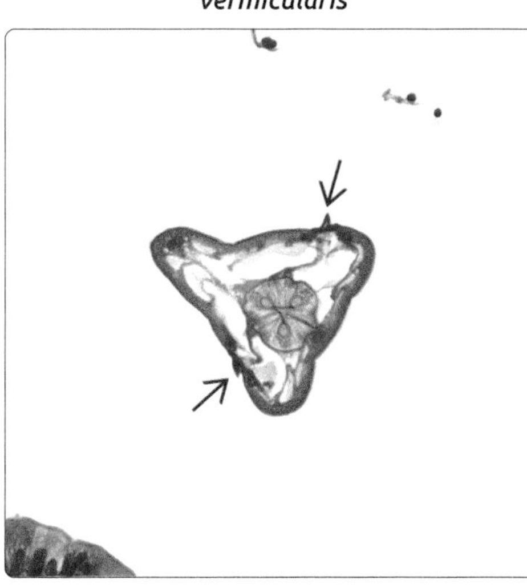

(Left) *Sections of E. vermicularis show a thin cuticle and underlying platymyarian muscle cells with minimal pseudocoelom. Prominent lateral alae* → *are present.* **(Right)** *This anterior cross section of E. vermicularis has a somewhat triangular shape and central esophagus but still exhibits characteristic lateral alae* → *seen in rounder cross sections.*

Gnathostomiasis

KEY FACTS

CLINICAL ISSUES

- Food-borne zoonotic parasitic infection caused by 3rd-stage larvae of spiruroid nematodes *Gnathostoma* spp.
- Endemic in Southeast Asia, Japan, China, Africa, Mexico, and South America
- Most commonly acquired by ingesting raw or poorly cooked fresh water fish
- Cutaneous gnathostomiasis is most common form and presents with nodular migratory panniculitis
- Migrating parasite can also invade stomach, lungs, urinary bladder, eye, ear, and CNS, causing visceral gnathostomiasis
- Surgical removal of larvae is most effective treatment

MACROSCOPIC

- L3 stage larvae of *Gnathostoma* spp. are ~ 3.5-4.0 mm long and have prominent cephalic bulb with 4 rows of hooklets

MICROSCOPIC

- Capture in biopsies is extremely difficult, and nonspecific findings are present in many cases
- Eosinophilic cellulitis/panniculitis, necroinflammatory tracts with prominent eosinophilic debris or "flame figures" should be interpreted as presumptive evidence in appropriate clinical context
- Cross sections of *Gnathostoma* spp. may show cuticular spines, coelomyarian musculature, prominent esophagus, &/or large lateral chords

TOP DIFFERENTIAL DIAGNOSES

- Sparganosis: Presents with subcutaneous masses; biopsy may show spargana with characteristic cestode features, including channel-rich matrix and calcareous bodies
- Angiostrongyliasis: May also present with eosinophilic meningitis; larvae are longer and lack spines
- Cutaneous larva migrans: Presents with superficial epidermal or near epidermal tracts with distinctive larvae

(Left) *Eggs are excreted in feces of definitive hosts and hatch in environment. Larvae develop in intermediate hosts but cannot complete their life cycle in humans, leading to aberrant migration.* **(Right)** *A horizontal erythematous chord ⇨ is present in the right posterior lower back of this patient, characteristic of migrating nodular cellulitis of cutaneous gnathostomiasis. Note a healing biopsy scar ➡, which corresponds to a pseudofuruncle developed after initiating treatment and which yielded an L3 larva diagnostic of gnathostomiasis.*

***Gnathostoma* spp. Life Cycle**

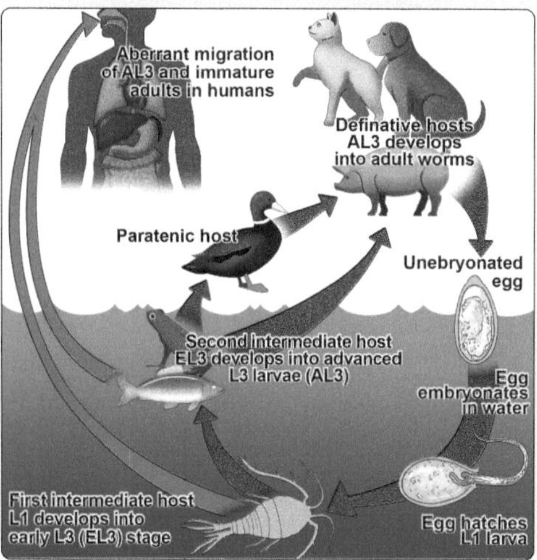

Migratory Cellulitis of Cutaneous Gnathostomiasis

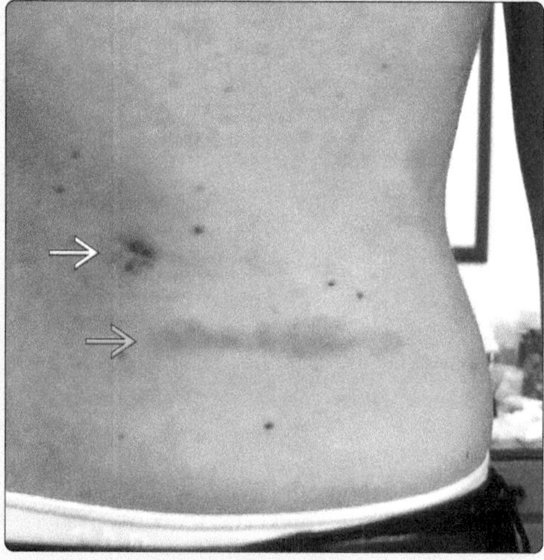

(Left) *Intact L3 larvae ⇨ of Gnathostoma spp. is labeled with numbers corresponding to histologic sections (CM = coelomic muscle; CS = cervical sacs; CU = cuticle; E = esophagus, H = hooklets, I = intestine; LC = lateral cords; RO = reproductive organs; S = spines). A cephalic segment shows 4 characteristic rows of hooklets ➡.* **(Right)** *Cross section of an L3 larvae shows spines in tegument ➡, large lateral chords ⇨, and pigmented intestine ➡.*

Gross and Microscopic Features of *Gnathostoma* spp. L3 Larva

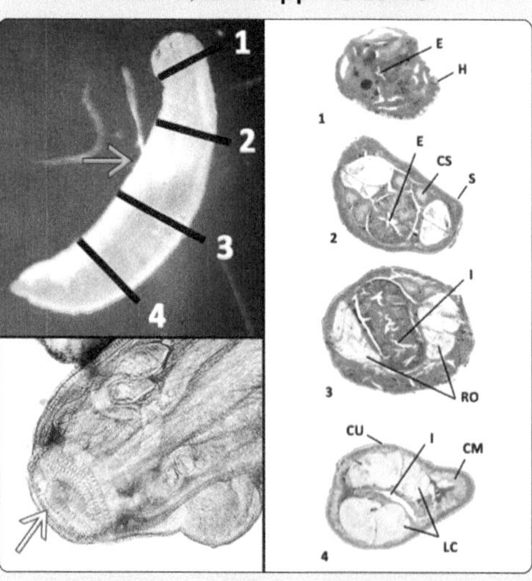

***Gnathostoma* spp. in Tissue**

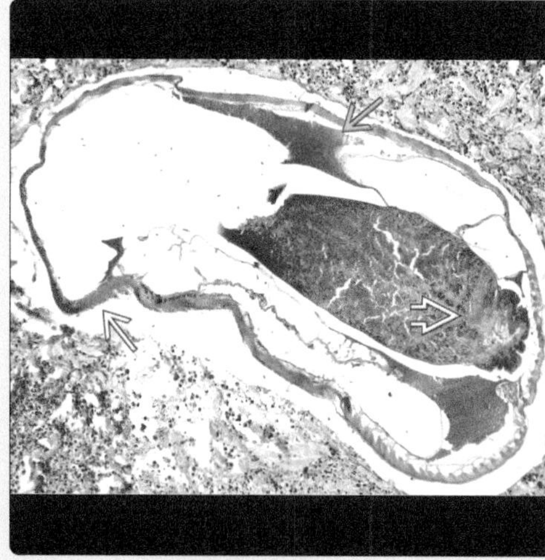

TERMINOLOGY

Synonyms

- Larva migrans profunda

Definitions

- Greek: "Gnathos" (jaw) + "stoma" (mouth)

ETIOLOGY/PATHOGENESIS

Infectious Agents

- Food-borne zoonotic infection caused by advanced 3rd-stage larvae (AL3) of spiruroid nematodes *Gnathostoma* spp.
- Most commonly acquired by ingesting raw or poorly cooked fresh water fish; chicken, snake, loach, and frog meat are other potential sources (incubation period: 3-4 weeks)
- Eggs excreted by host (e.g., carnivorous/omnivorous mammals) into environment where they hatch; larvae are ingested by copepod 1st intermediate host, molt twice, then ingested by 2nd intermediate host (e.g., fish, amphibians) where they develop into AL3 larvae
- AL3 larvae release lytic molecules, including cysteine proteases and matrix metalloproteinases to facilitate migration and penetration into organs
- 5 of 12 spp. of genus are known to infect humans (but do not reach full maturity): *G. binucleatum*, *G. doloresi*, *G. hispidum*, *G. nipponicum*, *G. spinigerum*

CLINICAL ISSUES

Epidemiology

- Endemic in Southeast Asia, Japan, China, Africa, Mexico, and South America
- ~ 5,000 cases reported worldwide

Presentation

- Cutaneous gnathostomiasis is most common form and presents with nodular migratory panniculitis
- Visceral gnathostomiasis caused by invasion of stomach, lungs, urinary bladder, eye, ear, and CNS

Laboratory Tests

- Blood/CSF eosinophilia
- Serologic testing performed in Thailand or Japan (not available in USA)

Treatment

- Surgical removal of larvae most effective treatment
- Several antiparasitic drugs have been used empirically, including thiabendazole, metronidazole, ivermectin, praziquantel, and diethylcarbamazine

Prognosis

- Patients with extracted or expelled larvae are cured
- Recurrences are common despite therapy with antiparasitic drugs if larvae not recovered
- Ocular, otic, and CNS involvement have worse prognosis with permanent sequelae

MACROSCOPIC

General Features

- L3 stage larvae: ~ 3.5-4.0 mm long and have prominent cephalic bulb with 4 rows of hooklets
- Numerous nondenticulated (single-pointed) cuticular spines are characteristic

MICROSCOPIC

Histologic Features

- Given migratory nature of larvae, capture in biopsies is extremely difficult, and, thus, nonspecific findings are present in many cases
- Presence of eosinophilic cellulitis &/or panniculitis, necroinflammatory tracts with prominent eosinophilic debris or "flame figures" should be interpreted as presumptive evidence in appropriate clinical context
- When captured on biopsy, cross sections of *Gnathostoma* spp. may show cuticular spines, coelomyarian musculature, prominent esophagus, &/or large lateral chords
- *Gnathostoma* spp. have been differentiated from each other by number of nuclei and morphologic features in intestinal cells, but lack of genomic studies makes their taxonomy controversial
- Dark granular pigment and prominent microvillous border in intestinal cells and RBCs within lumen are also helpful features

DIFFERENTIAL DIAGNOSIS

Sparganosis

- Sparganosis presents with subcutaneous masses; biopsy may show spargana with characteristic cestode features, including channel-rich matrix and calcareous bodies

Angiostrongyliasis

- Neuroangiostrongyliasis may also present with eosinophilic meningitis; larvae are longer and lack spines

Cutaneous Larva Migrans

- Caused by so-called hookworms (e.g., *Necator americanus*, *Ancylostoma duodenale*, among others)
- Tends to be more superficial, producing better demarcated cutaneous tracts in which larvae may be found and localized to epidermis or superficial dermis

SELECTED REFERENCES

1. Kongwattananon W et al: Intracameral gnathostomiasis: a case report and literature review. Ocul Immunol Inflamm. 1-5, 2022
2. Makino T et al: Cutaneous gnathostomiasis caused by Gnathostoma spinigerum. Br J Dermatol. 186(5):e198-9, 2022
3. Duong CM et al: Atypical gnathostomiasis-confirmed cutaneous larva migrans, Vietnam. BMJ Case Rep. 14(7), 2021
4. Thiangtrongjit T et al: Proteomics of gnathostomiasis: a way forward for diagnosis and treatment development. Pathogens. 10(9), 2021
5. Liu GH et al: Human gnathostomiasis: a neglected food-borne zoonosis. Parasit Vectors. 13(1):616, 2020
6. Schimmel J et al: An autochthonous case of gnathostomiasis in the United States. JAAD Case Rep. 6(4):337-8, 2020
7. Bravo F et al: Gnathostomiasis: an emerging infectious disease relevant to all dermatologists. An Bras Dermatol. 93(2):172-80, 2018
8. Laga AC et al: Cutaneous gnathostomiasis: report of 6 cases with emphasis on histopathological demonstration of the larva. J Am Acad Dermatol. 68(2):301-5, 2013
9. Ramirez-Avila L et al: Eosinophilic meningitis due to Angiostrongylus and Gnathostoma species. Clin Infect Dis. 48(3):322-7, 2009

Human Filariasis

KEY FACTS

ETIOLOGY/PATHOGENESIS

- Infection with filarial nematodes (i.e., *Wuchereria bancrofti*, *Brugia* spp., *Loa loa*, *Mansonella* spp., *Onchocerca volvulus*, and *Dirofilaria* spp.) spread by mosquitoes/flies

CLINICAL ISSUES

- Infections vary geographically due to reservoirs and vectors; rarely seen in travelers spending short periods of time in endemic regions
- Microfilariae evaluation in blood smears facilitates speciation; diagnostic yield increased at night for *W. bancrofti* and *Brugia* spp.
- Treated with surgery or anthelminthic drugs and good prognosis if recognized and treated early

MICROSCOPIC

- Intact male and female adult filariae can be seen in lymphatics, skin nodules, or pleural fluid; speciation may be difficult on worm cross section, especially if worm is dead
- Cross sections show smooth cuticle, few coelomyarian muscle cells, small intestinal lumen, and (in females) paired uterine tubes with eggs and developing microfilariae
- Microfilariae appear as coiled structures; presence or absence of sheath and pattern of nuclei in tails are main features used to distinguish various spp.
- Granulomatous reaction around dead and dying filariae, which may be calcified and lamellated

TOP DIFFERENTIAL DIAGNOSES

- Bacterial/fungal lymphadenitis: Organisms on Gram/GMS
- Edema secondary to nephrotic syndrome, congestive heart failure, cirrhosis
- Hydrocele: Loose connective tissue with mesothelial lining
- Malignancy of scrotum, testis, or kidney: Presence of neoplastic cells
- Nonfilarial elephantiasis: Reaction to mineral components rather than worms

Filariasis: Life Cycle

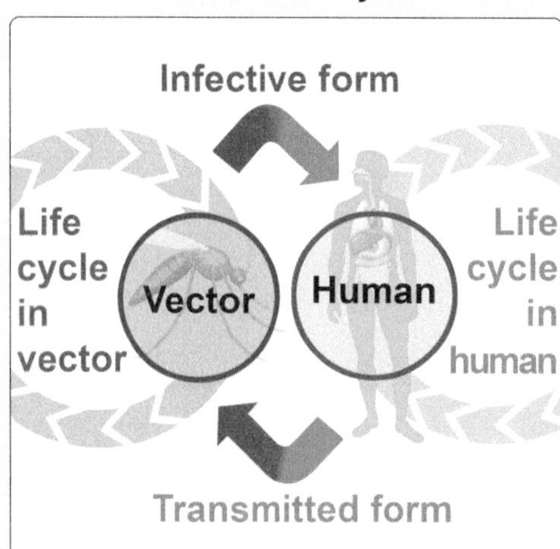

Mosquito With *Wuchereria bancrofti* Larva

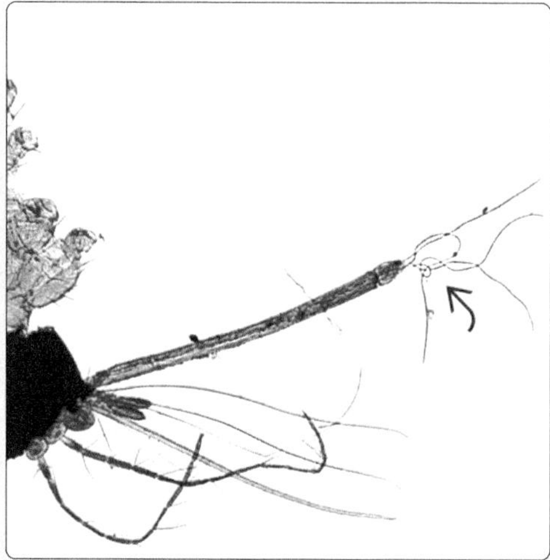

(Left) *Mosquitos and other biting insects inject 3rd-stage larvae into humans, which mature to adults and reside in lymphatics, leading to inflammation. Microfilaria are released, which can cause direct damage in some species and are ingested by biting insects to continue the life cycle.* **(Right)** *The 2nd stage of Wuchereria bancrofti larva is seen emerging from a mosquito stinger ➘. (Courtesy Franz von Lichtenberg Collection of Infectious Disease Pathology, BWH.)*

Lymphatic Filariasis

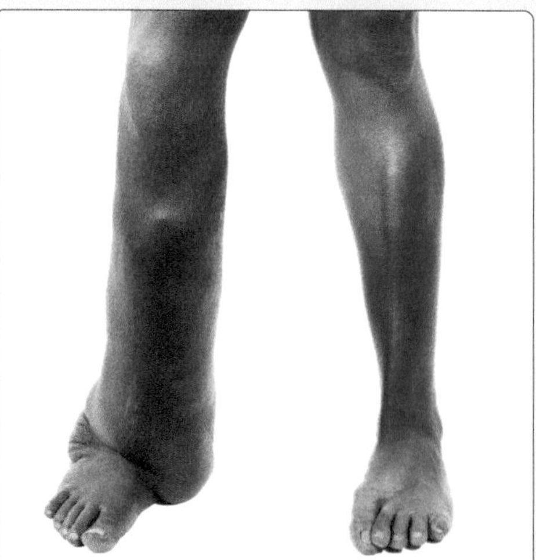

Lymphatic Filariasis Tissue Section

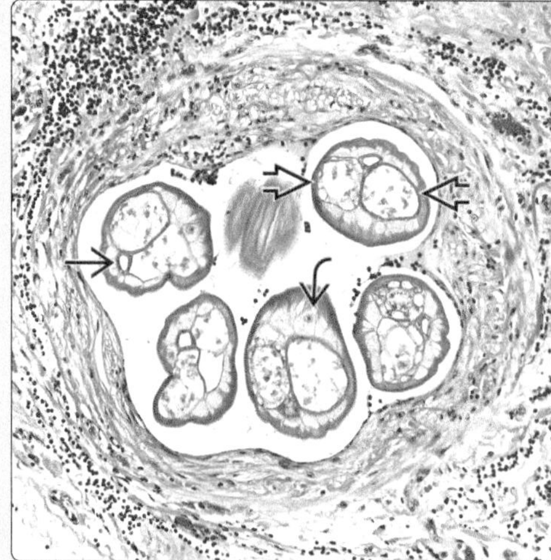

(Left) *Lymphatic filariasis, also referred to as "elephantiasis," results from edema caused by lymphatic damage due to nematode infection. (Courtesy R. Craig, CDC/PHIL.)* **(Right)** *This section of a neck mass in an 11-year old child shows multiple sections of a filarial nematode in the perinodal lymphatic space, surrounded by chronic inflammation and giant cell reaction. Identifiable features include intestine ➙, paired uterine tubes with developing microfilariae ➙, and broad muscle cells ➘.*

TERMINOLOGY

Definitions

- Latin: "Filum" (thread)
- *Wuchereria* from Otto Wucherer (German physician)
- *Brugia* from S. L. Brug (Dutch parasitologist)
- *Mansonella* from Sir Patrick Manson (English tropical medicine expert)
- *Loa* from word for "worm"
- *Dirofilaria* from "dīrus" (fearful; ominous)

ETIOLOGY/PATHOGENESIS

Infectious Agents

- Infectious disease caused by thread-like roundworms of *Filarioidea* superfamily
- Adult worms reside in lymphatics, peritoneal/pleural cavity, or subcutaneous tissue and cause symptoms through inflammation, tissue damage, and edema
- Adults produce microfilariae, which migrate to blood, are taken up by vector in blood meal, develop into L3 larvae, and are transmitted back into human host via blood meal through bite wound
- Lymphatic filariasis (elephantiasis) caused by *Wuchereria bancrofti*, *Brugia malayi*, and *Brugia timori*, transmitted by *Anopheles* (Africa), *Culex* (Americas), *Aedes*, and *Mansonia* (Pacific and Asia) mosquitos
- Subcutaneous filariasis caused by *Loa loa* (African eye worm; transmitted by *Chrysops* spp., day-biting flies), *Mansonella streptocerca* (transmitted by *Culicoides* spp., midges), and *Onchocerca volvulus* (transmitted by *Simulium* spp., blackflies)
- Serous cavity filariasis caused by *Mansonella perstans* (transmitted by midges) and *Mansonella ozzardi* (transmitted by midges and blackflies)
- *Dirofilaria immitis* (dog heartworm) dying worms lodge in lung vessels and cause infarcts; *Dirofilaria repens*/*Dirofilaria tenuis* manifest as wandering worms in subcutaneous tissue/conjunctiva or as granulomatous nodules

CLINICAL ISSUES

Epidemiology

- *W. bancrofti*, (> 90% of cases; sub-Saharan Africa, Southeast Asia, India, Pacific Islands, South America, Caribbean, *B. malayi* (China, India, Southeast Asia), *B. timori* (Timor)
  - 120 million infected worldwide (2/3 in Asia), 15 million of those infected have lymphedema of lower limbs, 25 million men have genital disease
  - 1st acquired in childhood, parasite burden increases over time spent in endemic areas
  - Mosquito not very effective at transmission; therefore, rarely seen in travelers spending short amounts of time in endemic regions
  - WHO has ranked disease as one of world's leading causes of permanent and longterm disability
- *L. loa* (West and Central Africa)
  - > 15 million infected; 20-40% in endemic areas report past history of eye worm
- *M. streptocerca* (Africa), *M. perstans* (sub-Saharan Africa and parts of Central and South America), *Mansonella ozzardi* (Central and South America)
  - > 100 million infected worldwide with gross underestimation due to asymptomatic/mild disease
- *D. immitis* (dogs in North and South America, Australia, Japan and Europe): Rare cause of human disease

Presentation

- *Wuchereria bancrofti* and *Brugia* spp.
  - Majority are asymptomatic but may have subclinical lymphatic and renal disease
  - Acute: Fever, lymphadenopathy (genital and axillary), orchitis/epididymitis, lymphedema of limbs &/or genitals
  - Chronic: Irreversible lymphedema
  - Florid eosinophilia found in peripheral blood counts; can present as tropical pulmonary eosinophilia
- *L. loa*
  - Calabar swellings: Localized, nontender swellings on arms and legs
  - Eye worm: Visible movement of adult worm across surface of eye with minimal damage
- *Mansonella* spp.
  - *M. perstans*/*M. ozzardi* cause body cavity filariasis: Calabar-like swellings, eosinophilia, abdominal pain, fever, headache, pruritus
  - *M. streptocerca* causes cutaneous nodules
- *Dirofilaria* spp.
  - Most pulmonary lesions diagnosed from biopsies of coin lesions

Laboratory Tests

- Antigen detection: Circulating filarial antigen can be detected using monoclonal antibodies raised against related spp. of nematodes
- Antibody detection: Can be used but may have overlapping cross reactivity with other nematodes
- Peripheral blood (also pleural fluid, CSF): Eosinophilia; microfilariae detection/speciation (maximal yield depends on blood collection timing)
- Large-scale prevalence studies are carried out using PCR

Treatment

- Diethylcarbamazine, albendazole, ivermectin, doxycycline, citronella essential oil
- Surgical excision of hydroceles may be option in some cases

Prognosis

- Chronic lymphedema is irreversible
- Good prognosis if recognized and treated early
- Secondary bacterial infection is common complication

IMAGING

Radiographic Findings

- Testicular ultrasound may show movement of echogenic particles, classically termed filarial dance
- Chest x-ray: "Coin lesion" (can be multiple) with *D. immitis*

MICROBIOLOGY

Parasite Features

- *W. bancrofti*
  - Adults are long and thread-like; females are 80-100 mm x 0.24-0.30 mm, and males are 40 mm x 1 mm; found predominantly in lymphatic vessels

  - Microfilariae (240-300 μm x 7.5-10 μm) are sheathed with gently curved body, tapered tail, and loosely packed nuclear column that does not extent to tail; circulate in blood and exhibit nocturnal periodicity
- *Brugia* spp.
  - *B. malayi* adult females are 43-55 mm x 130-170 μm, and males are 13-23 mm x 70-80 μm
  - *B. malayi* microfilariae (175-230 μm x 5-7 μm) are sheathed with tapered tails and gap between terminal and subterminal nuclei; circulate in blood and exhibit nocturnal periodicity
  - *B. timori* microfilariae (310 μm long) are sheathed and differentiated from *B. malayi* by longer cephalic space and sheath that does not stain with Giemsa; circulate in blood and exhibit nocturnal periodicity
- *L. loa*
  - Adult females are 40-70 mm x 45-60 μm, and males are 30-34 mm x 35-40 μm; exterior of cuticle contains irregularly spaced elevations (bosses); isolated from subconjunctiva
  - Microfilariae (250-300 μm x 6-8 μm) are sheathed with tapered tail and nuclei that extend to tip of tail; circulate in blood and exhibit diurnal periodicity
- *Mansonella* spp.
  - *M. perstans* adult female are 70-80 mm x 120 μm, and males are 45 mm x 60 μm
  - *M. perstans* microfilariae (190-200 μm x 4.5 μm) are unsheathed with blunt tail and paired nuclei that extend to tip of tail; circulate in blood
  - *M. ozzardi* adults are small and slender; females are 49 mm x 150 μm, and males are 26 mm x 70 μm
  - *M. ozzardi* microfilariae (160-205 μm) are unsheathed with pointed tail and single row of nuclei that end before tail; circulate in blood and rarely found in skin
  - *M. streptocerca* adult females are 27 mm x 50-85 μm, and males are 50 μm in diameter
  - *M. streptocerca* microfilariae (180-240 μm x 3-5 μm) are unsheathed with single row of nuclei that extend to end of tail; found in skin but can reach peripheral blood
- *Dirofilaria* spp.
  - *D. immitis* adult females are 230-310 mm x 350 μm, and males are 120-190 mm x 300 μm wide; found in heart; die and lodge in pulmonary arteries
  - *D. repens* adult females are 100-170 mm x 460-650 μm, and males are 50-70 mm x 370-450 μm
  - *D. tenuis* adult females are 80-130 mm x 260-360 μm, and males are 40-50 mm x 190-260 μm

Culture

- There is no role for culture in diagnosis of filarial worms

MICROSCOPIC

Histologic Features

- Intact male and female adult filariae can be seen in lymphatics, skin nodules, or pleural fluid; speciation may be difficult on worm cross section, especially if worm is dead
- Cross sections are up to 180 μm in diameter for females and exhibit smooth cuticle, few coelomyarian muscle cells, small intestinal lumen, and paired uterine tubes with eggs and developing microfilariae
- Microfilariae are diagnostic form, which may appear as coiled structures; presence or absence of sheath and pattern of nuclei in tails are main features used to distinguish various spp.
- Granulomatous reaction around dead and dying filariae, which may be calcified and lamellated
- Acute lymphangitis, chronic lymphatic dilatation/fibrosis, polypoid endolymphangitis, or eosinophilic lymphadenitis (Meyers-Kouwenaar syndrome) may be present

ANCILLARY TESTS

Histochemistry

- Microfilarial morphology is better appreciated with Giemsa stain

DIFFERENTIAL DIAGNOSIS

Bacterial or Fungal Lymphadenitis

- Presence of bacteria on Gram or silver stain; presence of fungal forms on silver stain

Edema Secondary to Nephrotic Syndrome, Congestive Heart Failure, Cirrhosis

- Correlation with clinical history

Hydrocele

- Diagnosed with transillumination
- Microscopically seen as loose connective tissue with mesothelial lining
- Chronic hydrocele may have inflammation and fibrosis

Malignancy of Scrotum, Testis, or Kidney

- Clinical correlation, serum tumor markers, histologic diagnosis

Nonfilarial Elephantiasis (Podoconiosis)

- Ascending and asymmetric
- Can begin as foot pain, plantar edema, and rigidity of toes
- Rarely involves groin
- Not caused by filarial reaction; rather, caused by reaction to mineral components in volcanic clay

Nonfilarial Lymphedema (Milroy Disease)

- Edema with dilated lymphatic spaces
- Lower limb edema present at birth or develops in early infancy

Onchocerciasis (*Onchocerca volvulus*)

- *Onchocerca* microfilaria are unsheathed with nuclei that do not extend to tip of pointed tail

SELECTED REFERENCES

1. Bottieau E et al: Human filariasis in travelers and migrants: a retrospective 25-year analysis at the Institute of Tropical Medicine, Antwerp, Belgium. Clin Infect Dis. 74(11):1972-8, 2022
2. Mischlinger J et al: Diagnostic performance of capillary and venous blood samples in the detection of Loa loa and Mansonella perstans microfilaraemia using light microscopy. PLoS Negl Trop Dis. 15(8):e0009623, 2021
3. Prasoon D et al: Wuchereria bancrofti and cytology: a retrospective analysis of 110 cases from an endemic area. J Cytol. 37(4):182-8, 2020
4. Mathison BA et al: Diagnostic identification and differentiation of microfilariae. J Clin Microbiol. 57(10), 2019
5. Flieder DB et al: Pulmonary dirofilariasis: a clinicopathologic study of 41 lesions in 39 patients. Hum Pathol. 30(3):251-6, 1999

Mansonella perstans Microfilaria

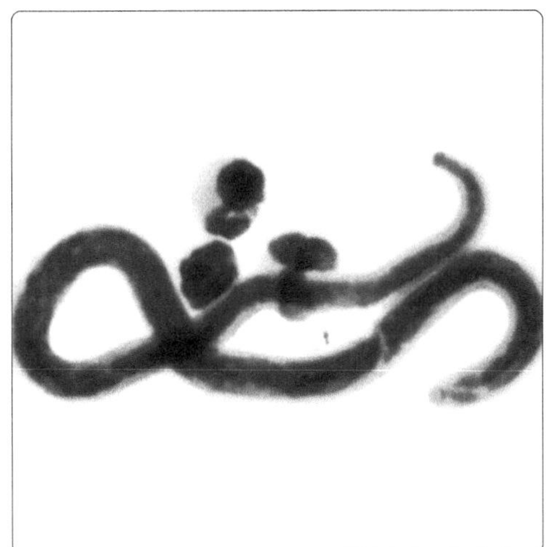

Brugia malayi Microfilaria

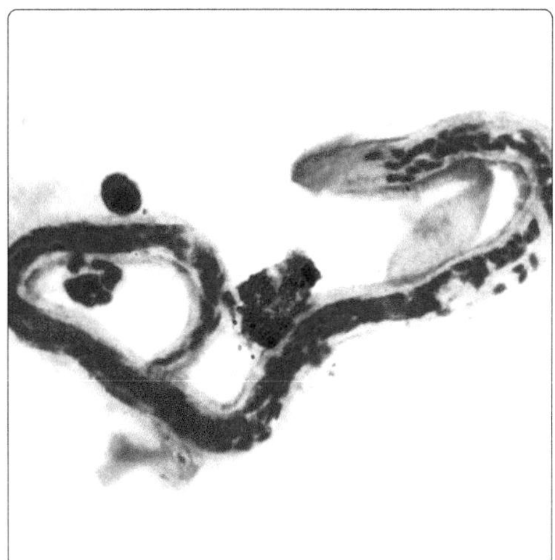

(Left) *This image of a blood smear shows an unsheathed microfilaria with a blunt tail and paired nuclei that extend to tip of the tail, features consistent with Mansonella perstans. (Courtesy M. Melvin, CDC/PHIL.)* **(Right)** *This image of a blood smear shows a sheathed microfilaria with a tapered tail and a gap between terminal and subterminal nuclei, features consistent with Brugia malayi. (Courtesy M. Melvin, CDC/PHIL.)*

Microfilariae in Kidney

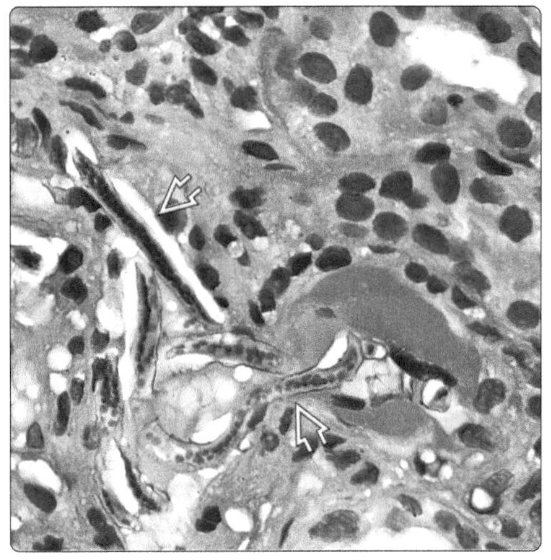

Dirofilaria immitis in Pulmonary Vessel

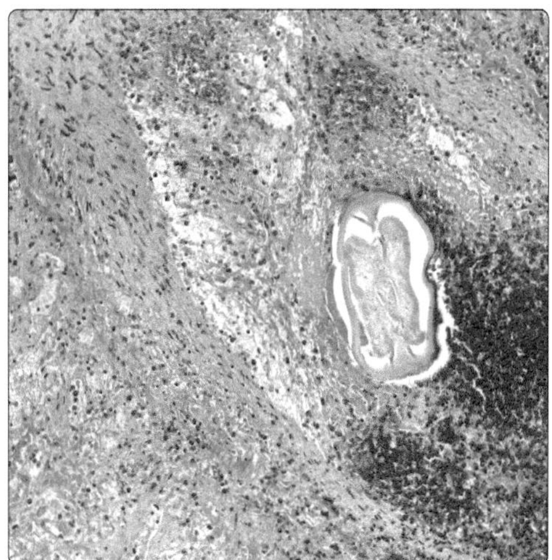

(Left) *Curved and elongated sections of microfilariae are shown within the arteriolar lumen of a glomerulus. Note the column of nuclei ➡ throughout the central portion of the microfilariae. (From DP: Kidney Diseases.)* **(Right)** *High-power view shows the larva of Dirofilaria immitis surrounded by necrotic material within a large pulmonary vessel. The salient feature of D. immitis here is the presence of a thick cuticle. (From DP: Thoracic.)*

Wuchereria bancrofti in Spermatic Cord

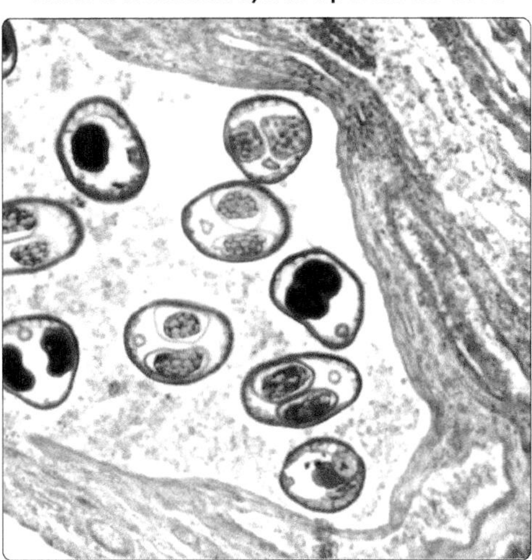

Calcified *Wuchereria bancrofti*

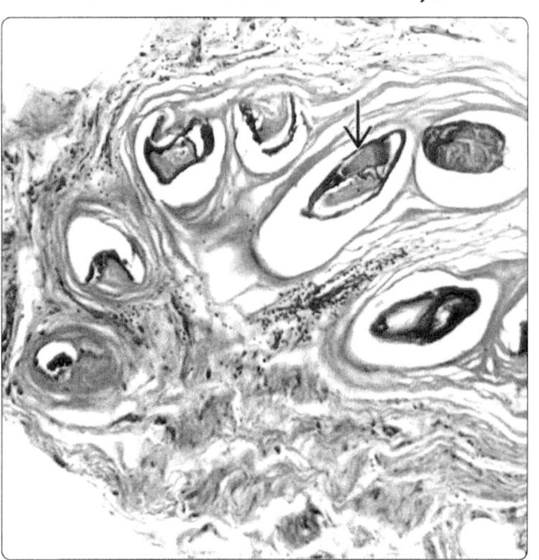

(Left) *Cross sections of dilated spermatic cord lymph vessels demonstrate male W. bancrofti. Note the lack of microfilaria. (Courtesy Franz von Lichtenberg Collection of Infectious Disease Pathology, BWH.)* **(Right)** *Pelvic lymphatics contain calcified W. bancrofti. Note the paired uteri remnants ➡. (Courtesy Franz von Lichtenberg Collection of Infectious Disease Pathology, BWH.)*

KEY FACTS

ETIOLOGY/PATHOGENESIS

- Nematode infection with *Onchocerca* spp., transmitted by blackflies (genus *Simulium)*

CLINICAL ISSUES

- Diffuse dermatitis with intense pruritus, ulceration, and bleeding followed by hypopigmented or atrophic skin lesions
- Subcutaneous nodules (onchocercoma)
- One of leading causes of blindness in developing world
- Laboratory tests: Amplification of *Onchocerca volvulus* parasite DNA from skin snips
- Ivermectin: Kills microfilaria and prevents blindness

MICROSCOPIC

- Skin: Hyperkeratosis, acanthosis, elongated rete ridges of epidermis, dermal edema, chronic lymphocytic and eosinophilic inflammation, and dilated lymphatics
- Microfilariae of (5-9 µm wide, 220-360 µm long) have have small nuclei that do not extend to tip of tail
- Onchocercoma: Fibrotic nodules formed by bundles of adult worms encased by lymphocytes and macrophages
- Adult worm has external ridges on longitudinal sectioning with 2 underlying striae per ridge
- Unsheathed microfilaria seen on skin snips or touch preps

TOP DIFFERENTIAL DIAGNOSES

- *Mansonella streptocerca*: Smaller microfilariae with nuclei extending to tail
- *Dirofilaria immitis*: Forms nodules (usually in lung) with no microfilariae
- Food allergies and vitamin A deficiency: Diffuse dermatitis mimicking onchocerciasis
- Tumors: Biopsy lacks microfilariae and shows tumor cells
- Inflammatory or reactive (subcutaneous nodules): Granulomatous, panniculitis, systemic vasculitis

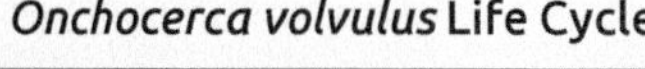

***Onchocerca volvulus* Life Cycle**

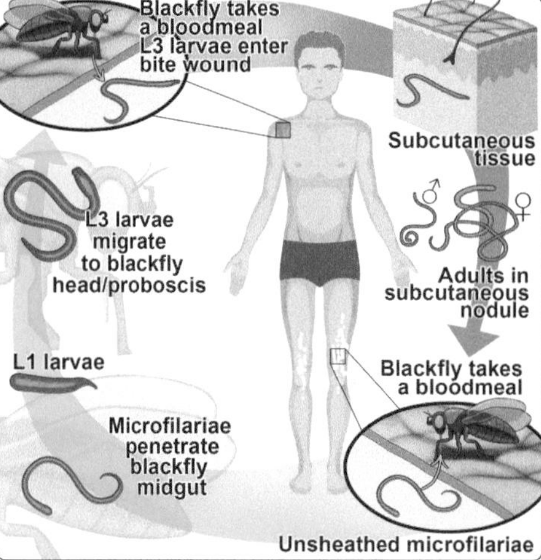

Filarial Skin Rash

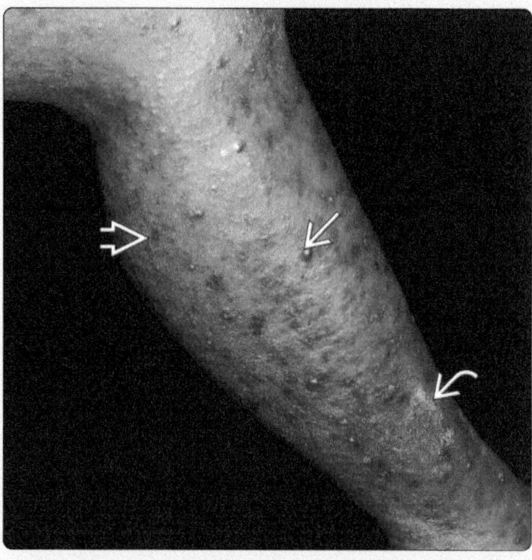

(Left) *Larvae enter skin during a blackfly bloodmeal and develop into adult filariae, which reside in subcutaneous tissue nodules. Microfilariae are typically found in skin and lymphatics, can be ingested by a blackfly during a bloodmeal, and develop through larval stages.* **(Right)** *Numerous hyperpigmented papules, lichenified plaques, and nodules diffusely involve the lower leg of a patient who recently returned from Africa. (From DP: Nonneoplastic Derm.)*

Onchocercal Nodule (Onchocercoma)

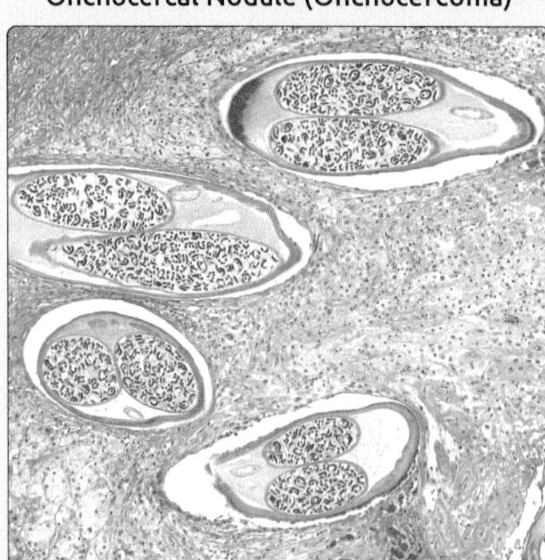

***Onchocerca volvulus* Microfilariae**

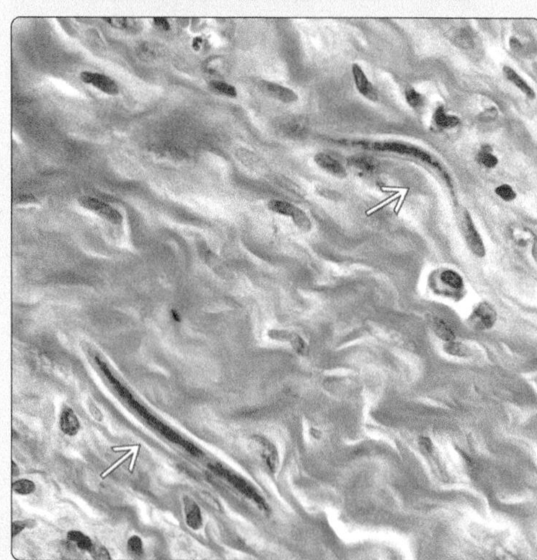

(Left) *This section of a mass-forming subcutaneous nodule shows multiple cross sections of an adult female Onchocerca volvulus containing numerous microfilariae within the uterus, surrounded by marked granulomatous inflammation.* **(Right)** *This section shows 2 microfilariae, which are unsheathed and contain small nuclei that do not extend to the tip of the pointed tail.*

TERMINOLOGY

Synonyms

- River blindness

Definitions

- From Greek terms, "onkos" (barbed) + "kerkos" (tail)

ETIOLOGY/PATHOGENESIS

Infectious Agents

- Nematode infection with *Onchocerca* spp., transmitted by blackflies (genus *Simulium*), which inhabit shores of rapidly flowing streams
- *Onchocerca volvulus* has 5-stage life cycle; humans are sole definitive host, and blackfly acts as obligate intermediate host
- Larva develops into adult female worm and sheds hundreds of microfilariae that migrate into skin and eyes of host
- Most symptoms of onchocerciasis are caused by bodily response to dead or dying larvae
- *Onchocerca lupi*: Extremely rare infection (reported in USA)

CLINICAL ISSUES

Epidemiology

- 25 million people are infected with *O. volvulus* worldwide
- Common in Africa, Middle East, and South/Central America

Presentation

- One of leading causes of blindness (estimated to affect 1.15 million), 2nd most important cause of infectious blindness worldwide after trachoma
- Skin: Acute stage with diffuse dermatitis with intense pruritus, ulceration, and bleeding followed by chronic stage with hypopigmented "leopard skin" or atrophic "lizard skin"
  - May also present as unilateral papular eruption with focal involvement (known as "sowda" in Yemen/Sudan)
  - Subcutaneous nodules over bony prominences of torso and hips in African cases and on head and shoulders in South American cases (onchocercoma)
- Ocular: Photophobia, conjunctivitis, and blindness
- Systemic: Fatigue, fever, and femoral/inguinal lymphadenitis
- Nodding syndrome: emerging evidence this is neuroinflammatory disorder caused by antibodies to *O. volvulus* cross reacting with neuron proteins

Laboratory Tests

- Serology, PCR, ELISA, and skin snip test
- Ocular infection can be diagnosed with slit-lamp examination of anterior part of eye where larvae are visible
- Amplification of *O. volvulus* parasite DNA from skin snips

Treatment

- No vaccine to prevent infection with *O. volvulus*
- Ivermectin: Kills microfilaria and prevents blindness
- Doxycycline: May sterilize female adults

Prognosis

- Chronic recurrent inflammation of eyes can lead to blindness

MICROBIOLOGY

General Features

- Adult females: 33-50 cm long, 270-400 μm in diameter; produce microfilariae for ~ 9 years
- Adult males: 1.9-4.2 cm long, 130-210 μm in diameter
- Microfilariae: 220-360 μm long, 5-9 μm in diameter, and unsheathed; 2-year life span

MICROSCOPIC

Histologic Features

- Skin: Hyperkeratosis, acanthosis, elongated rete ridges of epidermis, dermal edema, chronic lymphocytic and eosinophilic inflammation, and dilated lymphatics
  - Microfilariae of *O. volvulus* (5-9 μm wide, 220-360 μm long) have long anterior cephalic space (7-13 μm long) and nuclei that are adjacent to each other, while posterior end (9-15 μm long) has long caudal space that tapers to fine point
- Onchocercoma: Fibrotic nodules formed by bundles of adult worms encased by lymphocytes and macrophages
  - Adult worm has external ridges on longitudinal sectioning with 2 underlying striae per ridge

Cytologic Features

- Unsheathed microfilaria seen on skin snips or touch preps

DIFFERENTIAL DIAGNOSIS

Other Human Filariasis

- *Mansonella streptocerca*: Microfilariae are smaller in diameter (2.5-4.0 μm), contain shorter cephalic space coiled in shepherd's crook configuration and blunt tail with terminal round nuclei
- *Dirofilaria immitis*: Forms nodules (usually in lung) with no microfilariae

Food Allergies and Vitamin A Deficiency

- Can cause diffuse dermatitis mimicking onchocerciasis
- Careful clinical history and absence of organism easily differentiate from onchocerciasis

Tumors (Mesenchymal, Metastatic)

- Biopsy lacks microfilariae and shows tumor cells

Inflammatory or Reactive (Subcutaneous Nodules)

- Granulomatous: Rheumatoid arthritis, juvenile rheumatoid arthritis
- Panniculitis: Erythema nodosum, nodular panniculitis
- Systemic vasculitis: Polyarteritis nodosum, granulomatosis with polyangiitis

SELECTED REFERENCES

1. Tirados I et al: Vector control and entomological capacity for onchocerciasis elimination. Trends Parasitol. 38(7):591-604, 2022
2. Johnson TP et al: The pathogenesis of nodding syndrome. Annu Rev Pathol. 15:395-417, 2020
3. Mathison BA et al: Diagnostic identification and differentiation of microfilariae. J Clin Microbiol. 57(10), 2019
4. Unnasch TR et al: Diagnostics for onchocerciasis in the era of elimination. Int Health. 10(suppl_1):i20-6, 2018
5. Cantey PT et al: The emergence of zoonotic Onchocerca lupi Infection in the United States--a case-series. Clin Infect Dis. 62(6):778-83, 2016
6. Udall DN: Recent updates on onchocerciasis: diagnosis and treatment. Clin Infect Dis. 44(1):53-60, 2007

Strongyloidiasis

KEY FACTS

ETIOLOGY/PATHOGENESIS

- Infectious disease caused by *Strongyloides stercoralis*, intestinal nematode that infects humans through contact with soil that contains larvae

CLINICAL ISSUES

- Common in tropics, subtropics, and warm regions; affects ~ 30-100 million people worldwide
- Presence of rhabditiform larvae in stool examination is diagnostic (gold standard)
- Frequently asymptomatic; however, hyperinfection syndrome and disseminated strongyloidiasis occur in immunosuppressed patients

ENDOSCOPY

- Worms are not visualized during endoscopy due to small size of adults and localization within cells of small intestinal crypts but may produce discrete lesions (red, raised lesions), which are biopsied for diagnosis

CYTOPATHOLOGY

- Larvae can be seen by simple wet mount in fluid from bronchoalveolar lavage (BAL) or in other body fluids during hyperinfection

MICROSCOPIC

- Duodenal or jejunal biopsy may show no inflammatory reaction, eosinophilic microabscess, mixed cellular infiltrate of acute and chronic inflammation, or granulomatous inflammation to dead worms
- Adult females, eggs, rhabditiform larvae, and filarial larvae may be seen in small intestine

TOP DIFFERENTIAL DIAGNOSES

- Schistosomiasis (Katayama fever), amebiasis, balantidiasis, or infections by *Ancylostoma duodenale* or *Necator americanus*
- Ulcerative colitis and polyarteritis nodosa

***Strongyloides* Life Cycle**

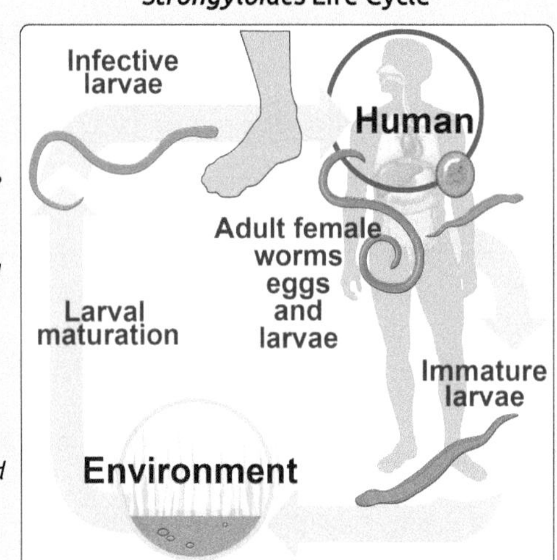

Filariform Larvae (L3)

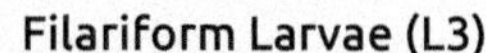

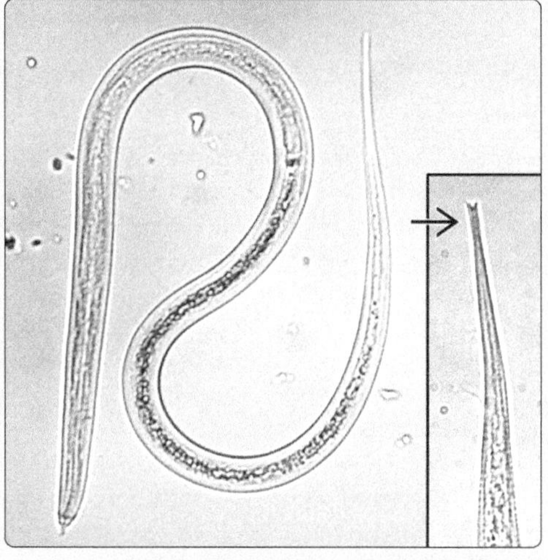

(Left) *Filariform larvae penetrate human skin. Adult worms lay eggs, which hatch quickly to produce rhabditiform larvae seen in stool. These larvae can mature and reinfect host directly, mature in the environment and replicate independent of a host, or mature and infect a new host.* **(Right)** *Strongyloides stercoralis filariform larvae have a 1:1 esophagus:intestine ratio and a forked tail ⇒, compared to shorter esophagus and pointed tail of hookworm filarial larvae. (Courtesy M. Melvin, PhD, CDC/PHIL.)*

Bronchoalveolar Lavage

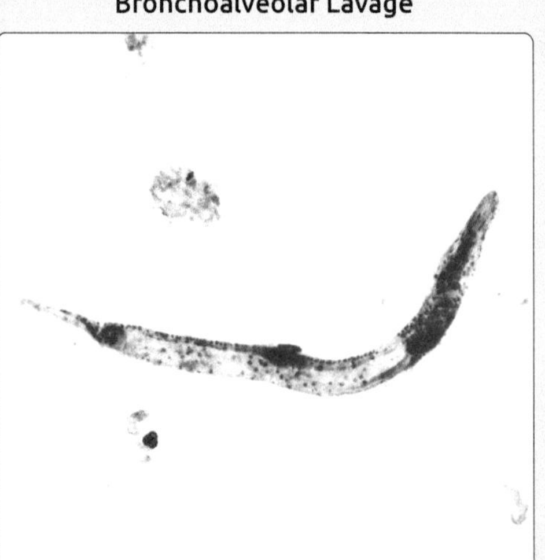

Intestinal Strongyloidiasis

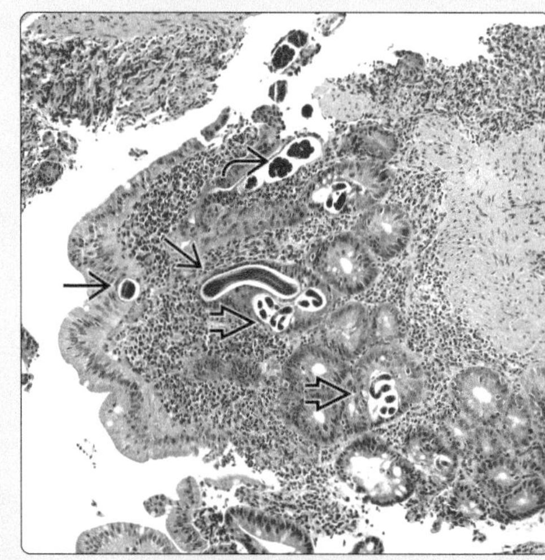

(Left) *Strongyloides larvae can be identified in bronchoalveolar lavage specimens from hyperinfected patients.* **(Right)** *Biopsy of small intestine shows numerous intraepithelial eggs ⇒, rhabditiform larvae ⇒, and sections of adult female S. stercoralis ⇒.*

TERMINOLOGY

Definitions

- From Greek terms, "strongylos" (round) + "eidos" (form)

ETIOLOGY/PATHOGENESIS

Infectious Agents

- Infectious disease caused predominantly by *Strongyloides stercoralis*, intestinal nematode that infects humans through contact with soil that contains larvae
- Zoonotic *Strongyloides fuelleborni* subspecies *fuelleborni* and *S. fuelleborni* subspecies *kellyi* are rare causes of human infection
- Filariform larvae directly penetrate skin, migrate via bloodstream/lungs and other routes to small intestine, where they mature and reside as adult females, which produce eggs via parthenogenesis, which hatch rhabditiform larvae
- Rhabditiform larvae can mature into filariform larvae in humans causing autoinfection

CLINICAL ISSUES

Epidemiology

- Common in tropics, subtropics, and warm regions; affects 30-100 million people worldwide

Presentation

- Frequently asymptomatic
- Acute infection shows cutaneous reaction "ground itch" as larvae penetrate skin, most commonly in foot
- Chronic infection larvae can migrate intradermally, which results in intense itchy red tracts, usually in perianal area
    - Larvae migration can cause respiratory symptoms
    - Loeffler syndrome: Fever, dyspnea, wheeze, pulmonary infiltrates with blood eosinophilia may be seen (rare)
    - Migration of larvae to gastrointestinal system can cause abdominal pain, diarrhea, vomiting, and anorexia
    - Up to 75% of people with chronic form have mild peripheral eosinophilia or elevated IgE levels
    - Upper thighs with larva migration (larvae currens) are pathognomic for strongyloidiasis
- Hyperinfection syndrome and disseminated strongyloidiasis occur in immunosuppressed patients
    - Infection with human T-cell leukemia/lymphoma virus type I (HTLV-I) is also major risk factor for *Strongyloides* hyperinfection syndrome, along with organ transplant and prolonged steroid therapy
    - Serologic testing prior to start of steroid therapy is strongly suggested for any patient with remote risk

Laboratory Tests

- Gold standard for diagnosis: Serial stool examination; presence of rhabditiform larvae is diagnostic
- Stool concentration techniques, such as Baermann technique and modified agar plate method, can be used to improve sensitivity
- Duodenal aspirates for identification of organisms
- Serologic testing for antibodies
    - For patients with potential exposure who are being placed on immunosuppression, serology should be used to determine pretreatment requirements
- Diagnostic sensitivity of qPCR is similar to conventional parasitology methods

Treatment

- Ivermectin or albendazole
- Moxidectin is veterinary antiparasitic drug that has FDA approval for treatment of human onchocerciasis and is in line for clinical trials in strongyloidiasis
- Apart from antiparasitic treatment, key management of complicated strongyloidiasis is restoring host immunity

Prognosis

- Acute symptomatic disease resolves with treatment
- Chronic disease with dissemination and immunosuppression (hyperinfection) has 80% mortality

MICROBIOLOGY

Parasite Characteristics

- Parasitic adult female worms are 2-3 mm long x 30-40 μm in diameter; free-living females 1 mm long
    - Long cylindrical esophagus in anterior 1/3 of body cavity
    - Intestine and reproductive organs posterior 2/3
- Parasitic adult male worms do not exist; free-living male worms measure up to 0.75 mm long
- Eggs are 50-60 μm x 30-40 μm
    - *S. stercoralis* eggs hatch in epithelium and absent in stool
    - *S. fuelleborni* eggs routinely shed in stool
- Rhabditiform larvae (L1) are 180-400 μm long x 15-20 μm in diameter and have short buccal canal, rhabditoid esophagus extending 1/3 of body length, and prominent genital primordium
- Filariform larvae (L3) are 500-600 μm long x 15-20 μm in diameter and have esophagus:intestine ratio of 1:1 and notched tail

MACROSCOPIC

Endoscopic Features

- Because of small size of adults and larvae, as well as localization within cells of small intestinal crypts, worms are not visualized during endoscopy but may produce discrete lesions (red, raised lesions), which are biopsied for diagnosis

MICROSCOPIC

Histologic Features

- Duodenal or jejunal biopsy may show no inflammatory reaction, eosinophilic microabscess, mixed cellular infiltrate of acute and chronic inflammation, or granulomatous inflammation to dead worms
- Hyperinfection: Larvae may be found in many tissues and fluids, including sputum, bronchial washings, cerebrospinal fluid, skin, and urine
- Adult females (30-40 μm in diameter) are present within small intestine submucosa; transverse sections show esophagus (anterior) or collapsed intestine with ovary or uterus often containing eggs (posterior)
- Oval embryonated eggs (60 μm in length) with thin shells are present in epithelium adjacent to adult females and rapidly hatch rhabditoid larvae (20 μm in diameter), which typically show intestine in transverse sections

- Filariform larvae (20 μm in diameter) show esophagus or intestine in transverse sections and double lateral alae (not always observed)

Cytologic Features

- Larvae can be seen by simple wet mount in fluid from bronchoalveolar lavage (BAL) or in other body fluids during hyperinfection

DIFFERENTIAL DIAGNOSIS

Other Parasitic Conditions

- Schistosomiasis (Katayama fever), amebiasis, balantidiasis, or infections by *Ancylostoma duodenale* or *Necator americanus*
- *Trichinella spiralis* larvae are more minute and primitive in structure; generally not seen in intestinal mucosa
- *Capillaria philippinensis* contains stichosome; eggs in uterus and adjacent tissue has distinctive morphologic features, including plugs
- Negative biopsy &/or serology/stool exam can differentiate strongyloidiasis from other parasitic infections

Ulcerative Colitis

- Mimics *Strongyloides* colitis, but obtaining travel and residence history is important
- Biopsy shows absence of larva or eggs with low eosinophilic infiltrates

Polyarteritis Nodosa

- Involvement of capillaries and venules in addition to arteriolar involvement seen in polyarteritis nodosa is major point of distinction

SELECTED REFERENCES

1. Luvira V et al: Strongyloides stercoralis: a neglected but fatal parasite. Trop Med Infect Dis. 7(10):310, 2022
2. Campo-Polanco LF et al: Strongyloidiasis in humans: diagnostic efficacy of four conventional methods and real-time polymerase chain reaction. Rev Soc Bras Med Trop. 51(4):493-502, 2018
3. Mendes T et al: Strongyloidiasis current status with emphasis in diagnosis and drug research. J Parasitol Res. 2017:5056314, 2017
4. Beknazarova M et al: Strongyloidiasis: a disease of socioeconomic disadvantage. Int J Environ Res Public Health. 13(5), 2016

Eggs

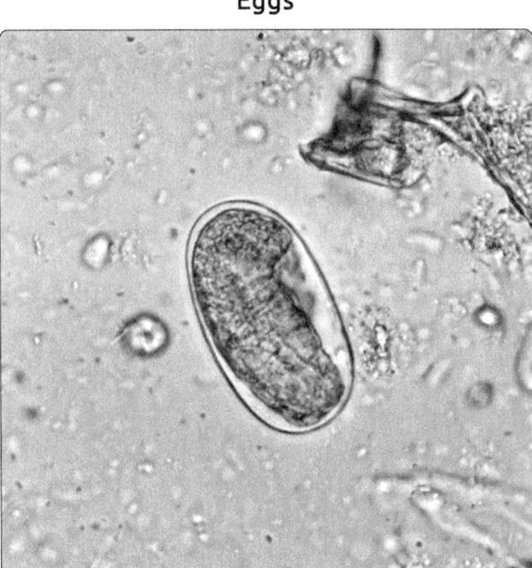

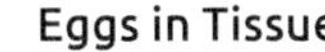

Eggs in Tissue

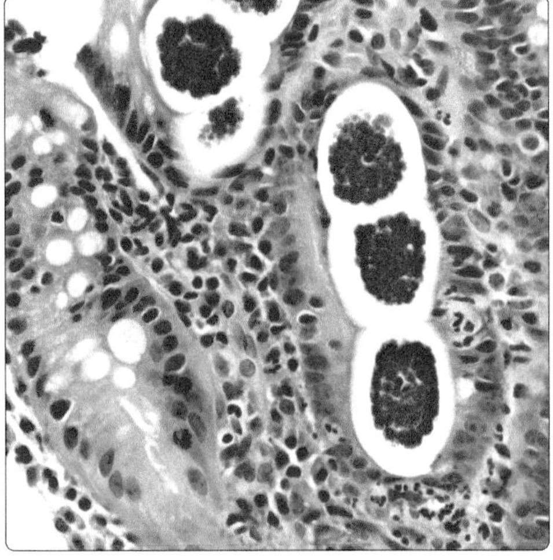

(Left) *Unlike S. stercoralis, Strongyloides fulleborni eggs are excreted in stool and are characterized by oval shape, thin shell, and presence of developing larvae. (Courtesy CDC/PHIL.)* **(Right)** *S. stercoralis eggs within the epithelium are up to 60 μm in length and contain a thin, barely visible shell.*

Rhabditiform Larvae (L1)

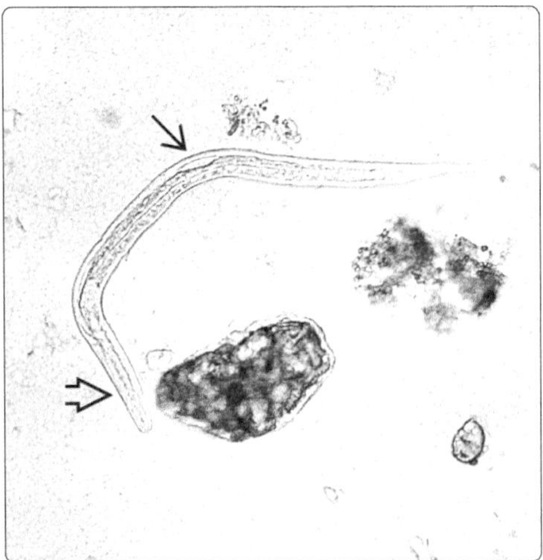

Rhabditiform Larvae in Tissue

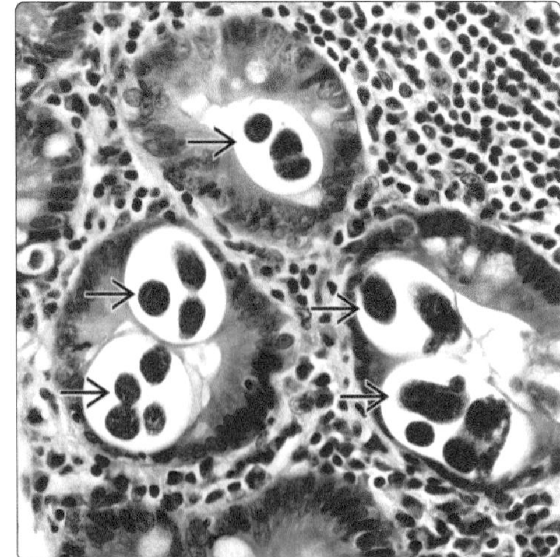

(Left) *S. stercoralis rhabditiform larvae are readily identified in stool by short buccal canal ➡, rhabditoid esophagus, and prominent genital primordium ⇨. (Courtesy M. Melvin, PhD, CDC/PHIL.)* **(Right)** *Transverse sections of rhabditiform larva ➡ are present within the epithelium of this small intestine biopsy.*

Filarial Larvae in Tissue

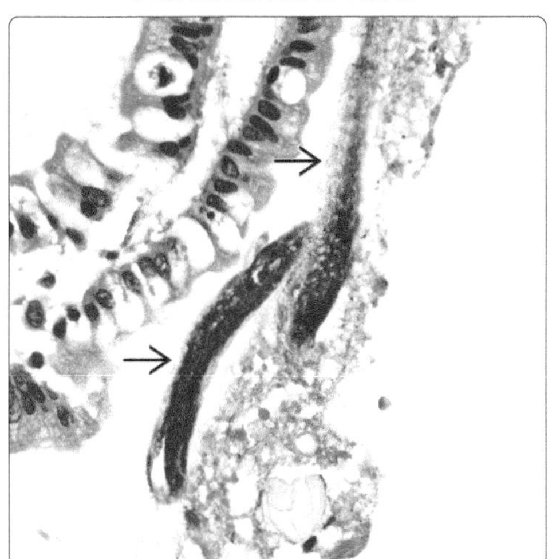

Adult Female in Tissue

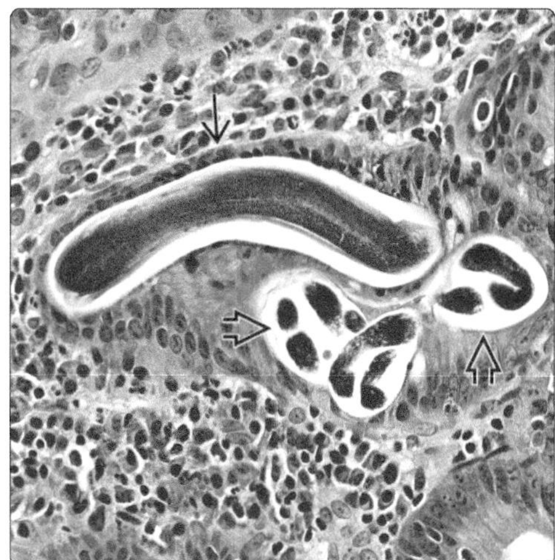

(Left) *This small intestine biopsy shows longitudinal sections of S. stercoralis filarial larva within the intestinal lumen* ➡. **(Right)** *A lateral section of an adult female S. stercoralis is present in this small intestine biopsy* ➡, *along with multiple rhabditiform larva* ⇨.

Transverse Sections of Adult Female

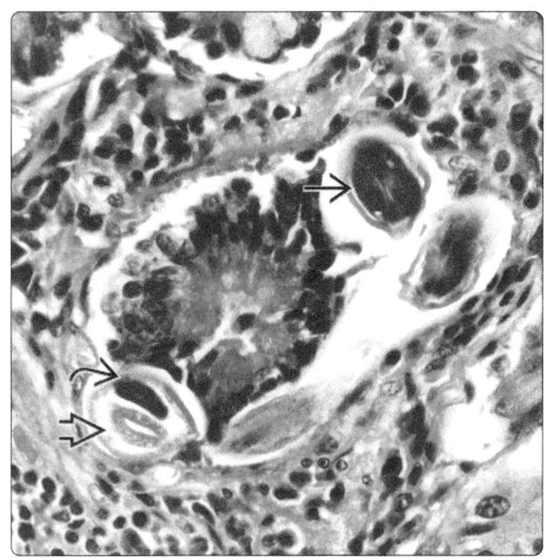

Transverse Sections of Adult Female

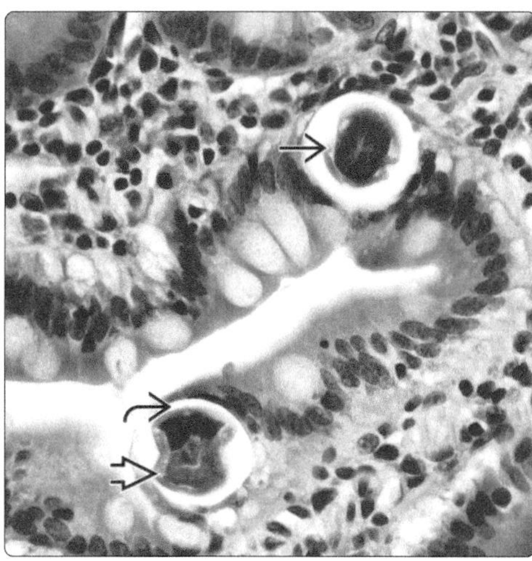

(Left) *Transverse sections of an adult female S. stercoralis in the small intestine submucosa show esophagus* ➡, *intestine* ⇨, *and ovary* ↗. **(Right)** *Transverse sections of an adult female S. stercoralis in the small intestine submucosa show esophagus* ➡, *intestine* ⇨, *and ovary* ↗.

Disseminated Strongyloidiasis Skin Lesion

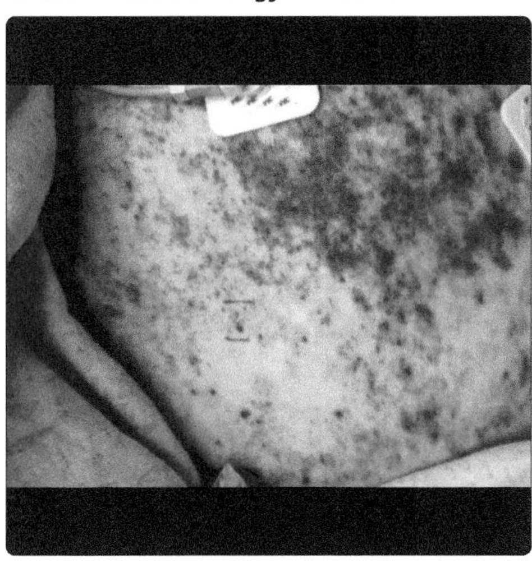

Disseminated Strongyloidiasis Skin Biopsy

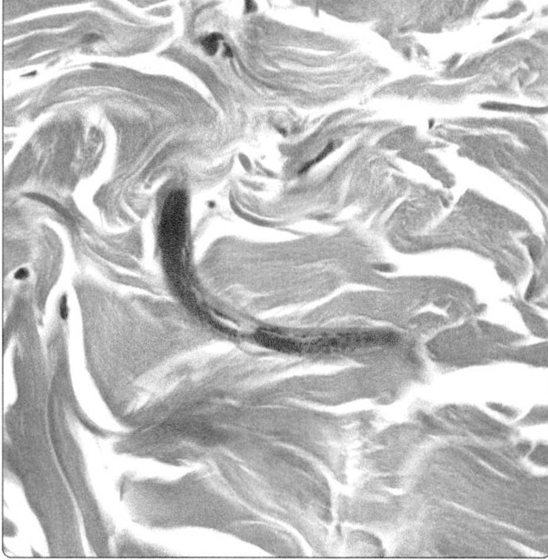

(Left) *Purpuric rashes can occur on the abdomen and thighs of immunocompromised individuals with disseminated strongyloidiasis due to vessel destruction.* **(Right)** *Punch biopsy of a skin lesion from an immunocompromised patient with disseminated strongyloidiasis shows scattered larva within the dermis.*

Trichuriasis

KEY FACTS

ETIOLOGY/PATHOGENESIS

- Soil transmitted nematode infection in setting of poor hygiene or lack of clean water
- Ingested eggs mature to adult worms and reside in colon

CLINICAL ISSUES

- Global prevalence of 17% with 800 million infections
- Worms are large and easily seen on endoscopy (single or multiple) but may mimic polyps (local inflammation)
- Heavy infestation in rectum leads to rectal prolapse
- Albendazole and mebendazole are 1st-line therapy

MICROBIOLOGY

- Eggs are barrel-shaped (50-55 x 20-25 μm), thick shelled, and possess pair of polar "plugs" at each end; unembryonated when passed in stool

MACROSCOPIC

- Worms visible (1.0-2.0 x 0.3-cm) adherent to mucosa ± colonic hyperemia and hyperplasia

MICROSCOPIC

- Colonic mucosa may show active colitis or hyperplasia of goblet cells (polyp-like hyperplasia)
- Narrow anterior head of worm contains stichosome and may be found between intestinal epithelial cells
- Posterior end of worm in lumen contains uterus with characteristic eggs (in females)
- Presence of spicule indicates specimen is male

TOP DIFFERENTIAL DIAGNOSES

- Hookworm infection: Attached directly to mucosa via cutting plates without burrowing, minimal inflammatory response
- Strongyloidiasis: Very small (not grossly visible) with raised red patches; microscopically shows collections of eosinophils with adult and larval forms within mucosal wall
- Capillariasis: Small nematode (< 5 mm) that produces eggs similar to *Trichuris* eggs and causes life-threatening, dysentery-like syndrome

Life Cycle of *Trichuris*

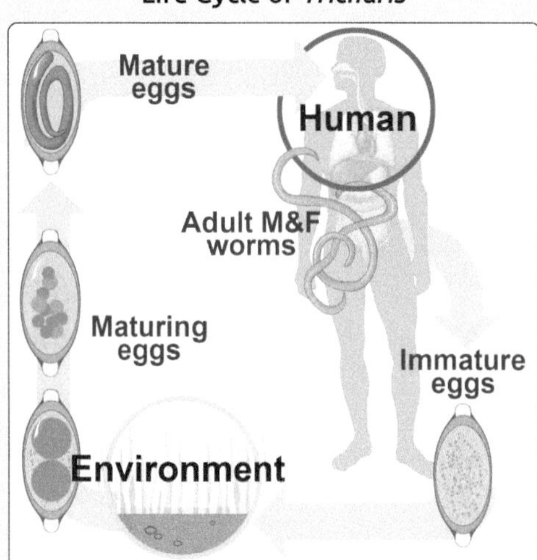

***Trichuris* Eggs: Stool**

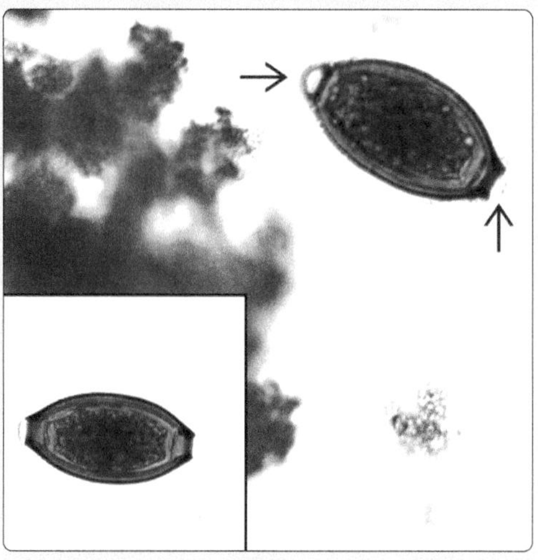

(Left) *Trichuris species has one of the simplest life cycles of the nematodes. Humans ingest mature eggs from the environment. Worms hatch in the intestine, and the adult worms live in the colon, producing eggs that are released into the stool. The eggs mature in the environment and are ingested.* **(Right)** *The eggs of the Trichuris species have a distinctive ovoid shape (rugby ball or American football) with bilateral mucus plugs ➙. They are only morphologically similar to the eggs in human infection capillariasis.*

***Trichuris* Eggs: Tissue Section**

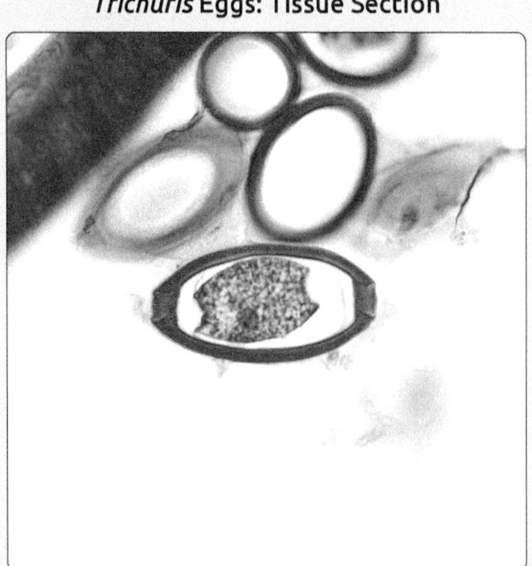

Adult *Trichuris* (Whipworm)

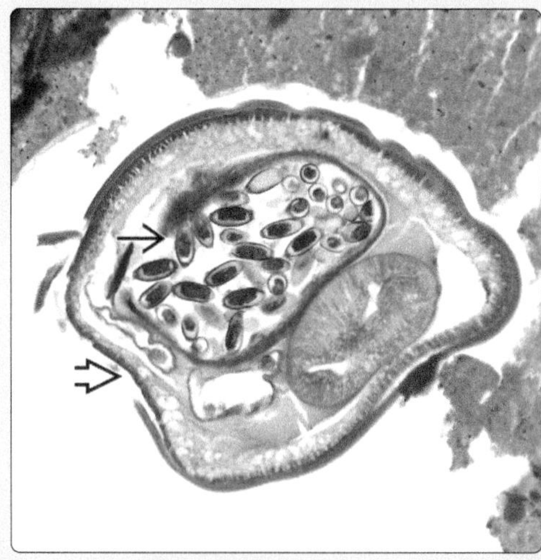

(Left) *Trichuris eggs can be identified in tissue sections by their characteristic ovoid shape and bilateral mucus plugs. However, eggs may appear circular and lack mucus plugs due to orientation and sectioning.* **(Right)** *Cross section from the posterior end of an adult female Trichuris worm shows a thick cuticle with annulations ⇨ with a thin underlying hypodermis and somatic muscle cells and numerous intrauterine eggs ➙.*

TERMINOLOGY

Synonyms

- Whipworm

Definitions

- Greek: "Tricho" (hair) + "oura" (tail)

ETIOLOGY/PATHOGENESIS

Infectious Agents

- Soil transmitted nematode infection with *Trichuris trichiura* via ingestion of eggs in setting of poor hygiene or lack of clean water
- Unembryonated eggs are excreted by host in stool where they mature to infective forms over 3-week period; ingested eggs hatch in small intestine, and worms mature and reside in colon
- Females lay up to 20,000 eggs per day (~ 65 days after infection), and adult worms survive in colon for 1 year
- Heavy infestation in rectum leads to rectal prolapse

CLINICAL ISSUES

Epidemiology

- Global prevalence: 17% with 800 million infections at any given time
- Specific community prevalence can be 30-40% and as high as 80% in subgroups (school-aged children)

Presentation

- Vast majority of patients are asymptomatic
- Symptomatic presentations include mild abdominal pain, rectal prolapse (young children), and dysentery-like syndrome with mucoid diarrhea, rectal prolapse, and anemia

Endoscopic Findings

- Adult worms are large and easily seen on endoscopy (single or multiple) but may mimic polyps (local inflammation)

Laboratory Tests

- Stool examination for ova and parasites reveals eggs
- In pregnant women and some other populations, anemia is related to intensity of egg burden

Treatment

- Albendazole and mebendazole are 1st-line therapy

Prognosis

- Chronic infection in childhood can lead to growth stunting and mental delays

MICROBIOLOGY

Parasite Features

- Adult males are 30-45 mm long with coiled posterior end, and females are 35-50 mm with straight posterior end; both have long, whip-like anterior end; reside in large intestine, cecum, and appendix
- Eggs are barrel-shaped (50-55 x 20-25 μm), thick shelled, and possess pair of polar "plugs" at each end; unembryonated when passed in stool

Culture

- No role in diagnosis of whipworm

MACROSCOPIC

Colonic Resection

- Either as rare indication or, more likely, when found incidentally, worms are visible as 1.0-2.0 x 0.3 cm white worms adherent to mucosa ± colonic hyperemia and hyperplasia

MICROSCOPIC

Histologic Features

- Sections from anterior end of adult worm shows stichosome with centrally located nucleus and subcuticle basal band; may be seen burrowed between intestinal epithelial cells
- Posterior sections of adult worms show thick cuticle with annulations, thin hypodermis, and layers of polymyarian muscle cells; presence of spicule indicates specimen is male; females are identified by egg-filled uterus
- Colonic mucosa may be benign or show active colitis or hyperplasia of goblet cells (polyp-like hyperplasia)

DIFFERENTIAL DIAGNOSIS

Hookworm Infection

- Attached directly to mucosa via cutting plates without burrowing, and they produce little (if any) inflammatory response

Strongyloidiasis

- Adults are very small (not grossly visible); produce raised red patches that microscopically show collections of eosinophils with adult and larval forms within mucosal wall (between intestinal epithelial cells)

Capillariasis

- Small nematode (< 5 mm) that produces eggs similar to *Trichuris* eggs and causes life-threatening, dysentery-like syndrome

SELECTED REFERENCES

1. Aiadsakun P et al: Comparison of the complete filtration method using an automated feces analyzer with three manual methods for stool examinations. J Microbiol Methods. 192:106394, 2022
2. Kupritz J et al: Helminth-induced human gastrointestinal dysbiosis: a systematic review and meta-analysis reveals insights into altered taxon diversity and microbial gradient collapse. mBio. 12(6):e0289021, 2021
3. Else KJ et al: Whipworm and roundworm infections. Nat Rev Dis Primers. 6(1):44, 2020
4. Gordon CA et al: Helminths, polyparasitism, and the gut microbiome in the Philippines. Int J Parasitol. 50(3):217-25, 2020
5. Ayana M et al: Comparison of four DNA extraction and three preservation protocols for the molecular detection and quantification of soil-transmitted helminths in stool. PLoS Negl Trop Dis. 13(10):e0007778, 2019
6. Mekonnen Z et al: Efficacy of different albendazole and mebendazole regimens against heavy-intensity Trichuris trichiura infections in school children, Jimma Town, Ethiopia. Pathog Glob Health. 107(4):207-9, 2013
7. Wang DD et al: Trichuriasis diagnosed by colonoscopy: case report and review of the literature spanning 22 years in mainland China. Int J Infect Dis. 17(11):e1073-5, 2013

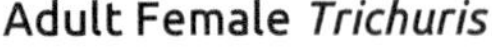

Adult Female *Trichuris*

Trichuris Worm in Colon

(Left) *This image of an adult female Trichuris trichiura measures 4 cm in length and demonstrates a wider posterior segment and narrower anterior segment reminiscent of a whip. (Courtesy M. Melvin, CDC/PHIL.)* (Right) *Multiple cross sections of the adult Trichuris worm ➔ are shown in the lumen or burrowed in intestinal cells. Note the lack of inflammatory response.*

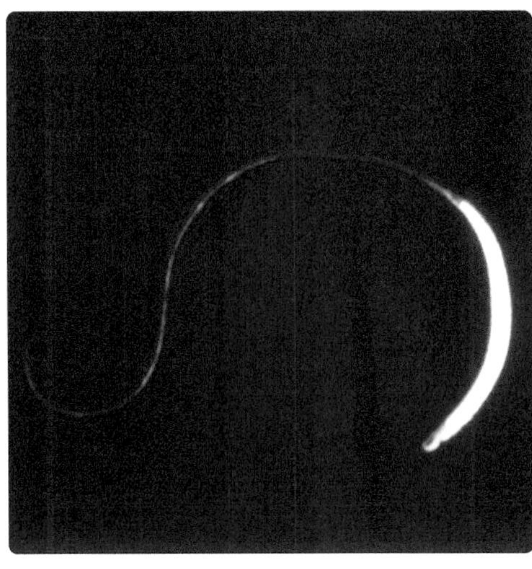

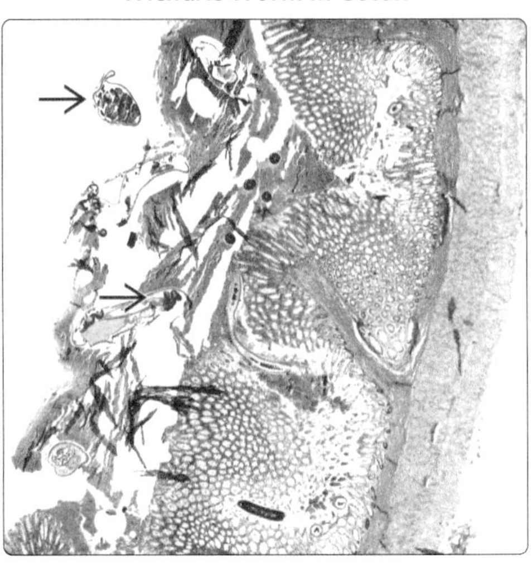

Trichuris Worm Embedding in Colon

Anterior Section and Eggs

(Left) *The long thin "head" ➔ of the Trichuris worm burrows in between intestinal epithelial cells, causing stimulation of nerves and the feeling of a full colon that leads to chronic pushing and prolapse.* (Right) *Scattered eggs ➔ are seen admixed with stool contents, adjacent to an anterior cross section of adult worm with bacillary band ➔.*

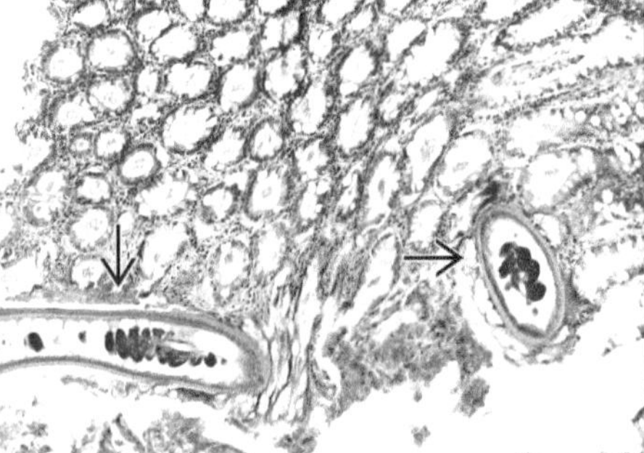

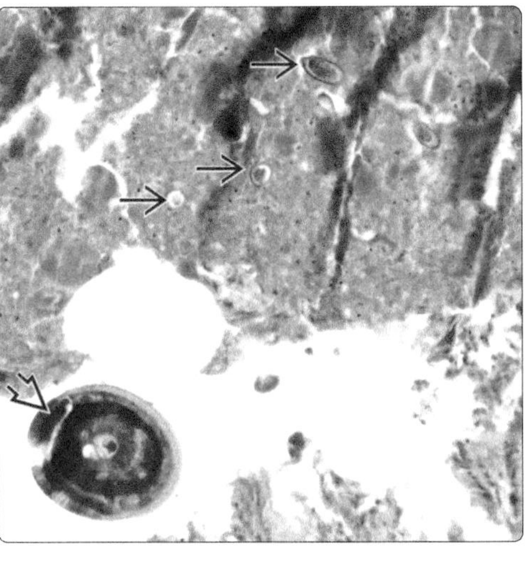

Longitudinal Anterior Section

Anterior Cross Section

(Left) *This longitudinal section of the anterior portion of an adult Trichuris worm shows stichocytes with a prominent nucleus ➔.* (Right) *This high-magnification image of a Trichuris worm anterior cross section shows a stichocyte ➔ with prominent nucleus.*

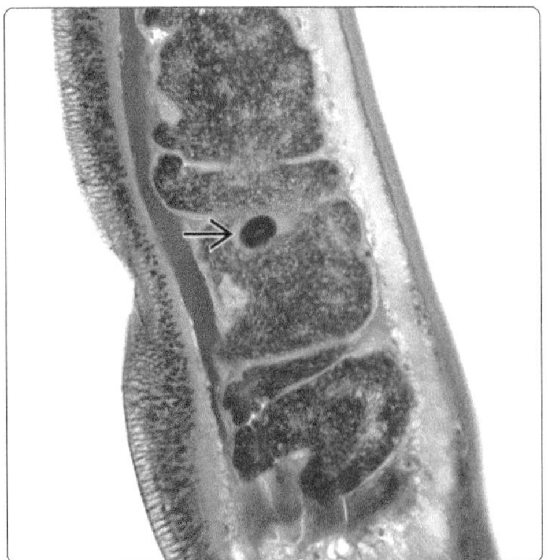

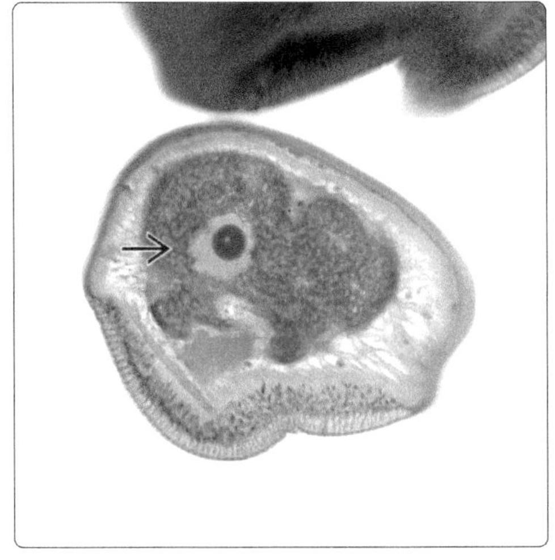

Anterior Sections

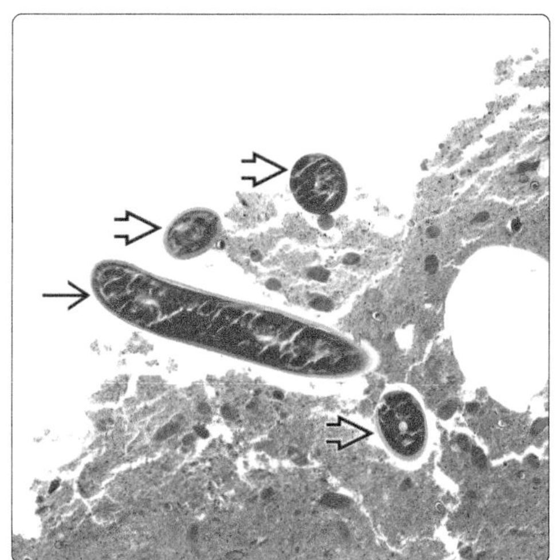

Longitudinal Section

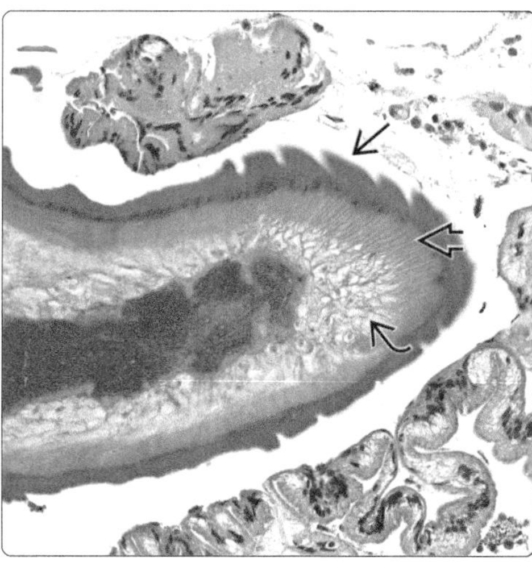

(Left) *A longitudinal section* ➔ *and multiple cross sections* ➩ *from the anterior portion of an adult Trichuris worm are present, admixed with stool content.* **(Right)** *A longitudinal section shows thick annulated cuticle* ➔*, a thin nucleate hypodermis* ➩*, and layers of polymyarian muscle cells* ➘*.*

Posterior Cross Section

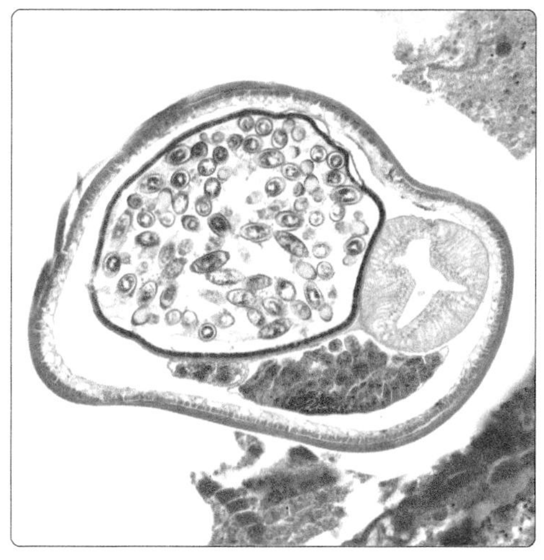

Posterior Longitudinal Section

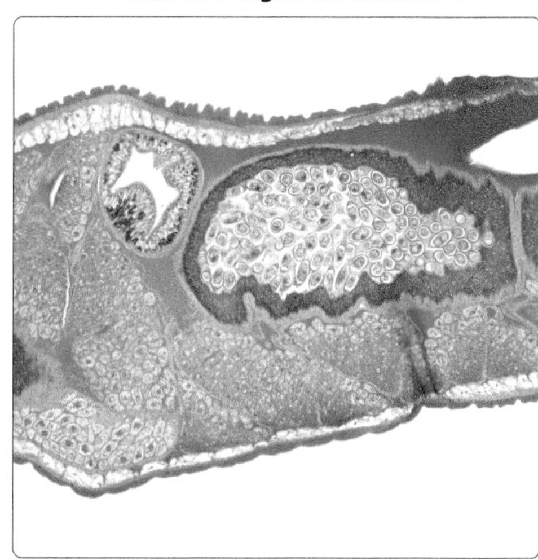

(Left) *This cross section through the wider posterior section of an adult female Trichuris worm shows a uterus containing numerous eggs. Up to 20,000 eggs per day may be shed.* **(Right)** *This longitudinal section through the posterior section of an adult female Trichuris worm shows a uterus containing numerous eggs.*

Intrauterine Eggs

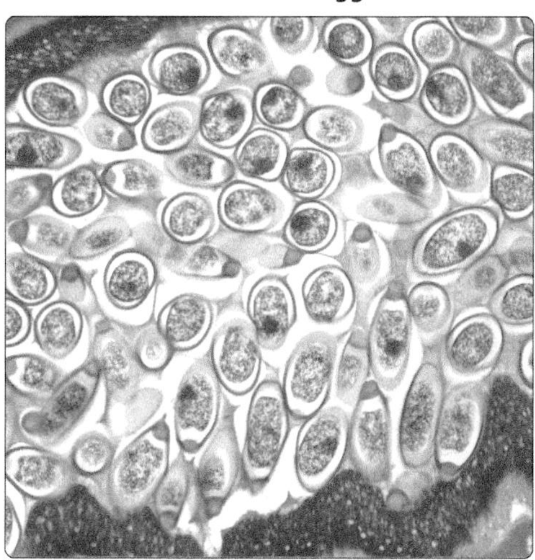

Intrauterine Eggs

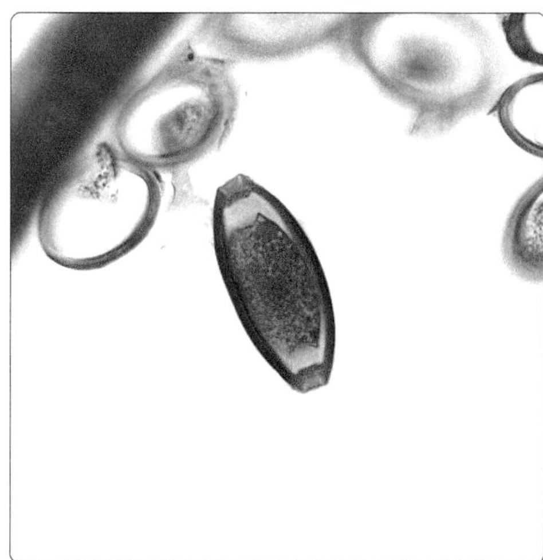

(Left) *Trichuris eggs in tissue sections can be oval or round and may exhibit 0, 1, or 2 mucus plugs, depending on the plane of section.* **(Right)** *The presence of eggs with characteristic barrel shape (50-55 x 20-25 µm) and bipolar plugs is very helpful in confirming the diagnosis of T. trichiura in tissue sections.*

KEY FACTS

ETIOLOGY/PATHOGENESIS

- Trichinellosis/trichinosis is parasitic zoonosis caused by *Trichinella* spp. via ingestion of undercooked meat
- Adult nematodes (roundworms) reside in intestinal tract; larvae encapsulate in muscle tissue and may persist for years before becoming calcified
- Worldwide distribution, outbreaks more common in regions of Eastern Europe and Southeast Asia
- *T. spiralis* infection associated with domestic pork consumption; sylvatic transmission of other species via wild game meats (wild boars, bear, hog, deer, moose, walrus)

CLINICAL ISSUES

- Suspicion of based on clinical symptoms, risk factors/epidemiology, and eosinophilia; confirmation via antibody detection &/or identification of encapsulated larvae in muscle tissue
- Serology useful for diagnosis; antibodies usually detectable 3-5 weeks post infection
- Clinical course divided between acute enteral (gastrointestinal symptoms) and systemic parental phases (allergic and inflammatory symptoms)
- Risk of neurotrichinellosis, myocarditis, heart failure, bronchopneumonia

MICROSCOPIC

- Visualization of intracellular encapsulated coiled larva (~ 1 mm in length) in striated muscle is diagnostic
- Cysts eventually undergo calcification and fibrosis

TOP DIFFERENTIAL DIAGNOSES

- Toxocariasis: Visceral and ocular larva migrans; invades multiple tissues, including skeletal muscle but does not encyst
- Anatrichosomiasis: Does not encyst; may be located in epithelium
- Haycocknemiasis: Extremely rare; adult females containing eggs present in muscle

(Left) *Ingestion of undercooked meat containing encysted Trichinella larvae results in maturation to adult worms that reside in the small intestine. New larvae are produced, which migrate to and encyst in skeletal muscle.* **(Right)** *Encysted ⇨ larvae of Trichinella spp. in this muscle section are variably associated with inflammation.*

Trichinella spp. Life Cycle

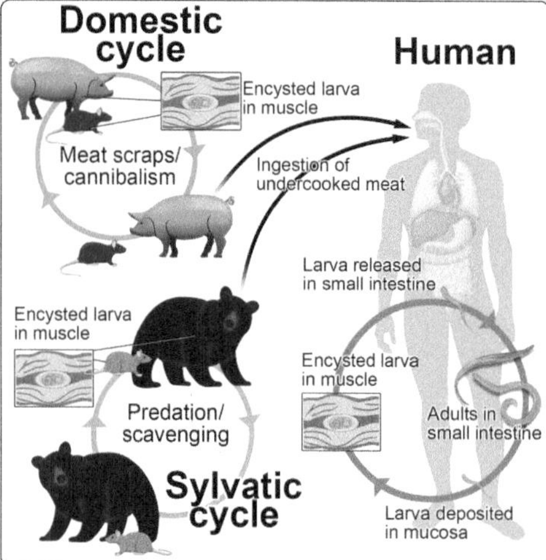

Striated Muscle With *Trichinella* spp. Larvae

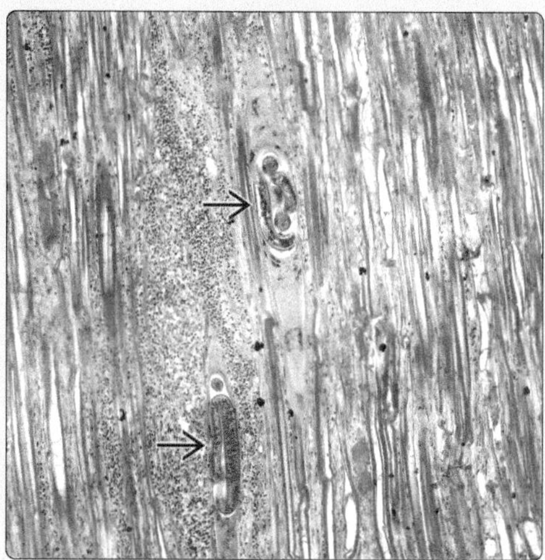

(Left) *Higher-magnification of encysted Trichinella larvae stained with hematoxylin and eosin shows a coiled larvae with stichosome ⇨ and surrounding nurse cell ⇨.* **(Right)** *This high-magnification image shows multiple cross sections as the coiled larva goes in and out of the plane of section.*

Encysted *Trichinella* spp. Larva

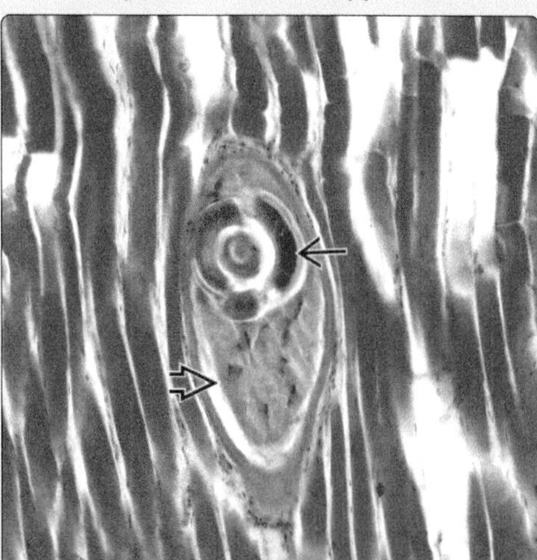

Cross Section of *Trichinella* spp. Larva

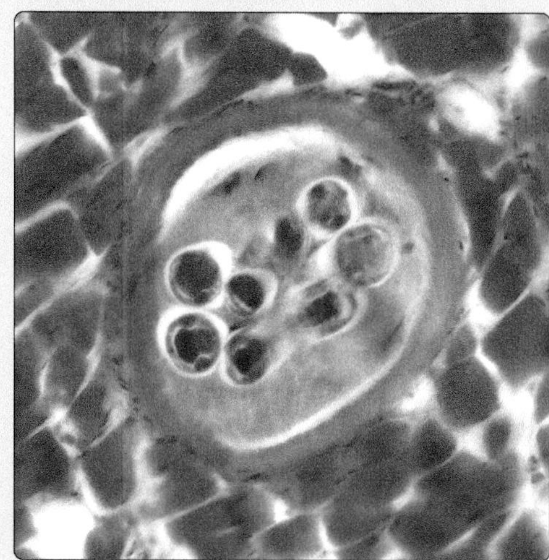

TERMINOLOGY

Definitions

- From Greek "tríkhinos" (of hair) and "ella" (dimutive); "spiralis" (spiral)

ETIOLOGY/PATHOGENESIS

Infectious Agents

- Zoonotic parasitic infection caused by nematodes of genus *Trichinella* via ingestion of undercooked meat containing encysted larvae
- *T. spiralis* (found worldwide in many carnivorous and omnivorous animals), *T. pseudospiralis* (mammals and birds worldwide), *T. nativa* (Arctic bears), *T. nelsoni* (African predators and scavengers), *T. britovi* (carnivores of Europe and western Asia), *T. papuae* (wild and domestic pigs of Papua New Guinea and Thailand)
- Prevention via adherence to hygienic practices when preparing wild game meats and cooking meats to recommended internal temperatures; *T. nativa* larvae (bear meat) are resistant to freezing

CLINICAL ISSUES

Epidemiology

- Estimated 10,000 cases occur worldwide annually
- Primarily affects adults; equal between men and women
- European region accounted for 87% of cases from 1990-1999 with 50% occurring in Romania; incidence in region ranged from 1.1-8.5 cases per 100,000 population

Presentation

- Lack of pathognomonic signs or symptoms; chronic disease difficult to diagnose
- Initial symptoms (days 2-7): Nausea, abdominal pain, anorexia, vomiting, diarrhea
- Systemic symptoms (days 9-28) due to larval migration into muscle tissues: Myalgias, weakness, fever, conjunctivitis, splinter hemorrhages, periorbital/facial edema, headaches
- Myositis peaks 5-6 weeks post infection and wanes as larva become encapsulated and calcified
- Elevated muscle enzymes; prolonged eosinophilia (degree of symptoms correlate with level of eosinophilia)
- Neurotrichinellosis: Encephalopathy, neuromuscular disturbances ± ocular involvement
    - Invasion of ocular musculature can cause conjunctival chemosis and hemorrhage, photophobia, retinal hemorrhages, and optic neuritis

Laboratory Tests

- Enzyme immunoassays (EIA) to detect *Trichinella*-specific antibodies (larval (TSL-1 group) or excretory-secretory (ES) antigens available in USA; IgG most sensitive
- Seroconversion often does not occur until after onset of acute stage (3-5 weeks); peaks in 2nd-3rd month and decline slowly for years
- Antibody levels related to infecting dose of larvae

Treatment

- Oral albendazole or mebendazole
- Corticosteroids to prevent allergic and severe manifestations

Prognosis

- Generally favorable; life-threatening manifestations occur in ~ 2% of cases (related to organ involvement)
- Risk of death or permanent sequelae highest with neurotrichinellosis and cardiovascular complications

IMAGING

Radiographic Findings

- Neurotrichinellosis: Nodular multifocal hypodensities

MICROBIOLOGY

Parasite Features

- Adult female worms measure 2-4 mm and males 1-1.5 mm (smallest nematode parasite of humans); reside in small intestine
- Microscopic identification of larva following partial digestion of tissue with pepsin and pressing meat between glass

MICROSCOPIC

Histologic Features

- Visualization of intracellular encapsulated coiled larva (~ 1 mm in length) in striated muscle is diagnostic
- Some species (*T. pseudospiralis* and *T. papuae*) do not encyst
- Cysts eventually undergo calcification and fibrosis with development of thick hyalinized capsules
- Eosinophilic and lymphocytic infiltrates
- Basophilic transformation and development of capillary network surrounding infected muscle cell ("nurse cell")

DIFFERENTIAL DIAGNOSIS

Toxocariasis

- Causes visceral and ocular larva migrans; invades multiple tissues, including skeletal muscle but does not encyst

Anatrichosomiasis

- Rare infection with trichuroid nematode *Anatrichosoma;* do not encyst and may be located in epithelium

Haycocknemiasis *(Haycocknema perplexum* Infection)

- Extremely rare infection reported in Australia; adult females containing eggs present in muscle

SELECTED REFERENCES

1. Harrison LB et al: Laboratory features of trichinellosis and eosinophilia threshold for testing, Nunavik, Quebec, Canada, 2009-2019. Emerg Infect Dis. 28(12):2567-9, 2022
2. Pritt BS et al: Imported haycocknema perplexum infection, United States(1). Emerg Infect Dis. 28(11):2281-4, 2022
3. Diaz JH et al: The disease ecology, epidemiology, clinical manifestations, and management of trichinellosis linked to consumption of wild animal meat. Wilderness Environ Med. 31(2):235-44, 2020
4. Bruschi F et al: Neurotrichinellosis. Handb Clin Neurol. 114:243-9, 2013
5. Murrell KD et al: Worldwide occurrence and impact of human trichinellosis, 1986-2009. Emerg Infect Dis. 17(12):2194-202, 2011
6. Neghina R et al: Reviews on trichinellosis (II): neurological involvement. Foodborne Pathog Dis. 8(5):579-85, 2011
7. Gottstein B, Pozio E, Nöckler K: Epidemiology, diagnosis, treatment, and control of trichinellosis. Clin Microbiol Rev 22(1):127-45, 2009
8. Crum-Cianflone NF: Bacterial, fungal, parasitic, and viral myositis. Clin Microbiol Rev. 21(3):473-94, 2008

KEY FACTS

ETIOLOGY/PATHOGENESIS

- Disease caused by liver flukes in genus *Opisthorchiidae* (class Trematoda) via ingestion of larval forms present in infected freshwater fish
- *Opisthorchis felineus*: Endemic to Europe and Russia
- *Opisthorchis viverrini*: Endemic in Southeast Asia
- *Clonorchis sinensis* (syn. *Opisthorchis sinensis*): Endemic in east Asia (e.g., China)

CLINICAL ISSUES

- Symptoms range from mild gastrointestinal complaints to malnutrition, recurrent pyogenic cholangitis, cholecystitis, hepatitis, and acute pancreatitis; cholangiocarcinoma
- *O. felineus* may present with acute syndrome resembling Katayama fever

IMAGING

- Mild diffuse dilatation of peripheral intrahepatic bile ducts without focal obstructing lesions in larger bile ducts

MICROBIOLOGY

- Examination of body fluids (stool, bronchoalveolar lavage fluid, or endoscopic biliary collection) for diagnostic eggs

MICROSCOPIC

- Liver and biliary system: Periductal fibrosis, adenomatous hyperplasia, intense inflammation, cholecystitis
- Ductal dilatation with identification of lancet-shaped adult worm (intra- and extrahepatic)
- Cholangiocarcinoma

TOP DIFFERENTIAL DIAGNOSES

- Fascioliasis: Eggs (130-150 μm x 60-90 μm) and adult worms larger (30-75 μm x 15 μm)
- Paragonimiasis: Eggs larger (85 μm x 53 μm), slightly flattened on one side, and more often found in sputum (occasionally in feces)
- Sclerosing cholangitis: Autoimmune disease, no intraluminal parasites

(Left) *Eggs shed by adult worms are passed in feces and ingested by freshwater snails. Following asexual reproduction, free-swimming cercariae penetrate the skin of freshwater fish, become encysted, and form metacercariae. Humans and other fish-eating mammals acquire infection by ingesting raw or inadequately cooked fish. Metacercariae excyst in the duodenum and migrate to the bile duct.* **(Right)** *Adult C. sinensis worm is a small trematode (fluke) with an average length of 10-25 mm with a large ventral sucker ➡.*

***Clonorchis sinensis* and *Opisthorchis* spp. Life Cycles**

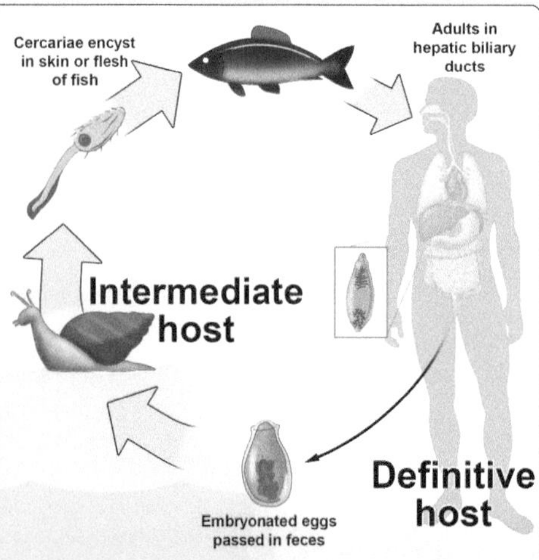

***Clonorchis sinensis*: Gross Specimen**

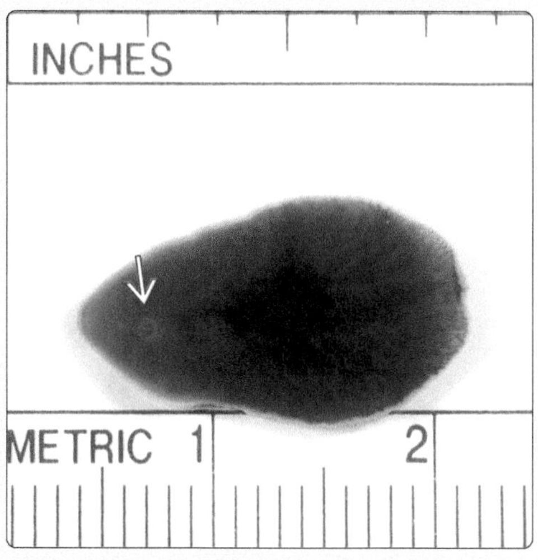

(Left) *Both C. sinensis and Opisthorchis spp. are hermaphroditic with both uterus ➡ and testes ➡. Also visible are the oral sucker ➡, branching cecum ➡, ventral sucker ➡, and vitellaria ➡. In this case, branched testes can be used to distinguish C. sinensis from Opisthorchis spp.* **(Right)** *Adult flukes can be seen in dilated intrahepatic bile ducts.*

***Clonorchis sinensis*: Adult Worm**

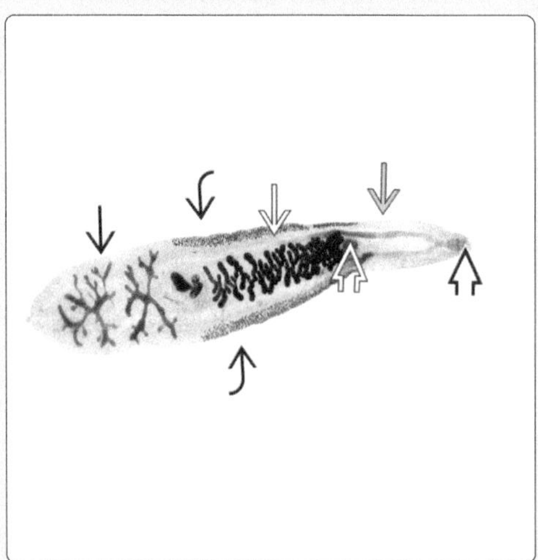

Liver With Intraductal *Clonorchis sinensis*

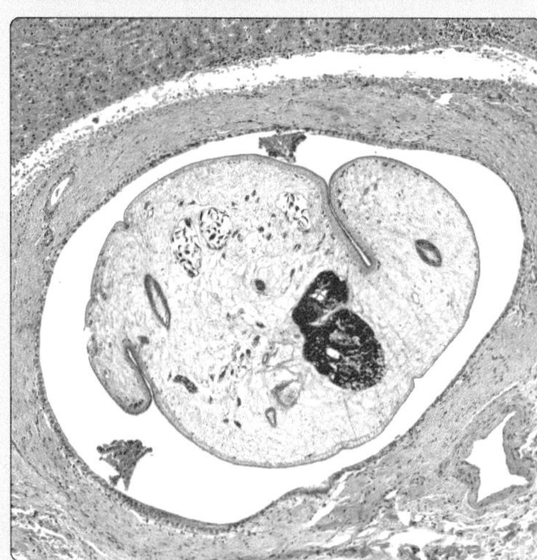

TERMINOLOGY

Synonyms

- "Chinese or oriental liver fluke" (*Clonorchis sinensis*)
- "Southeast Asian liver fluke" (*Opisthorchis viverrini*); "cat liver fluke" (*Opisthorchis felineus*)
- Trematodiasis, opisthorchiasis, clonorchiasis

Definitions

- *Clonorchis* from Greek "kln" (twig, spray, slip) + "órkhis" (testicle)
  - *sinensis* from Latin (from China)
- *Opisthorchis* from Greek "opisthen" (behind, at back) + "orkhis" (testicle)
  - *felineus* from Latin fēlīneus (of or pertaining to cat)
  - *viverrini,* representing host from which organism originally described, *Felis viverrinus* (fishing cat)

ETIOLOGY/PATHOGENESIS

Infectious Agents

- Trematode infections in which humans are accidental definitive hosts via consumption of infective metacercariae in improperly cooked infected fish (adequate freezing of fish prevents infection)
- All species have similar life cycle
  - Eggs ingested by fresh water snails (1st intermediate host); microscopic larvae (free-swimming cercariae) enter freshwater fish (2nd intermediate host)
  - Larva migrate to biliary tract, mature into adult worms (sexual stage), and attach to mucosal surface causing damage to biliary epithelium through both direct mechanical disruption and inflammatory-mediated changes
- *O. viverrini* and *C. sinensis* recognized as group 1A and *O. felineus* as group 3A biological carcinogens due to association with cholangiocarcinoma

CLINICAL ISSUES

Epidemiology

- *C. sinensis*: East Asia (China, Korea, Taiwan, Vietnam, Japan, and Asian Russia)
  - 15 million infected worldwide; 200 million living in endemic regions at risk of infection
- *Opisthorchis* species
  - *O. felineus*: Europe, mainly in Italy, Germany, Belarus, Russia, Kazakhstan, and Ukraine
    - Accounts for > 70% of helminth infestations in Russia
  - *O. viverrini*: Asia, mainly northeast Thailand, Laos, Cambodia, and central and southern Vietnam (Greater Mekong)
  - Estimated 20-40 million infected worldwide with prevalence rates > 50% in highly endemic regions (e.g., Thailand, Russia)

Site

- Hepatobiliary tract

Presentation

- Disease ranges from asymptomatic (~ 2/3) to severe
  - Up to 50% of people living in endemic regions are affected, but most do not show symptoms
  - Untreated infections can persist for lifespan of parasite (25-30 years)
- High blood eosinophilia and serum IgE
- **Mild symptoms**: Can be acute (fever, chills) or chronic (anorexia, fatigue, dyspepsia, nausea, indigestion, abdominal pain, diarrhea, constipation, malnutrition)
- **Severe disease**: Chronic infections may result in severe hepatobiliary disease; symptoms associated with infection intensity and related to inflammation and intermittent obstruction of bile ducts
  - Recurrent cholangitis, cholecystitis, hepatic abscesses, acute pancreatitis, bile peritonitis, hepatomegaly, fatty liver
  - Biliary fibrosis (portal cirrhosis and hypertension can occur) and bile duct cancers (e.g., cholangiocarcinoma)
  - Malnutrition and growth stunting in children with heavy infestation
- **Acute syndrome**: *O. felineus* may present with acute syndrome characterized by fever, facial edema, lymphadenopathy, arthralgias, and rash [resembling Katayama fever (schistosomiasis)]
- Hepatic mass/cholangiocarcinoma

Laboratory Tests

- Serologic testing
  - Considerable cross reactivity and low specificity
  - Not currently available in USA; serodiagnostics currently under development in Asia
- PCR: Amplification of parasite DNA from stool samples used in research and epidemiologic studies, not available commercially

Treatment

- Praziquantel (2 days) or albendazole (7 days, not FDA approved) are drugs of choice
- Reinfection occurs following treatment, lack of protective immune response

Prognosis

- Chronic, recurrent infection can lead to cholangiocarcinoma
- Published efficacy of treatment > 90%; unclear impact on risk of cholangiocarcinoma

IMAGING

General Features

- Cysts containing adult parasites can sometimes be detected by US, CT, or MR
- Mild diffuse, uniform dilatation of peripheral intrahepatic bile ducts with no or minimal dilatation of extrahepatic bile duct and without focal obstructing lesions in larger bile ducts
- Additional findings include periductal fibrosis, fatty liver, gallbladder enlargement, and stone formation
- Cholangiography usually shows many elliptical or filamentous filling defects within peripheral intrahepatic ducts
- Findings are considered pathognomonic in endemic regions

Ultrasonographic Findings

- Thickening of ductal wall with increased echogenicity
- Occasionally, flukes or aggregates of eggs seen as nonshadowing echogenic foci or casts within bile duct

MICROBIOLOGY

Ova and Parasite Stool Examination

- Identification of parasite eggs in stool specimens is diagnostic; multiple stool samples may be needed
  - Fecal preparations include unstained wet mount of concentrated stool, conventional iodine/saline and trichrome staining, Kato-thick smear, and formalin-ethyl acetate concentration techniques
- *C. sinensis*
  - Eggs are oval (27-35 µm x 12-20 µm), yellow brown with operculum with prominent shoulders at slender end and small spine-like prominence or "knob" at broad (abopercular) end
- *Opisthorchis* species
  - Eggs are 26-30 µm x 11-15µm, yellow brown, embryonated, and elongated with operculum on anterior end and pointed terminal "knob" on posterior end
- *Opisthorchis* species eggs are very similar morphologically to *C. sinensis* eggs but distinguished by lack of prominent operculum "shoulders"

MACROSCOPIC

Adult Worm

- Transparent or reddish-bile colored, leaf- or lancet-shaped with dorsoventrally flattening
- *Opisthorchis* species: 7-12 mm long, 1.5-2.5 mm in diameter
  - *O. viverrini* slightly larger, may infect pancreatic duct
- *C. sinensis:* 10-25 mm x 3-5 mm

MICROSCOPIC

Histologic Features

- Diagnosis via intraluminal identification of adult worm in bile ducts of liver, gallbladder, pancreas
  - Adult worm is hermaphroditic; *Clonorchis* and *Opisthorchis* species distinguished by shape and position of testes (located posterior to ovaries) and arrangement of highly branched vitelline glands
    - *Opisthorchis* species: Diagonal deeply lobed testes
    - *C. sinensis*: Highly branched (dendritic) testes
  - Attach to duct walls via small oral and ventral (acetabulum) suckers under regulatory function of circular and radius muscles
- Histologic changes may be focal or involve whole liver
- Early stage: Ductal ectasia, bile duct epithelial proliferation, adenomatous hyperplasia, periductal infiltrates of mononuclear cells, and eosinophil predominance
- Late stage: Intense bile duct inflammation (cholecystitis and cholangitis), periductal fibrosis, biliary and goblet cell hyperplasia, periductal proliferation and fibrosis
  - Mixed inflammatory infiltrate, including plasma cells, lymphocytes, and eosinophils
- Complications as result of biliary obstruction may include: Calculi, acute suppurative cholangitis, recurrent pyogenic cholangitis, cholecystitis, hepatitis, liver abscess, and acute pancreatitis
- Severe &/or chronic infection may lead to dysplasia and cholangiocarcinoma

DIFFERENTIAL DIAGNOSIS

Paragonimus westermani Infection

- Eggs are unembryonated, larger (85 µm x 53 µm), slightly flattened on one side, and more often found in sputum (occasionally in feces)

Fasciola hepatica Infection

- Eggs larger (130-150 µm x 60-90 µm), lack of "shouldered" operculum; adult worm larger *F. hepatica*: (30 µm x 15 µm); *F. gigantica*: (75 µm x 15 µm)

Metagonimus yokogawai or *Heterophyes heterophyes* Infections

- Adult flukes are minute (1-2.5 µm) and reside in small intestine; ventral sucker (genitoacetabulum) is present on side of midline and closely associated with genital pore

SELECTED REFERENCES

1. Pakharukova MY et al: Similarities and differences among the Opisthorchiidae liver flukes: insights from Opisthorchis felineus. Parasitology. 149(10):1306-18, 2022
2. Qian MB et al: Severe hepatobiliary morbidity is associated with Clonorchis sinensis infection: the evidence from a cross-sectional community study. PLoS Negl Trop Dis. 15(1):e0009116, 2021
3. Sripa B et al: Current status of human liver fluke infections in the Greater Mekong Subregion. Acta Trop. 224:106133, 2021
4. Cho PY et al: Serodiagnostic antigens of Clonorchis sinensis identified and evaluated by high-throughput proteogenomics. PLoS Negl Trop Dis. 14(12):e0008998, 2020
5. Qian MB et al: Rapid screening of Clonorchis sinensis infection: performance of a method based on raw-freshwater fish-eating practice. Acta Trop. 207:105380, 2020
6. Cheng N et al: Cs1, a Clonorchis sinensis-derived serodiagnostic antigen containing tandem repeats and a signal peptide. PLoS Negl Trop Dis. 12(8):e0006683, 2018
7. Petney TN et al: Taxonomy, ecology and population genetics of opisthorchis viverrini and its intermediate hosts. Adv Parasitol. 101:1-39, 2018
8. Suwannatrai A et al: Epidemiology of Opisthorchis viverrini Infection. Adv Parasitol. 101:41-67, 2018
9. Tangkawattana S et al: Reservoir animals and their roles in transmission of Opisthorchis viverrini. Adv Parasitol. 101:69-95, 2018
10. Kim TS et al: Clonorchis sinensis, an oriental liver fluke, as a human biological agent of cholangiocarcinoma: a brief review. BMB Rep. 49(11):590-97, 2016
11. Sithithaworn P et al: Roles of liver fluke infection as risk factor for cholangiocarcinoma. J Hepatobiliary Pancreat Sci. 21(5):301-8, 2014
12. Pozio E et al: Opisthorchis felineus, an emerging infection in Italy and its implication for the European Union. Acta Trop. 126(1):54-62, 2013
13. Lovis L et al: PCR Diagnosis of Opisthorchis viverrini and Haplorchis taichui Infections in a Lao Community in an area of endemicity and comparison of diagnostic methods for parasitological field surveys. J Clin Microbiol. 47(5):1517-23, 2009
14. Keiser J et al: Emerging foodborne trematodiasis. Emerg Infect Dis. 11(10):1507-14, 2005
15. Kaewkes S: Taxonomy and biology of liver flukes. Acta Trop. 88(3):177-86, 2003
16. Ditrich O et al: Comparative morphology of eggs of the Haplorchiinae (Trematoda: Heterophyidae) and some other medically important heterophyid and opisthorchiid flukes. Folia Parasitol (Praha). 39(2):123-32, 1992

Adult Worms in Biliary Tract

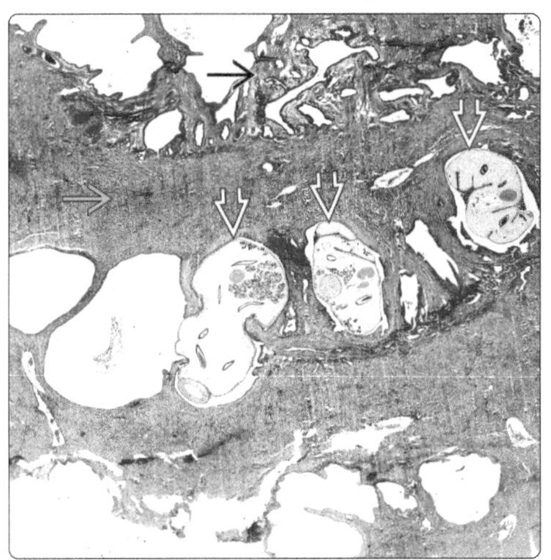

Clonorchis sinensis: Adult Worm in Bile Duct

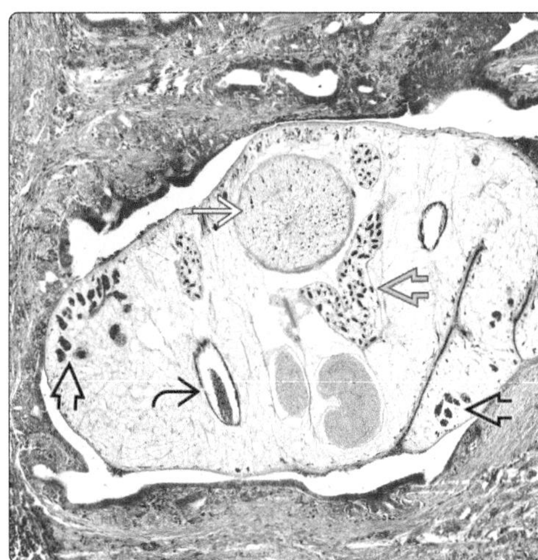

(Left) *Ductal ectasia with multiple adult worms ➡ within the ductal lumen and associated adenomatous hyperplasia ⇨ and periductal inflammation ⇨ is shown.* **(Right)** *Dilated bile duct with adult fluke is shown. Visible components of the worm include an egg-filled uterus ⇨, oral sucker ➡, intestinal cecum ⇨, and vitelline glands ⇨.*

Intrabiliary Adult Fluke

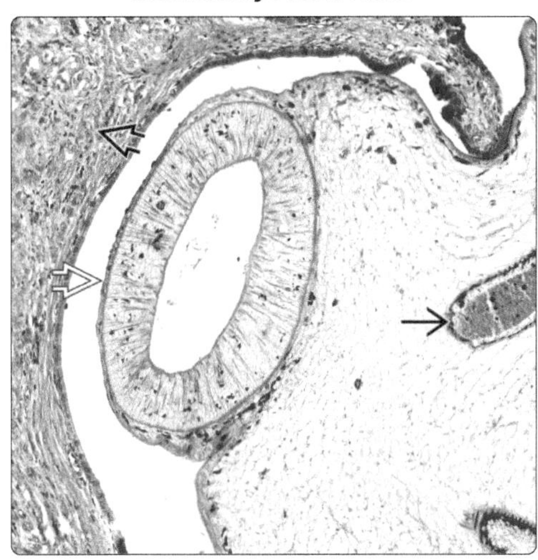

Clonorchis sinensis Eggs in Tissue

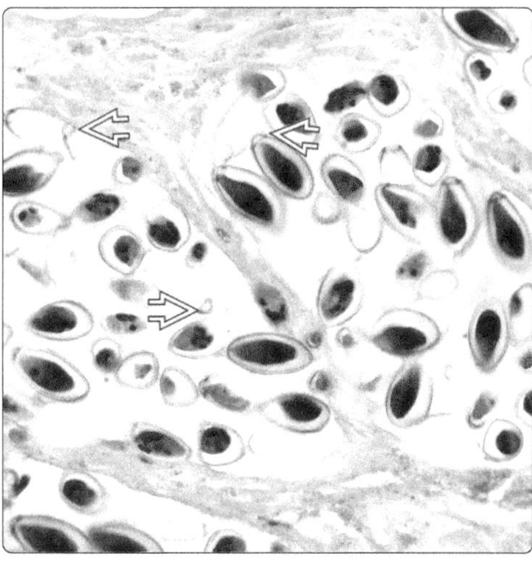

(Left) *Adult C. sinensis worm in biliary tract with surrounding adenomatous hyperplasia ⇨ is shown. Oral sucker ➡ and cecum are visible ⇨.* **(Right)** *This high-magnification image of intrauterine eggs (27-35 µm x 12-20 µm) demonstrates a shouldered opercula ➡ at the slender ends, the presence of which helps to distinguish C. sinensis from Opisthorchis spp.*

Clonorchis sinensis Egg: Stool Ova and Parasite Exam

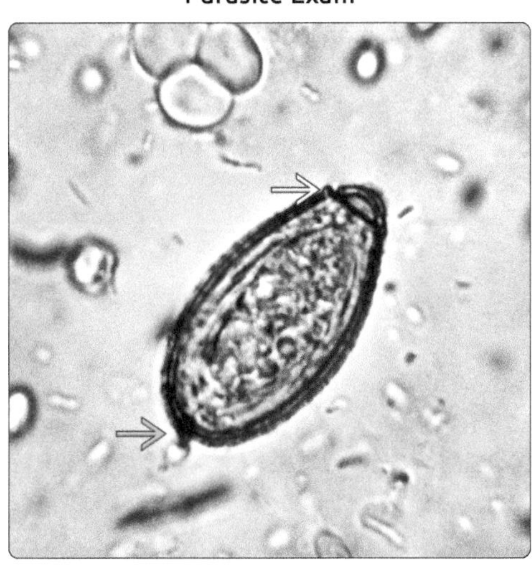

Opisthorchis Species Egg: Stool Ova and Parasite Exam

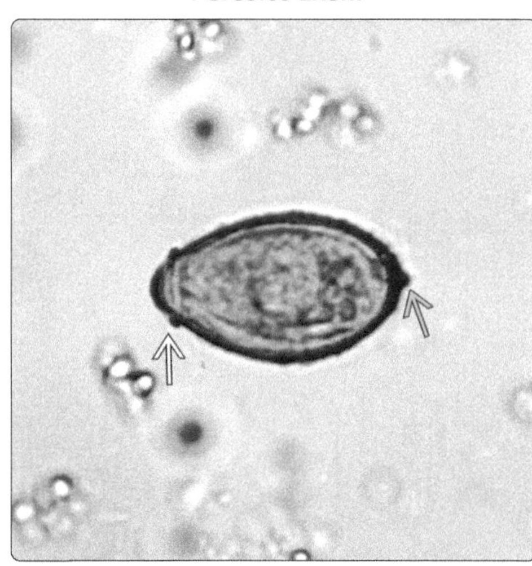

(Left) *Eggs are oval (27-35 µm x 12-20 µm) with an operculum ➡ at the slender end with prominent shoulders. The opposite (abopercular) end is broad and has a small spine-like prominence ⇨. (Courtesy CDC/PHIL.)* **(Right)** *Eggs are elongated (26-30 µm x 11-15µm) with operculum ➡ on the anterior end (without prominent "shoulders") and a pointed terminal "knob" ⇨ on the posterior end. (Courtesy M. Melvin, MD, CDC/PHIL.)*

KEY FACTS

ETIOLOGY/PATHOGENESIS

- Disease caused by liver (*Fasciola hepatica, Fasciola gigantica*) or intestinal (*Fasciolopsis buski)* flukes via ingestion of contaminated water or freshwater plants containing infective cercariae

CLINICAL ISSUES

- Acute-phase symptoms due to worm migration (fever, pain, gastrointestinal disturbances); stool O&P often negative, antigen/serology can be useful
- Chronic-phase symptoms due to longterm biliary obstruction (cholecystitis, cholangitis)

IMAGING

- Single or multiple lesions in liver or gastrointestinal system

MICROBIOLOGY

- *Fasciola* spp. and *F. buski* eggs morphologically similar (130-150 x 60-90 μm): Oval, thin shell, and operculated
- Adult *F. hepatica* (30 mm x 15 mm) have cone-shaped anterior end; adult *F. gigantica* (75 mm x 15 mm)
- Adult *F. buski* (20-75 mm x 8-20 mm) have rounded anterior end and poorly developed oral and ventral suckers

MICROSCOPIC

- Lancet-shaped adult fluke in liver parenchyma or biliary system; undulating, unbranched ceca, tandem dendritic testes, branched ovaries, and poorly developed oral and ventral suckers
- Liver: Necrosis and hemorrhage of ducts with abscess formation; fibrosis

TOP DIFFERENTIAL DIAGNOSES

- Paragonimiasis: Both eggs (85 μm) and adult worms (8-12 mm) are smaller; adults reside in lungs
- Opisthorchiasis/clonorchiasis: Also reside in biliary tree; both eggs (26-35 μm) and adult worms (7-25 mm in length) are smaller

(Left) *Miracidia hatch from eggs, infect freshwater snails (intermediate hosts), and develop into cercariae. Free-living cercariae encyst on aquatic vegetation. After ingestion by definitive host, metacercaria excyst in duodenum and develop into adult flukes in biliary ducts or small intestine.* **(Right)** *Liver flukes are flat and somewhat transparent with cone-shaped anterior and prominent oral and ventral suckers. (From DP: Hepatobiliary and Pancreas.)*

Fasciola **spp. and** ***Fasciolopsis buski*** **Life Cycles**

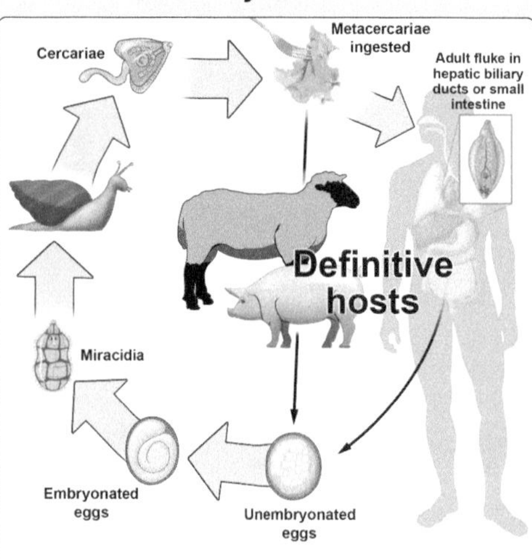

Fasciola hepatica **(Liver Fluke)**

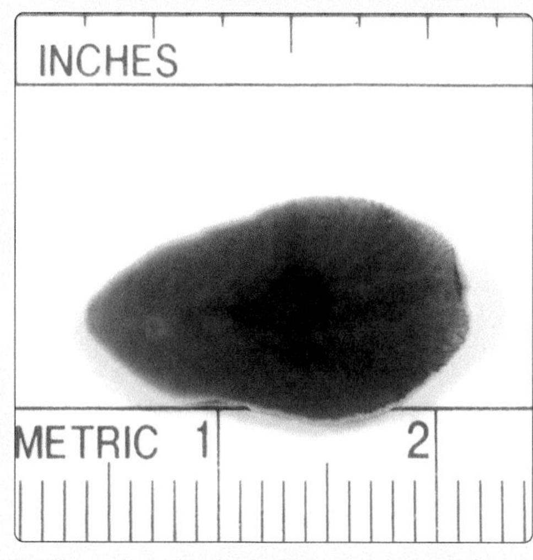

(Left) *Eggs of Fasciola hepatica are oval (130-150 μm long x 60-90 μm wide) and operculated and are passed unembryonated in feces. F. hepatica and Fasciola gigantica eggs cannot be distinguished morphologically. (Courtesy M. Melvin, CDC/PHIL.)* **(Right)** *Fasciolopsis buski eggs are oval (130-150 μm long x 60-90 μm wide), operculated, and are passed unembryonated in feces. Eggs are often reported as "Fasciola/Fasciolopsis" eggs due to morphologic overlap. (Courtesy M. Melvin, CDC/PHIL.)*

Fasciola hepatica **Eggs**

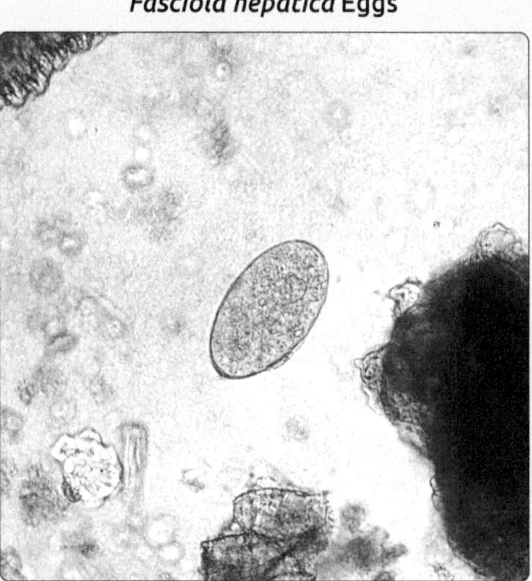

Fasciolopsis buski **Eggs**

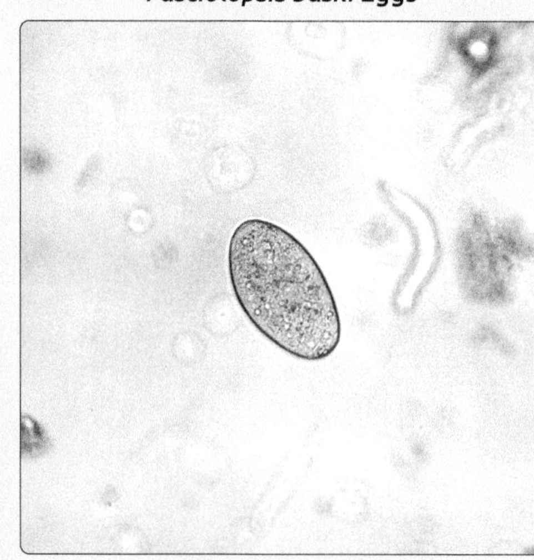

TERMINOLOGY

Definitions

- *Fasciola* from Latin "fascia" (band, bandage, swathe)

ETIOLOGY/PATHOGENESIS

Infectious Agents

- Infections with liver and intestinal flukes (class Trematoda, family *Fasciolidae*) via ingestion of contaminated water or raw or undercooked freshwater plants (e.g., bamboo shoots, watercress, water chestnuts)
- Immature eggs are passed in stool, become embryonated in freshwater, and release miracidia, which invade snail intermediate host and develop into sporocysts, rediae, and cercariae
- Cercariae are released from snail, encyst as metacercariae on aquatic vegetation, and ingested by humans or other mammals
- Metacercariae excyst in duodenum and attach to intestinal wall (*Fasciolopsis* spp.) or migrate through intestinal wall to liver (*Fasciola* spp.)

CLINICAL ISSUES

Epidemiology

- Global prevalence: 2.4-17 million confirmed (70 million estimated); higher in children and females
- *Fasciola hepatica*: Worldwide distribution, hyperendemic regions of South America, Middle East, and Southeast Asia; definitive hosts include sheep, cattle, goats
- *Fasciola gigantica*: Limited to tropical Asia and Africa
- *Fasciolopsis buski*: Southern Asia and Indian subcontinent; definitive hosts include humans and pigs

Presentation

- Variable, nonspecific symptoms; 15% asymptomatic
- Acute (migratory) phase: Fever, abdominal pain, nausea, vomiting, hepatomegaly, malaise, cough, eosinophilia, transaminitis
- Chronic phase (biliary/adult phase; months to years post exposure): Cholangitis, cholecystitis, pancreatitis, sclerosing cholangitis, hepatic fibrosis, obstructive jaundice due to inflammation or blockage of bile ducts or gallbladder
- "Halzoun": Allergy-like syndrome of eyes, ears, nose, or throat following ingestion of infected raw animal liver
- *F. buski*: Intestinal obstruction, ascites, appendicitis (rare), malabsorption, vitamin B12 deficiency, anemia

Laboratory Tests

- Serologic testing useful during acute stage (detectable at 2-4 weeks) and chronic stage (sporadic or low egg production); sensitivity ≥ 94%; specificity ≥ 98%; does not differentiate between current or past infection
- Antigen testing (stool and blood) useful during acute stage (positive as early as 8 weeks post infection); sensitivity and specificity > 93%; limited commercial availability

Treatment

- *Fasciola* spp.: Triclabendazole (some resistance)
- *F. buski*: Albendazole or praziquantel
- Extraction of adult flukes via ERCP for biliary obstruction

IMAGING

General Features

- Rim-enhancing or ill-defined hypodense or hypoechoic lesions in subcapsular and peripheral regions of liver
- Ultrasound: Dilated and thickened common bile duct, crescent-like parasites in gallbladder or bile ducts

MICROBIOLOGY

Parasite Features

- Adult *F. hepatica*: Up to 30 mm long x 15 mm wide; anterior end is cone-shaped; resides in liver bile ducts
- Adult *F. gigantica*: Up to 75 mm long x 15 mm wide
- Adult *F. buski*: 20-75 mm long x 8-20 mm wide; rounded anterior end, poorly developed oral and ventral suckers; resides in intestine
- *Fasciola spp.* and *F. buski* eggs are morphologically similar: Oval (130-150 µm x 60-90 µm) with thin shell and operculum

Stool Ova and Parasite Examination

- Eggs often not in stool during acute phase (not produced until 3-4 months), chronic phase (low-level or sporadic production), or in cases of ectopic migration or encapsulation of parenchymal liver abscess
- Pseudofascioliasis: False-positive following ingestion of liver containing noninfective eggs

MICROSCOPIC

Histologic Features

- Dorsoventrally flattened fluke with undulating, unbranched ceca, tandem dendritic testes, branched ovaries, and poorly developed oral and ventral suckers
- Liver: Necrosis and hemorrhage of ducts with abscess formation; fibrosis

Cytologic Features

- Detection of eggs in duodenal or biliary aspirates

DIFFERENTIAL DIAGNOSIS

Opisthorchiasis/Clonorchiasis

- Also reside in biliary tree; both eggs (26-35 µm x 11-20 µm) and adult worms (7-25 mm in length) are smaller

Paragonimiasis

- Both eggs (85 µm x 50 µm) and adult worms (8-12 mm in length) are smaller; adults reside in lungs

SELECTED REFERENCES

1. Mas-Coma S et al: Human and animal fascioliasis: origins and worldwide evolving scenario. Clin Microbiol Rev. 35(4):e0008819, 2022
2. Alba A et al: Towards the comprehension of fasciolosis (re-)emergence: an integrative overview. Parasitology. 148(4):385-407, 2021
3. Siles-Lucas M et al: Fascioliasis and fasciolopsiasis: current knowledge and future trends. Res Vet Sci. 134:27-35, 2021
4. Wu X et al: Case report: surgical intervention for Fasciolopsis buski infection: a literature review. Am J Trop Med Hyg. 103(6):2282-7, 2020
5. Robert W et al: Fascioliasis due to Fasciola hepatica and Fasciola gigantica infection: an update on this 'neglected' neglected tropical disease. Laboratory Medicine, 42(2):107-16, 2011

Paragonimiasis

KEY FACTS

ETIOLOGY/PATHOGENESIS

- Infection with *Paragonimus* species via consumption of raw crabs/crawfish
- Flukes become encysted in pulmonary tissue, eggs are coughed up, swallowed, and excreted in feces
- Global distribution, disease in endemic regions of Asia, Africa, North America, and South America

CLINICAL ISSUES

- Early symptoms due to gastrointestinal penetration and initial migration of parasite
- Pleuropulmonary symptoms due to presence of adult worm in lungs (often clinically misdiagnosed as tuberculosis)
- Brain is most common ectopic site of infection

MICROBIOLOGY

- Both stool and sputum samples should be submitted for ova and parasite examination
- Eggs: Unembryonated (68-118 μm x 39-67 μm), operculated, golden brown, ellipsoidal with thick shell

MICROSCOPIC

- Due to low incidence, may not be considered clinically; diagnosis often via histologic or cytologic identification of eggs or other parasite elements in respiratory and pulmonary specimens
- Operculated eggs birefringent and polarizable
- Portions of adult worm

TOP DIFFERENTIAL DIAGNOSES

- Strongyloidiasis: Larva transmigrate lung; seen in sputum
- Schistosomiasis: Eggs with lateral/terminal spine
- Other trematodes: Differentiated by size/shape of eggs and presence of opercular ridges
- Ascariasis: Larva transmigrate lung; seen in sputum
- Echinococcosis: Host-derived fibrous capsule or cyst containing protoscoleces

Paragonimus spp. Life Cycle

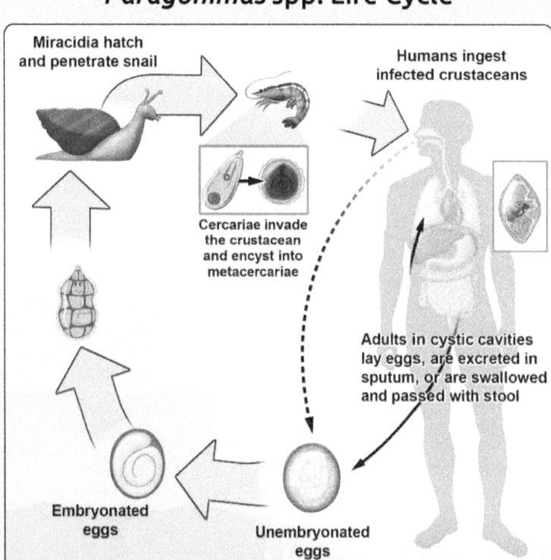

Miracidia hatch and penetrate snail
Humans ingest infected crustaceans
Cercariae invade the crustacean and encyst into metacercariae
Adults in cystic cavities lay eggs, are excreted in sputum, or are swallowed and passed with stool
Embryonated eggs
Unembryonated eggs

Cerebral Paragonimiasis

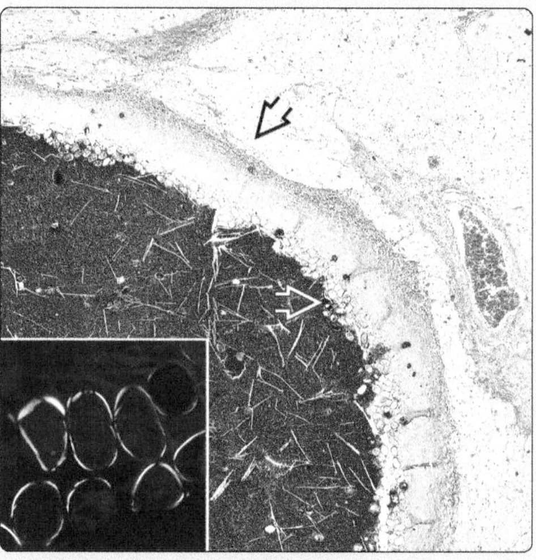

(Left) *Miracidia infect fresh water snails, develop into cercariae, then infect crustacean host, encyst, and become metacercariae. This infective form penetrates the intestinal wall of mammalian hosts and migrates to the lungs, maturing into adults.* **(Right)** *Low-power image shows a cerebral lesion surrounded by ➾ a well-organized fibrous capsule with numerous peripherally arranged degenerating Paragonimus westermani ova ➡, which are birefringent when viewed using plane-polarized light (inset).*

Ova and Parasite Exam

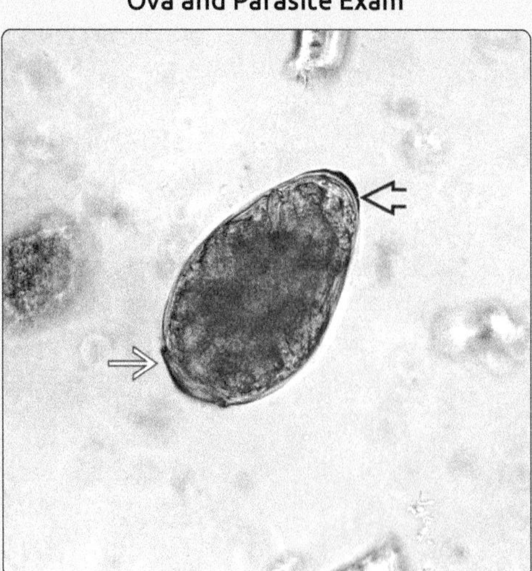

Paragonimus westermani Eggs in Tissue

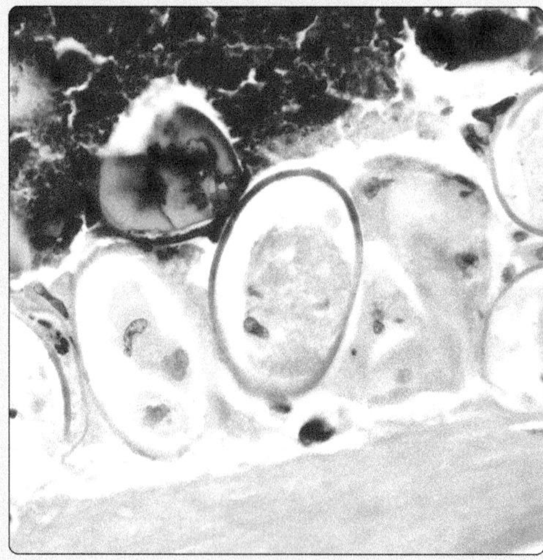

(Left) *P. westermani ova can be identified in both respiratory and stool samples, are operculated ➡, golden brown, and ellipsoidal with a thick shell. The opposite (abopercular) end ➾ is thickened. (Courtesy M. Melvin, MD, CDC/PHIL.)* **(Right)** *This high-power image of degenerating ova shows characteristic ellipsoidal thickened shells. Size, shape, identification of operculum, and birefringence to polarized light can be useful in confirming the diagnosis.*

TERMINOLOGY

Synonyms

- Lung fluke, pulmonary distomatosis, endemic hemoptysis

Definitions

- Greek words: "Para" (beside) and "gonimos" (productive, fertile)

ETIOLOGY/PATHOGENESIS

Infectious Agents

- Infection with *Paragonimus* species [phylum Platyhelminthes (i.e., flatworms), class Trematoda] via ingestion of raw or improperly cooked crustaceans
- Young flukes penetrate diaphragm and become encysted in pulmonary tissue, often in pairs; eggs are coughed up, swallowed, and excreted in feces

CLINICAL ISSUES

Epidemiology

- Global distribution; disease limited to endemic regions
- *P. westermani complex* and *P. heterotremus* (East and Southeast Asia), *P. skrjabini, P heterotremus complex* (India), *P. africanus, P. uterobilateralis* (Africa), *P. mexicanus* (Central America, South America), and *P. kellicotti* (North America)
- Estimate prevalence > 20 million and > 200 million at risk

Presentation

- Acute infection (2- to 15-day incubation) often asymptomatic; symptoms due to gastrointestinal penetration (abdominal pain, fever, urticaria, diarrhea) and migration to pleural cavity (dyspnea, pleuritic chest pain, pneumothorax)
- Chronic pleuropulmonary infection: Presence of paired adult worms (cough, recurrent hemoptysis, bronchiectasis, interstitial pneumonitis, pleuritic chest pain)
- Brain (2nd most common site): Eosinophilic meningitis and symptoms due to space occupying lesions
- Cutaneous &/or visceral larva migrans (tender, migratory skin nodules), breasts, heart, and genital organs (infertility)

Laboratory Tests

- Leukocytosis, eosinophilia, increased IgE
- Serology: Excellent sensitivity (96%) and specificity (≥ 99%); useful in ectopic disease when no eggs present in sputum/stool; can be performed on pleural fluid
- PCR/sequencing of ITS of ribosomal genetic complexes and mitochondrial cytochrome c oxidase gene (CO1)

Treatment

- Praziquantel (3 day course); triclabendazole

Prognosis

- 86-100% cure rates following treatment
- Coma in 15% of cases of cerebral paragonimiasis

IMAGING

General Features

- Lungs: Single (ring-enhancing) or multiple ("soap bubble") nodules or cystic lesions (5-30 mm), pneumothorax, effusions, pleural thickening
- Brain: Expansive, space-occupying lesion in cerebral cortex; late stage with solitary or clusters of amorphous calcifications (5-30 mm)
- Parasite migration results in "burrow tracts" (linear opacities, 0.5-1.0 cm in diameter)

MICROBIOLOGY

Parasite Features

- Adult worm: Ovoid (7.5-12 mm long x 4-6 mm wide x 3.5-5 mm thick); hermaphroditic with deeply lobed, paired testes and ovary with tightly coiled uterus on opposite sides of organism; occasionally present in sputum
- Eggs are unembryonated (68-118 μm x 39-67 μm), operculated, golden brown, ellipsoidal with thick shell; more commonly identified in respiratory than stool samples (11-15% sensitivity for single specimen)

MICROSCOPIC

Histologic Features

- Parasite may be predominantly parenchymal or pleural with mesothelial hyperplasia, fibrosis, entrapped eggs; surrounded by cyst capsule and dense infiltrate of eosinophils and nonnecrotizing granulomas
- Eggs are birefringent and operculated
- Portions of 1-2 adult worms in cystic or nodular lesion with cuticular spines

Cytologic Features

- Exudative fluids with numerous neutrophils, macrophages, and eosinophils; Charcot-Leyden crystals common
- Operculate ova often present in sputum and pleural fluid

DIFFERENTIAL DIAGNOSIS

Other Helminth Infections

- **Strongyloidiasis**: Larva transmigrate lung and can be seen in sputum
- **Schistosomiasis**: Unoperculated eggs may have lateral or terminal spine and are not birefringent
- **Other trematodes**: Differentiated by size/shape of eggs and presence of opercular ridges
- **Ascariasis**: Larva transmigrate lung and can be seen in sputum; eggs (in stool) are round with external mammillated layer (fertilized) or elongated with thinner shell (unfertilized)
- **Echinococcosis**: Produces parasitic lung disease with host-derived fibrous capsule or cyst; distinguished by protoscoleces and lack of cuticular spines

SELECTED REFERENCES

1. Ahn CS et al: Spectrum of pleuropulmonary paragonimiasis: an analysis of 685 cases diagnosed over 22 years. J Infect. 82(1):150-8, 2021
2. Fiorentini LF et al: Pictorial review of thoracic parasitic diseases: a radiologic guide. Chest. 157(5):1100-13, 2020
3. Boland JM et al: Histopathology of parasitic infections of the lung. Semin Diagn Pathol. 34(6):550-9, 2017
4. Xia Y et al: Cerebral paragonimiasis: a retrospective analysis of 27 cases. J Neurosurg Pediatr. 15(1):101-6, 2015
5. Procop GW: North American paragonimiasis (caused by Paragonimus kellicotti) in the context of global paragonimiasis. Clin Microbiol Rev. 22(3):415-46, 2009
6. Kim TS et al: Pleuropulmonary paragonimiasis: CT findings in 31 patients. AJR Am J Roentgenol. 185(3):616-21, 2005

KEY FACTS

ETIOLOGY/PATHOGENESIS

- Parasitic trematode worms (flukes) of *Schistosoma* genus
- 3 major species causing human infections: *S. mansoni*, *S. haematobium*, *S. japonicum*
- Host tissue reaction against egg antigens induces Th-2-predominant immune response

CLINICAL ISSUES

- Worldwide distribution; prevalence is highest in sub-Saharan Africa
- Mortality related to schistosomiasis is low
- Likelihood of complications and morbidity correlate with parasite burden, duration of infection, site(s) of infection
- Migratory infection or immediate manifestations occur
- Acute infection (Katayama fever) is symptomatic
- Chronic infection: Intestine, liver, spleen, urinary tract, genital systems, lungs, CNS

MICROSCOPIC

- Inflammatory granulomatous reaction and eosinophilic infiltration resulting in local tissue destruction and fibrosis
- *S. mansoni* (140 x 66 μm): Oval egg, lateral spine
- *S. haematobium* (143 x 60 μm): Oval egg, terminal spine
- *S. japonicum* (90 x 70 μm): Round egg, small lateral spine
- Adults worms rarely seen; in transverse sections, larger males surround more slender females

TOP DIFFERENTIAL DIAGNOSES

- Strongyloidiasis: Located in intestinal crypts and mucosa, more exuberant eosinophilic infiltration
- Tuberculosis: Positive for acid-fast stain, lacks ova and eosinophilic inflammation
- Coccidioidomycosis: Lacks ova and shows spherules with endospores
- Neoplasms, sarcoidosis: Lacks ova or significant eosinophilic inflammation

Schistosomasis Life Cycle

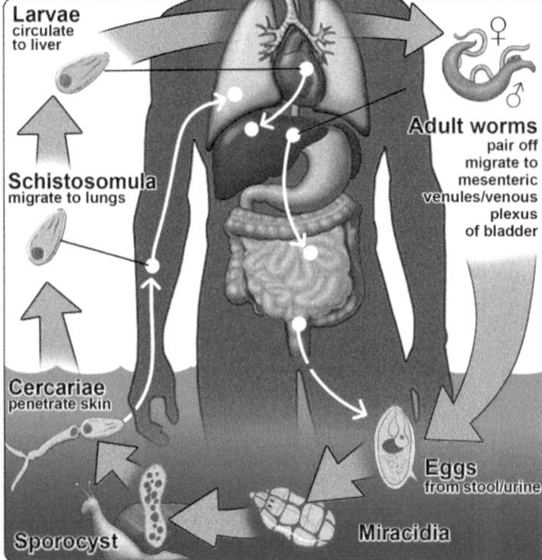

***Schistosoma* Eggs: Trichrome Stain**

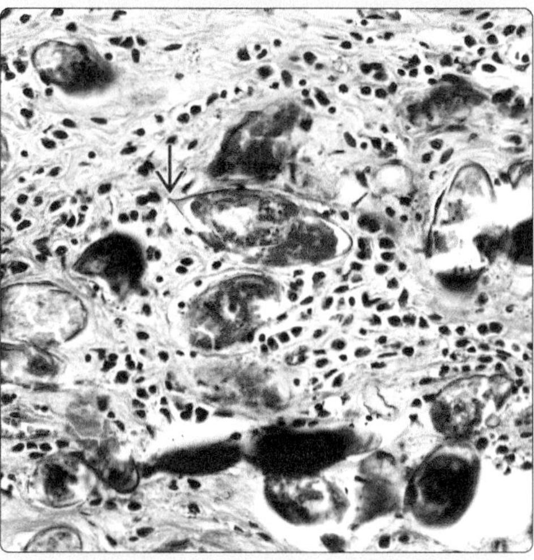

(Left) *Eggs are released into environment in stool or urine. Miracidia infect snails and develop into cercariae, which directly penetrate human skin. Schistosomulae circulate through lungs, heart, and liver, then mature into adults, which copulate and reside in mesenteric venules or venous plexus of bladder.* **(Right)** *Trichrome stain of bladder section shows oval and elongated eggs embedded. A terminal spine ➔ is present, consistent with Schistosoma haematobium.*

Adult *Schistosoma mansoni*

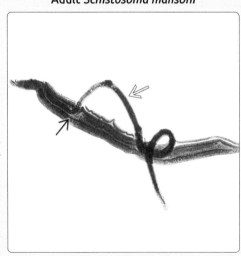

***Schistosoma* Adults in Tissue Sections**

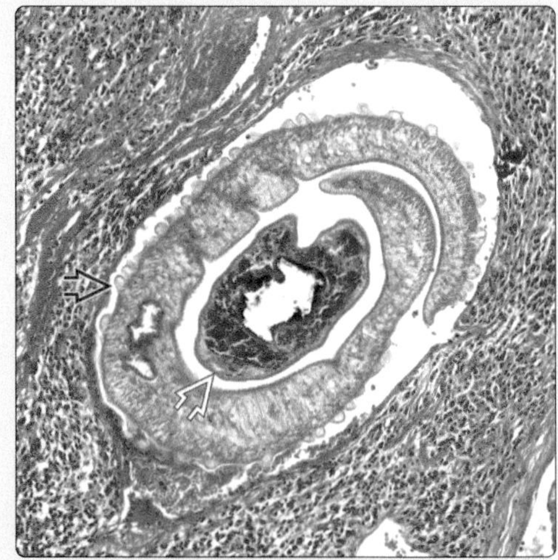

(Left) *This image shows an adult female ➔ residing within the gynecophoral canal ➔ of the thicker male. Paired adult worms migrate to mesenteric venules of bowel/rectum and lay eggs that circulate to liver and are shed in stool. (Courtesy L. Herring, CDC/PHIL.)* **(Right)** *This section from a rectal mass shows the tuberculate exterior ➔ of an adult male worm as well as sections of the more slender female adult worm ➔.*

TERMINOLOGY

Synonyms

- Bilharziasis, snail fever, Katayama fever

Definitions

- Greek: "Skhistos" (divided, cloven) + "soma" (body)

ETIOLOGY/PATHOGENESIS

Infectious Agents

- Infection with parasitic trematode worms (flukes) of *Schistosoma* genus
  - Pathology caused by host responses against egg antigens, which induce predominantly Th-2 immune response, resulting in eosinophilic granulomatous reaction, extent of which depends on worm burden, host genetic background, and parasite strains
  - Chronic egg deposition may lead to bladder, colorectal, renal, &/or prostate carcinoma
  - 3 major species cause disease: *S. mansoni, S. japonicum* (intestines and liver), and *S. haematobium* (genitourinary tract)
  - Less common species: *S. mekongi, S. intercalatum* can cause diseases in intestines and liver
- Life cycle
  - *Schistosoma* eggs, seeded into fresh water through urine or feces from infected humans or animals, release miracidia, which penetrate into snails (specific snail species determines geographic distribution) and produce cercariae (infectious larvae form), which are released into water
  - Cercariae penetrate human skin, become schistosomulae, and migrate through circulation until they reach liver, where they mature into adult worms and reside in bowel/rectum venules (*S. mansoni* and *S. japonicum*) or venous plexus in bladder (*S. haematobium*)
  - Eggs are deposited in tissue and move toward lumen of intestine or bladder and ureters and are then eliminated in feces or urine, respectively, but may embolize to liver, spleen, lungs, brain, or spinal cord, and, less commonly, skin and peritoneal surfaces

CLINICAL ISSUES

Epidemiology

- Worldwide distribution
- Prevalence is highest in sub-Saharan Africa, where 85% of total burden is found
- Endemic distributions of different *Schistosoma* spp.
  - *S. mansoni*: Mostly in Africa and South America
  - *S. haematobium*: Mostly in Africa and Middle East
  - *S. japonicum*: Mostly in East Asia
  - *S. mekongi*: Mostly in Laos, Cambodia
  - *S. intercalatum*: Mostly in West and Central Africa

Presentation

- Migratory infection or immediate manifestations
  - Maculopapular eruption at site of cercarial penetration
  - Cercarial dermatitis ("swimmer's itch")
    - Maculopapular skin eruption with pruritus after repeated contacts with parasites; mostly associated with larvae of bird schistosomes of *Trichobilharzia* spp.
- Acute infection (Katayama fever)
  - Hypersensitivity reaction to schistosome antigens and circulating immune complexes; occurs 3-8 weeks after exposure
  - Associated with eosinophilia
  - Symptoms are variable, e.g., fever, urticaria and angioedema, arthralgias, diarrhea, abdominal pain
- Chronic infection
  - Occurs in response to cumulative deposition of eggs in tissues and resulting host reactions
  - Intestinal infection
    - Most common symptoms: Abdominal pain, diarrhea (may mimic IBD)
    - Heavy infections: Intestinal bleeding and iron deficiency anemia
  - Hepatosplenic infection
    - In adults, chronic infection leads to periportal fibrosis, resulting in portal hypertension, splenomegaly, portocaval shunting, and gastrointestinal varices
    - Coinfection of hepatitis B/hepatitis C and schistosomiasis is reported to cause more severe disease and worse prognosis than those infected with either pathogen alone
  - Urinary tract infection
    - Early infection: Hematuria with eggs excreted in urine
    - Early chronic infection: Granulomatous inflammation and ulcerations result in development of pseudopolyps, which may mimic malignancy
    - Longstanding infection: Fibrosis and calcification of bladder wall, bladder neck obstruction; associated with bacterial superinfection, acute renal failure, and development of bladder cancer
  - Genital tract infection
    - Women: Hypertrophic &/or ulcerative lesions of cervix, vagina, or vulva; involvement of ovaries or fallopian tubes may lead to infertility
    - Men: Infection may involve epididymis, testicles, spermatic cord, or prostate
    - Reported to be risk factor for HIV infection in endemic areas
  - Pulmonary infection
    - Occurs mostly as complication in patients with hepatosplenic infection, which leads to embolization of *Schistosoma* eggs into pulmonary circulation
    - Progression of disease can result in granulomatous pulmonary endarteritis, pulmonary hypertension, and cor pulmonale
  - CNS infection
    - Results from embolization of eggs/egg-laying worms to spinal cord or cerebral microcirculation
    - Myelopathy is more common than cerebral disease
    - Brain involvement may present as single or multiple intracerebral lesions

Laboratory Tests

- Serologic testing
  - Commercial assays are available against various schistosome antigens, e.g., ELISA, radioimmunoassay, Western blot, complement fixation
  - Sensitivity and specificity depend on serologic technique, antigen used, and intensity of infection

- Tests are generally negative during acute infection and turn positive 6-12 weeks after exposure
- Cannot distinguish between prior infection and active disease
- Antigen testing
  - Qualitative assays that measure parasite antigens in blood, stool, &/or urine have been developed
  - Sensitivity and specificity vary with assay techniques and targeted antigens but are reported to be as good as or better than stool or urine concentration methods for egg detection
- Molecular diagnostics
  - PCR assays for stool, urine, and serum have been developed but largely remain as research tools
- Ova detection in clinical specimens
  - Eggs can be detected in urine and stool specimens by microscopy
  - Extent of egg shedding may vary widely; multiple specimens may be needed for diagnosis

Treatment

- Generally treated with praziquantel
- Reexamination of feces or urine after treatment is recommended to assess efficacy

Prognosis

- Mortality related to schistosomiasis is low
- Likelihood of complications and morbidity correlate with parasite burden, duration of infection, sites of infection

IMAGING

Radiographic Findings

- Chest: Fine miliary nodules corresponding to granulomatous reactions to *Schistosoma* eggs
- Bladder: Eggshell calcification in submucosa of bladder and ureteral wall in longstanding infection

CT Findings

- Liver: Septal calcifications aligned perpendicularly to liver capsule produce characteristic turtle-back appearance of hepatic schistosomiasis

MICROBIOLOGY

General Features

- Schistosoma adults typically found in copula
- Specific morphologic features vary with species
- Males are robust, 6-20 mm long, with ventral folding to form gynecophoral canal, grossly tuberculate tegument (most species), 2 small anterior suckers, and 4-9 testes posterior to ventral suckers
- Female are slender, 7-26 mm long, lack tegument tuberculation, and have single ovary near ventral sucker; uterus contains variable number of eggs

MACROSCOPIC

Gross Examination

- Liver: Symmer clay pipestem fibrosis: Enlarged fibrotic portal tracts with severe portal fibrosis due to schistosomiasis
- Bladder/intestines
  - "Sandy patches": Masses of calcified ova in mucosa
  - Polyps or masses: Arise due to granulomatous inflammation and subsequent fibrosis surrounding eggs

MICROSCOPIC

Histologic Features

- Tissue reactions
  - Inflammatory granulomatous reaction and eosinophilic infiltration, which result in local tissue destruction and fibrosis; entrapped ova eventually die and calcify
  - Recently laid eggs can cause acute inflammation
- Morphology of *Schistosoma* eggs can be used to identify species but requires careful interpretation due to irregular sectioning, which can obscure size/location of spines
  - *S. mansoni* (average:140 x 66 μm): Elongated/oval egg with lateral spine
  - *S. haematobium* (average: 143 x 60 μm): Elongated/oval egg with terminal spine
  - *S. japonicum* (average: 90 x 70 μm): Oval egg with small lateral spine/knob
  - *S. intercalatum* (average: 175 x 60 μm): Resembles *S. haematobium* egg, but it is longer, thinner, and has longer terminal spine
  - *S. mekongi* (average: 69 x 56 μm): Spherical egg with small lateral spine that is not always visible
- Adults worms are rarely seen but most commonly encountered in blood vessels; transverse sections show larger males surrounding more slender females

DIFFERENTIAL DIAGNOSIS

Strongyloidiasis

- *Strongyloides* worms and larvae are seen in intestinal crypts and mucosa, often associated with exuberant eosinophilic infiltration
- In intestinal infection, egg-laying *Schistosoma* worms are present in microvasculature, while ova are mainly in submucosa, associated with granulomatous reaction with less intense eosinophilic infiltrate

Coccidioidomycosis

- Lacks ova and shows spherules with endospores

Tuberculosis

- Positive for acid-fast stain and lacks ova and eosinophilic inflammation

Sarcoidosis

- Lacks presence of ova and eosinophilic inflammation

Neoplasms

- Lack ova and exhibit histologic morphologies consistent with malignant or benign neoplasms

SELECTED REFERENCES

1. Ebersbach JC et al: Matrix-assisted laser desorption/ionization time-of-flight mass spectrometry for differential identification of adult Schistosoma worms. Parasit Vectors. 16(1):20, 2023
2. Tamarozzi F et al: Diagnosis and clinical management of hepatosplenic schistosomiasis: a scoping review of the literature. PLoS Negl Trop Dis. 15(3):e0009191, 2021
3. Wilson RA: Schistosomiasis then and now: what has changed in the last 100 years? Parasitology. 1-9, 2020
4. McManus DP et al: Schistosomiasis. Nat Rev Dis Primers. 4(1):13, 2018

Schistosoma mansoni Ovum

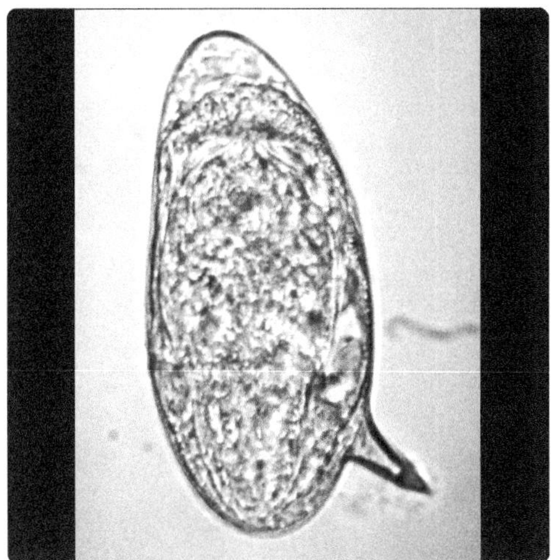

Schistosoma mansoni in Tissue Sections

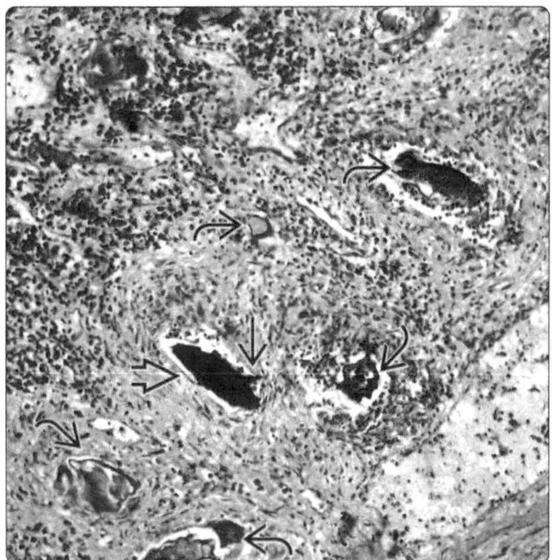

(Left) *Schistosoma mansoni ova are oval in shape, measuring 114-180 µm long x 45-70 µm wide, and can be identified by a prominent lateral spine near the posterior end. (Courtesy CDC/PHIL.)* **(Right)** *This liver section shows multiple S. mansoni eggs ➢ in different orientations, surrounded by granulomatous inflammation and fibrosis. One egg ➢ appears calcified and exhibits a prominent lateral spine ➢.*

Schistosoma haematobium Ovum

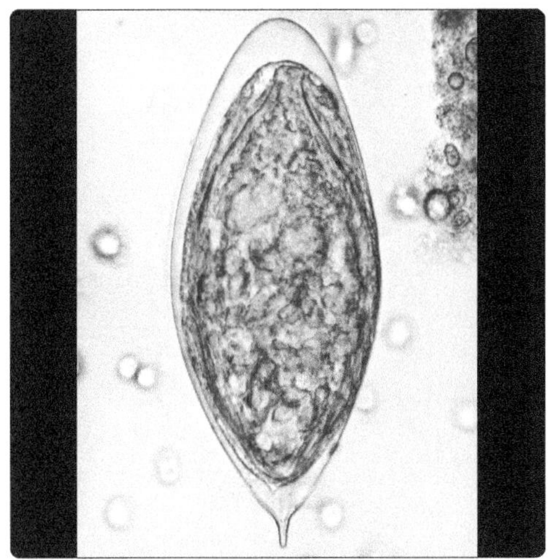

Schistosoma haematobium in Tissue Sections

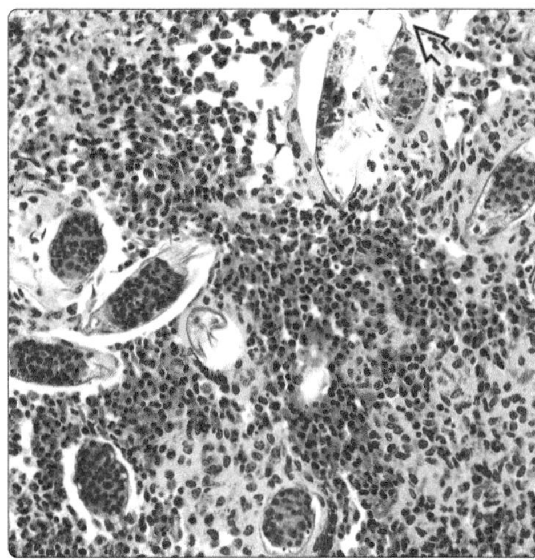

(Left) *S. haematobium ova are oval in shape, measuring 110-170 µm long x 40-70 µm wide, and contain a posteriorly protruding terminal spine. (Courtesy Dr. Martin, CDC/PHIL.)* **(Right)** *This bladder biopsy shows multiple elongated Schistosoma eggs containing viable miracidia. The abundance of eosinophils possibly suggests an acute infection. A terminal spine ➢ is present on an egg, consistent with S. haematobium.*

Schistosoma japonicum Ovum

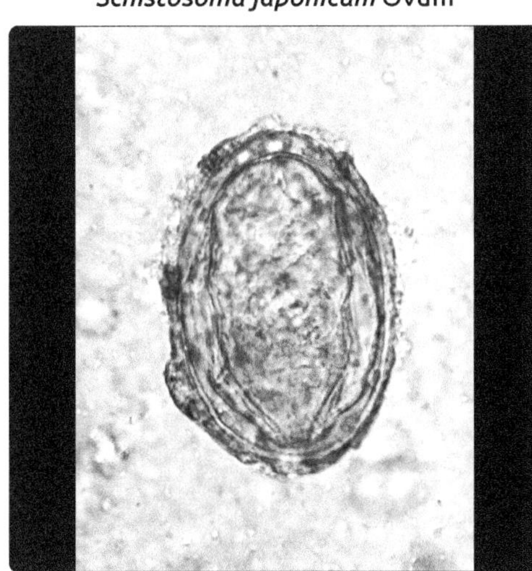

Schistosoma japonicum in Tissue Sections

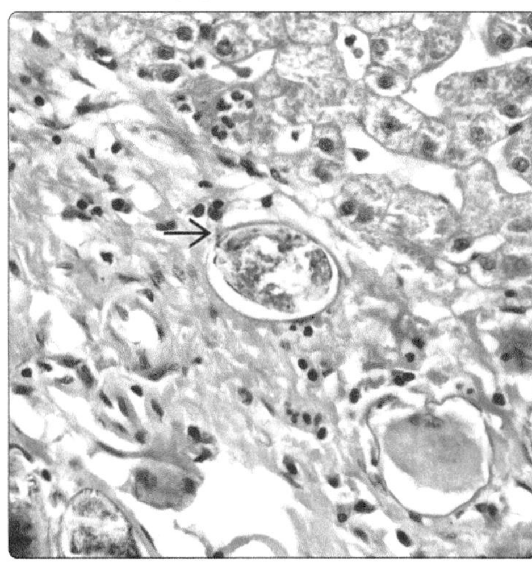

(Left) *Schistosoma japonicum ova are round, measuring 70-100 µm long x 55-64 µm wide, and contain vestigial, laterally protruding spines, which may be difficult to identify in tissue sections. (Courtesy CDC/PHIL.)* **(Right)** *This section shows a Schistosoma egg with a small lateral spine ➢, consistent with S. japonicum. (Courtesy A. Laga, MD, MMSc.)*

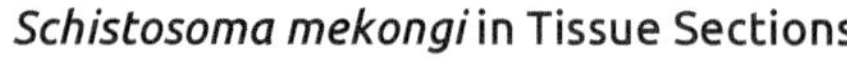

Schistosoma mekongi in Tissue Sections

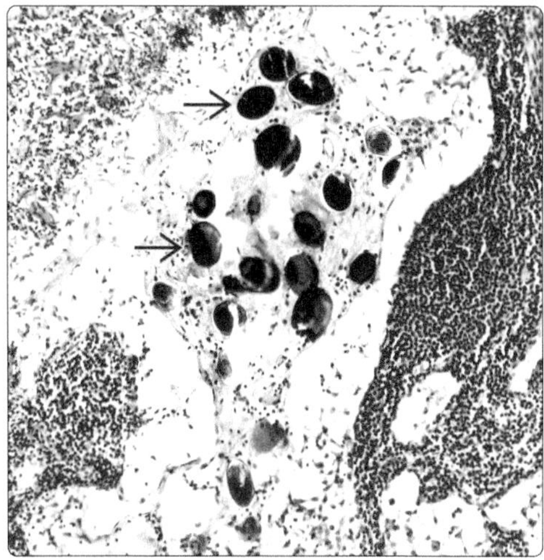

Pulmonary Granuloma

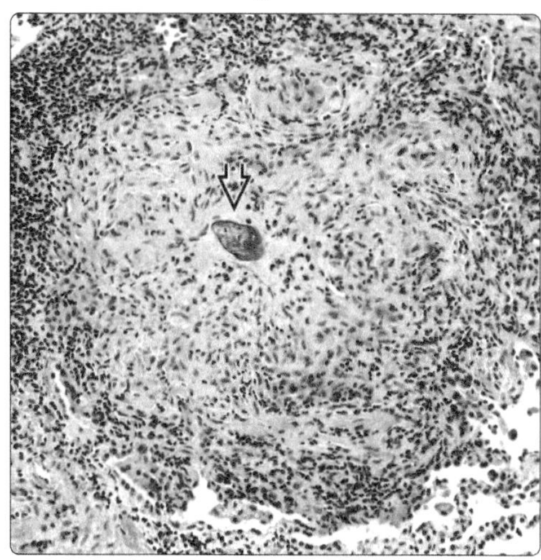

(Left) *This periintestinal lymph node section shows multiple small, spherical, calcified Schistosoma eggs → in a patient with infection of Schistosoma mekongi in the jejunal mucosa.* **(Right)** *A lung section shows a Schistosoma egg ⇨ in a granuloma surrounded by chronic inflammation with eosinophils.*

Schistosoma Eggs in Bowel

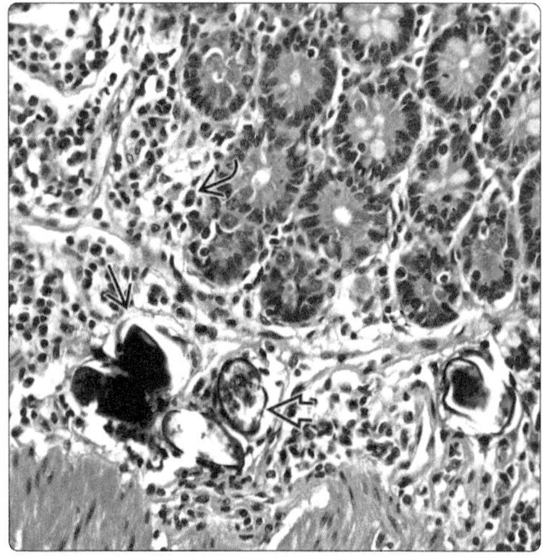

Schistosoma mansoni Lateral Spines

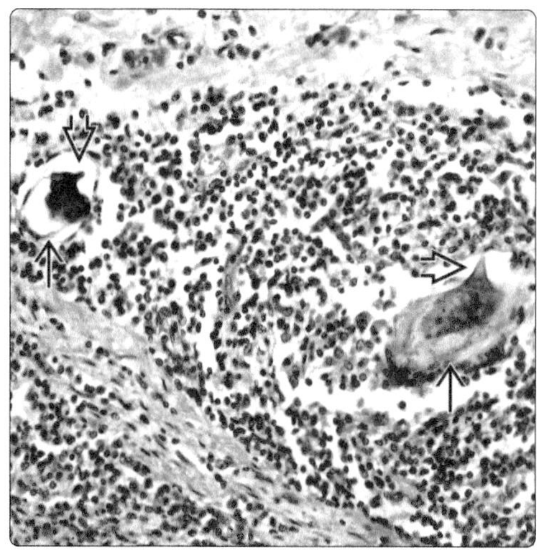

(Left) *Calcified → and noncalcified ⇨ eggs of Schistosoma are seen in the lamina propria of the bowel with scattered eosinophils ↷. Migrating eggs have a finite time to exit before they degrade and calcify.* **(Right)** *High magnification of this intestinal section shows 2 Schistosoma eggs ⇨ associated with confluent eosinophilic and chronic inflammation. Both ova exhibit prominent lateral spines →, consistent with S. mansoni.*

Liver With Chronic Schistosomiasis

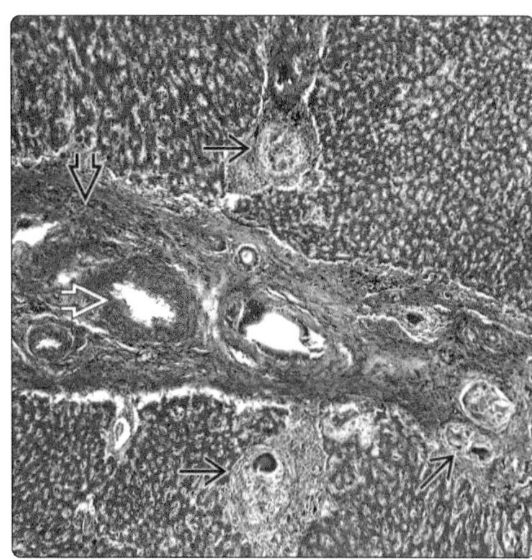

Omental *Schistosoma mansoni*

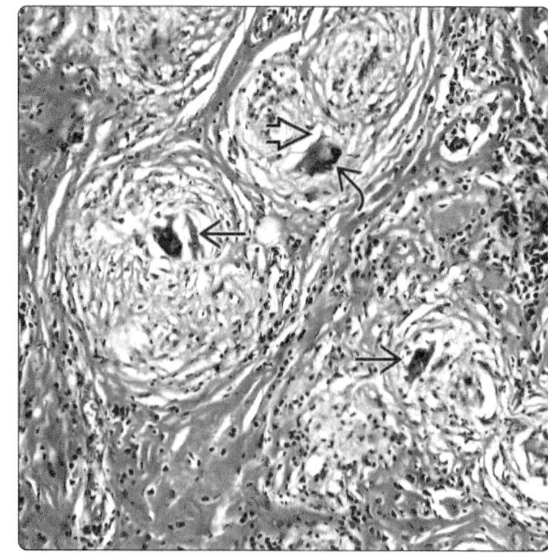

(Left) *This liver section shows periovular granuloma formation → against ova lodged in veins branching off from a medium-sized portal trunk, as well as periportal fibrosis ("pipestem fibrosis") ⇨ with arterial dilation ➡, consistent with advanced hepatic schistosomiasis.* **(Right)** *This omental mass shows a pseudotumor consisting of foamy histiocytes and inflammatory cells in whorled masses around S. mansoni eggs →. A lateral spine is seen on 1 of the eggs ⇨, which is being enveloped by a giant cell ↷.*

Bladder Schistosomiasis

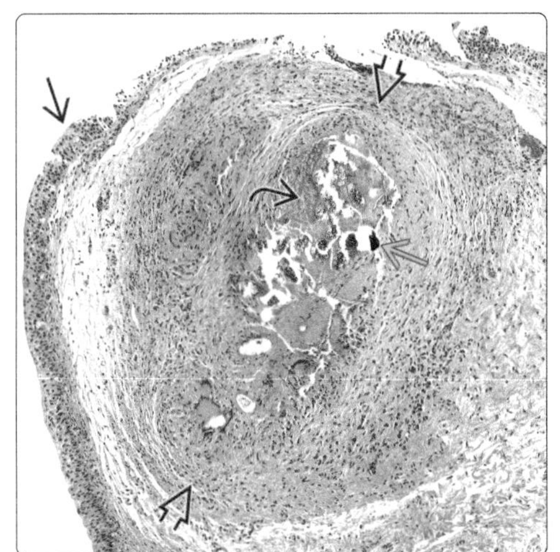

Bladder Schistosomiasis

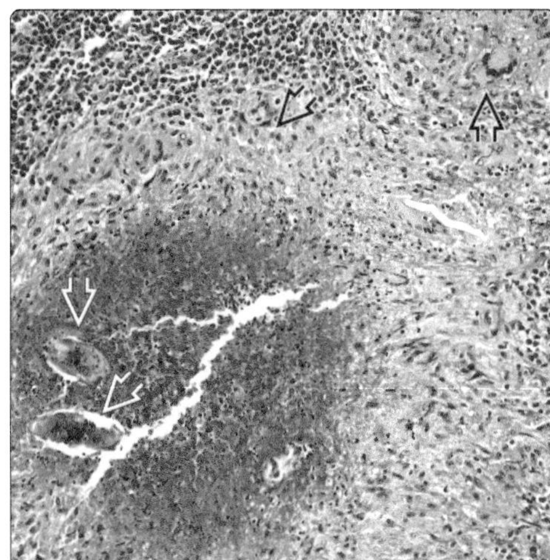

(Left) *Low magnification of a bladder wall with epithelium ➡ containing a large granuloma ➡ with giant cells, necrosis ➡, and calcified eggs ➡ is shown. Such a nodule may suggest tumor on cystoscopy.* **(Right)** *Medium magnification of this bladder section reveals 2 Schistosoma eggs ➡ associated with granulomatous reaction ➡ with central necrosis, eosinophils, and chronic inflammation.*

Cerebral Schistosomiasis

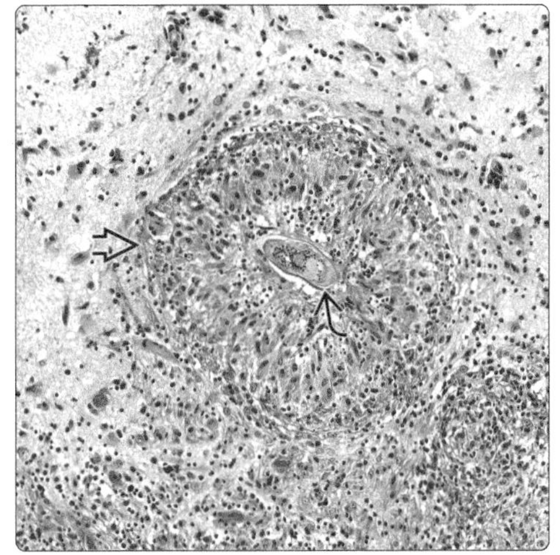

Uterine Schistosomiasis

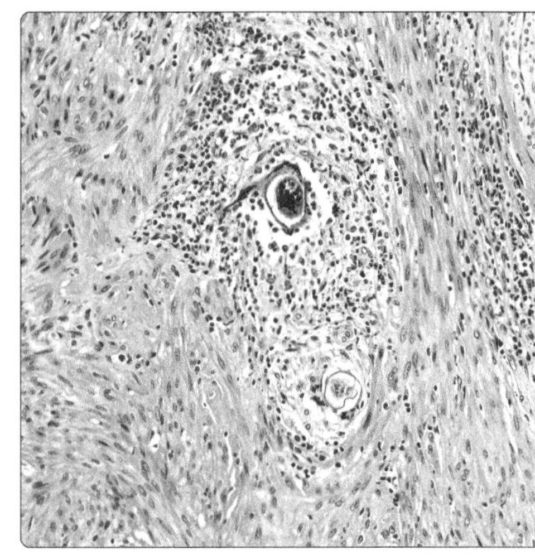

(Left) *A section of the brain with an active granuloma ➡ containing a Schistosoma egg ➡ is shown. Note that the brain is not a life cycle-supportive location for trematodes and represents aberrant pathology harmful to host and parasite.* **(Right)** *Schistosoma eggs in the female genitourinary tract are not uncommon in endemic areas and are often incidental in other surgical indications, as in these eggs seen in uterine fibroids. However, granulomas can precipitate surgical procedures for pain and bleeding.*

Cercarial Dermatitis (Swimmer's Itch)

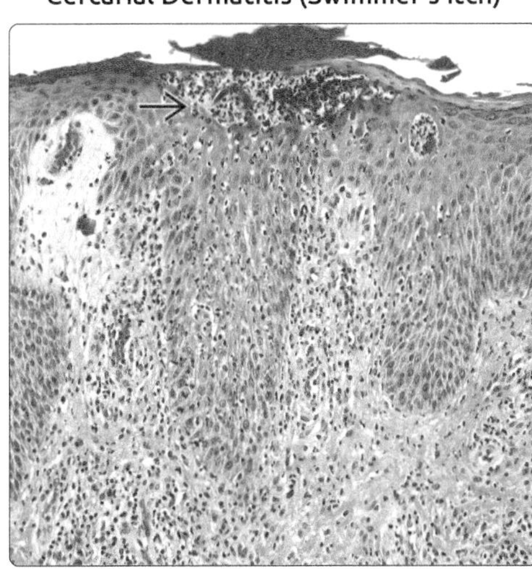

Cercariae in Tissue

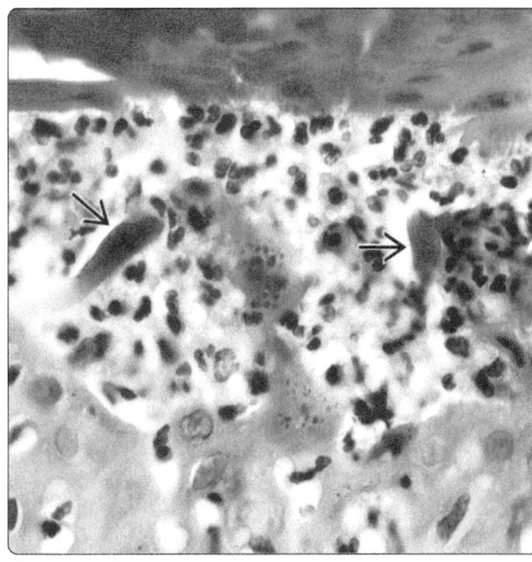

(Left) *Cercarial dermatitis is caused by penetration of skin by zoonotic schistosomes that do not complete their life cycle or mature into adults in humans. Immediately after emerging from water, exposed skin becomes itchy and red, indicative of cercariae penetration, which is shown here by a cercarial burrow ➡. (Courtesy A. Laga, MD, MMSc.)* **(Right)** *Tangential sections of 2 cercariae ➡ are present in this high-magnification image from a case of cercarial dermatitis. (Courtesy A. Laga, MD, MMSc.)*

KEY FACTS

ETIOLOGY/PATHOGENESIS

- Parasitic tissue infection caused by larval cysts (coenuri) of tapeworms *Taenia multiceps*, *Taenia serialis*, *Taenia brauni*, and *Taenia glomeratus*
- Transmitted by ingestion of eggs found in dog feces

CLINICAL ISSUES

- Rare infection in humans; occurs in areas with uncontrolled dog populations
- Majority of documented cases from Africa and sheep-raising areas of Europe, South America, USA, and Canada
- Occurs in any organ, particularly brain, eyes, and subcutaneous tissue

MACROSCOPIC

- Encapsulated, nodular mass consisting of inner parasitic cyst and outer host-generated capsule

MICROSCOPIC

- Body wall consists of outer tegument with papillae and microvilli, muscle cells, tegumental cells, and parenchyma with occasional calcareous corpuscles
- Invaginated protoscoleces present in irregular groups with birefringent and acid-fast hooklets
- Capsule consists of dense fibrous tissue infiltrated by plasma cells, lymphocytes, macrophages, and eosinophils
- Dying cysts associated with acute inflammation, followed by necrosis, chronic inflammation, fibrosis, and calcification

TOP DIFFERENTIAL DIAGNOSES

- Cysticercosis (*Taenia solium*) larvae
  - Single protoscolex and shorter hooklets
- Echinococcosis (*Echinococcus* spp.)
  - Smaller protoscoleces and hooklets; loose connecting cyst structures
- Sparganosis (*Spirometra* spp.) larvae
  - No protoscoleces

Coenurosis Life Cycle

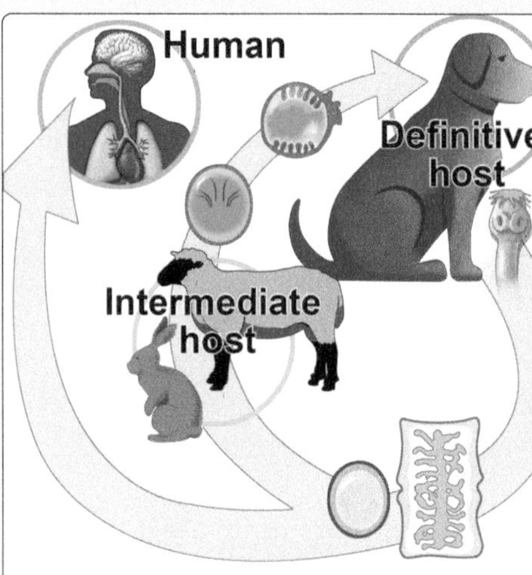

Coenurosis: Internal Structures

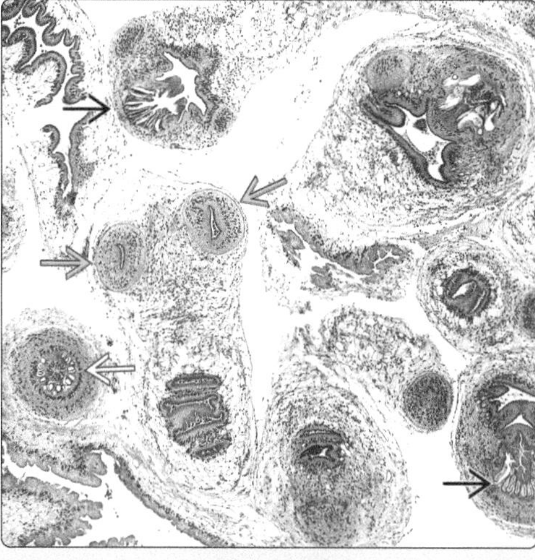

(Left) *Eggs and proglottids are passed in feces, where they may be ingested by intermediate hosts, develop from oncospheres into coenuri and complete life cycle after being consumed by definitive host. Humans can also develop tissue infections with coenur, but do not support maturation of worms into adults.* **(Right)** *A low-power image of a subcutaneous coenurus shows multiple invaginated protoscoleces ⇨. An armed rostellum ➡ and multiple suckers ⇨ are also present in this section.*

Coenurosis: Cyst Wall

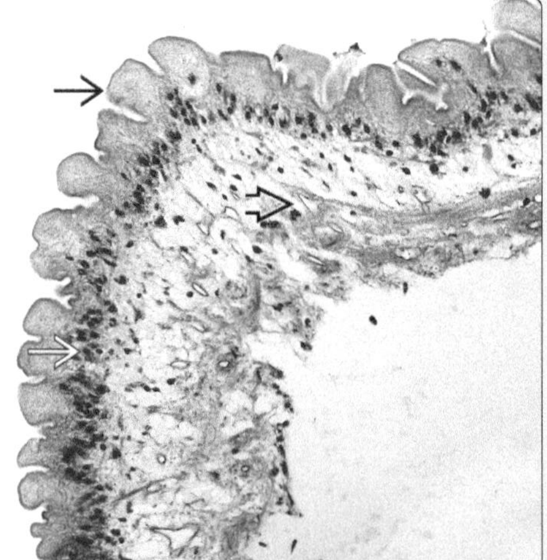

Coenurosis Protoscolex

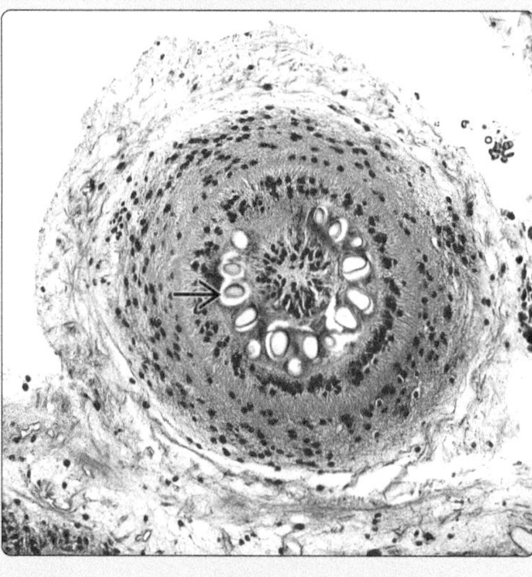

(Left) *A section of coenurus cyst wall shows the outer tegument with raised papillae ⇨ and a layer of tegumental cells ➡ separating the tegument from the underlying parenchyma containing haphazardly arranged muscle fibers ⇨.* **(Right)** *A coenurus protoscolex is shown with an armed rostellum with multiple hooklets ⇨. The hooklets are birefringent on polarized light, as are all cestode hooklets.*

TERMINOLOGY

Definitions

- "Coeno" (common) + "oura" (tail) from Greek, suggesting many heads with 1 tail

ETIOLOGY/PATHOGENESIS

Infectious Agents

- Parasitic tissue infection caused by larval cysts (coenuri) of tapeworms *Taenia multiceps*, *Taenia serialis*, *Taenia brauni*, and *Taenia glomeratus*
- Requires definitive host (canids) and intermediate host (e.g., sheep, rabbits) to complete life cycle; humans are accidental intermediate hosts
- Transmitted by ingestion of eggs found in dog feces
- Oncospheres hatch in intestine, invade intestinal wall, and migrate to brain, eyes, skeletal muscle, and subcutaneous tissue and develop into coenuri (~ 3 months after ingestion)

CLINICAL ISSUES

Epidemiology

- Wide distribution; predominantly in children (Africa and sheep-raising areas of Europe, South America, USA, Canada)

Site

- Occurs in any organ, particularly brain and eyes (*T. multiceps*) and subcutaneous tissue (*T. serialis*)

Presentation

- Skin/subcutaneous issues: Solitary painless nodules
- CNS: Headache, fever, vomiting, localized symptoms, hydrocephalus, arteritis with transient hemiparesis
- Eye infection: Intraocular and orbital infections, visual impairment, blindness

Laboratory Tests

- Exclude cysticercosis and echinococcosis with routine serology testing (IgG) for both organisms

Treatment

- Primary prevention
  - Avoidance of food/water that might be contaminated by feces from dogs or intermediate hosts
  - Regular treatment of dogs for tapeworms
- Surgical intervention preferred for single intracranial or eye coenurus
- Antihelminthic treatment with praziquantel effective in killing coenuri but associated with marked inflammation

Prognosis

- Generally good prognosis; recovery of sight
- Multiple neural coenuri associated with poor prognosis

IMAGING

MR Findings

- Isointense with cerebrospinal fluid

CT Findings

- Viable coenurus appears as thin-walled cyst
- Degenerating cyst with contrast-enhancing peripheral rim

MICROBIOLOGY

Parasite Features

- Coenurus (metacestode stage): Thin-walled, white, spherical, polycephalic cysts (< 1 cm to 6 cm) filled with jelly-like fluid and multiple protoscoleces (50-100 per cyst)
- Adult tapeworm: 20-70 cm in length; piriform scolex with 4 suckers and armed rostellum with double circle of 22-33 hooklets (only seen in canids)
- Gravid proglottids: Longer than broad; uterus with 18-26 lateral branches per site (*T. serialis* has well-developed vaginal sphincters compared to *T. multiceps*)
- Eggs: Spherical with thick, radially striated shell (29-37 μm in diameter); only seen in canid feces

MACROSCOPIC

General Features

- Encapsulated, nodular mass consisting of inner parasitic cyst and outer host-generated capsule

MICROSCOPIC

Histologic Features

- Body wall (50-150 μm thick): Outer tegument with papillae and microvilli, muscle cells, tegumental cells, and parenchyma with occasional calcareous corpuscles
- Invaginated protoscoleces: Attached to cyst wall by neck; present in irregular groups
- Hooklets (110-175 μm long) are birefringent and acid-fast
- Capsule consists of dense fibrous tissue heavily infiltrated by plasma cells, lymphocytes, macrophages, and eosinophils
- Dying cysts associated with acute inflammation, followed by necrosis, chronic inflammation, fibrosis, and calcification

DIFFERENTIAL DIAGNOSIS

Cysticercosis

- Larval form (cysticercus) of *Taenia solium*
- Similar morphologic features to coenurosis; contains single protoscolex
- Longer hooklets in *T. multiceps* and *T. serialis* (110-175 μm) vs. *T. solium* (100-130 μm)

Echinococcosis

- Larval form of *Echinococcus* spp.
- Contains multiple protoscoleces that arise from germinal membrane; protoscoleces and hooklets smaller than those of coenuri

Sparganosis

- Larval form (sparganum) of *Spirometra* spp.
- No protoscoleces

SELECTED REFERENCES

1. Nhlonzi GB et al: Clinicopathological review of human coenurosis in Kwazulu-Natal, South Africa: a retrospective single center study. Iran J Parasitol. 17(1):62-9, 2022
2. Varcasia A et al: Taenia multiceps coenurosis: a review. Parasit Vectors. 15(1):84, 2022
3. Kulanthaivelu K et al: Brain MRI findings in coenurosis: a helminth infection. J Neuroimaging. 30(3):359-69, 2020
4. Ali SM et al: Cerebral coenurosis masquerading as malignancy: a rare case report from India. J Neurosci Rural Pract. 10(2):367-70, 2019

Cysticercosis

KEY FACTS

ETIOLOGY/PATHOGENESIS

- Parasitic tissue infection; inflammatory response to dying larval cysts (metacestode stage) of *Taenia solium*

CLINICAL ISSUES

- Seizure disorder in 2.5 million people worldwide; 50,000 fatal cases/year
- Symptoms dependent on location, size, number, and stage of cysts (viable, degenerating, or calcified)
- Enzyme-linked immunoelectrotransfer blot detects serum or CSF antibodies
- Treat with anticonvulsants, corticosteroids, surgery, &/or antihelminthic drugs (albendazole, praziquantel)
- In patients with taeniasis, important to distinguish between *T. solium* and *Taenia saginata*

MACROSCOPIC

- Viable cysts (1 cm in diameter) are translucent and contain single invaginated protoscolex
- Racemose neurocysticercosis: Large, multiloculated, extraparenchymal cysts lacking identifiable scolex

MICROSCOPIC

- Cyst wall (100-200 μm thick): Outer tegument with papillae and microvilli, haphazardly arranged muscle fibers, tegumental cells, and parenchyma with occasional calcareous bodies
- Protoscoleces contain rostellum armed with double row of hooklets (birefringent and acid-fast) and spherical suckers
- Later stages of degeneration absent of larvae; fibrotic capsular abscess-like walls and chronic inflammation; remote infection with dystrophic calcified nodules

TOP DIFFERENTIAL DIAGNOSES

- Coenurosis: Similar morphology; multiple protoscoleces
- Echinococcosis: Larger; daughter cysts with multiple protoscoleces with smaller hooklets
- Other intraventricular cysts: Epithelium-lined cyst walls; no organism parts

Taenia solium Life Cycle

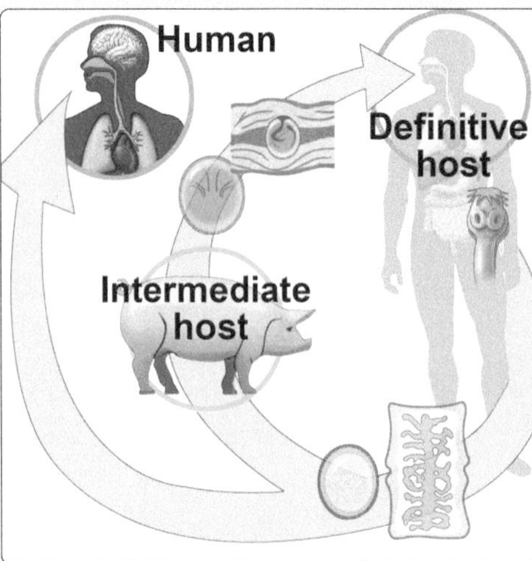

Single Cysticercus Involving Brain

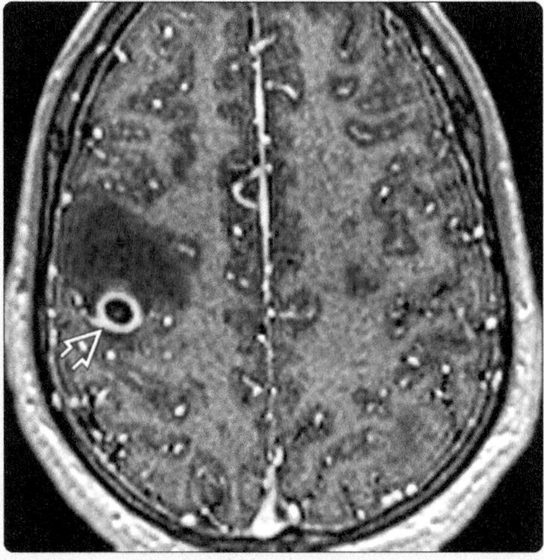

(Left) *Adult Taenia solium worms attach via scolex to the small intestine in humans, shedding proglottids and eggs in feces. Ingestion by pigs or humans results in hatching of oncospheres, which penetrate intestinal wall and migrate to muscles, brain, etc., and develop into cysticerci. Human tapeworm infection occurs with ingestion of undercooked pork containing cysticerci.* **(Right)** *MR of a patient with neurocysticercosis shows peripheral enhancement of the cyst wall ➡ with a central "dot" representing the scolex. (From DI: Brain.)*

Gross Photograph of Intact Cyst

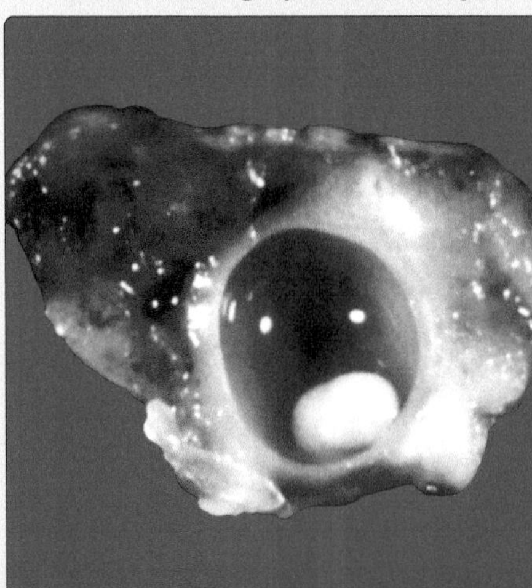

Viable Cysticercus With Inverted Scolex

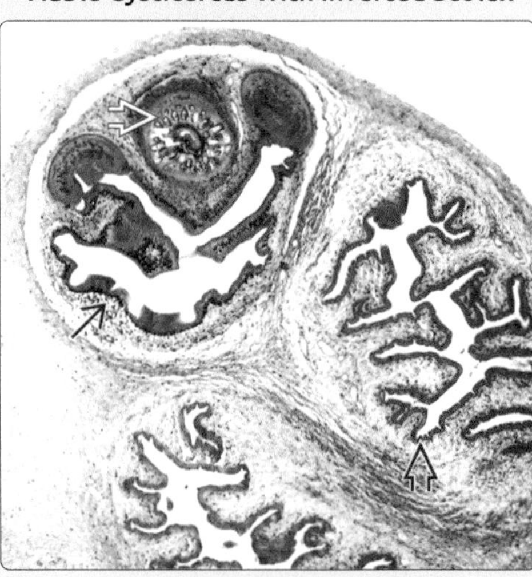

(Left) *Gross pathology shows a translucent cyst with a characteristic invaginated white scolex diagnostic of neurocysticercosis. This resected lesion came from a seizure patient. (Courtesy B. Cremin, MD.)* **(Right)** *Sections show a viable T. solium cysticercus with inverted protoscolex ⇨, armed rostellum with double row of hooklets ➡, and gastrodermis ⇨. (Courtesy Franz von Lichtenberg Collection of Infection Disease Pathology, BWH.)*

TERMINOLOGY

Definitions

- Derived from Greek: "Kystic" (bladder) and "kercos" (tail)

ETIOLOGY/PATHOGENESIS

Infectious Agents

- Parasitic tissue infection caused by cysticerci (metacestode stage) of tapeworm *Taenia solium*
- Transmitted by ingestion of eggs; oncospheres hatch in intestine, invade intestinal wall, migrate to tissues, and then develop into cysticerci
- Symptoms occur months to years after infection, typically when cysts start to die, releasing parasite antigens with acute inflammatory response

CLINICAL ISSUES

Epidemiology

- Occurs globally; highest rates of infection in areas of Latin America, Asia, and Africa with poor sanitation and free-ranging pigs that have access to human feces
- Seizure disorder in 2.5 million people worldwide; estimated 50,000 fatal cases per year

Site

- Brain, muscle, spine, eyes, skin, heart

Presentation

- Symptoms dependent on location, size, number, and stage of cysts (viable, degenerating, calcified, racemose)
- Neurocysticercosis: Usually presents with seizures (70-90%) or headaches; occasional confusion, difficulties with balance, or hydrocephalus; may be asymptomatic
- Muscle infection: Typically asymptomatic; may present with tender or nontender lumps
- Eye infection: Rarely causes blurry or disturbed vision

Laboratory Tests

- CSF: Lymphocytic or eosinophilic pleocytosis, low glucose, high protein
- EEG: Abnormal in 50% of cases; no specific pattern
- Serology, RT-PCR (serum, CSF)
  - Enzyme-linked immunoelectrotransfer blot (EITB): Serum or CSF
    - 100% specific; 90% sensitive for > 2 lesions
    - 50-60% sensitive for single or calcified lesions
  - Antibodies (IgG) detected by ELISA in serum or CSF
    - Decrease quickly with appropriate treatment so can be followed for response to therapy
  - Antibodies (IgG) detected by Western blot in serum
    - Positive tests to any of proteins of 50, 42-39, 24, 21, 18, or 14 kDa
    - Absence of 50 or 42-39 may indicate cross reaction from *Echinococcus*
  - Antigen detection not recommended except in special circumstances (consult with CDC)

Treatment

- Primary prevention
  - Treatment of tapeworm carriers and avoidance of food/water contaminated by human or pig feces
- Management of neurologic complications
  - Anticonvulsants, corticosteroids, surgical excision, ventricular shunting
- Antihelminthic treatment
  - Oral albendazole and praziquantel for symptomatic patients with multiple live (noncalcified) cysticerci
  - Used with caution due to inflammatory response induced by larval death; coadministration with corticosteroids

Prognosis

- Neurocysticercosis with > 50 parenchymal cysts or with extraparenchymal cysts (especially racemose) associated with poor prognosis

IMAGING

MR Findings

- More sensitive than CT at showing cysts in some locations (cerebral convexity, ventricular ependyma)
- Highlights surrounding edema and internal changes indicating cysticerci death

CT Findings

- Superior to MR for demonstrating small calcifications

MICROBIOLOGY

General Features

- Adult tapeworm: Up to 1,000 proglottids and 9 m in length; scolex with armed rostellum with double row of hooklets (22-36, 100-200 μm in length) and 4 large, cupped suckers
- Gravid proglottids: Longer than broad (11 x 5 mm); uterus with 7-13 lateral branches per side and single genital pore
  - *Taenia saginata* distinguished by greater number of uterine branches (15-20); does not cause human cysticercosis
- Eggs: Thick, radially striated shell (31-43 μm in diameter), not easily distinguished from other *Taenia* spp.

MACROSCOPIC

General Features

- Cysts intraparenchymal, in cortical sulci, or subarachnoid with grossly normal surrounding brain
- Viable cysts (1 cm in diameter) are translucent and contain single invaginated protoscolex
- Racemose neurocysticercosis: Large, multiloculated, extraparenchymal cysts lacking identifiable scolex

MICROSCOPIC

Histologic Features

- Cyst wall (100-200 μm thick): Outer tegument with papillae and microvilli, haphazardly arranged muscle fibers, tegumental cells, and parenchyma with occasional calcareous bodies
- Protoscoleces contain rostellum armed with double row of hooklets (birefringent and acid-fast) and spherical suckers
- Later stages of degeneration absent of larvae; fibrotic capsular abscess-like walls and chronic inflammation; remote infection with dystrophic calcified nodules

Distinguishing Cestodes in Human Tissue

Disease	Cysticercosis/Neurocysticercosis	Hydatid Disease	Coenurosis	Sparganosis
Species	*Taenia solium*	*Echinococcus granulosus, E. multilocularis, E. oligarthrus, E. vogeli*	*Taenia multiceps, T. serialis, T. brauni, T. glomeratus*	*Spirometra mansoni, S. ranarum, S. mansonoides, S. erinacei, Sparganum proliferum*
Exposure	Porcine or human tapeworm carriers of *T. solium*	Exposure to dogs/canids, foxes/canids, bush dogs/canids, felids (respectively)	Feces of canids feeding on intermediate hosts; pastoral (herding) exposures	Contaminated water or undercooked flesh of secondary intermediate host (fish/frog)
Radiology	Solitary cyst with fluid or internal structure or solid, calcified round to oval structure; can be multiple or aggregated (racemose)	Large (2- to 20-cm) cyst, largely fluid filled, with internal daughter cysts (grape-like appearance) or destructive, tumor-like lesions with daughter cyst formation	Single large (2- to 5-cm) cyst, hypoattenuating without central contrast enhancement (CT) with intensity of fluid (MR)	Variable (any body site)
Sampling	Surgical removal of 0.5- to 1.5-cm, whitish/gray, round to ovoid cyst (or solid calcified lesion)	Aspiration [(as part of puncture, aspiration, injection, reaspiration (PAIR)]; surgical resection of large, intact, thick-walled cyst (any size, usually much larger than other species) or ruptured with grape-like cystic structures	Surgical removal of 2- to 5-cm, whitish/gray, polypoid bladder structures	Surgical removal of 3- to 7-cm white, flat worms
Microscopy	Outer tegument containing calcareous corpuscles and single larval structure with 1 protoscolex with evident hooklets and suckers with supporting connective tissue	Outer tegument containing calcareous corpuscles and multiple protoscoleces with evident hooklets and suckers floating in clear fluid with thin connecting cyst walls	Outer tegument containing calcareous corpuscles and multiple protoscoleces with evident hooklets and suckers and cellular connective tissue	Outer tegument containing calcareous corpuscles, scattered nuclei, cystic spaces
Other helpful hints	Strong history of exposure to pigs or humans exposed to pigs; exposure may be 5-7 years prior to presentation	Grow ~ 1 cm per year in any body space (liver, lung, brain, etc.) with presentation timing related to body site	Most commonly seen in Africa or European settings with pastoral activities	Although worldwide in distribution, more common with consumption of undercooked/raw fish/frogs

Comparison of the most common cestodes found in human tissue with comparisons of the key features to distinguish them, which has implications for treatment.

Cytologic Features

- Aspiration/smear of solitary cyst or fluid from contaminated space may contain hooklets
    - Extreme caution should be used as persistent cysts large enough for aspiration are more likely *Echinococcus*, which has worse prognosis if disrupted

DIFFERENTIAL DIAGNOSIS

Coenurosis

- Metacestode larvae (*Taenia multiceps, T. serialis, T. brauni, T. glomeratus*)
- Similar morphologic features to cysticerci; distinguished by presence of multiple protoscoleces

Echinococcosis

- Larval stage of *Echinococcus* spp.
- Contains daughter cysts with multiple protoscoleces; grow at 1 cm per year until detection &/or rupture

Other Intraventricular Cysts

- Choroid plexus cysts, ependymal cysts, colloid cyst
- Cyst wall lined by epithelium; no organism parts

SELECTED REFERENCES

1. Stelzle D et al: Clinical characteristics and management of neurocysticercosis patients: a retrospective assessment of case reports from Europe. J Travel Med. 30(1):taac102, 2023
2. Del Brutto OH: Human neurocysticercosis: an overview. Pathogens. 11(10):1212, 2022
3. Garcia HH et al: New animal models of neurocysticercosis can help understand epileptogenesis in neuroinfection. Front Mol Neurosci. 15:1039083, 2022
4. Pineda-Reyes R et al: Neurocysticercosis: an update on diagnosis, treatment, and prevention. Curr Opin Infect Dis. 35(3):246-54, 2022
5. Del Brutto OH et al: The many facets of disseminated parenchymal brain cysticercosis: a differential diagnosis with important therapeutic implications. PLoS Negl Trop Dis. 15(11):e0009883, 2021
6. Gupta D et al: Cytomorphological spectrum of cysticercosis: a study of 26 cases. Cytopathology. 32(6):802-6, 2021
7. Centers for Disease Control and Prevention: Parasites. Cysticercosis. Updated September 22, 2020. Accessed January 3, 2023. http://www.cdc.gov/parasites/cysticercosis
8. Garcia HH et al: Laboratory diagnosis of neurocysticercosis (Taenia solium). J Clin Microbiol. 56(9):e00424-18, 2018
9. McClugage SG 3rd et al: Treatment of racemose neurocysticercosis. Surg Neurol Int. 8:168, 2017
10. Gonzales I et al: Pathogenesis of Taenia solium taeniasis and cysticercosis. Parasite Immunol. 38(3):136-46, 2016
11. Lichtenberg F: Pathology of Infectious Diseases. Raven Press, 1991

Egg of *Taenia* Species

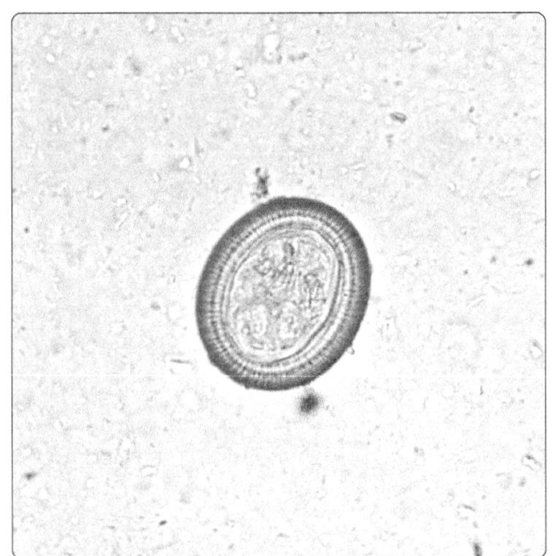

Taenia solium Scolex

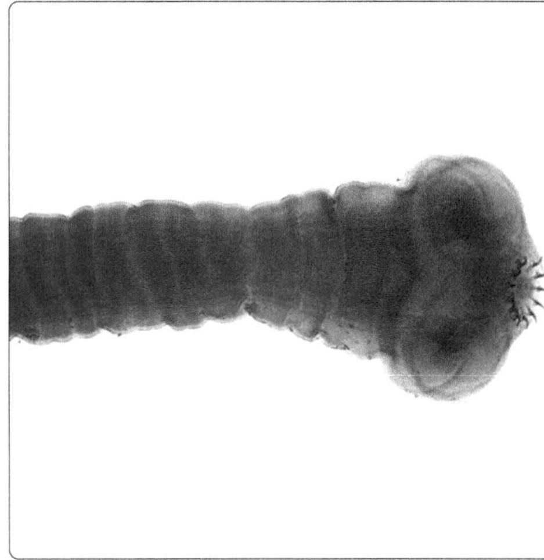

(Left) *Taenia species eggs are 30-35 μm in diameter, radially striated, and contain 6 refractile hooks in the internal oncosphere (unstained wet prep). Eggs are morphologically indistinguishable between Taenia species. (Courtesy M. Melvin.)* **(Right)** *The scolex of T. solium contains 4 large suckers and a rostellum with 2 rows of large and small hooks. (Courtesy M. Melvin.)*

Taenia solium Gravid Proglottid

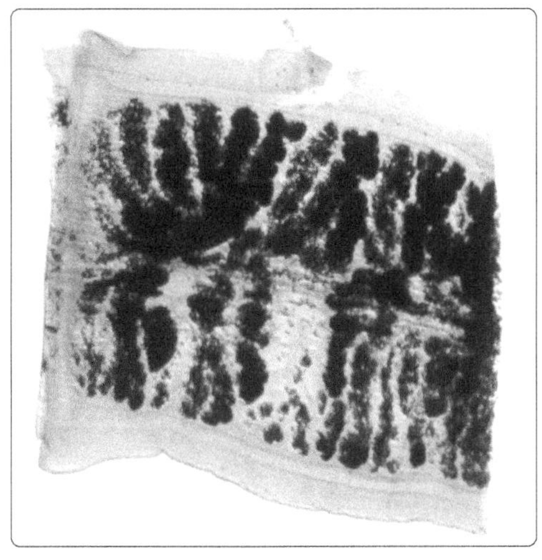

Taenia saginata Gravid Proglottid

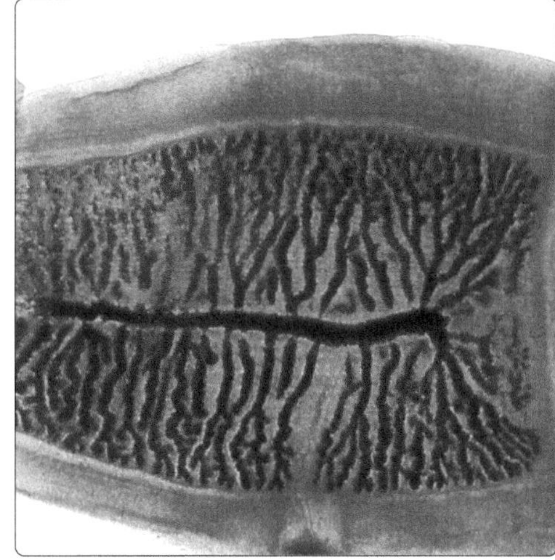

(Left) *T. solium proglottids contain 7-13 uterine primary lateral branches, which are visualized in this specimen by injection of India ink. The presence of eggs &/or proglottids is diagnostic of taeniasis (infection with adult pork tapeworm) rather than cysticercosis. (Courtesy CDC/PHIL.)* **(Right)** *In contrast to T. solium, Taenia saginata (beef tapeworm) proglottids contain 15-20 uterine primary lateral branches. (Courtesy CDC/PHIL.)*

Cysticercus in Striated Muscle

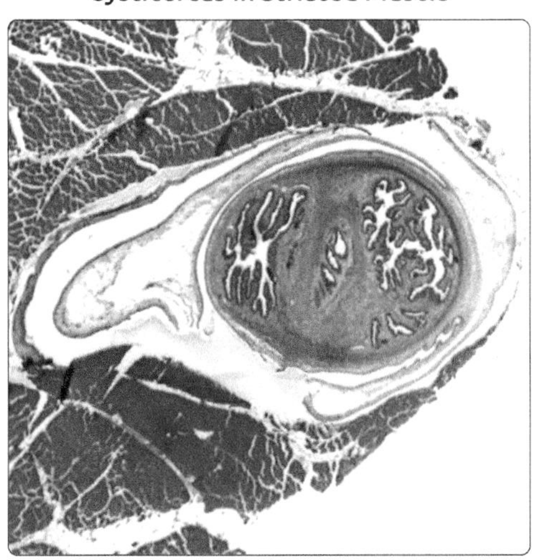

Multiple Skeletal Muscle Cysticerci

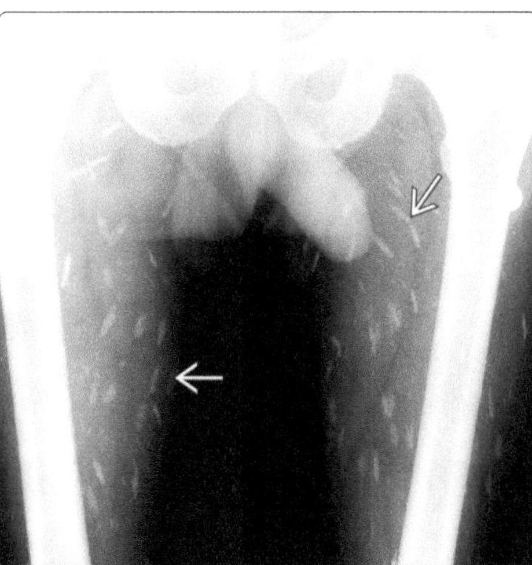

(Left) *Cysticerci in striated muscle can be numerous and are rarely symptomatic. (Courtesy Franz von Lichtenberg Collection of Infectious Disease Pathology, BWH.)* **(Right)** *AP radiograph reveals multiple ovoid calcifications oriented along the long axis of the muscle fibers of the thighs ➡. The appearance is classic for cysticercosis. (From DI: MSK Non-Trauma.)*

(Left) *Massive numbers of cysticerci are present in this autopsy brain section. This disseminated form of neurocysticercosis is rare and only seen in patients from endemic areas. (Courtesy Franz von Lichtenberg Collection of Infectious Disease Pathology, BWH.)* (Right) *MR shows innumerable cysts, each with a hyperintense scolex, in this patient from Mexico with neurocysticercosis. (From DI: Brain.)*

Neurocysticercosis in Autopsy Brain

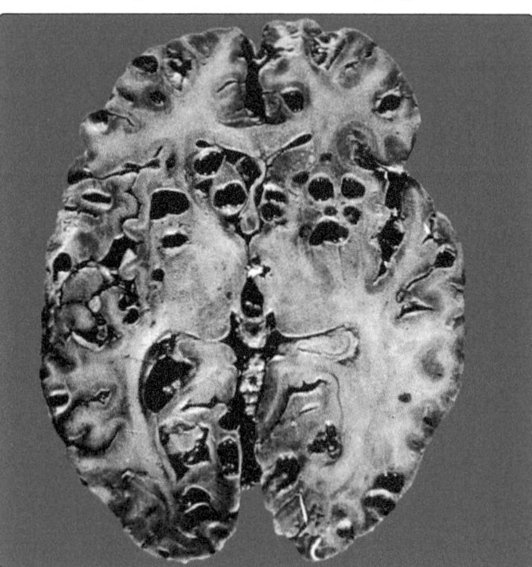

Multiple Cysticerci Identified by MR

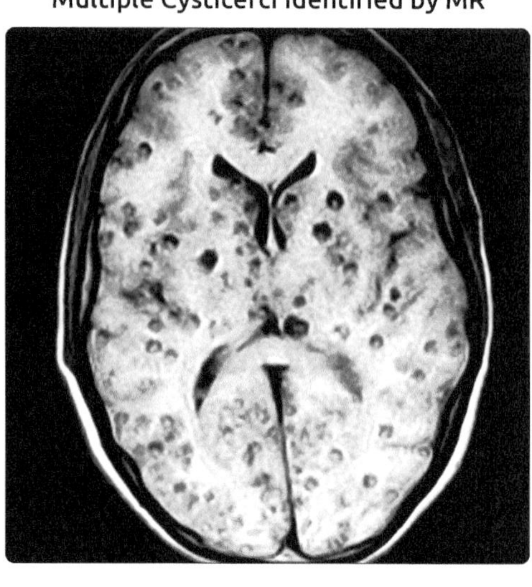

(Left) *Section of a cysticercus shows a scolex with armed rostellum →, gastrodermis ⇨, and suckers ↷. (Courtesy Franz von Lichtenberg Collection of Infectious Disease Pathology, BWH.)* (Right) *Acid-fast staining highlights hooklets, which are present in this section longitudinally and in cross section. (From DP: Neuro.)*

Histologic Features of Viable Cysticercus

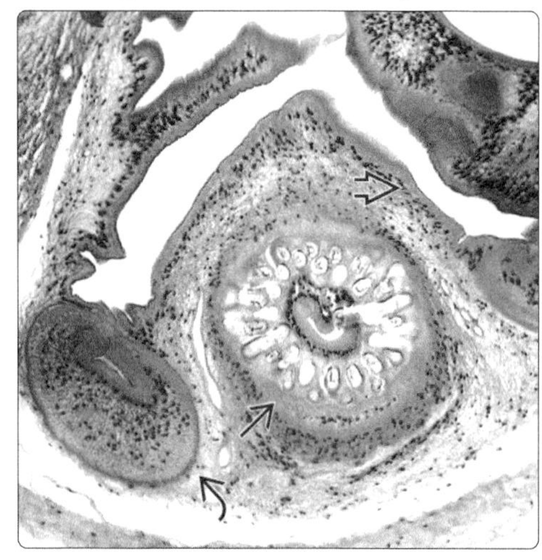

Acid-Fast Positivity of Hooklets

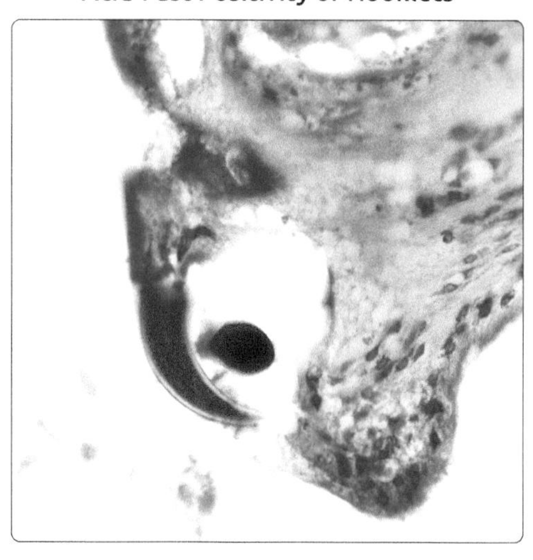

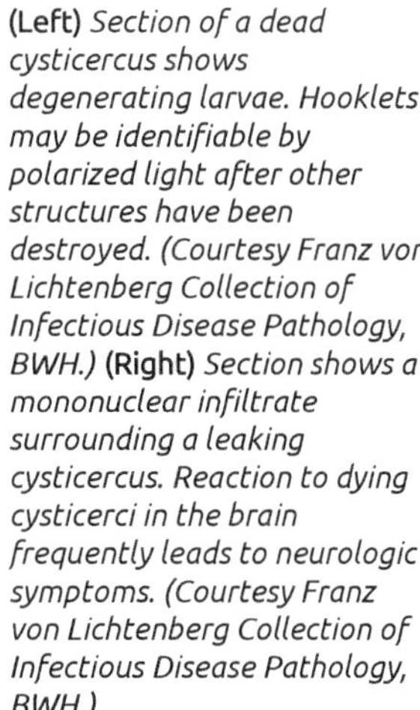

(Left) *Section of a dead cysticercus shows degenerating larvae. Hooklets may be identifiable by polarized light after other structures have been destroyed. (Courtesy Franz von Lichtenberg Collection of Infectious Disease Pathology, BWH.)* (Right) *Section shows a mononuclear infiltrate surrounding a leaking cysticercus. Reaction to dying cysticerci in the brain frequently leads to neurologic symptoms. (Courtesy Franz von Lichtenberg Collection of Infectious Disease Pathology, BWH.)*

Degenerating Cysticercus

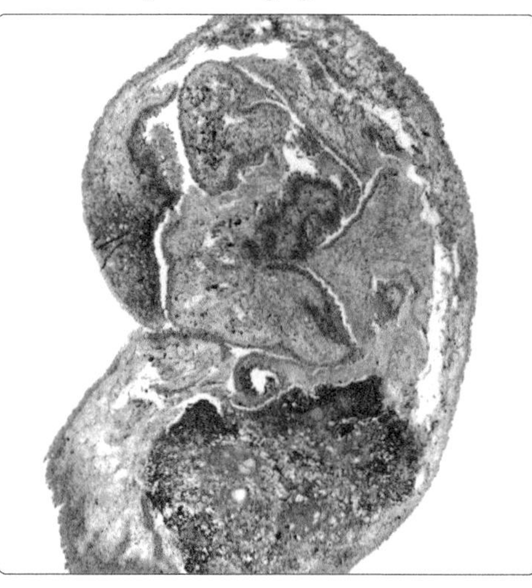

Inflammation Surrounding Degenerating Cysticercus

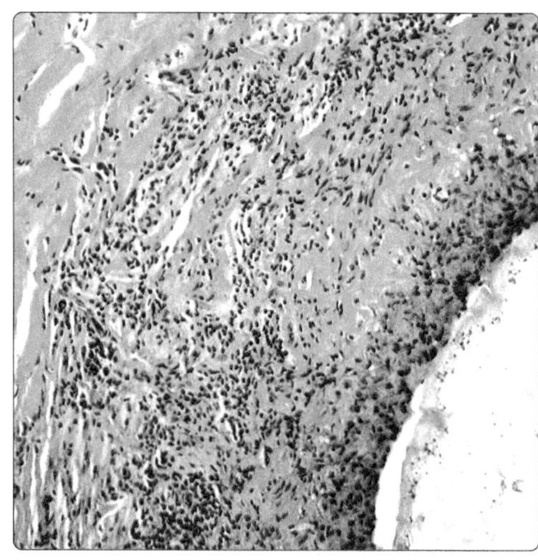

Encapsulated Degenerating Cysticercus

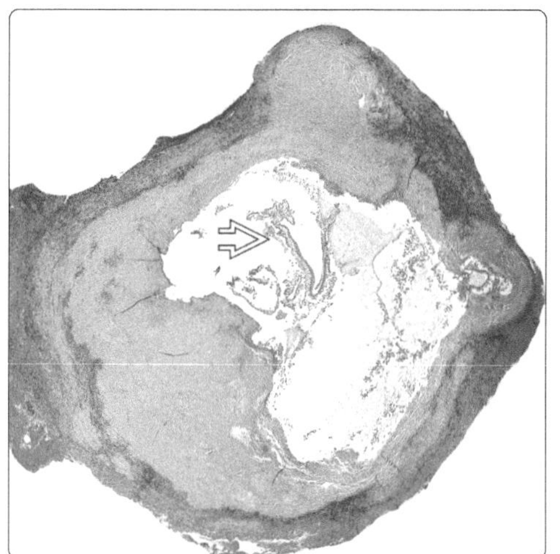

Fragments of Degenerating Cysticercus

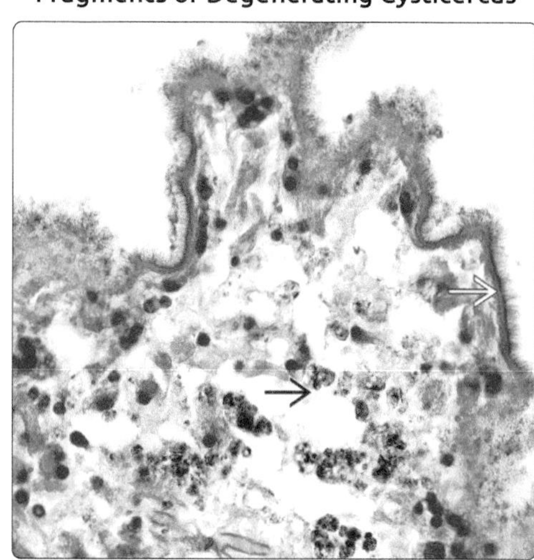

(Left) *This degenerating cysticercus exhibits fragments of bladder wall ➡ with surrounding reactive brain.* **(Right)** *High-power view of a degenerating cysticercus shows fragments of the bladder wall with microvilli ➡ and scattered pigmented cells ➡. Occasional hooklets (not shown) may be identified by polarization or acid-fast staining.*

Racemose Cysts

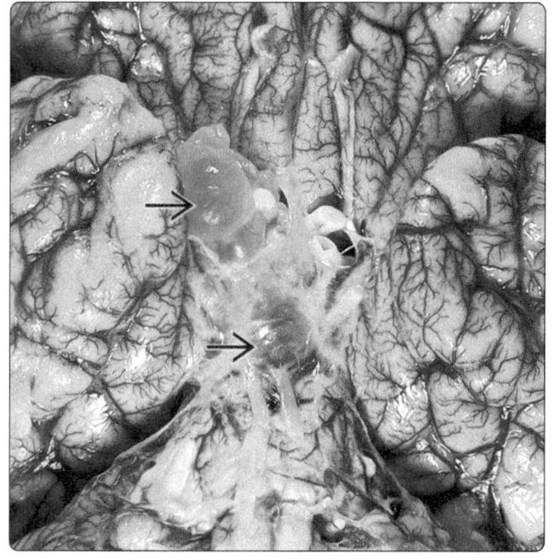

Racemose Neurocysticercosis

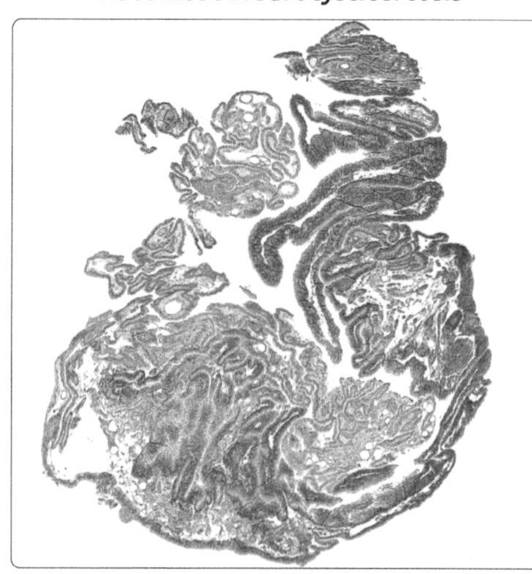

(Left) *Racemose neurocysticercosis consists of meningeal or intraventricular clear cysts without scolices ➡. Involvement of basal cisterns is commonly associated with hydrocephalus. (Courtesy R. Hewlett, PhD.)* **(Right)** *Section of a racemose neurocysticercosis (also referred to as "aberrant proliferating cestode larvae") shows numerous folds of a collapsed cyst wall without an identifiable protoscolex.*

Cyst Wall of Racemose Cysticercus

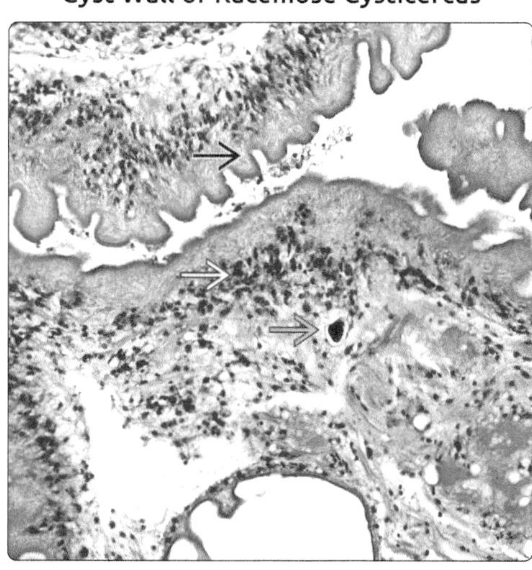

Cyst Wall Tegument

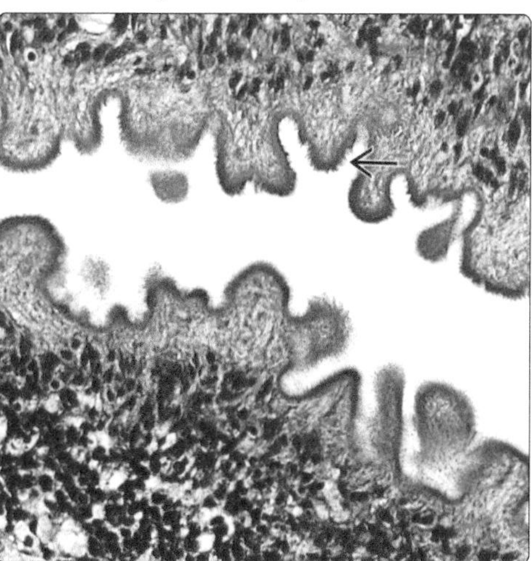

(Left) *Section of a racemose cysticercus cyst wall shows tegument with papillae ➡ and a layer of tegumental cells ➡ separating the tegument from the underlying parenchyma with occasional calcareous corpuscles ➡.* **(Right)** *Higher power view of a racemose cysticercus cyst wall highlights tegument microvilli ➡.*

Diphyllobothriasis and Hymenolepiasis

KEY FACTS

ETIOLOGY/PATHOGENESIS

- Intestinal parasitic zoonotic cestode infections, transmitted to humans via ingestion of marine or freshwater fish (diphyllobothriids) or insects (*Hymenolepis* spp.) that harbor infectious larvae (cysticercoids)
- Human-to-human transmission and autoinfection occurs with *Hymenolepis nana*

CLINICAL ISSUES

- Mild gastrointestinal symptoms common
- Rare complications include intestinal obstruction, aberrant migration of proglottids
- Laboratory testing largely nonspecific, may reveal eosinophilia, vitamin B12 deficiency, megaloblastic anemia, &/or pernicious anemia (diphyllobothriids)

MICROBIOLOGY

- Stool ova and parasite exam: Identification of characteristic eggs &/or proglottids (wider than long)
- Diphyllobothriid eggs: Ovoid (55-75), unembryonated, with thin shell
- *H. diminuta* eggs: Ovoid (70-85 μm), lack polar filaments
- *H. nana* eggs: Ovoid (30-50 μm) with polar filaments

MICROSCOPIC

- Proglottids and eggs may be identified in intestinal tissue
- Scolex attaches to mucosa via 2 lateral grooves (bothria) (diphyllobothriids) or suckers (*Hymenolepis*)

TOP DIFFERENTIAL DIAGNOSES

- Teniasis: Smaller (30- to 3-μm) round eggs with radial striations; proglottids longer than wide with numerous lateral uterine branches
- *Dipylidium caninum* infection: Round eggs (35-40 μm) with oncosphere that has 6 hooklets
- Intestinal round worm (nematode) infections: Fluid-filled cavity with intestinal tract; no proglottids
- Intestinal fluke (trematode) infections: Identified by ovoid, operculated eggs; no proglottids

Diphyllobothriid Life Cycle

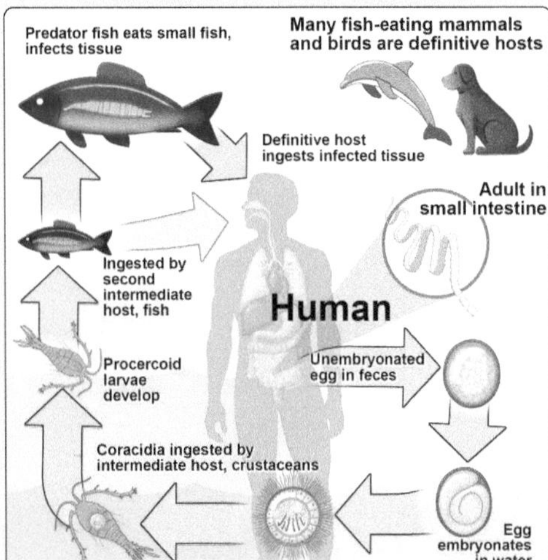

***Hymenolepis* Life Cycle**

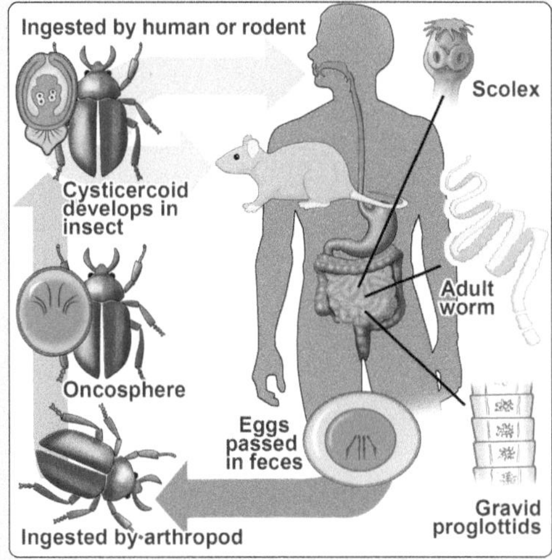

(Left) *Humans are infected via consumption of larvae in fish, which mature into adults in the small intestine. Eggs are excreted in feces and develop into free-swimming larva that are consumed by crustaceans, which are then ingested by fish.* **(Right)** *Humans are infected by consuming arthropod-containing cysticerci. Adult worm develops in small intestinal lumen and releases eggs into the environment in stool. Hymenolepis nana eggs are also directly infective, and can cause internal autoinfection within the small intestine.*

Diphyllobothriid Egg

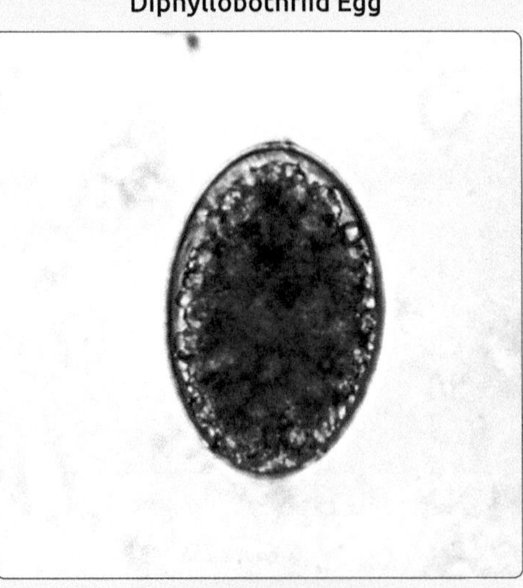

***Hymenolepis nana* Egg**

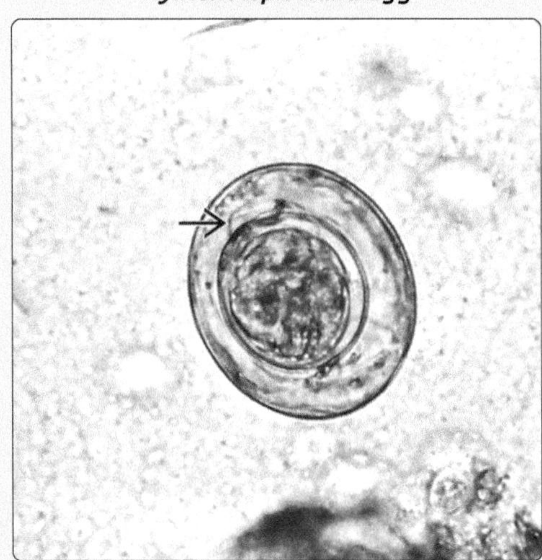

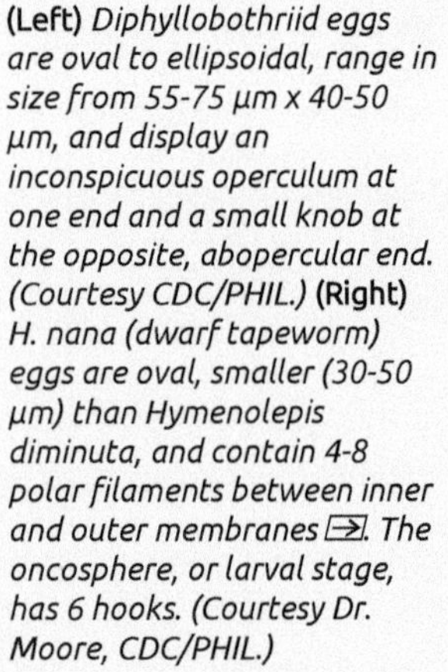

(Left) *Diphyllobothriid eggs are oval to ellipsoidal, range in size from 55-75 μm x 40-50 μm, and display an inconspicuous operculum at one end and a small knob at the opposite, abopercular end. (Courtesy CDC/PHIL.)* **(Right)** *H. nana (dwarf tapeworm) eggs are oval, smaller (30-50 μm) than Hymenolepis diminuta, and contain 4-8 polar filaments between inner and outer membranes ⇒. The oncosphere, or larval stage, has 6 hooks. (Courtesy Dr. Moore, CDC/PHIL.)*

TERMINOLOGY

Synonyms

- Diphyllobothriasis, *Dibothriocephalus*, broad fish tapeworm, flatworm
- Hymenolepiasis, dwarf tapeworm (*Hymenolepis nana*), rat tapeworm (*Hymenolepis diminuta)*

Definitions

- Greek: "Di" (two) + "phyllos" (leaf) + "bothrium" (groove)
- Greek: "Humen" (membrane) + "lepis" (eggshell) + "nana" (dwarf)

ETIOLOGY/PATHOGENESIS

Infectious Agents

- **Diphyllobothriasis**: Intestinal cestode (tapeworm) infection caused by consumption of infective larvae in undercooked marine or freshwater fish
  - Humans are accidental definitive hosts; lifespan of worm > 20 years
  - Most common human infections caused by 3 genera
    - *Dibothriocephalus*; terrestrial definitive hosts
      - *Dibothriocephalus latus* (formerly *Diphyllobothrium latum*): Most common species to cause human disease, endemic in northern Europe, Russia, and North America; infects freshwater fish (pikes, perches)
      - *Dibothriocephalus nihonkaiensis* (formerly *Diphyllobothrium nihonkaiense*): Endemic in northern Pacific, common in Japan (Salmon)
      - *Dibothriocephalus dendriticus* (formerly *Diphyllobothrium dendriticum):* Arctic distribution
    - *Diphyllobothrium*; marine definitive hosts
      - *Diphyllobothrium balaenopterae*: Whales
      - *Diphyllobothrium stemmacephalum*: Dolphins and porpoises
    - *Adenocephalus*
      - *Antrodiaetus pacificus* (formerly *Diphyllobothrium pacificum*): South America
  - Estimated 20 million people infected worldwide, more common in circumpolar regions
  - Changing distribution with regional reemergences (globalization and changes in culinary practices)
  - Infective larval forms readily killed by adequate cooking or freezing of fish
- **Hymenolepiasis**: Intestinal cestode (tapeworm) infection caused by consumption of infective larvae in insects (intermediate host); rodents are definitive host; lifespan of worm 4-6 weeks
  - *H. nana*
    - Human-to-human transmission and autoinfection cycle (eggs hatch in intestines without passage through intermediate host)
    - High prevalence, especially in regions with poor sanitation
    - Oncospheres invades intestinal villi and mature cysticercoids are released via villus rupture
  - *H. diminuta*
    - Relatively low prevalence, more common in children
  - Worldwide distribution

CLINICAL ISSUES

Presentation

- Adult tapeworms attach to mucosal surface of lower jejunum or upper ileum and extends to anus; do not invade
  - Patients may present due to passage of proglottids in stool
  - Single or multiple long, noodle-like, mobile worms may be observed during colonoscopy
- Often asymptomatic, nonspecific gastrointestinal symptoms common (diarrhea, abdominal pain, vomiting, diarrhea, constipation, dyspepsia)
- Rare complications include intestinal obstruction, allergic reactions, arthromyalgias, or symptoms due to aberrant migration of proglottides (cholecystitis, cholangitis)
- Puritis ani
- Mild eosinophilia and anemia
- Diphyllobothriasis: Minority of patients (2%) develop vitamin B12 deficiency and pernicious anemia
- Hymenolepis: Autoreinfection occurs (*H. nana)*

Laboratory Tests

- Speciation via PCR or sequencing techniques [often use mitochondrial marker (cox1)]; generally limited to research

Treatment

- Praziquantel (5-10 mg/kg), niclosamide, or nitazoxanide (*Hymenolepis*)
  - Occasionally, multiple doses required (repeat stool ova and parasite exam 5-6 weeks post treatment)
  - 2nd dose required for *H. nana* due to autoreinfection
- Intestinal purging or endoscopic removal of worm

Prognosis

- Untreated, diphyllobothriasis infections can last > 20 years
- Treatment generally effective and prognosis excellent

IMAGING

General Features

- Abdominal ultrasound: Hyperechoic strand-like structure
- Imaging with contrast: Longitudinal filling defect

MICROBIOLOGY

Stool Ova and Parasite Exam

- Identification of eggs and expelled proglottids in stool samples is diagnostic; however, species-level identification usually not possible
- Each proglottid contains sets of male and female reproductive organs; produces up to 1 million eggs per day per worm
- **Diphyllobothriasis**
  - Humans begin to pass eggs 15-45 days after ingestion of infective larvae
  - Eggs: Ovoid (55-75 x 40-50 µm), unembryonated, with thin shell
    - Inconspicuous operculum with minute terminal knob on opposite (abopercular) end
    - Eggs are usually numerous but are not directly infectious to humans
    - Species-level identification via egg morphology is unreliable

- Proglottids (worm segments)
  - Broader (0.82-10.0 mm) than long (0.13-2.1 mm) with concave lateral margins and more or less pointed projections formed bilaterally at each segmental junction
  - Central genital pore (joint opening of cirrus sac and vagina) and rosette-shaped uterus
- **Hymenolepiasis**
  - Eggs: Both species are embryonated with 6-hooked oncosphere
    - *H. diminuta*: Ovoid (70-86 x 60-80 μm) without polar filaments
    - *H. nana*: Ovoid (40-60 x 30-50 μm) with polar filaments
      - Immediately infective
  - Proglottids: Broader than long, overlapping (craspedote), trapezoidal

MACROSCOPIC

General Features

- **Diphyllobothriasis**: Elongated scolex with 2 sucking grooves (bothria)
  - Yellow, flat, ribbon-like worm with thin neck and 3,000-4,000 proglottids (segments)
  - Longest human tapeworm: 5-25 m in length, 10-20 mm in width
- **Hymenolepiasis**: Scolex with 4 suckers and rostellar hooks
  - *H. nana*: 15-40 mm in length
  - *H. diminuta*: 20-60 cm in length

MICROSCOPIC

Histologic Features

- Intestinal tissue may contain eggs or portions of gravid proglottids
- Each proglottid contains sets of male and female reproductive organs
- Speciation via differences in shape and size of scolex (head), neck, and male genital organs often not possible due to suboptimal condition of worm following expulsion and processing
- Scolex attaches to mucosa via 2 lateral grooves (bothria) (diphyllobothriids) or 4 suckers (*Hymenolepis* spp.)

DIFFERENTIAL DIAGNOSIS

Taeniasis

- Beef (*Taenia saginata*) or pork (*Taenia solium*) tapeworms
- Scolex attaches via 4 large suckers and central rostellum with hooks (*T. solium* only)
- Proglottids longer than wide with numerous uterine branches
- Eggs smaller (30-35 μm), round, with radial striations

Dipylidium caninum Infection

- Tapeworm infection of dogs and cats occasionally found in humans due to ingestion of cysticercoid contaminated fleas (also referred to as flea, cucumber, and double-pored tapeworm)
- Diagnosed by identification of proglottids or egg packets in stool or environment
- Eggs: Round to oval (35-40 μm) and contain oncosphere that has 6 hooklets
- Proglottids (12 mm x 3 mm) have 2 genital pores in middle of each lateral margin; contain round to ovoid packets with 5-15 eggs/each

Intestinal Roundworm (Nematode) Infections

- *Ancylostoma duodenale* and *Necator americanus* (hookworm); *Trichuris trichiura* (whipworm); *Ascaris lumbricoides*
- Round worms (nematodes) with intestinal tract; no proglottids
- Prolonged eosinophilia secondary to tissue invasion

Intestinal Fluke (Trematode) Infections

- e.g., echinostomiasis, fasciolopsiasis, gastrodiscoidiasis, metagonimiasis, heterophyiasis
- Diagnosis often made by identification of eggs in stool; size/shape varies with species but typically ovoid and operculated

SELECTED REFERENCES

1. Scholz T et al: Fish tapeworms (Cestoda) in the molecular era: achievements, gaps and prospects. Parasitology. 149(14):1876-93, 2022
2. Ando Y et al: Diphyllobothriasis from eating sushi. Am J Trop Med Hyg. 104(6):1953-4, 2021
3. Galán-Puchades MT: Human diphyllobothriasis. Lancet. 396(10253):755, 2020
4. Kitaoka H et al: Raw fish and diphyllobothriasis infection. QJM. 113(9):695-6, 2020
5. Panti-May JA et al: Worldwide overview of human infections with Hymenolepis diminuta. Parasitol Res. 119(7):1997-2004, 2020
6. Robert-Gangneux F et al: Dibothriocephalus nihonkaiensis: an emerging concern in western countries? Expert Rev Anti Infect Ther. 17(9):677-9, 2019
7. Ikuno H et al: Epidemiology of Diphyllobothrium nihonkaiense diphyllobothriasis, Japan, 2001-2016. Emerg Infect Dis. 24(8):1428-34, 2018
8. Yamasaki H et al: Complete sequence and characterization of the mitochondrial genome of Diphyllobothrium stemmacephalum, the type species of genus Diphyllobothrium (Cestoda: Diphyllobothriidae), using next generation sequencing. Parasitol Int. 66(5):573-8, 2017
9. Muehlenbachs A et al: Malignant transformation of Hymenolepis nana in a human host. N Engl J Med. 373(19):1845-52, 2015
10. Kuchta R et al: Tapeworm Diphyllobothrium dendriticum (Cestoda)–neglected or emerging human parasite? PLoS Negl Trop Dis. 7(12):e2535, 2013
11. Arizono N et al: Diphyllobothriasis associated with eating raw pacific salmon. Emerg Infect Dis. 15(6):866-70, 2009
12. Scholz T et al: Update on the human broad tapeworm (genus diphyllobothrium), including clinical relevance. Clin Microbiol Rev. 22(1):146-60, Table of Contents, 2009

Diphyllobothrium spp.: Adult Worm

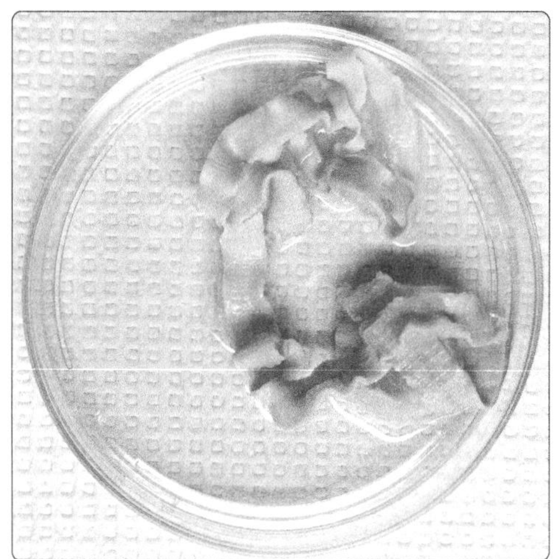

Diphyllobothriid Proglottids

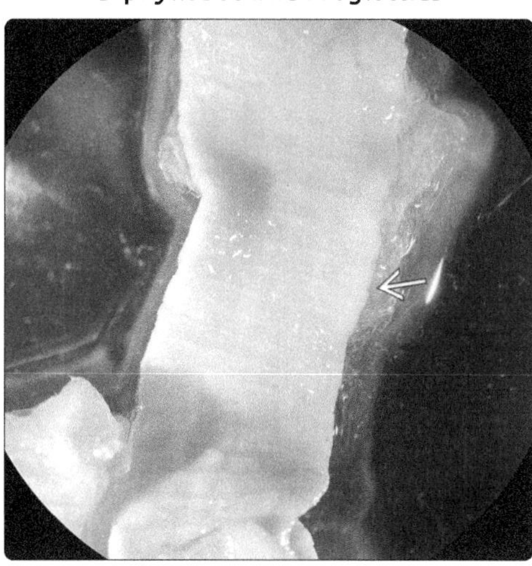

(Left) *This section of an adult diphyllobothriid tapeworm, passed by a human patient, contains numerous proglottides; however, the scolex was not present. Adult worms can reach up 15 m in length.* **(Right)** *This section of an adult diphyllobothriid worm shows proglottids* → *that are broader than they are long.*

Diphyllobothriid Proglottids

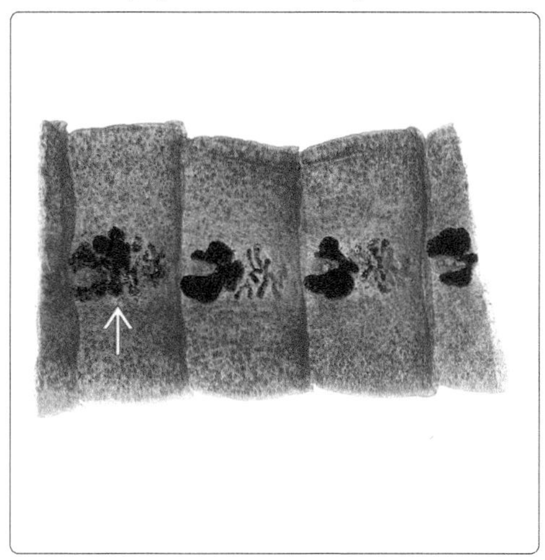

Hymenolepis diminuta Scolex

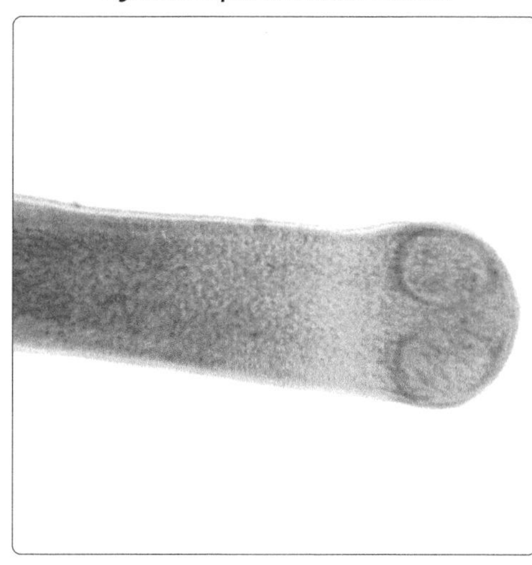

(Left) *This sections shows microscopic features of several gravid proglottids of Dibothriocephalus latus (formerly Diphyllobothrium latum), the "broad fish tapeworm," which are trapezoidal in shape and wider than long with centrally located rosette-shaped uteri* →*. (Courtesy M. Melvin, CDC/PHIL.)* **(Right)** *This image of a H. diminuta (rat tapeworm) scolex shows 2 suckers that allow the worm to secure itself on the host's intestinal mucosa. (Courtesy CDC/PHIL.)*

Hymenolepis diminuta Egg

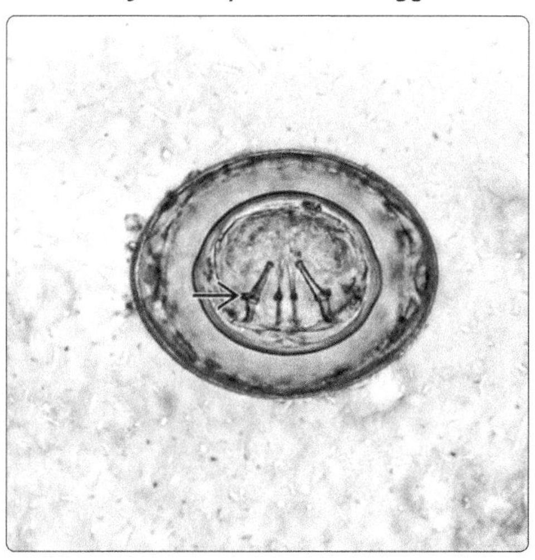

Hymenolepiasis nana Egg

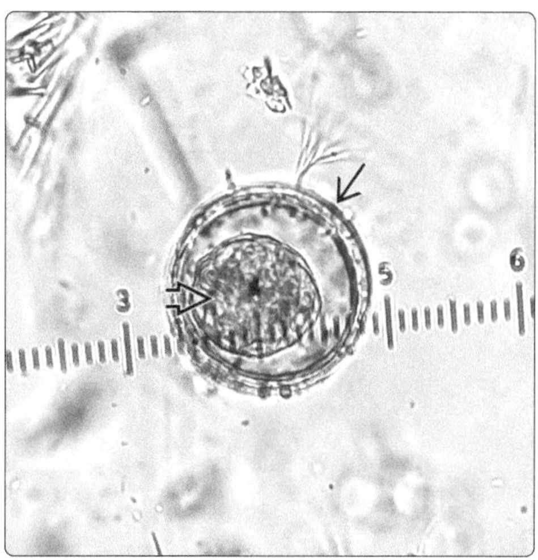

(Left) *H. diminuta (rat tapeworm) eggs measure 70-85 µm x 60-80 µm, are slightly round to oval with a striated outer and thin inner membrane with an inner oncosphere containing 6 hooks* →*, and has no polar filaments in the space between the oncosphere and the outer shell. (Courtesy M. Melvin, CDC/PHIL.)* **(Right)** *This H. nana egg, identified in an unstained wet mount, shows inner oncosphere* → *and outer shell* →*.*

KEY FACTS

ETIOLOGY/PATHOGENESIS

- Infection with *Echinococcus* species cestodes (tapeworms) incidentally found in humans through contact with infected animals

CLINICAL ISSUES

- Cystic echinococcosis: Abdominal pain, pleurisy, shortness of breath, bone pain, "tumor," headaches, or seizures
- Alveolar echinococcosis: Asymptomatic slow-growing, fibrotic mass with jaundice, right upper quadrant pain, or hepatic failure
- Polycystic echinococcosis (rare): Asymptomatic slow-growing, fibrotic mass (liver > pleura > mesentery)

IMAGING

- Radiograph: Chest or abdomen with solitary or multiple fluid-filled spaces in involved organs
- CT: Daughter cysts within larger cysts or reactive surrounding inflammation

MICROSCOPIC

- Cystic echinococcosis and polycystic echinococcosis: Thin to thick, fibrous response from human host, germinal matrix, and daughter cysts that contain protoscolices
- Rupture echinococcal disease: Fibrous response with varying amounts of identifiable necrotic helminth fragments
- Alveolar echinococcosis: Fibrous response with varying amounts of identifiable daughter cysts
- Fine-needle aspiration of solitary cysts should yield diagnostic hydatid sand/protoscolices

TOP DIFFERENTIAL DIAGNOSES

- Cysticercosis: *Taenia solium* larvae are small (1-2 cm) and contain single protoscolex with hooklets
- Coenurosis: Coenurus, or larval bladder, contains multiple protoscolices with hooklets within single lesion
- Noninfectious cystic/polycystic lesions

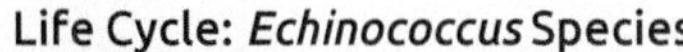

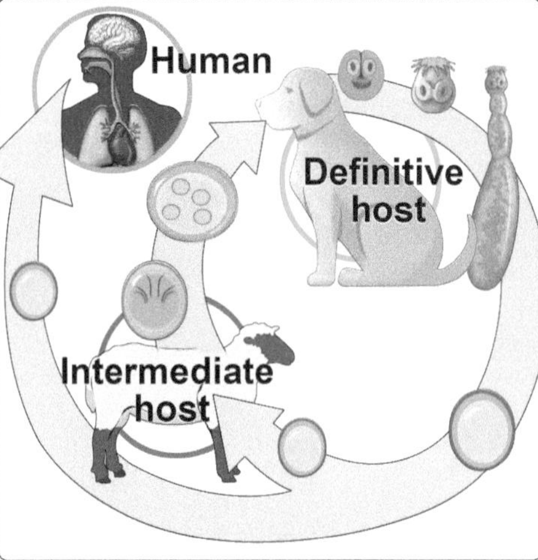

Adult *Echinococcus granulosus*

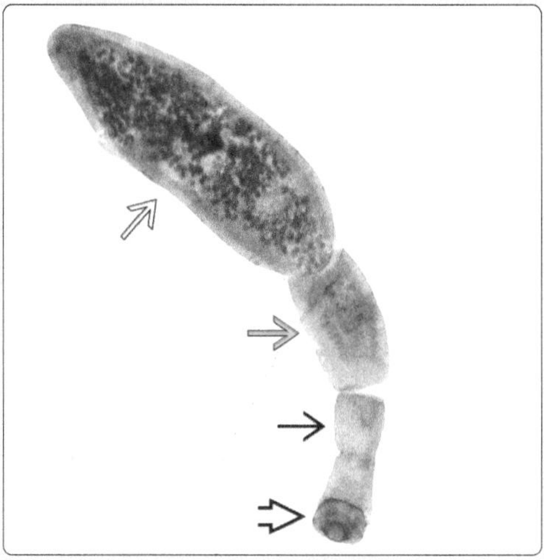

(Left) *Echinococcus species infect definitive hosts (tapeworm in gastrointestinal tract) and intermediate hosts (cysts in tissue) external to humans. When humans are exposed to the feces of definitive hosts (dogs, bears, foxes), they can become dead-end hosts with cyst forms found in intermediate hosts. Lesions can occur in any organ, but liver, lung, brain, and bone are common.* **(Right)** *Adult worms (not found in humans) consist of a scolex ⇨, immature proglottid ⇨, mature proglottid ⇨, and gravid proglottid ➡.*

Gross Intraoperative Photograph

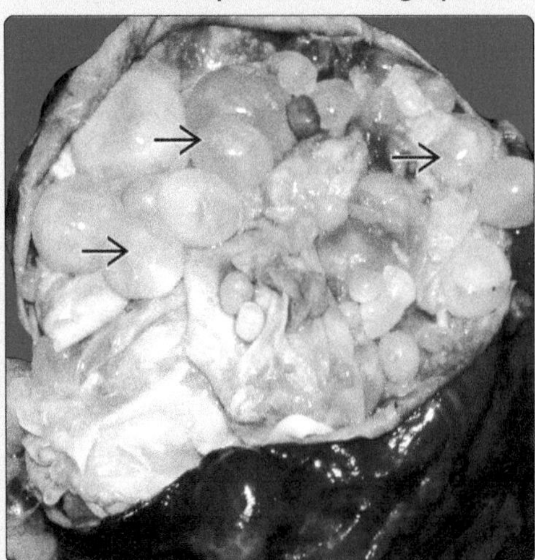

Viable Intact Cysts

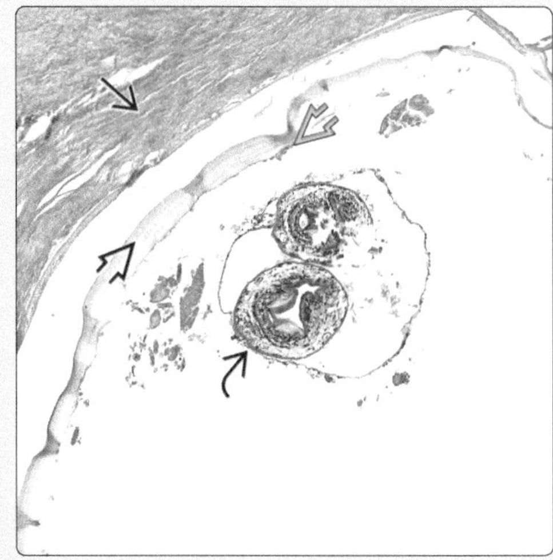

(Left) *This intraoperative photograph of the liver shows a large hydatid cyst due to Echinococcus granulosus, containing multiple daughter cysts ⇨, with a surrounding fibrous rim. (From DP: H&P.)* **(Right)** *Low-power view shows a cyst in tissue with an outer rim of fibrosis (or pericyst) ⇨, a laminated member ⇨, the germinal layer (living) ⇨, and viable daughter cyst with intact protoscolices ⇨.*

TERMINOLOGY

Synonyms

- Hydatid disease: From Greek "hudatís" (watery vesicle)

ETIOLOGY/PATHOGENESIS

Infectious Agents

- Infection with *Echinococcus* species cestodes (tapeworms)
  - Carnivorous predator [e.g., dog, (definitive host)] excretes proglottids &/or eggs into environment, which are ingested by herbivores (intermediate host)
  - Eggs hatch to oncospheres, which penetrate intestinal wall and migrate to final site of cyst development (brain, lung, liver, intestine, and bones most common)
  - Cyst stage is proliferative, grows 1 cm per year, and produces many protoscolices
  - Cysts and protoscolices are ingested by carnivorous predators when they eat meat of herbivores (does not occur in humans)
  - Protoscolices (inverted scolices) evert in gut lumen and attach to intestinal wall
  - Viable attached adult tapeworms in digestive tract produce proglottids and eggs
- 4 species (of 6 in genus) are zoonotic pathogens in humans
  - *E. granulosus* (cystic echinococcosis)
    - Broad geographic distribution
    - Definitive host: Canidae (dogs, wolves, foxes, jackals)
    - Intermediate host: Herbivores (sheep, goats, swine, kangaroos)
  - *E. multilocularis* (alveolar echinococcosis)
    - Predominantly northern hemisphere
    - Definitive host: Canidae and Felidae
    - Intermediate host: Small rodents
  - *E. vogeli* and *E. oligarthrus* (polycystic neotropic echinococcosis)
    - Central and South America; rare disease
    - Definitive host *E. vogeli*: Canidae (bush and domestic dogs); *E. oligarthrus*: Felidae (cats, cheetahs, lions)
    - Intermediate host: Rodents
- Humans are dead-end hosts and do not transmit infection

CLINICAL ISSUES

Presentation

- Cystic echinococcosis
  - Abdominal pain, pleurisy, shortness of breath, bone pain, "tumor," headaches, or seizures depending on site and size of cyst; any site in body may be involved, and isolated reports are numerous
  - Time course may be prolonged as primary cyst grows ~ 1 cm per year until detection or rupture (10-20 cm)
  - Rupture of cyst (iatrogenically or traumatically) can lead to immediate anaphylaxis
- Alveolar echinococcosis
  - Asymptomatic incubation (up to 15 years) with slow-growing, fibrotic mass (usually of liver), which can present with jaundice, right upper quadrant pain, or hepatic failure
- Polycystic echinococcosis
  - Asymptomatic incubation (~ 10 years) with slow-growing, fibrotic mass (liver > pleura > mesentery)
  - Present with jaundice, right upper quadrant pain, hepatic failure, shortness of breath, pleurisy, or abdominal pain, depending on location of cysts

Laboratory Tests

- Antibodies to *Echinococcus* spp. may be present in hosts with previous rupture
  - Cross reacts with other cestode antigens (e.g., *Taenia*)
  - Intact cysts may not have elicited antibody response
  - Multiple novel antigens derived from organism sequence are in development for improved detection
- Cytokine stimulation assays (IL-4) have shown promise experimentally
- Molecular testing: Multiple targets (mitochondrial, microRNAs, cell-free DNA) focused on diagnosis and differentiation of species are in development
- No role for culture or stool exam

Treatment

- Surgical removal of solitary cyst
  - Dangerous due to risk of anaphylaxis
  - Accidental rupture of intact viable cyst will lead to spilling of contents and infection of adjacent tissues leading to recurrence
- Drugs: Mebendazole (prolonged duration)
- Percutaneous aspiration, injection of chemicals, and reaspiration (PAIR): Preferred method for diagnosing and treating solitary cysts due to decreased anaphylaxis and spread of infection

Prognosis

- Ruptured cystic echinococcosis may require lifelong therapy with mebendazole to prevent recurrence
- Spread of cyst contents can create tumor-like conditions with local spread to other organs
- Anaphylaxis can lead to immediate death

IMAGING

Radiographic Findings

- Chest or abdomen examination will show solitary or multiple fluid-filled spaces in involved organs

Ultrasonographic Findings

- Multiple echogenic, clear to fluid-filled spaces within larger cyst of either liver, lung, or abdomen

CT Findings

- Higher resolution may reveal structure of daughter cysts within larger cysts (multiple densities)
- Reactive surrounding inflammation (in cases of rupture)

MICROBIOLOGY

Parasite Characteristics

- Adults (not found in humans): 1.2-7 mm in length with scolex containing 4 suckers and rostellum with 25-50 hooks and up to 6 proglottids, including terminal gravid proglottid
  - Hermaphrodites (have both male and female sex organs); mature proglottids do exchange spermatozoa through their genital pores within definitive host
  - Do not have digestive tract and absorb nutrients from environment through tegument

MACROSCOPIC

Intact Solitary Cysts (*E. granulosus*)

- Large, clear to milky, fluid-filled cysts
- Contain smaller white to yellow daughter cysts

Ruptured Cysts or Alveolar Echinococcosis

- Large, inflammatory to fibrotic masses
- Scattered cystic spaces ± daughter cyst contents

Polycystic Echinococcosis

- Multiple intact cysts (clusters of grapes) adjacent or scattered through involved organ

MICROSCOPIC

Histologic Features

- Cystic echinococcosis and polycystic echinococcosis
  - Intact cysts removed within organ (e.g., lobectomy) demonstrate thin to thick, fibrous response from human host, germinal layer, and daughter cysts that contain protoscolices with hooklets (20-40 µm long) and suckers
  - Lamellated cyst wall may be only visible portion in resection specimen
- Ruptured echinococcal disease
  - Fibrous response predominates with varying amounts of identifiable necrotic helminth fragments
  - Previously ruptured/traumatized cysts may include acute (neutrophilic) or granulomatous inflammation
  - Hooklets scanned for at low power with polarized light
- Alveolar echinococcosis
  - Fibrous response predominates with varying amounts of identifiable daughter cysts
  - Some cystic spaces may be empty due to natural rupture and progression of disease
- Because any body site may be involved, careful attention must be paid to any "cyst" or "tumor" for presence of cestode material (e.g., hooklets, intact protoscolices)

Cytologic Features

- Fine-needle aspiration of solitary cysts should yield diagnostic hydatid sand/protoscolices
  - Aspiration should only be conducted under medical/surgical guidance as part of treatment/removal procedure due to risk of contamination and spread
- Alveolar echinococcosis, due to natural creation of daughter cysts with fibrosis in tissue, may not produce hydatid sand on aspiration

DIFFERENTIAL DIAGNOSIS

Cysticercosis

- *Taenia solium* larvae are small (1-2 cm) and contain single protoscolex with hooklets
- More likely to have multiple scattered cysts

Coenurosis

- Coenurus, or larval bladder, contains multiple protoscolices with hooklets within single lesion (no daughter cysts)
- Caused by *Taenia multiceps*, *T. serialis*, *T. brauni*, and *T. glomerata*

Noninfectious Cystic/Polycystic Lesions

- Simple cortical cysts, congenital/developmental cysts, epidermal inclusion cysts, polycystic kidney disease, cystic primary or metastatic tumors, synovial cysts, etc.
- Diagnostic epithelial structures &/or lack of echinococcal elements separate on morphologic criteria

SELECTED REFERENCES

1. Darabi E et al: Evaluation of a novel Echinococcus granulosus recombinant fusion B-EpC1 antigen for the diagnosis of human cystic echinococcosis using indirect ELISA in comparison with a commercial diagnostic ELISA kit. Exp Parasitol. 240:108339, 2022
2. Ghasemirad H et al: Echinococcosis in immunocompromised patients: a systematic review. Acta Trop. 232:106490, 2022
3. Knapp J et al: Molecular diagnosis of alveolar echinococcosis in patients based on frozen and formalin-fixed paraffin-embedded tissue samples. Parasite. 29:4, 2022
4. Wan Z et al: Targeted sequencing of genomic repeat regions detects circulating cell-free Echinococcus DNA. PLoS Negl Trop Dis. 14(3):e0008147, 2020
5. Eckert J et al: Historical aspects of echinococcosis. Adv Parasitol. 95:1-64, 2017

Protoscolex: Smear

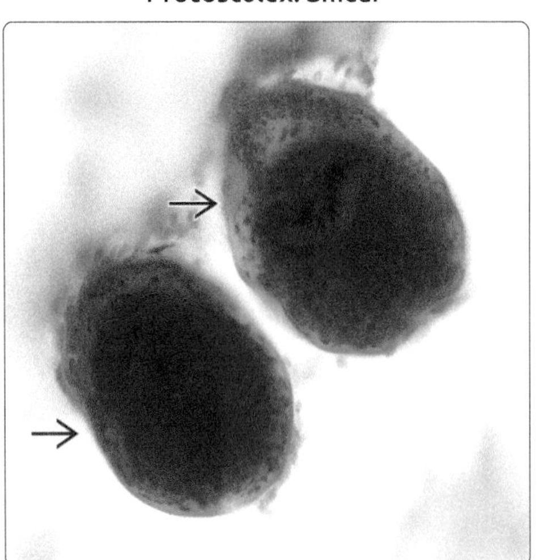

Protoscolex: Histology

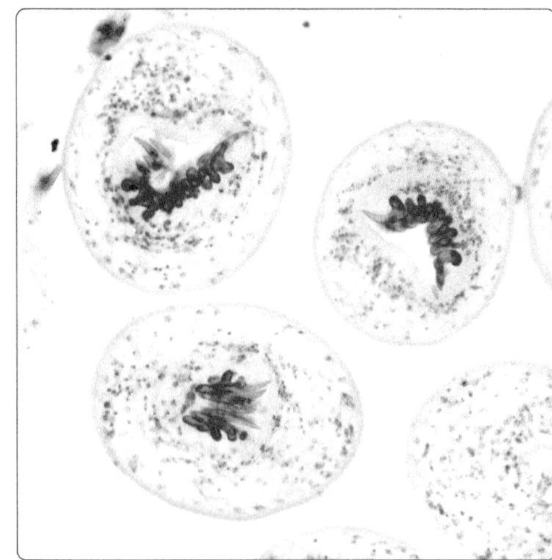

(Left) *Protoscolices ⮕ of Echinococcus in a cyst (smear) show the so-called hydatid sand is due to the invaginated "head" with hooklets.* **(Right)** *E. granulosus hydatid cyst in tissue section contains protoscolices, identified by hooklets and mouth located inside the structure and will evaginate when they enter the next host (canine).*

Alveolar Echinococcosis

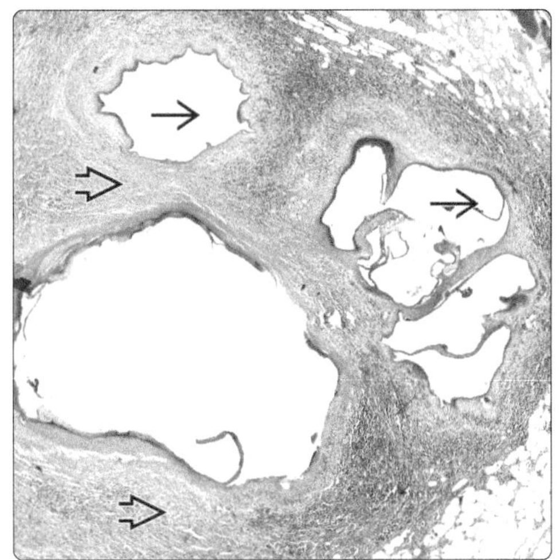

Germinal Layer

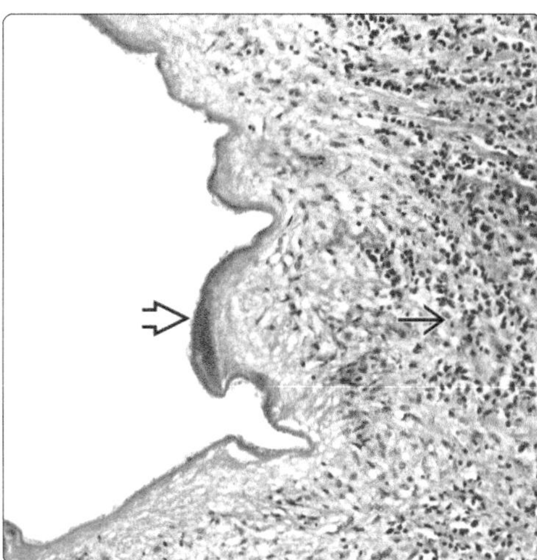

(Left) *Alveolar echinococcosis is a form of the disease with natural rupture and generation of new cysts ➡ in tissue, which leads to dense scarring ⇨.* **(Right)** *High magnification of the cyst lining in alveolar echinococcosis shows the lining germinal layer ⇨ and the host chronic inflammatory response ➡ (due to sequential rupture).*

Cyst Components

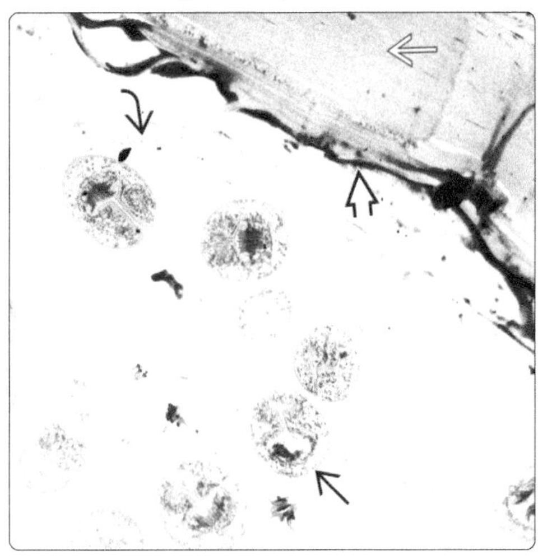

Cyst Components: Polarized

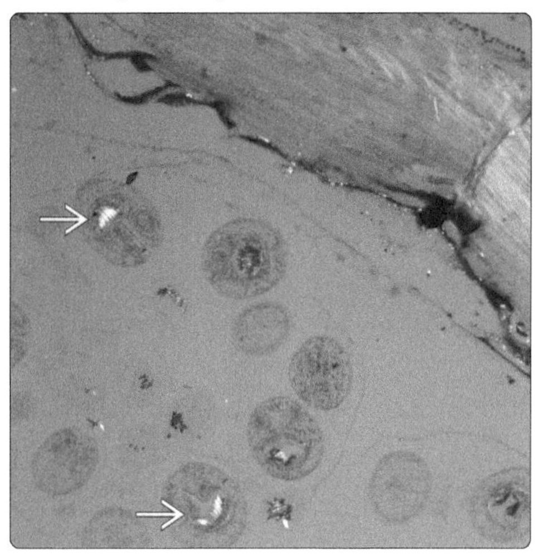

(Left) *The germinal layer ⇨ and protoscolices ➡ of an echinococcal cyst within the lung of an affected patient demonstrate the daughter cyst lining ⇨ from which the organisms form. The lamellated wall ➡, sometimes the only feature seen in resections, has bland layers.* **(Right)** *An echinococcal cyst under polarized light highlights the refractile hooklets ➡ buried within the protoscolex, a property that is retained in intact or dead organisms.*

Nonviable Disrupted Cysts

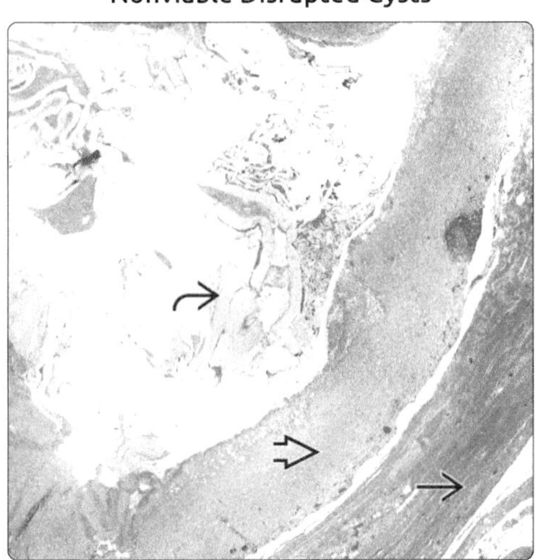

Necrotic Cyst With Hooklets

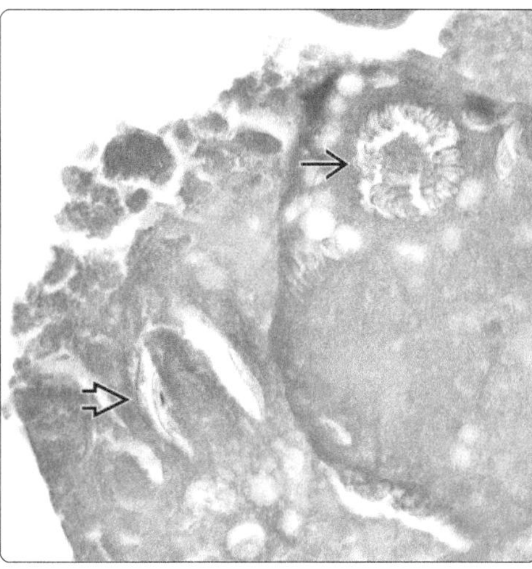

(Left) *Low-power view shows a cyst in tissue with an outer rim of fibrosis ➡, the laminated and germinal layers (dead) ⇨, and debris from dead daughter cysts ⇨.* **(Right)** *Necrotic debris from a previously damaged/dead echinococcal cyst still contains diagnostic hooklets in original configuration ➡ and floating within debris ⇨.*

KEY FACTS

ETIOLOGY/PATHOGENESIS

- *Spirometra* spp. and *Sparganum proliferum* larvae infection via ingestion of copepod-contaminated water or undercooked meat

CLINICAL ISSUES

- Worldwide, but majority of cases reported in Asia
- Presents as slow-growing migratory subcutaneous mass
- CNS involvement with weakness, headache, seizure, paraesthesia
- Definitive diagnosis by examination of surgically removed specimen; curative for nonproliferating sparganum

IMAGING

- CT: Punctate calcifications "calcospherules"
- Brain MR: Tunnel signs seen post contrast

MICROBIOLOGY

- White, flat, ribbon-like worms (0.1 cm thick x < 1-5 cm in length); lack suckers/hooklets

MICROSCOPIC

- Minimal histopathologic changes to marked tissue eosinophilia and abscess formation; granuloma formation and caseating necrosis with worm disintegration
- Spherical sections with microvilli-lined tegument, parenchyma with smooth muscle cells, branching excretory channels, and calcareous corpuscles; no reproductive organs, cystic formation, or scolex/protoscoleces

TOP DIFFERENTIAL DIAGNOSES

- Cysticercosis: ~ 1-cm fluid-filled cyst with single invaginated scolex surrounded by convoluted spiral canal; marked granulomatous inflammation with degeneration
- Gnathostomiasis: Immature adult with large, cavernous lateral chords, multinucleated intestinal cells, pigmented granular material, cuticular spines
- Visceral larva migrans: 15-20 μm in diameter larvae with prominent lateral alae; prominent granulomatous reaction

***Spirometra/Sparganum* spp. Life Cycle**

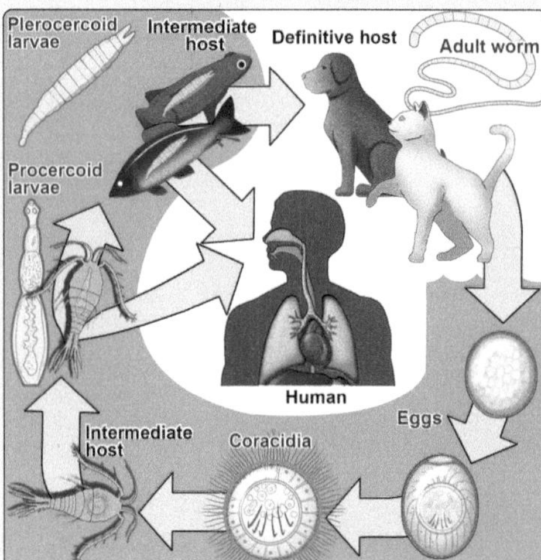

Subcutaneous Sparganosis

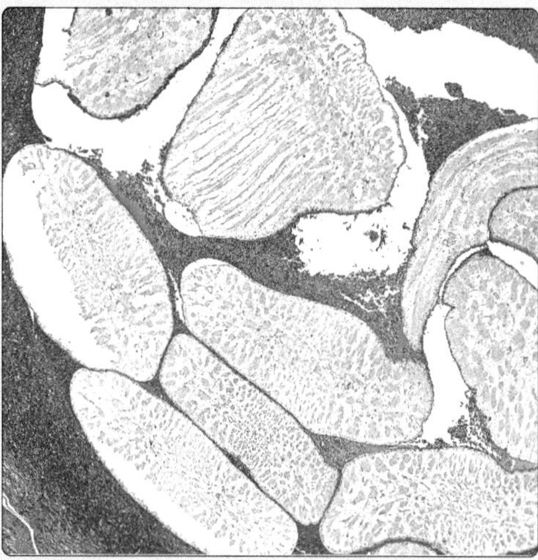

(Left) *Eggs are shed in feces, hatched in water releasing coracidia, which are ingested by copepods, develop into procercoid larvae consumed by fish, reptiles, and amphibians, and developed into plerocercoid larvae consumed by a dog or cat. Humans cannot serve as definitive hosts and develop sparganosis.* **(Right)** *This low-magnification image of a surgically removed soft tissue mass shows multiple tangential sections through a Spirometra spp. larva with dense intervening mixed inflammation.*

***Spirometra* spp. Histologic Features**

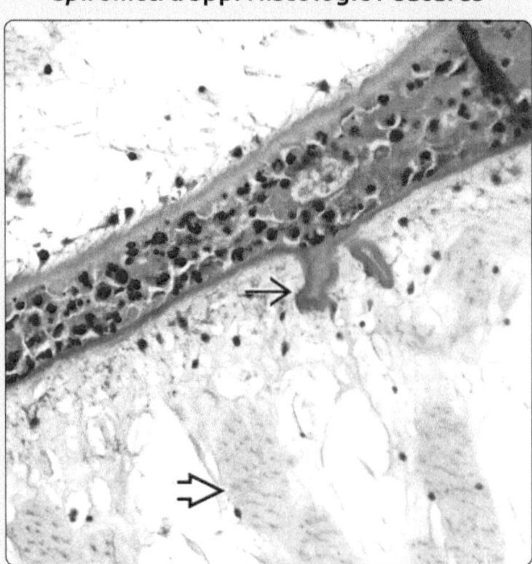

Calcareous Corpuscles

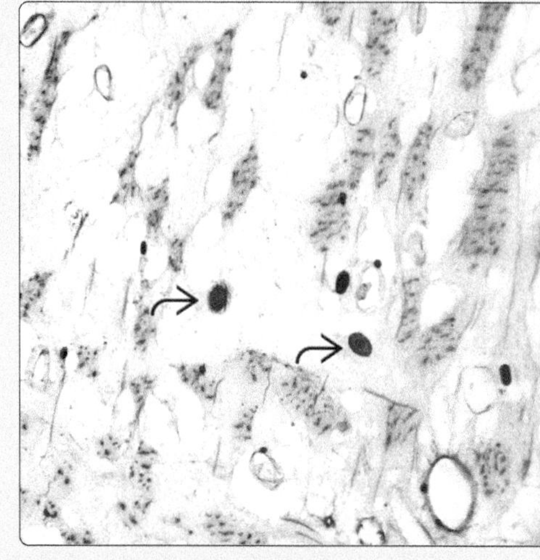

(Left) *Spirometra spp. contain an undulating microvilli-lined tegument* ➔ *overlying loose stroma with smooth muscle cells* ➩ *and branching excretory channels.* **(Right)** *Spirometra spp. stroma contains scattered calcareous corpuscles* ↷*, which aid in the identification of cestodes and can be differentiated based on lack of a cystic formation or scolex/protoscoleces.*

TERMINOLOGY

Definitions

- *Spirometra*: Greek "speira" (coil) + "metra" (uterus)
- *Sparganum*: Greek "sparganon" (swaddling clothes)

ETIOLOGY/PATHOGENESIS

Infectious Agents

- Infections with 3rd-stage plerocercoid larva (sparganum) of *Spirometra* spp. (*S. mansoni*, *S. ranarum*, *S. mansonoides*, *S. erinacei*) and *Sparganum proliferum* via ingestion of copepod-contaminated water or undercooked meat
- Adult *Spirometra* living in intestines of dogs/cats (definitive hosts) produce eggs that are shed in feces, embryonate, and hatch in water releasing coracidia
- Coracidia are ingested by copepods (intermediate host), develop into procercoid larvae, and are consumed by fish, reptiles and amphibians (2nd intermediate hosts), where they develop into plerocercoid larvae and are eventually consumed by predator (dog or cat)
- Humans serve as paratenic or 2nd intermediate hosts (but not definitive host) with larvae living up to 20 years

CLINICAL ISSUES

Epidemiology

- *Spirometra* spp. are present worldwide; majority of human cases reported from Asian countries where frogs or snakes are eaten or used for traditional medicinal practices
- Sparganosis is endemic in animals throughout North America; human cases are rare (typically *S. mansonoides*)

Presentation

- Usually presents as slow-growing subcutaneous or intramuscular mass; migration may be painless or associated with pain and pruritus
- Breast, orbit, urinary tract, pleural cavity, lungs, abdominal viscera, CNS may be involved
- Neurologic symptoms include weakness, headache, seizure, paraesthesia
- *S. proliferum* cause proliferative lesions with multiple plerocercoids in single site

Laboratory Tests

- Eosinophilia (blood)
- Enzyme-linked immunosorbent assay (serum, CSF) is sensitive and specific
- DNA sequencing of complete mitochondrial cytochrome c oxidase subunit I (*COI*) gene

Treatment

- Limited effect of antiparasitic medications (e.g., praziquantel) in peripheral sparganosis; no effect in CNS
- Surgical removal curative for nonproliferating sparganum

Prognosis

- Surgical removal is usually unsuccessful for proliferative sparganosis (*S. proliferum*), which may be fatal

IMAGING

General Features

- CT: Punctate calcifications "calcospherules"
- Brain MR: Tunnel signs seen post contrast

MICROBIOLOGY

Parasite Features

- White, flat, ribbon-like worms (0.1 cm thick x < 1-5 cm in length) that usually have vertical groove at anterior end but lack suckers and hooklets; spargana may crawl out of surgical incision
- Speciation of living sparganum via infection of definitive host and identification of adult after maturation (not clinically warranted)
- No role for stool examination

MACROSCOPIC

General Features

- Subcutaneous nodules contain cyst with flat, thread-like worm

MICROSCOPIC

Histologic Features

- Tissue reaction varies from minimal histopathologic changes to tissue eosinophilia and abscess formation; granuloma formation with worm disintegration progressing to caseating necrosis
- Spargana may appear as spherical sections with microvilli-lined tegument overlying parenchyma of loose stroma with smooth muscle cells, branching excretory channels, and calcareous corpuscles; no reproductive organs, cystic formation, or scolex/protoscoleces

DIFFERENTIAL DIAGNOSIS

Cysticercosis

- *Taenia solium* cysticerci: ~ 1-cm fluid-filled cystic structure with single invaginated scolex surrounded by convoluted spiral canal; degeneration with marked granulomatous inflammation

Gnathostomiasis

- Immature adult *Gnathostoma* spp.: Large, cavernous lateral chords, multinucleated intestinal cells containing pigmented granular material, and cuticular spines

Visceral Larva Migrans

- *Toxocara* spp. larvae: 15-20 μm in diameter with prominent lateral alae; prominent granulomatous reaction

SELECTED REFERENCES

1. Alvarez P et al: Four case reports of cutaneous sparganosis from Peruvian Amazon. Am J Dermatopathol. 44(7):510-4, 2022
2. Kuchta R et al: Sparganosis (Spirometra) in Europe in the molecular era. Clin Infect Dis. 72(5):882-90, 2021
3. Kikuchi T et al: Human proliferative sparganosis update. Parasitol Int. 75:102036, 2020
4. Carlson AL et al: The brief case: central nervous system sparganosis in a 53-year-old Thai man. J Clin Microbiol. 55(2):352-5, 2017
5. Eberhard ML et al: Thirty-seven human cases of sparganosis from Ethiopia and South Sudan caused by Spirometra Spp. Am J Trop Med Hyg. 93(2):350-5, 2015
6. Johnson G et al: Cutaneous sparganosis: a rare parasitic infection. J Cutan Pathol. 42(3):159-63, 2015
7. Meric R et al: Disseminated infection caused by Sparganum proliferum in an AIDS patient. Histopathology. 56(6):824-8, 2010

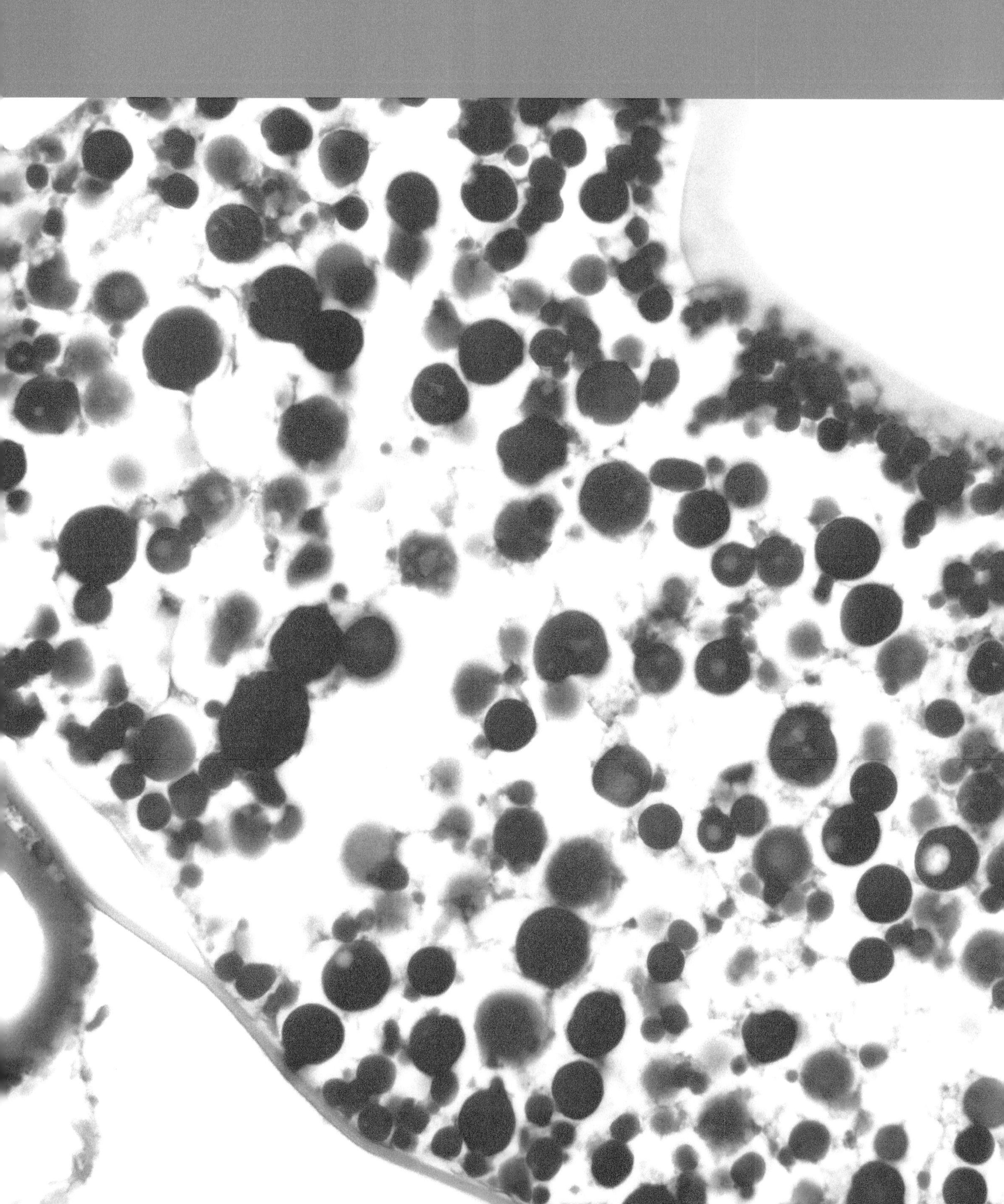

SECTION 8

Infestations and Other Invertebrate-Related Maladies

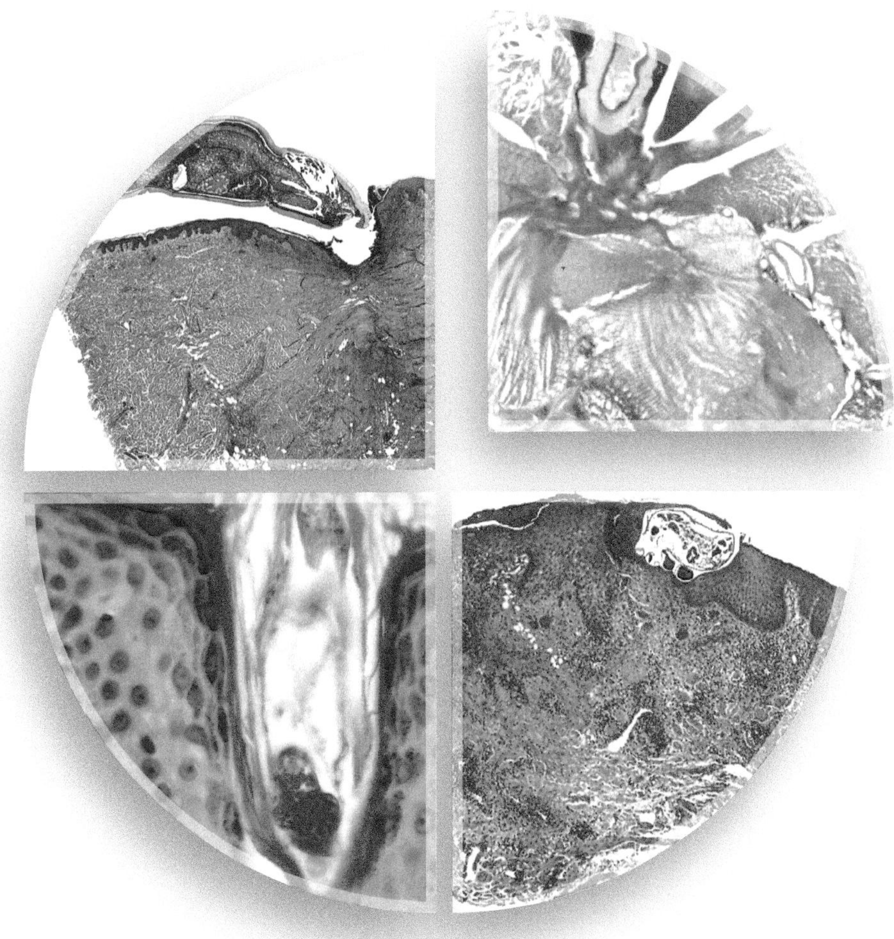

Tissue Damage From Arachnids and Insects

KEY FACTS

ETIOLOGY/PATHOGENESIS

- Insects and arachnids are found worldwide in all climates with seasonal variation in activity
- Important common organisms: Mosquitoes, biting flies, bees, wasps, hornets, ants, spiders, scorpions, bedbugs, chiggers, puss caterpillars, ticks, mites, lice

CLINICAL ISSUES

- Hallmark of most bites is local irritation of skin/mucosa: Erythema, edema, swelling, breaks in skin with bleeding, crusting, pruritus, pattern irritation, tissue necrosis/breakdown
- Insects and spiders have access to human skin in specific zones related to clothing, time and number of exposures

MICROSCOPIC

- Insect lesions may contain physical structures embedded in tissue (e.g., tick mouthparts, bot flies, Tunga fleas)
- Hypersensitivity reactions: Intercellular edema with perivascular lymphocytes and eosinophils
- Tissue necrosis: Necrosis with minimal inflammation or collaret of neutrophils; dense inflammation typically due to secondary infection
- Chronic/persistent reactions: Lymphoid aggregates with plasma cells and eosinophils
- Scarring: Increased collagen or dense dermal collagen

TOP DIFFERENTIAL DIAGNOSES

- Primary methicillin-resistant *Staphylococcus aureus* skin infections: Local erythema, edema, tissue breakdown, and purulence; gram-positive cocci present; confirmed by culture, PCR
- Secondary bacterial skin infections: Presence of bacteria, speciated by culture, PCR
- Drug reaction: May appear identical with eosinophils and edema; clinical history of new drug treatment
- Contact dermatitis: Associated with many irritants in distribution related to contact

Arthropod Assault Reaction

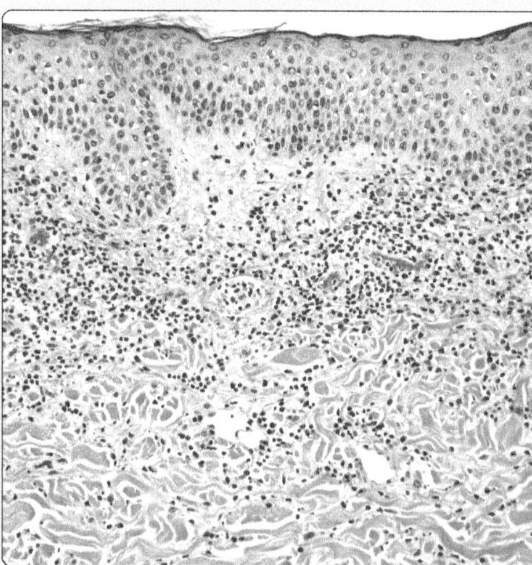

Clinical Appearance of Arthropod Lesions

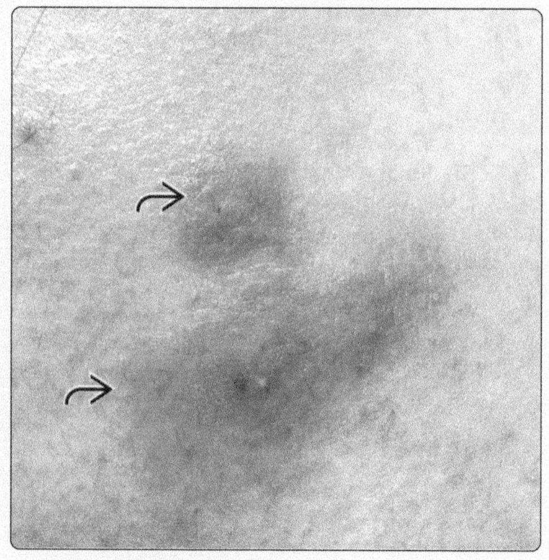

(Left) *Epidermal spongiosis, perivascular and interstitial lymphocytes, and frequent eosinophils typify type IV hypersensitivity reactions (e.g., arthropod bite). Similar findings are seen in scabies and tick bite reactions.* **(Right)** *Clinical features vary depending on the arthropod species. Most commonly, lesions appear as excoriated pruritic erythematous papules ⇗, but vesicles, bullae, nodules, erosions, and ulcers can also occur. (From DP: Nonneoplastic Derm.)*

Blister Response to Bites

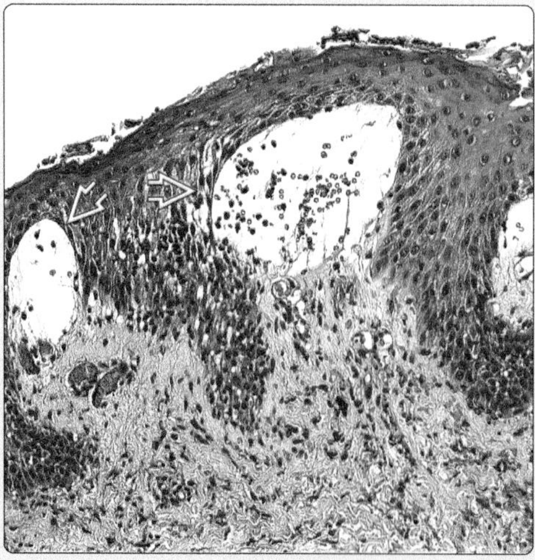

Tick Attached to Skin

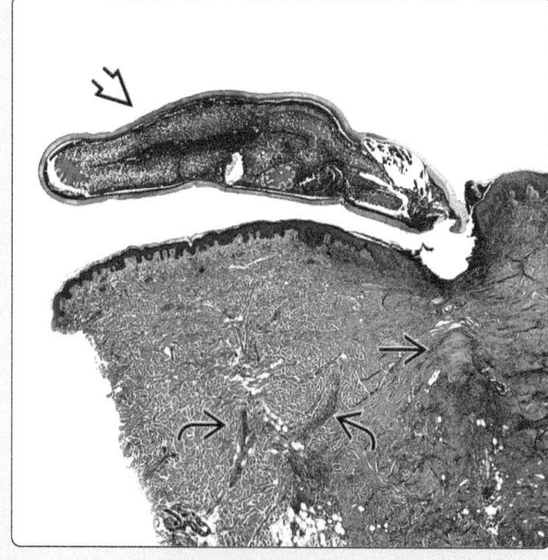

(Left) *Spongiosis, intraepidermal blister ➡ formation, and prominent papillary dermal edema may be seen in bites. Wedge-shaped, perivascular, moderate to dense lymphocytic infiltrate with eosinophils is typical. (From DP: Nonneoplastic Derm.)* **(Right)** *A tick ⇨ attached to the skin is shown. Moderately dense, perivascular mixed cell infiltrate ⇗ is seen. An intradermal cavity and necrosis ➡ are also visible, below which mouthparts may be seen. (From DP: Nonneoplastic Derm.)*

TERMINOLOGY

Definitions

- Latin: "Insectum" (cut into sections); pertains to organisms of class Insecta (invertebrates)
  - Adults: Antennae, 3 pairs of legs, compound eyes, 3-part body (head, thorax, and abdomen)
  - 7-10 million species (1/2 of known living organisms on Earth), including beetles, flies, moths, and wasps
- Greek: "Arachne" (spider); pertains to organisms in class Arachnida; 8 jointed legs
  - 100,000 species, including spiders, scorpions, solifuges, mites, harvestmen, and ticks

ETIOLOGY/PATHOGENESIS

Environmental Exposure

- Insects and arachnids are found worldwide in all climates with seasonal variation in activity
- Important common organisms: Mosquitoes, biting flies, bees, wasps, hornets, ants, spiders, scorpions, bedbugs, chiggers, puss caterpillars, ticks, mites, lice
- Probability of exposure increases in environments where control of insects and arachnids is limited: Poverty, rural settings, occupational exposure, poor environmental hygiene

CLINICAL ISSUES

Presentation

- Hallmark of most insect or spider bites is local irritation of skin or mucosa: Erythema, edema, swelling, breaks in skin with bleeding, crusting, pruritus (sometimes with secondary infection), pattern irritation (mirroring contact with organism), tissue necrosis/breakdown
- Exposure zones and lesion number; insects and spiders have access to human skin in specific zones related to clothing, time of exposure, and number of exposures
  - Bedbugs may produce row of bites on exposed skin, but most bites are not linear
  - Mosquitoes often bite exposed skin (ankles, neck, arms, face) but may bite through clothing and produce multiple identical lesions, depending on length and density of exposure
  - Ticks often feed beneath clothing but need exposed areas to access skin
  - Spiders, irritating insects (puss caterpillars), venomous organisms (centipedes), and painful biting horse flies or tsetse flies, in general, produce single lesion
- Although tissue biopsy is not necessary for diagnosis or treatment, tissue samples may be taken as part of debridement (e.g., spider bite necrosis) or in unclear clinical scenarios (persistent itchy nodules, history of insect exposure)
  - Biopsy or scraping may reveal scabies mites
  - Bites or infestations are often accompanied by infiltration of eosinophils &/or basophils

Laboratory Tests

- In cases of exposure to organisms that carry disease, range of laboratory tests specific to symptomatology may be warranted
- Mosquito exposure in malaria-endemic areas: Malaria testing, serology for arboviruses
- Tsetse fly exposure: Screening for African sleeping sickness
- Tick exposure: Screening for Lyme disease, babesiosis, anaplasmosis, Rocky Mountain spotted fever
- Ticks grossly identified morphologically (color, shape/size of scutum, mouthparts, presence of eye spots and festoons, and location/shape of anal canal); scutal index (body length divided by scutum width)
- Matrix-assisted laser desorption/ionization time-of-flight mass spectrometry (MALDI-TOF MS) may be used for identification of ticks and other arthropods

Treatment

- For embedded organisms, such as ticks, careful rapid removal is key to prevent further reaction and reduce risk of transmission
- For organisms that cause tissue destruction as result of venom, e.g., spiders, close attention to wound with possible treatment for secondary bacterial infection (rare) is necessary
- For organisms that transmit infections, empiric therapy for specific infections may be warranted if symptoms are begin
  - Presumptive/prophylactic treatment for tick that has fed for > 2 days
  - Erythema migrans in tick bites (indicating Lyme disease)
  - Fever in mosquito bites (indicating malaria or arbovirus infection)

Prognosis

- Although some spider bites may very rarely lead to death, vast majority of insects cause self-limited local irritation that may progress to fibrosis and scarring
- Rare reported cases of severe systemic complications (including death) have occurred related to bee stings, wasp stings, and other insect bites
- Some pathogens transmitted by interaction with insects may lead to fatality without treatment (e.g., African sleeping sickness)

MACROSCOPIC

Necrosis

- Insect or arachnid lesions that produce tissue necrosis (e.g., spider bites) may show ulceration, secondary purulence formation, or cavitation

Embedded Parts

- Insect lesions may contain physical structures embedded in tissue (e.g., tick mouthparts, bot flies, Tunga fleas) with swelling and obvious foreign material

MICROSCOPIC

Histologic Features

- Hypersensitivity reactions
  - Penetration of skin by insects or spiders may introduce foreign substances
  - Elicit response characterized by intercellular edema (epidermal spongiosis) and perivascular infiltrate of lymphocytes and eosinophils
- Tissue necrosis

Features of Ticks Commonly Biting Humans in USA

Species	Pathogen(s)	Distribution in USA	Morphologic Features
Ixodes scapularis (black-legged tick, deer tick)	*Borrelia burgdorferi*, *Babesia* spp., *Anaplasma phagocytophilum*, *Borrelia miyamotoi*, Powassan virus (lineage II)	Eastern and upper midwestern USA, including southern and Gulf Coast states	Red abdomen, black scutum (1/3 length in females; most of dorsum in males), capitulum, and, legs; narrow and elongated mouthparts with straight club-like palpi; no eye spots or festoons; inverted anterior-located U-shaped anal groove
Dermacentor variabilis (American dog tick)	*Rickettsia rickettsii*, *Francisella tularensis*	East, south, and along West Coast	Pale brown to gray dorsum with silvery white pattern over scutum (1/3 length in females; most of dorsum in males, patterned); mouthparts short with thick palpi, angular, rhomboidal shape; eye spots and festoons present; chalice-shaped posterior-located anal groove in males (absent in females)
Amblyomma americanum (lone star tick)	*Ehrlichia chaffeensis*, *Francisella tularensis*, *R. rickettsii*, *Coxiella burnetii*, Heartland virus	South, central, and east	Reddish brown with bronze iridescent appearance and angular-shaped scutum, eyes at lateral apices, and characteristic white spot in females; mouthparts much longer than basis capitulum; bulbous hypostome; eye spots and festoons present; chalice-shaped posterior-located anal groove
Rhipicephalus sanguineus (brown dog tick)	Mostly nuisance, *R. rickettsi*	Southwestern USA and Mexico	Red-brown with angular-shaped scutum and eyes at lateral margin; mouthparts short with thick palpi; hexagonal basis capituli; eye spots and festoons present; chalice-shaped posterior-located anal groove; anal plates and accessory plates on either side of anus in males

Adapted from Laga et al. Am J Dermatopathol. 44:163-9, 2022.

    - Toxic substances from insects or spiders may destroy tissue and produce necrosis with minimal inflammation or collaret of inflammation (neutrophils)
    - Dense inflammation, including numerous neutrophils, abscess formation, and crust, may indicate secondary infection and should warrant special stains for bacteria
- Chronic/persistent reactions: Persistence of antigens or allergens may produce lymphoid aggregates with plasma cells and eosinophils
- Scarring: Chronic lesions that have resolved may leave increased or dense collagen within dermis

DIFFERENTIAL DIAGNOSIS

Primary Methicillin-Resistant *Staphylococcus aureus* Skin Infections

- Produces local erythema, edema, tissue breakdown, and purulence that may be confused with spider bites
- Presence of gram-positive cocci confirmed by culture, PCR

Secondary Bacterial Skin Infections

- Breaks in skin (often from excoriation) from any cause may become secondarily infected
- Bacteria identified by special stains, culture, PCR

Drug Reaction

- May appear identical with eosinophils and edema
- Clinical history of new drug treatment

Contact Dermatitis

- Many irritants can lead to contact dermatitis, which usually has distribution related to contact with irritant but may mimic bites or insect/spider exposures

Factitious Disorders

- Picking or other forms of chronic irritation of skin may produce mimics of insect or spider bite lesions
- Psychologic evaluation for delusional parasitosis or other mental conditions leading to picking should be considered
- More common when patients present with multiple lesions in different exposure zones

"Junkie Itch"

- Opiate addicts/users may suffer from delusions of insects on skin, leading to aggressive scratching and excoriations

SELECTED REFERENCES

1. Laga AC et al: Identification of hard ticks in the United States: a practical guide for clinicians and pathologists. Am J Dermatopathol. 44(3):163-9, 2022
2. Sevestre J et al: Matrix-assisted laser desorption/ionization time-of-flight mass spectrometry: an emerging tool for studying the vectors of human infectious diseases. Future Microbiol. 16:323-40, 2021
3. Bernard Q et al: In vitro models of cutaneous inflammation. Methods Mol Biol. 1690:319-27, 2018
4. Haddad V Jr et al: Skin manifestations of tick bites in humans. An Bras Dermatol. 93(2):251-5, 2018
5. Pritt BS: Scutal index and its role in guiding prophylaxis for Lyme disease following tick bite. Clin Infect Dis. 67(4):617-8, 2018
6. Glatz M et al: Characterization of the early local immune response to Ixodes ricinus tick bites in human skin. Exp Dermatol. 26(3):263-9, 2017
7. Hadanny A et al: Nonhealing wounds caused by brown spider bites: application of hyperbaric oxygen therapy. Adv Skin Wound Care. 29(12):560-6, 2016
8. Milman Lde M et al: Acute generalized exanthematous pustulosis associated with spider bite. An Bras Dermatol. 91(4):524-7, 2016
9. An JY et al: Hemichorea after multiple bee stings. Am J Emerg Med. 32(2):196, 2014
10. Goddard J: Cutaneous reactions to bed bug bites. Skinmed. 12(3):141-3, 2014
11. Mathison BA et al: Laboratory identification of arthropod ectoparasites. Clin Microbiol Rev. 27(1):48-67, 2014
12. Fernando DM et al: Necrotizing fasciitis and death following an insect bite. Am J Forensic Med Pathol. 34(3):234-6, 2013
13. Kumar L et al: Autopsy diagnosis of a death due to scorpion stinging–a case report. J Forensic Leg Med. 19(8):494-6, 2012
14. Lin CJ et al: Multiorgan failure following mass wasp stings. South Med J. 104(5):378-9, 2011
15. Goddard J et al: Bed bugs (Cimex lectularius) and clinical consequences of their bites. JAMA. 301(13):1358-66, 2009

Brown Recluse Spider

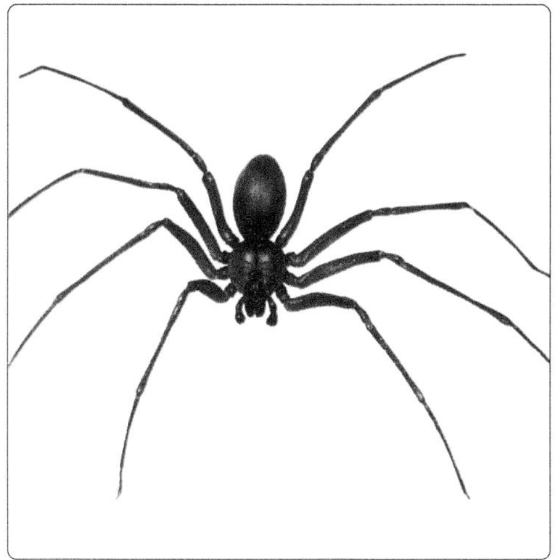

Brown Recluse Spider Bite

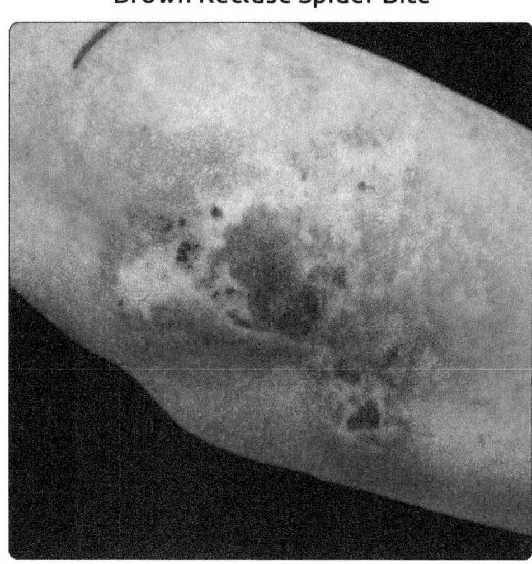

(Left) *Brown recluse spider bites elicit a strong reaction in 10% of those bitten. Such bites produce red, white, and blue lesions with tissue necrosis. (Courtesy A. Brooks, CDC/PHIL.)* **(Right)** *The red, white, and blue sign is seen in a patient with a brown recluse spider bite. The sign is identified by dry necrotic eschar or ulceration surrounded by pale then erythematous patches. (From DP: Nonneoplastic Derm.)*

Ulcer and Necrosis

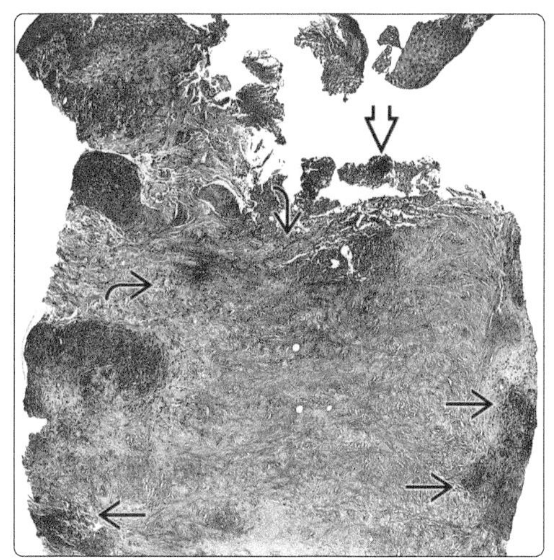

Coagulative Necrosis

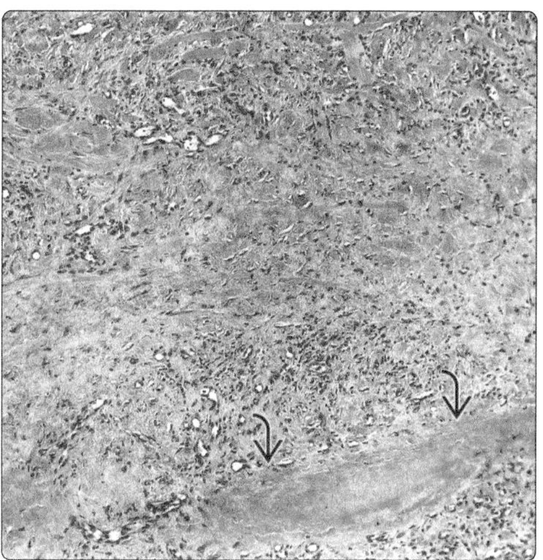

(Left) *The ulcer and coagulative necrosis in the epidermis and dermis, as well as neutrophilic, band-like infiltrate ➔ around the edge of the eschar/ulcer ➔, are shown. Note thrombosed blood vessels ➔ from vasculitis. (From DP: Nonneoplastic Derm.)* **(Right)** *Zone of eosinophilic staining is recognizable as "mummified" coagulative necrosis ➔ surrounded by neutrophilic infiltrate in the deep dermis, resulting in total necrosis of the skin. (From DP: Nonneoplastic Derm.)*

Chronic Inflammatory Response

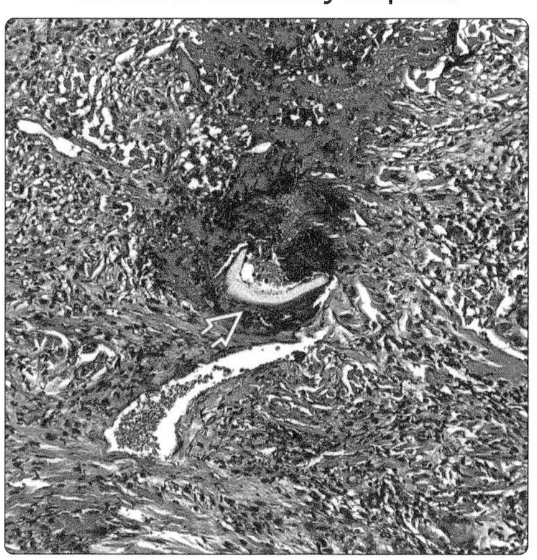

Nodular Scarring

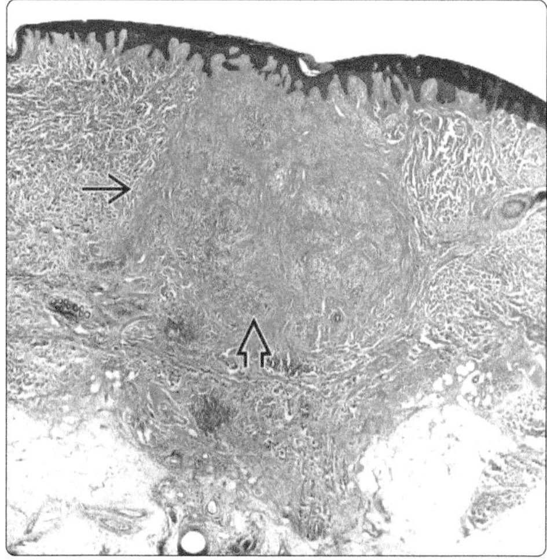

(Left) *A chronic bite lesion shows mouthparts ➔ of the tick in the intradermal necrotic tract, surrounded by dense, diffuse, superficial, and deep mixed cell infiltrate of fewer neutrophils and more lymphocytes. Fibrin thrombi may be seen in dermal capillaries. (From DP: Nonneoplastic Derm.)* **(Right)** *Low-power view shows a skin biopsy from a patient with a remote history of an insect bite (presumably a tick) that healed as a nodular scar ➔ with chronic infiltrates ➔.*

(**Left**) *This lesion was seen on the abdomen of a patient who had an adult tick attached, which was removed forcefully (leaving tick mouthparts behind), producing the red erythematous lesion. (Courtesy S. Granter, MD.)* (**Right**) *An adult female deer tick was dismembered in the process of removal, a common occurrence. The engorgement suggests feeding for ~ 2 days. (Courtesy R. Pollack, PhD.)*

Incomplete Tick Removal

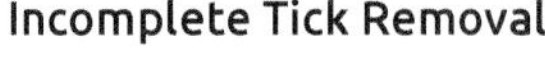

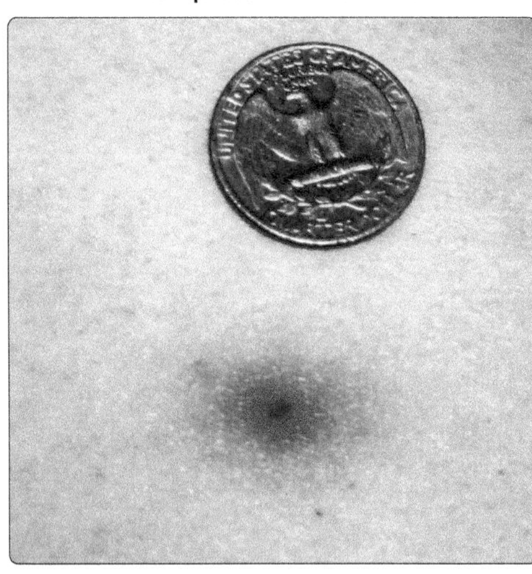

Fragmented Deer Tick

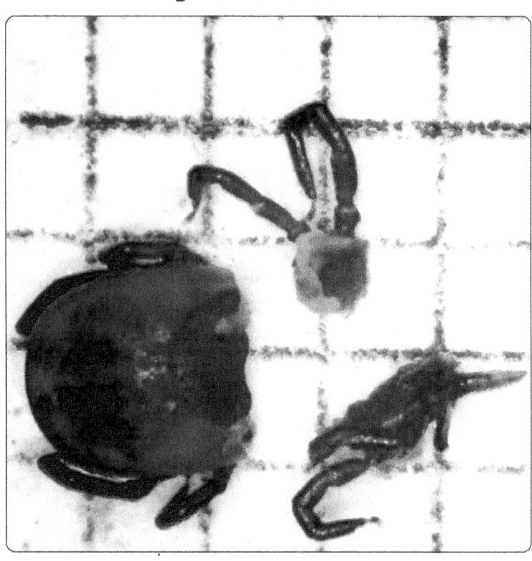

(**Left**) *A 10-mm skin punch biopsy with an embedded, partially engorged female lone star tick is shown. This method is not recommended and does not prevent tick-borne infections, but it does entirely remove the mouthparts. (Courtesy R. Pollack, PhD.)* (**Right**) *This image of a female Amblyomma americanum shows the characteristic lone star marking located centrally on its dorsal surface, at the distal tip of its scutum. (Courtesy C. Paddock, MD, J. Gathany, CDC/PHIL.)*

Inappropriate Tick Removal

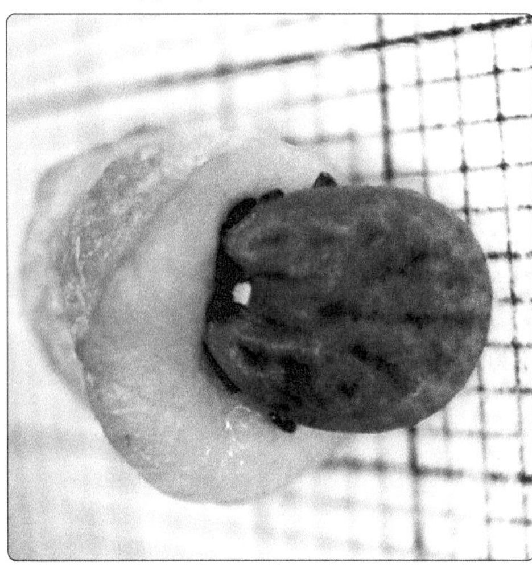

***Amblyomma americanum* (Lone Star Tick)**

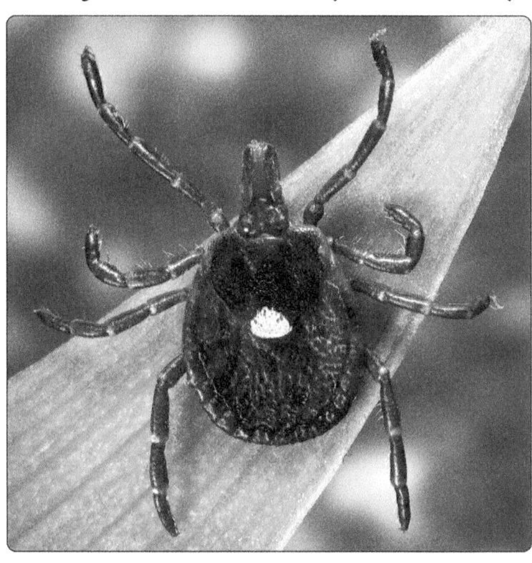

(**Left**) *An adult female lone star tick that fed for ~ 1 week demonstrates the characteristic spot* ➔ *on the scutal plate. (Courtesy R. Pollack, PhD.)* (**Right**) *This image of a female Amblyomma maculatumtium exhibits a red body with bright, white markings on the dorsal shield. (Courtesy C. Paddock, MD, CDC/PHIL.)*

Engorged Lone Star Tick

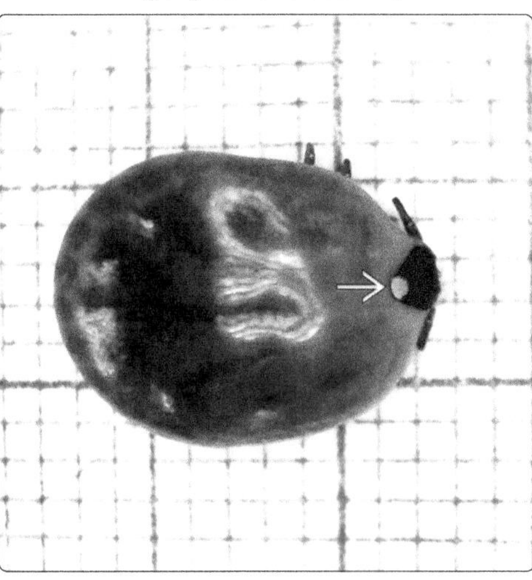

***Amblyomma maculatum* (Gulf Coast Tick)**

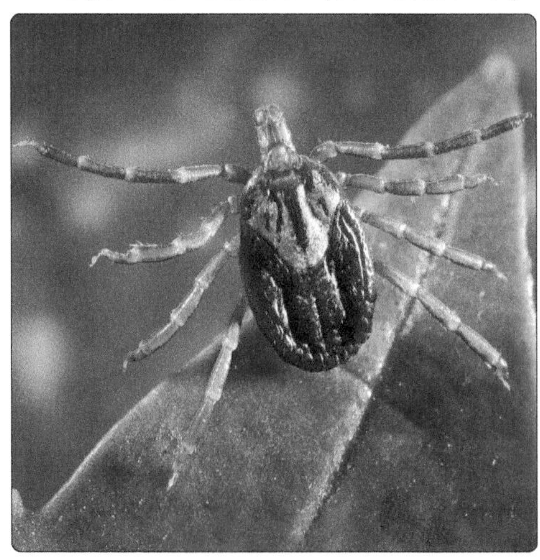

Ixodes scapularis (Deer Tick)

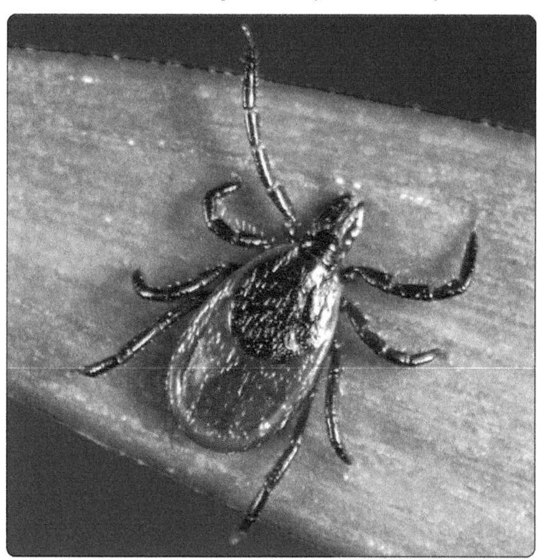

Engorged Deer Tick

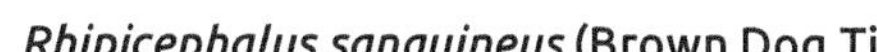

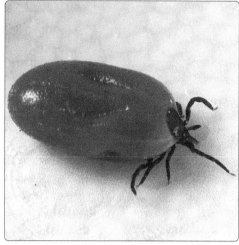

(Left) *This image of a female Ixodes scapularis (black-legged tick; deer tick) exhibits a red body with inverted U-shaped anal groove and black scutum. (Courtesy M. Levin, PhD, J. Gathany, CDC/PHIL.)* **(Right)** *This image depicts a lateral view of a female Ixodes scapularis, its abdomen engorged with a host blood meal. (Courtesy G. Alpert, PhD, CDC/PHIL.)*

Ixodes pacificus (Western Black-Legged Tick)

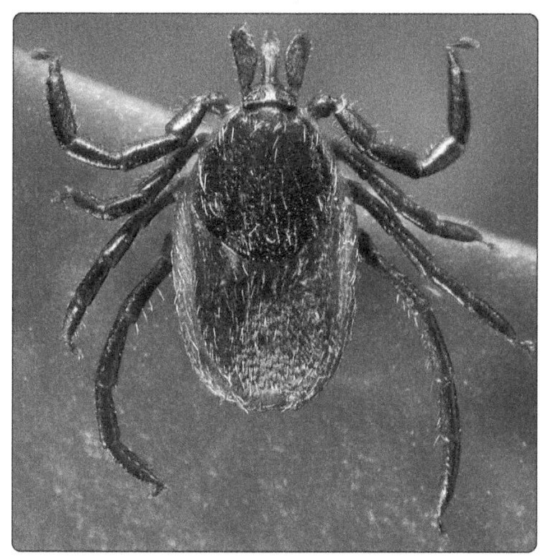

Rhipicephalus sanguineus (Brown Dog Tick)

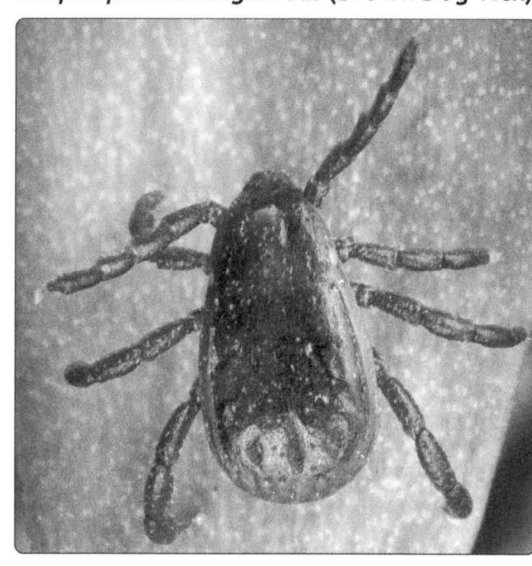

(Left) *This image shows a female Ixodes pacificus, which can be differentiated from I. scapularis by lack of festoons. (Courtesy C. Paddock, MD, J. Gathany, CDC/PHIL.)* **(Right)** *This image of a male Rhipicephalus sanguineus contains an angular-shaped scutum and accessory plates on either side of the anus. (Courtesy W. Nicholson, PhD, J. Gathany, CDC/PHIL.)*

Dermacentor variabilis (American Dog Tick)

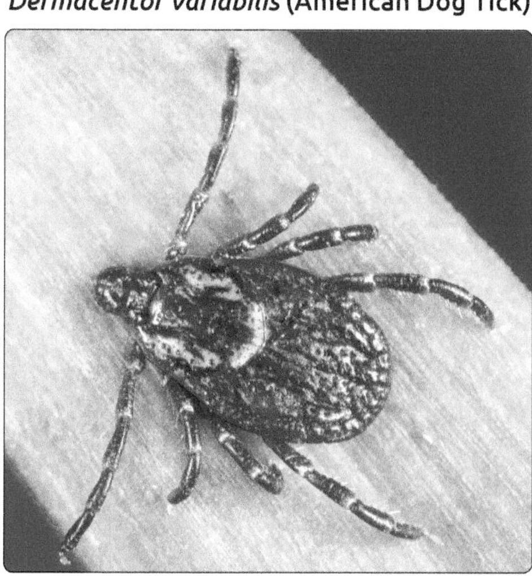

Dermacentor andersoni (Wood Tick)

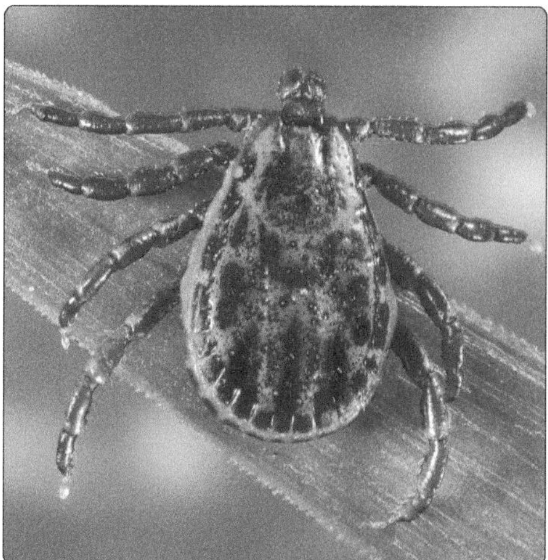

(Left) *This image of a female Dermacentor variabilis shows a brown and red dotted body with silvery white scutum 1/3 of the length and lacks an anal groove. (Courtesy G. Maupin, MS, J. Gathany, CDC/PHIL.)* **(Right)** *This image of a male Dermacentor andersoni shows a red teardrop-shaped body, distinguishing it from D. variabilis, with gray and white spots. (Courtesy C. Paddock, MD, J. Gathany, CDC/PHIL.)*

Anopheles gambiae **Mosquito**

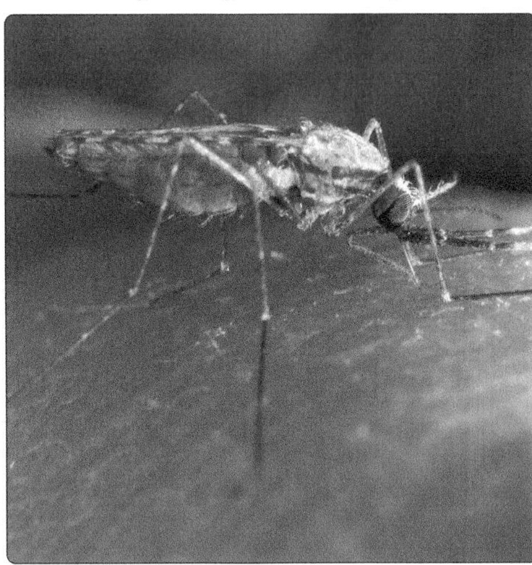

Aedes aegypti **Mosquito**

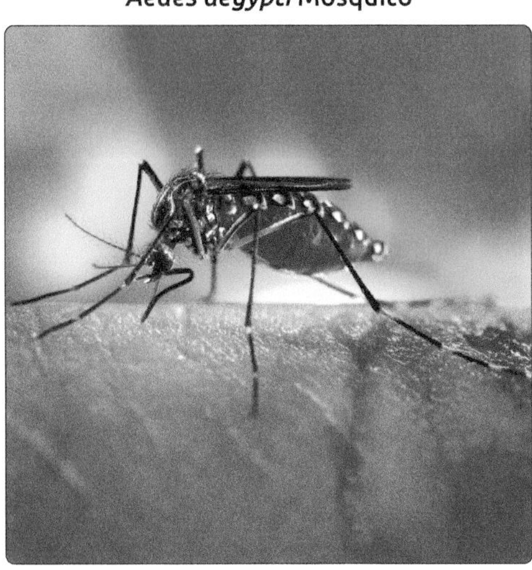

(Left) *Anopheles gambiae mosquitoes are identified by discrete blocks of black and white scales on their wings, and resting position with their abdomen sticking up in the air. (Courtesy J. Gathany, CDC/PHIL.)* **(Right)** *This female Aedes aegypti mosquito is identified by black and white markings on its legs and a marking in the form of a lyre on the upper surface of its thorax (not shown). The abdomen exhibited a red coloration, due to the insect's blood meal. (Courtesy F. Collins, PhD and J. Gathany, CDC/PHIL.)*

Culex quinquefasciatus **Mosquito**

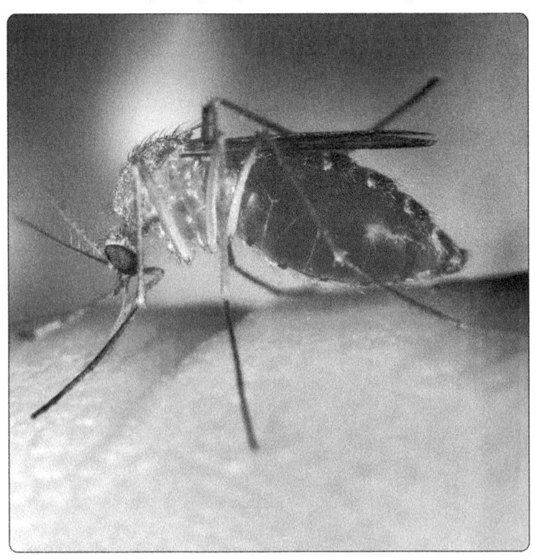

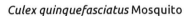

Black Widow Spider

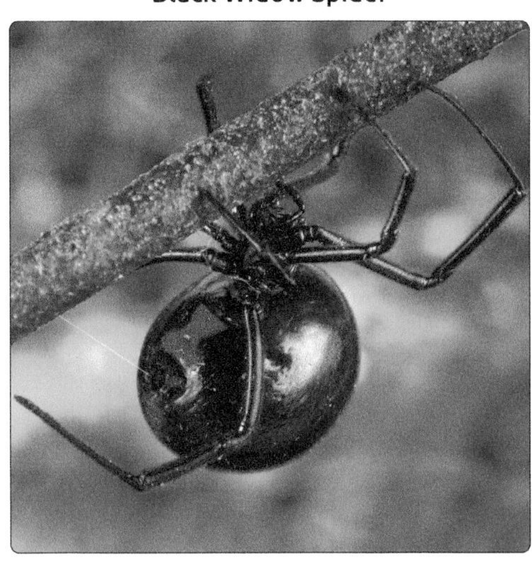

(Left) *Culex quinquefasciatus mosquitoes have brown bodies with darker brown proboscis, thorax, wings, and tarsi. This mosquito exhibits a red distended abdomen due to a blood meal. (Courtesy J. Gathany, CDC/PHIL.)* **(Right)** *The black widow spider is easily recognized by its dark, black, shiny body and legs and the characteristic red mark on its abdomen. (Courtesy P. Smith, CDC/PHIL.)*

Bedbug

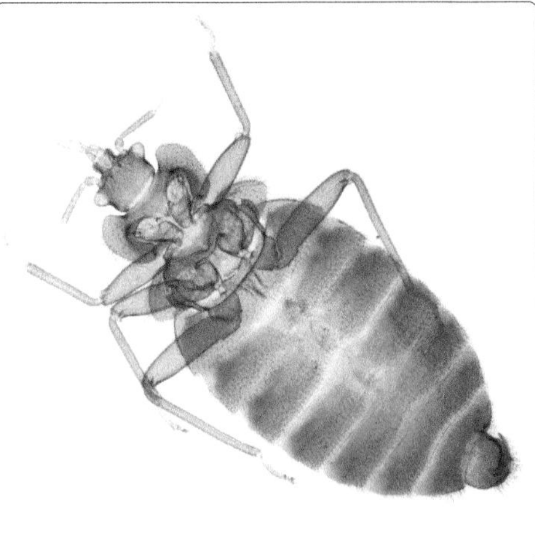

Common Flea

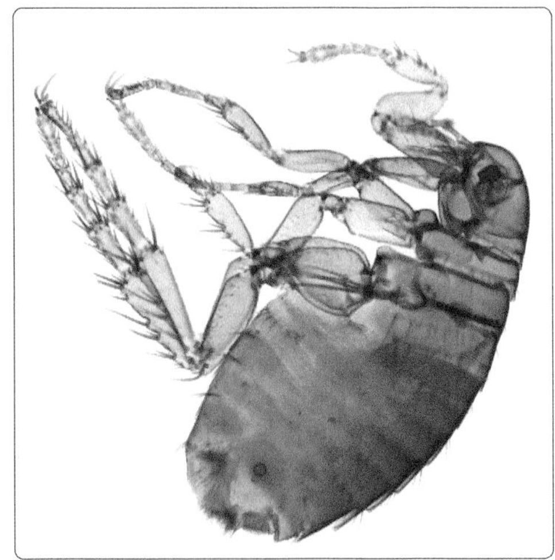

(Left) *An adult bedbug (Cimex lectularius) is shown with 3 pairs of legs, antennae, and the typical head, thorax, and abdomen of a bug. Although they do not transmit disease, infestations produce multiple bites and skin lesions for individuals exposed to them.* **(Right)** *A whole mount of a common flea (Pulex irritans) demonstrates the flat body and 3 pairs of legs. In addition to the bites that leave skin lesions, transmission of cat-scratch disease and plague is attributed to fleas.*

Pubic Lice

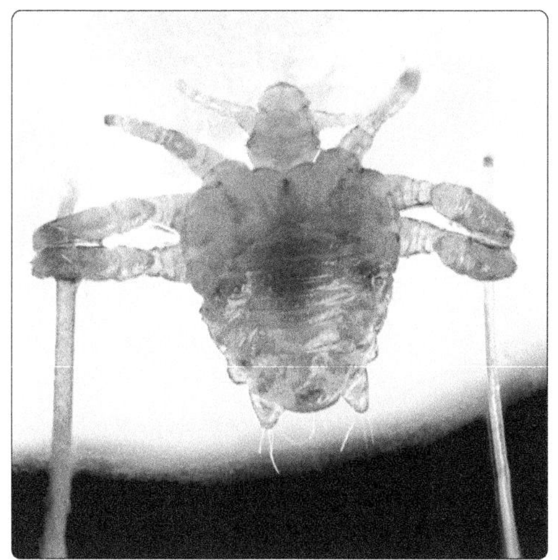

Body Lice

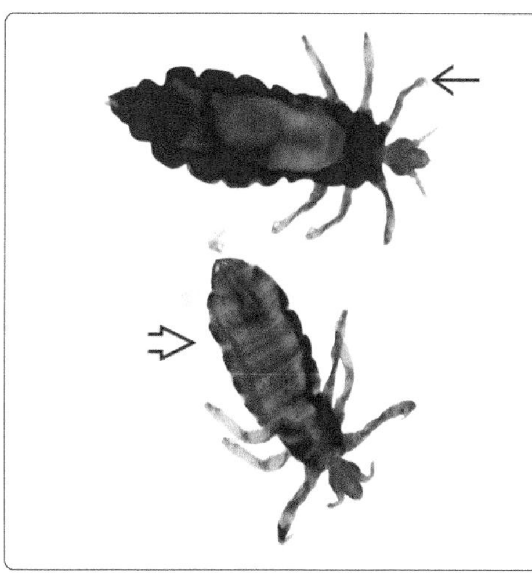

(Left) *An adult Pthirus pubis (crab or pubic louse) is shown attached to hairs, which may be any hair on the body (axilla, facial hair, chest hair, eyelashes, or, commonly, genital hairs). (Courtesy R. Pollack, PhD.)* **(Right)** *Whole mounts of preserved body lice demonstrate the 3 pairs of legs with clasping ends ➙ and the wide, flat abdomen ⇨.*

Mites

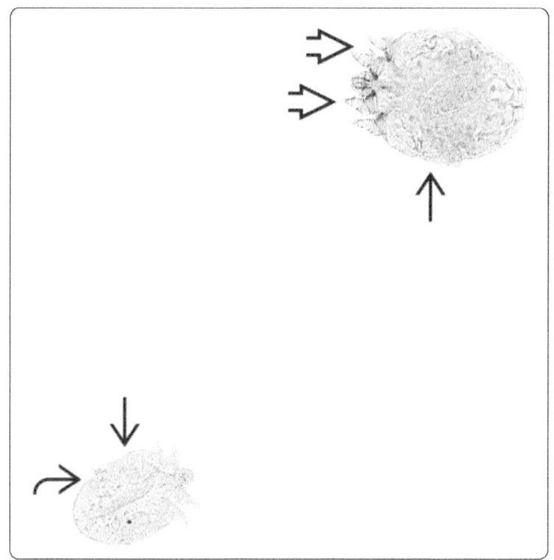

Wasp

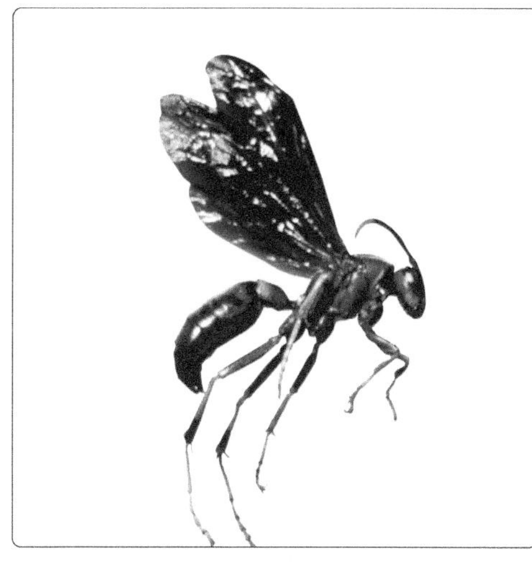

(Left) *Two mites ➙ are shown in which the 8 legs can be seen: 4 in the front ⇨ and 2 in the back ↪.* **(Right)** *Wasps, ants, and bees all have 4 life cycle stages, 2 paired membranous wings, chewing mouthparts, and colonial lifestyle. The bite or sting of these creatures occurs when threatened and may cause local irritation or necrosis, depending on the host reaction. (Courtesy CDC/PHIL.)*

Centipede

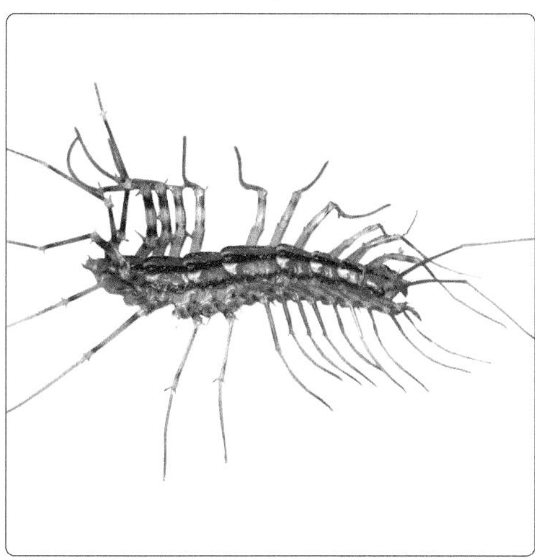

Scorpion

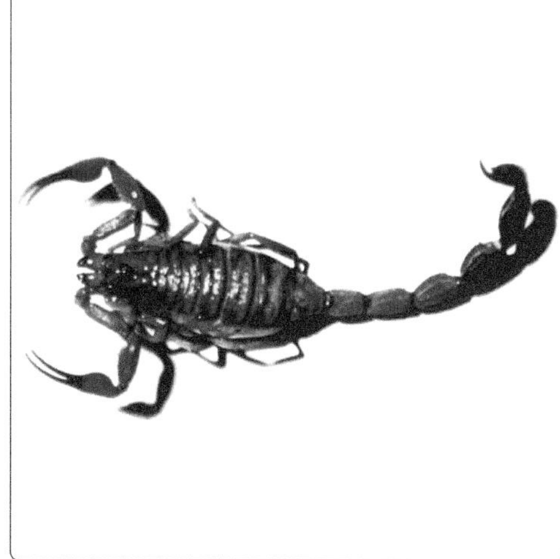

(Left) *Scutigera coleoptrata, or common house centipede, demonstrates its many pairs of legs. The bite of a centipede is venomous and causes extreme pain to human recipients, although it is generally nontoxic. (Courtesy Dr. G. Alpert, CDC/PHIL.)* **(Right)** *Tityus trinitatis, a black scorpion native to Trinidad, is shown. The sting of a scorpion is venomous and may cause a range of reactions, including, for this species, pancreatitis due to hyperstimulation. (Courtesy CDC/PHIL.)*

Myiasis

KEY FACTS

ETIOLOGY/PATHOGENESIS

- Infestation of human or animal tissue by Diptera "2-winged true fly" larvae (maggots) that are attracted to preexisting suppurative lesions

CLINICAL ISSUES

- Among 5 most common dermatologic conditions in travelers, representing 7.3-11.0% of cases
- Cutaneous and wound myiasis are most common forms
- Tissue invasion by maggots is generally well-recognized complication of neglected wounds
- Cavitary myiasis corresponds to infection of body cavities
- Orbital myiasis, or ophthalmomyiasis profunda, is infection of any anatomic structure of eye

MACROSCOPIC

- Larvae ~ 15 mm long; subclassification relies on examination anterior and posterior spiracles, mouthparts and cephalopharyngeal skeleton, and cuticular spines

MICROSCOPIC

- Ulcerated epidermis ± hyperkeratosis; dermis contains mixed acute and chronic inflammatory infiltrate
- Dipteran larva is seen in cross section but may not be possible to subclassify
- Cuticular spines, spiracles, striated muscle, and other internal organs may be identified

TOP DIFFERENTIAL DIAGNOSES

- Cellulitis, furunculosis, ruptured epidermoid cyst: Absence of larvae parts in tissue can rule out myiasis
- Leishmaniasis: Amastigotes (1-5 µm) with prominent kinetoplast within macrophages
- Onchocerciasis: Microfilariae (300-315 µm long), lack striated muscle, cuticular spines
- Tungiasis: Flea that resides at dermal-epidermal junction; contains numerous eosinophilic eggs

Dermatobia hominis **Gross Features**

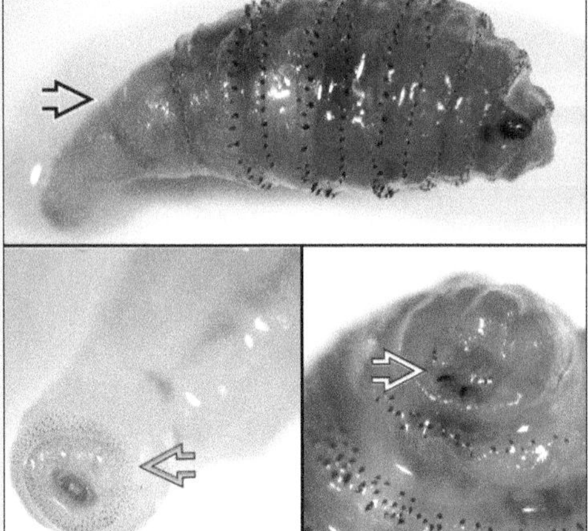

Cochliomyia hominivorax **Larvae in Tissue**

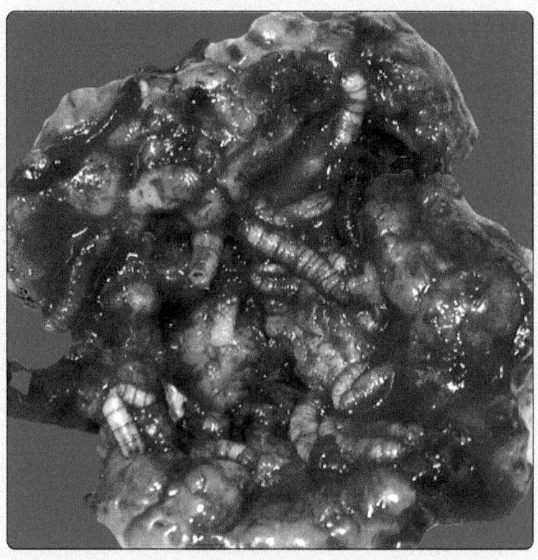

(Left) *Dermatobia hominis larva are ~ 15 mm in length and contain coarse cuticular spines, which are absent in the terminal 3 body segments ➡. The posterior end shows respiratory spiracles ⇨, while the anterior end shows mandibles ➡. (Courtesy B. Quattrochi, MD, PhD.)* **(Right)** *Many large Cochliomyia hominivorax larvae are shown in a basal cell carcinoma case where necrotic tissue has created fertile ground for maggot growth. (Courtesy O. Lupi, MD, PhD.)*

Bot Fly Larva Histologic Features

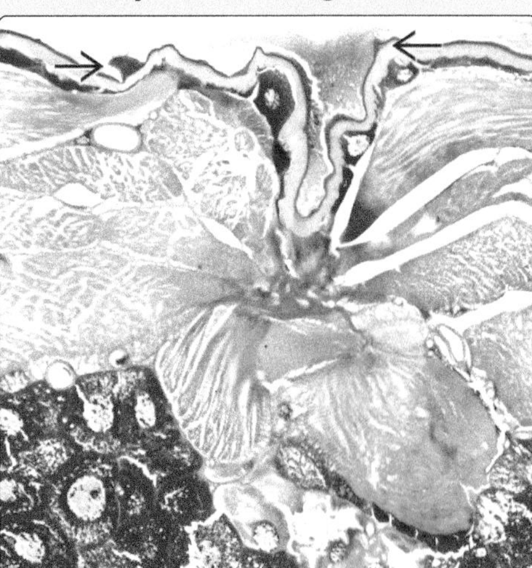

Bot Fly Anterior Spiracles

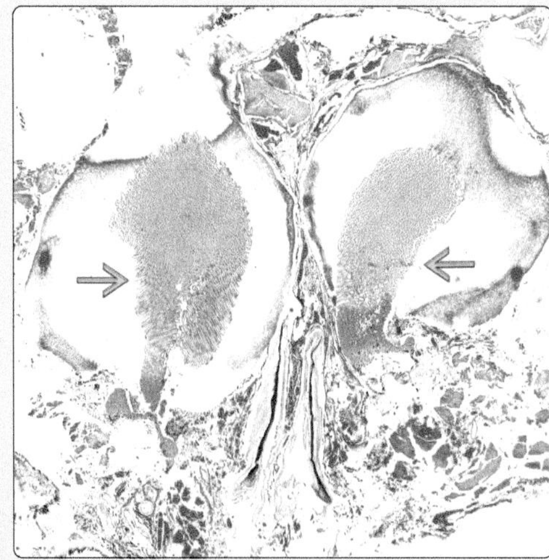

(Left) *Section of a bot fly shows cuticular spines ➡ and underlying skeletal muscle, the presence of which can distinguish from helminth infections. Further classification can be aided by prior gross examination and travel history. (Courtesy A. Laga, MD, MMSc.)* **(Right)** *Sagittal section of a bot fly through the cephalic end shows anterior spiracles ⇨. (Courtesy A. Laga, MD, MMSc.)*

TERMINOLOGY

Synonyms

- Flystrike, blowfly strike, fly blown

Definitions

- Greek: "Myia" (fly)

ETIOLOGY/PATHOGENESIS

Infectious Agents

- Infestation of human or animal tissue by Diptera "2-winged true fly" larvae (maggots) that are attracted to preexisting suppurative lesions
- Some species lay eggs on surface of blood-sucking vector (e.g., mosquitoes), which then enter host after blood meal
- *Dermatobia hominis*, bot fly, American warble fly (torsalo): Southeastern Mexico to northern Argentina, Chile, Uruguay
- *Chrysomya* species, screwworm, Old World screwworm: Asia, Africa, India, Papua New Guinea
- *Cochliomyia hominivorax*, blowflies, New World screwworm fly: Central and South America
- *Cordylobia anthropophaga*, tumbu fly, mango fly, putzi fly: East and Central Africa
- Sarcophagidae (e.g., *Wohlfahrtia* species), flesh flies: Worldwide; cause myiasis in sheep but also carry leprosy and cause intestinal pseudomyiasis if ingested by humans
- Species of maggots that feed only on dead tissue do not typically cause myiasis (e.g., common house fly)

CLINICAL ISSUES

Epidemiology

- Risk factors include poor hygiene and low socioeconomic status and travel to endemic regions without proper precautions
- Myiasis is among 5 most common dermatologic conditions in travelers, representing 7.3-11.0% of cases
- Leprosy is endemic in countries where myiasis-causing flies are highly prevalent
- Head and neck cancer patients represent risk group for development of myiasis in neoplastic wounds

Presentation

- Cutaneous and wound myiasis are most common forms
  - Furuncular myiasis occurs after skin penetration of larva
    - Papule or nodule with central punctum, which causes pruritus and pain
    - *D. hominis*, *C. anthropophaga*, *Cuterebra* species, *Wohlfahrtia vigil*, and *Wohlfahrtia magnifica*
    - Number of larvae within lesion varies with species
- Migratory myiasis occurs when dipteran maggot burrows in skin, producing migratory creeping pattern
  - Larvae of *Gasterophilus* (horse botfly) and *Hypoderma* (cattle botfly) cause this pattern in humans
- Wound myiasis occurs when fly larvae infest open wounds
  - *C. hominivorax*, *Chrysomya bezziana*, and *W. magnifica* are most common flies for wound myiasis
- Cavitary myiasis corresponds to infection of body cavities
- Orbital myiasis, or ophthalmomyiasis profunda, is infection of any anatomic structure of eye
- Other uncommon forms include ENT myiasis, urogenital myiasis, intestinal myiasis, cerebral myiasis, tracheopulmonary myiasis, and umbilical cord myiasis
- Recent report of extranodal NK-/T-cell lymphoma case presented as extensive myiasis

Treatment

- Surgical removal/debridement required for wound myiasis but not for simple cutaneous myiasis (requested by patient)
- Occlusion/oxygen depletions: Nonrestrictive cover (oil, animal fat, meat, petroleum jelly) forces larvae to migrate for oxygen supply after few hours; reduces scarring from surgical removal
- Alternative therapy (especially for oral or orbital) includes oral or topical ivermectin

Prognosis

- Self-limited disease in simple form (5-7 weeks)
- Wound with debridement and management of secondary infections is excellent

MACROSCOPIC

General Features

- Larvae are ~ 15 mm long, and identification to genus or species level relies on examination of features, including anterior and posterior spiracles, mouthparts and cephalopharyngeal skeleton, and cuticular spines

MICROSCOPIC

Histologic Features

- Ulcerated epidermis ± hyperkeratosis; dermis contains mixed acute and chronic inflammatory infiltrate
- Dipteran larva is seen in cross section but may not be possible to subclassify
- Cuticular spines, spiracles, striated muscle, and other internal organs may be identified

DIFFERENTIAL DIAGNOSIS

Cellulitis, Furunculosis, Ruptured Epidermoid Cyst

- Absence of larvae parts in tissue can rule out myiasis

Leishmaniasis

- Amastigotes (1-5 μm) with prominent kinetoplast present in macrophages in skin

Onchocerciasis

- Microfilariae (300-315 μm long) frequently present in skin; lack striated muscle, cuticular spines

Tungiasis

- Flea that resides at dermal-epidermal junction; contains numerous eosinophilic eggs

SELECTED REFERENCES

1. Chih Wong EH et al: A case report of extranodal natural killer / T-cell lymphoma presenting as extensive myiasis. Ann Med Surg (Lond). 75:103419, 2022
2. Gonçalves KKN et al: Head and neck cancer associated with myiasis. Int J Oral Maxillofac Surg. 51(7):847-53, 2022
3. Solomon M et al: Cutaneous myiasis. Curr Infect Dis Rep. 18(9):28, 2016
4. Singh A et al: Incidence of myiasis among humans-a review. Parasitol Res. 114(9):3183-99, 2015
5. Francesconi F et al: Myiasis. Clin Microbiol Rev. 25(1):79-105, 2012

Scabies

KEY FACTS

ETIOLOGY/PATHOGENESIS

- Acquired skin infestation of *Sarcoptes scabiei* var. *hominis* mites via direct skin to skin contact or, less frequently, via fomites, such as bedding or clothing

CLINICAL ISSUES

- 100 million affected worldwide (most common in children)
- Intense pruritus with nocturnal worsening
- Skin scrapings to detect mites, eggs, or mite fecal matter
- Treatment with topical permethrin or oral ivermectin
- With appropriate treatment, resolves with little scarring

MACROSCOPIC

- Mites are 0.5 mm in length and appear as white spots
- Skin: Linear or curved burrows appear red and possibly excoriated

MICROSCOPIC

- Identification of scabies mites, eggs, or feces (scybala) in subcorneum or superficial epidermis is pathognomonic
- Classic scabies
  - Ovoid mite containing chitinous exoskeleton, dorsal spines, and 4 pairs of legs
  - Spongiotic epidermis with exocytosis of eosinophils
- Nodular scabies: Identification of mites is less common
- Norwegian/crusted scabies: Innumerable mites and keratotic scale

TOP DIFFERENTIAL DIAGNOSES

- Demodex: Mites associated with hair follicles; typically involves face
- Arthropod bite: Rarely, insect mouthparts are identified in dermis; more prominent perivascular distribution with eosinophils
- Eczematous dermatitis: Similar appearance but absence of scabies mites, eggs, or scybala
- Cutaneous larva migrans: Nematode larval rarely identified; similar eosinophilic spongiotic and perivascular chronic dermatitis

Classic Scabies Skin Lesion

Crusted or Norwegian Scabies

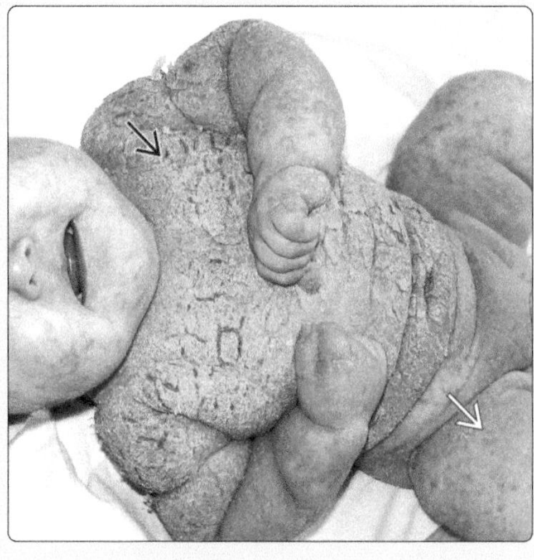

(Left) *Scabies presented in this patient as multiple excoriated papules ⇨ and burrows ⇨ on the hand. (From DP: Nonneoplastic Derm.)* **(Right)** *Norwegian scabies is characterized by crusted lesions ⇨ and scaly plaques ➡ infected with hundreds to millions of female mites. (Courtesy R. Alarcon, MD.)*

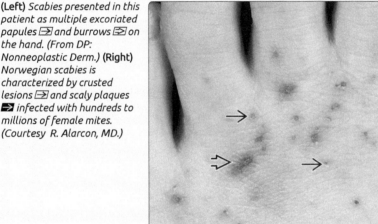

Intracorneal Burrow

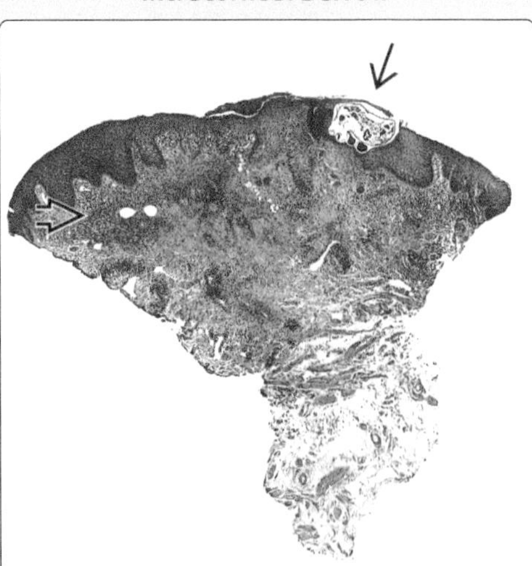

Chitinous Exoskeleton With Dorsal Spines

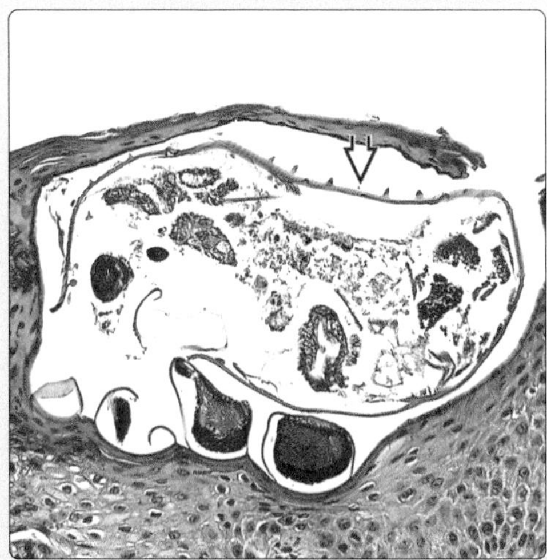

(Left) *Low-magnification view of a punch biopsy shows an intracorneal burrow containing a Sarcoptes mite ⇨ and florid dermatitis ⇨, which is frequently associated with an infestation.* **(Right)** *High-power magnification shows an intracorneal mite with a chitinous exoskeleton bearing multiple dorsal spines ⇨. Eggs are ovoid to curvilinear in shape.*

TERMINOLOGY

Synonyms

- 7-year itch
- Crusted scabies (Norwegian scabies)

Definitions

- Latin: "Scabere" (to scratch)

ETIOLOGY/PATHOGENESIS

Infectious Agents

- Acquired skin infestation of *Sarcoptes scabiei* var. *hominis* mites via direct skin to skin contact or, less frequently, via fomites, such as bedding or clothing
- Primary infection induces clinical symptoms only 4-8 weeks after inoculation
- Considered water-washed disease due to lack of proper sanitation and hygiene

CLINICAL ISSUES

Epidemiology

- Incidence: 100 million affected worldwide (most common in children)

Presentation

- Intense pruritus with nocturnal worsening
  - Classic scabies
    - Burrows: Wavy, gray-brown lines on epidermal surface
    - Predilection for palms, soles, wrists, nipples, inframammary folds, waist, and male genitalia
  - Nodular scabies
    - Subcutaneous nodules
    - Predilection for lower trunk, thighs, and scrotum
    - More prevalent in young/pediatric populations
  - Norwegian/crusted scabies
    - Diffuse epidermal crusts; extremely high mite load; more prevalent in immunocompromised and debilitated populations

Laboratory Tests

- Skin scrapings to detect mites, eggs, or mite fecal matter

Treatment

- Drugs: Topical permethrin or oral ivermectin

Prognosis

- With appropriate treatment, resolves with little scarring
- Recurrence may occur from close contacts (requires treatment)
- Crusted scabies requires prolonged course of therapy and may be difficult to eradicate without thorough environmental cleaning

MACROSCOPIC

General Features

- Mites are 0.5 mm in length and appear as white spots
- Skin: Linear or curved burrows appear red and possibly excoriated

MICROSCOPIC

Histologic Features

- Epidermal intracorneal presence of female scabies mite, eggs, or feces (scybala) is pathognomonic
- Ovoid mite containing chitinous exoskeleton, dorsal spines, and 4 pairs of legs
- Classic scabies
  - Intracorneal mites typically found at edge of cutaneous burrow
  - Associated nonspecific inflammatory response with eosinophils
- Nodular scabies
  - Histologic identification of mites is less common
  - Dense superficial and deep dermal lymphohistiocytic infiltrate with numerous eosinophils
- Norwegian/crusted scabies
  - Psoriasiform hyperplasia
  - Massive epidermal hyperkeratosis and parakeratosis
  - Massive orthokeratotic and parakeratotic scales containing innumerable mites and keratotic scale
  - Multilayered burrows

DIFFERENTIAL DIAGNOSIS

Demodex

- Mites associated with hair follicles and typically involve face
- Lack cuticular spines

Arthropod Bite

- Rarely, insect mouthparts are identified in dermis
- Dermatitis with eosinophils more prominent perivascular distribution at early stages
- Older lesions may show diffuse or nodular inflammation

Eczematous Dermatitis

- Exuberant dermatitis may be difficult to differentiate in absence of scabies mites, eggs, or scybala

Cutaneous Larva Migrans

- Similar spongiotic and perivascular chronic dermatitis with numerous eosinophils
- Rarely identified nematode larval forms 0.5 mm thick and up to 10 mm long in deep dermis

SELECTED REFERENCES

1. Grodner C et al: Crusted scabies in children in France: a series of 20 cases. Eur J Pediatr. 181(3):1167-74, 2022
2. Niode NJ et al: Crusted scabies, a neglected tropical disease: case series and literature review. Infect Dis Rep. 14(3):479-91, 2022
3. Siddig EE et al: Laboratory-based diagnosis of scabies: a review of the current status. Trans R Soc Trop Med Hyg. 116(1):4-9, 2022
4. Cassell JA et al: Scabies outbreaks in ten care homes for elderly people: a prospective study of clinical features, epidemiology, and treatment outcomes. Lancet Infect Dis. 18(8):894-902, 2018
5. Gopinath H et al: Tackling scabies: novel agents for a neglected disease. Int J Dermatol. 57(11):1293-8, 2018
6. Rosumeck S et al: Ivermectin and permethrin for treating scabies. Cochrane Database Syst Rev. 4:CD012994, 2018
7. Shmidt E et al: Dermatologic infestations. Int J Dermatol. 51(2):131-41, 2012

Demodex Infestations

KEY FACTS

TERMINOLOGY

- Demodicosis, *Demodex* folliculitis

ETIOLOGY/PATHOGENESIS

- Overpopulation of *Demodex* species, small mites that typically live in hair follicles as commensals
- Mites are transferred between hosts through contact of hair, eyebrows, and sebaceous glands on nose

CLINICAL ISSUES

- *Demodex* species-induced pathologic changes can cause dry eye conditions and chalazia formation and play important role in pityriasis folliculorum
- *Demodex* blepharitis: Ocular irritation, itching, and scaling of lids
- Patients with rosacea had significantly higher prevalence and degrees of *Demodex* mite infestation
- *Demodex* can proliferate in immunodeficiency states, such as HIV infection
- *Demodex* mite should be considered as causative agent for number of dermatoses for early diagnosis and appropriate treatment

MICROSCOPIC

- Organisms have chitin exoskeleton
- *D. folliculorum* measures 0.3-0.4 mm in length, whereas *D. brevis* measures 0.15-0.20 mm with similar structure of head and thorax but shorter abdomen
- Both mites produce inflammatory changes, epithelial hyperplasia, and follicular plugging

TOP DIFFERENTIAL DIAGNOSES

- Scabies: Mites in epidermis (not follicle associated); not usually on face
- Chalazion: Granulomatous and chronic inflammation of meibomian glands; no mites present in biopsy
- Blepharitis: Caused by bacterial colonization of eyelid
- Dry eye syndrome: Multifactorial disease of tears and ocular surface; no mites present in histologic section

Demodicosis

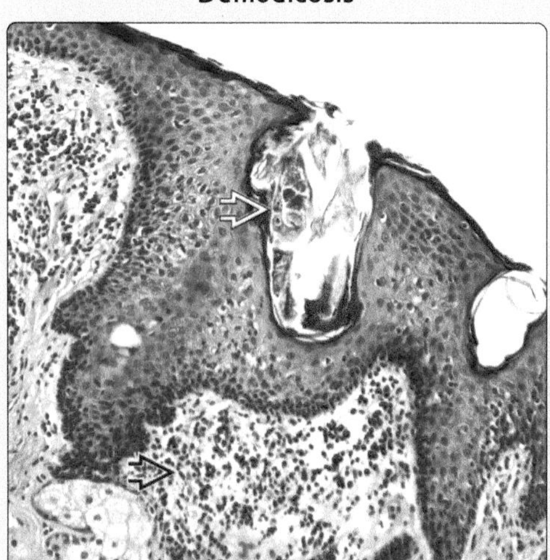

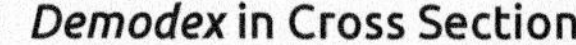

***Demodex* in Cross Section**

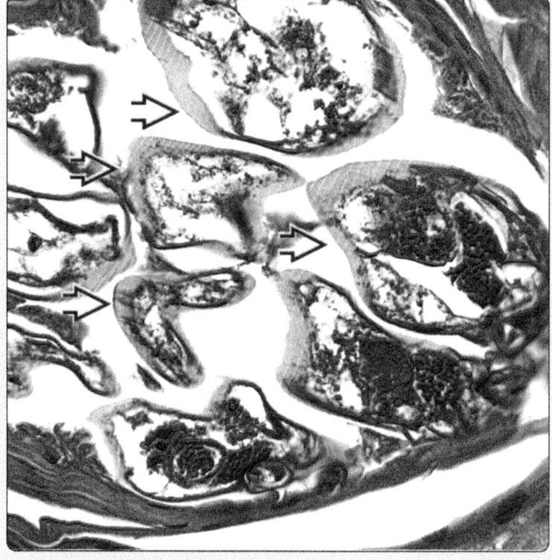

(Left) *H&E-stained skin biopsy shows a dense inflammatory infiltrate ⇨ around a sebaceous gland with Demodex mites* ➡*.* **(Right)** *Cross section of a skin biopsy stained with H&E shows Demodex mites ⇨.*

***Demodex* in Hair Shaft**

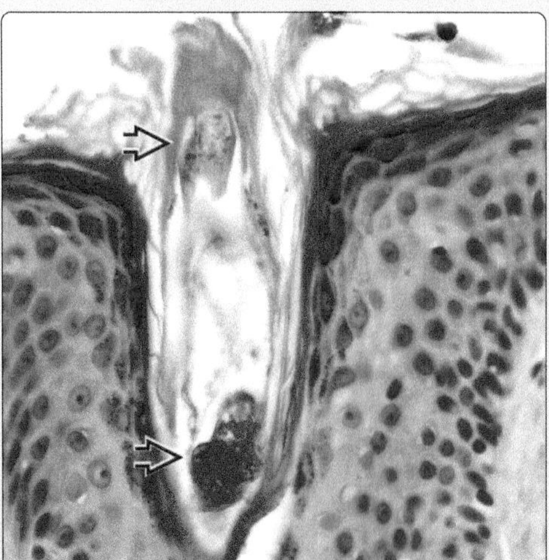

***Demodex* in Dense Keratin**

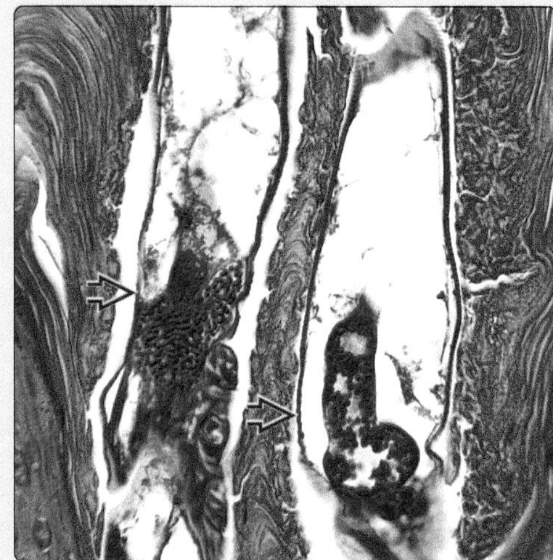

(Left) *An example of Demodex on histology is shown, which closely mimics a hair shaft. Note the substructure ⇨ of the organism. Below the organisms, there will be no typical hair structures seen.* **(Right)** *High-power view shows a cross section of Demodex folliculorum ⇨ in a skin biopsy stained with H&E.*

TERMINOLOGY

Synonyms

- Demodicosis, *Demodex* folliculitis
- Demodectic mange or red mange (in canids)

Definitions

- Greek: "Demos" (tallow) + "dex" (woodworm)

ETIOLOGY/PATHOGENESIS

Infectious Agents

- Overpopulation of *Demodex* species, small mites that typically live in hair follicles as commensals
- Mites are transferred between hosts through contact of hair, eyebrows, and sebaceous glands on nose
- 2 species: *Demodex folliculorum* and *Demodex brevis*
  - *D. folliculorum* (all stages) is found in small hair follicles and eyelash hair follicles
  - *D. brevis* (all stages) is present in eyelash sebaceous glands, small hair sebaceous glands, and lobules of meibomian glands
  - Life cycle of *D. folliculorum* estimated to be only 14.5 days from ovum to adult stage

CLINICAL ISSUES

Epidemiology

- Worldwide distribution; very common to find on human skin
- Prevalence of *Demodex* species infestation in recent study was 41% and was highest among inpatients and older adults
- In general population, 20-30 year olds have highest colonization due to rate of sebum production
- No racial or sex predilections have been observed

Presentation

- Very frequently are simply incidental findings, which are unrelated to underlying pathology generating biopsy
- Demodicidosis
  - Pruritic, erythematous, papulopustular lesions
  - Variations include pityriasis folliculorum, rosacea-like demodicidosis, or demodicidosis gravis
- Madarosis (loss of lashes) is associated with heavy infestation by mites
  - *Demodex* species-induced pathologic changes can cause dry eye conditions and chalazia formation
- *Demodex* blepharitis: Ocular irritation, itching, and scaling of lids
- Rosacea: Number of *Demodex* mites in rosacea patients higher than in control subjects
- Pityriasis folliculorum: Facial burning, fine follicular plugs and scales
- *Demodex* infestation also related to other dermatologic conditions, such as pustular folliculitis, perioral dermatitis, and hyperpigmented patches of face
- *Demodex* can proliferate in immunodeficiency states, such as HIV infection
- *Demodex* recently reported in pediatric patients with previous history of Langerhans cell histiocytosis
- *Demodex* mites reported more prevalent and quantitative in children with chalazia

Laboratory Tests

- Skin scraping with KOH examination

Treatment

- Tea tree oil with *Macadamia* nut oil are commonly used
- Topical insecticides in heavy infestation
- Oral ivermectin in severe cases, e.g., HIV patients

Prognosis

- No major morbidity or mortality

MICROSCOPIC

Histologic Features

- Organisms are mites and have chitin exoskeleton
- *D. folliculorum* measures 0.3-0.4 mm in length, whereas *D. brevis* measures 0.15-0.20 mm with similar structure of head and thorax but shorter abdomen
- Demodicidosis shows papulopustular lesions with neutrophils in/around glands with organisms
- *D. folliculorum* adult and immature forms consume epithelial cells and cause follicular hyperplasia and marked keratinization
- *D. brevis* adult and immature forms consume sebaceous and meibomian gland cells when infestations are heavy
- Both mites produce inflammatory changes, epithelial hyperplasia, and follicular plugging

DIFFERENTIAL DIAGNOSIS

Scabies

- Burrow through skin, not usually on face; mites in epidermis (not follicle associated)

Chalazion

- Granulomatous inflammation of meibomian glands composed of epithelioid cells and histocytes and chronic inflammation; no mites present in biopsy
- Demodicidosis should be considered in adults presenting with recurrent chalazia

Blepharitis

- Caused by bacterial colonization of eyelid

Dry Eye Syndrome

- Multifactorial disease of tears and ocular surface that causes discomfort and tear film instability; no mites present in histologic section

SELECTED REFERENCES

1. Xiao Y et al: High load of demodex in young children with chalazia. J Pediatr Ophthalmol Strabismus. 1-7, 2022
2. Álvarez-Salafranca M et al: Demodicosis in two patients with a previous history of Langerhans cell histiocytosis. Pediatr Dermatol. 34(6):e299-301, 2017
3. Chang YS et al: Role of Demodex mite infestation in rosacea: a systematic review and meta-analysis. J Am Acad Dermatol. 77(3):441-7.e6, 2017
4. Cheng AM et al: Recent advances on ocular Demodex infestation. Curr Opin Ophthalmol. 26(4):295-300, 2015
5. Chen W et al: Human demodicosis: revisit and a proposed classification. Br J Dermatol. 170(6):1219-25, 2014
6. Elston CA et al: Demodex mites. Clin Dermatol. 32(6):739-43, 2014
7. Wesolowska M et al: Prevalence of Demodex spp. in eyelash follicles in different populations. Arch Med Sci. 10(2):319-24, 2014

KEY FACTS

ETIOLOGY/PATHOGENESIS

- Cutaneous infestation by female sand flea *Tunga penetrans*
- Parasite enlarges up to 1 cm in diameter and sheds ~ 100 eggs over 2-week period prior to death and sloughing

CLINICAL ISSUES

- Itching and irritation usually start to develop as female fleas become fully developed into engorged state
- Dermoscopy (direct skin microscopy) may be helpful in identifying organism
- Surgical extraction of flea and application of topical antibiotic if secondary bacterial infection is suspected

MACROSCOPIC

- Differentiated from other human-biting fleas by shorter, rounder body; long, serrated mouthparts; compressed thoracic region; and lack of genal or pronotal combs
- Skin lesion: Whitish disc that varies in size with dark point in middle that darkens with time

MICROSCOPIC

- In most cases, sections show portions of exoskeleton, hypodermal layer, trachea, digestive tracts, striated muscles, and developing round eosinophilic eggs, all located below stratum corneum
- Biopsy may contain macerated or tangentially oriented flea
- Epidermis is usually hyperplastic and shows papillomatosis, parakeratosis, and hyperkeratosis with inflammatory infiltrate in underlying dermis

TOP DIFFERENTIAL DIAGNOSES

- Scabies: Smaller, present in subcorneum or superficial epidermis, and lack characteristic eggs
- Myiasis: Significantly larger, contain cuticular spines, and lack eggs
- Tick bite: Tick mouthparts often associated with intradermal cavity and necrosis
- Cutaneous larva migrans: Larvae rarely seen in skin lesion tracks; extensive eosinophilic infiltration

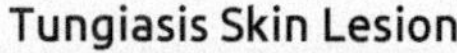

Tungiasis Skin Lesion

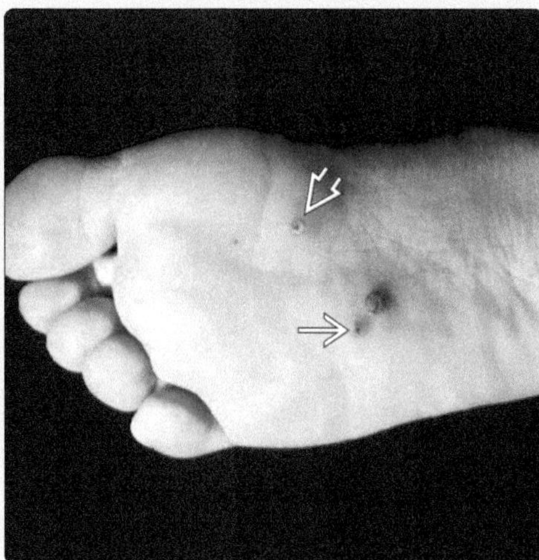

***Tunga penetrans* Below Stratum Corneum**

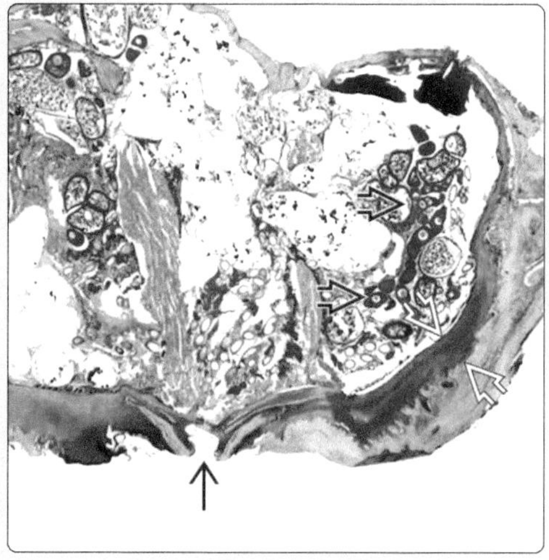

(Left) *Wart-like lesions caused by the female sand flea on the sole of a patient's foot are shown. Note the raised lesions with the central pore. (Courtesy K. Mumcuoglu, PhD.)* **(Right)** *Biopsy section shows viable Tunga penetrans below the thickened corneal layer and central epidermal pit. Note the egg-containing uterus underneath the plantar epidermis.*

Eosinophilic Cuticle and Hypodermal Layer

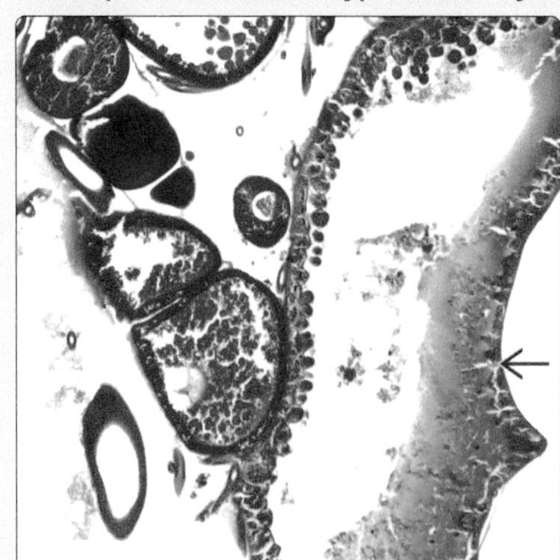

***Tunga penetrans* Developing Eggs**

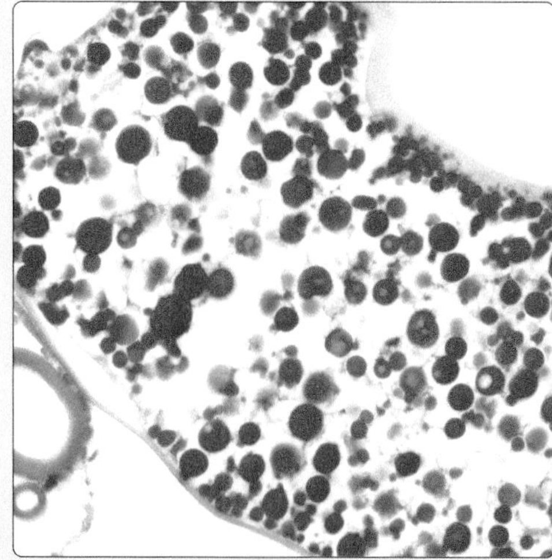

(Left) *Outermost layer in a skin biopsy shows an eosinophilic cuticle and hypodermal layer. The histologic findings are most consistent with tungiasis.* **(Right)** *This high-magnification image shows a uterus with round, variably sized eosinophilic developing eggs characteristic of T. penetrans. (Courtesy A. Laga, MD, MMSc.)*

TERMINOLOGY

Definitions

- Origin of *Tunga* is probably from Brazil from local word for infection, although there is word in almost every country where tungiasis exists for infection &/or flea

ETIOLOGY/PATHOGENESIS

Infectious Agents

- Cutaneous infestation by female sand flea *Tunga penetrans* (jigger, chigre, nigua, pico, chigoe flea)
- Main habitat is warm, dry soil and sand of beaches, stables, and stock farms
- Sand fleas (length of 1 mm) penetrate stratum corneum then burrow into stratum granulosum
- As parasite becomes engorged by host blood, it can enlarge up to 1 cm in diameter and shed ~ 100 eggs over 2-week period prior to death and sloughing by host skin
- In addition to humans, reservoir hosts include pigs, dogs, cats, cattle, sheep, horses, mules, rats, mice, and wild animals

CLINICAL ISSUES

Epidemiology

- Distributed in tropical and subtropical countries
- Occurs more frequently in travelers, riverside communities, slums in large urban centers, indigenous communities, and rural communities; related to poor hygiene
- No racial predisposition is apparent

Presentation

- Itching and irritation usually start to develop as female fleas become fully developed into engorged state
- Inflammation and ulceration may become severe, and multiple lesions in feet can lead to difficulty in walking
- Lesions usually appear on plantar, interdigital, or periungual regions of foot, but lesions in leg, hand, breast, wrists, elbow, and buttocks have also been reported

Laboratory Tests

- Dermoscopy (direct skin microscopy) may be helpful in identifying organism

Treatment

- Surgical extraction of flea and application of topical antibiotic if secondary bacterial infection is suspected
- Antimicrobial susceptibility testing for patients with resistant secondary bacteria
- Tetanus prophylaxis

Prognosis

- Excellent if proper sterile methods are followed for extraction of fleas

MACROSCOPIC

General Features

- Differentiated from other human-biting fleas by shorter, rounder body; long, serrated mouthparts; compressed thoracic region; and lack of genal or pronotal combs
- Skin lesion: Whitish disc that varies in size with dark point in middle that darkens with time

Fortaleza Classification System

- Stage 1: Penetration of epidermis by female flea's proboscis (within moments)
- Stage 2: Penetration is complete, and female flea is burrowed into host with only 4 air holes, reproductive organs, and anus exposed, feeding on blood and expanding her midsection (24-48 hours)
- Stage 3a: Midsection has reached its maximum size, and skin of host is stretched thin over it (3 days after penetration)
- Stage 3b: Surface appearance resembles caldera as thickness of exoskeleton increases and eggs or feces may be released (variable)
- Stage 4a: Flea begins to die (or has died), and lesion becomes smaller, darkened, and folded inward (2-3 weeks)
- Stage 4b: Resulting lesion is being expelled by host's body, and inflammatory repair mechanisms are at work (day 25 after penetration)
- Stage 5: Flea is fully expelled with only keratinized sloughing skin layers remaining (variable)

MICROSCOPIC

Histologic Features

- In most cases, sections show portions of exoskeleton, hypodermal layer, trachea, digestive tracts, striated muscles, and developing round eosinophilic eggs, located below stratum corneum
- Biopsy may contain macerated or tangentially oriented flea
- Epidermis is usually hyperplastic and shows papillomatosis, parakeratosis, and hyperkeratosis with inflammatory infiltrate in underlying dermis

DIFFERENTIAL DIAGNOSIS

Scabies

- Smaller than fleas (0.5 mm vs. 1.0 mm), present in subcorneum or superficial epidermis, and lack characteristic eggs

Myiasis

- Fly larvae (~15 mm) contain cuticular spines; typically associated with preexisting lesions

Tick Bite

- Refractile tick mouthparts often associated with intradermal cavity and necrosis

Cutaneous Larva Migrans

- Larvae rarely seen in skin track lesions with extensive eosinophilic infiltration (biopsy not recommended)

SELECTED REFERENCES

1. Tardin Martins AC et al: The efficacy of topical, oral and surgical interventions for the treatment of tungiasis: a systematic review of the literature. PLoS Negl Trop Dis. 15(8):e0009722, 2021
2. Nyangacha RM et al: Secondary bacterial infections and antibiotic resistance among tungiasis patients in Western, Kenya. PLoS Negl Trop Dis. 11(9):e0005901, 2017
3. Vasievich MP et al: Got the travel bug? A review of common infections, infestations, bites, and stings among returning travelers. Am J Clin Dermatol. 17(5):451-62, 2016
4. Louis SJ et al: Tungiasis in Haiti: a case series of 383 patients. Int J Dermatol. 53(8):999-1004, 2014
5. Maco V et al: Histopathological features of tungiasis in Peru. Am J Trop Med Hyg. 88(6):1212-6, 2013

INDEX

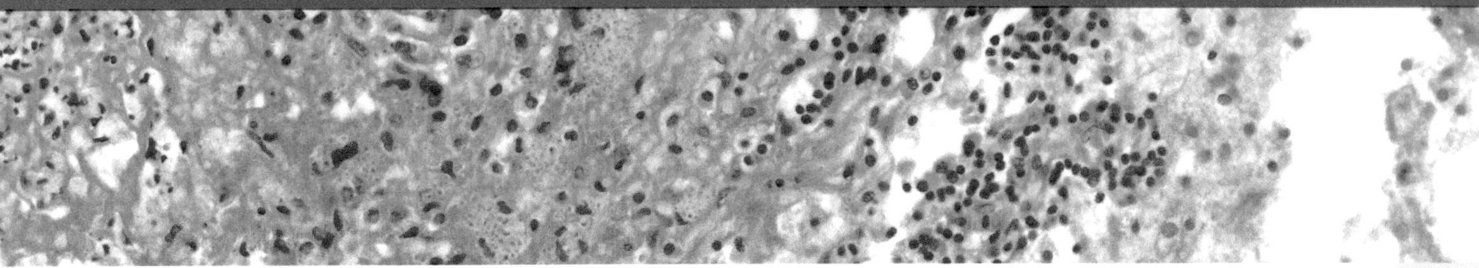

A

INDEX

B

INDEX

INDEX

C

INDEX

INDEX

INDEX

D

E

INDEX

INDEX

G

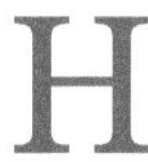

INDEX

INDEX

INDEX

I

INDEX

J

INDEX

M

INDEX

N

INDEX

P

INDEX

INDEX

Q

R

S

INDEX

INDEX

T

U

V

INDEX

W

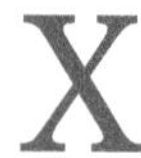

Y

Z